INTENSITY MODULATED RADIATION THERAPY

A Clinical Perspective

INTENSITY MODULATED RADIATION THERAPY

A Clinical Perspective

Arno J. Mundt, MD
Associate Professor
Department of Radiation and Cellular Oncology
University of Chicago
University of Illinois at Chicago
Chicago, Illinois

John C. Roeske, PhD
Associate Professor
Department of Radiation and Cellular Oncology
University of Chicago
University of Illinois at Chicago
Chicago, Illinois

2005
BC Decker Inc
Hamilton • London

BC Decker Inc
P.O. Box 620, L.C.D. 1
Hamilton, Ontario L8N 3K7
Tel: 905-522-7017; 800-568-7281
Fax: 905-522-7839; 888-311-4987
E-mail: info@bcdecker.com
www.bcdecker.com

BC Decker

06 07 08 09 10/WPC/9 8 7 6 5 4

ISBN 1-55009-246-4
Printed in the United States of America

Sales and Distribution

United States
BC Decker Inc
P.O. Box 785
Lewiston, NY 14092-0785
Tel: 905-522-7017; 800-568-7281
Fax: 905-522-7839; 888-311-4987
E-mail: info@bcdecker.com
www.bcdecker.com

Canada
BC Decker Inc
50 King Street East
P.O. Box 620, LCD 1
Hamilton, Ontario L8N 1A6
Tel: 905-522-7017; 800-568-7281
Fax: 905-522-7839; 888-311-4987
E-mail: info@bcdecker.com
www.bcdecker.com

Foreign Rights
John Scott & Company
International Publishers' Agency
P.O. Box 878
Kimberton, PA 19442
Tel: 610-827-1640
Fax: 610-827-1671
E-mail: jsco@voicenet.com

Japan
Igaku-Shoin Ltd.
Foreign Publications Department
3-24-17 Hongo
Bunkyo-ku, Tokyo, Japan 113-8719
Tel: 3 3817 5680
Fax: 3 3815 6776
E-mail: fd@igaku-shoin.co.jp

UK, Europe, Scandinavia, Middle East
Elsevier Science
Customer Service Department
Foots Cray High Street
Sidcup, Kent
DA14 5HP, UK
Tel: 44 (0) 208 308 5760
Fax: 44 (0) 181 308 5702
E-mail: cservice@harcourt.com

Singapore, Malaysia,Thailand, Philippines,
Indonesia, Vietnam, Pacific Rim, Korea
Elsevier Science Asia
583 Orchard Road
#09/01, Forum
Singapore 238884
Tel: 65-737-3593
Fax: 65-753-2145

Australia, New Zealand
Elsevier Science Australia
Customer Service Department
STM Division
Locked Bag 16
St. Peters, New South Wales, 2044
Australia
Tel: 61 02 9517-8999
Fax: 61 02 9517-2249
E-mail: stmp@harcourt.com.au
www.harcourt.com.au

Mexico and Central America
ETM SA de CV
Calle de Tula 59
Colonia Condesa
06140 Mexico DF, Mexico
Tel: 52-5-5553-6657
Fax: 52-5-5211-8468
E-mail: editoresdetextosmex@prodigy.net.mx

Brazil
Tecmedd Importadora E Distribuidora De Livr
Ltda.
Avenida Maurílio Biagi, 2850
City Ribeirão, Ribeirão Preto – SP – Brasil
CEP: 14021-000
Tel: 0800 992236
Fax: (16) 3993-9000
E-mail: tecmedd@tecmedd.com.br

India, Bangladesh, Pakistan, Sri Lanka
Elsevier Health Sciences Division
Customer Service Department
17A/1, Main Ring Road
Lajpat Nagar IV
New Delhi – 110024, India
Tel: 91 11 2644 7160-64
Fax: 91 11 2644 7156
E-mail: esindia@vsnl.net

Notice: The authors and publisher have made every effort to ensure that the patient care recommended herein, including choice of drugs and drug dosages, is in accord with the accepted standard and practice at the time of publication. However, since research and regulation constantly change clinical standards, the reader is urged to check the product information sheet included in the package of each drug, which includes recommended doses, warnings, and contraindications. This is particularly important with new or infrequently used drugs. Any treatment regimen, particularly one involving medication, involves inherent risk that must be weighed on a case-by-case basis against the benefits anticipated. The reader is cautioned that the purpose of this book is to inform and enlighten; the information contained herein is not intended as, and should not be employed as, a substitute for individual diagnosis and treatment.

Contents

III. Clinical Topics and Case Studies

22A Intact Prostate Cancer: Overview 436
Alan Pollack, MD, PhD, Robert Price, PhD, Lei Dong, PhD, Steven J. Feigenberg, MD,
Eric M. Horwitz, MD

22B Postoperative Prostate Cancer: Overview..449
Bin S. Teh, MD, Thomas M. Schroeder, MD, Wei-Yuan Mai, MD, E. Brian Butler, MD

22.1 Intact Prostate Cancer: Case Study...459
Robert A. Price Jr, PhD, Eric M. Horwitz, MD, Steven J. Feigenberg, MD, Alan Pollack, MD, PhD

22.2 Hypofractionated IMRT: Case Study...464
Patrick Kupelian, MD, Twyla Willoughby, MS

22.3 Targeted Lymph Node Irradiation: Case Study...467
Steven L. Hancock, MD, Todd Pawlicki, PhD, Raymond Tan, MD

22.4 ProstaScint-Guided IMRT: Case Study...475
Ashesh B. Jani, MD, John C. Roeske, PhD

22.5 Intra-Prostatic Boost: Emerging Technology 481
Maria T. Guerrero Urbano, FRCR, MRCPI, Catharine Clark, PhD, MIPEM,
Chris M. Nutting, MD, MRCP, FRCR, ECMO, David P. Dearnaley, MD, MRCP, FRCR

22.6 Repair of Unacceptable Implants: Emerging Technology 486
X. Allen Li, PhD, Jian Z. Wang, PhD

23 Gynecologic Cancer: Overview 492
Loren K. Mell, MD, John C. Roeske, PhD, Neil Mehta, MD, Arno J. Mundt, MD

23.1 Cervical Cancer: Case Study...506
Tracey E. Schefter, MD, Brian D. Kavanagh, MD

23.2 Endometrial Cancer: Case Study 513
Anuja Jhingran, MD, Mohammad Salehpour, PhD, Brooke Brooks, RT, CMD

23.3 Cervical Cancer Not Suitable for Brachytherapy: Case Study 518
Philip Chan, MBBS, Michael Milosevic, MD, Janet Paterson, MRT (T), CMD,
Inhwan Yeo, PhD, Anthony W. Fyles, MD

23.4 Bone Marrow-Sparing IMRT: Emerging Technology...523
John C. Roeske, PhD, Anthony E. Lujan, PhD, Arno J. Mundt, MD

23.5 Applicator-Guided IMRT: Emerging Technology...531
Daniel A. Low, PhD

24 Lymphoma: Overview..535
Billy W. Loo Jr, MD, PhD, Richard T. Hoppe, MD, FACR

24.1 Hodgkin's Disease: Case Study...547
Billy W. Loo Jr, MD, PhD, Richard T. Hoppe, MD, FACR

FOREWORD

This is a remarkably comprehensive and timely book on intensity modulated radiation therapy (IMRT). It is very difficult to write a book about a field while that field is rapidly changing and being refined. However, dealing with IMRT is like learning to utilize much of new technology; we must make an assessment at a point in time with special attention to the important questions and emerging principles of these technologies as they are being developed. It is a moving train not likely to stop or even slow down so this may be the best time to get on board.

IMRT is a part of the revolution in medical technology. I believe that the impact of technology on medical care has been even greater than that from the revolution in tumor and molecular biology. IMRT is at the leading edge of technological innovation. As shown in this book, it is the confluence of major technologic saltations in both imaging and computer controlled radiation treatment. The resulting radiation treatment methods have far greater current applications as well as potential implications for evolving treatment paradigms than better tumor assessment or computer controlled treatment would be expected to have individually.

This book suggests we need to reconsider a number of the currently accepted principles underlying radiation treatment. These include principles concerning the definition of tumor volume and its relationship to the irradiated volume. We also need to consider whether we desire the tumor volume to receive a homogeneous dose distribution. The notion that extensive fractionation is the desired method for maximizing the tolerance of normal tissues and therefore improves therapeutic ratio is a foundation pillar of conventional radiation therapy but it may be entirely different for IMRT. A single fraction or hypofractionation in some circumstances may be the desired method of treatment delivery.

Very important are considerations of the unwanted radiation outside the target volume. The IMRT dose-volume configurations are quite different than those seen with more conventional treatment with there being a larger volume irradiated using IMRT but it receives lower doses. The consequences of these very different dose distributions are significant and a functioning model of how to deal to with this must be determined. The editors own elegant work on minimizing bone marrow integral dose is a model of utilizing sophisticated constraints in treatment planning in order to limit the hematopoietic damage caused by radiation therapy and thus allow effective chemotherapy dosing. On the other hand, there is concern for the potential increased carcinogenic and leukemogenic consequences of IMRT, since a greater volume of tissue receives potential cancer causing radiation than with most conventional radiation therapy. Finally, with regard to old paradigms, one must re-evaluate the goal of given treatment; which patients are curable and which patients are to be treated for palliation only? Further, the technical advances in imaging and radiation therapy raise the possibility that there may be intermediary patients for whom IMRT delivered palliative treatment can result in long-term survival and potential cure of oligometastases. This becomes even more important today at a time when more effective systemic treatments are being made available.

New principles for IMRT will require reconsideration of the tumor volume to include: increased accuracy of delineation; an attempt to determine tumor cell concentration within the target volume; the biologic characteristics of different anatomic regions of the tumor with regard to such things as oxygenation, vascularity, proliferation, and repair of radiation damage. These data provide the necessary foundation for dose sculpting within the target volume.

With IMRT, we need to consider how and why we extend the treatment volume beyond the identifiable tumor. Is it in order to treat occult tumor cells? Is it to compensate for movement either between treatments or during a single treatment? Does it have to do with reproducibility of set-up or physiologic motions such as breathing and movement of gas in the bowel? Can the irradiated volume be reduced by immobilization, gating, fiducial markers, and real-time feed back and control? We must reconsider the basic principles of fractionation, which were developed at a much earlier time in the development of radiation therapy. Much has changed since these principles were formulated. Those were times when the radiation energy used for treatment did not penetrate very deeply nor did it provide skin sparing. The assessment of tumor location was limited and the accuracy and reproducibility of treatment was uncertain. Protraction, fractionation, tumor volume, and dose limiting normal tissues should all be approached with fresh eyes. IMRT provides the impetus for such a re-evaluation and this book provides a discussion of these principles, as they may apply to the evolving technology. The practical applications of IMRT in a variety of anatomic regions are explored using individual cases from different clinics. Most of the important questions are posed in this book and tentative answers formulated. It seems clear that precise, reproducible sculpting of the radiation dose is available. IMRT will open new horizons for more effective and less toxic treatment but will also bring to us issues and concerns not faced before in radiation oncology.

Samuel Hellman, MD
November 2004

***

Although in its relative infancy, IMRT has already had considerable impact on the practice of radiation oncology, having improved the clinical outcomes of many patients. *Intensity Modulated Radiation Therapy: A Clinical Perspective* presents the theoretical background as well as practical insights in the development, implementation and application of this novel technology. The text opens with a thorough review of the physical and biological basis of IMRT as well as the medical considerations of target delineation. As a basic science researcher, I particularly enjoyed the inclusion of a chapter focusing on the radiobiological issues in IMRT, an area of growing interest and importance. While many of the topics are complex, the chapters in this section (and throughout the entire book) are clearly written; comprehensible for the beginner while thought-provoking for the expert.

The various technologies for the planning, delivery and clinical implementation of IMRT are explored in the second section, along with an unbiased overview of all the commercially available inverse planning and delivery systems. Theoretical issues described in the initial section are integrated with practical aspects of IMRT clinical implementation, including simulation, immobilization and patient localization. Additionally, seemingly more esoteric topics such as image fusion and the applications of PET-CT in IMRT planning are discussed. These topics are, however, far from esoteric, having emerged on the cutting edge of IMRT research. A superb chapter on respiratory motion and its management follows with a description of its benefits and potential pitfalls. Included are chapters on commissioning and quality assurance, issues essential to the successful clinical implementation of IMRT. Excellent chapters on billing and reimbursement as well as on IMRT in the community setting complete this section, helping to broaden the scope of the book to all involved in the practice of radiation oncology.

The third section provides the reader with an overview of the application of IMRT in all clinical sites. Each disease is discussed in detail accompanied by considerations in treatment planning and a review of the published IMRT literature. This section will prove of particular interest to the practicing radiation oncologist for it integrates the clinical, radiobiological and physics issues with practical scenarios. I found it particularly valuable that renowned IMRT experts have contributed actual case studies along with a detailed description of their individual approach to simulation, immobilization, target delineation, plan optimization and delivery and quality assurance. In some, these cases provide class solutions; in others, specific clinical problems are addressed.

The final section consists of commentaries on selected topics in IMRT, including proton IMRT and the combination of IMRT and biological modifiers. This section ends with some final thoughts on the pros and cons of IMRT, addressing the state of the art as well as potential problems and pitfalls in applying IMRT to specific diseases.

In my opinion, this is a superb textbook that includes the very latest theoretical and practical underpinnings of IMRT. It is destined to become the standard text in the field. The editors are to be congratulated on a remarkable job.

Ralph R. Weichselbaum, MD
November 2004

PREFACE

While available at only a few institutions a mere decade ago, intensity modulated radiation therapy (IMRT) is used today at an increasing number of centers worldwide. The growing interest in this technology is reflected in its inclusion in the new editions of major radiation and oncology textbooks. We thus felt that the time was right for a new comprehensive IMRT textbook. Conversations with countless physicians and medical physicists in the United States and abroad taught us that a traditional textbook format would be of limited value. What was needed instead was a text conveying both the "how" and the "why", the art and the science of IMRT. It is our sincere hope that *Intensity Modulated Radiation Therapy: A Clinical Perspective* has met these goals.

This text is divided into four separate (but inter-related) parts. Part I introduces the overall IMRT "process" and includes in-depth overviews of the Physics, Biology and Medicine of IMRT, illustrating the basic principles underlying this technology. Expanding on concepts and issues introduced in Part I, Part II systematically explores the various steps and technologies involved in the planning and delivery of IMRT, including imaging, organ motion and its management, plan optimization, treatment delivery and quality assurance. Of practical interest, chapters focusing on the unique issues of IMRT in the community setting along with billing and reimbursement are also included in this section. Organized anatomically, Part III provides a comprehensive overview of the clinical application of IMRT. Within each section, overview chapters are paired with case studies highlighting the use of IMRT in specific diseases. Contributed by respected IMRT experts, each includes detailed descriptions of the simulation, immobilization, target delineation, plan optimization, delivery and quality assurance of an *actual* patient. An effort was made to include all major commercial planning and delivery systems in these cases, illustrating their unique features. Reflecting the rapidly evolving nature of IMRT, Emerging Technology reports are also included, illustrating cutting edge research approaches; some currently in use, others still under development. Part IV consists of invited commentaries on selected topics, including proton IMRT and biologic modifiers.

From its conception, it was our sincere wish to produce a textbook illustrating the depth and breadth of IMRT. While the purists amongst us may argue that IMRT is synonymous with *inverse* planning, we chose to adopt a broader definition and intentionally included *forward* planning approaches. Our goal was to provide an overview of the current level of knowledge in the field in a format accessible to the wide variety of individuals involved in IMRT planning and treatment, including radiation oncologists, medical physicists, radiation therapists, nurses, and administrators, as well as students and residents.

It was also never our intention to produce a textbook focusing on the viewpoint of a single institution using a particular planning system, and we thus solicited contributors from a wide variety of institutions with experience in a myriad of planning and delivery systems.

In fact, even within specific disease sites, we sought out experts from different institutions to provide the reader with diverse approaches. In the prostate cancer and head and neck cancer sections alone, there are 49 contributors from 14 centers. We also desired to highlight the international flavor of IMRT and thus populated this text with experts from around the globe. In all, there are 178 contributors from 43 centers in 9 countries including Belgium, Canada, China, Germany, Great Britain, Japan, Spain, Switzerland, and the United States. From the United States alone, there are 143 contributors from 35 institutions, including many of the major cancer centers performing IMRT research.

Such a project as this clearly could not have been accomplished without the help of many individuals. We benefited from the advice of Ralph Weichselbaum and Samuel Hellman. Our gratitude is extended to the many contributors who went far beyond what they had originally agreed upon, notably Todd Pawlicki, and to those who, on short notice, graciously offered to fill in gaps in the text, including John Buatti, Tim Fox, Ashesh Jani, Russell Hamilton, Eugene Lief, Shidong Li, Anthony Lomax, Yulin Song, Allen Li, Fang-Fang Yin, Wei-Yuan Mai and Brian O'Sullivan. Given the unconventional format, we wish to thank all our contributors for putting up with our constant emails and phone calls requesting seemingly endless changes and additions. Warm thanks goes out to Eli Glatstein for agreeing to present the "other side" of the IMRT story. It never was our intention to produce a propaganda pamphlet and his well reasoned arguments provide welcome balance.

We also wish to thank Brian Decker, Colleen Petrick, Petrice Custance and colleagues at B.C. Decker for their encouragement, help and patience, without which this project would never have been completed. Our gratitude is also extended to the representatives from various companies for their valuable input on their products and services, including (in alphabetical order) BrainLAB, CMS, Elekta, MedImmune, North American Scientific, Philips, Prowess, RAHD, Siemens, Southeastern Radiation Products, TomoTherapy, and Varian. Finally, we are truly appreciative and grateful to our students, residents, colleagues and, most of all, to our families for their encouragement and endless patience with us over this last year.

We are extremely pleased with the final product and sincerely hope that it will not only meet the needs of our readers but also contribute to the advancement of the field of radiation oncology as a whole.

Arno J. Mundt, MD
John C. Roeske, PhD
University of Chicago
University of Illinois at Chicago
November 2004

CONTRIBUTORS

KALED M. ALEKTIAR, MD
Department of Radiation Oncology
Memorial Sloan-Kettering Cancer Center
New York, New York

JAVIER ARISTU, MD, PhD
Department of Radiation Oncology
University of Navarre
Pamplona, Spain

BENJAMIN ARMBRUSTER, BS
Department of Mathematics
University of Arizona
Tucson, Arizona

DOUGLAS ARTHUR, MD
Department of Radiation Oncology
William Beaumont Hospitals
Royal Oak, Michigan

KOMANDURI M. AYYANGAR, PhD
Department of Radiation Oncology
University of Nebraska Medical Center
Omaha, Nebraska

JUAN D. AZCONA, MSc
Department of Radiation Oncology
University of Navarre
Pamplona, Spain

JAMES BALTER, PhD
Department of Radiation Oncology
University of Michigan
Ann Arbor, Michigan

STANLEY H. BENEDICT, PhD
Department of Radiation Oncology
Virginia Commonwealth University Medical Center
Richmond, Virginia

ANTHONY M. BERSON, MD
Department of Radiation Oncology
Saint Vincent's Comprehensive Cancer Center
New York, New York

STEPHEN BILTON, CMD
Department of Radiation Oncology
M.D. Anderson Cancer Center
Houston, Texas

YERKO BORGHERO, MD
Department of Radiation Oncology
M.D. Anderson Cancer Center
Houston, Texas

ARTHUR L. BOYER, PhD
Department of Radiation Oncology
Stanford University School of Medicine
Stanford, California

BROOKE BROOKS, RT, CMD
Department of Radiation Oncology
M. D. Anderson Cancer Center
Houston, Texas

PHILIP M. BRUCH, MS, CMPE
Department of Radiation Oncology
University of Nebraska Medical Center
Omaha, Nebraska

JOHN M. BUATTI, MD
Department of Radiation Oncology
Roy J. and Lucille A. Carver College of Medicine
University of Iowa
Iowa City, Iowa

ELIZABETH BUTKER, MS
Department of Radiation Oncology
Emory University School of Medicine
Atlanta, Georgia

E. BRIAN BUTLER, MD
Department of Radiation Oncology
Baylor College of Medicine
Houston, Texas

LUIS CANOVAS, CPC
Department of Radiation and Cellular Oncology
University of Chicago
Chicago, Illinois

ROBERT M. CARDINALE, MD
Department of Radiation Oncology
Princeton Medical Center
Princeton, New Jersey

PHILIP CHAN, MBBS
Department of Radiation Oncology
Princess Margaret Hospital
University Health Network
Toronto, Ontario, Canada

K. S. CLIFFORD CHAO, MD
Department of Radiation Oncology
M. D. Anderson Cancer Center
Houston, Texas

GEORGE T. Y. CHEN, PhD
Department of Radiation Oncology
Massachusetts General Hospital
Boston, Massachusetts

STEVEN J. CHMURA, MD, PhD
Department of Radiation and Cellular Oncology
University of Chicago
Chicago, Illinois

CARMELITA CHOTIPRADIT, RN
Department of Radiation and Cellular Oncology
University of Chicago Hospitals
Chicago, Illinois

WILLIAM W. CHOU, MD
Department of Radiation Oncology
Memorial Sloan-Kettering Cancer Center
New York, New York

CATHARINE CLARK, PhD, MIPEM
Department of Radiotherapy
Royal Marsden Hospital
London, England

FILIP CLAUS, MD, PhD
Department of Radiation Oncology
Ghent University Hospital
Ghent, Belgium

PHILIP P. CONNELL, MD
Department of Radiation and Cellular Oncology
University of Chicago
Chicago, Illinois

DÖLF CORAY, PhD
Department of Radiation Medicine
Paul Scherrer Institute
Villgen PSI, Switzerland

WILFRIED DE NEVE, MD, PhD
Department of Radiation Oncology
Ghent University Hospital
Ghent, Belgium

DAVID P. DEARNALEY, MD, MRCP, FRCR
Department of Radiotherapy
Royal Marsden Hospital
London, England

JOSEPH O. DEASY, PhD
Department of Radiation Oncology
Siteman Cancer Center
Washington University
St. Louis, Missouri

JÜRGEN DEBUS, MD, PhD
Department of Radiation Oncology
University of Heidelberg
Heidelberg, Germany

XIAO-WU DENG, PhD
Department of Radiation Oncology
Sun Yat-sen University
Guangzhou, China

J. KEITH DEWYNGAERT, PhD
Department of Radiation Oncology
New York University School of Medicine
New York, New York

LEI DONG, PhD
Department of Radiation Physics
M. D. Anderson Cancer Center
Houston, Texas

KENNETH J. DORNFELD, MD, PhD
Department of Radiation Oncology
Roy J. and Lucille A. Carver College of Medicine
University of Iowa
Iowa City, Iowa

WIM DUTHOY, MD
Department of Radiation Oncology
Ghent University Hospital
Ghent, Belgium

AVRAHAM EISBRUCH, MD
Department of Radiation Oncology
University of Michigan
Ann Arbor, Michigan

ERIC ELDER, PhD
Department of Radiation Oncology
Emory University School of Medicine
Atlanta, Georgia

BAHMAN EMAMI, MD, FACR
Department of Radiation Oncology
Loyola University Medical Center
Maywood, Illinois

RICHARD EMERY, MS, DABR
Department of Radiation Oncology
Saint Vincent's Comprehensive Cancer Center
New York, New York

NATIA ESIASHVILI, MD
Department of Radiation Oncology
Emory University School of Medicine
Atlanta, Georgia

KARL FARREY, MS
Department of Radiation and Cellular Oncology
University of Chicago
Chicago, Illinois

STEVEN J. FEIGENBERG, MD
Department of Radiation Oncology
Fox Chase Cancer Center
Philadelphia, Pennsylvania

JOHN B. FIVEASH, MD
Department of Radiation Oncology
University Hospital
Birmingham, Alabama

SILVIA C. FORMENTI, MD
Department of Radiation Oncology
New York University School of Medicine
New York, New York

KENNETH M. FORSTER, PhD
Department of Radiation Oncology
University of Texas Southwestern
Dallas, Texas

JACK F. FOWLER, DSc, PhD
Department of Human Oncology
University of Wisconsin-Madison
Madison, Wisconsin

TIM FOX, PhD
Department of Radiation Oncology
Emory University School of Medicine
Atlanta, Georgia

ANTHONY W. FYLES, MD
Department of Radiation Oncology
Princess Margaret Hospital
University Health Network
Toronto, Ontario, Canada

MICHAEL C. GAROFALO, MD
Department of Radiation Oncology
University of Maryland
Baltimore, Maryland

JASON GENG, PhD
Genex Technologies Inc.
Kensington, Maryland

ELI GLATSTEIN, MD
Department of Radiation Oncology
University of Pennsylvania
Philadelphia, Pennsylvania

GUDRUN GOITEIN, MD
Department of Radiation Medicine
Paul Scherrer Institute
Villgen PSI, Switzerland

MARIA T. GUERRERO URBANO, FRCR, MRCPI
Department of Radiotherapy
Royal Marsden Hospital
London, England

THOMAS GUERRERO, MD, PhD
Department of Radiation Oncology
M.D. Anderson Cancer Center
Houston, Texas

NATHAN C. HALL, MD, PhD
Department of Radiology
University of Tennessee
Knoxville, Tennessee

RUSSELL J. HAMILTON, PhD
Department of Radiation Oncology
University of Arizona
Tucson, Arizona

STEVEN L. HANCOCK, MD
Department of Radiation Oncology
Stanford University Medical Center
Stanford, California

DANIEL J. HARAF, MD
Department of Radiation and Cellular Oncology
University of Chicago
Chicago, Illinois

ROBERT HEATON, PhD
Department of Radiation Oncology
Princess Margaret Hospital
Toronto, Ontario, Canada

MARTIN J. HESLIN, MD
Department of Radiation Oncology
University Hospital
Birmingham, Alabama

LINDA HONG, PhD
Department of Radiation Oncology
Memorial Sloan-Kettering Cancer Center
New York, New York

RICHARD T. HOPPE, MD, FACR
Department of Radiation Oncology
Stanford University
Stanford, California

ERIC M. HORWITZ, MD
Department of Radiation Oncology
Fox Chase Cancer Center
Philadelphia, Pennsylvania

GEOFFREY HUGO, PhD
Department of Radiation Oncology
William Beaumont Hospital
Royal Oak, Michigan

MOHAMMAD ISLAM, PhD
Department of Radiation Physics
Princess Margaret Hospital
Toronto, Ontario, Canada

WELLS JACKSON, MS, CMD
Department of Radiation and Cellular Oncology
University of Chicago
Chicago, Illinois

ASHESH B. JANI, MD
Department of Radiation and Cellular Oncology
University of Chicago
Chicago, Illinois

HAZIM A. JARADAT, PhD
Department of Human Oncology
University of Wisconsin-Madison
Madison, Wisconsin

MARTIN JERMANN
Department of Radiation Medicine
Paul Scherrer Institute
Villgen PSI, Switzerland

ANUJA JHINGRAN, MD
Department of Radiation Oncology
M. D. Anderson Cancer Center
Houston, Texas

STEVE JIANG, PhD
Department of Radiation Oncology
Harvard Medical School
Boston, Massachusetts

BRAD KAHL, MD
Department of Medicine
University of Wisconsin
Madison, Wisconsin

SHALOM KALNICKI, MD
Department of Radiation Oncology
UPMC Cancer Centers
Pittsburgh, Pennsylvania

JOHNNY KAO, MD
Department of Radiation and Cellular Oncology
University of Chicago
Chicago, Illinois

BRIAN D. KAVANAGH, MD
Department of Radiation Oncology
University of Colorado Hospital
Denver, Colorado

LARRY KESTIN, MD
Department of Radiation Oncology
William Beaumont Hospitals
Royal Oak, Michigan

JAE HO KIM, MD, PhD
Department of Radiation Oncology
Henry Ford Hospital
Detroit, Michigan

CHRISTOPHER KING, MD, PhD
Department of Radiation Oncology
Stanford University Medical Center
Stanford, California

STEPHANIE KING, CMD
Department of Radiation Oncology
Loyola University Medical Center
Maywood, Illinois

ERIC E. KLEIN, MS, FAAPM, FACMP
Department of Radiation Oncology
Washington University
St. Louis, Missouri

MARY KOSHY, MD
Department of Radiation Oncology
Emory University School of Medicine
Atlanta, Georgia

KOMANDURI V. KRISHNA, PhD
Department of Radiation Oncology
UPMC Cancer Centers
Pittsburgh, Pennsylvania

JONG H. KUNG, PhD
Department of Radiation Oncology
Massachusetts General Hospital
Boston, Massachusetts

PATRICK KUPELIAN, MD
Department of Radiation Oncology
M.D. Anderson Cancer Center
Orlando, Florida

MARTIN E. LACHAINE, PhD
Department of Radiation Oncology
University of Arizona
Tucson, Arizona

PETER LAI, MD, PhD
Department of Radiation Oncology
Lakeland Hospital
St. Joseph, Michigan

JEROME LANDRY, MD
Department of Radiation Oncology
Emory University School of Medicine
Atlanta, Georgia

ROBERT S. LAVEY, MD, MPH
Department of Pediatrics
Department of Radiation Oncology
University of Southern California
Los Angeles, California

QUYNH-THU LE, MD
Department of Radiation Oncology
Stanford University Medical Center
Stanford, California

NANCY Y. LEE, MD
Department of Radiation Oncology
Memorial Sloan-Kettering Cancer Center
New York, New York

NORMAN LEHTO, MS
Advanced Radiotherapy Consulting, Inc.
Kalamazoo, Michigan

SHIDONG LI, PhD
Department of Radiation Oncology
John Hopkins University
Baltimore, Maryland

X. ALLEN LI, PhD
Department of Radiation Oncology
Medical College of Wisconsin
Milwaukee, Wisconsin

EUGENE P. LIEF, PhD
Department of Radiation Oncology
New York University School of Medicine
New York, New York

TONY LOMAX, PhD
Department of Radiation Medicine
Paul Scherrer Institute
Villgen PSI, Switzerland

BILLY W. LOO JR, MD, PhD
Department of Radiation Oncology
Stanford University
Stanford, California

DANIEL A. LOW, PhD
Department of Radiation Oncology
Barnes Jewish Hospital
Washington University School of Medicine
St. Louis, Missouri

TAI-XIANG LU, MD
Department of Radiation Oncology
Sun Yat-sen University
Guangzhou, China

ANTHONY E. LUJAN, PhD
Department of Radiation Oncology
Northwestern University
Chicago, Illinois

STELLA C. LYMBERIS, MD
Department of Radiation Oncology
New York University School of Medicine
New York, New York

C.-M. CHARLIE MA, PhD
Department of Radiation Oncology
Fox Chase Cancer Center
Philadelphia, Pennsylvania

GIKAS S. MAGERAS, PhD
Department of Medical Physics
Memorial Sloan-Kettering Cancer Center
New York, New York

WEI-YUAN MAI, MD
Department of Radiation Oncology
Baylor College of Medicine, Houston, Texas
Sun Yat-sen University, Guangzhou, China

RAFAEL MARTÍNEZ-MONGE, MD, PhD
Department of Radiation Oncology
University of Navarre
Pamplona, Spain

NEIL MEHTA, MD
Department of Radiation and Cellular Oncology
University of Chicago
Chicago, Illinois

LOREN K. MELL, MD
Department of Radiation and Cellular Oncology
University of Chicago
Chicago, Illinois

MICHAEL T. MILANO, MD, PhD
Department of Radiation and Cellular Oncology
University of Chicago
Chicago, Illinois

STEFANIE MILKER-ZABEL, MD
Department of Clinical Radiology
University of Heidelberg
Heidelberg, Germany

MICHAEL MILOSEVIC, MD
Department of Radiation Oncology
Princess Margaret Hospital
University Health Network
Toronto, Ontario, Canada

RADHE MOHAN, PhD
Department of Radiation Physics
M. D. Anderson Cancer Center
Houston, Texas

MARTA MORENO, MD
Department of Radiation Oncology
University of Navarre
Pamplona, Spain

REGINALD MUNDEN, MD
Department of Diagnostic Radiology
M.D. Anderson Cancer Center
Houston, Texas

ARNO J. MUNDT, MD
Department of Radiation and Cellular Oncology
University of Chicago
Chicago, Illinois

MICHAEL T. MUNLEY, PhD
Department of Radiation Oncology
Wake Forest University School of Medicine
Winston-Salem, North Carolina

MARC W. MÜNTER, MD
Department of Radiation Oncology
University of Heidelberg
Heidelberg, Germany

BRENT MURPHY, MS
Advanced Radiotherapy Consulting Inc.
South Bend, Indiana

YASUMASA NISHIMURA, MD, PhD
Department of Radiology
Kinki University School of Medicine
Osaka-Sayama, Japan

CHRIS M. NUTTING, MD, MRCP, FRCR, ECMO
Department of Radiotherapy
Royal Marsden Hospital
London, England

MASAHIKO OKUMURA, MP
Department of Radiology
Kinki University School of Medicine
Osaka-Sayama, Japan

ARTHUR J. OLCH, PhD
Department of Pediatrics
Department of Radiation Oncology
University of Southern California
Los Angeles, California

GUSTAVO OLIVERA, PhD
Department of Medical Physics
University of Wisconsin
Madison, Wisconsin

BRIAN O'SULLIVAN, MD, FRCPC
Department of Radiation Oncology
Princess Margaret Hospital
Toronto, Ontario, Canada

JANET PATERSON, MRT(T), CMD
Department of Radiation Oncology
Princess Margaret Hospital
University Health Network
Toronto, Ontario, Canada

TODD PAWLICKI, PhD
Department of Radiation Oncology
Stanford University Medical Center
Stanford, California

EROS PEDRONI, PhD
Department of Radiation Medicine
Paul Scherrer Institute
Villgen PSI, Switzerland

CHARLES A. PELIZZARI, PhD
Department of Radiation and Cellular Oncology
University of Chicago
Chicago, Illinois

CHRISTOPHER PETERSON, MD
Department of Human Oncology
University of Wisconsin
Madison, Wisconsin

GUY PETRUZZELLI, MD, PhD
Department of Otolaryngology
Loyola University Medical Center
Maywood, Illinois

ANDREA PIRZKALL, MD
Department of Radiation Oncology
University of California
San Francisco, California

ALAN POLLACK, MD, PhD
Department of Radiation Oncology
Fox Chase Cancer Center
Philadelphia, Pennsylvania

RICHARD A. POPPLE, PhD
Department of Radiation Oncology
University Hospital
Birmingham, Alabama

ROBERT A. PRICE JR, PhD
Department of Radiation Oncology
Fox Chase Cancer Center
Philadelphia, Pennsylvania

RAMANI RAMASESHAN, PhD
Department of Medical Physics
Peel Regional Cancer Centre
Mississauga, Ontario, Canada

GREGORY M. RICHARDS, MD
Department of Radiation Oncology
Saint Vincent's Comprehensive Cancer Center
New York, New York

JOHN C. ROESKE, PhD
Department of Radiation and Cellular Oncology
University of Chicago
Chicago, Illinois

SAMUEL RYU, MD
Department of Radiation Oncology
Henry Ford Hospital
Detroit, Michigan

JOSEPH K. SALAMA, MD
Department of Radiation and Cellular Oncology
University of Chicago
Chicago, Illinois

MOHAMMAD SALEHPOUR, PhD
Department of Radiation Physics
MD Anderson Cancer Center
Houston, Texas

ROBERTO J. SANTIAGO, MD
Department of Radiation Oncology
University of Pennsylvania
Philadelphia, Pennsylvania

CHENG B. SAW, PhD
Department of Radiation Oncology
UPMC Cancer Centers
Pittsburgh, Pennsylvania

TRACEY E. SCHEFTER, MD
Department of Radiation Oncology
University of Colorado Comprehensive Cancer Center
Aurora, Colorado

THOMAS M. SCHROEDER, MD
Department of Radiation Oncology
Baylor College of Medicine
Houston, Texas

ANIL SETHI, PhD
Department of Radiation Oncology
Loyola University Medical Center
Maywood, Illinois

DANNY SONG, MD
Department of Radiation Oncology and Molecular
  Radiation Sciences
John Hopkins University School of Medicine
Baltimore, Maryland

YULIN SONG, PhD
Department of Medical Physics
Memorial Sloan-Kettering Cancer Center
New York, New York

GEORGE STARKSCHALL, MD
Department of Radiation Oncology
M.D. Anderson Cancer Center
Houston, Texas

CRAIG W. STEVENS, MD, PhD
Department of Radiation Oncology
M.D. Anderson Cancer Center
Houston, Texas

VOLKER W. STIEBER, MD
Department of Radiation Oncology
Wake Forest University School of Medicine
Winston-Salem, North Carolina

MINORU SUZUKI, MD, PhD
Department of Radiation Oncology Research
Kyoto University
Kumatori-cho, Osaka, Japan

CHET SZERLAG, MBA, FACHE, CMPE
Department of Radiation and Cellular Oncology
University of Chicago
Chicago, Illinois

RAYMOND TAN, MD
Department of Radiation Oncology
Stanford University Medical Center
Stanford, California

SCOTT P. TANNEHILL, MD
Department of Radiation Oncology
Columbia-St. Mary's Hospital
Milwaukee, Wisconsin

BIN S. TEH, MD
Department of Radiation Oncology
Baylor College of Medicine
Houston, Texas

JOSEPH TING, PhD
Carolinas Healthcare System
Charlotte, North Carolina

DAVID W. TOWNSEND, PhD
Department of Medicine and Radiology
University of Tennessee
Knoxville, Tennessee

FRANK A. VICINI, MD
Department of Radiation Oncology
William Beaumont Hospitals
Royal Oak, Michigan

JIAN Z. WANG, PhD
Department of Radiation Oncology
University of Maryland
Baltimore, Maryland

STEVE WANG, PhD
Department of Radiation and Cellular Oncology
University of Chicago
Chicago, Illinois

JAMES S. WELSH, MS, MD
Department of Human Oncology
University of Wisconsin
Madison, Wisconsin

TWYLA WILLOUGHBY, MS
Department of Radiation Oncology
M.D. Anderson Cancer Center
Orlando, Florida

JOHN W. WONG, PHD
Department of Radiation Oncology
William Beaumont Hospital
Royal Oak, Michigan

SHIAO Y. WOO, MD, FRCP, FACR
Department of Radiation Therapy
Baylor College of Medicine
Houston, Texas

ANDREW WU, PHD
Department of Radiation Oncology
UPMC Cancer Centers
Pittsburgh, Pennsylvania

QIUWEN WU, PHD
Department of Radiation Oncology
William Beaumont Hospital
Royal Oak, Michigan

BRENDA WYMAN, RTT
Santa Fe Cancer Center
Santa Fe, New Mexico

LEI XING, PHD
Department of Radiation Oncology
Stanford University School of Medicine
Stanford, California

YULONG YAN, PHD
Department of Radiation Oncology
University of Arkansas for Medical Sciences
Little Rock, Arkansas

THOMAS YANG, MD
Department of Radiation Oncology
M. D. Anderson Cancer Center
Houston, Texas

YONG YANG, PHD
Department of Radiation Oncology
Stanford University School of Medicine
Stanford, California

JEFFREY T. YAP, PHD
Department of Medicine and Radiology
University of Tennessee
Knoxville, Tennessee

INHWAN YEO, PHD
Department of Radiation Oncology
Princess Margaret Hospital
University Health Network
Toronto, Ontario, Canada

FANG-FANG YIN, PHD
Department of Radiation Oncology
Wayne State University
Detroit, Michigan

ELLEN D. YORKE, PHD
Department of Medical Physics
Memorial Sloan-Kettering Cancer Center
New York, New York

PIOTR ZYGMANSKI, PHD
Department of Radiation Oncology
Brigham and Women's Hospital
Boston, Massachusetts

I. Fundamentals

Chapter 1

IMRT PROCESS

ARNO J. MUNDT, MD, PHILIP M. BRUCH, MS, CMPE, BRENDA WYMAN, RTT,
CARMELITA CHOTIPRADIT, RN, JOHN C. ROESKE, PhD

Intensity-modulated radiation therapy (IMRT) represents a fundamentally new approach to the planning and delivery of radiation therapy (RT). As such, IMRT should not simply be thought of as a new procedure or technique but instead as a process. Moreover, it should be thought of as a multistep process involving every aspect of patient care and every member of the radiation oncology team, including radiation oncologists, medical physicists, dosimetrists, radiation therapists, nurses, and administrators. Close cooperation between each team member is essential throughout the entire process to ensure its success.

The purpose of this chapter is to provide an overview of the important steps in the IMRT process, from the development of a new IMRT program to the treatment of the first patient. More detailed discussions of the concepts and issues presented here are provided in subsequent chapters throughout the "Fundamentals" and the "Technology and Implementation" sections. These issues are also discussed in many of the clinical site overview chapters, case studies, and emerging technology reports in the "Clinical Topics and Case Studies" section. Interested readers should also refer to the recent joint document of the American Society for Therapeutic Radiology and Oncology (ASTRO) IMRT Scope Committee and the American Association of Physicists in Medicine (AAPM) IMRT Subcommittee on Implementing IMRT in Clinical Practice.[1] Issues regarding the clinical implementation of IMRT were also recently presented at the AAPM summer school.[2]

Implementing an IMRT Program

The IMRT process commences long before the planning and treatment of the first patient. In fact, it begins with the simple desire to do so. It is important to realize, however, that multiple steps lay between such a desire and patient treatment. Table 1-1 summarizes the major steps involved in the implementation of a new IMRT program. Each step is discussed in detail below. Readers who have already clinically implemented IMRT at their center may wish to proceed to the subsequent section on patient treatment.

Identification of a Team Leader and Core Team

Implementation of an IMRT program is a complex undertaking, requiring considerable planning, coordination, patience, and time. It is thus worthwhile to identify a team leader to oversee the entire process. Among the responsibilities of this team leader are setting priorities, developing timelines, and organizing meetings. The leader must also be willing to arbitrate between the various team members if problems arise. The adoption of IMRT requires everyone in the department to learn new approaches and alter their daily routine. It is possible that problems and even disputes may develop. Such problems should be addressed early to prevent them from impeding program development.

The team leader at most centers is the most senior physician in the department. However, the leader need not be senior or a physician. A junior attending physician may be a good choice, particularly because most current radiation oncology residents are now exposed to IMRT technology

TABLE 1-1. Intensity-Modulated Radiation Therapy Program Implementation

Identify team leader and core team
Define program scope and goals
Evaluate staffing needs
Identify space and necessary equipment
Develop a budget and purchase equipment
Perform acceptance testing and commissioning
Develop written policies and procedures
Train personnel
Develop and implement quality assurance program
Develop marketing and educational materials

Adapted from Galvin JM et al[1] and Shostak C. Implementation strategies for IMRT. Palo Alto (CA): Varian Medical Systems; 2003.

during their training.[3] A medical physicist may also be an excellent choice, given the tremendous software and hardware requirements of IMRT planning and treatment. More important than the individual's position, however, is his or her commitment to the overall success of the project and ability to lead and work with the group as a whole.

An initial responsibility of the team leader is to identify a "core team" selected from the various sections of the department (physicians, physicists, dosimetrists, therapists, nurses, and administrators). Their primary responsibility is to represent their individual sections. The team approach is particularly useful in a large department to facilitate communication. However, it may be worthwhile even in smaller departments because it instills a sense of teamwork and inspires ownership in the IMRT process, hopefully avoiding the feeling of various members of the department that change is being "forced" on them.

Another important responsibility of the core team is education. First, they must initially educate themselves. Nearly all aspects of IMRT planning and treatment differ from conventional RT procedures. Consequently, even experienced radiation oncologists, medical physicists, and radiation therapists are faced with learning new approaches and techniques. Administrators must understand new billing codes and procedures; nurses must be ready to answer questions about IMRT posed by patients and families. Consequently, the adoption of IMRT may be somewhat humbling and even frustrating for many (if not all) members of the radiation oncology team.

IMRT education takes considerable time and effort. Early on, it may thus be helpful for the core team to attend an IMRT seminar. Given the increasing popularity of IMRT,[4] numerous IMRT "schools," seminars, and workshops have appeared, catering to practicing radiation oncologists and physicists sponsored by academic centers[5–10] and professional societies, including ASTRO,[11] AAPM,[12] and the American College of Radiation Oncology.[13] Educational seminars are also sponsored by vendors[14] and private companies.[15] Such programs provide invaluable educational opportunities for practicing clinicians, physicists, and dosimetrists interested in developing (or expanding) an IMRT program. In addition, many programs include lectures directed at radiation therapists and administrators. As noted above, most radiation oncology residents today are exposed to IMRT and have hands-on experience treating a variety of sites.[3] The growing number of medical physics residencies in this country will also increase the exposure to and education of IMRT in the medical physics community.[16] Radiation oncology training courses are also sponsored by the Oncology Nursing Society.[17]

It is important to realize, however, that IMRT education is an ongoing process because new approaches and indications are constantly being developed and introduced. The published IMRT literature is extremely large. By far, physics studies represent the majority of the published studies (see

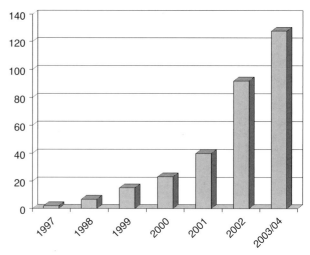

FIGURE 1-1. Intensity-modulated radiation therapy studies by publication year. Analysis was performed in May 2004.

Chapter 2, "Physics of IMRT"). However, reports focusing on the radiobiologic aspects of IMRT are increasing (see Chapter 3, "Radiobiology of IMRT"), and in many centers that have adopted IMRT, clinical studies are now being published, focusing on specific diseases (see Chapter 4, "Medicine of IMRT"). Figure 1-1 illustrates the number of published clinical IMRT reports. Although primarily focused on head and neck tumors and prostate cancer, IMRT studies have been published on nearly every disease site (Table 1-2). The authors of many of these reports have contributed representative cases to this text describing their approaches in detail. These studies were designed by experts around the world to provide the reader with insights on how IMRT is beneficial to these various tumor sites.

TABLE 1-2. Intensity-Modulated Radiation Therapy Clinical Studies

Category	Planning*	Outcome[†]	Total
Central nervous system	24	10	34
Head and neck	26	45	71
Lung[‡]	16	3	19
Breast	35	6	41
Gastrointestinal	11	5	16
Genitourinary[§]	33	29	62
Gynecology	12	8	20
Lymphoma	2	0	2
Sarcoma	5	2	7
Pediatrics	3	4	7
Metastatic/palliative	1	3	4
Total	168	115	283

*Dosimetric studies (no outcome data).
[†]Studies that describe the outcome of patients treated with intensity-modulated radiation therapy (many also include dosimetric comparisons with conventional treatment).
[‡]Includes mesothelioma studies.
[§]All but one study focuses on prostate cancer.

Given this large (and growing) number of IMRT applications and studies, it is impractical (and, in fact, impossible) for any one person to stay abreast of the use of IMRT in every disease site. Instead, the core team should identify a particular disease (or diseases) that they plan to treat at their center. It may be helpful for the team leader to select a few publications related to these diseases, allowing each team member to focus on the relevant areas (eg, immobilization, planning, quality assurance [QA]) and to report back to the group as a whole. Such a "study list" should not be a complete bibliography of all published IMRT reports in that site but instead should focus on reports highlighting important aspects of planning and treatment. An example study list of publications in prostate cancer IMRT is summarized in Table 1-3.[18–26] Review articles on IMRT in general[27–31] and its use in specific diseases[32–35] are also invaluable educational aids. Several IMRT texts have also been published.[36–40]

Once the core team members have educated themselves, it is then their responsibility to educate their colleagues. Staff meetings can serve as an excellent forum for this purpose. Radiation therapists should meet and review immobilization techniques and treatment regimens. Dosimetrists should present and discuss relevant IMRT planning studies. Such meetings serve not only to educate the individuals in the department on various IMRT techniques but also to identify any potential problems and concerns. One should always remember, however, that the "experts" do not have all of the answers.

Define Program Scope

One of the first decisions facing the core team is to define the scope of the IMRT program. Which patients and disease sites should receive IMRT? How many IMRT patients should be treated per day? It is not prudent to simply plan to switch to IMRT for all new patients. Such an attempt is not only destined to fail but also will most likely compromise patient care. An IMRT learning curve exists for all members of the team, and a more gradual approach to implementation is recommended. Moreover, as is discussed below, not all patients can or should receive IMRT. The team should focus on a particular disease site and, at first, limit the number of patients receiving IMRT. At many centers, the first IMRT case is often a patient with prostate cancer or a head and neck tumor. A clear benefit of this is that considerable experience exists worldwide using IMRT in these sites, allowing one to learn from the experience of others.[41] Moreover, in head and neck cancer, consensus guidelines are being developed regarding target delineation.[42] Whatever site is selected, however, it should be one commonly seen at the center, ensuring that each team member already has experience in the treatment of that disease with conventional RT techniques.

Once experience is gained, the IMRT program can be expanded, gradually increasing the number of patients and sites treated. It should be noted, however, that there is no ideal number of IMRT patients that a center should treat per day. The percentage of IMRT cases is a function of the diseases treated and the experience of the staff. An experienced staff at a center with a large prostate cancer referral base would naturally treat a higher percentage of IMRT cases than one treating a large number of palliative cases that has only recently adopted IMRT. It is always important to remember that the decision to use IMRT should be based on its clinical, not economic, advantages.

After a disease site has been selected, the next decision to make is how IMRT is to be used. Should it be used solely as a boost? Or should be it used throughout the entire treatment course? Many centers elect to initially use IMRT solely as a boost. Once experience is gained, more of the treatment in subsequent patients is then delivered with IMRT. Although there are certainly benefits to such an approach, it should be recognized, however, that less clinical benefit may be seen using IMRT in this fashion owing to a decrease in normal tissue sparing.[43] In addition, if this approach is used, it is important to create a composite plan that combines both portions of treatment. Some planning systems will include the conventional dose distribution during the IMRT optimization process (see Chapter 10, "Treatment Planning").

TABLE 1-3. Example Intensity-Modulated Radiation Therapy Study List: Prostate Cancer

Study	Topics/Issues
Zelefsky et al[18]	Immobilization, positioning, simulation, target/tissue delineation, dose escalation, optimization, plan evaluation, QA, outcome
Nutting et al[19]	Immobilization, simulation, target/tissue delineation, whole-pelvis IMRT, optimization, plan evaluation
Hancock et al[20]	Target/tissue delineation, whole-pelvis IMRT, outcome
Xia et al[21]	Immobilization, simulation, target/tissue delineation, dose escalation, incorporation of MRI/MRS, optimization, plan evaluation, QA, EPID, outcome
Teh et al[22]	Immobilization, simulation, target/tissue delineation, organ motion, rectal balloon, plan optimization, outcome
Shu et al[23]	Target/tissue delineation, incorporation of MRI/MRS, dose escalation, simultaneous integrated boost
Kupelian et al[24]	Immobilization, simulation, target/tissue delineation, dose escalation, plan evaluation, BAT, outcome
Buyyounouski et al[25]	Target/tissue delineation, MRI simulation, penile bulb sparing, plan evaluation
Kao et al[26]	Target/tissue delineation, penile bulb sparing, optimization

BAT = B-mode acquisition and targeting; EPID = electronic portal imaging; IMRT = intensity-modulated radiation therapy; MRI = magnetic resonance imaging; MRS = magnetic resonance spectroscopy; QA = quality assurance. Several of these authors contributed case studies and overview chapters to this text.

The team must also decide whether IMRT should be used primarily to spare normal tissue or to escalate the dose. Dose escalation is a common motivation for adopting IMRT,[4] most likely owing to promising IMRT studies in prostate cancer.[44,45] However, it should be recognized that dose escalation remains experimental in most disease sites, particularly when delivered using an integrated boost[46–50] or hypofractionated approaches.[40,51,52] A more reasonable approach would be to focus initially on normal tissue sparing without dose escalation, allowing experience to be gained in the various aspects of IMRT planning and treatment. A commonly held misconception is that IMRT is synonymous with dose escalation. However, a large number of disease sites are well treated with conventional doses. In such sites, the primary role of IMRT may not be dose escalation but instead sparing of normal tissues in an attempt to reduce treatment toxicity, improving patient quality of life.

Decisions also need to be made regarding the incorporation of more sophisticated imaging modalities. At present, IMRT is based primarily on computed tomography (CT) data (see Chapter 5, "CT Simulation"). However, increasing interest is focused on the incorporation of positron emission tomography (PET) in the IMRT planning process.[50,53] Other imaging studies, including ProstaScint (Cytogen Corporation, Princeton, NJ) scanning[54] and single-photon emission computed tomography,[55] may be useful in select patients. Magnetic resonance imaging (MRI) is also receiving interest as an IMRT planning tool.[25] Nonetheless, it is wise to focus first solely on CT-based planning. Once experience is gained, more sophisticated imaging can later be incorporated as desired. The role of other imaging modalities in IMRT planning is highlighted in many chapters throughout this book (see Chapter 7, "Imaging and Fusion Technologies"; Chapter 8, "PET-CT in IMRT Planning"; Chapter 18.6, "Functional Imaging in Head and Neck Cancer: Emerging Technology"; and Chapter 22.4, "ProstaScint-Guided IMRT: Case Study").

Evaluate Staffing Needs

Given the time-intensive nature of IMRT, it may be necessary to hire additional personnel. This is particularly true in a small center with a limited staff. As described in the subsequent section, IMRT planning is more time consuming, particularly initially, than conventional approaches. Moreover, commissioning and QA procedures place additional demands on the physics staff (see below). The medical physics section respresents the primary area in which additional staffing will be needed. Depending on the current staffing level and the anticipated IMRT patient volume, it may be necessary to hire one to two additional full-time equivalents or perhaps more depending on the size of the center and the IMRT caseload. Fortunately, the additional reimbursement of IMRT may help offset the financial burden of hiring additional staff (see Chapter 16, "Billing and Reimbursement").

Although the physics section is the most likely section in need of additional staffing, each member of the core team will need to evaluate his or her area in terms of staffing requirements. A gradual implementation of IMRT should help identify additional staffing needs and avoid major problems in this area.

Identify Space and Necessary Equipment

A major focus of the core team should be identifying the equipment (hardware and software) needed for implementing IMRT. Equipment needs are a daunting task for a center adopting IMRT. Vendors are all too willing to sell the latest IMRT "tool," but many of their products may not be necessary or worthwhile for a center embarking on a new IMRT program. It is important to note that no consensus exists regarding which equipment is truly necessary to perform IMRT. IMRT planning can be performed off-site (obviating the need for planning software), and treatment beams can be modulated with compensators (obviating the need for a multileaf collimator [MLC]). However, if one desires to perform on-site planning and deliver MLC-based treatment, it will be necessary to acquire a variety of software and hardware (see Chapter 10 and Chapter 12, "Delivery Systems").

It is important to recognize that as an IMRT program grows, so do its equipment needs. Hardware and software that would not have been used initially may later become important. Good examples are a PET-CT scanner (see Chapter 8) and respiratory gating software (see Chapter 9, "Respiratory Motion Management"). It is wise, however, not to attempt to purchase every possible piece of equipment but instead focus on one's more immediate needs.

With the proliferation of commercial software and hardware IMRT systems, there are now a considerable variety of available choices. The core team thus needs to become knowledgeable in what each commercial system can and cannot do. It is helpful to schedule a series of departmental "in-services" inviting representatives of the various companies to present their products. The core team should prepare in advance questions and evaluation guidelines, allowing them to critically compare different products and vendors. The currently available IMRT planning software products are described in Chapter 10. Chapter 12 highlights the various IMRT delivery systems.

At present, it appears that no one system or vendor is superior to the rest. In fact, a system that works well for one center may not be ideal for another. Nevertheless, whichever system is chosen, it is important to establish a good working relationship with the vendor to facilitate the necessary training and acquisition of upgrades and new equipment in the future (see below).

As decisions regarding equipment are made, one should bear in mind where the new equipment will be located. The simulator room may be adequate for a conventional simulator but too small for a CT simulator. The size of the treatment room or vault is also important. All new vaults should be designed to accommodate any special IMRT applications that the department will potentially use in the future. Additional shielding may be needed in an existing treatment vault. IMRT plans often result in three to four times the number of monitor units (MUs) as conventional plans, thus increasing the exposure outside the treatment room. Treatment vaults designed more than 10 years ago (before IMRT was considered) may no longer provide sufficient shielding to meet current regulatory requirements.

Members of the core team should address the issue of space relevant to their section and report back to the team as a whole to help anticipate future problems and issues. Additional space considerations for implementing IMRT include associated work space for medical physicists and clinicians. Additional office space should be allocated for the increase in staff, in addition to the storage needs for the related QA equipment and immobilization devices.

To perform IMRT, additional computer workstations most likely will be needed. The current computer setup should be evaluated and decisions made whether additional workstations are necessary. Included in the basic system package is a treatment planning computer and other networking equipment linking the linear accelerator with the main treatment planning system. The core team must also decide on which method of position verification equipment should be used. The choice between analog (film) or digital technology may necessitate revision of any room requirements to accommodate the imaging equipment.

QA equipment involved with IMRT is varied but necessary to provide verification of the treatment being delivered. If QA equipment has not already been purchased, the acquisition of a film reader, dose map system, ion chamber, thermoluminescent dosimeter reader, and several phantoms will be needed for commissioning and ongoing quality checks (see Chapter 13, "Commissioning and Dosimetric Quality Assurance" and Chapter 14, "Quality Assurance Processes and Future Directions").

The core team must also decide on which immobilization devices are most useful. A variety of vendors offer immobilization devices (see Chapter 6, "Immobilization and Localization") and the core team must determine which devices are best suited to their needs. The core team must also evaluate how extensive the immobilization system used should be. There are various degrees of immobilization, and the costs involved with the higher degree of devices will be a factor in the decision. Given that IMRT produces steep dose gradients around the target, accurate patient setup is important to minimize marginal misses and the subsequent irradiation of normal tissue. This is a good time to review the department's immobilization devices and quantify the setup uncertainty for the disease site that will be treated. If the immobilization is not adequate, and a new system is needed, it can be included as part of the IMRT budget.

Develop a Budget and Purchase Equipment

Once the space requirements and ancillary equipment needs are determined, a budget must be developed. Development of a realistic and functional budget will provide the institution with a template and projections by which progress of the new service or technology can be monitored. Institutions will normally develop a budgetary timeline with revenue and expense projections to determine the time element associated with the profitability for this new procedure (see Chapter 16).

Financial considerations involved with the budget process include the areas of capital equipment, fixed costs, and variable costs. The capital equipment cost is the major upfront institutional cost. Included in the capital cost is the linear accelerator and associated ancillary equipment, along with the cost of construction or renovation. A variety of plans and options associated with the most effective method to implement IMRT should be considered, as well as the disbursement of funds financing all purchases. Leasing options versus full purchase contracts may help minimize the financial burden on the institution, but revenue projections will be affected as well. Leasing a piece of capital equipment is financially feasible if the technology of the unit is projected to have a short timeline revision related to technologic improvement. Linear accelerators do not represent a technology with a short-term life span, so leasing should be considered only if a move is anticipated within 3 to 5 years. The capital equipment amortization schedule for a linear accelerator will differ from region to region, but the average schedule for a linear accelerator is in the range of 8 to 10 years.

The next area to be considered is the fixed costs. Most hospitals will delineate a standard list of fixed costs, including the utilities and services associated with performing all departmental services. Some institutions include personal costs into this category. With the development of an IMRT program, as noted above, an increase in the medical physics personnel is most likely necessary. Fixed costs are usually difficult to modify or change and will represent that relatively constant element in the monthly ledgers.

The other area associated with the budget is variable cost elements. This budgetary area deals with the associated costs involved with the day-to-day operations, including disposable items used during the normal operations of the system or equipment. This area allows for more financial control than the fixed costs area, but the individuals involved must be educated in the financial responsibilities of pertinent management of resources. Variable costs can greatly affect the net contribution to the institution.

All three areas create the internal budget that the institution will review and critique or analyze on a monthly basis. It is essential that the department creates a reasonable and logical budget, taking into consideration a variety of factors that influence the budget. The variable costs associated with a new technology can provide difficulty in managing the profitability of a new treatment option.

The next step in the process is to proceed with the request for purchase. The core team may work with the purchasing department in sending out qualifying letters to the vendors announcing the intention for purchase. Basic elements and additional add-ins are elements that should be included in the request for purchase. Industry vendors will have an opportunity to present a variety of options to the institution. Modifications to the options list will determine the final purchase price. Group purchasing organizations may have preferred vendors, which will allow for preferential pricing on high-priced pieces of equipment.

Once the core team has reviewed the equipment offers and has determined the list of options and accessories, it is imperative that the terms and conditions of the contract are reviewed. There are opportunities for the institution to manage the cash flow associated with this project by negotiating a payment plan that is tied to the delivery, installation, and acceptance of the equipment. Based on the time element involved with the decision to purchase and the actual implementation of the equipment, the institution can potentially use this capital money in a more fiscally responsible manner, prior to making the final payment. The purchase of equipment is the final stage of a long period of analysis and overview. Note that it is always easier to negotiate with vendors upfront regarding service contracts and training than at a later date. Economic and budgetary issues regarding IMRT implementation and treatment are discussed in detail in Chapter 16.

Perform Acceptance Testing and Commissioning

Once the purchased equipment is installed, it is the responsibility of the medical physicist to perform acceptance testing and commissioning (see Chapter 13). Acceptance testing is often performed in conjunction with the installer or another representative from the manufacturer. Its purpose is to verify that the equipment performs as specified. Many acceptance tests are functional in nature. For example, one may involve verifying that the planning software calculates and displays a dose distribution. Others may be more quantitative, such as verifying that the MLC positioning accuracy is within a certain tolerance. It is important to have a copy of the contract to verify that all equipment is functioning as specified, especially if upgrades were part of the purchase order. It is much easier to resolve these issues during acceptance testing because vendors often receive payment only after the acceptance test document is signed.

As part of acceptance testing, it is important to verify that the network connections between imaging devices (eg, CT, PET), treatment planning computers, and the linear accelerator are functional and perform appropriately. Scanning, planning, and treating a phantom would test the integrity of data transfer through the entire system. The cooperation of network services personnel is essential.

Once the acceptance testing procedure is complete, the commissioning process begins. Commissioning includes acquiring the necessary data for treatment planning and delivery and validating the planned dose distribution. AAPM task groups 40[56] and 53[57] have produced guidelines for commissioning a conventional treatment planning system. Several reports also describe the commissioning of an IMRT planning system.[58–62] One methodology involves progressing from open fields (nonmodulated) through more complex treatments, ultimately simulating an IMRT treatment.[62] The equipment needed for commissioning includes a phantom, an ion chamber, and film. Often a water tank system is needed for acquiring initial beam data. Analysis software for film dosimetry is also useful and may streamline the process. It is critical that enough time is allowed for commissioning and that one does not rush to treat a patient until the system is thoroughly tested. The commissioning process is discussed in Chapter 13.

Develop Written Policies and Procedures

The next step in implementing an IMRT program involves the development of written policies and procedures. If the department does not have a formal policy and procedure manual, one should be developed and continually updated. The basic elements of this manual cover the areas of human relations and personnel issues, institutional requirements, and a variety of department-specific policies and procedures. Delineation of the policies and procedures should reflect the normal business environment and maintain the principles outlined by the institution's vision and mission.

The core team should develop IMRT-specific procedures, serving as a template for personnel to follow in a majority of treatment regimens. Such procedures provide the necessary documentation to ensure quality control in the setup and delivery of IMRT. The critical factors associated with these procedures should be emphasized, and physician verification of treatment can be assigned prior to treatment delivery. IMRT is an extremely precise methodology, and it is imperative that review and verification of patient positioning be outlined in a procedure, ensuring that all personnel are cognizant of the need to check all parameters before treatment begins. Once the procedure is in place and a work flow has been established, the sequence of events will provide an efficient process for all personnel. Templates should also be developed for billing to avoid mistakes and claim rejections.

In-service meetings are useful to inform and educate the staff in all processes that have been developed. The advantage of any policy and procedure is that it will provide a medium for which individuals can be trained and provide a resource for further reference. Policies and procedures also provide useful information to all accreditation organizations.

It is also important to review all documentation performed at one's center, including how prescriptions are written and how treatments are recorded. Given the current increased reimbursement levels for IMRT, it is imperative to document the reason(s) why IMRT was selected and the necessary components of planning and treatment. These issues are further discussed in Chapter 15, "IMRT in the Community Setting" and Chapter 16.

Train Personnel

Ensuring that all personnel receive hands-on training is essential for the safe implementation of IMRT. Training can be performed in a number of venues. For example, prior to implementing IMRT, it may be useful to visit a department that has the same equipment that is being purchased. Participating in treatment planning, discussing evaluation methods, and observing patient treatments and billing procedures can alert the core team to issues that may have not been previously considered.

Most hands-on training will be conducted by personnel from the equipment vendor. Training typically lasts 1 to 2 weeks, and the scope varies by vendor. It is important that all groups—therapists, physicists, dosimetrists, and physicians—participate in their portion of the training. Additionally, one member of the core team (usually a medical physicist) should participate in all aspects of the training. Undoubtedly, there will be numerous questions after the trainer leaves, and having an individual who understands "the big picture" and can serve as a resource person is helpful. The first half of training usually consists of learning how to use the planning system, whereas the second half focuses on the treatment of an actual patient. Having the trainer present when the first patient is treated reassures the staff that they have a thorough understanding of the process and provides a "safety net."

On completion of training, the core team should schedule a follow-up visit in 2 to 3 months. The purpose of this visit is for the trainer to address new issues that surfaced after a number of patients had been treated. It is also an ideal time for the team to step back and evaluate the overall progress of their IMRT program.

Additional training can also be achieved off-site through third-party vendors. One such group, Advanced Radiotherapy Consultants ([www.arcphysics.net] South Bend, IN), provides off-site training for the *XiO* IMRT system (Computerized Medical Systems, St. Louis, MO).[15] During this intensive 5-day course, attendees receive didactic and hands-on training. One of the advantages of such a course is that staff can concentrate on learning the IMRT system without clinical distractions.

Develop and Implement a QA Program

A comprehensive QA program should be in place before IMRT is implemented. AAPM Task Group 40 has published a description of linear accelerator QA.[56] It is important to note that the Task Group 40 report was prepared prior to the widespread implementation of IMRT. As such, many of the tolerances, although adequate for conventional RT, may need to be modified to meet the stringent requirements of IMRT. Palta and colleagues provide a proposed set of tolerances based on the type of delivery method used.[63]

In addition to the requirements placed on the linear accelerator, IMRT demands accurate positioning of the MLC leaves. A detailed description of the characteristics of individual MLCs is provided in Chapter 12. It is important to note that MLC tests should be designed based on the type of IMRT delivery: static versus dynamic. Items that should be tested as part of conventional MLC use include carriage skew, gap between carriages, lead offset of light versus radiation field, leaf positioning and accuracy, and leaf transmission. Specific tests for IMRT delivery include leaf speed, dose rate evaluation, leaf position tolerance, leaf acceleration, rounded tip transmission, beam stability for low MUs, and effects of treatment interruptions. A number of test patterns are available from the individual vendors. As part of the QA program, the MLC should be tested on a daily basis. In addition, thresholds should be agreed on such that if the threshold is exceeded, patients should not be treated on that particular machine.

Given the complex nature of IMRT planning, the QA program should address the entire IMRT planning process, including QA of the CT scanner or simulator (see Chapter 5), target and normal tissue contouring, treatment planning, and evaluation. It is essential that treatment plans be reviewed on a slice-by-slice basis. This review should be performed with the dosimetrist, physicist, and physician together at the workstation. Once the plan is agreed on, patient-specific QA should be performed initially for all patients receiving IMRT (see below). Enough time should be allowed to account for unexpected findings. At the beginning, as much as 1 to 2 weeks should be allowed between the time a patient is simulated and treated. As staff become more proficient, this time can be significantly shortened.

A filming protocol should also be established. Some centers verify the isocenter positioning using only an anterior and a lateral radiograph. Others validate the fluence patterns and maximum leaf settings for each gantry angle. The frequency of this validation should also be established. A conservative approach involves filming each field prior to the initiation of treatment. The isocenter location is then validated every day during the first week of treatment and twice per week thereafter. Once the staff feels comfortable, the frequency of filming can be decreased. At many centers, isocenter validation is performed on the same frequency as in conventional treatment.

Develop Marketing and Educational Materials

Given increasing media interest in IMRT,[64,65] patients are becoming increasingly aware of IMRT and are seeking institutions and centers offering this technology. Unsurprisingly, a common motivation for adopting IMRT is competition. In fact, in a recent practice survey, desires to gain a competitive advantage or to remain competitive were cited as reasons for adopting IMRT by 38% and 36% of IMRT users surveyed, respectively. Corresponding percentages stated by non-IMRT users planning to adopt IMRT were 39% and 59%, respectively.[4]

Patient awareness is a vital component of a new IMRT program. Institutions with marketing or public relations departments should work with appropriate representatives to coordinate information related to IMRT and disseminate details to a variety of media venues. If the institution's marketing budget allows, information should be provided to the television media, local and regional newspapers, and the general public through informational flyers. The information provided to these venues should be on a level of understanding that allows the general public to appreciate the benefits of this new technology. The amount of information provided should allow the individual to compare and become more informed as to the benefits of IMRT. Industry vendors can help provide marketing references and assorted informational resources. An effective tool to publicize a new IMRT program is a press release.[66–68] An "open house" is also an excellent venue.[69,70]

An increasing number of patients seek health care information on-line.[71] This is true for cancer patients in general[72,73] and radiation oncology patients in particular.[74,75] Consequently, an excellent marketing tool for a new IMRT program is the Internet. In fact, many centers using (or planning to adopt) IMRT sponsor a Web site. Such sites vary considerably in size and scope. Many simply acknowledge the use of IMRT at a particular hospital or center[76,77]; others strive to educate the patient on the use and benefits of IMRT.[78,79] It is imperative that information be accurate and balanced. Recently, concerns have been raised about the quality of IMRT information on the World Wide Web.[80] In fact, a recent survey of IMRT Web sites found that nearly half contain false and/or misleading information.[81] Unfortunately, patients often fail to bring up information that they have gleaned from the Internet to their physicians, already accepting its veracity. It behooves all centers sponsoring an IMRT Web site to strive for accuracy and balance.[73]

Along with the marketing material provided to the general public, patient educational materials are also important. Supervision of the development of such materials is an excellent role for the radiation oncology nurse on the core team because nurses are often asked questions regarding IMRT by patients and families. In fact, it is frequently the nurse who fields telephone calls regarding IMRT by prospective patients and their families. As with the Web site, the accuracy and balance of all educational materials are important. Disease-specific informational materials can be developed to educate the patient as to the clinical ramifications of IMRT therapy and the associated risks and benefits. Head and neck tumors and prostate cancer are the main areas that have shown benefits to IMRT treatment; thus, many patients seek treatment options in these diseases.

Patient educational materials should focus on the methodology of IMRT, along with its potential benefits. Patients are always concerned about the side effects asso-

ciated with any treatment option, so information related to the potential side effects is very useful. Informational materials should indicate the time element involved with IMRT treatment and how the treatment is delivered. Providing the basic information regarding IMRT to the patient in a concise and detailed format will greatly enhance the experience of the patient and lessen apprehensions.

Education is also important for referring physicians. IMRT studies are being increasingly published in non–radiation oncology journals,[51,82–87] exposing more and more surgeons and medical oncologists to this technology. Like patients, referring physicians need to understand what IMRT is, what it is used for, and what benefits may be expected from its use. Longer simulation treatment intervals are common, particularly initially, resulting in apparent delays in initiating treatment. Involvement of referring physicians early on in the IMRT process can help avoid misunderstandings and other potential problems. Educational seminars and/or grand rounds are ideal venues for the education of non–radiation oncologists regarding IMRT. An open house focusing on referring physicians (eg, urologists, gynecologic oncologists, medical oncologists) may be beneficial.

IMRT Planning and Treatment

The next phase of the IMRT process involves the planning and delivery of IMRT treatment. The various steps involved in this phase, from patient selection to patient treatment and follow-up, are summarized in Figure 1-2. Each step is discussed in detail below. Interested readers are encouraged to refer to specific case studies throughout the clinical top-

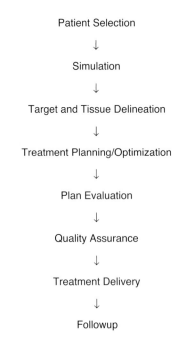

Patient Selection
↓
Simulation
↓
Target and Tissue Delineation
↓
Treatment Planning/Optimization
↓
Plan Evaluation
↓
Quality Assurance
↓
Treatment Delivery
↓
Followup

FIGURE 1-2. Schematic diagram of the steps involved in intensity-modulated radiation therapy planning and treatment.

ics and case studies section of this text for an in-depth overview of IMRT planning and treatment in particular disease sites.

Patient Selection

The initial step in IMRT planning is patient selection. An important caveat of IMRT is that not all patients can receive (nor should they receive) this therapy option. Many patients are treated well with three-dimensional conformal radiation therapy (3DCRT), and the benefits achieved using IMRT may be minimal at best (or even nonexistent). In fact, it is best not to think of IMRT as a replacement for conventional approaches but as a means of augmenting them in selected tumors and patients.

Table 1-4 summarizes the patient and tumor characteristics of an ideal IMRT patient. Such patients are cooperative and able to participate in the various aspects of IMRT planning and treatment. Each of these steps requires, at least initially, increased time for staff and the patient. Involvement of the patient throughout this process increases the likelihood that misunderstandings can be avoided and that treatment is optimally delivered. It is essential that patients be able to tolerate potentially increased time on the treatment table for both planning and treatment. Fortunately, with experience, time requirements will decrease considerably in future patients. Poor candidates for IMRT are clearly patients in considerable pain unless their pain can be effectively managed.

Poor IMRT candidates are also patients requiring urgent or emergent treatment. A possible approach in such patients, however, is to begin with conventional treatment and switch to IMRT as soon as the IMRT plan is ready. However, in many planning systems, it is difficult to generate a composite of the conventional and IMRT plans. It is imperative that IMRT be initiated as soon as possible; otherwise, the benefits of increased normal tissue sparing may be lost.[43]

Few patients are unable to receive IMRT, apart from the morbidly obese undergoing treatment to abdominal or pelvic sites, owing to the inability to capture their external contour on the planning CT scan. Without the external contour, IMRT planning cannot be performed. Patients in whom a limited portion of the external contour is not captured, however, may be treated with IMRT, with judi-

cious selection of beam angles avoiding missing tissues. However, markedly obese patients may also not be ideal due to difficulties in immobilization and daily setup accuracy. Some investigators even feel that such patients are less likely to benefit from IMRT.[88]

As shown in Table 1-4, ideal tumors for IMRT are irregularly shaped and in close proximity to normal tissues, particularly when higher than conventional doses are indicated. In contrast, regularly shaped targets located far from critical structures can be treated equally well with conventional approaches.

Given the inherent rapid dose gradients of IMRT plans, tumors in body sites that are poorly immobilized may not be appropriate candidates. Ideal sites in terms of immobilization include brain and head and neck tumors. Less ideal sites are the abdomen and pelvis. Adequate repositioning is particularly problematic in the treatment of extremity tumors. However, immobilization and repositioning issues are not insurmountable, and most can be overcome with creativity and experience, allowing the delivery of IMRT in most tumor sites. Interested readers should refer to the case studies section of this text for detailed descriptions of immobilization approaches used in various disease sites at centers throughout the world.

An ideal tumor site for IMRT is also one located in a part of the body with little or no organ motion concerns. Analogous to patient setup uncertainty, organ motion may result in lower than expected doses to target tissues (poorer tumor control) and higher than expected doses to normal tissues (increased toxicity) owing to the rapid dose gradients of IMRT. Sites with considerable organ motion concerns include the lung and upper abdomen owing to respiratory motion. Organ motion is also a concern in cervical and prostate cancers due to their proximity to the bladder and rectum. To date, most attention has been focused on the management of respiratory motion in thoracic and breast tumors (see Chapter 9 and Chapter 19.4, "Intrafractional Organ Motion and Planning: Emerging Technology"). However, methods to account for and/or manage organ motion have been developed in other disease sites (see Chapter 22A, "Intact Prostate Cancer: Overview," and Chapter 23.2, "Endometrial Cancer: Case Study").

A patient with a tumor recurrence within a prior treatment field is a possible candidate for IMRT, delivered with either palliative or curative intent. The highly conformal nature of IMRT planning may allow the delivery of sufficient doses in such patients with acceptable risk. Examples include reirradiation with IMRT in the treatment of recurrent spinal metastases[89] and recurrent nasopharyngeal cancer.[90] An overview of IMRT in patients with metastatic and/or recurrent disease is presented in Chapter 27, "Metastatic and Recurrent Tumors: Overview" and accompanying case studies (see Chapter 27.1, "Recurrent Spinal Metastasis: Case Study", Chapter 27.2, "Recurrent Nasopharyngeal Cancer: Case Study," and Chapter 27.3,

TABLE 1-4. Patient and Tumor Characteristics: Ideal Patient for Intensity-Modulated Radiation Therapy

Patient characteristics
  Cooperative
  Able to tolerate prolonged planning and treatment sessions
  Nonemergent treatment required
Tumor characteristics
  Irregularly shaped
  Near-critical structures
  Good immobilization and repositioning are possible
  Few or no organ motion concerns
  Higher than conventional doses indicated

"Intensity-Modulated Radiosurgery for Spinal Metastasis: Emerging Technology."

Simulation

Although differing considerably from conventional two-dimensional approaches, the simulation of an IMRT patient is similar to that performed in patients undergoing 3DCRT. At many centers, IMRT patients are simulated on a dedicated CT simulator (see Chapter 5.) However, if a CT simulator is not available, a diagnostic CT scan can be obtained in the radiology department and the data transferred to the treatment planning computer. However, care should be given to ensure that a flat table insert and external laser system are used. Furthermore, radiopaque markers should be placed on the patient to help reproduce the CT position on the conventional simulator. At some centers, MRI simulation is performed.[25] Increasing attention is also being focused on the use of PET-CT simulators (see Chapter 8).

Proper positioning is important in all patients undergoing IMRT. Interestingly, the position selected may differ from that used with conventional methods depending on the beam angles chosen. For example, whereas a chin-tuck position is often used in the conventional treatment of a parasellar meningioma, a neutral head position may be preferable with IMRT. Comfortable positioning is important in light of potentially longer treatment times.

Contrast is useful in the planning of IMRT patients, aiding in the delineation of both the target and normal tissues. This is the case, for example, in patients with head and neck tumors and lung cancer. However, the ability to fuse appropriate diagnostic images (eg, CT, PET, MRI) may obviate the need for contrast at simulation (see Chapter 7). Intravenous contrast is particularly useful in identifying regional lymph node sites, given the association of lymphatic and vascular vessels throughout the body. Other types of contrast used depend on the tumor site treated and may include rectal, bladder, and oral contrast. However, if one plans to use heterogeneity corrections within the treatment plan, a second CT scan (without contrast) may be required because regions of high contrast will be interpreted as having a high electron density by the planning system. Care must also be taken to ensure that the planning CT scan encompasses the entire external contour and all of the organs of interest. As noted earlier, without the external contour, IMRT planning cannot be performed. And without inclusion of the entire organ of interest, dose-volume histograms (DVHs) cannot be meaningfully interpreted.

As noted earlier, "protocols" should be developed for each disease site to improve efficiency and to decrease unnecessary mistakes. Such protocols should include detailed information on immobilization, positioning, contrast administration, and scan parameters.

Target and Tissue Delineation

After the simulation is complete and the data are transferred to the computer workstation, the target and normal tissues must be delineated. It is important to remember that unless a tissue is delineated, it will not be included in the optimization process. Target and tissue delineation is quite time-consuming for all targets, and normal tissues must be delineated on all axial slices of the planning CT scan. Initially, this task may be daunting because few practicing radiation oncologists were trained in this manner, unlike current radiation oncology residents.[3] Time can be saved by contouring on every other (or every third) slice and then interpolating the contours. However, unless thin slices are obtained, this approach can result in significant errors. Moreover, even when thin slices are obtained, this approach may not be appropriate in regions in which the target and/or normal tissues contours are rapidly changing. Whenever one uses interpolation, it is essential to review the resultant contours and edit them as necessary.

Use of a CT atlas is invaluable in target and tissue delineation, and one should be kept at the workstation for frequent reference. Assistance should also be obtained from the diagnostic radiologists. In selected cases, particularly in patients treated postoperatively, it may be worthwhile to review the treatment volume with the referring surgeon. Such an approach helps ensure that high-risk areas are included and provides an opportunity for education on the IMRT process. Fortunately, increasing resources are now available to assist the radiation oncologist in the clinical target volume (CTV) design.[91,92] Moreover, several IMRT seminars specifically focus on this issue.[7,11,13] With experience, target and tissue delineation should become considerably easier and more efficient. Moreover, the workload can be distributed between other team members, for example, normal tissues can be outlined by the dosimetrist and checked by the physician. However, the delineation of all target volumes remains the responsibility of the treating radiation oncologist and should not be delegated to other team members.

According to guidelines established by the International Commission on Radiation Units and Measurements (ICRU),[93,94] the gross tumor volume (GTV) and the CTV should be contoured. The GTV consists of all demonstrable tumor on imaging studies and physical examination. It comprises the primary tumor and all involved nodes or other metastases. An example GTV in a patient with head and neck cancer is shown in Figure 1-3. In general, most patients have a single GTV. However, multiple GTVs may be delineated in selected patients. In the future, areas within the GTV may be separately designated, for example, the hypoxic GTV based on functional imaging (see Chapter 18.6).[53]

The CTV includes the GTV and all regions of subclinical disease. The definition of the CTV should follow clinical knowledge about the spread of the disease and should not include margins to account for organ motion or setup uncertainty. In patients treated following surgery, one may

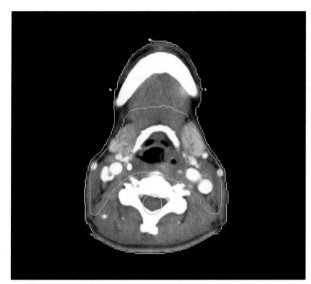

FIGURE 1-3. Axial slice of a planning computed tomography scan of a patient with head and neck cancer undergoing definitive intensity-modulated radiation therapy. The gross tumor volume is highlighted in orange. The clinical target volume was expanded by 3 mm, producing the planning target volume (*blue*). (To view a color version of this image, please refer to the CD-ROM.)

TABLE 1-5. Example Clinical Target Volume Components

Study	Disease Site	CTV
Duthoy et al[96]	Ovary	Entire peritoneal cavity (including pelvic and para-aortic lymph node regions), 0.5 cm rim of liver adjacent to peritoneum
Huang et al[114]	Medulloblastoma	Boost: primary tumor bed plus 2 cm
Kupelian et al[24]	Prostate	Prostate only (low-risk patients), prostate and seminal vesicles (high-risk patients)
Lee et al[115]	Nasopharynx	GTV (primary, enlarged neck nodes) plus base of skull, pterygoid fossae, RP nodal region, posterior third of maxillary sinuses, clivus, sphenoid sinus, posterior half of uninvolved nasal cavity
Roeske et al[103]	Cervix	Upper half of vagina, uterus/cervix (if present), parametria, presacral region, pelvic lymph nodes (common, internal, and external iliacs)
Pirzkall et al[108]	Meningioma	Contrast enhancement on MRI plus hyperostotic changes on CT
Suzuki et al[51]	Glioblastoma	GTV (contrast-enhanced tumor) plus 2 cm; enlarged to include areas of edema and decreased if adjacent to anatomic barriers

CT = computed tomography; CTV = clinical target volume; GTV = gross target volume; MRI = magnetic resonance imaging; RP = retropharyngeal.
Several of these authors contributed case studies and overview chapters to this text, including detailed descriptions of their clinical target volume designs.

contour only a CTV if the tumor has been completely resected. It is imperative to take advantage of all available imaging modalities (eg, MRI, PET), pathology reports, and the physical examination when contouring the GTV or CTV.

CTV delineation is a complex process. First, one must decide on which tissues to include. It is important to realize that the tissues included are often simply those sites included within a conventional treatment field. Such fields were derived over many years by detailed analyses of sites of spread and patterns of failure. However, it should be noted that in some cases, the CTV used in IMRT may include more sites than a conventional field owing to the inability of conventional planning to encompass all areas at risk. For each disease, radiation oncologists should compile a list of tissues that they wish to irradiate. In some sites, this list may be quite complex; in others, it may be fairly straightforward. Examples of the CTV components in representative tumor sites from published IMRT reports are shown in Table 1-5. Fortunately, an increasing number of investigators are including detailed descriptions of their CTV in their published reports.[95,96]

Selection of the components of the CTV is only half of the battle, however, for the physician is next faced with deciding on how to contour them. As noted above, a good CT atlas is essential, along with a working relationship with a diagnostic radiologist. In addition, all physicians implementing IMRT should show other radiation oncologists their contours. In centers with multiple physicians, an "IMRT round" evaluating target and normal tissue design is an invaluable education tool for the entire team.

It may be surprising to some that although two physicians may agree on the components of a CTV, they may disagree on how to contour them. Figure 1-4 illustrates this issue. Three physicians wish to irradiate a GTV plus two sites of microscopic disease (see Figure 1-4A and 1-4B) while avoiding a nearby normal structure or tissue (see Figure 1-4C). Nevertheless, these physicians may draw fundamentally different CTV contours. Physician 1 adopts the most aggressive approach, contouring only the sites of interest. Physician 2 is moderately aggressive and includes "bridges" between each of the structures. Finally, physician 3 adopts the most conservative approach, including a large margin around each structure, barely excluding the normal tissues (see Figure 1-4C). Although the components of each CTV are the same, the likelihood of both tumor control and normal tissue toxicities markedly differs between these three approaches.

A reasonable approach is to start conservatively with CTV design. Aggressive CTV contouring may simply result in higher local recurrence rates owing to underdosage of tumor and microscopic disease extensions. Radiation oncologists should also not be resistant to then modify their CTVs as more clinical experience is gained. Unfortunately, at the present time, the ideal CTV design is not known for any tumor

CTV Design

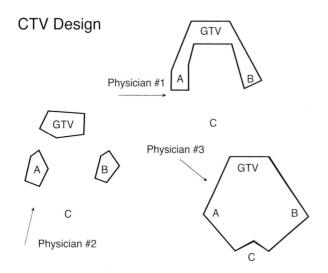

FIGURE 1-4. Schematic diagram of the potential differences in clinical target volume (CTV) delineation by three different radiation oncologists: gross tumor volume (GTV), sites of microscopic tumor involvement (*A* and *B*), and critical normal tissue (*C*).

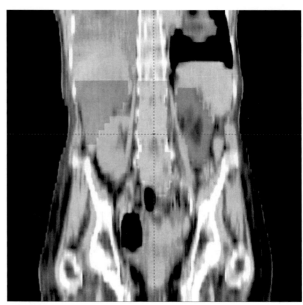

FIGURE 1-5. Clinical target volume (CTV) design in a previously irradiated patient with cervical cancer with lumbar spine metastases treated with palliative intensity-modulated radiation therapy. Eight years previously, she underwent whole-pelvic radiation therapy (45 Gy) extending to the top of the L4 vertebral body. Two CTVs were delineated: CTV$_1$ consisted of the L2–L4 vertebrae (*light purple*), and CTV$_2$ consisted of L5–S1 (*pink*). A simultaneous integrated boost technique was used to treat CTV$_1$ to 37.5 Gy in 2.5 Gy daily fractions and CTV$_2$ to 30 Gy in 2 Gy daily fractions while minimizing the dose to the small bowel and cauda equina within the prior radiation field. (To view a color version of this image, please refer to the CD-ROM.)

site. It is hoped that, with time, consensus guidelines will be developed for most tumor sites treated with IMRT.[42,97]

As with GTV design, it is often the case that multiple CTVs are delineated. This is the case if one is initially treating a large area followed by a boost to a smaller area. Multiple CTVs are also contoured if one is delivering a simultaneous integrated boost (SIB).[98] In a patient with head and neck cancer, for example, three CTVs may be contoured: CTV$_1$ comprises the GTV plus a 0.5 cm margin, CTV$_2$ consists of the adjacent high-risk lymph nodes, and CTV$_3$ includes the low-risk nodes. IMRT allows one to prescribe different total doses and fraction sizes to each CTV. For example, the total doses (and fraction sizes) to CTV$_1$, CTV$_2$, and CTV$_3$ might be 66 Gy (2.2 Gy), 60 Gy (2 Gy), and 56 Gy (1.8 Gy), respectively. A detailed discussion of the SIB approach in patients with head and neck cancer is provided in Chapter 18.7, "Simultaneous Integrated Boost: Emerging Technology." Interested readers should also refer to the case studies section of this text for descriptions of the SIB approach in a variety of tumor sites (see Chapter 20.2, "Accelerated Concomitant Boost: Emerging Technology," and Chapter 22.5, "Intra-Prostatic Boost: Emerging Technology"). An example case with multiple CTVs is shown in Figure 1-5.

After the GTV and CTV are delineated, the normal tissues must be contoured. Fortunately, most normal tissues are easily seen on the planning CT scan, particularly with judicious use of contrast. Some tissues, however, may be more challenging to contour, for example, the coronary artery region in a patient with left-sided breast cancer. Of note, normal tissue delineation should be approached in the same manner as target delineation, namely with patience

and a willingness to learn. Again, a good CT atlas and a good relationship with a diagnostic radiologist are invaluable. It is important to avoid the tendency to contour too many tissues. This practice is not only quite time-consuming but also unduly constrains the optimization program, resulting in inferior treatment plans. Above all, one should strive for consistency. Only then can one correlate clinical results with normal tissue DVHs, improving future treatment plans and patient outcome.[99,100]

Treatment Planning

Once the CTV is completed, the next step of the IMRT process is to specify a planning target volume (PTV), accounting for patient setup uncertainty and internal organ motion. It is important to remember that the PTV is the target used in IMRT planning, and unless the PTV is covered with prescription dose, the CTV is not.

The PTV is formed by a geometric expansion of the CTV and includes a margin accounting for setup uncertainties and organ motion. In ICRU 62,[94] these factors have been separated into an internal margin (IM) and a setup margin (SM). The IM is the expansion of the CTV required to account for expected physiologic changes in organ size, shape, and position relative to the geometry obtained during treatment planning. Such changes may arise from respiration, differential fillings of the rectum and bladder, heartbeat, swallowing, and peristalsis. The CTV plus the IM defines the internal target volume. These margins are defined based on changes relative to the patient geometry obtained at treatment planning.

Random errors arising from daily patient repositioning and alignment of the treatment beams must also be accounted for in treatment planning. A margin sufficient to account for these setup uncertainties is designated the SM. Careful setup and immobilization of the patient, coupled with imaging techniques, can minimize but not entirely eliminate the need for the SM. Setup uncertainties should be investigated at each institution to properly form an adequate (but not overly large) SM.

The combination of the IM and SM added to the CTV defines the PTV. Many investigators simply expand the CTV by 1 cm to generate a PTV. But in some sites, 1 cm may be too large; in others, it may be too small. One must always keep in mind that the larger the PTV, the larger the volume of normal tissues irradiated to the prescription dose and thus the higher the likelihood of untoward toxicity. Conversely, the smaller the PTV, the greater the probability the CTV (and GTV) will be underdosed and thus the higher the likelihood of a tumor recurrence. Issues of PTV design in various tumors are discussed in the disease-specific chapters throughout this book. Examples of CTV-to-PTV expansions in a variety of sites from the published literature are shown in Table 1-6. Interested readers should refer to the clinical case studies section for descriptions of CTV-to-PTV expansions used by various investigators in different tumor sites.

One should resist the temptation to directly contour the PTV on the planning CT scan. Although it may appear to save time and effort, it may result in inaccurate target design. A three-dimensional CTV-PTV expansion accounts for changes in the CTV contour above and below the CT slice in question; thus, individual slice portions of the CTV may need to be expanded by a larger margin to account for such changes. Contouring the PTV by simply drawing a larger CTV may thus result in underdosage of the CTV, increasing the likelihood of a tumor recurrence.

An increasing number of investigators are expanding normal tissues as well, generating planning organs at risk volumes.[94] To date, however, even less is known about normal tissue organ motion than tumor motion. Fortunately, current work is focused on deriving appropriate margins based on serial CT scans.[101] Incorporation of the planning organs at risk volume concept in the treatment planning process is illustrated in several case studies in this text (see Chapter 18.2, "Ethmoid Sinus Cancer: Case Study," and Chapter 26.1, "Retinoblastoma: Case Study").

It should be noted that in many patients, multiple PTVs are specified. For example, the CTV_1 may include the tumor (GTV) and regional lymph nodes, whereas the CTV_2

TABLE 1-6. Clinical Target Volume–Planning Target Volume Expansions

Author	Sites/Tumors	CTV-to-PTV Expansion
Central nervous system		
Pirzkall et al[108]	Meningioma	1–2 mm
Sultanem et al[116]	Glioblastoma	1.5 cm
Suzuki et al[51]	Glioblastoma	5 mm
Head and neck		
Claus et al[117]	Ethmoid sinus	3 mm
Hunt et al[118]	Nasopharynx	1 cm (except 0.6 cm posteriorly)
Munter et al[119]	Various	3 mm
Gastrointestinal		
Chmura et al[120]	Anal	1 cm
Milano et al[121]	Pancreas	1 cm
Landry et al[122]	Pancreas	2.5 cm
Genitourinary		
Zelefsky et al[18]	Prostate	1 cm (except 0.6 cm posteriorly)
Kupelian et al[24]	Prostate	5 mm (except 4 mm posteriorly and 8 mm laterally)
Teh et al[27]	Prostate	5 mm
Gynecology		
Duthoy et al[96]	Ovary	5 mm
Mundt et al[84]	Cervix/endometrium	1 cm
Heron et al[85]	Cervix/endometrium	5 mm
Other		
Fiveash et al[123]	Retroperitoneal sarcoma	1–1.5 cm

CTV = clinical target volume; PTV = planning target volume.
Several of these authors contributed case studies and overview chapters to this text, including detailed descriptions of their planning approaches.

includes the GTV. Expansions of both can then be done, producing a PTV_1 and a PTV_2, respectively.

Once PTV delineation is complete, the number, angle, and energy of the various treatment beams are selected. It is often a surprise to many adopting IMRT that these variables are not included in the optimization process. Although beam configuration optimization approaches have been proposed,[102] this step currently remains at the discretion of the treatment planner. At many centers, five to nine equally spaced coplanar beams are selected for most patients. Others use more individualized approaches based on their center's experience. It is always prudent, however, to explore a variety of beam configurations, particularly in disease sites that are less commonly treated at one's center.

Low-energy photon beams (6 MV) are often used and typically produce superior dose distributions, even in obese patients.[103] Higher-energy beams are also less desirable owing to the production of neutrons, increasing total-body radiation doses.[104] Current work is focused on the use of intensity-modulated electron beams, particularly in superficial tumors (see Chapter 18.8, "Modulated Electron Radiation Therapy: Emerging Technology."[105] As described in Chapter 28, "Intensity-Modulated Proton Therapy,"

IMRT approaches can also be applied to proton beams.[106]

Commercial inverse planning systems are now widely available. In the past, selected academic centers used home-grown planning software. Detailed descriptions of the various commercial planning systems are included in Chapter 10. Regardless of the commercial system selected, however, the treatment planner must enter input planning constraints for the target and normal tissues to be used in the inverse planning process, typically in the form of DVHs. These input parameters generally represent the desired DVHs for PTV and all normal organs.

Given that few radiation oncologists were trained to think of DVHs as an input parameter, selection of such parameters represents another potentially frustrating and humbling step of IMRT. However, with experience, the inverse approach becomes increasingly intuitive and straightforward. Examples of input DVHs used in treatment planning and resultant output DVHs are shown in Figure 1-6.

In terms of the PTV, one should strive for near-complete coverage by the prescription dose. However, attempts at covering the PTV with 100% of the prescription dose, especially in a highly irregularly shaped target, result in large inhomogeneities (hot spots) within the PTV. Instead, it is best to allow some cold spots, particularly along the periphery of the PTV. However, cold spots should be avoided within the CTV (and particularly within the GTV). Moreover, the magnitude of all cold spots should be small. Most investigators select a percentage of the PTV to receive the prescription, for example, ≥ 95% or ≥ 98%, in the planning process. Compared with conventional planning, IMRT is often associated with hot spots of larger magnitude and volume. This is particularly true with highly conformal plans. It is important to evaluate the magnitude, size, and location of all hot spots relative to normal tissues.

A reasonable planning approach, at least initially, is to enter the PTV and normal tissues and generate a conventional plan. The resultant normal tissues DVHs then provide a baseline or starting point for the inverse planning process. One should try to cover the PTV with the prescription dose while "beating" the normal tissue DVHs achieved with conventional planning. One should allow a modest degree of inhomogeneity in the PTV dose (small cold and hot spots), especially if one desires considerable dose conformity. It is essential not to choose impossible goals, for example, no dose to a nearby critical structure. Fortunately, more and more centers are publishing their input parameters in their methods section of the IMRT articles. Interested readers should refer to the individual case studies throughout this text for specific input parameters used in example cases.

Plan Evaluation

Evaluation of potential IMRT treatment plans requires considerable time and attention from the radiation oncologist, medical physicist, and dosimetrist. Close cooperation

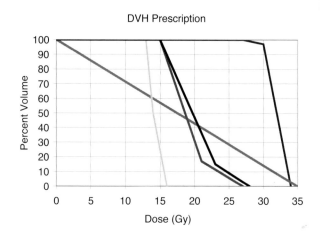

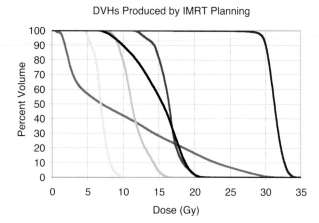

FIGURE 1-6. Input (*upper*) and output (*lower*) dose-volume histograms (DVHs) of the planning target volume (*blue*), tissue (*pink*), and other critical structures in a patient undergoing intensity-modulated radiation therapy. (To view a color version of this image, please refer to the CD-ROM.)

between each team member is also imperative in this phase. Potential IMRT plans should be evaluated both quantitatively and qualitatively. Quantitative evaluation involves an assessment of both the PTV and normal tissue DVHs. Qualitative evaluation involves a slice-by-slice evaluation of the dose conformity and of all hot and cold spots. As noted above, the magnitude, size, and location of hot and cold spots need to be evaluated and their clinical significance weighed in the selection of the treatment plan for an individual patient.

A lesson quickly learned during IMRT plan evaluation is the trade-off between conformity and dose homogeneity. The greater the conformity, the less homogeneity there is. Conversely, the less conformity there is, the greater the homogeneity. It is important to strike a balance between homogeneity and conformity for each patient. In general, if a high degree of conformity is desired, for example, in a patient undergoing reirradiation of a metastasis in the lumbar spine, a high degree of inhomogeneity must be accepted. On the other hand, if homogeneity is a priority, for example, in a patient with a pituitary tumor encasing the optic chiasm, less conformity must be accepted. A detailed description of the plan evaluation process is included in Chapter 11, "Plan Evaluation."

Quality Assurance

As discussed previously, a comprehensive QA program is an essential component of an IMRT program. Broadly speaking, a QA program encompasses the linear accelerator, MLC, CT scanner or simulator, target and tissue delineation, plan evaluation, and delivery. Well-defined thresholds should be set above which action needs to be taken.

Although there are no standards for IMRT QA, a widely recognized component is patient-specific QA. The most common implementation of this approach involves casting the IMRT plan onto a CT scan of a phantom. Ion chamber and film measurements are performed and compared with the results of the treatment planning system. Typically, ion chamber measurements agree within ±3%, whereas film is often evaluated as a percent discrepancy or distance to agreement (typically 3% or 3 mm). Initially, this type of analysis should be performed for all IMRT patients. It is useful to maintain a database of values so that outliers can be easily identified. As more patients are treated, and confidence is gained, it may be possible to eliminate or reduce the frequency of some tests. Some centers have eliminated film dosimetry after verifying several hundred patient plans.[107] Others perform phantom measurements only on certain cases (ie, pediatric patients) and have standard plans for each disease site that are routinely evaluated.

A frequently used QA tool is monitor unit verification (MUV) software. Such software uses the fluence maps and MUs generated by the treatment planning system to independently calculate the dose to the isocenter. The advantage of MUV software is that it uses the treatment depths from the patient (phantom plans do not), providing an additional level of patient-specific IMRT QA. When used in conjunction with phantom measurements, MUV software can often alert the physicist to problems before the phantom irradiation, thereby making the process more efficient. A commercial version of this software is available from LifeLine Software Inc. (Tyler, TX; http://www.lifelinesoftware.com/).

Treatment and Follow-up

It is important that all IMRT patients be closely followed during and after treatment. Doses are being distributed differently than one may be used to; thus, one must remain alert not only for less standard toxicities but also for potential new toxicities. Unexpected toxicities have been reported in several IMRT outcome reports, for example, conjunctivitis in patients with meningioma owing to the inclusion of beams entering or exiting through the orbit.[108] Unexpected reductions in other toxicities may also occur, for example, less hematologic toxicity in gynecology patients due to the unintentional sparing of the pelvic bone marrow.[109] It is imperative that such events be reported so that the field of IMRT can be advanced.

An important concern with IMRT is that whereas the volume of normal tissues irradiated with high doses is reduced, the volume of normal tissues receiving low doses is often increased. This is particularly the case when patients are treated with equally spaced beams around the patient or with helical tomotherapy. Unsurprisingly, concerns regarding the potentiation of second malignices owing to this low-dose spread have been raised.[110] In the future, beam angle configuration optimization programs should help reduce the use of such beam arrangements. Normal tissue radioprotectors, for example, amifostine (Ethyol, MedImmune Inc., Gaithersburg, MD), may also minimize this risk if combined with IMRT (see Chapter 29 "Biologic Modifiers and IMRT").[111] Nonetheless, careful follow-up is needed with all patients treated with IMRT in light of these concerns. Concerns regarding the risk of second malignancies with IMRT are discussed in Chapter 3 and Chapter 30, "Pros and Cons of IMRT: What's Been Swept Under the Rug?"

Radiation oncologists adopting IMRT should strive to optimize treatment by closely evaluating treatment toxicity in treated patients. Although normal tissue DVHs may be better than those achieved with conventional approaches, it is unclear whether such dosimetric differences translate into clinical benefits. With experience, the individual physician will determine what a normal tissue DVH needs to look like to achieve less toxicity. Moreover, the individual physician must carefully assess patient outcome. Only with experience will physicians know whether their targets are adequate. Unexpected sites of failure (particularly on the margin of the target) need to be carefully assessed, and targets should be modified accordingly.[95,112,113]

Conclusion

IMRT is clearly a fundamentally new approach to the planning and delivery of RT. As such, its adoption and routine use represent major changes for the RT department and staff. Not since the introduction of megavoltage linear accelerators has such a radically novel approach to RT treatment been introduced. IMRT represents a unique opportunity to learn new approaches, improve the quality of treatment, and, most importantly, improve the outcome of our patients.

Acknowledgment

We wish to acknowledge Carol Shostak (Varian Medical Systems, Palo Alto, CA) for sharing her ideas regarding IMRT program development and marketing.

References

1. Galvin JM, Ezzell G, Eisbruch A, et al. Implementing IMRT in clinical practice: a joint document of the American Society for Therapeutic Radiology and Oncology and the American Association of Physicists in Medicine. Int J Radiat Oncol Biol Phys 2004;58:1616–34.

2. Ezzell GA. Clinical implementation of IMRT treatment planning. In: Palta JR, Mackie TR, editors. Intensity modulated radiation therapy: the state of the art. Madison (WI): Medical Physics Publishing; 2003. p. 475–93.

3. Malik R, Oh JL, Roeske JC, et al. Resident education in intensity modulated radiation therapy (IMRT). Presented at the 46th Annual Meeting of the American Society for Therapeutic Radiology and Oncology (ASTRO), 3-7 October 2004, Atlanta, GA.

4. Mell LK, Roeske JC, Mundt AJ. A survey of intensity-modulated radiation therapy use in the United States. Cancer 2003;98:204–11.

5. Stanford University IMRT short course. Available at: http://www.ipomoea.stanford.edu /~lei/symposium/agenda.pdf (accessed 5/1/04).

6. Emory University IMRT school. Available at: http://www.knownexus.com/imrtschool.html (accessed 5/1/04).

7. M. D. Anderson Cancer Center. Second International Target Delineation Symposium for IMRT/3DCRT Treatment Planning. Available at:http://www.varian.com/onc/shared/pdf/040213_trainingagenda.pdf (accessed 5/1/04).

8. Memorial Sloan-Kettering Cancer Center Workshop on IMRT treatment and dosimetry. Available at: www.varian.com/onc/imr023.html (accessed 5/1/04).

9. University of Massachusetts IMRT school. Available at: http://www.knownexus.com/ IMRTSchool.html (accessed 5/1/04).

10. Indiana University IMRT seminar. Available at: http://www.cme. medicine.iu.edu/courses/05-095.pdf (accessed 5/1/04).

11. American Society for Therapeutic Radiology and Oncology (ASTRO). IMRT practicum. Available at: http://www.astro.org (accessed 5/1/04).

12. American Association for Physicists in Medicine (AAPM). AAPM summer school: IMRT. Available at: www.aapm.org/meetings/03SS/programinfo.asp (accessed 5/1/04).

13. American College of Radiation Oncology (ACRO). Available at: http://www.acro.org (accessed 5/1/04).

14. Varian Oncology Systems. IMRT school. Available at: www.varian.com/onc/imr023h.html (accessed 5/1/04).

15. Advanced Radiotherapy Consulting (ARC). Available at: http://www.physics-arc.com/corporate.pdf (accessed 5/1/04).

16. Commission on Accreditation of Medical Physics Educational Programs. Available at: http://www.campep.org (accessed 5/1/04).

17. Oncology Nursing Society (ONS). Available at: http://www.ons.org/nursinged/trainercourses.shtml (accessed 5/1/04).

18. Zelefsky MJ, Fuks Z, Happersett L, et al. Clinical experience with intensity modulated radiation therapy (IMRT) in prostate cancer. Radiother Oncol 2000;55:241–9.

19. Nutting CM, Convery DJ, Cosgrove VP, et al. Reduction of small and large bowel irradiation using an optimized intensity-modulated pelvic radiotherapy technique in patients with prostate cancer. Int J Radiat Oncol Biol Phys 2000;48:649–56.

20. Hancock S, Luxton G, Chen Y, et al. Intensity modulated radiotherapy for localized or regional treatment of prostatic cancer: clinical implementation and improvement in acute tolerance [abstract]. Int J Radiat Oncol Biol Phys 2000;48:252.

21. Xia P, Pickett B, Vigneault E, et al. Forward or inversely planned segmental multileaf collimator IMRT and sequential tomotherapy to treat multiple dominant intraprostatic lesions of prostate cancer to 90 Gy. Int J Radiat Oncol Biol Phys 2001;51:244–54.

22. Teh BS, Mai WY, Uhl BM, et al. Intensity-modulated radiation therapy (IMRT) for prostate cancer with the use of a rectal balloon for prostate immobilization: acute toxicity and dose-volume analysis. Int J Radiat Oncol Biol Phys 2001;49:705–12.

23. Shu HK, Lee TT, Vigneault E, et al. Toxicity following high-dose three-dimensional conformal and intensity-modulated radiation therapy for clinically localized prostate cancer. Urology 2001;57:102–7.

24. Kupelian PA, Reddy CA, Carlson TP, et al. Preliminary observations on biochemical relapse-free survival rates after short-course intensity-modulated radiotherapy (70 Gy at 2.5 Gy/fraction) for localized prostate cancer. Int J Radiat Oncol Biol Phys 2002;53:904–12.

25. Buyyounouski MK, Horwitz EM, Price RA, et al. Intensity-modulated radiotherapy with MRI simulation to reduce doses received by erectile tissue during prostate cancer treatment. Int J Radiat Oncol Biol Phys 2004;58:743–9.

26. Kao J, Turian J, Meyers A, et al. Sparing of the penile bulb and proximal penile structures with intensity-modulated radiation therapy for prostate cancer. Br J Radiol 2004;77:129–36.

27. Teh BS, Woo SY, Butler EB. Intensity modulated radiation therapy (IMRT): a new promising technology in radiation oncology. Oncologist 1999;4:433–42.

28. Tubiana M, Eschwege F. Conformal radiotherapy and intensity-modulated radiotherapy—clinical data. Acta Oncol 2000;39:555–67.

29. Verhey LJ. Issues in optimization for planning of intensity-modulated radiation therapy. Semin Radiat Oncol 2002;12:210–8.

30. Guerrero Urbano MT, Nutting CM. Clinical use of intensity-modulated radiotherapy: part I. Br J Radiol 2004;77:88–96.

31. Guerrero Urbano MT, Nutting CM. Clinical use of intensity-modulated radiotherapy: part II. Br J Radiol 2004;77:177–82.

32. Ozyigit G, Yang T, Chao KS. Intensity-modulated radiation therapy for head and neck cancer. Curr Treat Options Oncol 2004;5:3–9.

33. Krueger EA, Fraass BA, Pierce LJ. Clinical aspects of intensity-modulated radiotherapy in the treatment of breast cancer. Semin Radiat Oncol 2002;12:250–9.

34. Jani AB, Roeske JC, Rash C. Intensity-modulated radiation therapy for prostate cancer. Clin Prostate Cancer 2003;2:98–105.

35. Salama JK, Roeske JC, Mehta N, et al. Intensity-modulated radiation therapy in gynecologic malignancies. Curr Treat Options Oncol 2004;5:97–108.

36. Webb S, editor. Intensity-modulated radiation therapy. London: Institute of Physics Publishing; 2002.

37. Staff of Memorial Sloan-Kettering Cancer Center. A practical guide to intensity-modulated radiation therapy. Madison (WI): Medical Physics Publishing; 2003.

38. Chao KSC, Ozyigit G, editors. Intensity modulated radiation therapy for head and neck cancer. Philadelphia (PA): Lippincott Williams & Wilkins; 2003.

39. Gregoire V, Scalliet P, Ang KK, editors. Clinical target volumes in conformal and intensity modulated radiation therapy. Heidelberg (Germany): Springer Verlag; 2003.

40. Palta J, Rockwell T, editors. Intensity modulated radiation therapy: the state of the art. Madison (WI): Medical Physics Publishing; 2003.

41. Dawson LA, Anzai Y, Marsh L, et al. Patterns of local-regional recurrence following parotid-sparing conformal and segmental intensity-modulated radiotherapy for head and neck cancer. Int J Radiat Oncol Biol Phys 2000;46:1117–26.

42. Gregoire V, Levendag P, Ang KK, et al. CT-based delineation of lymph node levels and related CTVs in the node-negative neck: DAHANCA, EORTC, GORTEC, NCIC, RTOG consensus guidelines. Radiother Oncol 2003;69:227–36.

43. Cavanaugh SX. Acute toxicity in prostate cancer patients treated by high dose IMRT. Presented at the 86th Annual Meeting of the American Radium Society; 2004 May 1–5; Napa Valley, CA.

44. Zelefsky MJ, Fuks Z, Hunt M, et al. High-dose intensity modulated radiation therapy for prostate cancer: early toxicity and biochemical outcome in 772 patients. Int J Radiat Oncol Biol Phys 2002;53:1111–6.

45. Djemil T, Reddy CA, Willoughby TR, et al. Hypofractionated intensity-modulated radiotherapy (70 Gy at 2.5 Gy per fraction) for localized prostate cancer. Int J Radiat Oncol Biol Phys 2003;57:S275–6.

46. Wu Q, Mohan R, Morris M, et al. Simultaneous integrated boost intensity-modulated radiotherapy for locally advanced head-and-neck squamous cell carcinomas. I: dosimetric results. Int J Radiat Oncol Biol Phys 2003;56:573–85.

47. Amosson CM, Teh BS, Van TJ, et al. Dosimetric predictors of xerostomia for head-and-neck cancer patients treated with the smart (simultaneous modulated accelerated radiation therapy) boost technique. Int J Radiat Oncol Biol Phys 2003;56:136–44.

48. Lief EP, DeWyngaert J, Formenti SC. IMRT for concomitant boost to the tumor bed for breast cancer radiotherapy. Int J Radiat Oncol Biol Phys 2003;57:S366.

49. Kavanagh BD, Schefter TE, Wu Q, et al. Clinical application of intensity-modulated radiotherapy for locally advanced cervical cancer. Semin Radiat Oncol 2002;12:260–71.

50. Mutic S, Malyapa RS, Grigsby PW, et al. PET-guided IMRT for cervical carcinoma with positive para-aortic lymph nodes—a dose-escalation treatment planning study. Int J Radiat Oncol Biol Phys 2003;55:28–35.

51. Suzuki M, Nakamatsu K, Kanamori S, et al. Feasibility study of the simultaneous integrated boost (SIB) method for malignant gliomas using intensity-modulated radiotherapy (IMRT). Jpn J Clin Oncol 2003;33:271–7.

52. Floyd NS, Woo SY, Teh BS, et al. Hypofractionated intensity-modulated radiotherapy for primary glioblastoma multiforme. Int J Radiat Oncol Biol Phys 2004;58:721–6.

53. Chao KS, Bosch WR, Mutic S, et al. A novel approach to overcome hypoxic tumor resistance: Cu-ATSM-guided intensity-modulated radiation therapy. Int J Radiat Oncol Biol Phys 2001;49:1171–82.

54. Jani AB, Spelbring D, Hamilton R, et al. Impact of radio-immunoscintigraphy on definition of clinical target volume for radiotherapy after prostatectomy. J Nucl Med 2004;45:238–46.

55. Roeske JC, Lujan AE, Reba RC, et al. Incorporation of SPECT bone marrow imaging into intensity modulated whole-pelvic radiation therapy treatment planning for gynecologic malignancies. Radiother Oncol 2004. [In press]

56. Kutcher GJ, Coia L, Gillin M, et al. Comprehensive QA for radiation oncology: report of AAPM Radiation Therapy Committee Task Group 40. Med Phys 1994;21:581–618.

57. Fraass BK, Doppke K, Hunt G, et. al. American Association of Physicists in Medicine Radiation Therapy Committee Task Group 53: quality assurance for clinical radiotherapy treatment planning. Med Phys 1998;25:1773–829.

58. Intensity Modulated Radiation Therapy Collaborative Working Group. Intensity modulated radiotherapy: current status and issues of interest. Int J Radiat Oncol Biol Phys 2001;51:880–914.

59. Ezzell GA, Galvin JM, Low D, et al. Guidance document on delivery, treatment planning, and clinical implementation of IMRT. Report of the IMRT Subcommittee of the AAPM Radiation Therapy Committee. Med Phys 2003;30:2089–115.

60. Sharpe MB. Commissioning and quality assurance for IMRT treatment planning. In: Palta JR, Mackie TR, editors. Intensity-modulated radiation therapy: the state of the art. Madison (WI): Medical Physics Publishing; 2003. p. 495–514.

61. Essers M, deLangen M, Dirkx MLP, et al. Commissioning of a commercially available system for intensity-modulated radiotherapy dose delivery with dynamic multileaf collimation. Radiother Oncol 2001;60:215–24.

62. Xing L, Curran B, Hill R, et al. Dosimetric verification of a commercial inverse treatment planning system. Phys Med Biol 1999;44:463–78.

63. Palta JR, Kim S, Li JG, et al. Tolerance limits and action levels for planning and delivery of IMRT. In: Palta JR, Mackie TR, editors. Intensity-modulated radiation therapy: the state of the art. Madison (WI): Medical Physics Publishing; 2003. p. 593–612.

64. Carmichael M, Murdock J, Rappleye C. "Your next…" Newsweek 2002;139:64–6.

65. Brown E. Cancer in the crosshairs. Forbes 2002;170:361–4.

66. University of Nebraska Medical Center. Department of Radiation Oncology. Available at: http://www.unmc.edu/radonc/imrt_release.htm (accessed 3/1/04).

67. White Plains Hospital Center. News Release Available at: http://www.wphospital.org/whatsnew/intensemod.htm (accessed 3/1/04).

68. Cooper University Hospital. Press Release. Available at: http://www.cooperhealth.org/press/2002/02_04_01.htm (accessed 3/1/04).

69. BC Cancer Agency. News Release. Available at: http://www.bccancer.bc.ca/abcca/newscentre/2004/viopenhouse.htm (accessed 3/1/04).

70. Mary Bird Perkins Cancer Center. Newsletter. Available at: http://www.marybird.org/admin/newsletters/files/pp2002_winter.pdf (accessed 3/1/04).

71. Pew Internet and American Life Project. The online health care revolution: how the Web helps Americans take better care of themselves. Available at: http://www.pewinternet.org.

72. Bierman JS, Golladay GJ, Greenfield ML, et al. Evaluation of cancer information on the Internet. Cancer 1999;86:381–90.

73. Chen X, Siu LL. Impact of the media and the Internet on oncology: survey of cancer patients and oncologists in Canada. J Clin Oncol 2001;19:4291–7.

74. Metz JM, Devine P, DeNittis A, et al. A multi-institutional study of Internet utilization by radiation oncology patients. Int J Radiat Oncol Biol Phys 2003;56:1201–5.

75. Vordemark D, Kolbl O, Flentje. The Internet as a source of medical information: investigation in a mixed cohort of radiotherapy patients. Strahlenther Onkol 2000;176:532–5.

76. Northeast Health System.Available at: http://www.nehealth. com/html/neh sam ctc imrt.asp (accessed 3/1/04).

77. Valley Radiotherapy Associates Medical Group Inc., Available at: http://www.valley-radiotherapy.com/technology/imrt.html (accessed 3/1/04).

78. Palo Alto Medical Foundation. Department Of Radiation Oncology. Available at: http://www.pamf.org/radonc.

79. Dale and Frances Hughes Cancer Center. Pocono Medical Center. Available at: http://www.intensitymodulatedradiation.com (accessed 3/1/04).

80. Glatstein E. The return of the snake oil salesmen. Int J Radiat Oncol Biol Phys 2003;55:561–2.

81. Schomas D, Milano M, Roeske JC, et al. Intensity modulated radiation therapy and the Internet: evaluation of the content and quality of patient-oriented information. Cancer 2004;101:412–20.

82. Eisbruch A, Ship JA, Dawson LA, et al. Salivary gland sparing and improved target irradiation by conformal and intensity modulated irradiation of head and neck cancer. World J Surg 2003;27:832–7.

83. Bai YR, Wu GH, Guo WJ, et al. Intensity modulated radiation therapy and chemotherapy for locally advanced pancreatic cancer: results of feasibility study. World J Gastroenterol 2004;9:2561–4.

84. Mundt AJ, Roeske JC, Lujan AE, et al. Initial clinical experience with intensity-modulated whole-pelvis radiation therapy in women with gynecologic malignancies. Gynecol Oncol 2001;82:456–63.

85. Heron DE, Gerszten K, Selvaraj RN, et al. Conventional 3D conformal versus intensity-modulated radiotherapy for the adjuvant treatment of gynecologic malignancies: a comparative dosimetric study of dose-volume histograms. Gynecol Oncol 2003;91:39–45.

86. Ahamad A, Stevens CW, Smythe WR, et al. Promising early local control of malignant pleural mesothelioma following postoperative intensity modulated radiotherapy (IMRT) to the chest. Cancer J 2003;9:476–84.

87. Zelefsky M, Fuks Z, Hunt M, et al. High dose radiation delivered by intensity modulated conformal radiotherapy improves the outcome of localized prostate cancer. J Urol 2001;166:876–81.

88. Ahamad A, D'Souza W, Salehpour M, et al. Intensity modulated radiation therapy (IMRT) for post-hysterectomy pelvic radiation: selection of patients and planning target volume (PTV). Int J Radiat Oncol Biol Phys 2002;54:42.

89. Ryu S, Fang Yin F, Rock J, et al. Image-guided and intensity-modulated radiosurgery for patients with spinal metastasis. Cancer 2003;97:2013–8.

90. Lu TX, Mai WY, Teh BS, et al. Initial experience using intensity-modulated radiotherapy for recurrent nasopharyngeal carcinoma. Int J Radiat Oncol Biol Phys 2004;58:682–7.

91. Som PM, Curtin HD, Mancuso AA. An image-based classification for the cervical nodes designed as an adjunct to recent clinically based nodal classification. Arch Otolaryngol Head Neck Surg 1999;125:388–96.

92. Nowak PJCM, Wijers OB, Lagerwaard FJ, et al. A three-dimensional CT-based target definition for elective irradiation of the neck. Int J Radiat Oncol Biol Phys 1999;45:33–9.

93. International Commission on Radiation Units and Measurements. Prescribing, recording and reporting photon beam therapy. Report 50. Washington (DC): International Commission on Radiation Units and Measurements; 1993.

94. International Commission on Radiation Units and Measurements. Prescribing, recording and reporting photon beam therapy (supplement to ICRU report 50). Report 62. Bethesda (MD): International Commission on Radiation Units and Measurements; 1999.

95. Chao KS, Wippold FJ, Ozyigit G, et al. Determination and delineation of nodal target volumes for head-and-neck cancer based on patterns of failure in patients receiving definitive and postoperative IMRT. Int J Radiat Oncol Biol Phys 2002;53:1174–84.

96. Duthoy W, De Gersem W, Vergote K, et al. Whole abdominopelvic radiotherapy (WAPRT) using intensity-modulated arc therapy (IMAT): first clinical experience. Int J Radiat Oncol Biol Phys 2003;57:1019–32.

97. Mell LK, Fyles AW, Small W, et al. Adjuvant intensity modulated pelvic radiation therapy in gynecologic malignancies: Survey of the Gynecologic IMRT Working Group. Presented at the 46th Annual Meeting of the American Society for Therapuetic Radiology and Oncology, 3-7 October 2004, Atlanta, GA.

98. Mohan R, Wu Q, Manning M, et al. Radiobiological considerations in the design of fractionation strategies for intensity-modulated radiation therapy of head and neck cancers. Int J Radiat Oncol Biol Phys 2000;46:619–30.

99. Eisbruch A, Ten Haken RK, Kim HM, et al. Dose, volume, and function relationships in parotid salivary glands following conformal and intensity-modulated irradiation of head and neck cancer. Int J Radiat Oncol Biol Phys 1999;45:577–87.

100. Roeske JC, Bonta D, Mell LK, et al. A dosimetric analysis of acute gastrointestinal toxicity in women receiving intensity-modulated whole-pelvic radiation therapy. Radiother Oncol 2003;69:201–7.

101. Muren LP, Ekerold R, Kvinnsland Y, et al. On the use of margins for geometrical uncertainties around the rectum in radiotherapy planning. Radiother Oncol 2004;70:11–9.

102. Pugachev A, Li JG, Boyer AL, et al. Role of beam orientation optimization in intensity-modulated radiation therapy. Int J Radiat Oncol Biol Phys 2001;50:551–60.

103. Roeske JC, Lujan A, Rotmensch J, et al. Intensity-modulated whole pelvic radiation therapy in patients with gynecologic malignancies. Int J Radiat Oncol Biol Phys 2000;48:1613–21.

104. Waller EJ. Neutron production associated with radiotherapy linear accelerators using intensity modulated radiation therapy mode. Health Phys 2003;85(5 Suppl):S75–7.

105. Ma CM, Ding M, Li JS, et al. A comparative dosimetric study on tangential photon beams, intensity-modulated radiation therapy (IMRT) and modulated electron radiotherapy (MERT) for breast cancer treatment. Phys Med Biol 2003;48:909–24.

106. Lomax AJ, Cella L, Weber D, et al. Potential role of intensity-modulated photons and protons in the treatment of the breast and regional nodes. Int J Radiat Oncol Biol Phys 2003;55:785–92.

107. Klein E, Li Z, Jin J. Reduction of IMRT patient quality assurance by means of independent dose calculations [abstract]. Med Phys 2003;30:1496.

108. Pirzkall A, Debus J, Haering P, et al. Intensity modulated radiotherapy (IMRT) for recurrent, residual, or untreated skull-base meningiomas: preliminary clinical experience. Int J Radiat Oncol Biol Phys 2003;55:362–72.

109. Brixey CJ, Roeske JC, Lujan AE, et al. Impact of intensity-modulated radiotherapy on acute hematologic toxicity in women with gynecologic malignancies. Int J Radiat Oncol Biol Phys 2002;54:1388–96.

110. Hall EJ, Wuu CS. Radiation-induced second cancers: the impact of 3D-CRT and IMRT. Int J Radiat Oncol Biol Phys 2003;56:83–8.

111. Grdina DJ, Kataoka Y, Basic I, et al. The radioprotector WR-2721 reduces neutron induced mutations at the hypoxanthine-guanine phosphoribosyl transferase locus in mouse splenocytes when administered prior to or following irradiation. Carcinogenesis 1992;13:811–4.

112. Eisbruch A, Marsh LH, Dawson LA, et al. Recurrences near base of skull after IMRT for head-and-neck cancer: implications for target delineation in high neck and for parotid gland sparing. Int J Radiat Oncol Biol Phys 2004;59:28–42.

113. Kochanski J, Roeske JC, Mell LK, et al. Outcome of FIGO stage I-II cervical cancer patients treated with intensity modulated pelvic radiation therapy [abstract]. Proc Am Soc Clin Oncol 2004;23:454.

114. Huang E, Teh BS, Strother DR, et al. Intensity-modulated radiation therapy for pediatric medulloblastoma: early report on the reduction of ototoxicity. Int J Radiat Oncol Biol Phys 2002;52:599–605.

115. Lee N, Xia P, Fischbein NJ, et al. Intensity-modulated radiation therapy for head-and-neck cancer: the UCSF experience focusing on target volume delineation. Int J Radiat Oncol Biol Phys 2003;57:49–60.

116. Sultanem K, Patrocinio H, Lambert C, et al. The use of hypofractionated intensity-modulated irradiation in the treatment of glioblastoma multiforme: preliminary results of a prospective trial. Int J Radiat Oncol Biol Phys 2004;58:247–52.

117. Claus F, De Gersem W, De Wagter C, et al. An implementation strategy for IMRT of ethmoid sinus cancer with bilateral sparing of the optic pathways. Int J Radiat Oncol Biol Phys 2001;51:318–31.

118. Hunt MA, Zelefsky MJ, Wolden S, et al. Treatment planning and delivery of intensity-modulated radiation therapy for primary nasopharynx cancer. Int J Radiat Oncol Biol Phys 2001;49:623–32.

119. Munter MW, Thilmann C, Hof H, et al. Stereotactic intensity modulated radiation therapy and inverse treatment planning for tumors of the head and neck region: clinical implementation of the step and shoot approach and first clinical results. Radiother Oncol 2003;66:313–21.

120. Chmura SJ, Milano M, Garofalo M, et al. Initial outcome with intensity-modulated radiation (IMRT) and chemotherapy (CTX) in anal cancer [abstract]. Proc Am Soc Clin Oncol 2003;22:368.

121. Milano MT, Chmura SJ, Garofalo MC, et al. Intensity-modulated radiotherapy in treatment of pancreatic and bile duct malignancies: toxicity and clinical outcome. Int J Radiat Oncol Biol Phys 2004;59:445:53.

122. Landry JC, Yang GY, Ting JY, et al. Treatment of pancreatic cancer tumors with intensity-modulated radiation therapy (IMRT) using the volume at risk approach (VARA): employing dose-volume histogram (DVH) and normal tissue complication probability (NTCP) to evaluate small bowel toxicity. Med Dosim 2002;27:121-9.

123. Fiveash J, Hyatt MD, Caranto J, et al. Preoperative IMRT with dose escalation to tumor subvolumes for retroperitoneal sarcomas: initial clinical results and potential for future dose escalation [abstract]. Int J Radiat Oncol Biol Phys 2002;54:140.

Chapter 2

Physics of IMRT

Lei Xing, PhD, Qiuwen Wu, PhD, Yong Yang, PhD, Arthur Boyer, PhD

Radiation therapy (RT) as a means of managing cancer has its roots in the discipline of radiology. From the time Roentgen first discovered x-rays, two-dimensional transmission images of the human body provided unprecedented imagery of bony landmarks, allowing radiologists to deduce the location of internal organs. Using planar radiographs, radiologists planned cancer treatments by collimating rectangular fields encompassing the presumed tumor location. Additional blocks placed daily to match marks on the patient's skin and later the use of low-temperature melting dense alloys provided a cookie-cutter approach to treating the two-dimensional projections of the tumor volumes.

Human anatomy and tumor shapes, however, are inherently three-dimensional. By treating a large amount of nearby normal tissue, physicians were limited by the tolerance of the normal tissue they were treating. Additionally, it was not possible to take the three-dimensional structures into consideration because of the limitations of early dose calculations. The advantage of being able to treat a tumor target conformally can be appreciated by a simple example. Assume that the tumor is a sphere of 5 cm in diameter; it would have a volume of 65.4 cc. If one irradiates it with square fields, directed at the six faces of the cube containing the sphere (an anatomic impossibility that we will allow for the sake of making a theoretical point), a high-dose volume would be created within the sphere containing 125 cc. This represents the three-dimensional nonconformal situation. If one were to treat the volume with circular fields, directed toward the sphere from all directions (which, again, is anatomically impossible), the high dose would be limited to the sphere itself. Approximately 60 cc of normal tissue would be spared. The reduction of tissue irradiated is a factor of $6/\pi$ or about half. This reduction in normal tissue irradiation should theoretically improve the therapeutic ratio and allow the tumor target volume to be treated to a higher dose, thereby improving the probability of tumor control. Other factors play critical roles as well. Tumor biology has a great deal to do with the actual tumor control achieved, but the basic idea of reducing normal tis-

sue irradiation is a valid strategy and the goal for managing local tumor control with a minimum of normal tissue complications. The details on radiobiology are discussed in Chapter 3, "Radiobiology of IMRT."

Three-dimensional conformal radiation therapy (3DCRT) is a method of irradiating target volume defined in a three-dimensional anatomic image of the patient with a set of x-ray beams individually shaped to conform the two-dimensional beam's eye view projection of the target. 3DCRT became feasible with the development of computed tomography (CT). The development of spiral and multislice CT scanners has made the acquisition of large data sets practical. The reconstructed images, acquired with patients in the treatment position, provide a model on which geometric and dosimetric computations can be applied. These data sets can be acquired with spiral scanners capable of recording the transmission data needed to reconstruct 50 to 100 transverse image planes spaced 2 to 5 mm apart. Given adequate immobilization devices to help patients achieve and hold their treatment position for the duration of the image acquisition, these fast scanners provide excellent data sets that can be used for treatment planning. The transmission data are used to reconstruct a three-dimensional data set consisting of Hounsfield numbers associated with voxels. The development of the Digital Imaging and Communication in Medicine (DICOM) standard and its various extensions for data exchange has made possible the use of CT data sets acquired with the equipment from one vendor with treatment planning systems from another vendor and the ability to treat patients with equipment from yet another vendor. The transfer of these data over computer networks has improved the efficiency and accuracy of the entire treatment planning and delivery process.

Evolution from 3DCRT to IMRT

Intensity-modulated radiation therapy (IMRT) emerged in clinical practice as a result of the development of 3DCRT in the 1980s. Although the exact beginning of the modality depends on one's definition of IMRT, it is generally agreed on that the widespread implementation and realization of the technique occurred in the United States in the early 1990s with the commercially available Peacock IMRT planning system and MIMiC fan beam delivery device (North American Scientific, NOMOS Radiation Oncology Division, Cranberry Township, PA).[1,2] This was then followed by the cone beam multileaf collimator (MLC)-based IMRT in the mid-1990s. MLC allows the rapid and controllable adjustment of field aperture and is thus ideally suited for dynamic radiation beam modulation. In Figure 2-1, different IMRT modalities currently available or under intense investigation are summarized. Physically, a common feature of these IMRT techniques is that they all attempt to enhance control over the three-dimensional dose distribution through the superposition of a large number of independent segmented fields from either a number of fixed directions or from directions distributed on one or multiple arcs.

Intensity modulation adds a new degree of freedom to RT planning and provides a more effective means to produce tightly conformal dose distributions in complex treatment situations. The objective of this chapter is to provide an overall comprehension of IMRT and to review the physics aspect of this technology. In Figure 2-2, the overall treatment process of IMRT is illustrated. The key steps involved in the process are discussed in separate sections. In the remainder of this introductory section, we briefly describe the IMRT delivery modes listed in Figure 2-1. Given that fixed-gantry IMRT is by far the most popularly implemented technique, emphasis is given to this mode first.

Fixed-Gantry IMRT

Fixed-gantry IMRT is similar to 3DCRT in that a number of fixed beam directions are used (Figure 2-3A). In this mode, treatment planning is generally done in two steps. First, the dose optimization engine generates a set of intensity profiles, one for each incident beam. Depending on the treatment planning system, the optimized beam profile can be continuous or in a form that is discretized in space and intensity. Without loss of generality, an incident beam is assumed to be already divided into a grid of beamlets, and each beamlet can take a fixed number of intensity levels. The beamlet width (dimension perpendicular to the leaf travel direction) is limited to the MLC leaf width. The beamlet length, or the step size of MLC leaf movement defined as the smallest step in the leaf travel direction, is a parameter specified by the user. A smaller beamlet size or a larger number of intensity levels offers better spatial or intensity

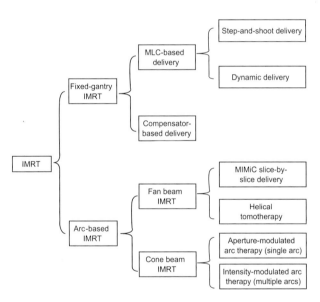

FIGURE 2-1. Currently available intensity-modulated radiation therapy (IMRT) techniques. MLC = multileaf collimator.

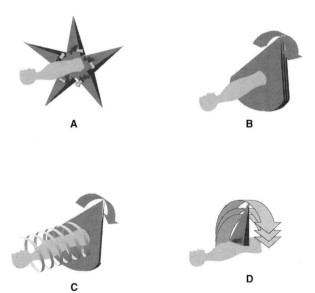

FIGURE 2-3. A schematic drawing of (A) fixed-gantry intensity-modulated radiation therapy (IMRT); (B) slice-by-slice fan beam delivery; (C) tomotherapy delivery; and (D) cone beam–based IMRT.

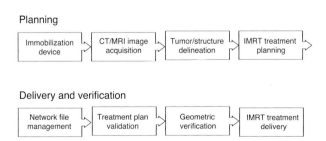

FIGURE 2-2. The intensity-modulated radiation therapy (IMRT) treatment process. CT = computed tomography; MRI = magnetic resonance imaging.

resolution but requires more MLC segments for delivery. Typically, the size of the beamlet and the number of intensity levels in current IMRT treatment are set to 1 × 1 cm and 10, respectively. Figure 2-4 shows an example of an intensity map for a head and neck IMRT treatment, obtained using the *CORVUS* (North American Scientific) inverse planning system. Occasionally, the beamlet size or the number of intensity levels is varied to meet a specific clinical requirement.

There are many ways to produce a desired fluence map. Conceptually, physical compensators are the most straightforward. The most popular delivery technique is, however, based on computer-controlled MLC. In this approach, an intensity map is decomposed into a set of MLC-formed apertures by using a leaf sequencing algorithm. The MLC sequences are recorded in a computer file, which is then used to control the MLC movement for plan delivery. It is important to note that an intensity map, regardless of its shape, can always be expressed as a superposition of a number of segmented fields (for a given intensity map, generally, a number of ways exist for this decomposition, leading to numerous leaf sequencing algorithms). Depending on the relationship between MLC leaf movements and radiation dose delivery, the delivery can generally be divided into step-and-shoot delivery and dynamic modes. The former is the simplest computer-controlled delivery scheme of the fixed-gantry IMRT, in which MLC leaf movements and dose deliveries are done at different instances. A leaf sequence file consists of alternatives of dose-only and motion-only instances. Dynamic delivery differs from a step-and-shoot mode in that leaf movement and dose delivery are realized simultaneously.

Arc-Based IMRT

Arc-based treatment delivery has a long history in RT. An early implementation of this method was the so-called Takahashi arc, in which the beam aperture dynamically follows the beam's eye view projection of the target. Stereotactic radiosurgery based on cylindric cones or micro-MLC often uses the arc delivery technique to "spread" the radiation dose to different regions of the brain to avoid overdosing the normal brain tissue. Conformal arc therapy can produce excellent dose conformation to a simple target. However, the target volumes often exhibit significant deviation from the ideal spherical or ellipsoidal shape. In this case, arc-based IMRT treatment, which was first proposed by Yu,[4] provides a viable option to improve the dose distributions through intensity modulation. The three different forms of arc-based IMRT deliveries are schematically shown in Figure 2-3, B to D, and their features are summarized below.

Fan Beam IMRT

A schematic drawing of the fan beam IMRT is shown in Figure 2-3B. The delivery is realized on a slice-by-slice manner, in which each slice covers 2 to 4 cm in the longitudinal direction and 20 cm in diameter. North American Scientific's

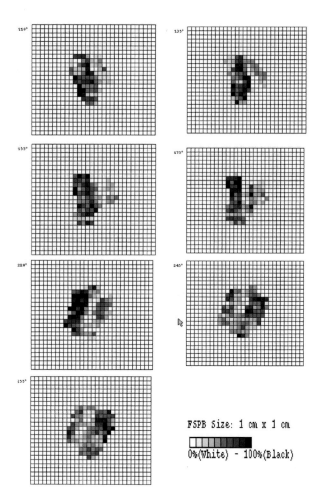

FIGURE 2-4. Intensity patterns of a seven-field intensity-modulated radiation therapy (IMRT) head and neck treatment obtained using the *CORVUS* IMRT planning system.

Peacock system, which includes the *PEACOCK* inverse treatment planning system and the MIMiC collimator, is used for this type of treatment. The planning system uses 54 equally spaced beams and optimizes the beamlet maps of each beam. The nominal beamlet sizes on the isocenter plane are 1 × 0.4 cm, 1 × 1 cm, and 1 × 2 cm. An advantage of this modality is that the MIMiC collimator can be retrofitted to an existing linear accelerator without an MLC, allowing IMRT treatment without a substantial hardware upgrade. Use of the arc delivery mode often results in a superior dose distribution in comparison with fixed-gantry IMRT with five to nine beams for deep-seated tumors because of the involvement of a large number of beams in an arc-based treatment.[3]

Tomotherapy

The tomotherapy machine has recently become commercially available (TomoTherapy Inc., Madison, WI). The delivery is also achieved slice by slice but in a helical (or spiral) fashion in which the couch moves at a constant speed during the gantry rotation (see Figure 2-3C). Radiation from the linear accelerator first passes through a single set of primary collimator jaws, which shape the beam into a rectangular slit that is 40 cm long and up to 5 cm wide at the isocenter. The MLC that is used to modulate the beam intensity consists of 64 tungsten leaves that move across a narrow opening to control the radiation passing through to the target. The computer-controlled MLC has two sets of interlaced leaves that move in and out very rapidly to constantly modulate the beam.

Cone Beam–Based IMRT

To date, the majority of work on arc-based IMRT has been focused on modulated fan beams, and little development has been done using cone beams. The concept of intensity-modulated arc therapy (IMAT) was first proposed in 1995 (see Figure 2-3D), and manufacturers have provided the technical capability for dynamic arc delivery.[4] However, IMAT has not been widely implemented. The lack of enthusiasm for IMAT stems in part from the shortage of effective planning tools and reliable quality assurance (QA) procedures. Reports from several institutions, however, support the notion that a cone beam–based arc technique can generate superior dose distributions, at least for some deep-seated tumors.[5–8]

Cone beam arcs use the arc feature of fan beam IMRT yet take advantage of the cone beam modulation of the fixed-gantry IMRT. To compute dose distributions, an arc is approximated by many fixed fields at small intervals of gantry rotation. Physically, however, the achievement of intensity modulation for cone beam delivery is less straightforward in comparison with its fan beam counterpart. Unlike a slice-by-slice delivery, in which the radiation across the slice can be segmentally blocked from the side by multiple independent vanes, the MLC-shaped aperture cannot change from one shape to another fast enough as the gantry rotates. This problem can be solved, at least in principle, by lowering the gantry rotation speed because, in reality, it is the relative speed between the gantry rotation and MLC leaf movement that determines the level of achievable intensity modulation.

An alternative approach is to use multiple cone beam arcs, as proposed by Yu.[4] At each gantry angle, the beam is considered to be a superposition of a series of subfields, each with uniform intensity from these arcs. When a single arc is used for treatment, the technique is sometimes called aperture-modulated arc therapy. At this time, there are no studies defining how many arcs are sufficient for any disease sites. In Figure 2-5, a comparison of average dose-volume histograms (DVHs) of 3DCRT, IMRT, and IMAT prostate plans for ten patients with prostate cancer is shown.[9] The solid line is IMAT, the dotted line is IMRT, and the dot-dash line is 3DCRT. It is evident that IMAT yields better target coverage and improved bladder and rectum sparing in comparison with fixed-gantry IMRT. Finally, being able to modulate the dose rate while the gantry rotates is a desirable feature, further enhancing the performance of the cone beam arc–based IMRT. To date, however, no linear accelerator manufacturers have provided such technical capability in the clinical mode.

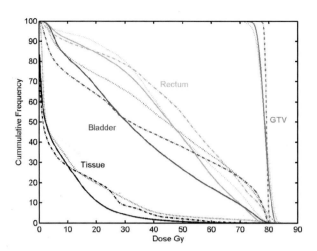

FIGURE 2-5. Average dose-volume histograms for 10 patients with prostate cancer planned using three-dimensional conformal radiation therapy (*dot-dash line*), intensity-modulated radiation therapy (*dotted line*), and intensity-modulated arc therapy (*solid line*). GTV = gross tumor volume. (To view a color version of this image, please refer to the CD-ROM.)

Treatment Planning

RT planning requires the calculation of a set of parameters for the delivery of a radiation dose to the patient. Although manual forward planning may be possible in some simple cases (see the examples below), computer optimization of the beam parameters is almost always used for IMRT treatment planning because of the vast size of search space involved in the problem. In general, this is realized using an inverse treatment planning technique, which derives the optimal beam parameters by starting from a prescribed or desired dose distribution. Although the details of the inverse planning calculation depend on the delivery method, the principle behind the algorithms is essentially the same. Inverse treatment planning is, in fact, a special case of general inverse problem encountered in the sciences and engineering, which attempt to derive the optimal input parameters that will produce the desired output. Before discussing the inverse planning algorithms in detail, it is illustrative to briefly summarize the features of the forward planning approach.

Forward Planning for Segment-Based Treatment

There are two aspects in RT planning: dose conformity and dose uniformity inside the target. What it takes to accomplish the two goals may be different. When the shape of the target is regular and/or when only two or three incident beams are employed, the isodose shaping can often be achieved by beam shaping with an MLC. To achieve a uniform dose distribution within the target volume, one only needs to accommodate the geometric variation of the external contour. Physical or dynamic wedges are usually used if the patient contour changes monotonically or in some simple hinge field arrangements. In a more general situation, additional MLC-shaped field segments can be introduced to boost a "cold" region or reduce a "hot" region. Examples of this type of case include but are not limited to opposed tangent field breast treatment and anterior-posterior treatment of Hodgkin's disease. For illustration purpose, a forward multisegment breast treatment plan is considered.

The multisegment breast plan starts with the standard opposed tangent fields. In many cases of breast cancer, obtaining a uniform dose within the target volume could be problematic when this approach is used. To improve on this, one may proceed to sequentially introduce additional MLC field segments to one or both beam directions to boost the cold region(s) under the guidance of dose distribution in the plane perpendicular to the incident beam direction. Figure 2-6 illustrates the three segments of the

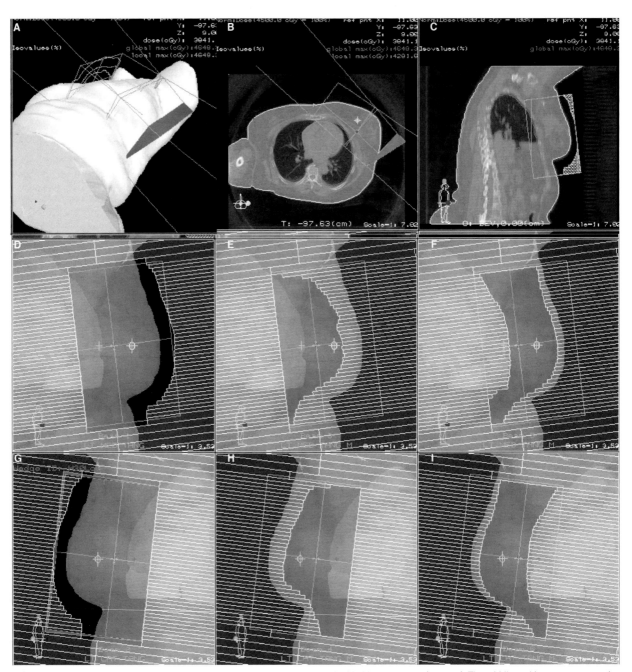

FIGURE 2-6. Opposed tangential fields for the treatment of a patient with left-sided breast cancer (*top row*). The middle and bottom rows are the multileaf collimator shapes of the three segments of the medial and lateral fields chosen to improve dose uniformity within the treatment volume. (To view a color version of this image, please refer to the CD-ROM.)

lateral and medial fields. In this plan, the first segments in the lateral and medial fields and their relative weights are determined using conventional techniques. A physical wedge of 30° is placed on the lateral beam. The two additional segments in each beam direction are then introduced sequentially, and their weights and apertures are adjusted using trial and error to achieve a more uniform dose distribution. The isodose distributions for both plans are shown in Figure 2-7. The maximum dose and the volume receiving a high dose in a multisegment plan are significantly reduced.

Multisegment-based forward planning techniques can be applied only to some relatively simple cases in which the high-dose region is primarily defined by the conventional treatment fields. When isodose conformity to an irregularly shaped target is needed, multiple beams (typically more than five) with a higher level of intensity modulation are needed. In this situation, it becomes tedious to use forward planning–based approaches, and more sophisticated inverse planning techniques become necessary.

Inverse Planning

Inverse planning uses a computer optimization algorithm to determine the optimal beam parameters that lead to a solution as close as possible to the desired output. Mathematically, the problems of image reconstruction, image restoration, signal process, and investment portfolio management can all be formulated as an inverse problem. Roughly speaking, inverse problems can be described as problems in which the output or consequences are known but not the cause. The difference between various treatment planning systems lies in the specifications of the input and output parameters and the criteria used to select the final solution. Specific to RT, the output is generally specified by a desired dose distribution, a set of desired DVHs, or even the tumor control probability (TCP) and normal tissue complication probability (NTCP) for the involved structures. The input parameters to be optimized depend on the delivery scheme. Typically, the number of beams and their incident directions are determined empirically before dose optimization. Each incident beam is discretized into a bixel map (the bixel or beamlet size is typically $1 \times 1\ cm^2$). The task of inverse planning is then to determine the optimal bixel map or the relative weights of all of the beamlets.

To better appreciate the problem, assume that six incident beams are used for an IMRT treatment. If each beam is divided into 100 beamlets and each beamlet has 10 permissible intensity levels, there would be $10^6 \times 100$ physically realizable plans. It can be shown that the number of physically realizable solutions for a six-field 3DCRT plan is much less than this number. When wedges are not used, there are 10^6 physically feasible solutions (many of these can be immediately eliminated from being a candidate treatment plan because they do not produce clinically acceptable dose distributions). For a given desired dose distribution D_0, the task is to find a solution D in the physically feasible solution pool {D} that is the same as D_0 or, more appropriately, differs the least from D_0. There are many ways to pick a D that is a "good" representation of the prescribed dose D_0. A commonly used approach for plan optimization is to minimize the distance between D and D_0 in the L^2 norm. For therapeutic applications, it is common to introduce an importance factor r_σ to control the relative importance of the structure σ. This leads to the following quadratic objective function:

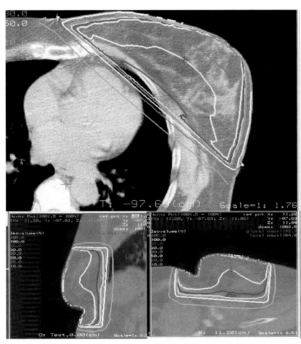

FIGURE 2-7. Conventional opposed tangential breast (*left*) and multisegment (*right*) plans. The isodose lines are (from inside to outside) 105, 100, 95, 90, 80, 50, 20, and 10%. A dose of 50.4 Gy was prescribed to the 90% line. Note that the use of multiple segments improves the dose uniformity to the breast. (To view a color version of this image, please refer to the CD-ROM.)

$$F = \frac{1}{N} \sum_n r_\sigma [D_c(n) - D_0(n)]^2,$$

(1)

where r_σ is the importance factor that weights the importance of the structure σ and parameterizes our clinical trade-off strategy and D_0 and D_n are prescribed and calculated doses, respectively. Optimization of this function is essentially a least squares type of estimation in statistical analysis. In addition to equation 1, many other types of objective functions have been proposed for plan optimization. The construct of the objective function plays a crucial role for the success of IMRT treatment and is worthy of detailed discussion.

Models and Model Parameters of Inverse Planning

A common feature of all inverse problems is that they are generally underdetermined and ill-posed. The selection of the final solution depends on the underlying assumption of the model. The objective function quantitatively ranks a candidate treatment plan, and the optimization of the function yields the optimal parameters. In conventional treatment planning, the objective function depends on beam weights, wedge angles, and orientations, whereas in IMRT, it is a function of the beamlet weights. Ideally, an objective function would mimic the decision-making of experienced oncologists and planners. It would rank a given solution (corresponding to a set of parameters) in a way consistent with clinical judgment. In practice, however, a gap exists between mathematical modeling and clinical decision-making, and much effort is being devoted to derive clinically meaningful objective functions for inverse planning. Because the optimization results depend strongly on the objective function, there is inevitably subjectivity associated with the various dose optimization schemes. Therefore, it is essential for physicians to carefully evaluate a treatment plan after optimization to ensure that the "optimal" solution makes clinical sense. Otherwise, the success of an optimization is, at best, mathematical.

If an optimization algorithm is to have a genuine impact on clinical practice, it should incorporate all of the dosimetric and radiobiologic knowledge plus an algorithm for modeling the way in which radiation oncologists and patients balance the risks and benefits. Despite the availability of high-speed computers, state-of-the-art inverse planning algorithms, and improved imaging modalities, we are still a long way from generating truly optimized IMRT treatment plans. For convenience, it is appropriate to classify the currently available dose optimization methods into four categories: (1) dose based, (2) clinical knowledge based, (3) equivalent uniform dose (EUD) based, and (4) TCP or NTCP based. The underlying difference between these models lies in which end points are used to evaluate the treatment plan or which fundamental quantities are used to define the optimal plan. In reality, each type of inverse planning formalism has its own pros and cons in coping with the clinical decision-making process and in practical implementation. These are briefly summarized below.

Dose-Based Formalism

The dose and/or dose volume–based optimization is concerned with accurate dose distributions or DVHs of the involved structures. The quadratic objective function given in equation 1 represents an example of this type. Frequently, DVHs and other physical constraints are imposed to describe certain clinical requirements. The dose or dose volume prescriptions are used implicitly as surrogates of the desired clinical outcome. At this point, the dose-based approach is the most widely employed method, as is evidenced by the fact that all commercial IMRT planning systems have chosen dose-based ranking as the starting point. There are several reasons for this. First, the physical dose objectives reflect the majority of the clinical practice. Although biologic models are available in both research and clinical systems, the uncertainty associated with the predictions often outweighs their guidance. Dose-based objectives will remain the dominant modality of optimization and evaluation for some time. Second, the physical dose is closely related to the optimization parameters, and simple mathematical models, such as the quadratic dose difference expressed in equation 1, can be effectively used.

Clinical Knowledge–Based Formalism

It is highly desirable to incorporate clinical end points in guiding the treatment plan optimization process. The currently available dose-based objective functions do not truly reflect the nonlinear relationship between dose and the response of tumors and normal tissues. In reality, the dose dependence of the clinical end point of a structure may be degenerate in the sense that a given clinical end point may be caused by a variety of dose distributions or DVHs. For the parotid glands, for instance, it is known that the clinical end point is the same if 15 Gy is delivered to 67% of the volume, if 30 Gy is delivered to 45% of the volume, or if 45 Gy is delivered to 24% of the volume. If the dose-based objective function, equation 1, is used, the rankings for the three different scenarios would be different. Even with the use of dose-volume constraints, it is difficult, if not impossible, to incorporate this type of knowledge to correctly model the behavior of the organ in response to radiation. Indeed, a constraint in optimization acts as a "boundary condition" during the optimization (there are methods of treating constrained optimization problem into an equivalent unconstrained one, with a different objective function) and does not change the rankings of dosimetrically different plans.

To overcome these dilemmas, a clinical knowledge–based optimization scheme has recently been developed by Yang and Xing.[10] The central theme of the approach is that clinical outcome data should be used to direct the plan optimization process. In this approach, the quality of a treatment plan is measured by a heuristically constructed objective function that depends not only on the dosimetric properties but also the dose-volume status, which makes it possible to take advantage of the existing outcome data of the involved organs. For the parotid glands, for instance, the three different DVHs mentioned above will be scored equally by the objective function. The final dose distribution or DVHs of the glands will be determined by the optimization algorithm with the consideration of the requirements of other structures. If one of the three possibilities needs to be selected, the one that yields better scores in other involved structures will be favored by the algorithm. The specifics of the plan selection process will, of course, depend on the geometric and dosimetric details of the particular patient.

It is important to emphasize that, at this point, clinical outcome data are sparse and underdetermined and may have large uncertainties. By "underdetermined," we mean that there are not enough clinical data points available to objectively rank all realizable plans. Thus, it is necessary to produce an interpolation/extrapolation scheme for plan ranking. A sensible approach has also been provided in Yang and Xing's work based on the well-known dose response model.[10] The clinical knowledge–based model allows one to more objectively rank treatment plans according to their clinical merits without relying on biological index-based or EUD-based prescriptions.

EUD-Based Formalism

Optimization of the dose distributions can also be cast into the realm of EUD, which is one level higher in terms of the use of biologic information.[11,12] The EUD is defined as the biologically equivalent dose, which, if given uniformly, leads to the same cell kill as the actual nonuniform dose distribution. It can be expressed as follows:

$$EUD = \left(\frac{1}{N} \sum_i D_i^a \right)^{\frac{1}{a}}$$

(2)

In this expression, N is the number of voxels in the anatomic structure of interest, D_i is the dose in the i'th voxel, and a is the tumor- or normal tissue–specific parameter that describes the dose-volume effect. This formulation of EUD is based on the power law dependence of the response of a complex biologic system to a stimulus.

EUD exhibits a dose-response relationship similar to that of the traditional biologic indices. Therefore, it can be a surrogate for them and, in the meantime, is closely related to the physical dose. The objective function based on EUD can be expressed in the following:

$$F = \prod_j f_j$$

(3)

where the component subscore f_j may be either

$$f_T = \frac{1}{1 + \left(\frac{EUD_0}{EUD} \right)^n}$$

for tumors or

$$f_{OAR} = \frac{1}{1 + \left(\frac{EUD}{EUD_0} \right)^n}$$

for normal tissues. There are several advantages of EUD-based optimization approaches: (1) the formulae are simple, (2) the formulae can be applied to both tumors and organs at risk (OAR) using different parameters, and (3) there are fewer planning parameters than dose volume–based or other biologic indices–based optimization. It has been shown that EUD-based optimization can provide the same or better coverage of targets as dose volume–based optimization and that it offers significantly better protection of OAR. These improvements in the dose distributions to OAR may be due to the fact that there is a larger search space available in EUD optimization because the constraint, or the objective, is determined on the basis of the whole organ rather than the partial volume of the structure. Thus, EUD optimization can be used to search for and evaluate multiple plans that may have different DVHs but the same EUDs. Figure 2-8 shows the dose distributions for IMRT plans optimized using dose volume–based and EUD-based objective functions for a patient with prostate cancer. The OAR are the rectum and bladder. All plans used identical configurations of five coplanar 18 MV photon beams placed at equally spaced gantry angles. The plans were normalized to deliver the prescription dose of 70 Gy to 99% of the target volume. It is clear that, for the same minimal target dose, sparing of the OAR is greatly improved in the EUD-based plan. Furthermore, a sharp dose gradient at the interface between the target and OAR is realized.

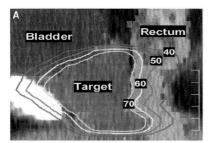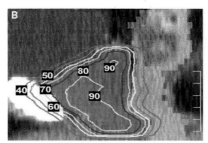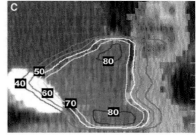

FIGURE 2-8. Sagittal isodose distributions for prostate intensity-modulated radiation therapy plans designed using (*A*) dose volume–based criteria; (*B*) equivalent uniform dose (EUD)-based criteria; and (*C*) EUD-based criteria with target inhomogeneity constraints. (To view a color version of this image, please refer to the CD-ROM.) Reproduced with permission from Wu Q et al[12].

The EUD concept can also be incorporated into the framework of physical dose optimization, such as the method of projection over the convex set.[13] In this method, EUD is implemented as an optimization constraint. At each iteration of the optimization, if an organ violates an EUD constraint, a new dose distribution is calculated by projecting the current one onto the convex set of all dose distributions fulfilling the EUD constraint. The cost is slightly more iterations than pure physically constrained optimization. This algorithm is easy to implement and provides better dose sparing of parallel structure organs for which physical constraints may be difficult to define.

Biologic Model–Based Formalism

Biologic model–based optimization proponents argue that plan optimization should be guided by estimates of biologic effects. The biologic effect and the radiation parameters are linked by the radiation dose through the use of a dose-response function. The relationship between the two is not, however, a one-to-one correspondence. A given biologic end point may be produced by many possible dose distributions, which would generally not be equally scored if a dose-based model was used. In principle, biologically based models are most relevant for RT plan ranking.[11,14–21] However, the dose-response function of various structures is not sufficiently understood, and at this point, there is considerable controversy about the models for computing dose-response indices and their use in optimization.

The treatment objective in biologic model–based inverse planning is usually stated as the maximization of the TCP while maintaining the NTCP to within acceptable levels.[22,23] Physical constraints on dose and dose volume are often introduced to ensure that the results are consistent with the clinical judgment of the physicians. Brahme and Kallman and colleagues used the probability of uncomplicated control, P+, in their formalism.[14,24] Practically, the use of dose-response indices for optimization might also pose some problems. For instance, dose response–based optimization may lead to very inhomogeneous target dose distributions. Furthermore, it is difficult for clinicians to specify the optimization criteria in terms of certain dose-response indices (eg, TCP, NTCP, and P+). This difficulty becomes even more significant when two or more independently optimized plans are to be combined because it is impractical to specify the desired TCP and NTCP of the component plans. Because of these problems, the use of biologic model–based dose optimization has mainly been limited to the research setting and little effort has been made to implement these into commercial IMRT planning systems.

Model Parameters

Any dose optimization framework must deal with trade-offs between the target and OAR.[25] Generally, the objectives of different structures are multifaceted and incommensurable. A combination of the objectives is usually done to form a single objective function. In this process, a set of importance factors is often incorporated into the objective function to parameterize trade-off strategies and prioritize the dose conformity in different anatomic structures. Whereas the general formalism remains the same, different sets of importance factors characterize plans of obviously different flavor and thus determine the final plan. One of the major difficulties is that the influence of these weighting factors on the final solutions is not known until the dose optimization is done, necessitating a trial-and-error determination of the parameters. In most (if not all) of the currently available planning systems, the values of the weighting factors are presented to the user as optimization parameters. A good understanding of the role of these parameters and suitable training on how to empirically determine the parameters are required.

It is possible to use an iterative algorithm to estimate the weighting factors numerically.[25] Plan selection is done in two steps. First, a set of importance factors is chosen, and the beam profiles are optimized under the guidance of a quadratic objective function using an iterative algorithm. The "optimal" plan is then evaluated by a decision function, in which the corresponding trade-off parameters are more easily determinable based on some simple considerations.[25] The importance factors in the objective function are adjusted iteratively toward the direction of improving the ranking of the plan. For every change in the importance factors, the beam parameters are reoptimized. Even though further refinement of the plan may still be needed in selected cases, the technique provides a good starting point for planning.

Dose Optimization Algorithms

Although the modeling of RT treatment is of paramount importance, the optimization of the selected multidimensional objective function provides a vehicle to obtain the optimal solutions. The task of an optimization algorithm is to find the combination of beam parameters that optimize the chosen objective function, possibly subject to some constraints. Numerous algorithms have been developed for the optimization of a multidimensional function in the sciences and engineering over the years, and there is a vast literature on the subject. Generally speaking, the selection of an optimization technique depends on the specific form of the objective function and the imposed constraints. In practice, even for the same class of problem, more than one algorithm may exist for achieving the same goal, and the detailed implementation of different algorithms can be quite different. Many optimization techniques have been used for RT inverse planning. Here we briefly describe a few approaches to illustrate how a multiobjective objective function is optimized and the pros and cons of these common techniques (see Chapter 10, "Treatment Planning").

Iterative Algorithms

The iterative method is perhaps the most widely implemented technique in RT optimization. Starting with an initial approximate solution, it generates a sequence of solutions that converge on the optimal one. For large systems, especially large linear systems, iterative methods prove to be efficient in terms of computer storage and computational time. The available iterative techniques can generally be grouped as non–derivative-based and derivative-based methods. The former incorporates only an objective function value calculation with some systematic method to search the solution space. This technique is generally intuitive, easy to implement, and particularly suitable for simple systems and educational illustration. For a complex system, the convergence behavior may not be as good as more sophisticated gradient-based search techniques. The computational cost and poor convergence in this situation may outweigh the benefit of avoiding derivative calculations.

As an example, Figure 2-9 illustrates the flowchart of an algebraic iterative inverse planning technique (AIIPT) described by Xing and colleagues.[26,27] A schematic drawing of calculation pixels and bins in the AIIPT calculation is shown in Figure 2-10. The algorithm was generalized from the algebraic reconstruction technique (ART) based on the analogy between rotational RT optimization and tomographic image reconstruction. In the AIIPT algorithm, voxels are examined in sequence, and corrections are made immediately after a pixel is addressed. The successive treatment of the system eventually leads to an optimized solution. A geometric interpretation of ART has been published.[28]

The iterative process is described by the following operations: (1) assume an initial set of beam profiles; (2) compute the dose at a voxel; (3) compare the calculated and prescribed doses; (4) obtain correction factors to the beamlets that irradiate the voxel; and (5) apply the corrections to the contributing beamlets and then repeat from step 2 for the next voxel (go back to the first voxel and increase the iteration index by one after all voxels are addressed). This process is repeated until the desired accuracy is achieved. The simultaneous iterative inverse planning and least squares inverse treatment planning algorithms also fall into the same category of the nonderivative method.[26,27] A similar algorithm with a multiplicative beamlet updating scheme was described by Jones and Hoban.[29]

Various gradient-based methods have been successfully applied to RT plan optimization and implemented in commercial IMRT planning systems. A general class of iterative algorithms can be written as

$$\mathbf{I}^{new} = \mathbf{I}^{old} - \lambda \mathbf{M}^{old} \nabla F(\mathbf{I}^{old}) \tag{4}$$

where $\mathbf{I}$ is the fluence vector, $\mathbf{M}^{old}$ is a matrix, and λ is a positive parameter. When $\mathbf{M}^{old}$ is a unit matrix, equation 4 is the well-known steepest descent algorithm, whereas when $\mathbf{M}^{old} = \mathbf{H}^{old}$, it describes Newton's method, in which $\mathbf{H}^{old}$ is the inverse of the Hessian matrix.[30] In the steepest descent algorithm, from a set of fluence functions, $\mathbf{I}^{old}$, we search along the direction of the negative gradient, $-\nabla F(\mathbf{I}^{old})$, to a minimum on this line; this minimum is taken to be $\mathbf{I}^{new}$.

It is fair to say that the choice of a specific algorithm

Algebraic iterative method:

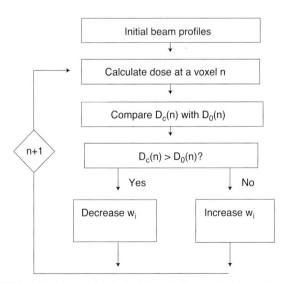

FIGURE 2-9. Flowchart of the algebraic iterative inverse planning technique.

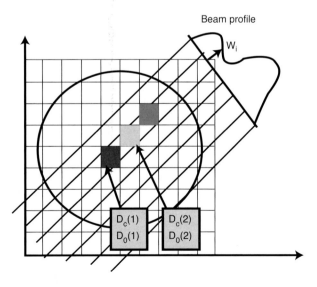

FIGURE 2-10. Pixel and bin configurations used in the algebraic iterative inverse planning technique. In this figure, w_i is the beamlet weight and D_c and D_0 represent the calculated and prescribed doses, respectively. Reproduced with permission from van Dyk J and Purdy JA.[147]

to solve the inverse planning problem is not unique and is determined by the problem at hand and, to a certain extent, by personal preference. Generally, the iterative approach works well for a nonconvex objective function, and the solution can be trapped in local minima for systems with a complicated form of the objective function. Several commercial systems provide both iterative and stochastic optimizers so that users have the tool to compare the functionality of different approaches and, more importantly, to independently check an optimization calculation.

Computer-Simulated Annealing

The simulated annealing method[31] is an extension of the original Monte Carlo simulation algorithm introduced by Metropolis and colleagues.[32] It attempts to find the optimal solution by mimicking the behavior of a system of interacting particles that are progressively cooled and allowed to maintain thermal equilibrium while reaching the ground state. In physical annealing, the system is heated, thereby conferring randomness to each component. As a result, each variable can temporarily assume a value that is energetically unfavorable, and the system explores configurations that have a higher energy. The fundamental principle here is that even at moderately high temperatures, the system slightly favors regions in the configuration space that are overall lower in energy and hence more likely to contain the global minimum. The algorithm employs a random search that not only accepts changes that decrease objective function but also some changes that increase it. The probability for accepting a trial configuration is controlled by the temperature and is given by

$$P = \begin{cases} 1 & \text{If } \Delta F < 0 \\ \exp(-\dfrac{\Delta F}{T}) & \text{Otherwise} \end{cases} \quad (5)$$

where ΔF is the increase of the objective function and T is the system temperature. The temperature is gradually lowered according to an empirically chosen cooling schedule.[33,34] As the temperature is slowly reduced, the probability of accepting a trial configuration with a higher objective function value is reduced. The starting temperature is chosen to be higher than the largest value of objective function calculated for a random set of variable configurations. In principle, this algorithm is capable of finding the global minimum of a multidimensional objective function even when local minima exist. For more details about the simulated annealing algorithm, readers are referred elsewhere.[34–36]

Other Optimization Algorithms

In addition to the iterative and simulated annealing algorithms, many other types of optimization approaches have been employed for therapeutic plan optimization. Linear programming was applied to the dose optimization of 3DCRT plans and cyberknife plans. The utility of filtered backprojection from CT image reconstruction has also been explored by several researchers.[37–39]

The constrained least square algorithm[40] was employed to optimize 3DCRT plans[41,42] and IMRT plans. Constrained optimization of a linear system can be viewed in two ways. One involves transformation of the problem into a reduced space. Another approach is to work with the lagrangian function and to obtain the solution of the system by a direct matrix manipulation. In this way, a priori knowledge of the variance of the system variables can be included as a lagrangian multiplier. Without repeatedly invoking the dose calculation, this algorithm allows one to obtain the optimal solution of the system with significantly increased computational speed, providing a fast interactive planning environment for IMRT planning.

Mixed integer programming technique was used to generate treatment plans for linear accelerator–based radiosurgery,[43] IMRT,[44] and 3DCRT.[45] Lee and Zaider also applied integer programming for permanent prostate implant planning.[46] The mixed integer programming models incorporate strict dose restrictions on the tumor volume and constraints on the desired number of beams, isocenters, couch angles, and gantry angles. The goal is to deliver the full prescription dose uniformly to the tumor volume while minimizing excess radiation to the surrounding normal tissue. Hou and colleagues used simulated dynamics in a classic system of interacting particles for IMRT optimization.[47] In this approach, an analogy is established between intensity profile optimization in IMRT and relaxation to the equilibrium configuration in a dynamic system. Dose-volume constraints are handled by placing hard constraints on partial volumes. The genetic algorithm is another widely used approach in sciences and engineering and has found some preliminary application in RT dose optimization.[48–51]

For all of their complexity, the algorithms to optimize a multidimensional function are routine mathematical procedures. In general, simulated annealing and genetic algorithms are powerful approaches, but excessive computation time is a drawback to their clinical application. Treatment planning based on filtered backprojection and direct Fourier transformation have difficulty handling the negative fluence problem and are not generally applicable for an arbitrary dose prescription and kernel. Iterative methods are widely used to optimize a multidimensional objective function by starting with an initial approximate solution and generating a sequence of solutions that converge to the optimal solution of the system.

It is useful to note that much effort has also been devoted to formulate the problem into a more effective mathematical framework. For example, Xing and Lian and their colleagues introduced a new concept of a preference function and recast the problem into the framework of Bayesian statistical analysis.[35,52–54] In this approach, instead of a rigid prescription dose, a range of prescription doses prioritized by the preference function is allowed. The rationale here is that since a rigid prescription is not achievable and the final solution will deviate from it anyway, we would have much better chance to obtain what we want if we could inform the system with some a priori information about our preferences on different possible scenarios (instead of leaving the decision-making totally to the computer). The techniques developed over the years in statistical decision-making can be easily extended to RT plan optimization problem. The primary advantage of the technique is that it enables one to effectively incorporate the existing clinical knowledge or other prior knowledge into inverse planning. When the prescribed dose takes a single rigid value, the above formula becomes identical to the conventional least squares approach or alike. Maximum likelihood estimation[55,56] or the maximum entropy approach[57] also represents a special case of the formalism. Finally, it is interesting to point out that various techniques in related fields such as neural networks[58] and fuzzy logic[59] are also being translated for RT dose optimization.

Practical Aspects of IMRT Planning

Inverse planning is a computer-based decision-making technique that derives the optimal treatment plan by starting with a set of desired doses or DVHs prescribed to the target and normal tissues. To use an inverse planning system to generate a treatment plan, one must delineate the tumor volume and sensitive structures, for which dose avoidances are desired. This differs from conventional planning, in which the target volume is often defined directly on the portal films (see Chapter 11, "Plan Evaluation"). If target contours need to be altered after a conventional treatment plan is obtained or during a course of treatment, it is usually achieved by modifying the positions of the corresponding MLC (or by modifying a block). In inverse treatment planning, however, the beam profiles and beam apertures are derived by the system, and any change in the target volume requires reoptimization of the plan. Moreover, all of the tasks following IMRT planning, such as patient-specific QA and data entry, need to be repeated.

IMRT planning is still inherently a trial-and-error process owing to the large number of input parameters.[60] The trial-and-error process here is quite different from that in 3DCRT, in which intuition and previous experience can be easily used to guide the planning process. In an anterior-posterior treatment, for example, if the dose in the anterior region is higher than that of the posterior region, one can simply increase the weight of the posterior field. This type of guidance is lost in inverse planning, and, frequently, the trial-and-error process has to proceed in a "blind-guessing" fashion because the influence of most of the system parameters is not known until the dose optimization is complete. A good understanding of the effect of treatment planning parameters used

in optimization on the resultant dose distribution is necessary to carry out the planning and the plan "tweaking" process. Recently, tools for assisting the interactive planning have emerged. The dose shaping technique described below is one example. Hopefully, this type of research will make clinical inverse planning more straightforward in the future.

Plan review is an important aspect of IMRT. In inverse planning, an objective function is constructed based on general physical, dosimetric, and biologic considerations and is defined as a global quantity.[52] The translation of the treatment objectives to a single objective function is at best an approximation. Just like any data reduction or compression scheme, there is a loss of information with regard to the characteristic of the individual data point. Even with the best possible objective function, the optimal solution may still not represent the best clinical solution in every aspect. It is important to review the plan to ensure that the final solution is consistent with clinical judgment. IMRT plan evaluation tools vary from one commerical planning system to another. Typically, they include isodose distributions in axial, coronal, and sagittal planes; DVHs; and maximum, minimum, and average target and sensitive structure doses. A description of plan evaluation methods is presented in Chapter 12.

The dose inhomogeneity of an IMRT plan is usually higher than that in 3DCRT as a consequence of increased conformity. Any deviation from a conventional uniform dose scheme should be carefully evaluated to ensure its clinical acceptability. If hot or cold spots are unavoidable, efforts should be made to ensure that they are not located in undesirable locations. For example, a cold spot in the center of the target or a hot spot outside the target should be avoided. Even a hot spot inside the target volume may not be desirable. For example, for prostate cancer, a hot spot close to the urethra is usually not acceptable, particularly if the total dose is escalated. The dose gradient of an IMRT plan near the boundary of the target or OAR can be very high. If the structure(s) is susceptible to the setup uncertainty and/or organ motion, the actual dose received by the target or OAR may be significantly lower or higher than that shown in the plan.[61,62] In this case, an adequate margin for the structure is important to ensure that the planned dose distribution can be achieved in a clinical setting.[63]

Beam placement in IMRT is worth discussing. Generally speaking, the beam configuration may have significant influence on the quality of an IMRT plan even when a large number of incident beams (eg, nine beams) are used.[64–69] Clinically, however, beam orientations are selected on a trial-and-error basis. To obtain an optimal beam configuration, in principle, one can simply add the degree of freedom of beam angles into the objective function and optimize them together with the beamlet weights.[65,70] Although this does not pose any conceptual challenge, the computational time becomes excessive because of the greatly enlarged search space and the coupling between the beam profiles and the beam configurations. The beam intensity profiles have to be optimized for every trial beam configuration because the influence of a set of gantry angles on the dose distribution is not known until beam intensity optimization is performed. A computationally efficient optimization algorithm is necessary to have a clinically practical beam orientation optimization tool. Some progress has been made toward this goal.[71,72] But before commercial companies implement clinically practical tools for automated or semiautomated beam placement, alternative techniques or even some general guidelines would be useful to facilitate IMRT planning.

One of the appealing approaches is the class-solution method.[73] The basic idea is to construct a representative beam configuration based on previous experience for a given disease site and then use this "class-solution" for subsequent treatment planning. Schreibmann and Xing systematically investigated the issue and proposed a set of class-solutions for IMRT prostate treatment.[74] To derive a population-based beam orientation class-solution, a beam orientation optimization algorithm was used to derive the optimal solutions for each individual in a group of 15 patients with prostate cancer. Figure 2-11 shows the distributions of optimal beam angles for five, six, seven, and eight beams for the 15 patients studied. The colored short lines represent directions found in individual cases, and the red bold long lines represent the directions identified as the class-solutions. These results indicate that the beam orientations for a certain incident direction are confined in a certain range and that beam orientation class-solutions may be a reasonable compromise between what is practical and what is optimal for prostate IMRT. For other disease sites, beam orientation class-solutions may not exist because the geometric variations among the patient population are too large.

On approval of the plan by the physician, an RT plan file or a DICOM-RT file is generated containing all of the relevant machine parameters for IMRT treatment. The IMRT plan file can be complex. For example, it may contain hundreds of MLC segments. Consequently, manual delivery is not an option. Instead, delivery is usually accomplished by the computer-controlled systems, including the record and verify system, linear accelerator control, and MLC control software. The detailed treatment settings contained in the RT plan or DICOM file are transferred from the planning system to the record and verify system. Normally, redundant checksums are also in place for each record, ensuring the safe transfer of data over the computer network. Although it is perhaps not necessary to list all of the information about the treatment in the chart, the chart should contain concise information about the treatment that can be easily verified, for example, the treatment machine, energy, number of beams, gantry and couch angles, monitor units (MUs) for each beam, number of fractions, and fraction doses. The plan output, such as isodose lines for a selected plan in different views on CT images, DVHs, and the QA report, should also be documented. The intensity maps for each beam should be included if possible.

Advanced Topics in IMRT Treatment Planning

Inverse planning is at the foundation of IMRT, and its performance critically determines the success of an IMRT treatment. Unfortunately, the currently available inverse planning formalism is not satisfactory, and the solutions out of so-called "optimization" systems are often suboptimal. Considerable effort may be required to compute a clinically acceptable plan, and the final results may strongly depend on the planner's experience and understanding of the planning system. These shortcomings of the existing systems are familiar to anyone engaged in clinical IMRT treatment planning. In addition to the prescription doses, the current planning system requires the user to preselect the angular variables (gantry, couch, and collimator angles) and the weighting factors of the involved structures. These variables and parameters constitute an additional multidimensional space, which is coupled to the beam profiles.

A survey carried out by us indicates that there are five major problems with current inverse planning systems: (1) no effective mechanism for incorporating prior experience into plan optimization; (2) lack of direct control over the regional dose or, more generally, lack of interactive tools to guide the planning process; (3) no effective tools for aiding beam placement in IMRT planning; (4) inability to incorporate organ motion directly; and (5) inefficient inter-

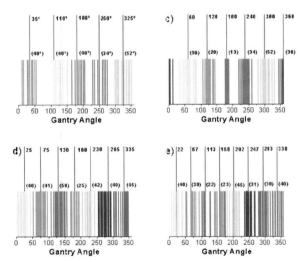

FIGURE 2-11. Distributions of beam angles for five, six, seven, and eight beams, respectively. The short colored lines represent directions found in individual cases, and the long red (bold) lines represent the directions identified as class-solutions. (To view a color version of this image, please refer to the CD-ROM.) Reproduced with permission from Van Dyk J and Purdy JA.

face between planning and delivery systems. Toward establishment of a clinically efficient and robust inverse planning system, many investigators have attacked the problems mentioned above, some of which are the subject of the following sections.

Statistical Analysis–Based Formalism for Therapeutic Plan Optimization

An important element that is missing in the current inverse planning formalism is a mechanism for incorporating prior knowledge into the dose optimization process. In image analysis and many other fields, it has proven valuable to include partial knowledge of the system variables into the optimization process[35,54,75] because it provides guidance in the search for the truly optimal solution. Statistical analysis formalism, which appears in virtually all branches of the sciences and engineering, affords a natural basis for this type of application and provides a powerful vehicle to achieve the goal of treatment plan optimization. Using this approach, Lian and colleagues demonstrated the feasibility of incorporating a range of prioritized dose prescriptions into the planning process.[52,76] The approach is based on a newly introduced concept of a preference function, whose role is to relax our requirement of a rigid dose prescription, to allow a range of doses to be considered, and to quantify the willingness to accept a dose in that range. In addition, to make the system less ill-defined, this new scheme can be used to formalize our clinical knowledge (such as outcome data[19,77]) and incorporate them into dose optimization. In Figure 2-12, we show the preference function derived using published data from Eisbruch and colleagues[78] for parotid glands (four different irradiation volumes). Coupled with the statistical inference techniques,[53,54] this should make the inverse planning process more computationally intelligent.

Another application of the formalism is to include model parameter uncertainties into dose optimization. For example, the radiobiologic formalism involves the use of model parameters that are of considerable uncertainty. Biologic "margins" have been used to account for the variability in radiation sensitivity. This method assumes the patient to be more sensitive than the mean value for normal tissues and more resistant than the tumor. EUD-based optimization with the incorporation of model parameters has been demonstrated through the use of a statistical inference technique.[79] Because currently available models for computing the biologic effects of radiation are simplistic and the clinical data used to derive the models are sparse and of questionable quality, the technique is valuable to minimize the influence of statistical uncertainties.

Multiobjective Optimization

Radiation dose optimization is intrinsically a multiobjective problem because of the existence of multiple conflicting objectives in the system. In the conventional

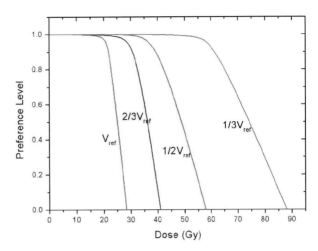

FIGURE 2-12. Preference function of parotid salivary glands for four fixed partial volumes (V_{eff}). In constructing the assumed dose-volume preference function, the preference level is assumed to be 1 for normal tissue complication probability (NTCP) < 5% and 0 for NTCP > 50%. The reference volume (V_{ref}) refers to the volume of the gland. Adapted from Eisbruch A et al.[78] (To view a color version of this image, please refer to the CD-ROM.)

approach, the multiple objectives are combined to form an overall objective function through the use of so-called importance factors.[25,80] Contrary to this, the dose delivered to each structure constitutes one of the objectives in multiobjective optimization, which is an alternative way to deal with the trade-offs of multiple conflicting objectives. The method attempts to obtain all efficient solutions and provide the planner with a more thorough picture of the possible options or the trade-offs between the different objectives. Here an efficient solution (often called the Pareto solution in multiobjective optimization theory) is defined as a plan with a good compromise of all of the objectives involved in the problem or, more precisely, a plan that cannot be further improved without significantly deteriorating the dose distribution in one or more organs. Mathematically, the multiobjective optimization (or vector optimization)[81–84] is to determine a set of decision variables that optimizes a vector function whose elements represent M objective functions without violating the system's constraints. The collection of all efficient solutions is named the Pareto front. Although the approach is conceptually appealing, practical issues, such as the enormous computing time required to obtain the Pareto solution and how to effectively select a plan from the Pareto front, must be resolved before it finds widespread application in RT plan optimization. Perhaps a hybrid of single- and multiobjective techniques is a viable option.

Integration of IMRT Planning and Delivery

IMRT planning is generally performed in two steps: calculation of the intensity maps of the incident beams and decomposition of each intensity map into a series of MLC-shaped segments using a leaf sequencing algorithm. In practice, the decoupling of dose optimization and leaf sequencing has a number of consequences. In addition to the need for the development of complicated MLC leaf sequencing software, the number of segments resulting from the approach is often unnecessarily large. The leaf sequencing algorithm sometimes has to go through additional steps to accommodate some special hardware constraints of the MLC delivery system that can be easily dealt with at the stage of dose optimization. To improve the efficiency of the interface between the inverse planning and the dynamic MLC delivery systems, attempts have been made to incorporate machine constraints and other physical aspects of the delivery system into dose optimization. The most effective method is perhaps the aperture- or segment-based optimization, which optimizes directly the objective function with respect to the shapes and weights of the segmented fields.[44,51,85,86] In this approach, the number of segments for each incident beam is prespecified instead of left "floating." Generally speaking, it is more computationally involved to optimize an objective function with respect to the segment shapes and weights because of the nonlinear dependence of the dose on the leaf coordinates. However, the benefits gained by eliminating the extra leaf sequencing step and the associated drawbacks outweigh the slight computational cost.

Interactive Planning Tools for IMRT

The interactive process of IMRT planning is less intuitive than that of forward planning because of the involvement of a large number of parameters whose roles in the final solution are not explicitly known until the completion of a dose optimization calculation. There is a need for the planner to adaptively modify or fine-tune a solution toward the desired direction. For example, frequently after optimization, the dose in only a few small regions is not satisfactory. Currently, plan modification is achieved by adjusting structure-dependent system parameters (eg, prescription, importance factors), which influence not only the dose in the region of interest but also in other areas. To modify the dose in a specific region, in principle, one can use ray-tracing to find the beamlets intercepting the area and adjust their intensities accordingly. The problem is that there are numerous ways to modify this intensity and the optimal arrangement of the beamlet intensities is not obvious. Cortrutz and Xing pointed out that local dosimetric behavior can be more effectively controlled by introducing a region-dependent penalty scheme and demonstrated the utility of this approach using a model system and clinical examples.[87,88] After the conventional planning is done, they identify the subvolumes on isodose layouts or the dose interval on the DVH curve in which the fractional volume needs to be changed. The local penalty (eg, local importance factor or local prescription) is then adjusted, and the dose is

reoptimized. The fine-tuning of doses is manually iterative in nature, and the process can be easily accomplished using a graphic user interface. Using this technique, it has been shown that one can eliminate hot and cold spots. Generally, in dose optimization, there is no net gain. That is, the improvement in the dose to a region is often accompanied by a dosimetrically adverse effect(s) at another point(s) in the same or different structures. Practically, however, some dose distributions are more acceptable than others. The important issue here is to find the solution that improves the dose(s) at the region of interest with a clinically insignificant or acceptable sacrifice.

It is useful to mention that some "hot spot editor" tools have recently been implemented in commercial systems. These editors rely primarily on a rudimentary ray-tracing, which is done as follows: (1) visually locating the hot/cold spot; (2) finding the corresponding beamlets that contribute to the dose at the point of interest (POI); (3) decreasing/increasing the intensities of one or more of the beamlets; and (4) updating the dose distribution. In reality, there are multiple beamlets contributing to the dose at the POI and the problem is determining the optimal way to modify them so that the doses at other points are compromised minimally. In the current commercial systems the hot/cold spot is improved by decreasing/increasing the beamlets with a pre-designed updating method, which is rarely optimal and often causes new cold/hot spots somewhere else within the patient. The approach described by Cortrutz and Xing allows optimal adjustment of the beamlet intensities, thus avoiding the aforementioned problem. Since the re-optimization is done on top of the existing solution, it requires only very limited additional computing time. Furthermore, it is done in the background (just like the recalculation of dose in step 4 is done in the background) and the user does not need to take any additional action.

Automated and Semiautomated Beam Placement

Clinically, gantry angles are selected empirically, and there is no guarantee that the beam configuration is optimal for a given patient. Many investigations are exploring the role of beam configuration selection in IMRT[39,65,69,89–91] and developing tools for beam placement. A promising technique uses beam's eye view dosimetrics (BEVD).[71,92] The central idea of this single-beam scoring technique is that the merit of a beam direction should be measured by what that beam could achieve dosimetrically without exceeding the dosimetric or dose-volume constraints of the system. For computational purposes, a beam portal is divided into a grid of beamlets. Each beamlet crossing the target is assigned the maximum intensity that could be used without exceeding the dose tolerances of the sensitive structures and normal tissue. A forward dose calculation using the "maximum" beam intensity profile is then performed, and the score of the given beam direction (indexed by i) is calculated according to[92]

$$S_i = \frac{1}{N_T} \sum_{n \in \text{Target}} \left(\frac{d_{ni}}{D_T^P} \right)^2 \qquad (6)$$

where d_{ni} is the maximum dose delivered to voxel n by the beam from the direction indexed by i, N_T is the number of voxels in the target, and D_T^P is the target prescription. The BEVD score function captures the main feature of a planner's judgment about the quality of a radiation beam and allows one to select beam orientations without excessive computational time. For a given patient, the score function for every possible beam direction is evaluated and the directions with the highest BEVD scores are identified. Although the technique does not yield the final beam configuration in a multifield IMRT treatment, it provides useful information with regard to which beam directions are potentially good or bad. During planning, the beams with the highest scores are considered favorable for the treatment. It is also illustrative to point out that the BEVD information can also be integrated into a beam orientation optimization program to improve the convergence behavior and computational speed.[72]

Hybrid Treatment of IMRT with Other Modalities

IMRT affords one the ability to produce not only spatially uniform but also purposely nonuniform doses. A natural application of the feature is to combine IMRT with other RT modalities to generate a dose distribution that would otherwise be impossible. Along this line, IMRT has been considered a method of salvaging suboptimal prostate implants.[93] The combination of IMRT with conventional electron beam(s) for improving the photon-electron field matching and for treatments of certain specially shaped targets has also been investigated.[94] Figure 2-13 illustrates a combined head and neck boost treatment using electron and intensity-modulated photon beams. In head and neck cancer, treatment initially involves the irradiation of the primary tumor and the cervical lymph nodes. After the tolerance dose of the spinal cord is reached using opposed lateral photon beams, the lateral fields are reduced off the spinal cord. The treatment of the anterior neck along with the primary tumor is continued using the reduced photon beams, whereas the posterior neck overlying the spinal cord is treated with lateral electron fields. This requires the matching of an electron field with two opposed photon fields. For comparison, the combined treatment using the conventional technique (electron + conventional photon beams) is shown in Figure 2-13. When the electron and unmodulated photon beams are matched directly, hot spots greater than 15% above the prescribed dose are seen in the abutting region. This is reduced to 5% when the proposed technique was used, with markedly better dose homogeneity in the abutting region. Furthermore, because of the broadened photon penumbra, the dose homogeneity in the junction region becomes less sensitive to patient setup errors.[94]

Gated or Synchronized IMRT

IMRT can produce highly conformal doses to targets and a sharp dose gradient between targets and surrounding critical structures.[60,95–98] Together with improved patient immobilization, the target margins can be reduced to facilitate dose escalation. However, margin reduction remains challenging for treatments in the thoracic regions and other sites in which intrafraction respiratory motion is significant.[99,100] The delivery of IMRT in either dynamic or static mode can cause unexpected high- and low-dose regions owing to the interplay between the movements of the tumor and the MLC leaves.[101] This issue can, in principle, be improved through the use of gating or respiration synchronization.[102–106] (See

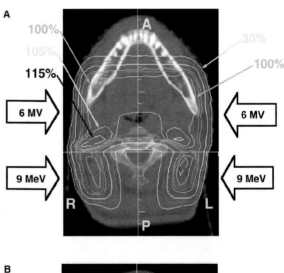

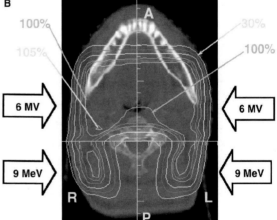

FIGURE 2-13. Comparison of the isodose distributions of the treatment plans in a transverse section of a patient with head and neck cancer when the electron and photon beams were matched directly (*A*) and when dynamic intensity modulation was used for the photon beams (*B*). Isodose levels are shown at 30%, 50%, 70%, 90%, 95%, 100%, 105%, 110%, and 115%. Note that the 110% and 115% isodose lines are not present in (*B*). (To view a color version of this image, please refer to the CD-ROM.) Reproduced with permission from Li JG et al[94].

Chapter 9, "Respiratory Motion Management," and Chapter 19.4, "Intrafractional Organ Motion and Planning: Emerging Technology".)

In gating, tracking, and breath-hold, the treatment machine is switched "on" or "off" in response to a signal that is representative of a patient's breathing motion. Both passive and active devices can be used to monitor the respiratory motion. Ideally, the beam is on only during portions of the breathing cycle when motion is small. The disadvantage of this technique is the prolonged treatment time compared with that of nongating approaches.

Motion-synchronized RT is based on two assumptions: (1) tumor motion is considered to be predictable, and the model of motion can be established prior to the treatment and is assumed to be the same (or at least adaptively predictable) throughout the treatment course, and (2) the treatment delivery system, either the MLC leaves or the treatment couch, can be instructed to precisely move to certain locations to adapt to the motion of the tumor. The main advantage of the motion-synchronized RT is that the radiation beam is on all of the time; therefore, there is no treatment time prolongation. However, several major technical difficulties must be overcome. Inverse treatment planning in this case must take into account the functionality of the delivery system.

Another issue is that respiratory motion exists in all stages of the RT process, including preplanning imaging and treatment planning and delivery. If respiratory motion is not accounted for during image acquisition, artifacts may arise during the image acquisition, leading to the distortion of the target volume. For gated treatment, the same window should be used for imaging and planning and delivery so that tumor positions and patient anatomy can be reproduced accurately. For motion-synchronized RT, several sets of CT images representing different phases of the breathing cycle need to be acquired through either a high-speed multislice CT scanner or by postprocessing software to sort the images. All of these images will be used for IMRT treatment planning, and the resulting MLC leaf sequences need to be multiplexed for delivery.

Biologically Conformal IMRT

Although the biology of tumors plays a crucial role in the success of RT, commonly used CT and magnetic resonance images provide few metabolic data and have significant shortcomings in characterizing benign and malignant tumors. Recent advancements in functional imaging make it possible to noninvasively obtain a patient's metabolic distribution. Coupled with the technical capability of IMRT in generating customized three-dimensional dose distributions with subcentimeter resolution, this may afford a significant opportunity to improve conventional RT by producing doses in accordance with biologic requirements.[107–110] Research effort is focused on integrating functional data into IMRT treatment planning to improve clinical cancer management. In general, functional imaging suggests nonuniform dose distributions to meet the heterogeneous biologic requirements. Xing and colleagues identified some relevant issues and developed a preliminary four-dimensional inverse planning scheme for functional imaging-guided IMRT.[109] The metabolic and functional data are incorporated effectively by modulating the prescription doses in the target voxels. This algorithm enables one to produce a high dose where there is resistance and/or where tumor burden is large and to differentially spare the sensitive structures with more emphasis on functionally important regions.

Delivery Techniques for Fixed-Gantry IMRT

IMRT delivery with MLC is based on the simple principle that moving jaws or leaves can be employed to control the dose delivered to a point. As mentioned previously, IMRT planning is currently performed in two steps: optimization of intensity maps and MLC leaf sequencing. The latter is to convert an intensity map into an MLC leaf sequence file, which specifies the leaf positions as a function of the fraction of MUs delivered. For the delivery, the two-dimensional beam fluence is divided into strips corresponding to the projection of each leaf pair of the MLC. Each MLC leaf pair is then required to modulate the fluence along its projection (see Chapter 12, "Delivery Systems"). For Varian linear accelerators (Varian Medical Systems, Palo Alto, CA), the leaf pairs are independent, reducing the conversion of two-dimensional fluence profiles into a collection of one-dimensional problems. As a result, the problem becomes finding a series of leaf positions (coordinates of leading and trailing leaves) to cover the area under a one-dimensional fluence function. There is no unique solution to this problem, leading to a number of ways to accomplish beam modulation.

MLC-based delivery is generally divided into static step-and-shoot[111–116] and dynamic modes.[117–119] A step-and-shoot leaf sequence file consists of alternatives of dose-only and motion-only instances. The step size of MLC movement in this mode is determined by the dimension of the beamlet in the leaf movement direction. Dynamic delivery differs from the step-and-shoot mode in that leaf movement and dose delivery are realized simultaneously. These algorithms are described below.

Step-and-Shoot Delivery

In step-and-shoot delivery, the total dose at a spatial point is the superposition of contributions from a series of segment fields (typically, the number of segments is between 20 and 100). The x-ray beam is off when the MLCs travel from one segment to another. This is perhaps the most intuitive technique to deliver intensity-modulated fields using MLC. The QA procedure for this delivery mode is relatively simpler (than dynamic delivery) because there is no correlation between the leaf speed and the dose. Instead of describing the algorithm generally, an example is used to illustrate how the step-and-shoot leaf sequencing methods work.[111]

Figure 2-14 depicts a simple example of an intensity pattern. The intensity in a 6 × 4 cm field is expressed using five discrete intensity levels. Four 1 cm–wide leaves (numbered 12, 13, 14, and 15) are to be used to generate the intensity pattern. The profiles that each leaf pair must generate are shown in the individual graphs (the profile required by leaf pair 12 in this example).

For a modulated field to be delivered at a gantry angle, each component profile along the center of the jth leaf pair must be rendered into a leaf trajectory. Intensity modulation along the profile, as shown in Figure 2-15, is obtained by sweeping the leading leaf, 12B, and the following leaf, 12A, from left to right along the x-axis. The first step in this procedure is to divide the total relative beam intensity into a number of equal intervals of width $\Delta\Phi$, as indicated in the illustration. The number of intervals selected to span the range of the intensity is NI. The second step in the procedure is to find the intersection of the centers of these profile increment bins with the profile. These points are indicated by circles in Figure 2-15. The algorithm requires

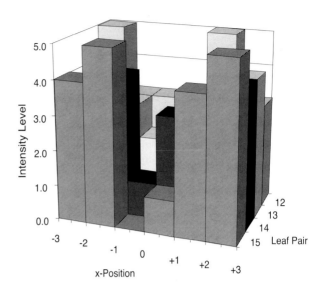

FIGURE 2-14. Intensity map used for illustrating the step-and-shoot leaf sequencing algorithm. (To view a color version of this image, please refer to the CD-ROM.)

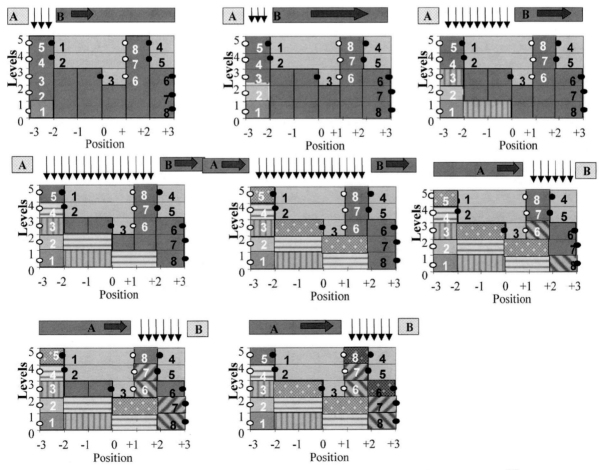

FIGURE 2-15. Intensity profile to be produced by leaf pair 12. Reproduced with permission from Van Dyk J and Purdy JA.[147]

that an even number of such points be found. The third step is to divide the coordinate points into two groups. One group consists of those points lying on an ascending slope of the profile in which there is a positive gradient (open circles in Figure 2-15), and the other group consists of those points lying on a descending slope of the profile in which there is a negative gradient (filled circles). The fourth step is to rank the points in each group. The numbers indicated are the i-index for the sequence for the twelfth pair of leaves. Pairing together the coordinates of equal rank order and assigning the coordinates to each pair of leaves produces the desired leaf sequence for the kth gantry angle position, $\{xA_{i,j,k}, xB_{i,j,k}\}$, where the index i ranges from 1 to NI_j. The number of steps required to create the trajectories will not be the same for all profiles that make up a field. Steps must be added to the shorter sequences with the leaves abutting beneath a jaw at one end of the profile so that all sequences for a field will have the same number of steps.

Another type of step-and-shoot delivery is based on the sequential reduction of intensities according to a prespecified scheme.[112,113,120] The pattern of integers in Figure 2-16 represents an intensity pattern to be delivered using this leaf setting sequence. The 5 × 5 cm field is to be delivered with a maximum beamlet intensity of 10 and a minimum beamlet intensity within the field of 1. The underlying principle of the algorithm for determining the sequence is that the most efficient way to subdivide a sequence is by halves. The sequence is to be delivered by increments that are powers of 2. In this case, the increments are 8, 4, 2, and 1. The first step is to set the leaves in a pattern that can deliver an exposure of 8. There are four beamlets with intensities of 8 or more. They are not contiguous, but leaves can be set to form two windows around the two regions that each deliver an intensity of 8. This is step 1 in Figure 2-17. After this exposure, all but one of the beamlet positions still require an exposure of 1 or more. A leaf pattern can then be found that exposes beamlets that require a residual exposure of 4 or more. However, two such regions exist that require two separate sets of leaf settings. These are steps 2 and 3 in Figure 2-17. The residual intensity then contains values up to 3, which can be reduced by exposures of 2. Again, to expose all of the beamlets, two leaf patterns are required, each delivering exposures of 2. These are steps 4 and 5 in Figure 2-17. Then all of the beamlet positions have either received their full exposure or have a residual value of 1. Two more leaf patterns are required to reach all of the 1 positions and reduce the residual intensity to zero. In all, seven steps are required to deliver the intensity pattern. The single-profile step-and-shoot leaf setting algorithm requires 13 steps to deliver this pattern.

Dynamic Delivery

Let $\Phi(x)$ be the fluence along the trajectory of the leaf pair. An example profile is shown in Figure 2-18. To deliver the fluence, one must determine the arrival times at x, $t_A(x)$ for leaf A and $t_B(x)$ for leaf B. The units of the arrival times can be seconds, or they can be expressed as MUs. The irradiation time interval at x between the opening of the ray by leaf B and the shielding of the ray by leaf A is indicated by

	5	7	2	4	7	
	4	1	3	10	5	
	4	5	2	9	8	
	3	2	5	7	3	
	4	7	9	2	4	

FIGURE 2-16. Example intensity map used for illustrating the "areal" leaf sequencing algorithm.

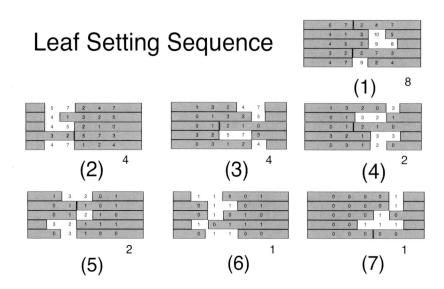

FIGURE 2-17. Leaf sequencing steps involved in decomposing the intensity map shown from Figure 2-16. The "areal" algorithm described by Xia and Verhey[112] is used here.

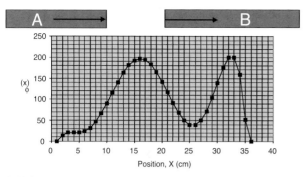

FIGURE 2-18. Example intensity map used for illustrating the dynamic leaf sequencing algorithm.

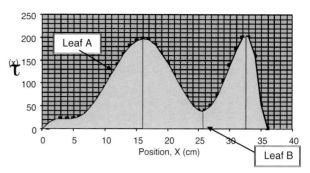

FIGURE 2-19. Time-position graph for the two leaves during the dynamic delivery process. Reproduced with permission from Van Dyk J and Purdy JA.[147]

$$\tau(x) = t_A(x) - t_B(x) = \Phi(x)/\Phi_0. \qquad (7)$$

Figure 2-19 can then be considered to be a time-position graph for the two leaves. The upper border of the shaded area is the leaf A trajectory, and the lower border, or x-axis, is the leaf B trajectory. The problem with this interpretation is that it requires leaf B to travel with infinite velocity and leaf A to travel backward in time! The dilemma can be resolved by applying a sequence of operations that transform the two trajectories such that they become deliverable. Note that there are four regions marked along the fluence profile in which the gradient is either positive or negative. To remove the time reversal from the continuous fluence profile, a reflection operator is introduced and is defined by

$$\tau' = \Delta\tau_{R1} \pm [\tau(x) - \Delta\tau_{R1}] \qquad (8)$$

$$\tau' = \Delta\tau_{R2} \pm [\tau(x) - \Delta\tau_{R2}] \qquad (9)$$

where $\Delta\tau_{R1}$ is the average value of the portion of the profile with a negative gradient within the R1 region around the first maxima and $\Delta\tau_{R2}$ is the average value of the portion of the profile with a negative gradient within the R2 gradient region around the second maxima. The positive sign is applied when there is a positive gradient and the negative sign when there is a negative gradient. The reflection operator is applied to the curves in the negative gradient regions to yield curves that do not require the leaves to travel backward in time. The results are shown in Figure 2-22.

The operations have introduced a discontinuity in the leaf sequence curves that can be removed by applying a translation operator defined in region R1 by

$$\tau''(x) = \tau'(x) + \Delta\tau \qquad (10)$$

where the increments are selected to remove the discontinuity between region R1 and R2, as illustrated in Figure 2-20. For the sake of generality, in region R1, the translation constant is zero. However, now there are still horizontal portions of the curves that represent infinite velocity of the leaves. There is always a horizontal segment occurring in either leaf A or leaf B trajectories across the entire sequence.

To remove the infinite velocity, some additional slope is introduced to each leaf trajectory. This can be achieved by applying a shear operator to the entire lengths of both leaf trajectories. The shear operator is defined by

$$\tau'''(x) = \tau''(x) + x/\upsilon_{max} \qquad (11)$$

This operator tilts the upper and lower horizontal bounds of each segment of the sequence by an amount determined by the maximum leaf velocity, resulting in a sequence that can be practically delivered. The slope of the shear is the inverse of the maximum velocity that the leaves can move, υ_{max}. The resulting leaf setting sequence is shown in Figure 2-20. The leaves begin the sequence closed at the left side of the field and end the sequence closed together at the right side of the field. In a region in which the original fluence gradient is positive, the leading leaf, leaf B, moves with a constant speed determined by the maximum velocity, and the trailing leaf A moves along the trajectory given in equation 11. In those regions in which the fluence gradient is negative, the trailing leaf, leaf A, moves with the maximum velocity, whereas the leading leaf moves along the trajectory given in equation 11.

The algorithm used to calculate the velocity modulation of the slower leaf can be derived by differentiating equation 12 with respect to distance:

$$d\tau'''/dx \equiv 1/\upsilon(x) = d\tau''/dx + 1/\upsilon_{max} \qquad (12)$$

The derivative of τ'' with respect to x can be obtained from equation 10 and is simply the derivative of τ' in all subdivisions of the trajectory. The derivative of τ' can be obtained from equations 8 and 9 and depends on the sign of the fluence gradient:

$$\nabla\Phi < 0 \Rightarrow d\tau'/dx = -d\tau/dx \qquad (13a)$$

$$\nabla\Phi > 0 \Rightarrow d\tau'/dx = +d\tau/dx \qquad (13b)$$

The derivative of τ can be seen in equation 7 to be

$$d\tau/dx = (d\Phi/dx)/\Phi_0 \qquad (14)$$

assuming that the variation in the incident fluence is negligible with respect to x. Using these results in equation 12, the velocity modulation equation becomes

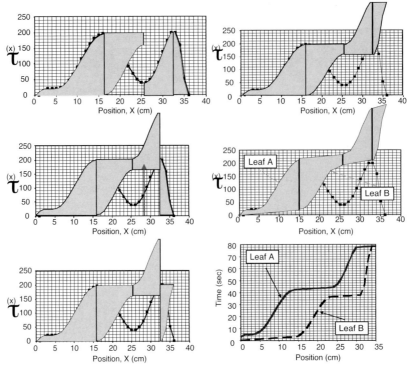

FIGURE 2-20. Trajectories of leaf A and leaf B during the dynamic delivery process. Reproduced with permission from Van Dyk J and Purdy JA.[147]

$$1/\upsilon(x) = \pm (d\Phi/dx)/\Phi_0 + 1/\upsilon_{max} \qquad (15)$$

where the positive sign applies to positive fluence gradient regions and the negative sign applies to negative fluence gradient regions. By rearranging, one arrives at

$$\upsilon(x) = \upsilon_{max}/[1\pm \upsilon_{max} \cdot (d\Phi/dx)/\Phi_0] \qquad (16)$$

This equation can be used to generate the velocity modulation required to deliver the fluence profile, starting with the leaves closed together at one side of the profile and ending with the leaves closed together again at the other. The leaf setting sequence computed by the velocity equation for the original fluence in Figure 2-18 is shown in Figure 2-20. The results are exact.

Our experience with both step-and-shoot and dynamic delivery indicates that there is no clear-cut advantage for any one of the methods except in some special situations. The main disadvantage of the step-and-shoot method is a sacrifice of accuracy in the delivery of beam profiles that have steep gradients. The dynamic method delivers the required distribution by sweeping the leaf pair across the beam and becomes inefficient in producing "large and flat" fluence segments.[121] It is possible to implement an algorithm combining the step-and-shoot and the dynamic deliveries to use the advantages of each.[122] This scheme would determine the slope of each segment of the intensity profile and then choose the suitable delivery method.

Related Issues in MLC-Based Delivery

Unlike conventional RT with static MLC fields, significant dosimetric issues must be addressed when IMRT delivery is used. Most of the algorithms in the literature, however, assume an ideal MLC and ignore the influence of many physical effects and the mechanical constraints of a realistic MLC, such as transmission and head scatter, tongue-and-groove effects, and collision constraints for adjoining leaf pairs.

Yang and Xing proposed an algorithm to account for the leaf transmission and head scatter effects in step-and-shoot leaf sequencing.[123] In their approach, an error function, defined as the least square difference between the desired and the delivered fluence maps, is introduced. Mathematically, this function is expressed as

$$F = \sum_{i,j}[\varphi(i, j) - \varphi_d (i, j)]^2 \qquad (17)$$

where $\varphi(i,j)$ and $\varphi_d(i,j)$ are the calculated and the desired fluences of beamlet (i,j), respectively. In equation 18, only those beamlets with nonzero fluences in the desired intensity map are considered because one cannot physically produce a beamlet with zero fluence.

The calculation starts with the MLC leaf sequence file derived from the desired fluence map without considering transmission and head scatter. The effects of transmission and head scatter are minimized by iteratively adjusting the fractional MUs in the initial MLC leaf sequences using a downhill simplex optimization method. A three-source model[124] is used to evaluate the relative head scatter contribution for each segment. The three effective sources are the source for the primary photons from the target and two extrafocal photon sources for the scattered photons from the primary collimator and the flattening filter, respectively. The algorithm has been assessed by comparing the dose distributions delivered by the corrected leaf sequence files and the theoretical predication, calculated by Monte Carlo simulation using the desired fluence maps and several clinical IMRT cases. The deviations between the desired fluence maps and the ones calculated using the corrected leaf sequence files are less than 0.3% of the maximum MU for the test field and less than 1.0% for the clinical IMRT cases. The experimental data demonstrate that both absolute and relative dose distributions delivered by the corrected leaf sequences agree with the desired ones within 2.5% of the maximum dose or 2 mm in high–dose gradient regions. It is found that the influence of the two effects is more pronounced in the absolute dose than in the relative dose. Figure 2-21 illustrates a measured absolute dose profile for a test field. In performing the measurements, MLC leaf sequences with different correction schemes described in the figure caption were used.

The influences of rounded leaf ends and interleaf transmission,[125] tongue-and-groove effect,[126] and the effect of back-scattered photons from the moving jaws and MLC leaves on the monitor chamber signal[127] have been studied using accurate models with realistic MLC geometries. It has been pointed out that the tongue-and-groove effect may be significant when underdosage occurs between two adjacent leaf pairs owing to the fact that the region between is always covered by the tongue, the groove, or both.[128,129] Algorithms have been developed to either minimize or remove this effect when MLC leaf sequences are generated.[114,130–133] Many researchers have shown that the tongue-and-groove effect can result in an underdose of as much as 10 to 15% in some special situations.[128,129,134,135] However, a Monte Carlo study by Deng and colleagues suggested that the difference between the dose distributions with and without the tongue-and-groove effect was hardly visible for an IMRT treatment with multiple gantry angles in a clinical setting.[126] More thorough investigations on the tongue-and-groove effect and other physical factors are needed to understand the system and to determine better solutions.

Finally, the inclusion of various physical factors is made simple if segment-based inverse planning is used. This represents one of the major advantages of the new type of inverse planning approach with integration of machine constraints.

Quality Assurance

IMRT adds a new degree of freedom to conventional RT and allows one to tune the dose distribution on an individual beamlet level. At the same time, it significantly increases the level of sophistication and complexity of the planning and delivery systems. With more and more institutions starting IMRT programs, it becomes increasingly important to have robust and efficient QA tools for clinical use. Otherwise, the gain from IMRT may be lost in a nonoptimal QA procedure and/or be offset by the increased cost of treatment. In general, IMRT QA has three aspects: commissioning and testing of the inverse treatment planning and IMRT delivery system, routine QA of the MLC delivery system, and patient-specific validation of each treatment plan. The first task is mainly concerned with the integrity of the IMRT system. The second involves the normal operation of the dynamic delivery system, and the third

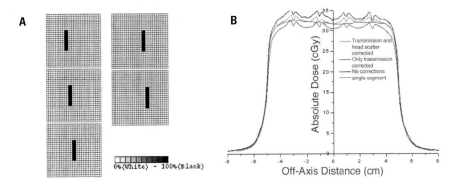

FIGURE 2-21. (A), A schematic diagram of the test field. The field includes five consecutive 2.0 × 10 cm^2 segments and attempts to produce a 10 × 10 cm^2 open beam. (B) The measured absolute dose profiles along the midline of leaf pair 21A–21B in the isocenter plane at a depth of 5 cm in solid water for the test field are shown on the left. The measured results of the single-segment 10 × 10 cm^2 open field with 30 monitor units are shown in the central black curve as a benchmark. The red curve is obtained with correction of head scatter and transmission. The top black and bottom blue curves represent the calculated dose profiles with only head scatter or transmission considered.[123] (To view a color version of this image, please refer to the CD-ROM.) Reproduced with permission from Yang Y and Xing L.[123]

task ensures accurate and safe treatment of the patient. Recently, there have been many excellent reports on IMRT QA–related issues.[60,136–139] Some practical aspects of IMRT QA are also discussed in Chapter 13, "Commissioning and Dosimetric Quality Assurance," and Chapter 14, "Quality Assurance Processes and Future Directions." In this section, the QA procedure and some recent advancements are summarized.

Commissioning and Testing

To ensure that the system can be used safely and accurately, the inverse treatment planning system must be commissioned prior to clinical use. Commissioning and testing consist of four separate but related steps. The first is concerned with the system's ability to accurately compute series of broad beam data. This type of testing is rudimental but useful to identify potential problems quickly. The second study tests the dose model and the delivery system with several specially designed intensity patterns. The accuracy of dose calculation for intensity-modulated beams can thus be assessed. The third type of study examines the system's functionality and dosimetric correctness for a number of hypothetical phantom cases. In addition to dose calculation, the functionality of dose optimization is evaluated at this level of tests. Figure 2-22 shows two examples of this type of measurement using a cylindrical water phantom and ion chamber.[140] The last type of study is to test the system using clinical cases to ensure the dosimetric accuracy and integrity of the system. This study evaluates the combination results of image acquisition and segmentation, geometric and dosimetric calibration of the planning system, planning and dose calculation, and data transfer. The dose distributions for single or multiple fields are usually done using an ion chamber and films in a phantom. Other dosimeters, such

as thermoluminescent dosimeters and semiconductor detectors, can also be employed. The American Association of Physicists in Medicine (AAPM) Task Group 40 and Task Group 53 reports provide guidelines on this topic and remain the benchmark documents on the subject.[141,142] This subject has also been discussed extensively in recent publications.[136,137,143]

Routine Machine QA

Intensity modulation is achieved with computer-controlled MLC using either static[112,144–146] or dynamic delivery techniques. To ensure that the planned dose distributions are safely and accurately delivered, an important requisition is the normal operation of the delivery system, which is warranted by routine machine QA. The principles and practice of QA for RT can be found in the classic documents of Van Dyk and Purdy,[147] as well as the report of AAPM Task Group 40.[141] For IMRT, several things specific to the IMRT MLC control system need to be checked periodically. Currently, the routine accuracy check of MLC leaf positioning in most clinics is performed using radiographic films with specially designed MLC leaf sequences.[148,149] Besides being time consuming, the results of film measurements are difficult to quantify and interpret. A few research groups have attempted to use an electronic portal imaging device (EPID) for quantitative verification of MLC leaf positions with edge detection algorithms.[150–153] The detection precision is limited to ~ 1 mm owing to the finite pixel size and the signal-to-noise ratio of the EPID, which is clearly insufficient for routine QA of the MLC delivery system. Here we describe a quantitative technique[154] for MLC leaf positioning QA developed recently at Stanford University. Given its simplicity, efficiency, and accuracy, we believe that the technique is ideally suitable for routine MLC QA and should have widespread clinical application in the future.

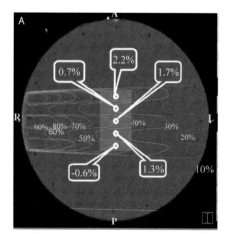 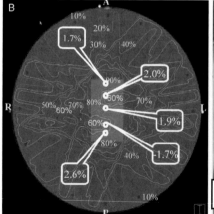 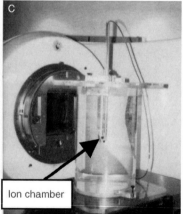

FIGURE 2-22. Hypothetical intensity-modulated radiation therapy plans generated for a cylindric water phantom and the measured dose distributions. The phantom is positioned with its axis perpendicular to the couch top and is supported by a bearing, allowing for rotation about its axis. This allows for measuring the dose of a multifield plan without gantry rotation. The measurements were made using the Varian dynamic multileaf collimator modulating 4 MV x-ray beams. The plans were generated using the *CORVUS* system. Reproduced with permission from Xing L et al.[140] (To view a color version of this image, please refer to the CD-ROM.)

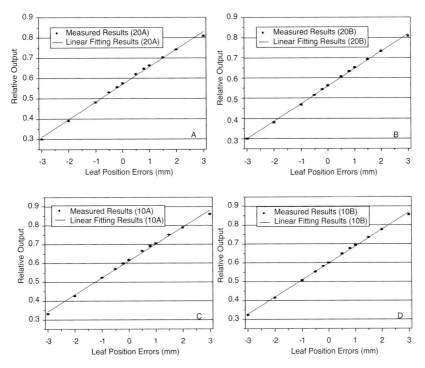

FIGURE 2-23. Relative output versus the displacement of leaves 20A, 20B, 10A, and 10B from their desired positions. The symbols are the measured data, and the solid lines are the least square fitting of the corresponding data sets. Reproduced with permission from Yang Y and Xing L.[154]

The Stanford MLC QA technique uses the fact that when a finite-sized detector is placed under a leaf, the relative output of the detector will depend on the relative fractional volume irradiated. A small error in leaf positioning would change the fractional volume irradiated and lead to a deviation of the relative output from the normal reading. For a given MLC and detector system, the relationship between the relative output and the leaf displacement can be easily established through experimental measurements and used subsequently as a quantitative means for detecting possible leaf positional errors. Figure 2-23 illustrates a set of calibration curves for different leaves obtained using an ion chamber and a Varian CL 2300C/D accelerator with an 80-leaf MLC.[154] Our results indicate that the method could accurately detect a leaf positional change of ~ 0.1 mm. The principle of the method is independent of the type of MLC and detector. The method overcomes the previously stated shortcomings of both film measurement and edge detection techniques and provides a reliable means for quantitative examination of MLC positional accuracy.

The principle has also been applied to MLC leaf positioning QA using an EPID,[155] which has the advantage of simultaneously detecting positional errors of any leaf at any point. In this technique, the active imaging region of an EPID is divided into a number of small rectangular regions of interest, each of which is centered at a point at which the leaf positioning accuracy is to be examined (Figure 2-24). Every region of interest here acts as a finite-sized detector,

and the integral signal from it can be processed based on the pre-established relation between the integral signal and the leaf displacement at the point. The EPID-based system also allows us to take the dosimetric influence of the adjacent leaves into account. For this purpose, the integral signal at a region of interest is expressed as a weighted sum of the contributions from the displacements of the leaf above the point and the adjacent leaves. The linear coefficients of the system equations are determined by fitting the integral signal data for a group of predesigned MLC leaf sequences to the known leaf displacements that are intentionally introduced during the creation of the leaf sequences. Once the calibration is done, the system can be used for routine MLC

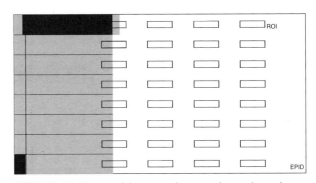

FIGURE 2-24. Diagram of the geometric setup using an electronic portal imaging device (EPID) to examine leaf positioning accuracy. (To view a color version of this image, please refer to the CD-ROM.)

leaf positioning QA to detect possible leaf errors. Table 2-1 shows a set of test data obtained using the technique. Overall, our results show that the proposed technique is superior to the conventional edge-detecting approach in two aspects. First, it deals with the problem in a systematic approach and allows one to take into account the influence of the adjacent MLC leaves effectively. Second, it has a much higher signal-to-noise ratio and is thus capable of quantitatively measuring extremely small leaf positional displacements. The technique can effectively detect a relative lead positional error as small as 0.1 mm at an arbitrary point within the field in the absence of an EPID setup error and 0.3 mm when this uncertainty is considered.

IMRT Treatment Plan Validation

The tasks of patient-specific QA can be divided into geometric and dosimetric verification. The former is concerned with the geometric accuracy of the IMRT beams, including isocenter and portal verification. The dosimetric verification includes a quantitative check of fluence maps, radiation doses at multiple points, and, in some cases, the dose distribution. Currently, the dosimetric verification is primarily done experimentally.

Geometric Verification

A pair of orthogonal simulation films (or digital reconstruction radiographs [DRRs]) is used to verify the patient position by comparison with portal films. In 3DCRT, a portal image is taken using the double-exposure technique, one with the customized radiation port and the other with

a larger rectangular open field, so that both the field boundary and selected patient anatomy can be visualized. A simulation image for an IMRT field can be created as well using the MLC boundary as the port of the radiation field. An example of such a portal image for an IMRT head and neck treatment is shown in Figure 2-25. For portal image exposure, an MLC field that defines the field boundary needs to be extracted from the IMRT leaf sequence file. The MLC-defined field aperture can be appended to the DRR to be displayed together with the patient's anatomy. The DRR in the beam's eye view, as shown on the left in Figure 2-25, is used as a reference for comparing with the portal image for target localization during the treatment.[156]

Dosimetric Verification and Independent Dose and Fluence Map Calculations

No consensus has emerged regarding what dosimetric quantities need to be examined to validate an IMRT treatment plan. Patient-specific dosimetric QA typically consists of dose measurements at multiple points and fluence map measurements. Some institutions also perform film dosimetry for each patient treatment. Because of the inherent complexity of the problem, it may be some time before definitive recommendations come from national organizations. In general, the goal of the dosimetric verifications is to ensure that the delivered dose distribution agrees with the one from the treatment planning system. The descriptions on equipment and procedure for these measurements have been the subject of a few recent review articles. The fundamental philosophy of IMRT QA and our experience with computer-based patient-specific QA are presented here.

First, one should note that the 3DCRT approach based on point dose verification is insufficient to validate an IMRT plan because of the independence of the involved beamlets. In 3DCRT, verification is mainly concerned with the MU calculation for each incident field. An independent

TABLE 2-1. Detected Leaf Positional Errors with Different Intentionally Introduced Errors for Different B-Bank Leaves at Two Locations

Location	Leaf Number	IIE, mm	DLPE, mm
X = –10 cm	16B	0.3	0.31
	20B	1.6	1.55
	23B	–0.5	–0.51
	31B	0.1	0.11
	33B	0.4	0.42
	34B	0.5	0.49
	37B	–0.4	–0.42
	44B	–0.2	–0.18
	45B	2.3	2.37
	50B	–0.5	–0.50
X = 0 cm	13A	0.8	0.76
	14A	–0.2	–0.19
	19A	–1.2	–1.20
	22A	–0.1	–0.09
	27A	2.7	2.66
	31A	0.1	0.11
	39A	–0.8	–0.79
	44A	0.2	0.22
	45A	–0.3	–0.28
	46A	–1.8	–1.81

DLPE = detected leaf positional error; IIE = intentionally introduced error.

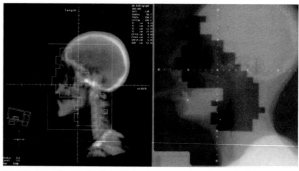

FIGURE 2-25. A left digitally reconstructed radiograph *left* with the field boundary of the IMRT field. A double-exposure portal image for the same field is shown on the right. These images are used by physicians to verify the maximum extent of the IMRT treatment fields.

calculation of the dose or MU at a point based on primitive machine data is recommended by AAPM Task Group 40.[141] Because the fluence of a uniform or wedged field is spatially correlated, information of the dose at a point can, in principle, be used to estimate the dose in other points provided that the off-axis information is known. However, this is not the case for intensity-modulated fields because the weights of the beamlets across a field are independent. The correctness of the dose at a spatial point warrants, at most, only the correctness of the beamlets passing through or nearby that point. To validate an IMRT treatment plan, the spatial distributions of the beamlets must be verified in addition to the point dosimetric check.

In practice, the above two tasks can be achieved by the verification of point dose(s) and fluence maps. The fluence map of an incident beam is usually normalized to the maximum beamlet weight in the beam. For a given intensity-modulated field, the verification of the fluence map or beamlet correlation ensures the correctness of the doses at other points once the dose(s) at one or more points inside the field is examined. Together with the point doses, they provide information on the integrity of the IMRT fields.

We now discuss how to efficiently carry out the two types of tests. Obviously, the most robust method is to measure the point doses and fluence maps to validate an IMRT plan. As depicted as the dashed lines in Figure 2-26, the approach checks both planning and delivery. Its drawback is that an intensive effort is needed to carry out the measurement for each field or patient. Alternatively, one can separate the QA of the delivery and planning systems, as illustrated by the solid lines at the bottom. Although QA of the delivery system is imperative, its goal should be practically achievable by periodical checks rather than actual measurement before each patient's treatment. The division of IMRT QA into machine QA and patient-specific QA allows us to check the integrity of an IMRT treatment plan by using computer

calculation, simplifying the pretreatment QA. In fact, the same philosophy has been used in 3DCRT over the years, in which a manual calculation is often used instead of actual point dose measurement to validate the patient-specific MU settings.

Algorithms to perform the independent point dose and fluence map calculations for IMRT have been reported recently.[157–162] Here a general formalism for the IMRT point dose check used at Stanford University Hospital (the software, *IMSure*, has been commercialized by Prodigm Inc., Chico, CA) is described. In this approach, the dose at an arbitrary spatial point is expressed as a summation of the contributions from all of the beamlets with the amplitude of each beamlet modulated by a dynamic modulation factor. The dynamic modulation factor represents the fractional time that the beamlet is "open" during the dynamic delivery process and can be computed once the MLC leaf sequences are known.[159] The dose at a point (x, y, z) is written as

$$D(x, y, z) = MU \sum_{m}^{M} C_m D_m^0$$

$$(18)$$

where the D_m^0 is the dose contribution to the calculation point per MU from the m-th beamlet when it is open, MU is the total monitor unit, and C_m is the dynamic modulation factor. When the MLC leaf transmission and head scatter effects are taken into account, C_m can be calculated by[160]

$$C_m = \sum_{k}^{K} [Sc_{m,k} + \alpha Sc'(1 - \delta_{m,k})] f_k$$

$$(19)$$

with

$$\delta_{m,k} = \begin{cases} 1 & \text{if} \quad m \in A_k \\ 0 & \text{if} \quad m \notin A_k \end{cases}$$

$$(20)$$

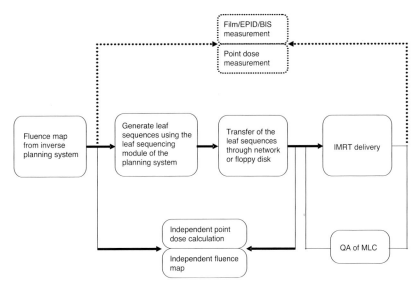

FIGURE 2-26. Intensity-modulated radiation therapy (IMRT) plan validation process. The fluence map/point dose verification is depicted by the dashed line on the top. The computer-based approach is outlined as the solid lines at the bottom of the figure. BIS = beam imaging system; EPID = electronic portal imaging device; MLC = multileaf collimator; QA = quality assurance. Reproduced with permission from Xing L et al.[163]

where f_k is the fractional MU of the k-th segment and A_k is the radiation field shape of the k-th segment. $Sc_{m,k}$ is the head scatter factor of the beamlet m in the k-th segment, Sc' is the head scatter factor for the rectangular field defined by the jaws, and α is the average transmission factor. The head scatter factor $Sc_{m,k}$ for each beamlet in a segment is calculated using the three-source model described earlier.[124]

Computer verification of the fluence maps or the MLC leaf sequences can be done similarly. The software reads in the leaf sequences and simulates the motion of the MLC leaves.[163] The computed fluence map is then compared quantitatively with the intended map from the treatment planning system. A set of predefined QA indices are introduced to measure the "closeness" between the computed and the reference maps. The implication of the simulation is twofold. By comparing the recalculated fluence map with that from the planning system, it examines the functionality of the leaf sequencer of the planning system and ensures that the leaf sequence is executable and correct. It can also detect possible errors that occur during the transfer process of the leaf sequence file from the planning computer to the MLC workstation. The goal of the simulation is to warrant that, assuming that a rigorous independent QA of the MLC system has been performed so that the dynamic MLC can accurately execute the instruction of a leaf sequence file, the execution of the leaf sequence will generate the desired fluence map should it pass the simulation test.

Because of the simplicity and reliability of computer-based IMRT plan validation, it becomes clinically practical to enforce QA of the point doses and fluence maps on an individual patient or field basis. Furthermore, the method is valid for both step-and-shoot and dynamic deliveries. The utility of the computer verification has been demonstrated by the many clinical IMRT cases at many institutions, and its widespread use should simplify the QA procedure. However, it is important to keep in mind that experimental measurement is the only reliable source for IMRT plan validation. Any computer-based validation tool must be validated by experimental means before its clinical use.

Special IMRT Techniques and Machine Limitations

Concurrent Boost

One of the advantages of IMRT is its ability to deliver different dose levels to different regions simultaneously so that target volumes with different prescription doses can be planned and delivered together (see Chapter 18.7, "Simultaneous Integrated Boost: Emerging Technology").[96,164] This approach has several potential advantages. Besides the efficiency of planning and delivery with a single plan, the resulting dose distribution can be more optimal. The conventional sequential boost strategy employs two or more independent plans in which the initial fields cover the elective regions and smaller boost fields focus on the primary target. The boost dose is often limited by the tolerances of nearby OAR, which have been given a significant amount of radiation. If planned simultaneously using IMRT, it is possible to distribute the dose evenly among fractions, and the system also has a greater degree of freedom to optimize the intensity among many beams. There are biologic advantages as well; for example, the shortened treatment course and increased dose per fraction to primary tumors can often be translated into a higher biologically equivalent dose, thus increasing the probability of local control.

Treatment of Large Tumors

The treatment of large tumors necessitates the use of large treatment fields. Depending on the implementation of the MLC by the linear accelerator vendors, the maximum field size formed by dynamic MLC may be different from those imposed by the collimators (jaws). Typically, the maximum field size is much smaller. For example, in the Varian MLC, the jaws and the MLC carriages do not move with the leaves. The leaf length in the current model of the MLC is 14.5 cm (projected at the isocenter). Given that each leaf pair must travel from the left boundary to the right boundary of the beam aperture and the back end of any leaf cannot travel past the edge of the jaw, the maximum width of the field aperture that can be accommodated in one sweep of leaves is also limited to 14.5 cm. The maximum IMRT field size that can be delivered in one sweep is 40×14.5 cm for an 80-leaf MLC (or a 120-leaf MLC) or 26×14.5 cm for a 52-leaf MLC.

To treat a target volume wider than 14.5 cm, an incident field must be split into two or more subfields unless some special techniques are used.[165] A simple step "break" in the middle, as is usually done for static treatments with MLC, may be implemented. Although this is certainly feasible, it could lead to field matching problems because uncertainties in patient setup and leaf positioning may cause undesirable hot or cold spots in the junctioning region. Given that the intensity varies across the field in IMRT anyway, it is natural to consider splitting the beam into components with overlap between them having variable intensity in the overlap region. A simple dynamic "feathering" technique for splitting large fields has been proposed by Wu and colleagues.[166] In this method, the intensity-modulated field is divided into two (or more) components. The components overlap each other, and the intensity gradually decreases in the overlap region for one component and increases for the other. The sum of intensities remains the same as for the original field. Each component is delivered using the sweeping window technique with the dynamic MLC. This method provides a smooth transition from one field component to the next, thereby eliminating the field junction problems. The dynamic feathering technique may also be applied to split large static fields to minimize the junction problem.[94,167] The feathering technique has been extended to treat the whole abdomen area, in which splitting into more than two beams in the leaf motion direction may be necessary. Also, field sizes larger than 40 cm may be required in the cephalad-caudad direction, leading to the use of multiple isocenters, and feathering (not splitting) is helpful.[168]

Dose Matching of an IMRT Plan with a 3DCRT or an IMRT Plan

One of the important problems in RT of breast cancer, Hodgkin's disease, head and neck cancer, and cervical cancer is the matching of an IMRT dose distribution for the treatment of part of the target volume(s) with a conventional 3DCRT or IMRT plan for the treatment of a different portion of target volume(s). Ideally, dose optimization of the second part should take into account the existing dose from the previous plan to optimally match the two dose distributions.[94,169]

The two treatment plans that need to be matched are generally produced sequentially. The first plan used for treating part of the tumor volume(s) is obtained with the consideration of the second plan. To reduce the sensitivity of potential setup errors, an attempt needs to be made to "blur" the penumbra or dose gradient in the direction perpendicular to the matchline. Specifically, instead of a sharp dose gradient, the dose is allowed to extend by an additional 1.5 to 5 cm in the direction perpendicular to the matchline. In this transition region, the dose is forced to fall off linearly. The overlap is generally determined by the desired sensitivity against setup error. After the first plan is done with the extended transitional dose gradient region, the second IMRT plan is optimized with consideration of the existing doses of the first plan. The goal of the second dose optimization is to obtain an IMRT plan that yields a uniform composite dose distribution in the target volume(s) and (including the transitional regions) while sparing the sensitive structures. The approach takes advantage of the state-of-the-art intensity modulation and dose optimization techniques and provides an effective solution to the timely clinical problem of IMRT dose matching. In addition to better dose uniformity in the target volumes in the matchline region, it reduces the sensitivity of the doses to setup uncertainties in the matchline region. The technique is not yet available in commercial planning systems but should be implemented in the near future.

Radiation Protection Issues

Generally speaking, IMRT tends to use more beams (than traditional approaches) to conform the isodose curves to the shape of the tumor volume. As a consequence, a larger volume of normal tissue is exposed to lower doses as opposed to a smaller volume of normal tissue irradiated by higher doses in 3DCRT. In addition, the number of MUs is often increased by a factor of 2 to 3 owing to dynamic intensity modulation, increasing the total-body exposure, which may increase the risk of secondary malignancies.[170,171] Hall and Wuu theoretically compared IMRT and 3DCRT and suggested that both factors tend to increase the risk of secondary cancers.[172] Altogether, IMRT is likely to almost double the incidence of secondary malignancies compared with conventional RT (from about 1 to 1.75% for patients surviving 10 years or more). The risk may be larger for patients with longer survival rates (and for younger patients), but the ratio should remain the same (see Chapter 3, "Radiobiology of IMRT," and Chapter 30, "Pros and Cons of IMRT").

Reduction of the number of segments using more advanced dose optimization techniques and/or appropriate shielding of the treatment room are crucial to reduce the potential risks to hospital personnel. The National Council on Radiation Protection and Measurements has developed an empiric method for designing shielding against ionizing radiation that will protect workers and the general public from harmful radiation exposures.[173,174] These methods have been used for several decades, and additional information that can be used in conjunction with these methods has since been published.[175–177] A thorough study of IMRT shielding design has been presented by Mutic and colleagues[178] and Low.[179]

Summary

Institutions worldwide are attempting or planning to integrate IMRT technology into their clinics. Before IMRT implementation, it is important to understand the physical principles behind the overall process of inverse planning and dynamic deliveries. This will help in making better decisions regarding which system best suits each clinical environment and facilitates the implementation process. The efficiency and quality of IMRT treatment depend on many factors. At this point, it seems that timely developments of inverse planning and QA techniques are highly desirable to make IMRT a truly superior and robust treatment modality. With these advancements, it is anticipated that IMRT will provide improved dose distributions with less effort in treatment planning, delivery, and verification.

Acknowledgments

We would like to thank J. G. Li, A. Pugachev, S. Crooks, C. Cotrutz, J. Lian, S. Hunjan, Z. Shou, E. Schreibmann, Y. Chen, G. Luxton, T. Pawlicki, Q. Le, S. Hancock, C. King, I. Gibbs, and B. Loo for many useful discussions. We also wish to acknowledge the support from the American Cancer Society (RSG-01-022-01-CCE), National Cancer Institute (5R01CA098523-02), Department of Defense (DAMD17-03-1-0023 and DAMD17-03-1-0019), and Vadasz Family Foundation. Last but not least, we wish to thank *International Journal of Radiation Oncology, Biology, Physics, Medical Physics,* and *Physics in Medicine and Biology* for permission to use their copyrighted materials.

References

1. Webb S. Intensity-modulated radiation therapy. Bristol (UK): Institute of Physics Publishing; 2001.

2. Webb S. Historical perspective on IMRT. In: Palta JR, Mackie TR, editors. AAPM intensity-modulated radiation therapy: the state of the art. Madison (WI): Medical Physics Publishing; 2003. p. 1–24.

3. Verhey LJ. Comparison of three-dimensional conformal radiation therapy and intensity-modulated radiation therapy systems. Semin Radiat Oncol 1999;9:78–98.

4. Yu CX. Intensity-modulated arc therapy with dynamic multileaf collimation: an alternative to tomotherapy. Phys Med Biol 1995;40:1435–49.

5. Yu CX, Li XA, Ma L, et al. Clinical implementation of intensity-modulated arc therapy. Int J Radiat Oncol Biol Phys 2002;53:453–63.

6. Wong E, Chen JZ, Greenland J. Intensity-modulated arc therapy simplified. Int J Radiat Oncol Biol Phys 2002;53:222–35.

7. Duthoy W, De Gersem W, Vergote K, et al. Whole abdominopelvic radiotherapy (WAPRT) using intensity-modulated arc therapy (IMAT): first clinical experience. Int J Radiat Oncol Biol Phys 2003;57:1019–32.

8. Crooks SM, Wu X, Takita C, et al. Aperture modulated arc therapy. Phys Med Biol 2003;48:1333–44.

9. Crooks S, King C, Pawlicki T, et al. Towards an optimal conformal technique for prostate radiotherapy: a dosimetric comparison between 3D CRT, IMRT, and IMAT. 2002. [In press].

10. Yang Y, Xing L. Clinical knowledge-based IMRT plan optimization. Phys Med Bio 2004;49:5101–17.

11. Niemierko A. Reporting and analyzing dose distributions: a concept of equivalent uniform dose. Med Phys 1997;24:103–10.

12. Wu Q, Mohan R, Niemierko A, et al. Optimization of intensity-modulated radiotherapy plans based on the equivalent uniform dose. Int J Radiat Oncol Biol Phys 2002;52:224–35.

13. Thieke C, Bortfeld T, Niemierko A, et al. From physical dose constraints to equivalent uniform dose constraints in inverse radiotherapy planning. Med Phys 2003;30:2332–42.

14. Brahme A. Optimized radiation therapy based on radiobiological objectives. Semin Radiat Oncol 1999;9:35–47.

15. Niemierko A, Goitein M. Modeling of normal tissue response to radiation: the critical volume model. Int J Radiat Oncol Biol Phys 1993;25:135–45.

16. Niemierko A. Radiobiological models of tissue response to radiation in treatment planning systems. Tumori 1998;84:140–3.

17. Schultheiss TE, Orton CG, Peck RA. Models in radiotherapy: volume effects. Med Phys 1983;10:410–5.

18. Schultheiss TE, Orton CG. Models in radiotherapy: definition of decision criteria. Med Phys 1985;12:183–7.

19. Martel MK, Ten Haken RK, Hazuka MB, et al. Estimation of tumor control probability model parameters from 3-D dose distributions of non-small cell lung cancer patients. Lung Cancer 1999;24:31–7.

20. Martel MK. NTCP modeling for normal lung and tumors: analysis of clinical data. 3D conformal and intensity modulated radiation therapy: physics & clinical applications. Middleton (WI): Advanced Medical Physics Publishing; 2001. p. 489.

21. Kwa SL, Lebesque JV, Theuws JC, et al. Radiation pneumonitis as a function of mean lung dose: an analysis of pooled data of 540 patients. Int J Radiat Oncol Biol Phys 1998;42:1–9.

22. Mohan R, Wang X, Jackson A, et al. The potential and limitations of the inverse radiotherapy technique. Radiother Oncol 1994;32:232–48.

23. Wang XH, Mohan R, Jackson A, et al. Optimization of intensity-modulated 3D conformal treatment plans based on biological indices. Radiother Oncol 1995;37:140–52.

24. Kallman P, Lind BK, Brahme A. An algorithm for maximizing the probability of complication-free tumour control in radiation therapy. Phys Med Biol 1992;37:871–90.

25. Xing L, Li JG, Donaldson S, et al. Optimization of importance factors in inverse planning. Phys Med Biol 1999;44:2525–36.

26. Xing L, Chen GTY. Iterative algorithms for inverse treatment planning. Phys Med Biol 1996;41:2107–23.

27. Xing L, Hamilton RJ, Spelbring D, et al. Fast iterative algorithms for three-dimensional inverse treatment planning. Med Phys 1998;25:1845–9.

28. Brooks RA, DeChiro G. Principles of computer assisted tomography (CAT) in radiographic and radioisotopic imaging. Phys Med Biol 1976;21:689–732.

29. Jones L, Hoban P. A method for physically based radiotherapy optimization with intelligent tissue weight determination. Med Phys 2002;29:26–37.

30. Luenberger D. Introduction to linear and nonlinear programming. Reading (MA): Addison-Wesley; 1973.

31. Kirkpatrick S, Gelatt C, Vecchi M. Optimization by simulated annealing. Science 1983;220:671–80.

32. Metropolis N, Rosenbluth A, Rosenbluth M, et al. Equation of state calculation by fast computing machines. J Chem Phys 1953;21:1087–91.

33. Rosen, II, Lam KS, Lane RG, et al. Comparison of simulated annealing algorithms for conformal therapy treatment planning. Int J Radiat Oncol Biol Phys 1995;33:1091–9.

34. Webb S. Optimization by simulated annealing of three-dimensional conformal treatment planning for radiation fields defined by a multileaf collimator. Phys Med Biol 1991;36:1201–26.

35. Winkler G. Image analysis, random field and dynamic Monte Carlo methods. Berlin: Springer-Verlag; 1995.

36. Webb S. Optimization by simulated annealing of three-dimensional, conformal treatment planning for radiation fields defined by a multileaf collimator: II. Inclusion of two-dimensional modulation of the x-ray intensity. Phys Med Biol 1992;37:1689–704.

37. Bortfeld T, Burkelbach J, Boesecke R, et al. Methods of image reconstruction from projections applied to conformation radiotherapy. Phys Med Biol 1990;35:1423–34.

38. Holmes T, Mackie TR. A filtered backprojection dose calculation method for inverse treatment planning. Med Phys 1994;21:303–13.

39. Pugachev AB, Boyer AL, Xing L. Beam orientation optimization in intensity-modulated radiation treatment planning. Med Phys 2000;27:1238–45.

40. Andrew HC, Hunt BR. Image restoration. Upper Saddle River (NJ): Prentice Hall; 1977.

41. Starkschall G. A constrained least-squares optimization method for external beam radiation therapy treatment planning. Med Phys 1984;11:659–65.

42. Starkschall G, Eifel PJ. An interactive beam-weight optimization tool for three-dimensional radiotherapy treatment planning. Med Phys 1992;19:155–63.

43. Lee EK, Fox T, Crocker I. Optimization of radiosurgery treatment planning via mixed integer programming. Med Phys 2000;27:995–1004.

44. Bednarz G, Michalski D, Houser C, et al. The use of mixed-integer programming for inverse treatment planning with pre-defined field segments. Phys Med Biol 2002;47:2235–45.

45. Langer M, Morrill SS, Brown R, et al. A comparison of mixed integer programming and fast simulated annealing for optimizing beam weights in radiation therapy. Med Phys 1996;23:957–964.

46. Lee EK, Zaider M. Intraoperative dynamic dose optimization in permanent prostate implants. Int J Radiat Oncol Biol Phys 2003;56:854–61.

47. Hou Q, Wang J, Chen Y, et al. An optimization algorithm for intensity modulated radiotherapy—the simulated dynamics with dose-volume constraints. Med Phys 2003;30:61–8.

48. Langer M, Brown R, Morrill S, et al. A generic genetic algorithm for generating beam weights. Med Phys 1996;23:965–71.

49. Ezzell GA, Gaspar L. Application of a genetic algorithm to optimizing radiation therapy treatment plans for pancreatic carcinoma. Med Dosim 2000;25:93–7.

50. Wu X, Zhu Y. A mixed-encoding genetic algorithm with beam constraint for conformal radiotherapy treatment planning. Med Phys 2000;27:2508–16.

51. Cotrutz C, Xing L. Segment-based dose optimization using a genetic algorithm. Phys Med Biol 2003;48:2987–98.

52. Xing L, Li JG, Pugachev A, et al. Estimation theory and model parameter selection for therapeutic treatment plan optimization. Med Phys 1999;26:2348–58.

53. Lian J, Cotrutz C, Xing L. Therapeutic treatment plan optimization with probalistic dose prescription. Med Phys 2003;30:655–66.

54. Winkler RL. An introduction to bayesian inference and decision. New York: Holt, Rinehart & Winston; 1972.

55. Llacer J. Inverse radiation treatment planning using the dynamically penalized likelihood method. Med Phys 1997;24:1751–64.

56. Llacer J, Solberg TD, Promberger C. Comparative behaviour of the dynamically penalized likelihood algorithm in inverse radiation therapy planning. Phys Med Biol 2001;46:2637–63.

57. Wu X, Zhu Y. A maximum-entropy method for the planning of conformal radiotherapy. Med Phys 2001;28:2241–6.

58. Wu X, Zhu Y. A neural network regression model for relative dose computation. Phys Med Biol 2000;45:13–22.

59. Li RP, Yin FF. Optimization of inverse treatment planning using a fuzzy weight function. Med Phys 2000;27:691–700.

60. Ezzel G. Clinical implementation of IMRT treatment planning. In: Palta JR, Mackie TR, editors. Intensity-modulated radiation therapy: the state of the art. Colorado Springs (CO): Medical Physics Publishing; 2003. p. 475–94.

61. Xing L, Lin Z, Donaldson SS, et al. Dosimetric effects of patient displacement and collimator and gantry angle misalignment on intensity modulated radiation therapy. Radiother Oncol 2000;56:97–108.

62. Manning MA, Wu Q, Cardinale RM, et al. The effect of setup uncertainty on normal tissue sparing with IMRT for head-and-neck cancer. Int J Radiat Oncol Biol Phys 2001;51:1400–9.

63. International Commission on Radiation Units and Measurements. Recording and reporting photon beam therapy. Report 50. Washington (DC): International Commission on Radiation Units and Measurements; 1993.

64. Bortfeld T, Schlegel W. Optimization of beam orientations in radiation therapy: some theoretical considerations. Phys Med Biol 1993;38:291–304.

65. Pugachev A, Li JG, Boyer AL, et al. Role of beam orientation optimization in intensity-modulated radiation therapy. Int J Radiat Oncol Biol Phys 2001;50:551–60.

66. Pugachev A, Xing L, Boyer AL. Beam orientation optimization in IMRT: to optimize or not to optimize? Presented at the XII International Conference on the Use of Computers in Radiation Therapy; 2000; Heidelberg, Germany.

67. Soderstrom S, Brahme A. Selection of suitable beam orientations in radiation therapy using entropy and Fourier transform measures. Phys Med Biol 1992;37:911–24.

68. Rowbottom CG, Nutting CM, Webb S. Beam-orientation optimization of intensity-modulated radiotherapy: clinical application to parotid gland tumours. Radiother Oncol 2001;59:169–77.

69. Djajaputra D, Wu Q, Wu Y, et al. Algorithm and performance of a clinical IMRT beam-angle optimization system. Phys Med Biol 2003;48:3191–212.

70. Stein J, Mohan R, Wang XH, et al. Number and orientations of beams in intensity-modulated radiation treatments. Med Phys 1997;24:149–60.

71. Pugachev A, Xing L. Computer assisted beam orientation selection in IMRT. Phys Med Biol 2001;46:2467–76.

72. Pugachev A, Xing L. Incorporating prior knowledge into beam orientation optimization. Int J Radiat Oncol Biol Phys 2002;54:1565–74.

73. Xing L, Pugachev A, Li JG, et al. A medical knowledge based system for the selection of beam orientations in IMRT. Int J Radiat Oncol Biol Phys 1999;45:246.

74. Schreibmann E, Xing L. Feasibility study of beam orientation class-solutions for prostate IMRT. Med Phys 2004;31:2863–70.

75. Kay S. Fundamentals of statistical signal processing: estimation theory. Upper Saddle River (NJ): Prentice Hall; 1993.

76. Wu Q, Mohan R. Algorithms and functionality of an intensity modulated radiotherapy optimization system. Med Phys 2000;27:701–11.

77. Emami B, Lyman J, Brown A, et al. Tolerance of normal tissue to therapeutic irradiation. Int J Radiat Oncol Biol Phys 1991;21:109–22.

78. Eisbruch A, Ten Haken RK, Kim HM. Dose, volume, and function relationships in parotid salivary glands following conformal and intensity-modulated irradiation of head and neck cancer. Int J Radiat Oncol Biol Phys 1999;45:577–87.

79. Lian J, Xing L. Incorporating model parameter uncertainty into inverse treatment planning. Med Phys 2004;31:2711–20.

80. Chen Y, Michalski D, Houser C. A deterministic iterative least-squares algorithm for beam weight optimization in conformal radiotherapy. Phys Med Biol 2002;47:1647–58.

81. Yu Y, Zhang JB, Cheng G, et al. Multi-objective optimization in radiotherapy: applications to stereotactic radiosurgery and prostate brachytherapy. Art Intel Med 2000;19:39–51.

82. Cotrutz C, Lahanas M, Kappas C, et al. A multiobjective gradient-based dose optimization algorithm for external beam conformal radiotherapy. Phys Med Biol 2001;46:2161–75.

83. Lahanas M, Schreibmann E. Multiobjective inverse planning for intensity modulated radiotherapy with constraint-free gradient-based optimization algorithms. Phys Med Biol 2003;48:2843–71.

84. Bortfeld T. Physical optimization. In: Palta JR, Mackie TR, editors. AAPM intensity-modulated radiation therapy: the state of the art. Madison (WI): Medical Physics Publishing; 2003. p. 51–76.

85. De Gersem W, Claus F, De Wagter C, et al. Leaf position optimization for step-and-shoot IMRT. Int J Radiat Oncol Biol Phys 2001;51:1371–88.

86. Shepard DM, Earl MA, Li XA, et al. Direct aperture optimization: a turnkey solution for step-and-shoot IMRT. Med Phys 2002;29:1007–18.

87. Cotrutz C, Xing L. Using voxel-dependent importance factors for interactive DVH-based dose optimization. Phys Med Biol 2002;47:1659–69.

88. Cotrutz C, Xing L. IMRT dose shaping using regionally variable penalty scheme. Med Phys 2003;30:544–51.

89. Rowbottom CG, Webb S, Oldham M. Improvements in prostate radiotherapy from the customization of beam directions. Med Phys 1998;25:1171–9.

90. Das S, Cullip T, Tracton G, et al. Beam orientation selection for intensity-modulated radiation therapy based on target equivalent uniform dose maximization. Int J Radiat Oncol Biol Phys 2003;55:215–24.

91. Bedford JL, Webb S. Elimination of importance factors for clinically accurate selection of beam orientations, beam weights and wedge angles in conformal radiation therapy. Med Phys 2003; 30:1788–881.

92. Pugachev A, Xing L. Pseudo beam's-eye-view as applied to beam orientation selection in intensity-modulated radiation therapy. Int J Radiat Oncol Biol Phys 2001;51:1361–70.

93. Holt R, Xing L. Salvage of suboptimal prostate seed implants using IMRT. Med Phys 2001;28:1308.

94. Li JG, Xing L, Boyer AL, et al. Matching photon and electron fields with dynamic intensity modulation. Med Phys 1999;26:2379–84.

95. Chao KS, Majhail N, Huang CJ, et al. Intensity-modulated radiation therapy reduces late salivary toxicity without compromising tumor control in patients with oropharyngeal carcinoma: a comparison with conventional techniques. Semin Radiat Oncol 2002;12(1 Suppl 1):20–5.

96. Wu Q, Mohan R, Morris M, et al. Simultaneous integrated boost intensity-modulated radiotherapy for locally advanced head-and-neck squamous cell carcinomas. I: dosimetric results. Int J Radiat Oncol Biol Phys 2003;56:573–85.

97. Mundt AJ, Lujan AE, Rotmensch J, et al. Intensity-modulated whole pelvic radiotherapy in women with gynecologic malignancies. Int J Radiat Oncol Biol Phys 2002;52:1330–7.

98. Forster KM, Smythe WR, Starkschall G, et al. Intensity-modulated radiotherapy following extrapleural pneumonectomy for the treatment of malignant mesothelioma: clinical implementation. Int J Radiat Oncol Biol Phys 2003;55:606–16.

99. Hanley J, Debois MM, Mah D, et al. Deep inspiration breath-hold technique for lung tumors: the potential value of target immobilization and reduced lung density in dose escalation. Int J Radiat Oncol Biol Phys 1999;45:603–11.

100. Murphy MJ, Martin D, Whyte R, et al. The effectiveness of breath-holding to stabilize lung and pancreas tumors during radiosurgery. Int J Radiat Oncol Biol Phys 2002;53:475–82.

101. Bortfeld T, Jokivarsi K, Goitein M, et al. Effects of intra-fraction motion on IMRT dose delivery: statistical analysis and simulation. Phys Med Biol 2002;47:2203–20.

102. Ramsey CR, Scaperoth D, Arwood D, et al. Clinical efficacy of respiratory gated conformal radiation therapy. Med Dosim 1999;24:115–9.

103. Wong JW, Sharpe MB, Jaffray DA, et al. The use of active breathing control (ABC) to reduce margin for breathing motion. Int J Radiat Oncol Biol Phys 1999;44:911–9.

104. Vedam SS, Keall PJ, Kini VR, et al. Determining parameters for respiration-gated radiotherapy. Med Phys 2001;28:2139–46.

105. Keall PJ, Kini VR, Vedam SS, et al. Motion adaptive x-ray therapy: a feasibility study. Phys Med Biol 2001;46:1–10.

106. Kini VR, Vedam SS, Keall PJ, et al. Patient training in respiratory-gated radiotherapy. Med Dosim 2003;28:7–11.

107. Ling CC, Humm J, Larson S, et al. Towards multidimensional radiotherapy (MD-CRT): biological imaging and biological conformality. Int J Radiat Oncol Biol Phys 2000;47:551–60.

108. Rosenman J. Incorporating functional imaging information into radiation treatment. Semin Radiat Oncol 2001;11:83–92.

109. Xing L, Cotrutz C, Hunjan S, et al. Inverse planning for functional image-guided IMRT. Phys Med Biol 2002;47:3567–78.

110. Alber M, Nusslin F. An objective function for radiation treatment optimization based on local biological measures. Phys Med Biol 1999;44:479–93.

111. Bortfeld T, Boyer AL, Schlegel W, et al. Realization and verification of three-dimensional conformal radiotherapy with modulated fields. Int J Radiat Oncol Biol Phys 1994;30:899–908.

112. Xia P, Verhey LJ. Multileaf collimator leaf sequencing algorithm for intensity modulated beams with multiple static segments. Med Phys 1998;25:1424–34.

113. Crooks SM, McAven LF, Robinson DF, et al. Minimizing delivery time and monitor units in static IMRT by leaf-sequencing. Phys Med Biol 2002;47:3105–16.

114. Siochi RA. Minimizing static intensity modulation delivery time using an intensity solid paradigm. Int J Radiat Oncol Biol Phys 1999;43:671–80.

115. Langer M, Thai V, Papiez L, et al. Improved leaf sequencing reduces segments or monitor units needed to deliver IMRT using multileaf collimators: the influence of irradiation and packaging on the quality of prepacked vegetables. Med Phys 2001;28:2450–8.

116. Beavis AW, Ganney PS, Whitton VJ, et al. Optimization of the step-and-shoot leaf sequence for delivery of intensity modulated radiation therapy using a variable division scheme. Phys Med Biol 2001;46:2457–65.

117. Convery DJ, Rosenbloom ME. Generation of intensity modulated fields by dynamic collimation. Phys Med Biol 1992;37:1359–74.

118. Svensson R, Kallman P, Brahme A. An analytical solution for the dynamic control of multileaf collimators. Phys Med Biol 1994;39:37–61.

119. Spirou SV, Chui CS. Generation of arbitrary intensity profiles by dynamic jaws or multileaf collimators. Med Phys 1994;21:1031–41.

120. Dai JR, Hu YM. Intensity-modulation radiotherapy using independent collimators: an algorithm study. Med Phys 1999;26:2562–70.

121. Beavis AW, Ganney PS, Whiton VJ, et al. Slide and shoot: a new method for MLC delivery of IMRT. In: Proceedings of the XIII International Conference on the Use of Computers in Radiation Therapy, Heidelberg, Germany, May 2000.

122. Beavis A, Ganney P, Whitton V, Xing L. Slide and shoot: a new method for MLC delivery of IMRT. The Use of Computers in Radiation Therapy, Heidelberg, Germany, 2000.

123. Yang Y, Xing L. Incorporating leaf transmission and header scatter corrections into MLC leaf sequences for IMRT. Int J Radiat Oncol Biol Phys 2003;55:1121–34.

124. Yang Y, Xing L, Boyer A, et al. A three-source model for the calculation of head scatter factors. Med Phys 2002;29:2024–33.

125. Chen Y, Boyer AL, Ma CM. Calculation of x-ray transmission through a multileaf collimator. Med Phys 2000;27:1717–26.

126. Deng J, Pawlicki T, Chen Y, et al. The MLC tongue-and-groove effect on IMRT dose distributions. Phys Med Biol 2001;46:1039–60.

127. Hounsell AR. Monitor chamber backscatter for intensity modulated radiation therapy using multileaf collimators. Phys Med Biol 1998;43:445–54.

128. Chui CS, LoSasso T, Spirou S. Dose calculation for photon beams with intensity modulation generated by dynamic jaw or multileaf collimations. Med Phys 1994;21:1237–44.

129. Wang X, Spirou S, LoSasso T, et al. Dosimetric verification of intensity-modulated fields. Med Phys 1996;23:317–27.

130. van Santvoort JP, Heijmen BJ. Dynamic multileaf collimation without 'tongue-and-groove' underdosage effects. Phys Med Biol 1996;41:2091–105.

131. Webb S, Bortfeld T, Stein J, et al. The effect of stair-step leaf transmission on the 'tongue-and-groove problem' in dynamic radiotherapy with a multileaf collimator. Phys Med Biol 1997;42:595–602.

132. Dirkx ML, Heijmen BJ, van Santvoort JP. Leaf trajectory calculation for dynamic multileaf collimation to realize optimized fluence profiles. Phys Med Biol 1998;43:1171–84.

133. Ma L, Boyer AL, Ma CM, et al. Synchronizing dynamic multileaf collimators for producing two-dimensional intensity-modulated fields with minimum beam delivery time. Int J Radiat Oncol Biol Phys 1999;44:1147–54.

134. Galvin JM, Smith AR, Lally B. Characterization of a multileaf collimator system. Comment in: Int J Radiat Oncol Biol Phys 1993 Jan 15;25(2):373–5. Int J Radiat Oncol Biol Phys 1993;25:181–92.

135. Sykes JR, Williams PC. An experimental investigation of the tongue and groove effect for the Philips multileaf collimator. Phys Med Biol 1998;43:3157–65.

136. IMRT Collaborative Working Group. Intensity-modulated radiotherapy: current status and issues of interest. Int J Radiat Oncol Biol Phys 2001;51:880–914.

137. Sharpe MB. Commissioning and quality assurance for IMRT treatment planning. In: Palta JR, Mackie TR, editors. Intensity-modulated radiation therapy: the state of the art. Madison (WI): Medical Physics Publishing; 2003. p. 449–74.

138. Xia P, Chuang C. Patient-specific quality assurance in IMRT. In: Palta JR, Mackie TR, editors. Intensity-modulated radiation therapy: the state of the art. Madison (WI): Medical Physics Publishing; 2003. p. 495–514.

139. Moran JM. Dosimetry metrology. In: Palta JR, Mackie TR, editors. Intensity-modulated radiation therapy: the state of the art. Madison (WI): Medical Physics Publishing; 2003. p. 415–38.

140. Xing L, Curran B, Hill R, et al. Dosimetric verification of a commercial inverse treatment planning system. Phys Med Biol 1999;44:463–78.

141. Kutcher GJ, Coia L, Gillin M, et al. Comprehensive QA for radiation oncology: report of AAPM Radiation Therapy Committee Task Group 40. Med Phys 1994;21:581–618.

142. Fraass B, Doppke K, Hunt M, et al. American Association of Physicists in Medicine Radiation Therapy Committee Task Group 53: quality assurance for clinical radiotherapy treatment planning. Med Phys 1998;25:1773–829.

143. Ezzell G, Galvin J, Low D, et al. Guidance document on delivery, treatment planning, and clinical implementation of IMRT: report of the IMRT Subcommittee of the AAPM Radiation Therapy Committee. Med Phys 2003;30:2089–115.

144. Bortfeld TR, Kahler DL, Waldron TJ, et al. X-ray field compensation with multileaf collimators. Int J Radiat Oncol Biol Phys 1994;28:723–30.

145. Ma L, Boyer AL, Xing L, et al. An optimized leaf-setting algorithm for beam intensity modulation using dynamic multileaf collimators. Phys Med Biol 1998;43:1629–43.

146. Crooks S, Pugachev A, King C, et al. Examination of the effect of increasing the number of radiation beams on a radiation treatment plan. Phys Med Biol 2002;47:3485–501.

147. Van Dyk J, Purdy JA. Clinical implementation of technology and the quality assurance process. In: Van Dyk J, editor. The modern technology of radiation oncology. Madison (WI): Medical Physics Publishing; 1999. p. 19–51.

148. Chui CS, Spirou S, LoSasso T. Testing of dynamic multileaf collimation. Med Phys 1996;23:635–41.

149. LoSasso TJ. IMRT delivery system QA. In: Palta JR, Mackie TR, editors. AAPM intensity-modulated radiation therapy: the state of the art. Madison (WI): Medical Physics Publishing; 2003. p. 561–91.

150. Herman MG, Balter JM, Jaffray DA, et al. Clinical use of electronic portal imaging: report of AAPM Radiation Therapy Committee Task Group 58. Med Phys 2001;28:712–37.

151. Chang J, Mueller K, Sidhu K, et al. Verification of multileaf collimator leaf positions using an electronic portal imaging device. Med Phys 2002;29:2913–24.

152. Samant SS, Zheng W, Parra NA, et al. Verification of multileaf collimator leaf positions using an electronic portal imaging device. Med Phys 2002;29:2900–12.

153. Vieira SC, Dirkx ML, Pasma KL, Heijmen BJ. Fast and accurate leaf verification for dynamic multileaf collimation using an electronic portal imaging device. Med Phys 2002;29:2034–40.

154. Yang Y, Xing L. Using the volumetric effect of a finite-sized detector for routine quality assurance of MLC leaf positioning. Med Phys 2003;30:433–41.

155. Yang Y, Xing L. Quantitative measurement of MLC leaf displacements using an electronic portal image device. Phys Med Biol 2004;49:1251-1533.

156. Chen Y, Xing L, Luxton G, et al. A multi-purpose quality assurance tool for MLC-based IMRT. ICCR, Heidelberg, Germany, May, 2000.

157. Boyer A, Xing L, Ma CM, et al. Theoretical considerations of monitor unit calculations for intensity modulated beam treatment planning. Med Phys 1999;26:187–95.

158. Kung J, Chen G. A monitor unit verification calculation in intensity modulated radiotherapy as a dosimetric quality assurance. Med Phys 2000;27:2226–30.

159. Xing L, Chen Y, Luxton G, et al. Monitor unit calculation for an intensity modulated photon field by a simple scatter-summation algorithm. Phys Med Biol 2000;45:N1–7.

160. Yang Y, Xing L, Li JL, et al. Independent dosimetric calculation with inclusion of head scatter and MLC transmission for IMRT. Med Phys 2003;30:2937–47.

161. Xing L, Yang Y, Li J, et al. Monitor unit calculation and plan validation for IMRT. In: Palta JR, Mackie TR, editors. Intensity-modulated radiation therapy: the state of the art. Madison (WI): Medical Physics Publishing; 2003. p. 3567–78.

162. Watanabe Y. Point dose calculations using an analytical pencil beam kernel for IMRT plan checking. Phys Med Biol 2001;46:1031–8.

163. Xing L, Li JG. Computer verification of fluence maps in intensity modulated radiation therapy. Med Phys 2000;27:2084–92.

164. Schefter TE, Kavanagh BD, Wu Q, et al. Technical considerations in the application of intensity-modulated radiotherapy as a concomitant integrated boost for locally-advanced cervix cancer. Med Dosim 2002;27:177–84.

165. Xing L, Yi BY, Li J, et al. Adaptive inverse planning with consideration of MLC field size constraint. Presented at the American Association of Physicists in Medicine Annual Meeting; 1999; Nashville, TN.

166. Wu Q, Arnfield M, Tong S, et al. Dynamic splitting of large intensity-modulated fields. Phys Med Biol 2000;45:1731–40.

167. Xing L, Boyer A, Kapp D, et al. Improving the matching of abutting photon fields by modulating photon beams. Med Biol Eng Comp 1997;35:921.

168. Hong L, Alektiar K, Chui C, et al. IMRT of large fields: whole-abdomen irradiation. Int J Radiat Oncol Biol Phys 2002;54:278–89.

169. Xing L, Yang Y, Li J, et al. Dose matching of an IMRT plan with an electron or 3D conformal treatment plan. Presented at the World Congress on Medical Physics and Biomedical Engineering; 2003 Aug 24–29; Sydney, Australia.

170. Followill D, Geis P, Boyer A. Estimates of whole-body dose equivalent produced by beam intensity modulated conformal therapy. Int J Radiat Oncol Biol Phys 1997;38:667–72.

171. Verellen D, Vanhavere F. Risk assessment of radiation-induced malignancies based on whole-body equivalent dose estimates for IMRT treatment in the head and neck region. Radiother Oncol 1999;53:199–203.

172. Hall EJ, Wuu CS. Radiation-induced second cancers: the impact of 3D-CRT and IMRT. Int J Radiat Oncol Biol Phys 2003;56:83–8.

173. Radiation protection design guidelines for 0.1-100 MeV particle accelerator facilities. Vol. 51. Washington (DC): National Council on Radiation Protection and Measurements; 1977.

174. Structural shielding design and evaluation for medical use of x-rays and gamma rays of energies up to 10 MeV. Vol 49. Washington (DC): National Council on Radiation Protection and Measurements; 1976.

175. McGinley PH. Shielding techniques for radiation oncology facilities. 2nd ed. Madison (WI): Medical Physics Publishing; 2002.

176. McGinley HM, Miner MS. A history of radiation shielding of x-ray therapy rooms. Health Phys 1995;69:759–65.

177. Rodgers JE. Radiation therapy vault shielding calculation methods when IMRT and TBI procedures contribute. J Appl Clin Med Phys 2001;2:157–64.

178. Mutic S, Low DA, Klein EE, et al. Room shielding for intensity-modulated radiation therapy treatment facilities. Int J Radiat Oncol Biol Phys 2001;50:39–46.

179. Low D. Radiation shielding for IMRT. In: Palta JR, Mackie TR, editors. AAPM intensity-modulated radiation therapy: the state of the art. Madison (WI): Medical Physics Publishing; 2003. p. 401–14.

Chapter 3

RADIOBIOLOGY OF IMRT

JOSEPH O. DEASY, PHD, JACK F. FOWLER, DSC, PHD

Intensity-modulated radiation therapy (IMRT) represents a fundamentally new approach to the planning and delivery of radiation therapy (RT). In this chapter, the radiobiologic issues of time, dose, and treatment volume relevant to the effective clinical implementation of IMRT are discussed. In addition, time-dose factors, data and models of dose-volume factors, and ways in which they may be used in IMRT treatment planning systems are reviewed. A shorter discussion of radiobiologic issues in IMRT has been presented by Fowler.[1] Goffman and Glatstein have also reviewed radiobiologic issues relevant to IMRT.[2]

Basic Principles of Clinical Radiobiology

Several decades of careful animal, clinical, cell culture, and biostatistical investigation have led to the crucial distinction between early and late radiation effects that remain entirely valid today. The books by Hall and Steel provide much more detailed information on the topics covered in this section.[3,4] The important difference between early and late effects is still being optimized by clinical trials. However, reliable quantitative tests in individual patients for known tumor and normal tissue characteristics are necessary for the true individualization of treatments. These factors are no less important now than they ever were. The overall effect of a fractionated course of RT depends primarily on overall dose, fraction size, overall treatment time, and volumes of the tissues or organs irradiated.

Fraction Size Factors

Fraction size effects are primarily controlled through two tissue-specific parameters:

1. Single-track cellular radiosensitivity, quantified using the exponential cell kill parameter α (in terms of $\log_e$ cell sterilization per Gy). Alpha represents the damage done by individual radiation particle tracks* and asso-

---

*In conventional RT, cell-kill effects are primarily due to the particle tracks of fast electrons either set in motion by photons, or other fast electrons, or originating in the accelerator head.

ciated indirect chemical damage. Consistent with that, α is independent of dose rate, fraction size, or interfraction time. Although α damage is partially repairable over time, it still represents the probability of cell sterilization owing to individual, noninteracting, particle tracks and is independent of interfraction interval.

2. Intertrack cellular radiosensitivity, β. Beta represents cell kill owing to interactions between individual particle tracks (normally two particle tracks but possibly more at very high fraction doses). Beta is therefore sensitive to fraction size, or dose rate if small enough, and time between fractions.

Together, these two factors specify the linear-quadratic (LQ) model of cell kill or fraction size effects according to

$$\text{cell survival} = \exp(-\alpha d - \beta d^2), \quad (1)$$

for cell survival owing to a single fraction of dose d, and

$$\text{fractionated cell survival} = \exp(-\alpha d - \beta d^2)^n$$
$$= \exp(-\alpha n d - \beta n d^2), \quad (2)$$

for n fractions, each of dose d.

The crucial point is that the β term is quadratic in fraction size only rather than quadratic in the overall dose. This is just what is expected owing to repair of particle track damage between fractions. However, this assumes that enough time is allowed between fractions (at least 6–8 hours) for repair processes to (nearly) finish.

The ratio of these two parameters, α/β, therefore defines the sensitivity to dose per fraction. This has led to significant advances in the basic understanding of therapeutic ratio and of the advantage of fractionated irradiation.[5–8] In short, smaller fraction sizes than the traditional 2 Gy usually give better therapeutic ratios, and larger fractions can be used only with great caution and in exceptional circumstances. Attempts to use larger and fewer fractions have the obvious attractions of brevity, convenience, and economy of resources but can be used only in carefully circumscribed conditions, which are discussed below.

Biologically Effective Dose

The LQ model provides for a simple way of comparing the effects of various fractionation schemes in terms of a biologically effective dose (BED), which is proportional to the number of logs of cells killed (sterilized) by any treatment. Only the number and size of dose fractions need be given, and the only biologic factor needed is the ratio α/β of the appropriate target cells. From equation 2 above,

$$\log \text{ cell kill} = \text{E} = \text{minus log cell survival} = n(\alpha d + \beta d^2), \tag{3}$$

where E stands for effect. This is the simplest and most obvious statement of the LQ formula.

Then if we take the d outside the parenthesis, we have

$$\text{E} = nd(\alpha + \beta d), \tag{4}$$

and dividing both sides by α leads to the BED:

$$\text{BED} = \text{E}/\alpha = nd(1 + d/(\alpha/\beta)). \tag{5}$$

The BED is conceptually the dose that would give the same log cell kill as the schedule of interest, if given at an infinitely low dose per fraction or infinitely low-dose rate, in the absence of repopulation. Different parts of a compound schedule can be added together to give the total effect in terms of log cell kill. BEDs for different tissues have to be kept separate from each other and are usually designated by the α/β ratio as a postfix, such as Gy3 for late and Gy10 for early biologic effects.

BED is equal to the total dose (nd) multiplied by the factor called relative effectiveness, which is a highly convenient term for investigating changes of fraction size in relation to different types of tissue:

$$\text{RE} = 1 + d/(\alpha/\beta). \tag{6}$$

Further, because BED = E/α, log cell kill is obviously equal to BED $\times$ α and can thus easily be estimated. BED can also be modified to include repopulation.[9]†

Normalized Tissue Dose

Although BEDs are basic, being proportional to log cell kill, convenient, and easy to calculate, they are not readily understood unless users calculate them often. Thus, a more complex substitute is preferred by many, called the normalized total dose (NTD). This is biologically equivalent to the dose

---

†The BED equation with repopulation is

$$\text{BED} = nd\left(1 + \frac{d}{\alpha/\beta}\right) - \frac{(\log_e 2)(T - T_k)}{\alpha T_p}$$

where n is the number of fractions at dose d, T is the overall treatment time, T_k is the delay before the onset of compensatory proliferation, and T_p is the cellular doubling time.

---

in 2 Gy fractions that would kill (sterilize) the same proportion of cells as the schedule under discussion.[10] NTD is therefore a function of the α/β ratio:

$$\text{NTD}_{\alpha/\beta} = D\frac{\alpha/\beta + d}{\alpha/\beta + 2 \text{ Gy}}, \tag{7}$$

where D is the total dose and d is the fraction dose, both in Gy. One can see that, for a given total dose D, the NTD increases with increasing fractional dose d (and correspondingly fewer fractions). Note also that NTD depends less on the fractional dose as the α/β ratio increases. The α/β subscript is specified when NTD is used, for example, NTD3. NTD is alternatively sometimes denoted EQD2 (equivalent dose in 2 Gy fractions).[11]

Treatment Time Factor

Treatment time effects can be understood through the use of two related parameters:

1. The approximate starting time of compensatory tumor cell repopulation after the beginning of treatment, T_k in days.
2. The rate of compensatory repopulation, quantified as the tumor clonogen potential doubling time, T_p, which continues from T_k to the overall treatment time T days. Note that T_p refers to doubling of tumor clonogens (stem cells) rather than all tumor cells, including differentiated cells. The pretreatment value of T_p, known as T_{pot}, may be significantly different from T_p owing to changes in tumor growth fractions or differences between the true clonogenic or stem cell population and the overall cell population that is assayed.

These two repopulation factors constitute an overall time factor, which implies, consistent with many clinical data, that more dose per day of prolongation must be delivered to maintain the isoeffect. For late-responding tissues, in which the late complications that may be life-threatening occur, there is little or no treatment time factor. Repopulation begins many months after irradiation, so there is no repopulation during the weeks of RT. Acutely responding normal tissues, however, are sensitive to overall treatment time and the treatment intensity (dose accumulated per day).

Apart from this absence of a time factor for most late complications, the above four factors are always in operation in RT and must be taken into account in any treatment planning to achieve an optimum (or near-optimum) effect, whether in increased tumor control probability (TCP) or decreased normal tissue complication probability (NTCP). Both tumors and normal tissues are also under the influence of volume factors, in obviously opposing ways (see below).

Fractionation Schedules

Most carcinomas contain rapidly proliferating cells and have been found to demonstrate high values of α/β such as 8, 14, 19, or 30 to 50 Gy or even larger.[12,13] Late complications, however, consistently have low α/β ratios,[8,12] typically in the range of 2 to 5 Gy. It then follows that smaller doses per fraction, for the same overall total dose, will spare late complications more than tumor damage. Hence, apart from volume factors, therapeutic ratios will be best for hyperfractionation, such as two fractions a day of 1.1 to 1.2 Gy to total doses of 77 to 82 Gy in about 7 weeks. This is exemplified in Figure 3-1.

The success of well-planned hyperfractionation schedules has been well demonstrated.[14] However, the inconvenience of delivering two fractions a day has resulted in continued attempts to obtain an optimum schedule by another strategy for improving results, namely, accelerated schedules that reduce the overall treatment time to overcome tumor clonogen repopulation. The principle is valid, but these approaches have sometimes been too "hot" at first and have then been modified to more and smaller fractions, for example, 35×2 Gy = 70 Gy in 35 days (treating 7 days a week), and then moderated to 39×1.8 Gy = 70.2 Gy in 39 days, avoiding the very long overall times with the 1.2 Gy fractions.[15,16]

The use of fewer and larger fractions, called hypofractionation, however, had been thought to be generally dangerous, with a diminished therapeutic ratio, leading to more late complications for a given tumor effect, as indicated on the left-hand side of Figure 3-1. Nonetheless, IMRT, stereotactic RT, and potentially protons, can be used to produce highly conformal and small-volume irradiations, which make hypofractionation feasible. The use of hypofractionation is further discussed below.

Overall Treatment Times

Most tumors contain a significant fraction of cells that are rapidly proliferating, with cell-cycle times of one to several days, with average tumor potential doubling times (T_{pot}, which neglects cell loss) of 4 or 5 days.[16] But the blood supplies of most types of tumors are so poorly organized and chaotic that spontaneous nutritional cell loss rates in human carcinomas can be 90 or 95% of all of those produced, so that gross volume doubling times are often 10 to 20 times longer than the mean T_{pot}.[17] Apoptosis is less but, of course, will add to the cell loss. This means that observed tumor volume doubling times are relatively meaningless, and so are most rates of volume shrinkage during treatment, although shrinkage sometimes correlates with tumor response.[17] Tumor regression during treatment is affected by the presence of both host cells and doomed tumor cells and therefore is not a reliable measure of tumor cell kill.

After several fractions of conventional RT, nonsterilized tumor cells comprise only a small proportion of metabolically active tumor clonogens. Following a time lag for resulting intermitotic cell death and the reabsorption of dead cells, viable cells move closer to blood capillaries, and the spontaneous cell loss falls. Consequently, surviving cells may become more oxygenated. Theoretically, one is then treating repopulating cells in the tumors (although attempts to observe the time course of reoxygenation during RT have given conflicting results).[18–22]

Clinical evidence from prolongation of RT demonstrates that most types of carcinoma can repopulate their surviving clonogenic cells at or above the rates measured as T_{pot} before treatment. For example, tumor clonogen number doubling time T_p during treatment of head and neck tumors is 2 to 3 days[23,24] versus mean T_{pot}s of 4 to 6 days before treatment.[25,26] It is now accepted worldwide that RT schedules should not be permitted to last longer than the planned 6 or 7 weeks for breaks related to either acute reactions or patients' convenience. Any lost treatment days should be compensated for with some fractions of increased dose by special rules.[13] Dramatic reductions in tumor control (eg, 10–25% or more absolute loss of local control per week) can potentially result from the prolongation of therapy beyond standard schedules.[27] This was a major change in RT strategy in the 1990s.[28]

Accelerated Hyperfractionation

Accelerated hyperfractionated schedules typically employ two fractions per day and are theoretically ideal at about the same overall time as T_k, the start of compensatory proliferation. For head and neck tumors, T_k has been estimated to be 32 days[29] or 21 days.[30–32]

Accelerated schedules range from 54 Gy in 11 days (CHART[33]), through 3 weeks,[34] through $3\frac{1}{2}$ weeks,[35] through 4 weeks,[36,37] through 5 weeks,[38] through $5\frac{1}{2}$ weeks,[15] through 6 weeks.[39,40] From all of these clinical trials, the best approach to an optimum overall time for head and neck tumors or other carcinomas should eventually emerge. Non–small cell lung tumors appear to repopulate about equally as fast as head and neck tumors. So a trend for shorter overall times is apparent for many carcinoma tumor types.

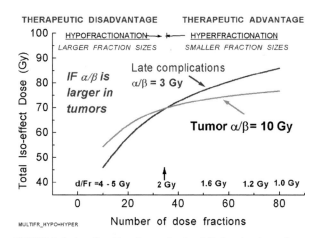

THERAPEUTIC DISADVANTAGE   THERAPEUTIC ADVANTAGE

HYPOFRACTIONATION → ←— HYPERFRACTIONATION
LARGER FRACTION SIZES   SMALLER FRACTION SIZES

IF α/β is larger in tumors

Late complications α/β = 3 Gy

Tumor α/β = 10 Gy

d/Fr = 4 - 5 Gy   2 Gy   1.6 Gy   1.2 Gy 1.0 Gy

MULTIFR_HYPO+HYPER

FIGURE 3-1. Isoeffect lines (normalized at 2 Gy fractions) as a function of total dose versus number of fractions (or dose per fraction). Late complications behave differently from tumor response (or early complications): more and smaller fractions increase the therapeutic ratio.

Hypofractionation ("Walk the Other Way")

The exceptions to the principles derived from the first two of the four parameters described above are now mentioned briefly here. First, it is obvious that in the exceptional circumstance of tumors with a smaller α/β ratio than late-responding tissues at risk, the general preference for hyper- over hypofractionation should obviously be reversed. There is much current discussion about this possibility for prostate tumor RT, in which the α/β ratio for tumors might be as low as 1.5 Gy but the ratio for late rectal and bladder complications is probably 3 Gy or higher.[41–48] The possibly low α/β ratio for the prostate may be due to the slow proliferation of tumor clonogens (similar to late-responding normal tissues).

The second situation, in which a few large fractions might be better than 2 Gy fractions given five times a week, is if the tumors proliferate very quickly, so that the standard overall times of 6 to 8 weeks allow too much tumor cell repopulation.[16,23,24] This situation can easily arise in some, but not all, tumors of the head and neck or the lung.[49] Here the two important parameters are the kickoff time T_k of compensatory proliferation of clonogenic cells in the tumors and their average doubling time T_p, neither of which is well known in any individual tumor. As noted above, this implies optimal fractionation schedules with overall treatment times similar to T_k (20–30 days).[50]

A third opening for hypofractionation is rather new and currently being investigated. For small target volumes, less than about 5 cm spherical diameter, therefore containing early-stage tumors, quite high doses and doses per fraction can be given, for example, three fractions of 15 to 23 Gy in 2 weeks if the tumors are in "parallel-type" tissues, such as the lung or liver.[49] This follows from clinical experience with well-tolerated, small, high-dose brain volumes in stereotactic radiosurgery.[51]

Late-Responding Normal Tissues

Two treatment limitations arise for late complications. One is for dose and the other for volume, and they are closely related, except for very small lesions (less than about 1 cm³) receiving high doses, which certain organs could tolerate. An extensive list of tolerance doses, estimated based on clinician experience, has been tabulated by Emami and colleagues for organs partially irradiated with hypothetical uniform doses to one-third of, two-thirds of, or the full organ volume.[52] Despite their usefulness, however, those values can be viewed only as rough estimates based on pre–three-dimensional treatment planning era clinical experience. Collection of dose-volume tolerance data and associated modeling is ongoing,[53,54] and dose-volume factors are discussed below for end points relevant to IMRT. For normal tissues nonuniformly irradiated, which is the usual situation, methods of reducing dose distributions to a single equivalent biologically effective uniform dose have been suggested, along with methods of estimating NTCP, which

is also discussed below. A long learning curve is essential for this study, but a good source of further information is the *Seminars in Radiation Oncology* issue edited by Ten Haken.[53]

Examples of dose values often thought of as limiting (before IMRT) have been the 35×2 Gy = 70 Gy in 7 weeks schedule for head and neck tumors, whose BED of 117 Gy3 is not regularly exceeded in any schedule throughout the world. The 70 Gy dose has been achieved only by coning down the irradiated volume toward the end of a treatment. Before the use of this technique, a standard head and neck treatment would be 30×2 Gy = 60 Gy, which was gradually increased to 66 Gy in Europe and to 70 Gy in the United States. Furthermore, a maximum late BED to the rectum of 110 to 125 Gy3 in treatments for cervical carcinoma has been found from a variety of low–, medium–, and high–dose rate schedules.[36] These rectal doses are restricted to 80 to 85% of the prescribed dose to the tumor edge at "point A."

Normal tissues have been classified into two types, series function or parallel function, depending on their functional construction.[55,56] Many series function organs are hollow, and their structural function can be destroyed (the most serious complication) by a high dose to a small (yet large enough) section of the wall, like a link in a chain being broken. The spinal cord, on the other hand, is not hollow and may be able to recover from a very small-volume injury.[57] Series-type organs include the spinal cord, small and large intestine, esophagus, rectum, peripheral nerves, and urethra. These organs cannot usually be given more than about 50 Gy (in NTD3) to any part, and the probability of damage increases very rapidly above that dose. For low rates of complications, the risk is expected to increase linearly with the volume given a high dose, that is, any dose over about 50 to 55 Gy. An exception to this expected behavior is when the hot spot is so small as to be repairable (analogous to repair of small skin lesions) or when the tissue also has a parallel function, as for absorption in the small intestine. Even a single "hot spot" in a series-type organ could cause a complication. Such complications can be serious, such as stenosis or fistulae, requiring surgical repair (if possible).

Three-dimensional conformal radiation therapy (3DCRT) and IMRT may significantly impact the type of complications observed and the absolute risk, as in the case of late rectal damage. The use of 3DCRT and IMRT has reduced the "all around the circumference" rectal irradiation to a narrow strip along the anterior surface of the rectal wall. The circumference is no longer irradiated to high doses, so complications have changed from stenoses—requiring serious surgical intervention—to bleeding from limited areas. As further discussed below, if the rectal surface area given a high dose is restricted to 25% (not circumferential), then doses up to 70 Gy are tolerated, with a limited incidence of bleeding, which, however, rises steeply for larger areas irradiated.[58,59] This is an example of the way in which 3DCRT or IMRT can change the nature of the late complications, with a reduction in serious consequences (Figure 3-2). The result is that stenoses have virtually disappeared as complications, being replaced by bleeding from irradiated areas of rectal wall, which can be treated without major surgery.[58,59]

Parallel function organs are quite different.[55] Parallel function organs each consist of many similar biologic subunits, such as alveoli in lungs, tubules in kidneys, and lobules in liver. Some function could be lost, but a complication would not result until function is reduced below a critical level. Complications for parallel function organs therefore move along a functional continuum in damage, which is typically categorized by the necessary medical intervention. Tolerance can be thought of as a high-dose volume which equals the reserve capacity volume; any further damage reduces function below what is physiologically required. Experience from accidents or from surgical removals has shown that one kidney can be removed, or more than half of the liver, or one lobe of a lung, with good survival of patients. Normal parallel function organs always have excess capacity. It has often been found that mean dose correlates well with complication rates in parallel function organs,[60,61] for reasons that are still unclear. In such organs, limited portions can be irradiated to very high doses provided that the mean dose to the whole organ is kept below tolerance, for example, about 20 Gy in 2 Gy fractions for both lungs considered as a pair but with the tumor volume excluded.[61–63] IMRT will have opportunities here as more knowledge of the limiting doses in those

terms and in models that use more features of the dose-volume histogram (DVH) is obtained.

Early-Responding Normal Tissues

A new proposal has recently been discussed for estimating acute mucosal reactions. This was derived from an overview of worldwide head and neck cancer RT schedules, some of which were intolerable, such that these schedules are no longer used. These tolerance BED levels have yet to be tested for mucosal tolerance in other parts of the body.[9] In this, $\alpha/\beta = 10$ Gy was assumed, $\alpha = 0.35$ Gy^{-1}, $T_k = 7$ days, and a doubling time T_p of 2.5 days, with a limiting tolerance BED of 59 to 63 Gy10 (Gy10 denotes the assumption of $\alpha/\beta = 10$ for early effects).

It appears that with some of the newly emerging schedules, acute tolerance might be reached at doses below those that cause late complications to be limiting, which has often been the case when conventionally long schedules of 6 to 8 weeks have been shortened. It is suggested that if the estimated Gy10 BEDs for a proposed schedule approach the range suggested above, then a dose escalation study should be carried out as an initial part of the project. The clinical data to obtain these values were analyzed before the advent of IMRT, so the treatment volumes are generally large, covering the whole of the mouth and pharynx. Relative volumes are considered quantitatively by Bentzen and colleagues.[64]

It was notable that a difference of 1 day altered the total mucosal BED by about 1 Gy10. This is close to the loss of BED by 1 Gy10 per day reported for head and neck tumors by Fu and colleagues,[23] which would lose about 2% of TCP per day of prolongation beyond T_k. Thus, a rough cost-benefit algorithm can be imagined for shortening schedules, which some radiation oncologists have operated by clinical judgment, consciously or not.

IMRT and 3DCRT: What Are the Main Radiobiologic Differences?

Technically, IMRT allows for dose shaping or sculpting, both in terms of isodose contour shape and the spatial placement of nonuniform doses within the target. IMRT can therefore be seen as minimizing the volume of the target that receives a lower than desired (prescribed) dose owing to required avoidance of normal tissues.[65] As implied, however, taking advantage of IMRT relies critically on our knowledge of tumor and normal tissue dose-volume factors. New (or rather increasingly important) radiobiologic issues include the following:

1. Increased involvement of quantitative clinical radiobiology in the prescription and treatment planning process (eg, in the specification of dose-volume constraints)
2. Increased need for reliable information on dose-volume effects to safely guide prescriptions
3. Increased need for information about the usefulness

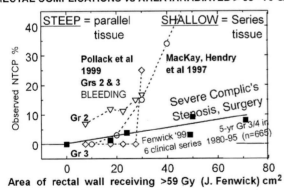

FIGURE 3-2. The major change in the type of late rectal reaction with the advent of three-dimensional conformal radiation therapy (3DCRT) and intensity-modulated radiation therapy: from stenosis, requiring major surgical repair (*full line and squares at bottom*, proportional to volume of rectum before 3DCRT, Fenwick et al; *squares* [Fenwick]), to bleeding from the high-dose volume in the rectal wall (*dashed curves*: Pollack et al,[161] *diamonds*, MacKay et al,[162] *circles*). The volume effect for bleeding is much steeper than the volume effect for stenosis and is more characteristic of a parallel function tissue. NTCP = normal tissue complication probability.

of nonuniform target dose distributions (ie, dose distributions with small cold volumes and/or large boost volumes)

These issues are further discussed in workshop proceedings reported by Deasy and colleagues.[54] Currently, data are sparse in all of these areas. As Paliwal and colleagues recently wrote, "the science of optimizing therapeutic gain lags significantly behind the capability to deliver IMRT."[66]

Because IMRT dose distributions vary greatly between individuals, it is impossible to run clinical trials that answer all of the relevant questions about the dose-volume factors needed for treatment planning. Any particular clinical trial is designed to, at best, answer one particular quantitative question. No clinical trial can be designed to determine the correct dose-volume NTCP model and additionally yield an accurate determination of the model parameters. The most powerful analyses will eventually be those that combine disparate data sets (single-institution and multi-institution clinical trial datasets) for combined analyses. Of course, many methodologic and technical issues will need to be addressed, not the least being differences in scoring complication end points.

Unfortunately, analyzing dose distributions versus outcomes produced in the 3DCRT era and then using those data to predict the effect of how improved (IMRT) dose distributions will affect patients is inherently risky, being highly extrapolative. Typically, in a 3DCRT-based dose-volume analysis, several dose-volume cutoff points will correlate with outcome (if any do at all). The selection of DVH constraints on which to base IMRT prescriptions is therefore usually uncertain. Ultimately, reliable dose-volume models must be based on dose distributions that are like those being considered for an individual patient, thereby moving closer to interpolation instead of extrapolation. For this reason, we are in a phase transition between pre-IMRT dose-volume data sets and IMRT dose-volume data sets. For the foreseeable future, therefore, most dose-volume outcome models must be considered relatively uncertain in details, although they may nevertheless be useful mathematical statements of how to improve IMRT dose distributions.

Dose-Rate Effects in IMRT

External beam RT is usually delivered with dose rates of 1 to 4 Gy/min delivered to several different fields within a 10-minute period. Experimental data, from both in vitro and clinical experience with brachytherapy treatment, demonstrate that fewer cells are killed per unit dose as the dose rate is reduced.[13] This is consistent with the two-track interpretation of the β component. Typically, the rate of lesion repair slows down with time. Hence, it cannot be modeled using a single exponential.[67,68] Recently, Fowler reported that measured residual damage owing to radiation in the form of single- or double-strand breaks (transections) of deoxyribonucleic acid (DNA) is repaired with

kinetics (time dependency), which is fairly well modeled as a reciprocal time term.[69] That is, the number of residual lesions is reduced in proportion to the inverse of the elapsed time: the same fractional reduction is seen in going from 10 to 20 minutes as in going from 30 to 60 minutes (a factor of 2 in both cases).

This effect is already operative at perhaps the 5 to 10% level when dose delivery is protracted from 5 up to 20 minutes, as seen in calculations and measured cell-kill experiments.[70,71] One potentially important implication for IMRT is that 2 Gy fractions delivered effectively in 1 to 2 minutes may be slightly more biologically effective than doses delivered in segments over, for example, 20 minutes.[72,73] This effect, predicted to be about 5 to 10% from repair kinetics models,[72] has also been observed in vitro.[73,74] Animal dose-rate studies also have shown a significant difference between 1 Gy/min and 0.1 Gy/min dose rates (Figure 3-3).[71] This implies that fast IMRT may be biologically more effective than slow IMRT, except for tumors with unusually low α/β ratios (possibly including prostate cancer).[41,43–45,47,48] (See Chapter 18.9, "Impact of Prolonged Treatment Times: Emerging Technology".)

Tumor Oxygenation

At partial oxygen pressures below about 20 mm Hg, cell survival is significantly enhanced owing to increasing repair of free radical damage.[‡] It may require two to three times more dose to reach the same level of cell kill compared with well-oxygenated conditions.[3] Tumor oxygenation varies on both microscopic and macroscopic scales and, at a given location, can either be acute (variable in time) or chronic. Compared with normal tissue vasculature, tumor vascula-

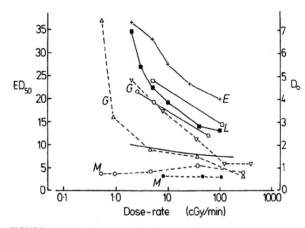

FIGURE 3-3. The dose-rate effect in normal tissues of the mouse, as compiled by Steel (used with permission). E = epilation; G = GI; L = lung; M = bone marrow. There is a significant increase in effect (and the fall in the dose required to reach an end point) between 10 cGy/min (2 Gy in 20 minutes) and 100 cGy/min (2 Gy in 2 minutes). This may have implications for slow deliveries of IMRT and stereotactic radiosurgery.

[‡]The presence of molecular oxygen frequently leads to the irreparable fixation of DNA damage.

ture and microvasculature are often geometrically chaotic and disorganized.[75] Molecular oxygen (O_2) delivered via hemoglobin diffuses away from capillaries and is absorbed by nearby cells. At large enough distances from all capillaries (greater than about 70 μm), the resulting oxygen content is low enough to reach hypoxic conditions. This is known as diffusion-limited oxygenation and is a chronic condition at least until substantial cell kill occurs. In addition, perfusion-limited oxygenation, whereby the local hemoglobin delivery system is simply inadequate, even near a capillary, is also common. Moreover, tumor blood flow varies temporally, resulting in acute hypoxia.[76] These effects together result in both chronic hypoxia (only slowly varying, on the order of days) and acute hypoxia (changing in seconds, minutes, or hours).

It is believed that several days after tumor irradiation, the preferential elimination of normoxic cells leads to a reoxygenation of hypoxic cells, which face reduced competition for resources. The mathematical effects of reoxygenation have been studied.[77] Recently, limited efforts have been made to study tumor reoxygenation during therapy using oxygenation probes and nuclear medicine markers (positron emission tomography),[18–22] and the results have been highly variable. Much further work will be needed to fully understand reoxygenation during RT.

Coleman and colleagues reviewed the present state of knowledge regarding the role of hypoxia and its relationship to treatment outcome (typically negative).[78] As reported by Chapman and colleagues, extreme hypoxia affects the α and β values differently.[79] They reported a reduction in α by a factor of 1.75 and a factor of 3.25 for β in Chinese hamster cells. The effect of hypoxia is therefore expected to decrease with fraction size. The greater effect on β may not seem surprising because β kill requires the interaction of two lesions, either of which can be affected by a lack of oxygen.

Recently, Nahum and colleagues modeled the dose-response curve for prostate treatment outcomes, including a fraction of (completely) hypoxic tumors, based on clinical hypoxia measurements.[80] These investigators found that although normoxic prostate tumors may be well controlled at doses of 70 Gy, only a fraction of hypoxic tumors are expected to be controlled at that dose. Mixed populations of hypoxic and normoxic tumors, for several different prostate-specific antigen patient groups, were chosen to produce good agreement with the clinical dose-response data (Figure 3-4). The Nahum and colleagues' results support the possibility that hypoxic tumors may, at least for prostate cancer, represent a significant fraction of clinical failures at high doses, possibly even the majority.

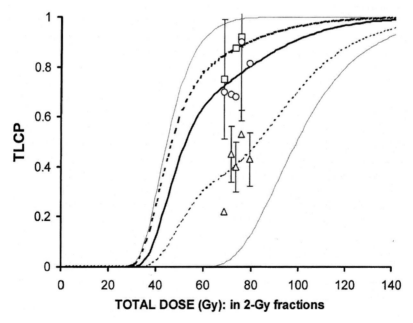

External-beam: Hanks' data vs *TLCP* model predictions

FIGURE 3-4. Local control versus total doses for external beam treatment of prostate cancer: the possible impact of hypoxic tumors on local control. Tumor control probability was modeled for well-oxygenated (*leftmost*) and hypoxic (*rightmost*) tumors whose clonogens otherwise have the same variable radiosensitivity parameters. "The three intermediate curves describe patient populations whose hypoxic tumor/aerobic tumor ratios are 15/85 (*dashed*), 25/75 (*full*), and 60/40 (*dotted*) from left to right, respectively." The data points are local control rates for patient groups with increasing prostate-specific antigen (PSA) levels (*squares* = lowest PSA levels; *circles* = intermediate; *triangles* = highest), taken from Hanks et al.[163] One standard deviation error bars are shown. Reproduced with permission from Nahum et al.[80]

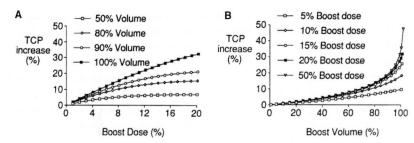

FIGURE 3-5. The modeled effect of boosting a significant fraction of a gross tumor volume, as taken from Goitein et al.[164] The tumor control probability (TCP) model is based on Poisson statistics and an assumed Gaussian interpatient spread in radiosensitivity values (the dose-response slope parameter, gamma 50, was set to 2.0). Parameters were chosen to yield 50% TCP with no boost. (*A*) shows that TCP increases (in absolute response percentage points) significantly as the boost dose (the extra dose to the boost volume) is increased, although the effect tends to saturate above 20% boost dose. The increase in TCP from the boost increases as the boost volume increases, as shown in (*B*).

Tumor Dose-Volume Effects
Hot Spots and Partial Tumor Boosts

Several authors have considered the effect of partially boosting tumor dose distributions when the entire volume cannot be given a high dose owing to normal tissue constraints, in an effort to improve TCP.[66,81,82] Modeling results have been very consistent in predicting that partial tumor (gross target volume [GTV]) boosts are likely to improve TCP if no more than a small fraction of the GTV must be left relatively "cold" (ie, unboosted). As shown in Figure 3-5, the boost volume dose needs to be no more than 20% greater than the cold spot dose to obtain maximum benefit (the predicted benefit saturates). Relatively hot boosts may be looked at as reducing the likelihood that a recurrence will be located only in the boost volume. The boost volume, if dosimetrically hot enough, effectively reduces the volume of tumor at which recurrence might occur to that of the nonboost region.

However, there are several reasons why leaving small cold spots on the edge of the planning target volume or even the clinical target volume may be even less detrimental, and tumor boosts may be even more beneficial than expected strictly from the modeling[65]: (1) after tumor regression, small cold spots may not overlap with tumor cells; (2) significant parts of the clinical target volume may, in fact, contain no tumor cells[65]; and (3) tumors are likely to be spatially heterogeneous with respect to various factors, such as hypoxia, tumor phenotype, and blood supply.[83] A spatially nonuniform tumor is likely to respond more favorably, on average, to a partial tumor boost than a uniformly resistant tumor.[65] Partial tumor boosts have become practical now owing to the advent of IMRT. IMRT can be said to be a technology for reducing the volume of necessary target underdosage (owing to nearby normal structures) to a minimum.

Effect of Cold Spots

The effect of cold spots on the edge of (or inside) a tumor (the GTV, not the planning target volume) has also been

mathematically modeled.[82,84,85] The potentially adverse effect on local control of a cold spot on the edge of a tumor is very difficult to estimate owing to tumor regression during therapy, patient geometric variations (setup changes and normal anatomy changes), and variations in radiosensitivity across the tumor.[86] These obstacles make treatment planning TCP calculations problematic unless the disease is highly indolent, imaging defines the target well, and the setup is highly reproducible. TCP models do warn that even small (< 10% volume) cold spots in GTVs need to be irradiated to a reasonably high dose to avoid reduced local control (Figure 3-6). The volume of any potential cold spot should be minimized, indeed, because the effect of a partial volume underdosage increases strongly with volume (see Figure 3-6).

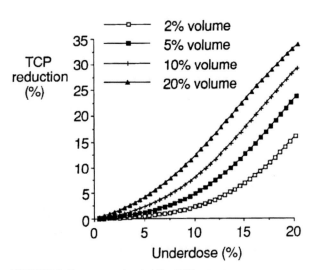

FIGURE 3-6. Tumor control probability (TCP) reduction owing to partial volume underdosage. The expected reduction in TCP (in absolute response percentage points) for a dose distribution that is uniform except for an underdosed region. Parameters were chosen such that TCP is 50% for a uniform dose. Modest dose variations (less than 5%) for underdosed volumes of 10% or less have only a small impact on TCP. However, even relatively small underdosed volumes can negatively affect outcome if the underdose exceeds 5%. Taken from Goitein et al.[164]

Tumor Clonogen Density near and outside Gross Disease

Pathology data, especially from surgical studies, form the basis for understanding the probability of local unimageable tumor extension. The International Commission on Radiation Units and Measurements provides a useful discussion of the problem of local tumor extension for the purposes of defining the region of possible subclinical disease.[87] Chao and colleagues recently presented a useful analysis of quantitative information regarding the probability of pathologically finding tumor cells at a given distance from the gross tumor margin.[88] For breast carcinoma, squamous cell carcinoma of the lung, and adenocarcinoma of the lung, the probability of observing a (usually isolated) microscopic tumor deposit was well fitted by an exponential falloff as a function of distance from the tumor edge (Figure 3-7).[§] Chao and colleagues also presented data showing the falloff of the likelihood of positive lymph nodes with approximate distance from the gross disease. The data clearly indicate that there is a greatly declining risk of microscopic extension of lymph node involvement as a function of distance from the tumor. These types of data provide some basis, for example, for increased sparing of the contralateral parotid gland in head and neck IMRT.

Dose Response of Subclinical Disease

How much dose is required to sterilize microscopic or subclinical tumor cell deposits? Withers and colleagues published a very useful summary of dose-response information for subclinical disease (Figure 3-8).[89,90] A nearly universal dose-response curve for microscopic disease was found that is very shallow, reaching zero control only at very low doses (0–20 Gy). They explained that this is expected based on the presumed logarithmic size distribution of microscopic deposits of disease owing to exponential growth. The clinical implication of the subclinical dose-response curve is that although 50 to 55 Gy is adequate to ensure sterilization of subclinical disease, delivering even lower doses (eg, to spare parotid function) will still reduce the risk of subclinical recurrence.

NTCP Models

The inclusion of NTCP models has two motivations: (1) many of the reports on dose-volume factors are in the form of models or dose-volume cutpoints such as those discussed here and (2) IMRT treatment planning is sometimes driven by radiobiologically relevant computerized goals (called radiobiologic optimization, which is further discussed below). The relationship between commonly used dose-volume constraints and complication probability models is also discussed.

The basic idea underlying NTCP modeling is that dose volume–based factors, and potentially other patient-related factors, are weighted together to form a "damage metric," which represents the x-axis of a dose-response curve, as shown in Figure 3-9. The goal of NTCP modeling is usually to find a function and corresponding parameters that best predict the risk of a given complication. Models that mix dose-based metrics with other patient- or disease-based prog-

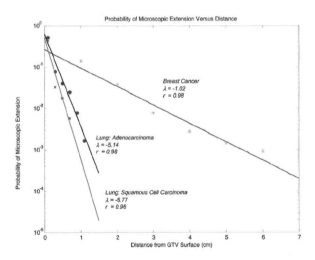

FIGURE 3-7. Data and exponential fits to the probability of microscopic extension, taken from Chao et al. The data, for lung and breast tumors, show that the falloff of microscopic extension is a steep function of distance from the edge of the gross tumor volume (GTV).

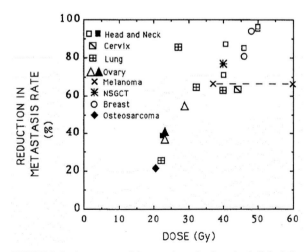

FIGURE 3-8. A summary of data on the reduction of subclinical disease as a function of dose, as compiled by Withers et al. The data show that even if less than the conventional regional irradiation dose of 50 to 55 Gy is given, owing to possible normal tissue constraints, the probability of controlling any subclinical disease can still be high. In particular, even doses as low as 40 Gy may sterilize nearly 70% of all subclinical disease deposits.

[§]However, the doubtful assumption is made that the probability of local microscopic disease is independent of the presence of other microscopic extension in the same patient. Although the data did not allow it, a more useful analysis would give the relative number of patients with microscopic extension beyond various distances rather than the raw number of microscopic foci.

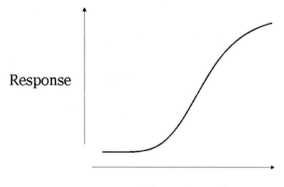

FIGURE 3-9. The fundamental idea of normal tissue complication probability (NTCP) modeling: a "damage metric" is constructed that serves as the input to a sigmoidal probability of response (NTCP). The damage metric can be a combination of dosimetric and clinical factors.

nostic factors are relatively new but have been published by Marks and colleagues[91] and Levegrun and colleagues.[92]

Any treatment side effect can present in graded severity.[||] A modeled binary end point is then often of a group of patients, such as "all patients with greater than or equal to grade 2 esophagitis." The probability of reaching such a defined end point needs to be estimated using actuarial methods if early post-treatment deaths might be correlated with one of the predictors.

Fraction-size effects can be included in an a priori fashion by using the LQ model to convert to 2 Gy fraction dose values (NTD values).[8,11] Alternatively, α/β ratios can be derived directly from the data.

Two commonly used NTCP models for estimating complication rates from the dose distribution are described here.

Lyman-Kutcher-Burman Model

In a slightly modified form to what is usually written, the three-parameter Lyman-Kutcher-Burman (LKB) model[93,94] can be expressed as

$$\text{NTCP}(\text{EUD}_a) = \frac{1}{\sqrt{2\pi}} \int_{-\infty}^{t} du \exp(-u^2/2) \quad (8)$$

where

$$t = (\text{EUD}_a - \text{TD}_{50})/(m\text{TD}_{50}) \quad (9)$$

TD_{50} is the 50% response dose, and the maximum slope of the response curve is inversely proportional to m. The equivalent uniform dose (EUD) is actually just the generalized mean value (as defined in Abramowitz and Stegun[95]) of the dose distribution:

[||]The Radiation Therapy Oncology Group (RTOG)/European Organization for the Research and Treatment of Cancer (EORTC) scale of toxicity grades is 0 = none, 1 = minor, 2 = requires treatment, 3 = requires hospitalization, 4 = life threatening, and 5 = lethal.[165]

$$\text{EUD}_a = \left(\sum_{i=1}^{} v_i d_i^a \right)^{1/a}. \quad (10)$$

The notation used here is that of Niemierko.[96] The important point is that the EUD tends toward the maximum dose when a is very large, toward the mean dose when a approaches 1, and toward the minimum dose when a is large in magnitude but negative.[95,97] The value of a can be optimized to give the best fit to the data. (Note that the traditional LKB notation uses a parameter, n, which is the inverse of the EUD's a.)

The LKB model may be viewed as a model in which average functional damage (represented by the surrogate EUD_a) must accumulate above a given level (TD_{50}) before a complication is likely.

Parallel Function Model

For some tissues, as noted, even very high doses to small volumes may not lead to a complication, although local function may be irreversibly affected. Correspondingly, a volume threshold effect may exist (ie, the volume irradiated to a high dose). This biologically based insight can be codified with the parallel function model suggested by Jackson and colleagues[98] (or a similar model suggested by Niemierko and Goitein[99]). Yorke and colleagues remarked that lung complications appear to have such a volume threshold.[100] The parallel function model first attempts to directly estimate functional damage by assuming that local functional damage follows a sigmoid curve. The volume-averaged mean functional damage (f_{dmg}) is then given by

$$f_{\text{dmg}} = \sum_{i=1}^{\text{voxels}} v_i p(d_i), \quad (11)$$

where $p(d_i)$ is the local function reduction curve and is the fractional volume of the ith voxel. The sigmoidal functional damage curve can be given, for example, by a simple logistic equation:

$$p(d) = \frac{1}{[1 + (d_{50}/d)^k]}, \quad (12)$$

where d_{50} is the dose to reach a 50% reduction in function, d again is the voxel dose, and k is a constant determining the slope of the response (higher k values imply steeper slopes). Again, following Jackson and colleagues,[98] we have

$$\text{NTCP}(f_{\text{dmg}}) = \frac{1}{\sqrt{2\pi\sigma_f^2}} \int_{0}^{f_{\text{dmg}}} \exp(-(f - f_{50})^2/2\sigma_f^2)df, \quad (13)$$

where f_{50} is the level for a 50% complication rate and σ_f is the standard deviation that determines the slope of the response curve. The parallel model could alternatively be interpreted as incorporating the probability of incapacitating functional subunits, but this mechanistic interpretation is unnecessary for its successful use.

The essential difference between the parallel function and LKB models is that in the LKB (power law) model, increasing the dose to one or more voxels will always increase the damage metric, whereas for the parallel function model, increasing the dose to one or more voxels eventually causes a saturation effect owing to the sigmoidal response function; therefore, any increase in dose to saturated or high-dose voxels will cause little increase in the damage metric (and therefore little change in response probability). If the local damage function $p(d)$ is very shallow (ie, nearly linear) to up to high doses (as is sometimes estimated for lung dose response), then, as Jackson and Yorke pointed out, the two models may give very similar predictions.[54]

Physiologically, the ability of some tissues to receive at least some very high doses of radiation without manifesting a clinical end point may correspond to either (1) eventual healing of a highly damaged but small volume (as for small-volume, partial-circumferential, high-dose irradiation of the rectum) or (2) reduction of functional capacity, but not beyond that needed to avoid a complication (ie, functional reserve), as may be the case for lung irradiation. Parallel-type tissues typically perform a physiologic function in parallel in repeated local subunits (eg, lung acini, nephrons in the kidney).

Use of Dose-Volume Cutpoints

Alternatively, dose-volume constraints are more intuitive and are predominantly used currently to prescribe IMRT. Conventional dose volume–based indices include, for example, the maximum dose or mean dose for normal tissues or the minimum dose or the D_{95} (the dose at the 95% volume level of the cumulative DVH) for a target volume.[#]

Dose-volume cutpoints, such as V_{20} for the relative volume exceeding 20 Gy, are often included in dose-volume effect analyses. This is equivalent to approximating the local damage function $p(d)$ in the parallel function model by an "off-on" step-function (ie, no damage below the threshold and complete damage above).[61] The use of a single cutpoint can therefore be referred to as the dose-volume threshold model.

The use of dose-volume constraints is best justified (1) when tissue damage is thought to occur only above some (approximate) dose threshold or (2) even when a dose threshold is not known accurately, a dose-volume constraint can be used to limit the high-dose part of the DVH. It is usually unreliable to use a single dose-volume con-

straint derived directly from an analysis of outcome data because, typically, many volume cutoffs will correlate with outcome (if any do).

Dose-Volume Data Relevant to IMRT Planning

This section examines complication end points with significant dose-volume effects relevant to IMRT planning, including chronic rectal injury, small bowel toxicity, and parotid salivary gland function (xerostomia). In the future, it is expected that more end points will become relevant to IMRT (particularly for lung treatment planning but also for other sites).

Rectal Complications

Clinical DVH-based analyses indicate that the probability of rectal bleeding is related to the volume of rectal wall that receives a high dose,[101–108] as already shown in Figure 3-2. Importantly, the probability of late rectal bleeding may also be correlated with the shape of the lesions created: high-dose regions that completely encompass the circumference of the rectum are thought to be more likely to cause chronic bleeding than lesions that do not encompass the rectal circumference. Such topologic dose features, which are not derivable from DVHs, may be crucial to the accurate estimation of the risk of late rectal complications. Investigators at Memorial Sloan-Kettering Cancer Center recently reported that the dichotomous variable "enclosure of the outer rectal contour by the 50% isodose line on the isocenter computed tomography (CT) slice" was significant in a logistic regression analysis of late rectal bleeding factors.[108]

Johannessen and colleagues reported on an attempt to model the probability of rectal stenosis for rat rectal (single fraction) partial volume irradiation.[109] For that end point, the tissue behaved like a parallel-type structure with a significant "functional reserve" and was well fit by the parallel tissue model. Computed DVHs were perhaps known with more confidence than for human data because single fractions were used. Their results support the concept that the human rectum can tolerate a small hot spot (if consistently positioned between fractions).

Huang and colleagues recently reported that late rectal complications at 6 years after 3DCRT were strongly correlated with the high-dose rectal volume: for patients with > 26.2% rectal volume irradiated to > 70 Gy, 54% had grade 2 or higher complications; for all other patients, only 13% had grade 2 or higher sequelae.[58]

In an analysis based on 331 patients, Vargas and colleagues noted that "rectal wall V_{60} and V_{70} are closely associated with chronic rectal toxicity [grade 2 and 3]."[59] Acute and chronic toxicity were significantly correlated.

Dale and colleagues recently fitted the LKB model to a questionnaire survey of rectal late effects for convention-

---

[#]The popularity of the D_{95} as a designation may be partly due to the technical aspects of current IMRT optimization algorithms, which tend not to significantly penalize very small cold spots.

al fractionation conformal prostate RT.[101] Interestingly, late effects (diarrhea, rectal mucous discharge, rectal bleeding, rectal pain, bowel cramps, or bowel gas) were correlated with the highest-dose part of the rectum DVH, including the rectal interior (EUD "*a*" parameter greater than 10). In this data set, complications were more highly correlated with the highest dose volume. In addition, better correlations were found if the entire rectal volume was used as the LKB volume reference rather than the restricted volume recommended by Emami and colleagues.[52]

As summarized by Jackson and colleagues,[54,103] most current DVH analyses have shown a correlation between the high-dose volume (> 65–70 Gy) and the probability of late rectal bleeding (Figure 3-10). It is possible, however, that lower-dose regions (40–50 Gy) also contribute to the probability of late rectal bleeding.

However, distention of the rectum (mostly owing to the presence of stool) commonly causes shifts of up to about 1 cm. Obviously, rectal motion depends strongly on immobilization techniques. The pretreatment-based DVH may be either hotter or colder than the true accumulated DVH, which is delivered. This "smearing" of the dose distribution probably affects the analysis of rectal complications. Little has been done to quantify the effect of rectal motion on modeled outcome parameters. Another problem, less recognized, is that single-institution DVH guidelines may depend critically on the setup and immobilization techniques used and therefore may have less prognostic significance elsewhere.

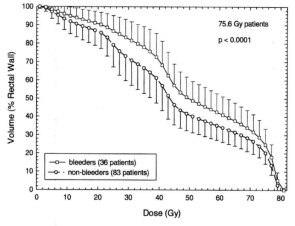

FIGURE 3-10. Late rectal bleeding from external beam radiation therapy treatment to 75.6 Gy, as reported by Jackson et al.[104] Average dose-volume histograms (DVHs) for patients with late rectal bleeding (*squares*) and without late rectal bleeding (*circles*) are shown. Bars show the standard deviation of the corresponding DVHs at each dose point. The *p* value is with respect to the null hypothesis that bleeders and nonbleeders have the same distribution of DVH shapes. This curve illustrates the difficulty of choosing a dose threshold below which the volume irradiated does not matter.

Small Bowel Complications

Chronic intestinal morbidity (radiation enteropathy) typically presents 6 months to 3 years post-therapy.[110] Characterized by dysmotility, malabsorption, and diarrhea, the symptoms are often recurrent. Long term, about 10% of patients may die as a direct result of radiation enteropathy. Some form of chronic intestinal dysfunction from RT is present in approximately 60 to 90% of patients. The number of cancer survivors in the United States living with long-term bowel symptoms can be estimated to be approximately 1 to 2 million people.[110] It may be surprising, therefore, that so little has been reported about small bowel toxicity as a function of treatment volume. Acute and late effects are not completely independent bowel injuries.[111]

Baglan and colleagues studied dose-volume factors for acute bowel toxicity for rectal cancer chemoradiotherapy (5-fluorouracil) for standard fractionation three-field pelvic RT to 45 Gy.[112] They did not fit an NTCP model to the results. Instead, they determined a DVH threshold, that is, a clear line (threshold DVH), which divided high-risk from low-risk patients. No other clinical factors were found to correlate with acute toxicity. The threshold DVH is not a direct determination of the effect of different parts of the DVH on radiation risk because the DVHs were very similar in shape (same treatment technique). The line merely divides the higher-risk treatments from the lower-risk treatments. Hence, it is not a direct determination of a dose-volume effect, only a start toward it.

Gallagher and colleagues reported on acute and late small bowel effects for 150 consecutive patients who received abdominal irradiation, most receiving 45 to 50 Gy in 1.8 to 2.0 Gy fractions.[113] The presence and severity of acute diarrhea correlated strongly with the volume of small bowel irradiated ($p < .001$): 43 patients with no diarrhea had mean in-field bowel volumes of 58 cc, 30 had mild diarrhea with a mean volume of 116 cc, 29 had responsive (to treatment) diarrhea with a mean volume of 342 cc, and 5 had unresponsive diarrhea with a mean volume of 485 cc. Pretreatment surgery, which often increased the volume of irradiated small bowel, was significantly correlated with the risk of both acute and chronic morbidity. Chronic diarrhea (mild or responsive to treatment) was associated with increased volumes irradiated to doses above 45 to 50 Gy.

Roeske and colleagues reported on acute gastrointestinal toxicity in 50 gynecology patients treated using IMRT.[114] They found a highly significant correlation between the volume of the small bowel receiving at least 45 Gy (in 1.8 Gy fractions) and clinically significant acute toxicity. As a function of the high-dose volume, the complication frequency reached 25% at about 300 cc. The proposed dose-response curve is shown in Figure 3-11.

Letschert and colleagues reported on late small bowel toxicity based on estimates of the volume of small bowel in the high-dose region (50 Gy in 25 fractions) in RT for

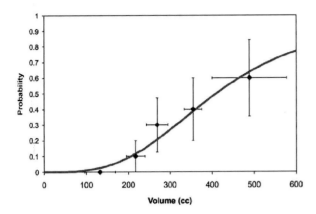

FIGURE 3-11. Acute gastrointestinal complications for whole-pelvis treatment delivered with intensity-modulated radiation therapy. Complications included "moderate to severe" grade 2 symptoms. The dose response is a function of the volume of small bowel receiving at least the prescription dose of 45 Gy. Data points consist of 10 patients each. Reproduced with permission from Roeske et al.[114]

rectal cancer.[115] They reported that chronic diarrhea was observed to increase in incidence when the treatment volumes exceeded about 178 cc (to a maximum of about 50% incidence at 5 years). The type of surgery also affected the risk.

Mundt and colleagues reported on the use of IMRT to reduce normal tissue irradiation while still covering pelvic clinical target volumes for gynecologic malignancies.[116] IMRT provides a reduced volume of small bowel irradiation, and this is reflected in a significant decrease in chronic small bowel toxicity (primarily diarrhea), 11% (IMRT) versus 50% (conventional pelvic RT).

Parotid Salivary Gland Damage (Xerostomia)

Xerostomia is the most prevalent late side effect of radiation to the head and neck area and is cited by patients as the primary cause of decreased quality of life after RT.[117,118] In addition to its effects on subjective well-being, decreased saliva output causes alterations in speech and taste and the potential for secondary nutritional deficiencies. Oral mucosal dryness creates a predisposition to fissures and ulcers, and changes in the composition of the oral flora lead to dental caries and infections. As Amosson and colleagues wrote, "Xerostomia affects every aspect of life including speech, nutrition, taste, and sleep. Patients live with a constant reminder of their diminished quality of life."[119]

The treatment of xerostomia has been unsatisfactory or expensive.[120,121] The major salivary glands produce 80 to 90% of salivary secretions, and the minor salivary glands produce the remainder.[60]

Recent advances in conformal RT, such as IMRT, enable partial sparing of the parotid gland.[122] IMRT allows the treatment planner to "sculpt the high-dose region to largely avoid the parotid glands. However, one or both of the parotid glands often abut the region that needs a high dose,

and some irradiation of the parotid glands is typically unavoidable. A quantitative model of the reduction of parotid function for varying possible dose distributions is therefore highly desirable as a guide to whether a dose distribution will be well tolerated.

Amosson and colleagues analyzed the subjective response of 30 patients to xerostomia-related questions.[119] They found that patients typically felt that they had "adequate" saliva when the contralateral (less irradiated) gland mean dose was 16.2 Gy or less in 25 fractions. They felt that they had "too little" saliva at a mean dose of 22.5 Gy or greater. This agrees qualitatively with our results, which are discussed below.

Eisbruch and colleagues reported the University of Michigan experience with contralateral sparing of parotid glands during head and neck RT.[123] The mean dose thresholds for both unstimulated and stimulated parotid saliva flow rates to reduce to < 25% of pretreatment levels (ie, the definition of xerostomia) were 24 and 26 Gy (in approximately 35 fractions), respectively. They recommend giving less than 26 Gy to a parotid gland to preserve substantial gland function.

Roesnik and colleagues modeled the reduction in individual parotid flow rates using the LKB model.[124] They originally derived an exponential parameter $a < 1$ but fixed it at one, for reasons that were not stated. From that NTCP analysis, they derived a TD_{50} mean dose of 35 to 39 Gy in 25 to 35 fractions.

The current Washington University xerostomia data set, building on previous work presented by Chao and colleagues[60] and Blanco and colleagues,[125] consists of 55 patients with pretreatment and post-treatment measurements of relative salivary function (at 6 months post-RT and a smaller data set at 12 months), primarily Peacock IMRT treatments (Nomos Corporation, Sewickley, PA).[60] Quality-of-life data were collected. Figure 3-12 summarizes measured stimulated salivary flow 6 months after the end of RT relative to pretreatment values and shows the main trend as a function of gland mean doses.

Analysis showed that the data could be described with a simple "mean-dose exponential" equation[60,126]:

$$\text{Relative total flow} = \frac{\left[\exp[-A \cdot \bar{d}_L] + \exp[-A \cdot \bar{d}_R]\right]}{2}.$$

(14)

This model simply says that salivary flow is reduced exponentially, for each gland individually, according to the value of that gland's mean dose ($\bar{d}_L$ or $\bar{d}_R$). The coefficient A was found to be 0.054/Gy (95% CI 0.046–0.067; $n = 55$). That is, parotid glands lose function at a rate of approximately 5% per Gy. This coefficient yields a threshold dose (25% function) of 25.8 Gy (in 35 fractions), which is consistent with Michigan's data (28 Gy, determined at 1-year follow-up) but lower than Roesnik and colleagues' value (35–39

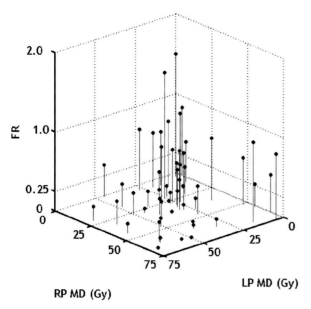

FIGURE 3-12. Salivary flow as a function of parotid gland mean doses. Data show total stimulated salivary flow (FR) 6 months after head and neck radiation therapy, relative to pretreatment values (Washington University data set), as a function of right and left parotid mean doses (RP MD and LP MD). The data imply that if one or the other parotid gland is shielded to below 15 to 20 Gy, xerostomia (a drop below 25% of the pretreatment level) is unlikely.

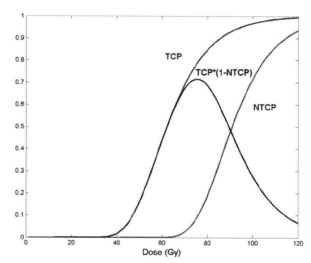

FIGURE 3-13. The basic principle of radiobiologic optimization. The leftmost sigmoid represents tumor response, and the rightmost sigmoid represents the probability of normal tissue complications (NTCP). The peaked curve is the result of multiplying the left curve (local control) by one minus the right curve (complication-free treatment) to yield the probability of complication-free local control. Ideally, by using favorable fractionation and highly conformal dose distributions to reduce the volume of critical normal tissue irradiated, the complication-free control can reach a high peak, resulting in the possibility of treating to a high local control rate with a low complication rate. TCP = tumor control probability.

Gy).[124] Figure 3-12 is consistent with the 26 Gy value: if both glands receive more than about 25 to 30 Gy, salivary flow is poor, whereas if both glands receive less, salivary flow is significantly higher. The mean dose exponential model also statistically significantly correlated with quality-of-life answers 6 months after the end of RT.

The data and model imply that attempting to minimize the parotid mean dose, ideally included in the IMRT objective function, consistent with desired target doses, may help protect salivary function.

Radiobiologic Optimization of Treatment Plans

What is radiobiologic optimization? Here we take it to mean the numeric attempt to produce the radiobiologically best treatment plan. Ideally, optimization would refer only to the actual attainment of optimal (ie, unimprovable) solutions. However, there is no good substitute for the usage as given here, which is at least consistent with current usage in medical physics. The basic idea is shown in Figure 3-13: we hope to choose a dose level that obtains a high TCP with a low NTCP. Radiobiologic criteria are typically quantified through NTCP dose-volume models but also through the EUD function, or DVH cutpoints, as discussed above. In addition to being used to judge or rank alternative dose distributions,

in radiobiologically optimized IMRT treatment planning, the equations themselves (or with modifications) are used to drive the optimization process: that is, there is a search for the best plan according to the equations. Each equation relating to a different end point can be referred to as an "objective function term," and the overall combination that is minimized to drive IMRT treatment planning is the "objective function." Sometimes dosimetric or radiobiologic terms are used in the solution as constraints not to be violated. Langer and colleagues give definitions of the basic terminology of IMRT treatment planning optimization.[127]

For reasons given above, TCP is typically unreliable when computed in treatment planning systems, so we focus on the use of NTCPs. As an example, the minimization of mean dose to each parotid salivary gland, constrained by target dose requirements, could be viewed as radiobiologically relevant. Another example might be to maximize the EUD value of a target volume (with a negative value of the parameter a to emphasize the lower dose part of the DVH), along with normal tissue constraints.

Given all of the uncertainties in the NTCP models available, one may fairly ask, "Why attempt radiobiologically driven IMRT treatment planning?" There is a straightforward, albeit two-part, answer: (1) outcomes models are continually improving and will not always be considered "unreliable," and (2) when an IMRT treatment plan is analyzed using outcomes-based model predictions (NTCP and TCP), the inevitable question is "Could another plan be produced that is better according to outcomes measures?" Answering this important question requires radiobiologically based optimized treatment planning. The Memorial Sloan-Kettering Cancer Center group made the case for radiobiologic optimization:

> ...for certain clinical situations, it is not sufficient to specify the objectives of optimization purely in terms of the desired pattern of the dose. The objectives must also include dose-volume effects and biological indices. ...it is imperative that the criteria of optimization be specified in a clinically relevant manner.[128]

The earliest reported use of radiobiologic criteria to drive IMRT treatment planning is from Miller[129] and is remarkably also the first report on either the planning or delivery of IMRT. Miller stated, "Beam modifications derived in this way...provide conformal isodose distributions which are related directly to the probabilities of disease control and treatment complications."[129] This is still the rationale for radiobiologic optimization. This section introduces the use of radiobiologic information directly in the IMRT optimization process (see Chapter 2, "Physics of IMRT").

Radiobiologic Objective Functions

Briefly, any of the TCP or NTCP models, or surrogates such as EUD or dose-volume metrics (eg, V_{20}), could be used as an objective function term. Sometimes these objective function terms are combined into a single equation, the probability of complication-free control or complication-free cure,** which can be written under the assumption of no correlation between normal tissue and tumor response as TCP × (1 − NTCP). A similar estimate is denoted P_+, referred to as a "complication-free cure" by Brahme and Kallman and colleagues.[130,131] This or a similar objective function can then be optimized using straightforward unconstrained optimization methods. However, such equations do not reflect the clinical reality that reductions in the probability of local control are considered by clinicians and patients quite differently from the risk of complications (some of which can be mild or very manageable). Lack of local control is (currently) almost always associated with death for the patient, whereas most RT complications are manageable despite being undesirable. In the other direction, some complications are almost always avoided (eg, radiation myelopathy), even at the cost of inferior target dose distributions, and this is not reflected in complication-free cure, as noted by Goitein.[132]

As noted above, dose-volume constraints are radiobiologically relevant in the sense that they can approximate the dose threshold, above which damage is assumed to be severe and below which damage is assumed to be negligible. For most tissues, it is still unknown whether the local tissue damage function is steep enough, as a function of dose, for the approximation to be valid. In this sense, the use of dose-volume constraints can be considered a simplified version of radiobiologic optimization. We briefly discuss two approaches: using only radiobiologic objective terms in the objective function and the addition of constraints, which can either be radiobiologic objective function terms or dose and dose-volume factors.

Unconstrained Optimization of the Probability of Complication-Free Local Control

As discussed above, these methods seek to optimize a single objective function using simple unconstrained optimization techniques, as chiefly used by the Stockholm group.[131,133–137] The basic approach has been developed into a commercial module in the *Pinnacle* treatment planning system (Philips Medical Systems, Andover, MA) by Lof and colleagues.[138] Various types of local search algorithms are used, including the gradient descent algorithm. The seriality NTCP model is used.[139] A potential correlation between complication and local control probability is also included. As recognized by Brahme, many of the input parameters need further clinical study.[133]

Compared with purely physical optimization techniques, optimizing the probability of uncomplicated control typically results in high doses to a large part of the target.[140] This occurs owing to the predicted favorable effect of partial tumor boosts previously discussed. However, as Vaarkamp and Krasin have noted, "The very fact that clinically unsuitable dose distributions are found signals that the biologic objective function is somehow an incomplete description of clinical reality."[141] Furthermore, they suggest that in the specific case of unacceptably high tumor doses, a new NTCP term could be introduced that "could model the probability of tissue matrix break down in the tumor." This is an approach also implemented by the Richmond group using EUD functions instead of NTCPs.[142] Compared with constrained optimization methods, unconstrained optimization of complication-free control will typically be faster. As mentioned, however, unintended trade-offs between incommensurate entities and end points are likely to occur.

An advantage of EUD-based optimization compared with optimization based solely on dose-volume constraints is that the search process may improve normal tissue doses beyond that which might be rather arbitrarily set prior to planning.[143] As a technical consideration, the search space for dose-volume constraint–based optimizations is inherently more complex than that defined by EUD-based problems, and the efficiency of a solution may reflect this.[144,145]

**This is a misnomer because it has always been the case that only the probability of locoregional control, not cure, is estimated. Distant disease may exist independently.

Constrained Optimization of Radiobiologic Objective Functions

Ideally, biologic indices could be used either as objective function terms or as constraints. However, when the (large scale) problem is formulated in this way, general nonlinear solvers are typically slow (ie, taking 10 minutes or much more on current hardware).[††] An interesting approach is that of the Tubingen group, who formulated the planning problem as a constrained optimization problem of a set of EUD-like functions.[138,146] A detailed sensitivity analysis of the problem is routinely obtained using Lagrange multipliers.[146] Thus, the EUD value of any given structure can be constrained to be less than or more than some clinically relevant value. In practice, however, EUD values cannot be made strictly responsive to the highest or lowest doses in a volume because EUD is inherently sensitive to many voxels unless the parameter is extremely large in magnitude.

Radiobiologically based objective functions and dose-based constraints (such as maximum and minimum permissible doses) can be combined into a single framework (see Stavrev and colleagues[147]). Wu and colleagues demonstrated a two-stage algorithm designed to produce a good plan according to both radiobiologic (ie, EUD) criteria and dose-volume criteria and reported good results.[143]

Another promising approach has been proposed by Chen and colleagues: they solve difficult nonlinear problems (potentially radiobiologically relevant) by repeatedly making quadratic approximations to the nonlinear objective function at the current dose estimate.[148] That is, there is an inner loop (solution of the quadratic approximation to the objective function) and an outer loop (approximation of the nonlinear objective functions based on the local dose distribution). This approach is consistent with the smooth nature of radiobiologic objective functions, especially if the logarithm of the model is used.

The main points concerning IMRT treatment planning with radiobiologically relevant objective functions can be summarized as follows:

- Radiobiologically relevant mathematical functions can be incorporated into the IMRT treatment planning process.
- Radiobiologically relevant objective functions may increase the quality of the treatment plans by driving plans further in the direction of improvements compared with dose-volume constraints fixed in an a priori fashion.
- Radiobiologically relevant objective functions can be mixed with dose-volume constraints (to prevent large hot regions or unacceptably cold spots in the target or small hot spots in serial function normal structures).

- Data collection and modeling to validate radiobiologically relevant objective functions are ongoing. Hence, their relevance will increase.
- Dose-volume constraints can be viewed as a type of radiobiologically relevant objective function that roughly separates volumes into "heavily damaged" versus "undamaged."
- In some cases, even simple mathematical functions, such as the mean dose, can be highly radiobiologically relevant, as when the mean dose to the parotid glands (or normal lung tissue) is included in the IMRT objective function.

Two (More) Unresolved Issues
Low-Dose Hyperradiosensitivity

Low-dose hyperradiosensitivity is a departure from the expected LQ cell survival behavior at low doses[149,150] consisting of a steeper than normal initial part to the LQ cell survival curve (denoted α_s) at doses below about 0.5 Gy, followed at higher doses by a plateau or hill and then the typical LQ shape, but with a lower (normal) α value (Figure 3-14). Contrary to impressions made by some recent reviews, this phenomenon was first found in experimental animals (renal damage in mice) and confirmed as being reproducible in small daily fractions.[149] As summarized in Figure 3-15, nearly 50 cell lines have now been investigated by Joiner and colleagues showing increases in α values by factors from 1 to 30, as quantified by the hyperradiosensitivity ratio, defined as α_s/α_r. The median ratio was 6.7.[151]

The implication is that even when α_s/α_r is not large, very small (< 0.25 Gy) fractional doses may be significantly

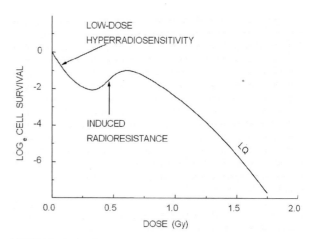

FIGURE 3-14. A schematic showing typical hyperradiosensitivity cell survival. The hyperradiosensitivity ratio is defined as the slope of the linear extrapolation to zero dose at very low doses, divided by the α coefficient of the linear-quadratic fit at relatively high doses (> 0.75 Gy). The transition zone may comprise a valley and a hill or be relatively flat.

[††]Our experience includes the use of standard packages, such as MINOS and the NAG solver.

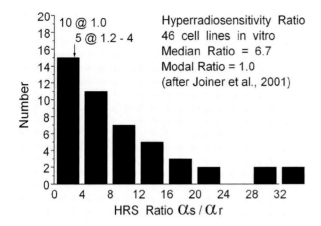

FIGURE 3-15. Summary of hyperradiosensitivity ratio data from Joiner's group. Although there are many cell lines with relatively low hyperradiosensitivity ratios, the median ratio is 6.7. Data have accrued that the effect is primarily related to an inactive G_2/M checkpoint in cycling cells. The checkpoint is activated only at high damage levels.

more cytotoxic than expected, whereas changes in fraction size above about 0.75 Gy are consistent with LQ behavior. Consequently, for a given total dose delivered in fractions, cell kill could be significantly enhanced if only very small fractions are used (termed "ultrafractionation"[152,153]).

In a recent publication, Joiner and colleagues plausibly attribute the phenomenon to the avoidance at very low doses of a checkpoint in the cell cycle (G_2/M) that, if not activated, could lead to premature entry into mitosis before repair can take place.[154] The implication is that "actively proliferating cell populations may therefore demonstrate a greater increase in radiosensitivity to very low radiation doses compared with quiescent populations."[155] That is, hyperradiosensitivity might affect only tumor and acutely responding normal tissue response, excluding late-responding normal tissues.

Based on mathematical modeling results, Redpath and colleagues concluded that when hyperradiosensitivity is significant, cell killing may suppress the rate of malignant transformation.[156] This might have implications for the likelihood of radiation-induced second malignancies but needs further clinical investigation.

Presumably, this hyperradiosensitivity at very low doses effect must have been present before it was identified.[149] It is surprising that we have not become further aware of its biologic effects, if significant, either before or after then. It may be that hyperradiosensitivity in human tissues is not a large or very common effect and is difficult to detect in volumes of tissue given low total doses except in those experiments especially designed to investigate it, such as top-up animal experiments or in vitro automated colony trackers.[149,150]

The only unambiguous clinical test of hyperradiosensitivity is that of Turesson and Joiner, who showed definitively that 0.45 Gy/fraction doses are much more potent than 1.1 Gy/fraction with an end point of basal cell density in skin.[157] Thus derived, the hyperradiosensitivity ratio was about 2. This result is far below the median hyperradiosensitivity of 6 from cell lines in vitro. The lower human value rightly leads to caution and the need for more observations.

If hyperradiosensitivity is further validated in human tissues, two potential treatment planning principles may then apply: first, in tissues in which hyperradiosensitivity is active (acutely responding normal tissues), some irradiated volumes receiving between 0.25 Gy/fraction and 0.75 Gy/fraction could just as well be increased to 0.75 Gy/fraction if a gain in tumor response might thereby be achieved or if irradiation of critical late-responding normal tissues could be thereby reduced. That is, in some instances, instead of spreading around very small-dose tails via rotational or many-beam IMRT therapy, fields or beamlets might beneficially be concentrated into volumes delivering up to about 0.75 Gy. Second, and in contrast, when the tumor is embedded in a late-responding normal tissue (eg, in brain), using very small fractional doses may confer a therapeutic advantage, a possibility that is being studied.[153]

Second Malignancies

Second malignancies many years after successful RT have been well investigated.[158,159] Although they do occur in irradiated volumes (and only in that way can they be distinguished from the normal risk of 25% of the population getting cancer in their lifetime), the frequency is not high, except in patients treated with adjuvant chemotherapy. Hall and Wuu recently concluded that the lifetime risk of a radiation-induced carcinoma following RT is approximately 1% for 3DCRT treatment and is predicted to increase to about 1.75% for IMRT (see Chapter 30, "Pros and Cons of IMRT: What's Been Swept Under the Rug?").[158] However, there were many large uncertainties involved in the estimates, including the dose-transformation curve, the method accounting for increased leakage radiation, potential reductions in integral dose with IMRT compared with 3DCRT because the high-dose volume is smaller, and the beam energy used (not considered). Based on the bladder cancer data reviewed by Hall and Wuu,[158] the risk of radiation-induced second malignancies may sometimes be surprisingly independent of dose. Future technical developments may decrease this risk, which depends on the particle type (eg, protons deliver smaller integral doses[160]), particle energy (photon fields below 12 MV do not produce neutrons), and leakage shielding designs. Overall, the imperative to control a tumor at the time of treatment far outweighs the small stochastic chance of a second tumor many years ahead.

References

1. Fowler JF. Radiobiological issues in IMRT. In: Paliwal BR, Fowler JF, Herbert DE, et al, editors. Sixth International Conference on Dose, Time and Fractionation in Radiation Oncology: Biological and Physical Basis of IMRT and Tomotherapy. Madison (WI): Medical Physics Publishing; 2001. p. 8–22.

2. Goffman TE, Glatstein E. Intensity-modulated radiation therapy. Radiat Res 2002;158:115–7.

3. Hall EJ. Radiobiology for the radiologist. 4th ed. Philadelphia: Lippincott; 1994.

4. Steel GG. Basic clinical radiobiology. London: Arnold; 2002.

5. Withers H, Thames, HD, Peters LJ. Differences in the fractionation response of acutely and late-responding tissues. In: Kärcher KH K, HD, Reinartz G, editors. Progress in radio-oncology. Vol II. 1992. p. 287–96.

6. Peters L, Ang KK, Thames HD. Accelerated fractionation in the radiation treatment of head and neck cancer. A critical comparison of different strategies. Acta Oncol 1988;27:185–94.

7. Thames H, Withers HR, Peters LJ, et al. Changes in early and late radiation responses with altered dose fractionation: implications for dose-survival relationships. Int J Radiat Oncol Biol Phys 1982;8:219–26.

8. Fowler J. The linear-quadratic formula and progress in fractionated radiotherapy. Br J Radiol 1989;62:679–94.

9. Fowler JF, Harari PM, Leborgne F, et al. Acute radiation reactions in oral and pharyngeal mucosa: tolerable levels in altered fractionation schedules. Radiother Oncol 2003;69:161–8.

10. Maciejewski B, Taylor JM, Withers HR. Alpha/beta value and the importance of size of dose per fraction for late complications in the supraglottic larynx. Radiother Oncol 1986;7:323–6.

11. Joiner MC, Bentzen SM. Time-dose relationships: the linear-quadratic approach. In: Steel GG, editor. Basic clinical radiobiology. London: Arnold; 2002. p. 120–33.

12. Thames HD, Hendry JH. Fractionation in radiotherapy. New York: Taylor & Francis; 1987.

13. Bentzen SM, Baumann M. The linear-quadratic model in clinical practice. In: Steel G, editor. Basic clinical radiobiology. London: Arnold; 2002. p. 134–46.

14. Stuschke M, Thames HD. Hyperfractionated radiotherapy of human tumors: overview of the randomized clinical trials. Int J Radiat Oncol Biol Phys 1997;37:259–67.

15. Skladowski K, Maciejewski B, Golen M, et al. Randomized clinical trial on 7-day-continuous accelerated irradiation (CAIR) of head and neck cancer—report on 3-year tumour control and normal tissue toxicity. Radiother Oncol 2000;55:101–10.

16. Withers H, Taylor JMG, Maciejewski B. The hazard of accelerated tumor clonogen repopulation during radiotherapy. Acta Oncol 1988;27:131–46.

17. Begg AC, Steel GG. Cell proliferation and growth rate of tumours. In: Steel GG, editor. Basic clinical radiobiology. London: Arnold; 2002. p. 8–22.

18. Cooper RA, West CM, Logue JP, et al. Changes in oxygenation during radiotherapy in carcinoma of the cervix. Int J Radiat Oncol Biol Phys 1999;45:119–26.

19. Koh WJ, Bergman KS, Rasey JS, et al. Evaluation of oxygenation status during fractionated radiotherapy in human non-small cell lung cancers using [F-18]fluoromisonidazole positron emission tomography. Int J Radiat Oncol Biol Phys 1995;33:391–8.

20. Lartigau E, Lusinchi A, Weeger P, et al. Variations in tumour oxygen tension (pO_2) during accelerated radiotherapy of head and neck carcinoma. Eur J Cancer 1998;34:856–61.

21. Stadler P, Feldmann HJ, Creighton C, et al. Changes in tumor oxygenation during combined treatment with split-course radiotherapy and chemotherapy in patients with head and neck cancer. Radiother Oncol 1998;48:157–64.

22. Dunst J, Hansgen G, Lautenschlager C, et al. Oxygenation of cervical cancers during radiotherapy and radiotherapy + cis-retinoic acid/interferon. Int J Radiat Oncol Biol Phys 1999;43:367–73.

23. Fu KK, Pajak TF, Trotti A, et al. A Radiation Therapy Oncology Group (RTOG) phase III randomized study to compare hyperfractionation and two variants of accelerated fractionation to standard fractionation radiotherapy for head and neck squamous cell carcinomas: first report of RTOG 9003. Int J Radiat Oncol Biol Phys 2000;48:7–16.

24. Fowler JF, Harari PM. Confirmation of improved local-regional control with altered fractionation in head and neck cancer. Int J Radiat Oncol Biol Phys 2000;48:3–6.

25. Begg AC, McNally NJ, Shrieve DC, et al. A method to measure the duration of DNA synthesis and the potential doubling time from a single sample. Cytometry 1985;6:620–6.

26. Wilson GD, Dische S, Saunders MI. Studies with bromodeoxyuridine in head and neck cancer and accelerated radiotherapy. Radiother Oncol 1995;36:189–97.

27. Fowler JF, Lindstrom MJ. Loss of local control with prolongation in radiotherapy. Int J Radiat Oncol Biol Phys 1992;23:457–67.

28. Hendry JH, Bentzen SM, Dale RG, et al. A modeled comparison of the effects of using different ways to compensate for missed treatment days in radiotherapy. Clin Oncol (R Coll Radiol) 1996;8:297–307.

29. Brenner D. Accelerated repopulation during radiotherapy: quantitative evidence for delayed onset. Radiat Oncol Invest 1993;1:167–72.

30. Roberts SA, Hendry JH. The delay before onset of accelerated tumour cell repopulation during radiotherapy: a direct maximum-likelihood analysis of a collection of worldwide tumour-control data. Radiother Oncol 1993;29:69–74.

31. Roberts SA, Hendry JH, Brewster AE, et al. The influence of radiotherapy treatment time on the control of laryngeal cancer: a direct analysis of data from two British Institute of Radiology trials to calculate the lag period and the time factor. Br J Radiol 1994;67:790–4.

32. Robertson C, Robertson AG, Hendry JH, et al. Similar decreases in local tumor control are calculated for treatment protraction and for interruptions in the radiotherapy of carcinoma of the larynx in four centers. Int J Radiat Oncol Biol Phys 1998;40:319–29.

33. Dische S, Saunders M, Barrett A, et al. A randomised multicentre trial of CHART versus conventional radiotherapy in head and neck cancer. Radiother Oncol 1997;44:123–36.

34. Slevin NJ, Hendry JH, Roberts SA, et al. The effect of increasing the treatment time beyond three weeks on the control of T2 and T3 laryngeal cancer using radiotherapy. Radiother Oncol 1992;24:215–20.

35. Bourhis J, De Crevoisier R, Abdulkarim B, et al. A randomized study of very accelerated radiotherapy with and without amifostine in head and neck squamous cell carcinoma. Int J Radiat Oncol Biol Phys 2000;46:1105–8.

36. Leborgne F, Fowler J, Leborgne JH, et al. Biologically effective doses in medium dose-rate brachytherapy of cancer of the cervix. Radiat Oncol Invest 1997;5:289–99.

37. Wang CC. Local control of oropharyngeal carcinoma after two accelerated hyperfractionation radiation therapy schemes. Int J Radiat Oncol Biol Phys 1988;14:1143–6.

38. McGinn CJ, Harari PM, Fowler JF, et al. Dose intensification in curative head and neck cancer radiotherapy—linear quadratic analysis and preliminary assessment of clinical results. Int J Radiat Oncol Biol Phys 1993;27:363–9.

39. Knee R, Fields RS, Peters LJ. Concomitant boost radiotherapy for advanced squamous cell carcinoma of the head and neck. Radiother Oncol 1985;4:1–7.

40. Overgaard J, Hansen, HS, Overgaard, M, et al. Conventional radiotherapy as primary treatment of squamous cell carcinoma of the head and neck. A randomized multicenter study of 6 vs 5 fractions per week—report from the DAHANCA 7 trial. Int J Radiat Oncol Biol Phys 1997;39:188.

41. Fowler JF, Ritter MA, Fenwick JD, et al. How low is the alpha/beta ratio for prostate cancer? In regard to Wang et al. IJROBP 2003;55:194–203. Int J Radiat Oncol Biol Phys 2003;57:593–5; author reply 595–6.

42. Fowler JF, Ritter MA, Chappell RJ, et al. What hypofractionated protocols should be tested for prostate cancer? Int J Radiat Oncol Biol Phys 2003;56:1093–104.

43. King CR, Fowler JF. Yes, the alpha/beta ratio for prostate cancer is low or "methinks the lady doth protest too much…about a low alpha/beta that is." Int J Radiat Oncol Biol Phys 2002;54:626–7; author reply 627–8.

44. Denham JW. Prostate cancer: low alpha/beta the only consideration? In regard to Fowler, Chappell, and Ritter: the prospects for new treatments for prostate cancer. Int J Radiat Oncol Biol Phys 2002;53:1394–5; author reply 1395.

45. Dale RG, Jones B. Is the alpha/beta for prostate tumors really low? In regard to Fowler et al., IJROBP 2001;50:1021–1031. Int J Radiat Oncol Biol Phys 2002;52:1427–8; author reply 1428.

46. King CR, Fowler JF. A simple analytic derivation suggests that prostate cancer alpha/beta ratio is low. Int J Radiat Oncol Biol Phys 2001;51:213–4.

47. Fowler J, Chappell R, Ritter M. Is alpha/beta for prostate tumors really low? Int J Radiat Oncol Biol Phys 2001;50:1021–31.

48. Brenner DJ, Martinez AA, Edmundson GK, et al. Direct evidence that prostate tumors show high sensitivity to fractionation (low alpha/beta ratio), similar to late-responding normal tissue. Int J Radiat Oncol Biol Phys 2002;52:6–13.

49. Timmerman R, Papiez L, McGarry R, et al. Extracranial stereotactic radioablation: results of a phase I study in medically inoperable stage I non-small cell lung cancer. Chest 2003;124:1946–55.

50. Mehta M, Scrimger R, Mackie R, et al. A new approach to dose escalation in non-small-cell lung cancer. Int J Radiat Oncol Biol Phys 2001;49:23–33.

51. Levegrun S, Ton L, Debus J. Partial irradiation of the brain. Semin Radiat Oncol 2001;11:259–67.

52. Emami B, Lyman J, Brown A, et al. Tolerance of normal tissue to therapeutic irradiation. Int J Radiat Oncol Biol Phys 1991;21:109–22.

53. Ten Haken RK, editor. Partial organ irradiation. Semin Radiat Oncol 2001;11.

54. Deasy JO, Niemierko A, Herbert D, et al. Methodological issues in radiation dose-volume outcome analyses: summary of a joint AAPM/NIH workshop. Med Phys 2002;29:2109–27.

55. Withers HR, Taylor JM, Maciejewski B. Treatment volume and tissue tolerance. Int J Radiat Oncol Biol Phys 1988;14:751–9.

56. Marks LB. The impact of organ structure on radiation response. Int J Radiat Oncol Biol Phys 1996;34:1165–71.

57. Bijl HP, van Luijk P, Coppes RP, et al. Dose-volume effects in the rat cervical spinal cord after proton irradiation. Int J Radiat Oncol Biol Phys 2002;52:205–11.

58. Huang EH, Pollack A, Levy L, et al. Late rectal toxicity: dose-volume effects of conformal radiotherapy for prostate cancer. Int J Radiat Oncol Biol Phys 2002;54:1314–21.

59. Vargas C, Kestin LL, Yan D, et al. Dose-volume analysis of predictors for chronic rectal toxicity following treatment of prostate cancer with high-dose conformal radiotherapy. Int J Radiat Oncol Biol Phys 2003;57:S398–9.

60. Chao KS, Deasy JO, Markman J, et al. A prospective study of salivary function sparing in patients with head-and-neck cancers receiving intensity-modulated or three-dimensional radiation therapy: initial results. Int J Radiat Oncol Biol Phys 2001;49:907–16.

61. Seppenwoolde Y, Lebesque JV, de Jaeger K, et al. Comparing different NTCP models that predict the incidence of radiation pneumonitis. Int J Radiat Oncol Biol Phys 2003;55:724–35.

62. Kwa SL, Lebesque JV, Theuws JC, et al. Radiation pneumonitis as a function of mean lung dose: an analysis of pooled data of 540 patients. Int J Radiat Oncol Biol Phys 1998;42:1–9.

63. Marks LB. Dosimetric predictors of radiation-induced lung injury. Int J Radiat Oncol Biol Phys 2002;54:313–6.

64. Bentzen SM, Saunders MI, Dische S, et al. Radiotherapy-related early morbidity in head and neck cancer: quantitative clinical radiobiology as deduced from the CHART trial. Radiother Oncol 2001;60:123–35.

65. Deasy JO. Partial tumor boosts: even more attractive than theory predicts? Int J Radiat Oncol Biol Phys 2001;51:279–80.

66. Paliwal BR, Brezovich IA, Hendee WR. POINT/COUNTERPOINT: "IMRT may be used to excess because of its higher reimbursement from Medicare." Med Phys 2004;31:1–3.

67. Foray N, Badie C, Alsbeih G, et al. A new model describing the curves for repair of both DNA double-strand breaks and chromosome damage. Radiat Res 1996;146:53–60.

68. Foray N, Monroco C, Marples B, et al. Repair of radiation-induced DNA double-strand breaks in human fibroblasts is consistent with a continuous spectrum of repair probability. Int J Radiat Biol 1998;74:551–60.

69. Fowler J. Repair between dose fractions: a simpler method of analyzing and reporting apparently bi-exponential repair. Radiat Res 2002;158:141–51.

70. Steel GG, Deacon JM, Duchesne GM, et al. The dose-rate effect in human tumour cells. Radiother Oncol 1987;9:299–310.

71. Steel GG, Down JD, Peacock JH, et al. Dose-rate effects and the repair of radiation damage. Radiother Oncol 1986;5:321–31.

72. Fowler JF, Welsh JS, Howard SP. Loss of biological effect in prolonged fraction delivery. Int J Radiat Oncol Biol Phys 2004;59(1):242–49.

73. Morgan WF, Naqvi SA, Yu C, et al. Does the time required to deliver IMRT reduce its biological effectiveness [abstract]? Int J Radiat Oncol Biol Phys 2002;54:222.

74. Ling CC, Spiro IJ, Stickler R. Dose-rate effect between 1 and 10 Gy/min in mammalian cell culture. Br J Radiol 1984;57:723–8.

75. Brown JM, Giaccia AJ. The unique physiology of solid tumors: opportunities (and problems) for cancer therapy. Cancer Res 1998;58:1408–16.

76. Dewhirst MW. Presented at the BIROW Workshop; 2003 Jan; Washington, DC.

77. Okunieff P, Hoeckel M, Dunphy EP, et al. Oxygen tension distributions are sufficient to explain the local response of human breast tumors treated with radiation alone. Int J Radiat Oncol Biol Phys 1993;26:631–6.

78. Coleman CN, Mitchell JB, Camphausen K. Tumor hypoxia: chicken, egg, or a piece of the farm? J Clin Oncol 2001;20:610–5.

79. Chapman JD, Gillespie CJ, Reuvers AP, et al. The inactivation of Chinese hamster cells by x-rays: the effects of chemical modifiers on single- and double-events. Radiat Res 1975;64:365–75.

80. Nahum AE, Movsas B, Horwitz EM, et al. Incorporating clinical measurements of hypoxia into tumor local control modeling of prostate cancer: implications for the alpha/beta ratio. Int J Radiat Oncol Biol Phys 2003;57:391–401. (See comment in Int J Radiat Oncol Biol Phys 2004;58:1637–39.)

81. Tome WA, Fowler JF. Selective boosting of tumor subvolumes. Int J Radiat Oncol Biol Phys 2000;48:593–9.

82. Goitein M, Niemierko A, Okunieff P. The probability of controlling an inhomogeneously irradiated tumour: a stratagem for improving tumour control through partial tumour boosting. In: Proceedings of the 19th L H Gray Conference: Quantitative Imaging in Oncology; 1997.

83. Molls M, Vaupel P. Blood perfusion and microenvironment of human tumors: implications for clinical radiooncology. Berlin; Springer; 1998.

84. Deasy JO. Tumor control probability models for non-uniform dose distributions. In: Paliwal BR, Fowler JF, Herbert DE, editors. Fifth International Conference on Dose, Time and Fractionation in Radiation Oncology: Volume and Kinetics in Tumor Control and Normal Tissue Complications. Madison (WI): Medical Physics Publishing; 1997. p. 65–85.

85. Tome WA, Fowler JF. On cold spots in tumor subvolumes. Med Phys 2002;29:1590–8.

86. Britten RA, Evans AJ, Allalunis-Turner MJ, et al. Intratumoral heterogeneity as a confounding factor in clonogenic assays for tumour radioresponsiveness. Radiother Oncol 1996;39:145–53.

87. International Commission on Radiation Units and Measurements. Prescribing, recording and reporting photon beam therapy. Report 62. Supplement to Report 50. Bethesda (MD): International Commission on Radiation Units and Measurements; 1999.

88. Chao KS, Blanco AI, Dempsey JF. A conceptual model integrating spatial information to assess target volume coverage for IMRT treatment planning. Int J Radiat Oncol Biol Phys 2003;56:1438–49.

89. Withers HR, Peters LJ, Taylor JM. Dose-response relationship for radiation therapy of subclinical disease. Int J Radiat Oncol Biol Phys 1995;31:353–9.

90. Withers HR, Suwinski R. Radiation dose response for subclinical metastases. Semin Radiat Oncol 1998;8:224–8.

91. Marks LB, Munley MT, Bentel GC, et al. Physical and biological predictors of changes in whole-lung function following thoracic irradiation. Int J Radiat Oncol Biol Phys 1997;39:563–70.

92. Levegrun S, Jackson A, Zelefsky MJ, et al. Analysis of biopsy outcome after three-dimensional conformal radiation therapy of prostate cancer using dose-distribution variables and tumor control probability models. Int J Radiat Oncol Biol Phys 2000;47:1245–60.

93. Kutcher GJ, Burman C, Brewster L, et al. Histogram reduction method for calculating complication probabilities for three-dimensional treatment planning evaluations. Int J Radiat Oncol Biol Phys 1991;21:137–46.

94. Lyman JT. Complication probability as assessed from dose-volume histograms. Radiat Res 985;8 Suppl:S13–9.

95. Abramowitz M, Stegun I. Handbook of mathematical functions. New York: Dover Publications, Inc; 1970.

96. Niemierko A. A generalized concept of equivalent uniform dose [abstract]. Med Phys 1999;26:1100.

97. Deasy JO. Comments on the use of the Lyman-Kutcher-Burman model to describe tissue response to non-uniform irradiation. Int J Radiat Oncol Biol Phys 2000;47:1458–60.

98. Jackson A, Ten Haken RK, Robertson JM, et al. Analysis of clinical complication data for radiation hepatitis using a parallel architecture model. Int J Radiat Oncol Biol Phys 1995;31:883–91.

99. Niemierko A, Goitein M. Modeling of normal tissue response to radiation: the critical volume model. Int J Radiat Oncol Biol Phys 1992;25:135–45.

100. Yorke ED, Jackson A, Rosenzweig KE, et al. Dose-volume factors contributing to the incidence of radiation pneumonitis in non-small-cell lung cancer patients treated with three-dimensional conformal radiation therapy. Int J Radiat Oncol Biol Phys 2002;54:329–9.

101. Dale E, Olsen DR, Fossa SD. Normal tissue complication probabilities correlated with late effects in the rectum after prostate conformal radiotherapy. Int J Radiat Oncol Biol Phys 1999;43:385–91.

102. Kupelian PA, Reddy CA, Klein EA, et al. Short-course intensity-modulated radiotherapy (70 GY at 2.5 GY per fraction) for localized prostate cancer: preliminary results on late toxicity and quality of life. Int J Radiat Oncol Biol Phys 2001;51:988–93.

103. Jackson A. Partial irradiation of the rectum. Semin Radiat Oncol 2001;11:215–23.

104. Jackson A, Skwarchuk MW, Zelefsky MJ, et al. Late rectal bleeding after conformal radiotherapy of prostate cancer. II. Volume effects and dose-volume histograms. Int J Radiat Oncol Biol Phys 2001;49:685–98.

105. Storey MR, Pollack A, Zagars G, et al. Complications from radiotherapy dose escalation in prostate cancer: preliminary results of a randomized trial. Int J Radiat Oncol Biol Phys 2000;48:635–42.

106. Teshima T, Hanks GE, Hanlon AL, et al. Rectal bleeding after conformal 3D treatment of prostate cancer: time to occurrence, response to treatment and duration of morbidity. Int J Radiat Oncol Biol Phys 1997;39:77–83.

107. Fenwick JD, Khoo VS, Nahum AE, et al. Correlations between dose-surface histograms and the incidence of long-term rectal bleeding following conformal or conventional radiotherapy treatment of prostate cancer. Int J Radiat Oncol Biol Phys 2001;49:473–80.

108. Skwarchuk MW, Jackson A, Zelefsky MJ, et al. Late rectal toxicity after conformal radiotherapy of prostate cancer (I): multivariate analysis and dose-response. Int J Radiat Oncol Biol Phys 2000;47:103–13.

109. Johannessen HO, Dale E, Hellebust TP, et al. Modeling volume effects of experimental brachytherapy in the rat rectum: uncovering the limitations of a radiobiologic concept. Int J Radiat Oncol Biol Phys 2002;53:1014–22.

110. Hauer-Jensen M, Wang J, Denham JW. Bowel injury: current and evolving management strategies. Semin Radiat Oncol 2003; 13:357–71.

111. Peck JW, Gibbs FA. Mechanical assay of consequential and primary late radiation effects in murine small intestine: alpha/beta analysis. Radiat Res 1994;138:272–81.

112. Baglan KL, Frazier RC, Yan D, et al. The dose-volume relationship of acute small bowel toxicity from concurrent 5-FU-based chemotherapy and radiation therapy for rectal cancer. Int J Radiat Oncol Biol Phys 2002;52:176–83.

113. Gallagher MJ, Brereton HD, Rostock RA, et al. A prospective study of treatment techniques to minimize the volume of pelvic small bowel with reduction of acute and late effects associated with pelvic irradiation. Int J Radiat Oncol Biol Phys 1986;12:1565–73.

114. Roeske JC, Bonta D, Mell LK, et al. A dosimetric analysis of acute gastrointestinal toxicity in women receiving intensity-modulated whole-pelvic radiation therapy. Radiother Oncol 2003;69:201–7.

115. Letschert JG, Lebesque JV, Aleman BM, et al. The volume effect in radiation-related late small bowel complications: results of a clinical study of the EORTC Radiotherapy Cooperative Group in patients treated for rectal carcinoma. Radiother Oncol 1994;32:116–23.

116. Mundt AJ, Mell LK, Roeske JC. Preliminary analysis of chronic gastrointestinal toxicity in gynecology patients treated with intensity-modulated whole pelvic radiation therapy. Int J Radiat Oncol Biol Phys 2003;56:1354–60.

117. Bjordal K, Kaasa S, Mastekaasa A. Quality of life in patients treated for head and neck cancer: a follow-up study 7 to 11 years after radiotherapy. Int J Radiat Oncol Biol Phys 1994;28:847–56.

118. Harrison L, Zelefski MJ, Pfitzer DG, et al. Detailed quality of life assessment in patients treated with primary radiotherapy for cancer of the base of the tongue. Head Neck 1997;19:169–75.

119. Amosson CM, Teh BS, Van TJ, et al. Dosimetric predictors of xerostomia for head-and-neck cancer patients treated with the SMART (simultaneous modulated accelerated radiation therapy) boost technique. Int J Radiat Oncol Biol Phys 2003;56:136–44.

120. Brizel D, Wasserman TH, Strand V, et al. Final report of a phase III randomized trial of amifostine as a radioprotectant in head and neck cancer [abstract]. Int J Radiat Oncol Biol Phys 1999;45:147.

121. Johnson J, Ferretti GA, Nethery WJ, et al. Oral pilocarpine for post-irradiation xerostomia in patients with head and neck cancer. N Engl J Med 1993;329:390–5.

122. Chao KS. Protection of salivary function by intensity-modulated radiation therapy in patients with head and neck cancer. Semin Radiat Oncol 2002;12:20–5.

123. Eisbruch A, Ten Haken RK, Kim HM, et al. Dose, volume, and function relationships in parotid salivary glands following conformal and intensity-modulated irradiation of head and neck cancer. Int J Radiat Oncol Biol Phys 1999;45:577–87.

124. Roesink JM, Moerland MA, Battermann JJ, et al. Quantitative dose-volume response analysis of changes in parotid gland function after radiotherapy in the head-and-neck region. Int J Radiat Oncol Biol Phys 2001;51:938–46.

125. Blanco A, Chao CK, Deasy JO, et al. Recovery kinetics of salivary function in patients with head and neck cancers receiving radiation therapy [abstract]. Int J Radiat Oncol Biol Phys 2002;54:166.

126. Blanco AI, Chao KSC, Deasy JO, et al. Dose-volume modeling of salivary function in patients with head and neck cancer receiving radiation therapy. 2004. [Submitted]

127. Langer M, Lee EK, Deasy JO, et al. Operations research applied to radiotherapy, an NCI-NSF-sponsored workshop February 7-9, 2002. Int J Radiat Oncol Biol Phys 2003;57:762–8.

128. Wang XH, Mohan R, Jackson A, et al. Optimization of intensity-modulated 3D conformal treatment plans based on biological indices. Radiother Oncol 1995;37:140–52.

129. Miller DW. Optimization of attenuator shapes for multiple field radiation treatment. In: Paliwal BP, Herbert DE, Orton CG, editors. Optimization of cancer radiotherapy: proceedings of the Second International Conference on Dose, Time, and Fractionation in Radiation Oncology. Madison (WI): American Institute of Physics; 1984. p. 493–7.

130. Brahme A. Treatment optimization using physical and radiobiological objective functions. In: Smith AR, editor. Radiation therapy physics. New York: Springer; 1995. p. 209–46.

131. Kallman P, Lind BK, Brahme A. An algorithm for maximizing the probability of complication-free tumour control in radiation therapy. Phys Med Biol 1992;37:871–90.

132. Goitein M. The comparison of treatment plans. Semin Radiat Oncol 1992;2:246–56.

133. Brahme A. Biologically based treatment planning. Acta Oncol 1999;38 Suppl 13:61–8.

134. Soderstrom S, Gustafsson A, Brahme A. The clinical value of different treatment objectives and degrees of freedom in radiation therapy optimization. Radiother Oncol 1993;29:148–63.

135. Soderstrom S, Brahme A. Optimization of the dose delivery in few field techniques using radiobiological objective functions. Med Phys 1993;20:1201–10.

136. Asell M, Hyodynmaa S, Soderstrom S, et al. Optimal electron and combined electron and photon therapy in the phase space of complication-free cure. Phys Med Biol 1999;44:235–52.

137. Mavroidis P, Lind BK, Brahme A. Biologically effective uniform dose (D) for specification, report and comparison of dose response relations and treatment plans. Phys Med Biol 2001;46:2607–30.

138. Lof J, Lind BK, Brahme A. ORBIT: optimization of radiation therapy beams by iterative techniques, a new optimization code. In: Schlegel W, Bortfeld T, editors. Proceedings of the XIIIth International Conference on the Use of Computers in Radiation Therapy. Heidelberg: Springer; 2000. p. 49–51.

139. Kallman P, Agren A, Brahme A. Tumour and normal tissue responses to fractionated non-uniform dose delivery. Int J Radiat Oncol Biol Phys 1992;62:249–62.

140. Jones L, Hoban P. A comparison of physically and radiobiologically based optimization for IMRT. Med Phys 2002;29:1447–55.

141. Vaarkamp J, Krasin M. Reduction of target dose inhomogeneity in IMRT treatment planning using biologic objective functions. Int J Radiat Oncol Biol Phys 2001;49:1518–20.

142. Wu Q, Mohan R, Niemierko A, et al. Optimization of intensity-modulated radiotherapy plans based on the equivalent uniform dose. Int J Radiat Oncol Biol Phys 2002;52:224–35.

143. Wu Q, Djajaputra D, Wu Y, et al. Intensity-modulated radiotherapy optimization with gEUD-guided dose-volume objectives. Phys Med Biol 2003;48:279–91.

144. Deasy JO. Multiple local minima in radiotherapy optimization problems with dose-volume constraints. Med Phys 1997;24:1157–61.

145. Choi B, Deasy JO. The generalized equivalent uniform dose function as a basis for intensity-modulated treatment planning. Phys Med Biol 2002;47:3579–89.

146. Alber M, Birkner M, Nusslin F. Tools for the analysis of dose optimization: II. Sensitivity analysis. Phys Med Biol 2002;47:N265–70.

147. Stavrev P, Hristov D, Warkentin B, et al. Inverse treatment planning by physically constrained minimization of a biological objective function. Med Phys 2003;30:2948–58.

148. Chen Y, Michalski D, Houser C, et al. A deterministic iterative least-squares algorithm for beam weight optimization in conformal radiotherapy. Phys Med Biol 2002;47:1647–58.

149. Joiner MC, Johns H. Renal damage in the mouse—the response to very small doses per fraction. Radiat Res 1988;114:385–98.

150. Marples B, Joiner MC. The response of Chinese-hamster V79 cells to low radiation-doses—evidence of enhanced sensitivity of the whole cell-population. Radiat Res 1993;133:41–51.

151. Joiner MC, Marples B, Lambin P, et al. Low-dose hypersensitivity: current status and possible mechanisms. Int J Radiat Oncol Biol Phys 2001;49:379–89.

152. Short SC, Mitchell SA, Boulton P, et al. The response of human glioma cell lines to low-dose radiation exposure. Int J Radiat Biol 1999;75:1341–8.

153. Krause M, Hessel F, Wohlfarth J, et al. Ultrafractionation in A7 human malignant glioma in nude mice. Int J Radiat Biol 2003; 79:377–83.

154. Marples B, Wouters BG, Joiner MC. An association between the radiation-induced arrest of G(2)-phase cells and low-dose hyper-radiosensitivity: a plausible underlying mechanism? Radiat Res 2003;160:38–45.

155. Short SC, Woodcock M, Marples B, et al. Effects of cell cycle phase on low-dose hyper-radiosensitivity. Int J Radiat Biol 2003;79:99–105.

156. Redpath JL, Short SC, Woodcock M, et al. Low-dose reduction in transformation frequency compared to unirradiated controls: the role of hyper-radiosensitivity to cell death. Radiat Res 2003;159:433–6.

157. Turesson I, Joiner MC. Clinical evidence of hypersensitivity to low doses in radiotherapy. Radiother Oncol 1996;40:1–3.

158. Hall EJ, Wuu CS. Radiation-induced second cancers: the impact of 3D-CRT and IMRT. Int J Radiat Oncol Biol Phys 2003;56:83–8.

159. Brenner DJ, Curtis RE, Hall EJ, et al. Second malignancies in prostate carcinoma patients after radiotherapy compared with surgery. Cancer 2000;88:398–406.

160. Miralbell R, Lomax A, Cella L, et al. Potential reduction of the incidence of radiation-induced second cancers by using proton beams in the treatment of pediatric tumors. Int J Radiat Oncol Biol Phys 2002;54:824–9.

161. Pollack A, Zagars GK, Starkschall G, et al. Prostate cancer radiation dose response: results of the M. D. Anderson phase III randomized trial. Int J Radiat Oncol Biol Phys 2002;53:1097–105.

162. MacKay RI, Hendry JH, Moore CJ, et al. Predicting late rectal complications following prostate conformal radiotherapy using biologically effective doses and normalized dose-surface histograms. Br J Radiol 1997;70:517–26.

163. Hanks GE, Schultheiss TE, Hanlon AL, et al. Optimization of conformal radiation treatment of prostate cancer: report of a dose escalation study. Int J Radiat Oncol Biol Phys 1997;37:543–50.

164. Goitein M, Schultheiss TE. Strategies for treating possible tumor extension: some theoretical considerations. Int J Radiat Oncol Biol Phys 1985;11:1519–28.

165. Cox et al. Toxicity criteria of the Radiation Therapy Oncology Group (RTOG) and the European Orgaanization for Research and Treatment of Cancer (EORTC). Int J Radiat Oncol Biol Phys 1995;31:1341–6.

Chapter 4

MEDICINE OF IMRT

BAHMAN EMAMI, MD, FACR

Historical Perspective

For a long time, the planning and execution of radiation therapy (RT) were based on portals designed using planar x-ray films. Moreover, prescription and documentation were based on the dose to a single point, namely, the central axis.[1] The development, clinical use, and incorporation of computed tomography (CT) in the planning of RT were major steps forward in the field of radiation oncology, which led to true two-dimensional treatment planning.[2] Although state of the art for nearly two decades, two-dimensional approaches had significant limitations, which are well described in the literature. Novel strategies in the use of CT, along with significant progress in the science of computers and graphics, facilitated extensive research to overcome these deficiencies, leading to the creation of three-dimensional conformal radiation therapy (3DCRT).

Following the development of the first 3DCRT planning system,[3] several university-based systems were implemented in clinical practice.[4–6] However, the quantum leap forward leading to the widespread availability of 3DCRT was a series of research contracts funded by the National Cancer Institute (NCI) between 1982 and 1994.[7] At that time, new terminologies and concepts were introduced, including beam's eye view, room view, dose-volume histograms, tumor control probabilities (TCPs), and normal tissue complication probabilities (NTCPs). In addition, the work of the International Commission on Radiation Units and Measurements (ICRU) proposed the concepts of gross tumor volume (GTV), clinical target volume (CTV), planning target volume (PTV), and treatment volume.[8] Furthermore, the introduction of new computer-controlled treatment delivery systems with multileaf collimation and on-line portal imaging has made 3DCRT feasible for community use. Widespread clinical use of 3DCRT, along with advances in diagnostic radiologic imaging, has allowed the development of precise delineation of target volumes and dose conformity to the intended tar-

get volume. Although the impact of this process in improving the cure rates of cancer patients needs further follow-up, the reduction in normal tissue complication has already been seen.[9]

In spite of revolutionary progress in the technology of RT planning and delivery, 3DCRT is "forward" planning and thus essentially a trial and error approach, which depends greatly on the experience of the operator. In this regard, the treatment planner attempts to create the "best" plan to achieve the desired dose coverage. This process has to be repeated until the optimal dose and coverage are achieved. Obviously, such an approach is not only time-consuming, but, in addition, sometimes an optimal plan cannot be generated.

Intensity-Modulated Radiation Therapy

Progress in computer technology has resulted in the next revolutionary step in the planning and delivery of external beam RT, namely, intensity-modulated radiation therapy (IMRT). IMRT combines two advanced concepts to deliver 3DCRT: inverse treatment planning with computerized optimization and computer-controlled intensity modulation of the treatment beams.[10] With this approach, the planner selects the desired input parameters, and the computer then calculates the optimal beam intensities to achieve the desired dose distribution. Treatment delivery is also computer controlled. In IMRT, beam intensity is varied across the entire treatment field, and the result is highly nonuniform intensity patterns, which deliver the prescription dose to the target while sparing normal structures. Figure 4-1 illustrates an example intensity profile of a treatment beam in a patient undergoing IMRT.

The physics and planning aspects of IMRT are described in detail elsewhere in this book. In this section, attention is focused on the physician's involvement in the IMRT process. In many ways, the IMRT process is basically the

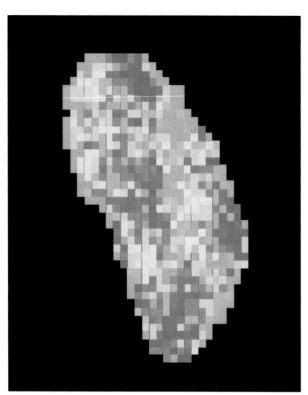

FIGURE 4-1. Intensity pattern of an intensity-modulated radiation therapy treatment beam. The red and yellow areas represent regions of high intensity, whereas the green area represents regions of low intensity. (To view a color version of this image, please refer to the CD-ROM.)

same as in conventional 3DCRT, which involves delineation of target volumes and normal tissues, optimization of treatment plans, and the delivery and documentation of treatment. The difference is that IMRT is less forgiving owing to sharp gradients between targets and normal tissues inherent in the treatment plans. Therefore, more accuracy is required in every step of the process.

Target Delineation

For delineation of target volumes, the recommendations of Report 50 of the ICRU should be followed.[8] At the present time, delineation of the GTV is primarily CT based. However, the results of recent research have confirmed the utility of other diagnostic modalities. In a recent analysis of 15 patients with nasopharyngeal cancer, Emami and colleagues demonstrated that magnetic resonance–CT fusion is important for the proper delineation of target volumes in these patients.[11] Erdi and colleagues showed that positron emission tomography (PET)-CT fusion in patients with lung cancer improves the accuracy of target delineation, thereby avoiding the inclusion of the uninvolved lungs.[12] By using ^{60}Cu-ATSM (Cu(II)-diacetyl-bis(N(4)-methyl-thiosemicarbazone) as a metabolic marker in head and neck cancers, Chao and colleagues identified hypoxic regions within the GTV.[13] Grosu and colleagues showed a significant improvement in GTV delineation in patients with

brain tumors by the fusion of ^{11}C-methionine PET and CT.[14] Multimodality imaging, as well as the ever-increasing use of fusion technology, is a focus of current research, which will have a profound impact on the practice of radiation oncology in the coming years (see Chapter 18.6, "Functional Imaging in Head and Neck Cancer: Emerging Technology"). The importance of accurate and precise delineation of the GTV, which is the basis for every subsequent step of the IMRT planning process, cannot be overemphasized.

Delineation of the CTV is more problematic. According to the recommendations of Report 50 of the ICRU, the CTV should encompass the microscopic extensions around the GTV and regional nodes potentially harboring microscopic disease.[8] Very little accurate information, however, is available regarding the latter, and the margins used to account for microscopic tumor extensions are usually based on traditional concepts. This is currently an area of active research. Inclusion of regional nodes within the irradiated volume is also under investigation. In some disease sites, such as lung cancer, routine inclusion of nodal stations within the target volume, in the absence of obvious radiographic nodal involvement, may no longer be necessary.[15] In other sites, traditional concepts on this issue are being challenged. However, when the inclusion of these nodal stations in the irradiated volume is indicated, accurate radiographic knowledge of the three-dimensional anatomy of these regions is required. Until recently, this information was not available. Several authors have made an attempt to address the issue of nodal delineation.[16] A recently published article on the delineation of nodal regions in the head and neck is an excellent sample of these efforts.[17] Similar research in other anatomic sites is desperately needed.

The PTV is designed to account for setup errors and internal organ motion. Extensive physics research has been devoted to this issue in recent years (see Chapter 6, "Immobilization and Localization"). Addressing respiratory motion in thoracic malignancies has gained considerable attention, resulting in a new technique of "gated" RT. Suffice it to say that physicians are intimately involved and should be knowledgeable in this approach (see Chapter 9, "Respiratory Motion Management").

In the delineation of normal structures, knowledge of three-dimensional radiographic representation of the anatomy is required. Although the dosimetrists may delineate some structures, such as the lungs or spinal cord, outlining other structures, including the brachial plexus, optic nerves, and optic chiasm, should be done by the physician. The recommendations of Report 62 of the ICRU on this issue are not used by most institutions.

Dose Prescription

Traditional dose prescriptions for 3DCRT are usually approximately 50 Gy to subclinical (microscopic) disease, 60 Gy to high-risk microscopic disease, and 70 to 75 Gy to the GTV. In most cases, the dose prescriptions are delivered in a conventional fractionation (1.8–2 Gy/fraction). Treatment is usually performed according to a long-standing practice of "shrinking fields" or, more appropriately, "shrinking volumes" (in the three-dimensional era). Concerns about normal tissue (with some exceptions on research projects) are focused on critical organs, such as the spinal cord, and the most severe sequelae, such as myelitis.

IMRT has introduced new opportunities and challenges. In principle, the same strategy can be used to design IMRT plans. At many institutions, the initial phase is delivered via conventional 3DCRT and the later (boost) phase with IMRT (the so-called "IMRT boost" technique). However, such a strategy defeats the principal purpose of IMRT and has not resulted in significant improvements. Moreover, as discussed by Mohan and colleagues, if a large portion of the total dose is delivered to a large volume, it will be difficult to achieve significant dose conformity with the remaining IMRT boost.[18] The superiority of IMRT planning lies in the simultaneous delivery of different doses to different tissues in a single treatment session, an approach known as a simultaneous integrated boost (see Chapter 18.7, "Simultaneous Integrated Boost: Emerging Technology"). It has been claimed that such a dose distribution and delivery is easier, more efficient, and perhaps less error prone.[18]

Given that each target volume and normal tissue require and receive different doses in a fixed time, different dose fractionation needs to be selected for each tissue. The adjusted dose and dose per fraction for each region depend on the number of fractions chosen. The importance of fractionation on TCP and/or NTCP cannot be overemphasized.[18] For evaluation of various IMRT fractionation strategies, the isoeffect relationship based on the linear-quadratic (LQ) model has been used. These relationships are the result of extensive work by Ang and colleagues and Withers and colleagues.[19,20] The important factor in these calculations is the values of the α/β ratios for each tissue. As discussed by Mohan and colleagues, there is considerable uncertainty in the available data and numerous assumptions in the LQ model and isoeffect formalism.[18] Therefore, until their validity is fully established, they should not be used in daily clinical decision-making. As emphasized by Ang and colleagues, "No isoeffect formula is sufficiently reliable to preempt clinical judgment and… in the final analysis, each new fractionation schedule must be tested clinically to establish safety."[19]

In IMRT dose prescriptions, one must prescribe dose to normal tissues. Most, if not all, commercial IMRT planning systems require precise dose prescription in terms of minimum dose, maximum dose, etc., which constitutes the essential constraints for inverse treatment planning. Unfortunately, there was a considerable lack of accurate data on the partial tolerance of normal tissues to radiation with a variety of end points.

During the process of research on National Institutes of Health/NCI 3DCRT contracts, the necessity of such knowledge resulted in the formation of a task force to update the available information. Based on this work, Emami and Lyman reported on the partial volume tolerance of normal tissues with limited end points.[21] As emphasized in that report, there were few or no hard data for many organs, and most of the "doses were the experience of radiation oncologists in a given disease site." Since then, owing to the recognition of the importance of such information and the increasing use of 3DCRT, reliable data of the partial tolerance of certain organs have become available (see "Clinical Studies").[22] Such information is critical to the implementation of IMRT.

Planning and Treatment Delivery

As mentioned earlier, the IMRT treatment planner selects the desired outcome, which could be physical, such as dose or dose-volume histograms, and/or biophysical models, such as TCP and/or NTCP. Using computerized optimization, the beam parameters (mainly the intensity) are adjusted in an attempt to achieve the desired outcome, a process known as inverse planning.

From the physician's point of view, several important issues need to be emphasized in regard to this process:
1. There is a lack of precise information on the optimal dose required to control different types of cancers.
2. With a few exceptions (lung, liver, and salivary glands), there is a lack of precise and complete information on the tolerance of normal tissues.
3. The concepts of TCP and NTCP are models and have never been clinically tested and validated using clinical data.

Lastly, after a review of the computer-optimized dose distribution, there is almost always a need for some modification of the desired outcome and adjustment of the relative importance of each end point. With experience, highly conformal treatment plans can be achieved (see Chapter 11, "Plan Evaluation"). Representative IMRT treatment plans in patients with head and neck, prostate, and gynecologic tumors are shown in Figures 4-2 to 4-4.

Clinical Studies

A voluminous (and growing) literature has appeared over the last few years demonstrating the dosimetric superiority of IMRT over conventional RT approaches. Such studies have been performed in nearly all of the major tumor sites, including central nervous system tumors,[23,24] head and neck cancers,[25,26] breast cancer,[27] lung cancer,[28] gastrointestinal tumors,[29] genitourinary tumors,[30,31] gynecologic cancers,[32,33] lymphomas,[34] and sarcomas.[35] These results are summarized in the clinical chapters of this book.

Although early clinical results have been encouraging, the impact of IMRT on tumor control and survival remains

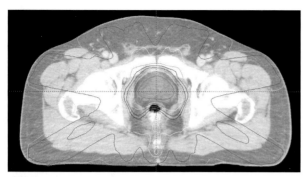

FIGURE 4-2. Dose distribution of an intensity-modulated radiation therapy plan in a patient with prostate cancer. Note that the high-dose lines conform to the shape of the prostate, reducing the volume of bladder and rectum receiving high doses. (To view a color version of this image, please refer to the CD-ROM.)

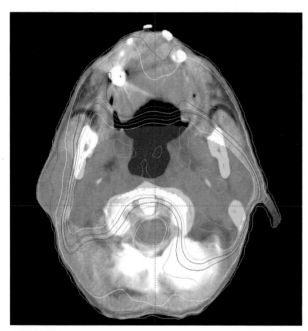

FIGURE 4-3. Dose distribution of an intensity-modulated radiation therapy (IMRT) plan in a patient with head and neck cancer. This patient had a recurrent left-sided oropharyngeal cancer. IMRT planning was used to minimize the dose to the contralateral parotid gland. (To view a color version of this image, please refer to the CD-ROM.)

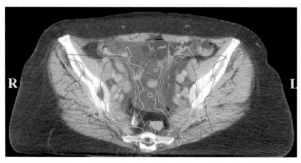

FIGURE 4-4. Dose distribution of an intensity-modulated radiation therapy plan in a patient with endometrial cancer. Note that the high-dose lines conform to the shape of the laterally situated lymph node regions, sparing the small bowel and rectum. (To view a color version of this image, please refer to the CD-ROM.)

to be seen. Ongoing clinical trials need to mature, with a larger number of patients and longer follow-up. To date, the most important contribution of IMRT technology in the management of patients with cancer has been in the reduction of short- and long-term complications. Moreover, IMRT has been a tremendous tool for studying the relationship between the radiation dose, volume, and various side effects and complications of RT. Although covered in other sections of this book, a brief overview of several noteworthy studies is presented here.

Prostate Cancer

Multiple investigators have evaluated the role of IMRT planning and treatment in patients with prostate cancer (see Chapter 22A, "Intact Prostate Cancer: Overview" and Chapter 22B, "Postoperative Prostate Cancer: Overview"). The largest clinical experience using IMRT in prostate cancer is from the Memorial Sloan-Kettering Cancer Center.[36,37] In their initial report, Zelefsky and colleagues reported on 171 patients with localized prostate cancer treated with IMRT and compared their outcome with that seen in 61 patients treated with 3DCRT.[36] A significant reduction in the volume of the rectum and bladder walls receiving high-dose levels ($p < .01$) was seen, indicating improved dose conformity with IMRT. Moreover, grade 2 rectal bleeding was significantly lower with IMRT. The 2-year actuarial risk of grade 2 bleeding was 2% for IMRT versus 10% for 3DCRT ($p < .001$).

Recently, Zelefsky and colleagues updated their experience reporting on 772 clinically localized patients undergoing IMRT.[37] Most (90%) received a total dose of 81 Gy; the remainder received 86.4 Gy. Overall, acute grade 2 or higher rectal toxicity was seen in 4.5% of patients. Grade 2 or higher acute genitourinary toxicity occurred in 28% of patients. At a median follow-up of 24 months, the 3-year actuarial risk of grade 2 or higher rectal and genitourinary complications was 4% and 15%, respectively. The 3-year actuarial biochemical control rates of the favorable-, intermediate-, and unfavorable-risk patients were 92%, 86%, and 81%, respectively.

Researchers at the Cleveland Clinic have reported the outcome of patients with prostate cancer treated with a hypofractionated IMRT approach.[38–41] Patients received a total dose of 70 Gy in 2.5 Gy daily fractions. In their most recent report, Djemil and colleagues reported on 100 patients with T1–T3 cancer treated between 1998 and 1999 with a median follow-up of 43 months.[41] The 6-year actuarial relapse-free survival rate of the entire group was 88%. The 6-year relapse-free survival was 100% in low-risk patients (T1–T2, prostate-specific antigen [PSA] ≤ 10, Gleason grade ≤ 6) versus 81% in high-risk patients (T3 or PSA > 10 or Gleason grade > 6). Treatment was well tolerated, with no patient experiencing grade 3 or higher acute toxicity. Moreover, the 4-year actuarial risk of grade 2 or higher rectal sequelae was 6%. Others have similarly reported promising experiences using a hypofractionated IMRT approach.[42] The hypofractionated IMRT approach developed by Kupelian and colleagues at the Cleveland Clinic is described in detail in Chapter 22.2, "Hypofractionated IMRT: Case Study."

Head and Neck Cancer

IMRT has received considerable attention in the treatment of head and neck cancer, particularly tumors of the nasopharynx and oropharynx (see Chapter 18, "Head and Neck Cancer: Overview"). In a review of the University of California, San Francisco (UCSF) experience, Lee and colleagues reported the outcome of 67 patients with nasopharyngeal carcinoma treated with IMRT.[43] Seventy percent of patients had stage III–IV disease, and 50 patients received concomitant chemotherapy. With a median follow-up of 31 months, there has been only one local failure and one nodal failure. Seventeen patients developed distant metastases. The 4-year actuarial local progression-free, locoregional progression-free, and distant metastasis-free survival rates were 97%, 98%, and 66%, respectively. The 4-year overall survival rate was 88%. Grade 3 to 4 late toxicities were seen in eight patients (seven grade 3, one grade 1).

An update of the UCSF experience in the treatment of 150 patients with head and neck cancer who underwent IMRT was recently reported by Lee and colleagues.[44] Most patients had tumors of the nasopharynx (86) and oropharynx (22). Of 107 patients treated with definitive IMRT, there were four local failures at a median follow-up of 25 months. The 2- and 3-year actuarial local control rates were 97% and 95%, respectively. Of 43 patients treated postoperatively, 7 failed locally, for a 2-year local control rate of 83% (see Chapter 18.1, "Nasopharyngeal Cancer: Case Study").

Chao and colleagues reported the outcome of 41 patients with head and neck cancer undergoing IMRT.[45] Salivary gland function and quality of life were studied in all patients. Objective and subjective improvement in both xerostomia and quality-of-life scores were noted. In a subsequent report, Chao and colleagues evaluated the outcome of 26 patients with oropharyngeal carcinoma treated with IMRT.[46] Fourteen were treated postoperatively, and 12 underwent definitive treatment. The 2-year locoregional control, disease-free survival, and overall survival rates for the postoperative group were 100%, 92%, and 100%, respectively. Corresponding results in the definitive group were 88%, 80%, and 100%, respectively. Two patients in the postoperative group and three patients in definitive IMRT group had grade 2 xerostomia. No grade 3 xerostomia was noted in either group.

Breast Cancer

Several investigators have shown the dosimetric advantages of IMRT planning in patients with either intact breast and/or postoperative breast cancer (see Chapter 20, "Breast Cancer: Overview").[47–50] All of these studies have shown improved target coverage with reductions in the dose to the heart (left-sided breast patients) and to the underlying normal lung.

In the largest clinical experience to date, Vicini and colleagues at William Beaumont Hospital presented the outcome of 281 patients with stage 0–II breast cancer treated with a static multileaf collimator IMRT technique to the whole breast following lumpectomy. Overall, treatment was well tolerated, with 56% of patients experiencing grade 0 or 1 acute skin toxicity. Grade 2 and 3 acute skin toxicity was seen in 43% and 1% of patients, respectively. Of 95 evaluable patients, 94 (99%) had good or excellent cosmesis at 12 months. No patient developed skin telangiectasias, significant fibrosis, or persistent breast pain.[51] A detailed description of the William Beaumont Hospital approach is described in Chapter 20.1, "Intact Breast Cancer: Case Study").

Gynecology

Increasing attention has been focused recently on the role of IMRT in gynecologic tumors (see Chapter 23, "Gynecologic Cancer: Overview"). In a series of reports, investigators at the University of Chicago reported lower rates of toxicity in gynecology patients undergoing IMRT compared with conventional approaches.[52–55] In their initial report, Mundt and colleagues reported on the results of 40 patients with gynecologic malignancies treated with intensity-modulated pelvic RT.[52] No patient developed grade 3 gastrointestinal toxicity. Grade 2 acute gastrointestinal toxicity was less common in IMRT patients compared with those undergoing conventional RT (60 vs 91%; $p = .002$). Less acute genitourinary toxicity was seen in IMRT patients (10% vs 20%); however, this difference did not reach statistical significance. The same group also reported that intensity-modulated pelvic RT in gynecologic patients resulted in less acute hematologic toxicity by reducing the volume of pelvic bone marrow irradiated.[53,54]

In their most recent report, Mundt and colleagues evaluated chronic gastrointestinal toxicity in 30 gynecology patients treated with intensity-modulated pelvic RT, with a median follow-up of 19.6 months.[55] Compared with a balanced cohort of conventional RT patients, IMRT was associated with fewer chronic gastrointestinal sequelae (11.1 vs 50%; $p = .001$). On multivariate analysis controlling for age, stage, chemotherapy, surgery, brachytherapy, and length of follow-up, IMRT remained correlated with fewer sequelae ($p = .01$).

Conclusions

Reviewing the clinical IMRT experience generally points to significantly improved dosimetry and marked reductions in acute and sometimes late toxicities of RT. Improvement in tumor control requires further research with a larger number of patients and a longer follow-up.

References

1. Johns HE, Cunningham JR. The physics of radiology. 4th ed. Springfield (IL): Charles C. Thomas; 1983. p. 382–407.

2. Emami B, Melo A, Carter BL, et al. Value of computed tomography in radiotherapy of lung cancer. AJR Am J Roentgenol 1978;131:63–7.

3. McShan DL, Silverman A, Lanza D, et al. A computerized three-dimensional treatment planning system utilizing interactive color graphics. Br J Radiol 1979;52:478–81.

4. Fraass BA, McShan DL. 3-D treatment planning. I. Overview of a clinical planning system. In: Proceedings of the 9th International Conference on the Use of Computers in Radiation Therapy, Scheveningen, Netherlands, 1987.

5. Purdy JA, Wong JW, Harms WB, et al. Three-dimensional radiation treatment planning system. In: Proceedings of the 9th International Conference on the Use of Computers in Radiation Therapy, Scheveningen, Netherlands, 1987.

6. Mohan R. Barest G, Brewster IJ, et al. A comprehensive three-dimensional radiation treatment planning system. Int J Radiat Oncol Biol Phys 1988;15:481–95.

7. Intensity Modulated Radiation Therapy Collaborative Group. Intensity-modulated radiotherapy: current status and issues of interest. Int J Radiat Oncol Biol Phys 2001;51:880–914.

8. International Commission on Radiation Units and Measurements. Prescribing, recording and reporting photon beam therapy. Report 50. Washington (DC): International Commission on Radiation Units and Measurements; 1993.

9. Morris D, Emami B, Mauch P. An evidence-based review of 3-dimensional conformal radiation therapy in localized prostate cancer: an ASTRO outcomes initiative. Int J Radiat Oncol Biol Phys 2004. [In press]

10. Teh BS, Woo SY, Butler EB. Intensity modulated radiation therapy (IMRT): a new promising technology in radiation oncology. Oncologist 1999;4:433–42.

11. Emami B, Sethi A, Petruzzelli G. Influence of MRI on target volume delineation and IMRT planning in nasopharyngeal carcinoma. Int J Radiat Oncol Biol Phys 2003;57:100–4.

12. Erdi E, Rosenzweig K, Erdi K, et al. Radiotherapy treatment planning for patients with non-small cell lung cancer using positron emission tomography (PET). Radiother Oncol 2002;62:51–60.

13. Chao KSC, Bosch WR, Mutic S, et al. A novel approach to overcome hypoxic tumor resistance: Cu-ATSM-guided intensity-modulated radiation therapy. Int J Radiat Oncol Biol Phys 2001;49:1171–82.

14. Grosu AL, Lachner R, Wiedenmann N, et al. Validation of a method for automatic image fusion (BrainLAB System) of CT data and 11C-methionine-PET data for stereotactic radiotherapy using a LINAC: first clinical experience. Int J Radiat Oncol Biol Phys 2003;56:1450–63.

15. Emami B, Mirkovic N, Scott C, et al. The impact of regional nodal radiotherapy (dose/volume) on regional progression and survival in unresectable non-small cell lung cancer: an analysis of RTOG data. Lung Cancer 2003;41:100–4.

16. Levendag P, Braaksma M, Coche E, et al. Rotterdam and Brussels CT-based neck nodal delineation compared with the surgical levels as defined by the American Academy of Otolaryngology-Head and Neck Surgery. Int J Radiat Oncol Biol Phys 2004;58:113–23.

17. Gregoire V, Levendag P, Ang KK, et al. CT-based delineation of lymph node levels and related CTVs in the node-negative neck: DAHANCA, EORTC, GORTEC, NCIC, RTOG consensus guidelines. Radiother Oncol 2003;69:227–36.

18. Mohan R, Wu Q, Manning M, et al. Radiobiological considerations in the design of fractionation strategies for intensity-modulated radiation therapy of head and neck cancers. Int J Radiat Oncol Biol Phys 2000;26:619–30.

19. Ang KK, Thames HD, Peters LJ. Altered fractionation schedules. In: Perez CA, Brady LW, editors. Principles and practice of radiation oncology. Philadelphia: Lippincott-Raven; 1997. p. 119–42.

20. Withers HR, Peters LJ, Taylor JMG, et al. Late normal tissue sequelae from radiation therapy for carcinoma of the tonsil: patterns of fractionation study of radiobiology. Int J Radiat Oncol Biol Phys 1995;33:563–8.

21. Emami B, Lyman J, Brown A, et al. Tolerance of normal tissue to therapeutic irradiation. Int J Radiat Oncol Biol Phys 1991;21:109–22.

22. Graham MV, Purdy JA, Emami B, et al. Clinical dose volume histogram analysis for pneumonitis after 3D treatment for non-small cell lung cancer. Int J Radiat Oncol Biol Phys 1999;45:323–9.

23. Thilmann C, Zabel A, Grosser KH, et al. Intensity-modulated radiotherapy with an integrated boost to the macroscopic tumor volume in the treatment of high-grade gliomas. Int J Cancer 2001;96:341–9.

24. Nakamura JL, Pirzkall A, Carol MP, et al. Comparison of intensity-modulated radiosurgery with gamma knife radiosurgery for challenging skull base lesions. Int J Radiat Oncol Biol Phys 2003;55:99–109.

25. Kam MK, Chau RM, Suen J, et al. Intensity-modulated radiotherapy in nasopharyngeal carcinoma: dosimetric advantage over conventional plans and feasibility of dose escalation. Int J Radiat Oncol Biol Phys 2003;56:145–57.

26. Nutting CM, Convery DJ, Cosgrove VP, et al. Improvements in target coverage and reduced spinal cord irradiation using intensity-modulated radiotherapy (IMRT) in patients with carcinoma of the thyroid gland. Radiother Oncol 2001;60:173–80.

27. Hong L, Hunt M, Chui C, et al. Intensity-modulated tangential beam irradiation of the intact breast. Int J Radiat Oncol Biol Phys 1999;44:1155–64.

28. Van Sornsen de Koste J, Voet P, Dirkx M, et al. An evaluation of two techniques for beam intensity modulation in patients irradiated for stage III non-small cell lung cancer. Lung Cancer 2001;32:145–53.

29. Nutting CM, Bedford JL, Cosgrove VP, et al. A comparison of conformal and intensity-modulated techniques for oesophageal radiotherapy. Radiother Oncol 2001;61:157–63.

30. Nutting CM, Corbishley CM, Sanchez-Nieto B, et al. Potential improvements in the therapeutic ratio of prostate cancer irradiation: dose escalation of pathologically identified tumour nodules using intensity modulated radiotherapy. Br J Radiol 2002;75:151–61.

31. Pickett B, Vigneault E, Kurhanewicz J, et al. Static field intensity modulation to treat a dominant intra-prostatic lesion to 90 Gy compared to seven field 3-dimensional radiotherapy. Int J Radiat Oncol Biol Phys 1999;44:921–9.

32. Roeske JC, Lujan A, Rotmensch J, et al. Intensity-modulated whole pelvic radiation therapy in patients with gynecologic malignancies. Int J Radiat Oncol Biol Phys 2000;48:1613–21.

33. Portelance L, Chao KS, Grigsby PW, et al. Intensity-modulated radiation therapy (IMRT) reduces small bowel, rectum and bladder doses in patients with cervical cancer receiving pelvic and para-aortic irradiation. Int J Radiat Oncol Biol Phys 2001;51:261–6.

34. Loo BW, Crooks SM, Xing LZ, et al. A dosimetric comparison of conventional and intensity modulated radiation therapies for the treatment of Hodgkin's disease [abstract]. Int J Radiat Oncol Biol Phys 2002;54:323.

35. Hong L, Alektiar K, Hunt M, et al. Intensity modulated radiotherapy for soft tissue sarcoma of thigh [abstract]. Int J Radiat Oncol Biol Phys 2002;54:139–40.

36. Zelefsky MJ, Fuks Z, Happersett L, et al. Clinical experience with intensity modulated radiation therapy (IMRT) in prostate cancer. Radiother Oncol 2000;55:241–9.

37. Zelefksy MJ, Fuks Z, Hunt M, et al. High-dose intensity modulated radiation therapy for prostate cancer: early toxicity and biochemical outcome in 772 patients. Int J Radiat Oncol Biol Phys 2002;53:1111–6.

38. Dasarahally SM, Kupelian PA, Willoughby TR. Short-course intensity-modulated radiotherapy for localized prostate cancer with daily transabdominal ultrasound localization of the prostate gland. Int J Radiat Oncol Biol Phys 2000;46:575–80.

39. Kupelian PA, Reddy CA, Klein EA, et al. Short-course intensity-modulated radiotherapy (70 Gy at 2.5 Gy per fraction) for localized prostate cancer: preliminary results on late toxicity and quality of life. Int J Radiat Oncol Biol Phys 2001;51:988–93.

40. Kupelian PA, Reddy CA, Carlson TP, et al. Preliminary observations on biochemical relapse free survival rates after short course intensity modulated radiotherapy (70 Gy at 2.5 Gy/fraction) for localized prostate cancer. Int J Radiat Oncol Biol Phys 2002;53:904–12.

41. Djemil T, Reddy CA, Willoughby TR, et al. Hypofractionated intensity-modulated radiotherapy (70 Gy at 2.5 Gy per fraction) for localized prostate cancer [abstract]. Int J Radiat Oncol Biol Phys 2003;57:275

42. Kitamura K, Shirato H, Shinohara N, et al. Reduction in acute morbidity using hypofractionated intensity-modulated radiotherapy assisted with a fluoroscopic real-time tumor-tracking system for prostate cancer: preliminary results of a phase I/II study. Cancer J 2003;9:268–76.

43. Lee N, Xia P, Quivey JM, et al. Intensity-modulated radiotherapy in the treatment of nasopharyngeal carcinoma: an update of the UCSF experience. Int J Radiat Oncol Biol Phys 2002;53:12–22.

44. Lee N, Xia P, Fischbein NJ, et al. Intensity-modulated radiation therapy for head-and-neck cancer: the UCSF experience focusing on target volume delineation. Int J Radiat Oncol Biol Phys 2003;57:49–60.

45. Chao KSC, Deasy JO, Markman J, et al. A prospective study of salivary function sparing in patients with head-and-neck cancers receiving intensity-modulated or 3-dimensional radiation therapy: initial results. Int J Radiat Oncol Biol Phys 2001;49:907–16.

46. Chao KSC, Majhail N, Huang CJ, et al. Intensity-modulated radiation therapy reduces late salivary toxicity without compromising tumor control in patients with oropharyngeal carcinoma: a comparison with conventional techniques. Radiother Oncol 2001;61:275–80.

47. Lo YC, Yasuda G, Fitzgerald TJ, et al. Intensity modulation for breast treatment using static multi-leaf collimators. Int J Radiat Oncol Biol Phys 2000;46:187–94.

48. Hurkmans CW, Cho BCJ, Damen E, et al. Reduction of cardiac and lung complications probabilities after breast irradiation using conformal radiotherapy with or without intensity modulation. Radiother Oncol 2002;62:163–71.

49. Cho BCJ, Hurkmans CW, Damen MF, et al. Intensity modulated versus non-intensity modulated radiotherapy in the treatment of left breast and upper internal mammary lymph node chain: a comparative planning study. Radiother Oncol 2002;62:127–36.

50. Krueger EA, Fraass BA, McChan DL, et al. Potential gains for irradiation of chest wall and regional nodes with intensity modulated radiotherapy. Int J Radiat Oncol Biol Phys 2003;56:1023–37.

51. Vicini FA, Sharpe M, Kestin L, et al. Optimizing breast cancer treatment efficacy with intensity-modulated radiotherapy. Int J Radiat Oncol Biol Phys 2002;54:1336–44.

52. Mundt AJ, Lujan AE, Rotmensch J, et al. Intensity-modulated whole pelvic radiotherapy in women with gynecologic malignancies. Int J Radiat Oncol Biol Phys 2002;52:1330–37.

53. Brixey CJ, Roeske JC, Lujan AE, et al. Impact of intensity-modulated radiotherapy on acute hematologic toxicity in women with gynecologic malignancies. Int J Radiat Oncol Biol Phys 2002;54;1388–96.

54. Lujan AE, Mundt AJ, Yamada SD, et al. Intensity-modulated radiotherapy as a means of reducing dose to bone marrow in gynecologic patients receiving whole pelvic radiotherapy. Int J Radiat Oncol Biol Phys 2003;57;516–21.

55. Mundt AJ, Mell LK, Roeske JC. Preliminary analysis of chronic gastrointestinal toxicity in gynecology patients treated with intensity-modulated whole pelvic radiation therapy. Int J Radiat Oncol Biol Phys 2003;56:1354–60.

II. Technology and Implementation

Chapter 5

CT SIMULATION

TIM FOX, PhD, ELIZABETH BUTKER, MS, ERIC ELDER, PhD

Over the past decade, many radiation oncology departments have incorporated the modern computed tomography (CT) simulator into their treatment process. In fact, many clinics are moving away from conventional simulators altogether and are relying primarily on CT simulators. Commercial CT simulators are available that combine many of the functions of an image-based, three-dimensional treatment planning system and a conventional simulator.[1–18] These systems attempt to integrate as much of the planning process as possible using exact anatomic information of the patient obtained at the time of CT scanning. The software used in conjunction with a CT simulator provides virtual representations of the patient and the geometric capabilities of a treatment machine. Often CT simulation is referred to as virtual simulation, and the two terms tend to be used interchangeably.[1]

The initial concept of the CT simulator was to emulate the conventional simulation process on a contiguous CT data set representing the patient. This idea was first proposed by Goitein and colleagues as beam's eye view (BEV) planning.[15] In BEV treatment planning, relevant segmented critical structures from CT contours are projected to a plane beyond the patient from the vantage point of the radiation source to ensure appropriate three-dimensional target coverage. This concept was further developed by Sherouse and colleagues, who introduced a system that could work like a simulator but used digital information derived from the patient imaging data set.[11–13] A patient treatment simulation could be completed on a virtual patient model with digitally reconstructed radiographs (DRRs). A DRR is simply a virtual radiographic projection of the CT data in a BEV and is analogous to the conventional simulation film. The DRR allows for verification of the treatment field using conventional port film techniques. Therefore, the simulation process can be completed in a virtual domain without having the patient in the simulator room. This method

not only improves the accuracy of target localization but also provides flexibility for radiation oncologists to complete the simulation process at a time that is more conducive to their schedule.

Intensity-modulated radiation therapy (IMRT) treatment planning uses dose-volume constraints as part of the optimization methods during the plan creation phase. CT simulation allows the anatomic segmentation of the target volumes and critical structures for IMRT planning. In addition to CT imaging, other imaging modalities, such as magnetic resonance imaging (MRI), positron emission tomography (PET), single-photon emission computed tomography (SPECT), or another CT scan, can be registered with the CT simulation scan to provide more anatomic or functional information during the process (see Chapter 8, "PET-CT in IMRT Planning").

The American Association of Physicists in Medicine (AAPM) created Task Group Report 66 (TG-66), "Quality Assurance for Computed-Tomography Simulators and the Computed Tomography-Simulation Process," which provides the medical physicist with a framework and guidance for the establishment of a comprehensive quality assurance (QA) program for CT scanners used for CT simulation, CT simulation software, and the CT simulation process.[1] A section is provided in this chapter that highlights the main tests to perform for a typical radiation oncology department. For detailed information, the reader is encouraged to review this report.

Technology and Process

A CT simulator consists of three main components: a CT scanner with a flat tabletop, an integrated laser marking system, and virtual simulation and visualization software. All three components form the package for simulating the treatment of an individual patient. The CT simulation scanner table must have a flat top similar to that of radiation therapy (RT) treatment machines (Figure 5-1). Even though the general shape of the CT simulation and treatment machine tables may be similar, the treatment machine table usually has components, such as removable panels and table support components, that are not reproduced on the simulator table. As described in the AAPM TG-66 report, treatment policies and planning target volumes should account for these differences.[1] Besides the flat tabletop, the scanners used for CT simulation are usually equipped with external patient marking or positioning lasers, which can be fixed or mobile. Mobile lasers allow easier marking of patients. In particular, the sagittal laser should be mobile because CT tables do not move in the lateral direction, and it allows marking away from the patient's midline.

Today, most devices used for CT simulation are capable of both conventional and spiral CT scanning for image acquisition. Conventional CT (sometimes called axial scanning) acquires data one slice at a time. Alternatively, spiral or helical CT, which became available in the late 1980s, allows data to be acquired while the table translates and the x-ray tube gantry rotates simultaneously. The path of the tube forms a helical pattern around the patient. The spiral mode is preferred for CT simulation owing to faster scan times.

Besides image acquisition techniques, the use of multislice CT scanners has been recently adopted in CT simulation, allowing projection data from multiple slices to be acquired simultaneously.[19–23] These multislice scanners use multiple rows of detectors to acquire image studies faster than single-slice scanners. In addition, the tube heat loading for a particular patient volume is lower for multislice than for single-slice scanners. Multislice technology can be especially beneficial for simulation of tumors in the thorax because breathing artifacts can be minimized. This technology is also valuable for simulation of respiratory-gated treatments.

Most conventional CT scanners use a 70 cm bore opening. This has been a weakness for CT simulation because patient positioning may be compromised with a small opening. Currently, two manufacturers (GE Healthcare and Philips Medical Systems) offer a CT scanner with an 85 cm bore opening, designed specifically for radiation oncology purposes. The larger opening allows for greater flexibility in patient positioning and use of immobilization devices.[24] These large-bore scanners also have an increased scan field of view, 60 cm compared with 48 cm on most 70 cm bore units. The large-bore scanner image quality is generally comparable to that of 70 cm units; however, some degradation in high-contrast resolution and image noise has been observed. The various systems offered by the commercial vendors are summarized in Table 5-1.

The CT simulation process has been divided into three major categories by the AAPM TG-66 report.[1] Methods for simulating specific anatomic sites have been described by several authors and are discussed here.[3,4,6,16–18]

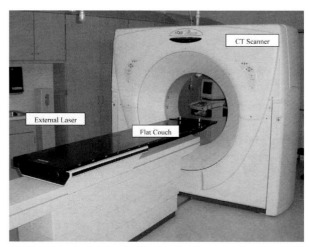

FIGURE 5-1. An AcQSim (Philips Medical Systems, Cleveland, OH) CT simulator equipped with a flat couch top to mimic the Varian (Varian Medical Systems, Palo Alto, CA) Exact Couch Top on a CL2100 EX. The external laser system, used for marking the patient, is located outside the scanner.

CT Scanning, Positioning, and Immobilization

The CT simulation scan is similar to a conventional diagnostic scan. However, the radiation oncology requirements must specify information in regard to patient positioning and immobilization, treatment-specific scan protocols, use of contrast, and placement of localization marks on the patient's skin. It is highly recommended that procedures and protocols be developed for most treatment sites to ensure consistency during the CT simulation process. In IMRT, one of the most critical issues is patient positioning and immobilization. All cranial patients, including patients with head and neck cancer, should use a head support system with a head mask or cast. For other regions of the body, either a Vac-Lok Bag (MED-TEC, Orange City, IA) or an Alpha Cradle (Smithers Medical Products, North Canton, OH) should be used. The use of a reliable and reproducible fixation system for the patient is important and should verify

TABLE 5-1. Technical Options for Commercial Computed Tomography Simulation Systems

| | CT Simulator Manufacturer | | |
Features	GE Healthcare	Siemens	Philips Medical Systems
Spiral CT option	Yes	Yes	Yes
Multislice CT option	Yes	Yes	Yes
Flat tabletop option	Yes	Yes	Yes
Bore size	85 cm	70 cm	85 cm
SFOV size	60 cm	48 cm	60 cm
Data transfer	DICOM-RT	DICOM-RT	DICOM-RT
Software platform	Advantage Sim	Virtual Simulation	AcQSim
4D simulation	Yes	Future product	Future product

CT = computed tomography; 4D = four-dimensional; DICOM = Digital Imaging Communications in Medicine; RT = radiation therapy; SFOV = scan field of view.

that patient movement is minimized during the CT simulation process.[3] The immobilization device should ideally register or fix to the treatment table. Using an immobilization device that is registered to the table, the record-and-verify system can monitor treatment table coordinates with tight tolerance limits. Contrast agents may also be used to improve visualization of the patient's normal (and abnormal) anatomy and may be desirable for certain situations. However, for heterogeneity-based calculations in IMRT planning, contrast can cause dose distribution errors owing to artificial CT numbers and corresponding tissue densities.

During CT simulation, patients are scanned using preset oncology-specific protocols for each treatment site. These protocols are designed to optimize both the transaxial CT and the DRR image quality. The imaging parameters include kilovolts peak, milliamperes, slice thickness, slice spacing, and total scan time. A small slice thickness and spacing are desirable for producing high-quality DRRs. In addition to the scan protocols, scan limits should be specified by the physician and should encompass a volume large enough to create DRRs with enough anatomic infor-

mation. The AAPM TG-66 report recommends that the scan volume should be at least 5 cm or greater in the superior and inferior directions from the anticipated treatment volumes and that larger scanning regions may be necessary for special situations.[1]

Treatment Planning and CT Simulation

Beam placement and treatment design are performed using virtual simulation software. The virtual simulation process typically consists of contouring the target and normal structures, placement of the treatment isocenter and beams, design of treatment portal shapes, generation of DRRs, and documentation. However, for IMRT planning, the design of treatment portal shapes is not performed at this time because an intensity map is created to deliver a nonuniform dose distribution from each treatment field. DRRs are created by the virtual simulation software but are mainly used for visual comparison and alignment of anatomic sites (Figure 5-2). Thus, CT simulation for IMRT planning relies more on anatomic segmentation and localization of the isocenter for treatment setup.

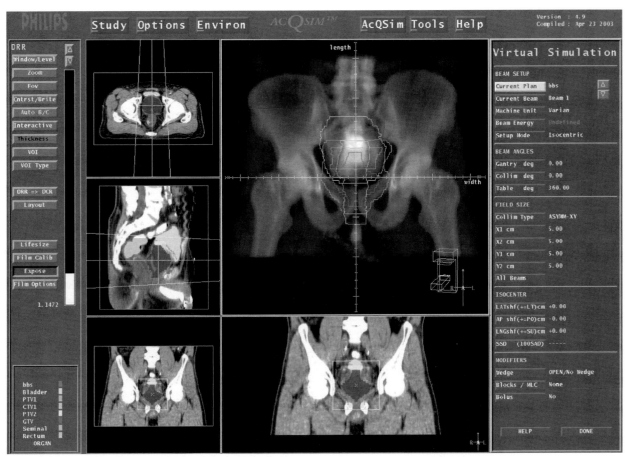

FIGURE 5-2. Philips virtual simulator software (*AcQSim*, Philips Medical Systems, Cleveland, OH). The large window shows a digitally reconstructed radiograph (DRR) from an anterior view. The contours drawn on individual axial slices are superimposed on this DRR. Other views are axial, sagittal, and coronal computed tomography slices through various planes intersecting the isocenter. (To view a color version of this image, please refer to the CD-ROM.)

The treatment planning portion of the CT simulation process begins with target and normal structure delineation. Other imaging studies (diagnostic CT, MRI, PET) may be registered to the planning CT scan to provide information for improved target and normal tissue delineation. After delineation of the target volumes, a treatment isocenter is created either manually or automatically in the CT study. The automated isocenter placement is performed by the software by computing the center of the mass of the target volume. After the isocenter has been identified in the virtual simulation software, these coordinates must be transferred to the external laser marking system for localizing on the patient's skin. These marks are required to ensure a daily reproducible setup at the treatment machine. There are two methods for localization of the marks on the patient, which are described as either final isocenter marking or reference point marking.[1]

When a final isocenter is marked, the patient is scanned, and the physician or physicist determines the isocenter location on the digital images while the patient remains on the CT scanner table. This requires that the target volume be delineated during this time by a clinician. Once the isocenter has been determined, these coordinates are transferred to the external laser system. The marks are then placed on the patient and are used for patient positioning on the first day of treatment at the linear accelerator.

The reference point method is typically used when the radiation oncologist is not available during the simulation process.[1,3] Prior to the scan procedure, the physician instructs the radiation therapist where to place a set of reference marks on the patient. These are marked on the patient, and radiopaque markers are placed on the skin. After the scan, the patient can leave, and images are transferred to the virtual simulation workstation. Subsequently, the treatment isocenter coordinates are determined after the target volumes are delineated. The distances in three directions between the initial reference marks and the final treatment isocenter (referred to as shifts) are then calculated. On the first day of treatment, the patient is aligned to the initial reference marks using the treatment machine's lasers and then shifted to the CT simulation isocenter using the calculated shifts. Initial reference marks are then removed, and the isocenter localization marks are placed on the patient. This process is conducive to IMRT planning because the isocenter is often determined by the planning system.

Treatment Setup

On the treatment machine, the patient is set up according to instructions created from the CT simulation software. Port films are acquired and are compared with CT simulation DRRs. In some cases, the patient may undergo treatment setup verification on a conventional simulator prior to treatment. Some radiation oncology departments use both a conventional simulator and a CT simulator during the planning process. The CT simulator is used for the initial CT scan, virtual simulation, and treatment planning

process. Once the plan has been completed, the patient is set up on the conventional simulator for treatment plan verification. Thus, the conventional simulator is being used for the final step of the planning process, which does not take dedicated time on the treatment machine. In certain cases, the fluoroscopic mode of the conventional simulator can also be used for verifying intrafraction motion of the target volume or critical structures. This can be important for treatment sites in the thorax and abdomen, for example, owing to the inability of the CT simulation process to display breathing motion.

Table 5-2 provides a representative step-by-step outline of a typical CT simulation process for a specific body site. This table provides a checklist for verifying the steps used in their CT simulation process, as well as identifying the roles of different clinical team members. In a well-designed CT simulation process for IMRT planning and delivery, all of these steps appear to be relatively seamless and the duration of the entire process relatively short.

TABLE 5-2. CT Simulation Step-by-Step Process for Intensity-Modulated Radiation Therapy

Description	Personnel
1. Patient enters room and the immobilization device is constructed	Therapist
2. Position patient on CT table in treatment position	Therapist
3. Acquire AP and lateral scout images of patient to ensure correct patient position	Therapist
4. Place preliminary alignment marks on patient using lasers	Therapist
5. Record CT couch position of preliminary lasers	Therapist
6. Choose appropriate scanning protocol	Therapist
7. Set CT scan limits to include region superior and inferior to treatment volume	Therapist
8. Administer prescribed contrast: eg, IV, oral, urethral, rectal	Therapist
9. Place external markers if desired on scars, tattoos, palpable mass, etc.	Therapist
10. Scan patient	Therapist
11. Transfer data to virtual simulation workstation	Therapist
12. Localize, compute, and lock in isocenter	Therapist and physician
13. Mark isocenter on patient using long laser lines in three orthogonal planes	Therapist and/or physician
14. Patient leaves CT suite	Therapist
15. Contour all critical organs for dose-volume constraints	Dosimetrist
16. Beam placement for treatment plan design	Dosimetrist and physician
17. Print hard copy of DRRs	Dosimetrist
18. Transfer data to treatment planning	Dosimetrist
19. Plan patient via computer-aided optimization	Dosimetrist and physicist
20. Verify patient setup according to plan	Therapist and physician
21. Perform routine QA to ensure accurate localization of port films	Physicist

AP = anterior-posterior; CT = computed tomography; DRR = digitally reconstructed radiograph; IMRT = intensity-modulated radiation therapy; IV = intravenous; QA = quality assurance.

Integration of CT Simulators with IMRT Planning Systems

Traditionally, radiology departments have implemented image acquisition, archive, and distribution systems in clinical diagnostic environments, referred to as picture archive and communication systems (PACS). However, radiation oncology departments have different needs and data than radiology departments. Thus, PACS for radiation oncology or radiation oncology information systems (ROIS) have been developed for handling the tasks of storing and sharing image, patient, and machine data.[25] A ROIS is a system for acquiring, transmitting, storing, and operating on images and image-related information specifically used in radiation oncology. The technical data objects used in CT simulation are three-dimensional image sets, anatomic volumes, target volumes, and treatment plan parameters (including multileaf collimator [MLC] settings). Anatomic and target volumes are the outlined contours of various organs and tumors used for visualization on DRRs and CT images. Treatment parameters are the machine settings for each individual treatment field, including the gantry angle, collimator angle, collimator jaw settings, and couch angle. CT simulation data may contain all or part of these technical data objects used for ROIS.

The ROIS data may be transmitted to both radiation treatment planning systems and record-and-verify database systems for sharing and reuse of these data. The communication system used for transmitting, converting, and associating medical imaging data is the Digital Imaging and Communications in Medicine (DICOM) standard.[26] This standard describes the methods of formatting and exchanging images and associated information. DICOM relies on industry standard network connections and effectively addresses the communication of digital images from CT simulation systems to various data systems. Over the past 5 years, an extension to DICOM was developed for RT objects, referred to as DICOM-RT. This extension handles the technical data objects in radiation oncology, such as anatomic contours, DRR images, treatment planning data, and dose distribution data. Many CT simulator and treatment planning vendors have begun to adopt DICOM-RT for ensuring a cost-effective solution for sharing technical data in a radiation oncology department. The DICOM-RT objects used for CT simulation are as follows:

- *CT images.* These are images taken during the CT simulation procedure consisting of transaxial CT slices.
- *RT structure sets.* These consists of contours of anatomic structures that have been segmented by physicians, dosimetrists, and/or physicists. Target volumes and normal structures are represented by these objects.
- *RT images.* DRRs that are created by the CT simulation software are stored in this data object.
- *RT plans.* Treatment plans that consist of treatment fields

(RT beams) are represented by this DICOM object. Static and dynamic MLCs can be stored with an RT plan. Dynamic MLCs used to represent IMRT treatment fields can support both step-and-shoot and sliding windows for data formats.

After the data have been transferred from CT simulation to IMRT treatment planning, the physicist and dosimetrist will generate the optimal IMRT plan for the patient. If the planning system needs to use any software features of the CT simulation software, the treatment planning system can transmit the DICOM-RT objects back to the CT simulation system. However, this process rarely happens because most treatment planning systems provide the same functionality of virtual simulation. Typically, once the IMRT plan is complete, the transfer of the treatment plan from the IMRT planning system to a record-and-verify system is performed for treatment verification and delivery.

Data transfer and communications among disparate technical systems were once a difficult feat to accomplish. However, the use of DICOM-RT has provided a more open standard for efficiently sharing data within the radiation oncology software systems. Most modern CT simulator vendors support the use of DICOM-RT, as reflected in Table 5-1.

CT Simulation QA

AAPM TG-66 provides a comprehensive QA program for CT scanners used for CT simulation, CT simulation software, and the CT simulation process.[1] Depending on the CT scanner location and primary use, acceptance testing, commissioning, and QA can be the responsibility of the therapy physicist, the diagnostic physicist, or a joint responsibility. The commissioning and periodic QA of the accompanying software and the QA of the CT simulation process are always the responsibility of the therapy physicist. AAPM TG-66 establishes a set of QA procedures that are applicable to scanners used for CT simulation regardless of their location and primary purpose. The report breaks the QA tests into three main areas: QA for CT scanners used for CT simulation, QA for CT simulation software, and evaluation of the CT simulation process.

QA for CT Scanners Used for Simulation

The TG-66 report addresses QA procedures for the CT scanners to ensure consistent operation and a successful CT simulation process. One of the important performance components for daily and monthly testing of the CT scanner is the external laser marking system. These laser systems are used to position the patient in the correct treatment position and place positioning marks on the patient. The accuracy of the lasers affects the reproducibility of patient positioning from the CT scanner to the treatment delivery machine.

Table 5-3 summarizes the laser QA tests recommended by the TG-66 report, including the frequency of the test and acceptable tolerance limits.[1] The external laser marking system for the CT scanner consists of three separate components: gantry lasers, wall-mounted lasers, and an overhead mobile sagittal laser. Besides the laser marking system, the other electromechanical components, such as the couch and tabletop, gantry tilt, and scan localization from the scout image, should be part of a comprehensive QA program. Table 5-4 summarizes the TG-66 recommendations for evaluating the image quality of CT simulators.

TABLE 5-3. American Association of Physicists in Medicine Task Group Report 66 Test Specifications for External Laser Marking System

Performance Parameter	Frequency	Tolerance Limits
Alignment of gantry lasers with the center of imaging plane	Daily	± 2 mm
Orientation of gantry lasers with respect to the imaging plane	Monthly and after laser adjustments	± 2 mm over the length of laser projection
Spacing of lateral wall lasers with respect to lateral gantry lasers and scan plane	Monthly and after laser adjustments	± 2 mm
Orientation of wall lasers with respect to the imaging plane	Monthly and after laser adjustments	± 2 mm over the length of laser projection
Orientation of the ceiling laser with respect to the imaging plane	Monthly and after laser adjustments	± 2 mm over the length of laser projection

Adapted from Mutic S et al.[1]

TABLE 5-4. American Association of Physicists in Medicine Task Group Report 66 Test Specifications for Image Quality Evaluation

Performance Parameter	Frequency	Tolerance Limits
CT number accuracy	Daily, monthly, annually	Water: 0 ± 5 HU
Image noise	Daily	Manufacturer's specifications
In-plane spatial integrity	Daily, monthly	± 1 mm
Field uniformity	Monthly, annually	± 5 HU
Electron density	Annually	Commissioning results and manufacturer's specifications
Spatial resolution	Annually	Manufacturer's specifications
Contrast resolution	Annually	Manufacturer's specifications

Adapted from Mutic S et al.[1]
HU = Houndsfield unit.

QA for CT Simulation Software

In addition to the CT scanner QA, TG-66 discusses testing features of the CT simulation software for verifying its accuracy. The QA program should verify the following features: image input test, structure delineation, multimodality image registration, machine definition, isocenter calculation and movement, and image reconstruction. One of the final products from the CT simulation process is the generation of DRRs used for verifying the patient's position at the treatment machine. The use of poor-quality DRRs can affect the patient positioning process owing to the inability to visualize anatomic details. The choice of slice thickness and spacing will affect the spatial resolution and image quality of the DRR. Figure 5-3 shows DRRs scanned with 10, 5, 2.5, and 1.25 mm slice spacing using a pelvic phantom, respectively. These figures illustrate the relationship between poor DRR spatial resolution and slice spacing. Figure 5-3A depicts a blurred and poor DRR image using 10 mm slice spacing. Figure 5-3B and Figure 5-3C indicate improved DRRs with smaller slice spacing of 5 and 2.5 mm, respectively. Figure 5-3D shows a DRR with excellent detail using 1.25 mm slice spacing. From these images, the use of 10 mm slice spacing would be inadequate for proper DRR images. The use of 1.25 mm slice spacing for DRRs may not show enough visual improvement compared with the 2.5 mm slice spacing to warrant using it for routine clinical scanning. A clinic should perform a similar test to determine the acceptable slice thickness and slice spacing to use for DRR generation.

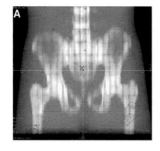
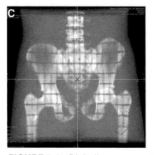
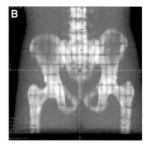
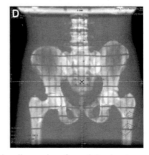

FIGURE 5-3. Digitally reconstructed radiographs of a pelvic phantom using various slice thicknesses to illustrate the effect of slice thickness on image quality: (A) 10 mm slice thickness; (B) 5 mm slice thickness; (C) 2.5 mm slice thickness; and (D) 1.25 mm slice thickness. (To view a color version of this image, please refer to the CD-ROM.)

Evaluation of CT Simulation Process

After testing the CT scanner components and virtual simulation software, the overall simulation process should be evaluated by the clinical team members. A CT simulation program should include a written set of procedures and be reviewed annually by the clinical staff. Procedures should be written for each treatment site to identify the scan protocol, scan limits, contrast, special instructions, and possible beam arrangements.

Emerging Technologies

A new method of CT simulation is evolving known as four-dimensional CT simulation (three dimensions + time = four dimensions). In four-dimensional CT simulation, retrospective gating of the CT simulation data is performed using the patient's respiratory breathing cycle. GE Medical Systems (Waukesha, WI) and Varian Medical Systems (Palo Alto, CA) have developed a system using the Real-Time Position Monitor (RPM) respiratory gating system (Varian Medical Systems) with a multislice CT scanner for analyzing and incorporating intrafraction motion management using tomographic data sets. The system provides retrospective gating of the tomographic data set by taking three-dimensional data sets at specific time intervals to create a time-dependent four-dimensional CT imaging study. The use of this four-dimensional imaging set allows one to accurately define the target and its trajectory with respect to normal anatomy and critical structures. This type of CT simulation tool can then be used with the respiratory gating system at the treatment machine to gate the beam delivery with the patient's breathing cycle. The use of four-dimensional CT simulation makes it possible to acquire CT scans that provide new information on the motion of tumors and critical structures. As this technology emerges within radiation oncology departments, IMRT treatment planning systems may begin to incorporate the dimension of time into the planning process.

In addition to CT simulation, some departments are using magnetic resonance scanners with virtual simulation software to create magnetic resonance simulation systems. Typically, CT scans have been used to provide a tomographic data map of the patient's anatomy. If MRI was incorporated for improved soft tissue delineation, the MRI set was often registered to the CT image data for the virtual simulation process. One reason for using CT data has been its use for heterogeneity information in the treatment planning process. Another reason is that portal films at the treatment machine are matched to DRRs for treatment verification of geometric patient setups. However, there are some areas in which magnetic resonance simulation may be used as the main imaging data set in a department. A magnetic resonance simulator consists of a magnetic resonance scanner with a flat tabletop along with an external laser marking system. Because this technology is relatively new, its clinical role has yet to be defined.

Conclusion

As with other components of IMRT planning and delivery, CT simulation is an evolving process. Much of the virtual simulation software is being incorporated into treatment planning systems, making it more difficult to distinguish between CT simulation and treatment planning. The overlap of these systems with seamless communication of data provides powerful tools to clinicians in visualizing the patient's anatomy. With IMRT treatment planning, anatomic segmentation and dose-volume constraints drive the final solution for the patient, which places more importance on accurate and precise delineation of anatomy. The medical physicist in RT must take on more responsibility for ensuring that an adequate QA process has been implemented for the CT simulation system and process. As new treatment planning and delivery systems are developed, the process of CT simulation will evolve and adapt to provide the clinician with accurate representations of patient anatomy.

References

1. Mutic S, Palta J, Butker E, et al. Quality assurance for computed tomography simulators and the computed tomography-simulation process: American Association of Physicists in Medicine, Radiation Therapy Committee Task Group 66. Med Phys 2003;30:2762–92.
2. Lichter AS, Lawrence TS. Recent advances in radiation oncology. N Engl J Med 1995;332:371–9.
3. Butker E, Helton D, Keller J, et al. Practical implementation of CT simulation: the Emory experience. In: Purdy JA, Starkschall G, editors. A practical guide to 3-D planning and conformal radiation therapy. Middleton (WI): Advanced Medical Publishing; 1999. p. 58–9.
4. Coia LR, Schultheiss TE, Hannks G, editors. A practical guide to CT simulation. Madison (WI): Advanced Medical Publishing; 1995.
5. Conway J, Robinson MH. CT virtual simulation. Br J Radiol 1997;70:S106–18.
6. Jani SK, editor. CT simulation for radiotherapy. Madison (WI): Medical Physics Publishing; 1993.
7. Kushima T, Kono M. New development of integrated CT simulation system for radiation therapy planning. Kobe J Med Sci 1993;39:197–213.
8. Michalski JM, Purdy JA, Harms W, et al. The CT simulation 3-D treatment planning process. Front Radiat Ther Oncol 1996;29:43–56.
9. Nagata Y, Nishidai T, Abe M, et al. CT simulator: a new 3-D planning and simulating system for radiotherapy: Part 2. Clinical application. Int J Radiat Oncol Biol Phys 1990;18:505–13.
10. Nishidai T, Nagata Y, Takahashi M, et al. CT simulator: a new 3-D planning and simulating system for radiotherapy: part 1. Description of system. Int J Radiat Oncol Biol Phys 1990;18:499–504.
11. Sherouse G, Mosher K, Novins K, et al. Virtual simulation: concept and implementation. In: Bruinvis IAD, van der

Giessen PH, van Kleffens HJ, Wittkamper FW, editors. Ninth International Conference on the Use of Computers in Radiation Therapy. North Holland; 1987. p. 433–6.

12. Sherouse GW, Bourland JD, Reynolds K. Virtual simulation in the clinical setting: some practical considerations. Int J Radiat Oncol Biol Phys 1990;19:1059–65.

13. Sherouse GW, Novins K, Chaney EL. Computation of digitally reconstructed radiographs for use in radiotherapy treatment design. Int J Radiat Oncol Biol Phys 1990;18:651–8.

14. Van Dyk J, Taylor JS. CT simulators. In: Van Dyk J, editor. The modern technology for radiation oncology: a compendium for medical physicists and radiation oncologists. Madison (WI): Medical Physics Publishing; 1999. p. 131–68.

15. Goitein M, Abrams D, Rowell H, et al. Multidimensional treatment planning: II. Beam's eye-view, back projection, and projection through CT sections. Int J Radiat Oncol Biol Phys 1983;9:789–97.

16. Van Dyk J, Mah K. Simulation and imaging for radiation therapy planning. In: Williams JR, Thwaites TI, editors. Radiotherapy physics in practice. 2nd ed. Oxford (UK): Oxford University Press; 2000. p. 118–49.

17. Mah K, Danjoux CE, Manship S, et al. Computed tomographic simulation of craniospinal fields in pediatric patients: improved treatment accuracy and patient comfort. Int J Radiat Oncol Biol Phys 1998;41:997–1003.

18. Butker EK, Helton DJ, Keller JW, et al. A totally integrated simulation technique for three-field breast treatment using a CT simulator. Med Phys 1996;23:1809–14.

19. Kalender WA. Principles and performance of spiral CT. In: Goldman LW, Fowlkes JB, editors. Medical CT and ultrasound: current technology and applications. Madison (WI): Advanced Medical Publishing; 1995. p. 379–410.

20. Kalender WA, Polacin A. Physical performance characteristics of spiral CT scanning. Med Phys 1991;18:910–5.

21. Klingenbeck-Regn K, Schaller S, Flohr T, et al. Subsecond multi-slice computed tomography: basics and applications. Eur J Radiol 1999;31;110–24.

22. Hu H. Multi-slice helical CT: scan and reconstruction. Med Phys 1999;26:5–18.

23. Fuchs T, Kachelriess M, Kalender WA. Technical advances in multi-slice spiral CT. Eur J Radiol 2000;36:69–73.

24. Garcia-Ramirez JL, Mutic S, Dempsey JF, et al. Performance evaluation of an 85 cm bore x-ray computed tomography scanner designed for radiation oncology and comparison with current diagnostic CT scanners. Int J Radiat Oncol Biol Phys 2002;52:1123–31.

25. Brooks K, Fox T, Davis L. A critical look at currently available radiation oncology information management systems. Semin Radiat Oncol 1997;7:49–57.

26. National Electrical Manufacturers Association. DICOM PS 3 (set). Digital Imaging Communications in Medicine (DICOM); 1998. Available at: www.nema.org/dicom.

Chapter 6

IMMOBILIZATION AND LOCALIZATION

JAMES BALTER, PhD

The steep dose gradients and small margins associated with modern conformal radiation therapy (RT) and intensity-modulated radiation therapy (IMRT) demand introspection into the concepts of patient positioning. This chapter attempts to aid in the quest to understand what is to be accomplished by the tools and procedures used to position a patient for treatment and what paradigms for positioning, including variations on methods of image guidance, may be needed. The reader is challenged to consider each anatomic target uniquely and to consider how a specific patient may be unique compared with others with the same disease site.

Immobilization Systems

Quite often, a vendor will describe the "reproducibility" of an immobilization system. Herein lies the first opportunity for consideration. It is necessary to both make a target immobile (ie, not moving during irradiation) and position the target correctly. It is a very complex task to achieve both goals simultaneously via a mechanical system. The most successful applications of this joint paradigm are found in the use of stereotactic head frames, which are invasive and rely on minimal organ motion within the skull.

Coordinate Systems Related to Patient Positioning

It is useful to consider at least three coordinate systems for patient positioning. The first set of axes defines the treatment room and is defined by the axes of gantry and collimator rotation. This system is known most precisely and is usually maintained (through positioning lasers) to an accuracy of 2 mm or better with routine physics quality assurance.

A second coordinate system is somewhat arbitrary but has been the standard tool for treatment setup verification for decades. The patient coordinate system defines the gross position of the anatomic section of the patient to be treated. This system is routinely assessed by marks placed on the patient's skin and/or immobilization device. Alignment

of external markers to room lasers remains the standard practice for patient positioning in the majority of centers performing conformal RT and IMRT.

The patient coordinate system may also be referred to by the position and orientation of the regional skeletal anatomy of the patient visible on radiographic film or on electronic portal and diagnostic images. Verification of bony landmark position is routinely performed at the initiation of treatment and subsequently throughout the treatment course on an infrequent basis (typically weekly). Although it is possible that some targets (eg, brain tumors and upper neck lesions) may maintain a fixed location with respect to regional skeletal anatomy, targets in the thorax, abdomen, and pelvis may vary significantly in position relative to the skeleton.

The third coordinate system is the target coordinate system. It is reasonable to define the target in this situation as the clinical target volume. This coordinate system is the most difficult to establish routinely over the course of treatment; however, target location is the dominant concern of immobilization and localization. Examples of technology for target localization include ultrasonography, radiography of implanted fiducial markers, and in-room computed tomography (CT) scanners.

By these definitions, it becomes clear that the primary goal of treatment verification is to register the target and treatment room coordinate systems. Although the patient coordinate system is more conveniently established, its relationship to the target coordinate system may be highly variable. Persistent use of skin marks or skeletal anatomy to position a patient requires establishment of this variation and incorporation of the residual uncertainty into the treatment planning process to ensure sufficient dose to the target.

Systems for Patient Positioning

The variety of systems developed for patient positioning is quite extensive, and a detailed list is beyond the scope of this chapter. For some details, the reader is referred to an excellent summary by Bentel.[1] To provide a framework for evaluation, an overview of the core technologies that have been used recently is summarized:

1. *Styrofoam cast with foaming agent for customized shaping.* Custom foam casts, or alpha cradles, are routinely used in RT treatments. The general process for creating an alpha cradle involves placing the patient on a Styrofoam mold encased in a plastic bag. A foaming agent is poured into the bag, which forms to the patient's regional anatomy as it solidifies. Custom foam immobilization has been applied to the concept of distal joint positioning through the use of very large casts and has been shown to positively impact reproducibility of positioning the thorax, abdomen, and pelvis.[2,3]

2. *Evacuated bean bags.* A similar concept of customized shaping to individual patients involves the use of large bean bags. These bags are sealed with a single access port containing a valve. As the patient is positioned in the bag for simulation, the air is evacuated, and the bag is formed to the patient's regional anatomy.[4,5]

3. *Thermoplastic material.* Thermoplastic sheets are either solid or perforated sheets of plastic. At relatively low temperatures, these plastics soften and can be formed around the patient. They quickly solidify at room temperature. Thermoplastic masks have been routinely used for immobilization of the head and neck[6] but have also been used as a component in immobilization systems for the pelvis.[7]

4. *Dental molds and bite blocks.* The hard palate is a unique fixation point for positioning the skull and, by extension, aiding in configuring the orientation of the upper neck. It is rigid with respect to the skull, does not move about as the skin over the skull does, and provides a relatively large surface area for matching with an immobilization system. Various devices have been designed to take advantage of this unique landmark, ranging from simple blocks to custom molds and even systems employing suction to affix the immobilization system to the upper palate.[8,9] A relocatable stereotactic frame relies heavily on the dental immobilization concept for positioning accuracy,[10,11] as does a slightly less invasive system employed initially at the University of Florida.[12]

5. *Pins and screws.* The highest accuracy routinely reported primarily through the use of a mechanical positioning system has been through the use of stereotactic frames affixed to the skull.

6. *Emerging systems.* Beyond these well-known systems, a few other systems have emerged. Many positioning systems used for thoracic, abdominal, and pelvic positioning are simpler in concept, providing flat or generically contoured surfaces with adjustable arm, head, and pelvic rests. Although these systems may, at the outset, appear to be less accurate than the previously mentioned systems because they minimally adapt to the individual patient, a further investigation of the role of these systems in positioning is worthwhile.

Indexed Systems

Some of the more significant developments in precision therapy over the past decade are related to the integration of computer-controlled systems in linear accelerators. These advancements have permitted a minor paradigm shift that is nonetheless highly significant in reducing the chance of gross errors in positioning and may improve the accuracy of routine patient setup.

The position of the treatment couch at setup can be recorded and used as an interlock with tolerance limits. This development permits the establishment of a reference couch position as an aid in setup. To take advantage of this development, some modern couch tops have labeled indents or other registration indices to which immobilization devices can be reproducibly affixed. The combination of placing the immobilization device in the same place on the couch and validating the couch position electronically serves as a significant adjunct to skin marks and lasers for positioning. It is possible that, for certain body sites, positioning the patient relative to the immobilization device and indexing the device to the digital couch readout may be as or more reproducible than attempting to set up the patient to the isocenter using skin marks and lasers. This concept needs to be approached with caution but is nonetheless promising. Exploration of the nature of position distributions in the subsequent section of this chapter elucidates this concept further.

Nature of Patient Positioning

Regardless of positioning equipment used, there is some variation in target position over multiple sessions of patient setup. The position of the target over the course of treatment can be described as a distribution with an average value and a spread about this average.

The process of simulation, typically performed using CT, involves one instance of patient positioning. It is unlikely that patients will be observed in their average position during simulation. Thus, there is an offset between the position of the target used for treatment planning and the average position realized through consistent use of the immobilization equipment and standard setup procedure. This difference has been labeled as "systematic" setup error in the literature. It is incorrect to assume that systematic error is attributed to differences in couch sag, laser calibration, or other components between simulation and treatment equipment. Owing to the random nature of setup variation, systematic error will persist, and a major goal of the localization process involves minimization of random variation and resolution of systematic offsets.

It is also important to understand a number of additional features about the patient position distribution. The random variation in position for the same immobilization technique may vary significantly between patients in the same population. Furthermore, these may vary based on the skill and experience of the therapist performing the setup. These variations can be ameliorated somewhat through extensive training and development of standard procedures for use of positioning systems. It is a critical, although typically neglected, part of the process of using a new immobilization system for an institution to establish its own population statistics of setup variation. In addition, these measurements should be used for rational decisions in localization strategy, as well as margins and treatment planning directives. The steep dose gradients seen in IMRT plans make such a process crucial to safe and effective treatment.

Localization Strategies

Table 6-1 shows examples of population setup variations for different body sites. These data were acquired via frequent portal imaging during a planned observation period. Although images were acquired daily, only a subset of weekly images was used for setup verification. Orthogonal portal images were acquired daily, and setup variations were measured retrospectively. The mean random variation is clearly a poor predictor of the range of random setup errors for the population.

Given these average and patient-specific variations, it is important to determine which strategy will most efficiently achieve the precision necessary for IMRT. A few strategies have been studied extensively. The methods described below present a trade-off of effort (and treatment time) expended versus accuracy achieved.

Weekly Verification

This strategy (or small variations thereof) is probably the predominant means of setup verification in use today. Evolved over the past decades from the advent of portal films,[13] this method involves acquiring portal images to verify patient position at the initiation of treatment and then infrequently through the course of treatment. Corrections are generally based on a threshold for action, and adjustment is made either on the treatment fraction during which images are acquired or on the subsequent treatment fraction.

This strategy is certainly acceptable for reduction of gross (eg, over 1 cm) systematic errors. It has no application in the reduction of random variation (as is described further). The potential for this strategy to reduce the magnitude of smaller systematic errors, for which it is generally believed to be acceptable, is discussed further here.

Figure 6-1 shows the actual data of daily position variation of a patient for whom daily imaging was performed. The patient had daily position adjustments. The images acquired following setup (to skin marks) but prior to adjustment of position were compared with the reference digitally reconstructed radiograph to establish position error. The data shown represent position variation in the cranial-caudal axis. A simulation is shown of the impact of weekly setup adjustment with "perfect" correction. Perfect correction is simulated by taking the error seen on the days of imaging (every fifth fraction) and applying that correction on all subsequent fractions until the next imaging session. It is clearly conceivable that no significant improvement is made to patient position by weekly adjustment. In fact, given the selection of the "day," the potential remains to increase setup error over doing nothing at all (in this example, both the average and the random variation increased slightly with ideal weekly adjustment).

Pretreatment (On-line) Setup Adjustment

One of the most labor- and time-intensive methods to improve setup accuracy involves daily pretreatment localization of the patient. In fact, this procedure is performed on almost all patients via the use of external marks and lasers, thus registering the patient coordinate system to some extent with the room coordinate system. As mentioned above, however, the veracity of surface localization is likely insufficient to achieve the accuracy necessary for most

TABLE 6-1. Average and Maximum Random Variations in a Population of Patients

	σ_{avg} (Maximum) Observed Random Variations, mm		
Site	Lateral	Anterior-Posterior	Cranial-Caudal
Pelvis	2.6 (6.2)	2.4 (6.3)	2.7 (7.0)
Chest	3.0 (7.9)	2.6 (7.0)	3.4 (11.8)
Abdomen	2.5 (9.1)	3.1 (9.1)	3.1 (12.4)
Head/neck	2.1 (8.4)	2.2 (8.6)	2.7 (5.8)

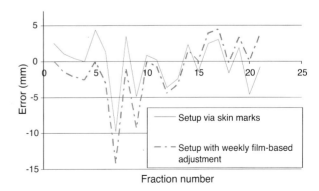

FIGURE 6-1. Measured cranial-caudal position offsets (*solid line*) and a simulation of setup error via exact implementation of weekly portal films and pretreatment correction (*dashed line*).

IMRT treatments.

The advent of electronic portal imaging saw a plethora of studies involving daily targeting of skeletal anatomy, as well as implanted fiducial markers. These studies showed a significant reduction in systematic and random variations, although with the associated cost of increased treatment time. Further advances of in-room imaging, including the use of an ultrasound system indexed to isocenter position, as well as in-room CT scanning and registration to reference CT data, have provided increased potential to realize the target position more directly than by conventional radiographic means. These developments are still quite dynamic, and at the time of writing, it is too early to state the expected accuracy of using in-room CT.

Within the daily verification paradigm, there are two subsets of strategies. Under one strategy, all measurements of target offset are used to correct patient position. Although seemingly the most accurate strategy, this process comes at the highest cost in time and needs some further thought prior to acceptance.

Consider the steps in the process of daily setup verification. A measurement is made of position (via imaging and some visual or computer-aided alignment technique). This measurement is then translated into instructions to adjust the treatment, typically by adjustment of the treatment table position. Both the measurement process and the couch adjustment are not perfect, and their combined error leads to a limit in the final accuracy that can be achieved (even assuming that the patient is completely immobile during the time of imaging, adjustment, and treatment). This means that even if every measured setup error is corrected, there is the potential to have a residual error that is, in fact, introduced by the correction process.

To better understand the magnitude of these residual errors, it is important to do a self-assessment. Any RT department that wishes to set margins based on the expected improvement from daily setup correction should first determine the accuracy of setup measurement and then attempt to understand the accuracy of adjustment. Setup measurement accuracy can be determined by having the observers (typically therapists) who will perform measurements go through a period of training and then perform multiple alignments of the same portal image to itself and multiple alignments of a series of portal images to a reference image. The spread of these distributions can give an estimate of measurement accuracy. Adjustment accuracy is more difficult to assess but may be possible to determine if measurements are acquired both before and after measurement-based adjustment (eg, on the first day of treatment). If a distribution of errors measured before and after adjustment can be acquired, then the change in positioning error can be compared with the expected measurement error to see whether table adjustment is a significant confounding factor. Both measurement and adjustment variation can vary with technology and body

site (possibly as well as user skill) and should be assessed for new systems.

Given this limit, it is reasonable to consider a slightly different strategy for adjustment in which measurements are acquired daily but adjustment is performed only if the measured position error exceeds a defined threshold. Using this strategy, the threshold can be selected by body site as a trade-off of the effort expended versus the accuracy achieved. An illustration of this trade-off is shown in Figure 6-2. It can be seen that as the residual error approaches the limit of accuracy for measurement and correction, dramatic increases in effort yield minimal gain in accuracy until, finally, no significant gain is realized, even with adjustment on every treatment fraction.

Thus, with daily adjustment, it is important to be realistic about expectations of effort and accuracy. One important thing to think about is whether the random variation in patient position is so large that it exceeds these accuracy limits and is also unacceptably large with respect to treatment planning directives. This area is still under exploration. For conformal therapy of the prostate, Remeijer and colleagues described a margin formula that denotes planning target volume (PTV) margin size as

$$\text{PTV margin} \approx 2.5\Sigma + 0.7\sigma$$

where Σ represents the population standard deviation for systematic error and σ is the random variation standard deviation.[14,15] It is important to note that the latest version of van Herk's formula includes a constant 3 mm reduction. This value was based on the equivalent uniform dose formalism, including an estimate of the influence of dose homogeneity on tumor control, and is not reproduced

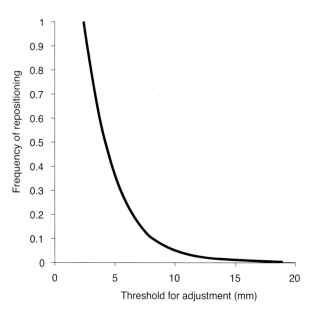

FIGURE 6-2. Trade-off of residual error versus effort with daily threshold-based setup adjustment.

here because it requires assumptions that are beyond the scope of this chapter. The key point of this finding is that systematic error plays a far more important role in dose coverage and margins than random variations and that attempts to reduce the magnitude of systematic variation achieve most of the benefit possible in positioning for the majority of patients.

Off-line Setup Correction Strategies

Although a reduction in systematic offset can be achieved through daily on-line setup measurement and adjustment, more efficient means of reducing systematic error have been realized. Given that the systematic error is the average difference between the reference and treated patient position, the combination of patient setup error measurements from multiple days will yield a better estimate of the average error than any single daily setup measurement. Such measurements do not need to take place completely while the patient is waiting on the treatment table and thus can decrease treatment time. The strategies that involve decisions about treatment made while the patient is not on the table are considered off-line methods.

There are a number of different off-line strategies of varying complexity, but the overall issue involves the question of how many measurements are needed to establish the systematic error.[16–18] Although the results of studies vary, it has generally been accepted that three to five measurements are sufficient for estimating the systematic component of setup variation with sufficient accuracy. There is some question as to whether the first treatment fraction should be considered one of these measurements because many factors, including patient discomfort, the length of the initial treatment session, and resolution of potentially complex gross errors (eg, improper communication of offsets to the isocenter from the simulated position of the patient), prior to initial treatment may come into play.

It is still somewhat difficult to implement off-line strategies in most clinics. Although the use of pretreatment localization involves training and use of software that is now becoming available on most commercial imaging systems, and the impact on clinic flow is easily seen, the most efficient use of off-line strategies is still open to discussion. Two leading strategies involve either (1) a designated therapist spending a fraction of his or her day analyzing all portal images acquired in preparation for off-line measurement (with experience, a single therapist can align all of the images for a 60 patient/day clinic in less than 2 hours per day for a four-measurement off-line protocol) or (2) having the therapist at the treatment unit analyze the images for a particular patient during or after the delivery of each fraction in the off-line protocol or analyzing all images immediately before the fraction on which action is to be taken. Either of these strategies can be implemented efficiently with sufficient planning. It is very useful to develop a database to record alignment results

and provide an average or predicted correction. Such tools are generally not available in imaging systems or record-and-verify software but are not too difficult to produce (a simple paper worksheet can suffice).

Intratreatment Movement

The subject of intratreatment movement is also critical to IMRT. Various means have been developed to account for movement owing to breathing. The most widespread of these technologies follows the concept of immobilization. Both active breath-hold[19–24] and gating[25–27] systems are designed to restrict the range of positions of internal anatomy to a fraction of that seen during normal breathing. Note that these systems do not eliminate the need for margins for movement. Given that the reproducibility of active breathing control is limited and the use of phase or amplitude windows for gating permits some intratreatment movement and some variation in position at the gated state, caution needs to be taken to understand the benefit of these systems prior to margin reduction. It is strongly recommended that these systems be evaluated locally via fluoroscopy or similar means prior to clinical use.[28–30]

Summary

Our understanding of position variation has evolved significantly over the past few years. Parallel developments in localization technology, computer control, immobilization technology, and theory of positioning have led to more rational and efficient means of achieving reasonable margins than previously thought possible. Adoption of these technology and concepts, however, requires significant introspection into the RT process and may require extensive training and infrastructure development. Nonetheless, it is likely that both technology and paradigms are necessary for efficient margin reduction on the order necessary to perceive a benefit from IMRT in most regions of the body.

References

1. Bentel GC. Patient positioning and immobilization in radiation oncology. New York: McGraw-Hill; 1998.
2. Bentel GC, Marks LB, Sherouse GW, et al. The effectiveness of immobilization during prostate irradiation. Int J Radiat Oncol Biol Phys 1995;31:143–8.
3. Sherouse GW, Bourland JD, Reynolds K, et al. Virtual simulation in the clinical setting: some practical considerations. Int J Radiat Oncol Biol Phys 1990;19:1059–65.
4. Dickens CW. Personalized fixation using a vacuum consolidation technique. Br J Radiol 1981;54:257–8.
5. Jakobsen A, Iversen P, Gadeberg C, et al. A new system for patient fixation in radiotherapy. Radiother Oncol 1987;8:145–51.
6. Verhey LJ, Goitein M, McNulty P, et al. Precise positioning of patients for radiation therapy. Int J Radiat Oncol Biol Phys

1982;8:289–94.

7. Akino H, Ohyama N, Mori H, et al. [Treatment of prostate cancer by radiotherapy]. Hinyokika Kiyo 1997;43:461–4.

8. Nelson TJ, Lindberg RD. Biteblock-head immobilizer system. Med Dosim 1989;14:147–51.

9. Schulte RW, Fargo RA, Meinass HJ, et al. Analysis of head motion prior to and during proton beam therapy. Int J Radiat Oncol Biol Phys 2000;47:1105–10.

10. Kooy HM, Dunbar SF, Tarbell NJ, et al. Adaptation and verification of the relocatable Gill-Thomas-Cosman frame in stereotactic radiotherapy. Int J Radiat Oncol Biol Phys 1994;30:685–91.

11. Havelka C, Nelson LP, Shusterman S, et al. Custom oral appliance for noninvasive immobilization during stereotactic radiotherapy. Pediatr Dent 1995;17:212–5.

12. Bova FJ, Buatti JM, Friedman WA, et al. The University of Florida frameless high-precision stereotactic radiotherapy system. Int J Radiat Oncol Biol Phys 1997;38:875–82.

13. Byhardt RW, Cox JD, Hornburg A, et al. Weekly localization films and detection of field placement errors. Int J Radiat Oncol Biol Phys 1978;4:881–7.

14. Remeijer P, Rasch C, Lebesque JV, et al. Margins for translational and rotational uncertainties: a probability-based approach. Int J Radiat Oncol Biol Phys 2002;53:464–74.

15. van Herk M, Remeijer P, Lebesque JV. Inclusion of geometric uncertainties in treatment plan evaluation. Int J Radiat Oncol Biol Phys 2002;52:1407–22.

16. de Boer JC, Heijmen BJ. A new approach to off-line setup corrections: combining safety with minimum workload. Med Phys 2002;29:1998–2012.

17. de Boer HC, Heijmen BJ. A protocol for the reduction of systematic patient setup errors with minimal portal imaging workload. Int J Radiat Oncol Biol Phys 2001;50:1350–65.

18. Yan D, Wong J, Vicini F, et al. Adaptive modification of treatment planning to minimize the deleterious effects of treatment setup errors. Int J Radiat Oncol Biol Phys 1997;38:197–206.

19. Balter JM, Brock KK, Litzenberg DW, et al. Daily targeting of intrahepatic tumors for radiotherapy. Int J Radiat Oncol Biol Phys 2002;52:266–71.

20. Dawson LA, Brock KK, Kazanjian S, et al. The reproducibility of organ position using active breathing control (ABC) during liver radiotherapy. Int J Radiat Oncol Biol Phys 2001;51:1410–21.

21. Wong JW, Sharpe MB, Jaffray DA, et al. The use of active breathing control (ABC) to reduce margin for breathing motion. Int J Radiat Oncol Biol Phys 1999;44:911–9.

22. Wong J, Sharpe M, Jaffray D. The use of active breathing control (ABC) to minimize breathing motion in conformal therapy. In: Proceedings of the XIIth ICCR. Medical Physics Publishing; 1997. p. 220–2.

23. Cheung PC, Sixel KE, Tirona R, et al. Reproducibility of lung tumor position and reduction of lung mass within the planning target volume using active breathing control (ABC). Int J Radiat Oncol Biol Phys 2003;57:1437–42.

24. Remouchamps VM, Letts N, Vicini FA, et al. Initial clinical experience with moderate deep-inspiration breath hold using an active breathing control device in the treatment of patients with left-sided breast cancer using external beam radiation therapy. Int J Radiat Oncol Biol Phys 2003;56:704–15.

25. Kubo HD, Hill BC. Respiration gated radiotherapy treatment: a technical study. Phys Med Biol 1996;41:83–91.

26. Ritchie CJ, Hsieh J, Gard MF, et al. Predictive respiratory gating: a new method to reduce motion artifacts on CT scans. Radiology 1994;190:847–52.

27. Wagman R, Yorke E, Ford E, et al. Respiratory gating for liver tumors: use in dose escalation. Int J Radiat Oncol Biol Phys 2003;55:659–68.

28. Ford EC, Mageras GS, Yorke E, et al. Evaluation of respiratory movement during gated radiotherapy using film and electronic portal imaging. Int J Radiat Oncol Biol Phys 2002;52:522–31.

29. Mageras GS, Yorke E, Rosenzweig K, et al. Fluoroscopic evaluation of diaphragmatic motion reduction with a respiratory gated radiotherapy system. J Appl Clin Med Phys 2001;2:191–200.

30. Vedam SS, Kini VR, Keall PJ, et al. Quantifying the predictability of diaphragm motion during respiration with a noninvasive external marker. Med Phys 2003;30:505–13.

Chapter 7

IMAGING AND FUSION TECHNOLOGIES

CHARLES A. PELIZZARI, PhD, ANTHONY E. LUJAN, PhD

From the early days of radiation therapy (RT), imaging has played an important role in diagnosis and treatment. Initially, RT was delivered with large unshaped fields using erythema as a gauge to limit the dose. Soon the importance of limiting the dose to normal tissues was recognized, and treatment began to be focused on regions in which disease was actually present (or was suspected to be present). The advent of computed tomography (CT) in the 1970s allowed physicians and physicists to begin to visualize the internal anatomy of patients. In turn, this information helped improve target localization, resulting in improved treatment planning. With advances in computing technology, it became possible for the radiation dose to be computed in three dimensions and for that information to be visualized using three-dimensional graphic tools.

Fundamental to the intensity-modulated radiation therapy (IMRT) planning process is the construction of an accurate and complete three-dimensional patient model that can be used for the computer-aided design of an optimized configuration of beams and IMRT beam intensities that satisfies as fully as possible an appropriate set of goals. Given the availability of IMRT delivery systems that can "sculpt" a three-dimensional dose distribution with a considerable degree of precision, it is a natural inclination to design dose distributions that conform ever more closely to target volumes, elegantly avoiding organs at risk (OAR). This places a premium on the accurate definition of all relevant volumes and the rational incorporation of all available estimates of uncertainty in the location of target and normal structures both as they are defined and as they are treated. Combining information from multiple modalities, each of which may have an advantage in defining a particular aspect of a structure, is often very helpful in this regard.

Target and Normal Tissue Volume Definition

The introduction of IMRT into the clinic has required better definition of both targets and normal tissue. Imaging technologies such as positron emission tomography (PET) and magnetic resonance imaging (MRI) are playing an increased role in treatment planning. New applications of these technologies can provide improved identification of macroscopic gross disease and allow one to identify disease progression that is too small to be visualized via conventional means. Use of these technologies coupled with IMRT may lead to overly aggressive target definitions, which may compromise patient treatment. Thus, it has become ever more important to follow guidelines for target and normal tissue definition.

The International Commission on Radiation Units and Measurement (ICRU) has published recommendations (Report 50) for the definition of target volumes in three-dimensional treatment planning that include the effects of organ motion and setup uncertainties.[1] In Report 62, the concepts in Report 50 are expanded on.[2] These concepts and definitions should be adopted by all institutions for a variety of reasons; the most essential is communication. Use of these concepts can allow clinical information about patient treatment (identification of disease, target definition, treatment geometry) to be conveyed between institutions and aid in developing appropriate clinical studies for new applications of imaging technology and IMRT. The ICRU concepts for target definition are described. For a complete description of the full recommendations for dose recording and reporting, the reader should refer to Reports 50 and 62.[1,2] Interested readers should also refer to Chapter 1, "IMRT Process," for an additional discussion of target and tissue delineation.

There are four major target definition concepts to consider: gross tumor volume (GTV), clinical target volume (CTV), planning target volume (PTV), and the planning organ at risk volume (PRV). Each should be kept in mind when applying imaging technologies to define targets and normal tissues for IMRT treatment planning. The GTV is the gross demonstrable extent and location of malignant growth. It comprises the primary tumor and all involved nodes or other metastases. Clinical examination may be used in conjunction with (or in lieu of) imaging to determine the GTV; however, usually, the region with the highest tumor cell density is designated as the GTV. Of note, the GTV may occupy a portion of an organ or involve an entire organ. Similarly, the GTV may extend outside the borders of the involved organ. From a clinical standpoint, the definition of the GTV should meet the criteria for staging the tumor according to the TNM and American Joint Commission on Cancer (AJCC) systems.[3,4]

In many instances, the GTV is not the only region of disease. Alternatively, in cases in which surgery has been performed, it may not be possible to define a GTV. In either case, microscopic extension of disease may be present that may not be clinically evident. The CTV is the tissue volume that includes the GTV and any regions of subclinical disease. All regions of suspected subclinical disease should be included in the definition of the CTV (eg, local lymph nodes). Some investigators designate multiple CTVs. Regions of subclinical involvement adjacent to the GTV should be designated CTV 1 to differentiate these areas from volumes of disease distal from the GTV (designated CTV 2, CTV 3, etc.). The definition of the CTV should follow clinical knowledge about the spread of disease and should not include margins to account for organ motion or setup uncertainty.

The PTV is formed by a geometric expansion of the CTV and includes a margin accounting for setup uncertainties and organ motion. In ICRU Report 62, these factors have been separated into an internal margin and a setup margin.[2] The internal margin is the expansion of the CTV required to account for expected physiologic changes in organ size, shape, and position relative to the geometry obtained during treatment planning. Such changes may arise from respiration,[5–8] differential fillings of the rectum and bladder,[9–11] heartbeat,[12] swallowing,[13,14] and peristalsis. These changes can be difficult (or impossible) to control and may depend on the setup orientation of the patient (eg, prone vs supine[15–17]). Because of the nature of these physiologic changes, the internal margin may be asymmetric around the CTV. The CTV plus the internal margin defines the internal target volume. These margins are defined based on changes relative to the patient geometry obtained at treatment planning. Various imaging techniques[18,19] can be used to observe and quantify these uncertainties to aid in the definition of the internal target volume.

Random errors arising from daily patient repositioning and alignment of the treatment beams must also be accounted for in treatment planning.[20–22] The margin sufficient to account for these setup uncertainties is designated the setup margin. Careful setup and immobilization of the patient, coupled with imaging techniques,[23–28] can minimize but not entirely eliminate the need for the setup margin. Setup uncertainties should be investigated at each institution to properly form an adequate (but not overly large) setup margin.

The combination of the internal margin and the setup margin added to the CTV defines the PTV. It is not straightforward as to how to combine the internal and setup margins. A purely linear addition of the margins often results in too large a PTV, which may, in turn, lead to additional complications or require compromising the necessary dose delivered. Because the margins account for both random and systematic uncertainties, the margins are often added in quadrature. This approach has been shown to provide margins that are both realistic and acceptable.[29] This method of combining the margins is possible only in situations in which the sources of uncertainties can be identified and quantified (eg, via a standard deviation). Appropriate margins should be generated based on clinical experience. The means used to generate these margins should be clearly identified when reporting results. Figure 7-1 illustrates these basic concepts.

It should be mentioned that the internal margin and PTV concepts were originally conceived in the context of three-dimensional conformal rather than IMRT planning and require additional thought when intensity-modulated beams are involved. The elegant sculpting of dose distributions, which is one of the defining characteristics of IMRT, depends on the correct superposition (at high spatial resolution) of doses from numerous fields, each with spatially varying intensity. It is important to keep in mind that this superposition can be seriously compromised by target motion and that the agreement of a dose distribution delivered to a stationary phantom with calculation may not

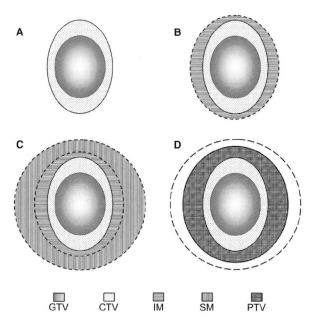

FIGURE 7-1. (*A*) A single contour representing the gross tumor volume (GTV) is shown along with a margin added to account for microscopic spread of disease to form the clinical target volume (CTV). (*B*) The internal margin (IM) is added to account for organ motion. (*C*) A setup margin (SM) in addition to the IM accounts for setup uncertainty. (*D*) The SM and IM are combined in a nonlinear fashion to form the planning target volume (PTV) around the CTV. The dashed line represents the size of the PTV contour if the IM and SM were linearly combined.

reflect the dose to moving anatomy. The same is, of course, true for three-dimensional conformal therapy, but the spatial variation of intensity in the IMRT beams exacerbates the situation. One must bear in mind that the irradiated tissue integrates the dose from multiple fields, and when that tissue moves during and between fields into nearby regions of different doses, the resulting dose distribution can deviate considerably from what is intended. Although practical implementations are not presently available in commercial radiation therapy planning (RTP) systems, it may be more appropriate to account for organ motion (and perhaps estimated setup uncertainty as well) using a method that models the accumulation of dose by a moving tissue volume. Several researchers have proposed methods of doing this by convolving a model of the moving organ with the calculated dose[30] or fluence[31,32] distributions. Methods for optimizing treatments based on organ motion models from serial imaging studies have been described.[33,34] The same considerations apply, of course, when considering motion of OAR, as discussed below.

The definition and delineation of normal tissue are also critical in the treatment process. The location and type of normal tissue can be a limiting factor in the prescribed dose. To that end, it is important to define the OAR in the treatment planning process. The radiation sensitivity of an OAR (eg, spinal cord, lung) and whether it is arranged to operate in a serial, parallel, or mixed-type fashion may influence treatment planning. Because of the uncertainties described above in CTV localization (organ motion and setup uncertainty), a PRV should be considered. The PRV is created by a margin expansion of the OAR. As with the PTV, the margins can be asymmetric and depend on any physiologic variation for that specific OAR. Like the PTV, the PRV is a geometric concept and represents a region that includes the potential positions of the OAR based on organ motion and setup uncertainty. The dose received by the PRV should be interpreted to be the dose that the OAR may receive during treatment. Figure 7-2 illustrates the potential relationships between the PTV and the PRV. The PTV and the PRV may overlap, and in inverse planned IMRT, this overlap may limit the ability of the treatment planning system to obtain an optimal solution. Nonoverlapping structures may be defined for the planning process, but when evaluating the output from the treatment planning system, the actual PRV and OAR volumes should be considered.

Anatomic Modalities
Computed Tomography

Since the late 1970s, the most commonly used anatomic modality in RTP has been x-ray CT. This modality offers a number of advantages, some of which are briefly summarized here. A properly calibrated CT scanner produces images with consistent and reliable three-dimensional spa-

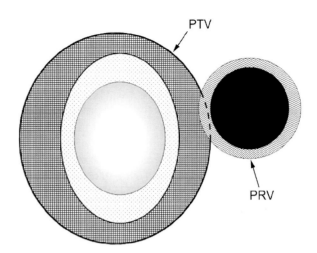

FIGURE 7-2. The relationship between the planning target volume (PTV) and the organ at risk volume (shown in black) and the planning organ at risk volume (PRV) is illustrated. Note that the PTV and PRV may overlap in some cases.

tial coordinates, without the distortions that may occur in MRI. Thus, CT remains the "gold standard" for spatial fidelity in the construction of a three-dimensional patient model. CT numbers are proportional to x-ray attenuation coefficient at each point. Digitally reconstructed radiographs (DRRs) can readily be produced from three-dimensional CT data for comparison with diagnostic radiographs from a simulator or an in-room x-ray imaging system. This has remained one of the strong motivations for reliance on CT in RTP. It is also fairly straightforward to derive from a set of CT images an approximate three-dimensional map of Compton interaction coefficients that can be used in a dose calculation for photon beams[35] or to produce megavoltage DRRs for comparison with portal images.[36] CT scanners are typically less expensive than MRI units, and they can readily be installed in rooms originally designed for RT simulators. Thus, it has become common for RT clinics to have their own dedicated CT scanners. One interesting development that has occurred in the past several years is the introduction of a CT scanner (AcQSim CT, Philips Medical Systems, Andover, MA) designed specifically for the RTP application (see Chapter 5, "CT Simulation").

A number of characteristics of CT scanners affect their suitability for RTP purposes. Spiral data acquisition, in which the gantry rotates continuously while the patient couch moves through the aperture, allows collection of the complete projection data set in a shorter time compared with the axial mode, in which the couch stops and the gantry makes a complete rotation at each slice position. This is useful in helping to minimize respiratory motion artifacts if the projection data set can be acquired during one or more patient breath-holds in a reproducible state of respiration. Multislice scanners that have multiple rows of detectors can acquire projections for several (eg, 4, 8, 16, 32, 40) slices simultaneously, further reducing the time required to scan. Many scanners also allow gated imaging, in which projection data are acquired only when a gating signal is within a certain range. This signal might be derived from a respiratory monitoring system, in which case, only projections within a certain range around some point in the breathing cycle would be used to reconstruct the image. The image would then represent a "snapshot" of the patient's anatomy at that point in the cycle. In addition, retrospective gating in which images are acquired very rapidly and sorted in time according to a gating signal can allow the derivation of a dynamic model of the patient's anatomy.[37] Gated or breath-hold image acquisition must, of course, be done in a way that can be related to the way in which the treatment will be delivered (see Chapter 9, "Respiratory Motion Management," and Chapter 19.4, "Intrafractional Organ Motion and Planning: Emerging Technology"). Slice thickness (the axial extent of the patient over which the slice is averaged) and index (the separation between slice centers along the direction of couch motion) for RTP applications can vary over a wide range of values, from 1 mm or less for high-precision intracranial plans up to 5 to 10 mm for thoracic or pelvic scans. It is noteworthy that to produce the highest-quality DRRs, a small slice spacing is important. In fact, a scan with a small slice separation and a low x-ray tube current can produce better-quality DRRs than a less noisy scan with larger slice separation.[38] Compared with diagnostic applications, the degree to which identification of extremely fine detail in CT images is needed in RTP is somewhat less. Thus, the spatial resolution of most modern CT scanners is more than adequate for RTP purposes. CT scans for RTP are frequently done with continuous injection of iodinated contrast during image acquisition. This typically improves the visualization of vessels, certain glands, and lymph nodes, which are often important in defining the CTV, and areas of increased vascularity or vascular leakage, which may be associated with tumor.

A number of tumor types are well visualized on CT. For example, primary and metastatic tumors in the liver frequently appear with lower intensity than the surrounding parenchyma, as seen in Figure 7-3. It is still often the case, however, that CT images cannot provide adequate discrimination of adjacent soft tissue structures or of tumor from

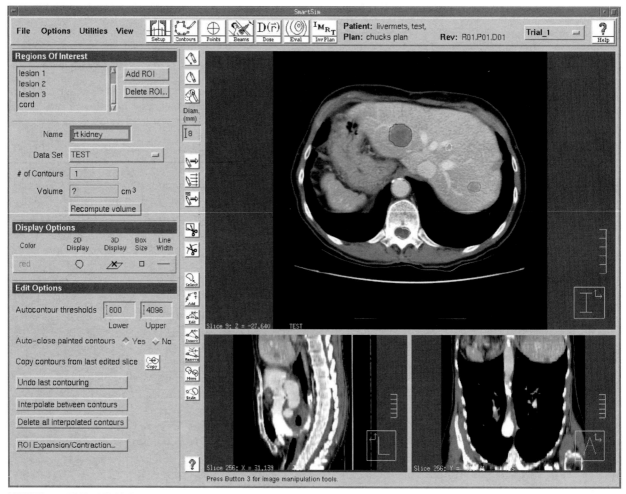

FIGURE 7-3. Philips/ADAC *Pinnacle* screen capture illustrating a computed tomography slice from a patient with liver metastases with the target and normal structures being defined. ROI = region of interest. (To view a color version of this image, please refer to the CD-ROM.)

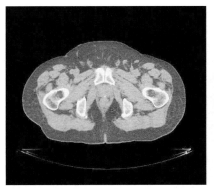 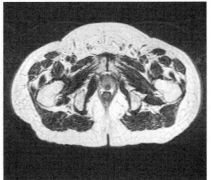 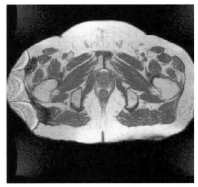

FIGURE 7-4. Corresponding slices through the prostate from computed tomography (*left*), 1.5 Tesla closed magnetic resonance imaging (MRI) (*center*), and 0.23 Tesla open MRI (*right*).

surrounding tissue. In these cases, the inclusion of MRI into the process of anatomy definition is frequently useful. For example, Figure 7-4 shows CT and MRI slices through the prostate. On CT, it is somewhat difficult to differentiate between the prostate gland and the surrounding musculature, whereas on MRI, the margin of the prostate can be clearly identified. Note that, as mentioned earlier, owing to the use of intravenous contrast, blood vessels and lymph nodes in the anterior subcutaneous fat are clearly visible in CT. Merging information from these two studies requires image registration and fusion techniques, which are discussed in another section. Note that the patient couch for treatment planning CT is flat and for diagnostic CT or MRI is usually curved. The distortion of the patient anatomy owing to this difference complicates the image fusion process.

Magnetic Resonance Imaging

Unlike CT, in which image intensity is determined by x-ray attenuation, the MRI signal is generated by precessing proton spins because nuclear magnetization induced by an initial radiofrequency pulse decays owing to interactions of the polarized nuclei with their environment. Two characteristic decay times determine the time dependence of the signal: T_1, which characterizes the overall decay of the initially perturbed spin system to its equilibrium state, and T_2, which characterizes the loss of coherence of the originally polarized spins in the transverse plane owing to various dephasing processes. In addition, the signal intensity depends directly on the local proton spin density. The relaxation times depend on the physical and chemical properties of the local environment, including, among others, water content, viscosity, and diffusion coefficient. Local variations in the magnetic field owing to the presence of paramagnetic species or other effects also lead to dephasing of the transverse magnetization. The overall effective transverse decay time owing to both the intrinsic T_2 and these other effects is called T_2^*. Using spin-echo techniques, T_2 and T_2^* effects can be separated. T_2^*-weighted images are useful in functional imaging, which are discussed later.

In a spin-echo imaging technique, image contrast between tissues with different T_1 and T_2 values can be manipulated by varying the time between pulse repetitions (TR) and the echo time (TE). If TE is short relative to T_2, then image contrast will not be strongly affected by the T_2 variation. If TR is comparable to T_1, then the T_1 variation will affect image contrast. If the TR is relatively long and the TE is comparable to T_2, image contrast will be mainly due to T_2 variations. Some practical implications for several common types of images are summarized in Tables 7-1 and 7-2.

TABLE 7-1. Magnetic Resonance Spin-Echo Image Weighting

TR (ms)	TE (ms)	Image Type	Fat Intensity	Water Intensity
400–800	< 30	T_1 weighted	High	Low
400–800	> 90	Proton density	Intermediate	Intermediate
> 1,500	< 30	Proton density	Intermediate	Intermediate
> 1,500	> 90	T_2 weighted	Intermediate to low	High

Adapted from Li A and Bluemke D.[110]

TABLE 7-2. Relative Intensity of Several Tissues in T_1- and T_2-Weighted Magnetic Resonance Images

Tissue	Image Weighting	
	T_1	T_2
Adrenal gland	3	4
Cervix	2	2
Cortical bone	1	1
Brain		
CSF	2	5
Gray	2–3	3–4
White	4	2–3
Water	2	4
Fat	4	2–3
Muscle	2	2
Lung	1	1
Liver	3–4	2–3
Pancreas	3–4	2–3
Prostate	3	4
Spleen	3	4

Adapted from Li A and Bluemke D.[110]
CSF = cerebrospinal fluid. 1 = darkest; 5 = brightest.

Owing to the generally superior visualization of soft tissues and tumors in MRI, a considerable amount of effort has been directed toward incorporation of MRI into the treatment planning process. One of the original motivations for the development of image registration and fusion methods, discussed later, was to allow importing MRI-defined tumor volumes into an overall CT-based treatment planning process.[39,40] However, entirely MRI-based treatment planning has not become widespread owing to several of the desirable characteristics of CT mentioned earlier. Recently, commercial MRI simulation systems analogous to CT simulation systems have been introduced. The Philips MRI simulation product, which uses a low-field open MRI system, is shown in Figure 7-5. The low-field magnet is relatively inexpensive, so the overall system cost can be comparable to that of a CT simulator. The open system will

alleviate problems in scanning patients immobilized in the treatment position, which would complicate use of a conventional closed magnetic resonance scanner. Considerable effort has been expended in correcting distortions to address the problem of lower spatial accuracy, which has traditionally been associated with MRI in treatment planning.[41,42] Whether the use of dedicated MRI simulation systems in RT departments will become widespread remains to be seen.

Frequently, MRI contrast agents containing gadolinium, a paramagnet, are used. At relatively low concentrations, gadolinium shortens T_1. Thus, regions of contrast uptake appear brighter on T_1-weighted images, as seen in Figure 7-6. As in the case of CT contrast, this improves visualization of regions of blood-brain barrier disruption, increased vascular permeability, and other effects that may reflect the presence of a tumor. However, even with contrast, the specificity of MRI alone in identifying tumor is less than ideal, and it is frequently difficult to differentiate image changes owing to necrosis from tumor recurrence. Additional information from functional imaging is valuable in such cases, as discussed below. A bolus of paramagnetic contrast in relatively high concentration may decrease the image signal, and this effect may be used as the basis of flow-sensitive imaging techniques.

Functional Modalities
Emission Tomography

Frequently, it is difficult to identify tumor volumes with as much specificity and sensitivity as one would wish based on anatomic images alone. In addition, the CTV concept is explicitly intended to include microscopic extensions of disease beyond that visible on anatomic images. Functional imaging holds promise to aid in defining these volumes. The potential for IMRT to produce three-dimensional dose distributions with controlled inhomogeneities to both irradiate and avoid complicated three-dimensional regions rais-

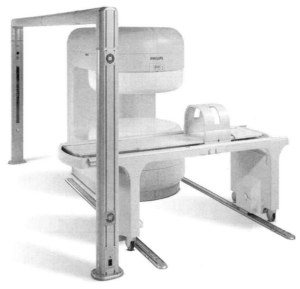

FIGURE 7-5. Low-field, open magnetic resonance imaging simulator used for radiation therapy planning. Courtesy of Philips Medical Systems.

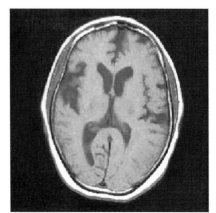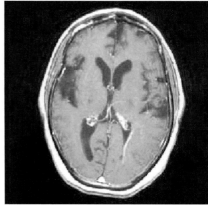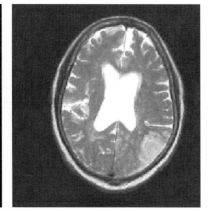

FIGURE 7-6. T_1-weighted pre- (*left*) and post- (*center*) contrast and T_2-weighted (*right*) images in a patient with a brain tumor. Note regions of contrast enhancement in the center image. Courtesy of P. MacEneaney, MD, University of Chicago.

es the possibility of designing a dose distribution to place more dose where the tumor burden is higher and vice versa. Regions to be avoided might also be rationally defined with the addition of information on the location of important functional regions, as in the brain, or of the level of function of different regions of an organ, as in the lung. The inclusion of functional imaging modalities into the treatment planning and assessment process, with the definition of a biologic target volume (BTV) to which dose can be tailored, potentially with different doses delivered to more or less malignant or radioresistant regions,[43] seems highly promising in moving toward these goals.[44,45] Here we briefly describe several functional imaging modalities that are in relatively widespread use in RTP and some that seem likely to become more widely used in the near future.

Emission tomography provides information on the three-dimensional distribution of a radiolabeled substance in the body. In PET, the isotopic label is a positron-emitting nucleus such as ^{18}F, ^{15}O, or ^{11}C. When the positron annihilates with an electron, two 511 keV photons are emitted, traveling in nearly opposite directions. The signature of these events is detection by two detectors nearly simultaneously, providing an electronic collimation that helps to discriminate true events from random counts or scattered photons. In addition, the total energy of the two detected photons depends to first order not on depth but on the line integral of attenuation through the patient, along the path connecting the two detectors. Thus, an attenuation correction can be made based on a separate measurement of these line integrals for each detector pair, which is typically made using an external source of 511 keV photons in a transmission geometry. For this reason, information from PET images is usually considered to have more quantitative potential than from single-photon emission computed tomography (SPECT), in which radioisotopes are used that decay by photon rather than positron emission. However, the variety of tracers available for SPECT is larger, and SPECT scanners are more widely available, so inclusion of functional information from SPECT into RTP is of considerable interest as well. A few PET isotopes and tracers relevant to oncologic imaging are listed in Table 7-3.

Two radioisotopes dominate clinical uses of SPECT: ^{99m}Tc and ^{111}In. Tc is the more commonly used of the two because many pharmaceutical agents can be labeled with generator-produced Tc in the nuclear medicine department using commercially available kits. A few of the tracers that have proven useful in oncologic imaging with SPECT are listed in Table 7-4. A particularly successful application of SPECT in radiation oncology has been the identification of regions of healthy and damaged lung, both for assessment of radiation-induced lung complications and for adjusting treatment plans in an attempt to spare healthy lung regions.[46–48]

Application of nuclear medicine images in RTP requires registration and fusion of the functional information with CT scans and/or MRIs because the anatomic location of each functional region is critical to beam targeting. Example applications of the use of SPECT imaging in RTP for prostate and gynecologic cancers are discussed in the image registration section. The advent of combined CT-PET scanners is having a major impact on the use of PET for RTP because accurate registration is, if not guaranteed, at least greatly simplified (Figure 7-7). A detailed discussion of combined CT-PET imaging in oncology is given in Chapter 8, "PET-CT in IMRT Planning."

Functional Imaging from Magnetic Resonance Contrast

With appropriate analysis, dynamic changes in MRIs can yield qualitative or quantitative information concerning aspects of physiology in a number of settings. The most commonly used forms of functional MRI are blood oxygen level–dependent (BOLD) contrast, which yields information concerning local oxygen concentration and/or oxygen use, and perfusion imaging, which yields information such as regional blood volume and blood flow and tissue perfusion or diffusion.

TABLE 7-4. Single-Photon Emission Computed Tomography Tracers Used in Radiation Therapy Planning and Evaluation

Isotope	Tracer	Application
^{111}In	Somatostatin receptor	Lung, neuroendocrine tumors Binding agents (octreotide, pentreotide)
^{111}In	OncoScint	Colorectal, ovarian cancer
^{111}In	ProstaScint	Prostate cancer
^{99}Tc	Macroaggregated albumen	Lung perfusion
^{99}Tc	Anti-CEA	Colorectal cancer
^{99}Tc	DTPA	Lung ventilation
^{99}Tc	MDP	Bone metastases
^{99}Tc	HMPAO	Brain perfusion
^{99}Tc	Sulfur colloid	Bone marrow activity
^{67}Ga	Gallium citrate	Lymphoma
^{123}I	IMP	Cerebral blood flow
^{201}Tl	Thallium chloride	Tumor detection—brain, head and neck

CEA = carcinoembryonic antigen; DTPA = diethylenetriamine pentaacetic acid; HMPAO = hexamethylpropyleneamine oxime; IMP = iodoamphetamine; MDP = ^{99m}Tc medronate.

TABLE 7-3. Positron Emission Tomography Tracers Used in Oncologic Imaging

Isotope	Tracer	Physiology
^{15}O	Water, CO_2	Blood flow
^{15}O	O_2	Necrosis
^{13}N	Ammonia	Blood flow
^{11}C	Acetate	Oxidative metabolism
^{11}C	Methionine, leucine	Protein synthesis (tumor viability)
^{18}F	F-	Osteoblastic activity (bone scan)
^{18}F	Fluorodeoxyglucose	Glucose metabolism (tumor activity)
^{60}Cu, ^{64}Cu	ATSM	Hypoxia

ATSM = Cu(IT)-diacetyl-bis(N4-methylosemicarbazone).

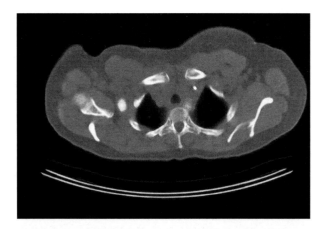

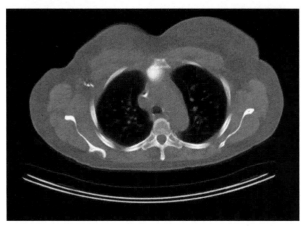

FIGURE 7-7. ^{18}F-labeled fluorodeoxyglucose (^{18}FDG)–positron emission tomography (PET) images overlaid on axial computed tomography (CT) slices as acquired from a PET-CT scanner. The yellow colorwash represents regions of high ^{18}FDG uptake. (To view a color version of this image, please refer to the CD-ROM.)

The BOLD effect is due to differences in the magnetic properties of oxygenated and deoxygenated hemoglobin. Deoxyhemoglobin is paramagnetic, and its presence in tissue leads to dephasing of precessing proton spins and consequent shortening of the effective transverse relaxation time T_2^*. Regions with higher levels of deoxyhemoglobin show decreased intensity on appropriately weighted MRIs. BOLD signal intensities can then be directly interpreted in terms of local tissue oxygenation, although only qualitatively. Differences in BOLD images in two conditions can be used to identify regions in which oxygenation changes, for example, between a resting and a task state,[49] and thus yield information as to which brain regions are involved in a specific activity. This type of information has not been widely used in RTP, although Hamilton and colleagues described the potential for including important functional brain regions as avoidance structures in planning for stereotactic radiosurgery.[50]

Perfusion-weighted imaging is based on the analysis of time dependence of image intensity changes following the introduction of a contrast agent. The contrast agent may be endogenous, for example, saturated spins in flowing blood, or exogenous, such as a gadolinium-containing material. In the most basic technique, multiple T_1-weighted images are acquired in rapid succession following a bolus injection of gadolinium contrast. Analysis of the time dependence of image intensity in a particular region can yield measurements of blood volume, blood-brain barrier integrity, diffusion, perfusion, blood flow, and other parameters. Incorporation of perfusion maps from dynamic imaging has been reported to improve specificity in the identification of active tumor areas in brain lesions, for example, in the differentiation of tumor from necrosis.[51] Information on local diffusion coefficients from MRIs has also been reported to be useful in identifying active regions in brain tumors.[52] Such information should be useful in the definition of a BTV.

Functional Information from Magnetic Resonance Spectra

The actual magnetic field experienced by each proton in an MRI study is influenced by the electrons in the molecule of which the proton is a part. Different molecules introduce different degrees of shielding of the applied field, leading to a chemical shift in the proton resonance frequency for the various molecules—water, fat, etc. Thus, analysis of the spectrum of resonant frequencies can yield information concerning the relative abundance of the different molecules. This, in turn, can be interpreted in terms of physiologic processes that may be associated with the presence of some molecules in greater or lesser abundance relative to that observed in normal tissue. For example, choline, a metabolite that is associated with cell membrane turnover, has been observed to have a higher abundance in malignant prostate tissue compared with either a normal or a benign hypertrophic prostate.[53] Magnetic resonance spectroscopy can map the location of tissue with abnormal ratios of choline to citrate peaks, and this spatial information can be used in the definition of a BTV. Thus, potentially higher doses can be delivered to regions that are spectroscopically more likely to be malignant.[54] Spectroscopic information can also be used to identify active tumor regions in the brain. Figure 7-8 shows the same T_2-weighted brain slice as in Figure 7-6, with spectra from normal (left) and tumor (right) regions. The relative heights of several peaks on the left, as shown with a dashed line in Figure 7-8, are a signature of normally functioning brain tissue. In the tumor region on the right, the spectrum is considerably altered, with the relative intensities of the peaks owing to choline and creatine reversed. Magnetic resonance spectroscopy may also be used to identify hypoxic tumor regions, which may be useful in designing a BTV.

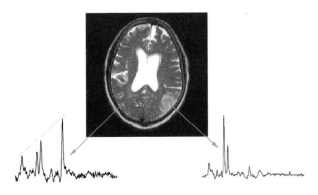

FIGURE 7-8. T_2-weighted brain image with spectra from normal and tumor regions. The normal linearly increasing relationship between several spectral peaks on the left is absent on the right, indicative of tumor. Courtesy of P. MacEneaney, MD, University of Chicago.

Image Import into RTP Systems: DICOM and DICOM-RT

One of the key technologies that has led to the ubiquitous use of image data sets in RTP is the industry standard Digital Imaging and Communications in Medicine (DICOM) protocol. DICOM is the registered trademark of the National Electrical Manufacturers Association (NEMA) for its standards publications relating to digital communications of medical information. It provides a consistent format and a set of protocols by which images may be communicated between computers and applications and stored. The American College of Radiology and NEMA developed DICOM to facilitate standardized image communication. Several versions of the basic standard were developed in the late 1980s,[55,56] and the current version of the standard, version 3.1, was released in 2001. DICOM is based on a number of key notions, a few of which are described here. Quoted definitions are from the draft standards documents.[57]

An Information Object is "an abstraction of a real information entity (e.g., CT Image, Study, etc.) which is acted upon by one or more DICOM Commands." An Information Object Instance is "a representation of an occurrence of a real-world entity, which includes values for the attributes of the Information Object Class to which the entity belongs" (eg, a specific CT image). An Information Object Definition (IOD) "is an object-oriented abstract data model used to specify information about Real-World Objects. An IOD provides communicating Application Entities with a common view of the information to be exchanged."

IODs are thus a common language by which different computers and programs may communicate images. IODs must exist for each data set type that is to be communicated using DICOM. IODs are defined in the 2001 standard for CT, nuclear medicine, MRI, PET, ultrasonography, secondary capture (eg, digitized film, screen dump), RT image, RT dose, RT structure set, RT plan, RT beams treatment record, RT brachytherapy treatment record, visible light image, and numerous others.

A Service Class is "a structured description of a service which is supported by cooperating DICOM Application Entities using specific DICOM commands acting on a specific class of Information Object." Examples include storage, query, retrieval, and print service classes. A Service-Object Pair (SOP) Class is "the union of a specific set of...Services and one related Information Object Definition (as specified by a Service Class Definition) which completely defines a precise context for communication." For example, CT Image (the object) Storage (the service) is a Service-Object Pair. A Service Class User is "the role played by a DICOM Application Entity...which invokes operations and performs notifications on a specific Association." A Service Class Provider is "the role played by a DICOM Application Entity...which performs operations and invokes notifications on a specific Association."

As an example, CT images are frequently "pushed" from a scanner console to an RTP system. In this case, the scanner is actually requesting that the RTP system act as a service class provider of CT image storage, for which the scanner console will be the service class user. If the RTP system queries the scanner console or picture archive and communications system (PACS) to find a particular study and then "pulls" the study, the RTP system is a service class user of first the CT image query and then CT image retrieve services, provided by the scanner or the PACS.

The IOD for a particular information object defines a set of data elements that make up the object. DICOM communication involves some initial negotiation between the service class user and the provider, followed by a stream of messages containing a tag, (sometimes) the number of bytes of data to be transmitted, (sometimes) information about how the data are represented, and, finally, the data corresponding to the current tag's data element. Most RTP systems today can import images directly from a scanner or PACS system via DICOM query and retrieve or by reading DICOM files saved on disk by a local storage server.

Of particular importance in RTP are the so-called DICOM-RT extensions to the original standard, developed in the 1990s and now part of the base standard. These include the IODs for RT Image (a simulator image, portal image, or DRR, with optional curve overlays for collimator jaws, beam apertures, etc.); RT Structure Set (any number of three-dimensional structures, defined as multiple contours); RT Dose (dose information, expressed as lists of point doses, two- or three-dimensional dose grids, isodose curves, or dose-volume histograms), and RT Plan (eg, beam definitions, fractionation information, brachytherapy application information, multileaf collimator [MLC] control information). These are the information objects that are usually used, for example, to transmit structures contoured on a CT simulation workstation to an RTP system, an MLC sequence from an IMRT planning system to an RT information system, or a DRR to a portal image processing workstation. In the case of structures, another mechanism for transfer is also available. Image information objects in DICOM may also include data elements called curves, which can be used to store contours of structures or regions, among other uses. CT and MRI IODs include curve modules for this purpose. Images transferred from a CT simulation workstation to an RTP system may include these curves for contours that have been defined on each image. If they do, the planning system may support extracting the curves associated with each image slice and using them to create three-dimensional planning structures.

Multimodality Imaging, Image Registration, and Fusion

Rationale for Multimodality Imaging in RTP

Incorporation of information from more than one image study into RTP is motivated by the desire to use the most complete information available on each anatomic or functional region that affects the plan. In many instances, this involves the combination of anatomic information from multiple modalities. In other instances, combinations of anatomic and functional information can serve to improve the definition of a target or avoidance region.

Registration and Fusion

Several terms that are frequently used interchangeably but that, in fact, have distinct meanings are useful in this discussion. The combination of multiple images or, more generally, the transfer of information from one image study to another is correctly termed *image fusion*. Taking the example of multiple tomographic image studies of a single patient, accurate image fusion clearly requires knowledge of how the patient is oriented with respect to the image planes of the two studies. The process of establishing a coordinate transformation between the coordinates of multiple image spaces, such that homologous points in the two spaces are mapped accurately onto each other, is termed *image registration*. Several review articles have surveyed the field of medical image registration.[58–60] Once the interscan coordinate transformation is known, it may be used to transfer any information from one scan to another, which is the process of data fusion.

Clinical Applications of Image Registration and Fusion

The earliest applications of multimodality fusion in RTP addressed the problem of locating brain lesions, which were better visualized using MRI, in the coordinates of CT scans being used for planning.[39,61] This continues to be the dominant application of this technology today. An example from a prostate planning case is shown in Figure 7-9. It is also frequently useful to merge multiple scans of the same

modality, for example, a treatment planning CT with preoperative or prechemotherapy diagnostic CT, to allow inclusion of suspected microscopic disease extension around a no longer visible tumor to be included in the CTV.[62] Fusion of serial imaging studies is also useful in the assessment of tumor response to therapy and for the analysis of organ motion and patient setup uncertainties.

Fusion of PET and SPECT images with CT and MRI was developed initially for the purpose of allowing more accurate analysis of the functional images and to facilitate anatomically based interpretation, diagnosis, and surgery planning.[63–68] The potential for using a set of anatomic images as a reference coordinate frame in which multiple functional images could be combined was recognized as useful early on. For example, combining images reflecting metabolic, blood flow, and blood-brain barrier breakdown status was used to assist in the differential diagnosis of recurrence versus necrosis.[69] Fusion of functional lung images with CT and analysis of temporal changes in fused serial lung images have been useful in analysis and in attempts to limit lung toxicity, as mentioned earlier. In addition, registration of SPECT images with CT was proposed for use in planning for radioimmunotherapy.[70]

Inclusion of functional imaging in IMRT planning may allow optimization of dose distributions to minimize irradiation of identified functional regions. One such application is briefly described here. Originally, intensity-modulated whole-pelvic RT was developed to limit small bowel irradiation when treating whole-pelvis fields in gynecologic cases.[71,72] Recent work has investigated means to reduce hematologic toxicity owing to irradiation of bone marrow in the pelvis.[73] Active bone marrow regions identified on ^{99m}Tc sulfur colloid SPECT images can be transformed into the CT scan coordinate system used for IMRT planning. These functional bone marrow regions can then be used as avoidance structures in IMRT optimization. A more detailed discussion of this technique is presented in Chapter 23.4, "Bone Marrow–Sparing Approaches: Emerging Technology."

Methods of Multimodality Fusion

An important distinction between registration methods involves the class of coordinate transformations that they are capable of using in matching one data set onto another. The simplest transformation is the rigid body transformation, which permits only translation and scaling in the mapping between the two coordinate spaces. Clearly, such simple transformations are limited in their applicability because few parts of any patient's anatomy actually move as rigid bodies. As might be expected, considerable success has been achieved in registration of brain images using rigid body transformations and less so in other areas of the body. A slightly more complex transformation is the affine or general linear transformation, which includes anisotropic scaling and shearing. Progressively more complex and with correspondingly more ability to model distortion of anato-

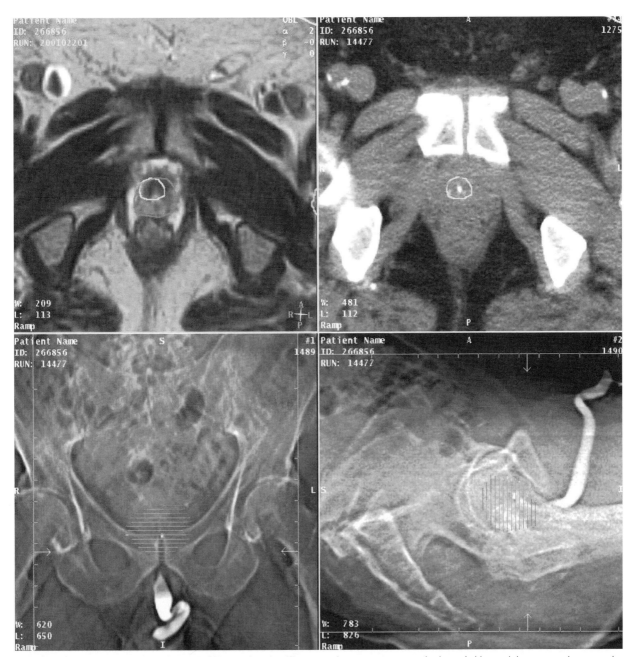

FIGURE 7-9. Image capture from a Philips AcQPlan workstation. The magnetic resonance contour is shown in blue and the computed tomography (CT) contour in yellow for one slice on magnetic resonance imaging (MRI) (*left*) and CT (*right*). The change in volume is seen on the digitally constructed radiographs below, with the MRI in blue and the CT in green. (To view a color version of this image, please refer to the CD-ROM.) Courtesy of Philips Medical Systems.

my between two sets of images are polynomial warping, elastic warping (of which a particularly widespread variant is thin plate spline warping[74]), and viscous fluid deformation. Each of these warping techniques allows every image voxel to effectively have its own coordinate transformation, slightly different from its neighbors. This allows for continuous shape changes of tissues between scans, as would be caused by patient positioning on a flat instead of a curved couch, or of internal organ shape changes, such as bladder and rectal filling or even tumor growth or resection. Furthermore, coordinate transformations may be either global (ie, a single transformation is applied to every voxel in the image spaces) or local (ie, a different coordinate transformation may apply at different locations in the image spaces). Local transformations can be used to account for differences in the motions or distortions of different organs.

Feature-Based Registration

Given that image registration requires the knowledge of a coordinate transformation between the two image studies that relates the patient position in each of them, it is necessary to understand the orientation of the slices of each study with respect to some coordinate system fixed to the patient. The basis of this coordinate system can be intrinsic to the patient, that is, defined by some aspect of the patient's anatomy, or it can be extrinsic, added to the patient. The stereotactic localizer frame generally used in planning radiosurgery cases is a classic example of an extrinsic coordinate basis. To be useful in image registration, of course, the frame must be visible in all image sets of interest; frames have been designed over the years that are compatible with CT, MRI, angiography, and nuclear medicine images[66] and for extracranial localization. The position in the image slices of the coordinate apparatus is used to solve for the orientation of the image coordinate system of each separate modality relative to the frame. The relationship of the two relative orientations then defines the interscan coordinate transformation required for image registration.

The use of extrinsic registration methods with MRI-compatible frames or fiducial markers requires either elimination of or correction for distortions that may be present in MRIs.[75,76] It has been argued that under certain circumstances, errors of several millimeters may be inherent in uncorrected MRIs.[77] Even when corrections are made, registration based on an external stereotactic frame in MRI may still be subject to errors on the order of several millimeters.[78] One approach to addressing this problem is to use an intrinsic rather than an extrinsic registration basis, that is, to use the patient's anatomy as the basis of registration.

Many registration methods using patient-intrinsic information as their basis have been developed, differing in one or more of several key areas. Most methods identify anatomic homologies between the two image studies and attempt to find an interscan coordinate transformation that matches the homologous structures. The characteristics of the structures used and the particular mathematical algorithms used to maximize the interscan homology are the factors that generally differentiate one method from another. The structure to be matched may be three-dimensional "point" landmarks, either manually or, in some cases, automatically identified. Alternatively, "curve" landmarks, such as the three-dimensional trajectory of vessels, may be used. "Plane" landmarks are not frequently used, but the interhemispheric plane in the brain has, indeed, been used as a constraint in several registration methods. The use of all or portions of three-dimensional surfaces, such as the surface of the brain, as elements to be matched is also common.

An illustrative example of a surface-based registration method is the chamfer matching method developed by Kooy and van Herk and their colleagues[78,79] and integrated into the Radionics XKnife planning system (Radionics Inc, Burlington, MA). Chamfer matching is a calculational technique for minimizing the average or mean squared distance between two models of the same surface, in which one model might be the surface of some organ or bony structure as defined from CT and another the same surface as defined from MRI. In fact, identification of the surfaces to be matched may be done semiautomatically or even fully automatically, depending on the particular registration method. It is not even necessary to uniquely identify the three-dimensional objects of which the surfaces are to be matched; one may simply locate the positions of high gradients, intensity ridges, points of maximum curvature, or other mathematically defined features in the two scans and use those features for registration. The object of image registration is, of course, to find the transformation between these two coordinate systems, which, when applied to one of the models (eg, the MRI brain model), matches it most closely with the other (CT). Numerous methods for characterizing how well the two models fit together and for finding the transformation that optimizes the match have been developed. Chamfer matching involves precalculation of a three-dimensional distance field that defines for each point (eg, in CT space) the distance from that point in space to the nearest point that is on the brain surface. If the surface was an electrically charged object, the distance field would be analogous to a potential. Once the distance field is calculated, the evaluation of the goodness of fit of the MRI with the CT consists simply of adding up the value (or the square) of the distance field at each point on the MRI. The procedure then consists of iteratively moving the MRI around in CT space, evaluating the distance sum at each reorientation, and using some search procedure to find the reorientation of the MRI model that results in the minimum distance sum. Many matching procedures allow the definition of multiple homologous structures in the two scans, which are all used simultaneously in the matching process.

Intensity-Based Registration

A final step up in the complexity of features to be matched involves methods in which the entire volume of image data, that is, the intensities of the image voxels themselves, is used for matching. Understanding such methods is simplest in the context of single-modality registration. Consider the simple case of a single CT scan of a head and a copy of the same data set that has been deliberately translated and rotated. To register these two data sets, the second (transformed) data set must be translated and rotated in an attempt to match it with the first (original). When the data sets are perfectly registered, every voxel of the second data set (which is just the original data set transformed away and then transformed back) should map onto an original voxel of exactly the same intensity. Thus, a potential registration strategy might be to attempt to maximize the correlation in intensities between the original and the transformed data sets. Interestingly, the same type of strategy is useful for multimodality registration, even including functional images. This is true because although anatomic regions may appear with different relative intensities in different image modalities, their intensities are still highly correlated. For example, air is very dark in both CT and MRI; bone is bright in CT and dark in MRI, although not as dark as air; and brain is intermediate in intensity in both modalities but with a considerable range of intensities in MRI. Let the intensities of air, tissue, and bone in CT and MRI be $\{A_c, T_c, B_c\}$ and $\{A_m, T_m, B_m\}$, taking a single value for brain in MRI. If the entire image volumes are perfectly registered with each other, then there is a high probability that bright CT bone voxels of intensity B_c will map onto dark MRI bone voxels of intensity B_m, and tissue CT voxels of intensity T_c will likewise have a high probability of mapping onto brain MRI voxels of intensity T_m. If the volumes are less than perfectly registered, some bright CT bone voxels may map onto MRI brain voxels and some dark MRI bone voxels onto CT brain voxels, and bone or tissue voxels in either scan may map onto air voxels in the other. Mathematically, we can say that when the registration is best, the joint distribution of intensity pairings in the overlapped volumes is most highly ordered.

A useful concept that quantifies the extent to which intensities are correlated, as evidenced in properties of the joint intensity distribution, is mutual information. Formally, mutual information expresses the extent to which knowledge of the value of one random variable allows prediction of the value of another. In the registration example, when the volumes are perfectly registered, then knowing that a CT voxel has a bone intensity should mean that there is a high probability that the corresponding MRI voxel also has a bone intensity, likewise for tissue and air voxels. Registration methods based on maximization of mutual information in the registered data sets have proven useful for a wide range of single- and multimodality problems, including both anatomic and functional images, in two and in three dimensions.[80–82] Several commercial image registration software systems provide mutual information–based registration capability, and the use of mutual information–based registration on a routine basis in RTP has been reported.[83]

It has frequently been found useful in clinical practice to use an interactive intensity-based registration tool in which the operator manipulates the interscan coordinate transformation and is immediately presented with fused slices from the two registered data sets. The user adjusts the interscan transformation until the match of the fused images appears to be acceptable. The Philips AcQSim system, among others, offers such an interactive matching capability.

Assessment of Registration Accuracy

Ideally, every image registration and fusion system should provide uncertainty estimates on the accuracy with which information can be transferred from one image set to another. This uncertainty would logically be incorporated into the design of treatment plans, for example, by adding a margin around fused anatomic structures to indicate the uncertainty in their position relative to the planning scans. Unfortunately, useful uncertainty estimates are seldom available. Evaluation of registration methods using data with known truth[84] is useful in characterizing performance but does not provide an accuracy estimate for any individual case of interest. Point-to-point feature matching is the only registration technique in which it is at all clear how to make a quantitative uncertainty estimate. In that case, one may simply calculate the mean squared distance between the nominally matched homologous point pairs and use this as an estimate of accuracy either globally or locally. Of course, there is uncertainty as well in the identification of the points, which must also be taken into account. This is particularly true when point matching is used to register functional images with anatomic images; in this case, point landmark localization is liable to be subject to significant error. In any event, it is nearly always necessary and always a good idea to review the fused image volumes visually before using any fused information in treatment planning.

Image Segmentation

An essential step in the use of image information to create the "virtual patient" model used in RTP is image segmentation, which is the process of identification and localization of each region of interest, both target and nontarget, that is to be considered in the treatment planning process. As discussed earlier, regions of interest may be either anatomic or functional and may need to be identified and located in any number of image modalities. Techniques for performing these segmentation tasks have been the topic of intensive research for decades, and a complete, satisfactory set of methods for use in RTP still does not exist. The situation is much the same in other areas of medicine in which quantitative use is made of image data for modeling or analysis, such as surgical planning.

Requirements for Image Segmentation

Not very much attention has been devoted to formally characterizing the performance requirements for segmentation in RTP in terms such as specificity and sensitivity, which are widely used to evaluate image processing algorithms used in diagnostic radiology. As pointed out by Jolesz, "Diagnosis needs specificity, but it is less susceptible to accuracy of localization. For therapy, sensitivity should be a fundamental feature."[85] One may question to what extent the importance of sensitivity should be stressed at the expense of specificity, but, certainly, it is intuitive that if we desire to identify a target volume, it is necessary to identify all of the image voxels that correspond to tumor, thus avoiding the possibility of leaving tumor cells inadequately treated, and perhaps less important not to include some nontumor voxels in the target. Analogously, if one is identifying an OAR, one might prefer to use a technique that errs in the direction of a more generous definition rather than miss some voxels at risk, which then might not be accorded all of the dose sparing one had wished. In any given treatment situation, there will be some trade-off between the desires for complete identification of all of the voxels that belong in a particular structure and for leaving out voxels that are not, in fact, part of the structures. This, of course, applies to the imaging modalities used in RTP, as well as to the segmentation methods used to process them. There may also inevitably be ambiguities as to which region (target or OAR) certain voxels belong. Another point of view concerning accuracy requirements for segmentation is that such requirements are context dependent, varying from one anatomic site or treatment technique to another. If uncertainties owing to segmentation are insignificant compared with expected physiologic motion or patient setup uncertainty, then the segmentation may be "good enough," whereas for high-precision treatments with rigid immobilization and minimal margins, more accuracy may be required of segmentation.

As with registration methods, it is useful to classify segmentation techniques according to what type of knowledge they use and what type of image features they operate on. One such classification, similar to that suggested by Udupa,[86] is shown in Table 7-5. Methods are broadly divided as to whether they identify regions by delineation, that is, by identifying portions of the image with some specified properties (intensity, texture, gradient) and calling those the segmented objects, or by recognition, that is, by looking for patterns or shapes known to be associated with the desired objects in the image. Delineation is by nature a more low-level, image processing–oriented approach. Recognition is a more high-level, computer vision–oriented approach.

Manual and Semiautomated Methods

The majority of image segmentation for RTP continues to be done using manual or semiautomated software tools for structure delineation. Direct tracing of contours on an image

TABLE 7-5. Semiautomatic and Automatic Segmentation Methods

Delineation
Boundary based (eg, edge detection)
Region based (eg, region growing)
Recognition
Automatic
Knowledge based
Operator assisted
Specification of seed point
Specification of search region
Accept or reject delineated objects

Adapted from Udupa J.[86]

display workstation remains by far the most common technique. A selection of flexible tools for freehand drawing, editing, copying from slice to slice, and so on is included in nearly every RTP system. The *Pinnacle* (Philips Medical Systems, Cleveland, OH) screen shown in Figure 7-3 provides an example. A number of enhancements to the basic slice-by-slice contouring technique have been introduced in recent years. Several systems, for example, the GE Advantage Sim (GE Medical Systems, Waukesha, WI), permit contouring on multiple planes, that is, sagittal and coronal as well as transaxial, and visualizing the intersection of each contour with the other planes. This provides a valuable context for the operator in identifying the extrema of structures, such as the apex of the prostate. Interpolation of structures between planes is also supported by many systems. Most systems include some form of semiautomatic structure delineation. As indicated in Table 7-5, such methods may be contour based, as in the case of isodensity threshold or edge following beginning near a point indicated by the operator, or region based, as in the case of a region growing around a seed point indicated by the operator. In some cases, these tools are able to propagate the identified region from slice to slice, allowing rapid definition of an entire three-dimensional region. The combination of two- and three-dimensional semiautomated tools to improve the efficiency of segmentation was the thrust of the Medical Anatomy Segmentation Kit (MASK) project at the University of North Carolina in the early 1990s.[87] Less commonly used in RTP but quite popular in other areas of medical image analysis are parametrically deformable or active contour models, which can be initialized in the region in which a structure is to be segmented and allowed to find the contour or three-dimensional surface location, which minimizes some combination of "image energy" (having to do with image intensity, gradient, or texture properties) and "shape energy" (having to do with shape descriptors such as curvature, size, and smoothness).[88–91]

Knowledge-Based Methods

A particularly promising class of segmentation methods includes those that use an atlas containing a statistical description of the shape, location, and image properties of tissues to be segmented and attempts to recognize or find these structures in the image data space.[92,93] These methods have proven quite successful in brain image segmentation.[94–98] Ultimately, one may hope that such knowledge-based methods will allow nearly automated segmentation of an extensive set of normal tissues and even perhaps of tissues that are severely distorted by tumors or surgery (by implication, possibly also labeling tumor voxels).[99] Recently, the University of North Carolina group presented a method based on a deformable multiscale medial shape descriptor, which incorporates statistical shape variability explicitly in a user-guided segmentation method.[100,101] This method has shown good agreement with segmentation by human experts and has improved reproducibility.[102]

A number of modality-specific methods for automatically segmenting high-contrast surfaces in CT by isosurfacing[103] or for brain structure segmentation in MRI using multispectral feature space discrimination and connected component analysis[104] have been successfully used in diagnostic and three-dimensional display applications. Considerable progress has been made in automated segmentation of a number of normal and pathologic structures in the brain from MRI[105] and the atlas-based approaches discussed earlier. A recent review of segmentation methods by Pham and colleagues provides an introduction to a large number of methods.[106] Given that RTP demands that a number of different types of structures must be segmented from several different modalities, no single technique or tool is adequate to the entire task.

Segmentation of PTVs

Unfortunately, even if all tumor and normal structures are correctly labeled in the image data sets, the segmentation task in RTP still requires the addition of margins to account for subclinical disease (CTV) and position uncertainty (PTV). Usually, the PTV is developed via simple expansion, either isotropic or anisotropic, of the GTV using suitably chosen margins for a given treatment type. Automation of the process of identifying these volumes is also the subject of research. At the University of Washington, knowledge-based tools have been developed to create PTVs based on identified tumor location using a rule-based system[107] and compared with PTVs developed by humans using semi-automated tools (simple expansions).[108] Another important application of knowledge-based systems in this area is in the prediction of disease spread for particular anatomic sites,[109] which, ultimately, may aid in CTV definition.

Acknowledgments

We are grateful to Himanshu Shukla of Philips Medical Systems and Peter MacEneaney, MD (Radiology), of The University of Chicago, for providing images.

References

1. International Commission on Radiation Units and Measurements. Prescribing, recording and reporting photon beam therapy. Report 50. Washington (DC): International Commission on Radiation Units and Measurements; 1993.

2. International Commission on Radiation Units and Measurements. Prescribing, recording and reporting photon beam therapy. Report 62. Supplement to ICRU report 50. Washington (DC): International Commission on Radiation Units and Measurements; 1999.

3. Sobin JH, Wittekind C, editors. TNM classification of malignant tumors. 5th ed. New York: Wiley-Liss and Sons; 1997

4. Greene FL, Page DL, Fleming ID, et al. AJCC cancer staging manual. 6th ed. New York: Springer-Verlag; 2002.

5. Davies SC, Hill AL, Holmes RB, et al. Ultrasound quantitation of respiratory organ motion in the upper abdomen. Br J Radiol 1994;67:1096–102.

6. Balter JM, Ten Haken RK, Lawrence TS, et al. Uncertainties in CT-based radiation therapy treatment planning associated with patient breathing. Int J Radiat Oncol Biol Phys 1996;36:167–74.

7. Ahmad NR, Huq MS, Corn BW. Respiration-induced motion of the kidneys in whole abdominal radiotherapy: implications for treatment planning and late toxicity. Radiother Oncol 1997;42:87–90.

8. Shimizu S, Shirato H, Ogura S, et al. Detection of lung tumor movement in real-time tumor-tracking radiotherapy. Int J Radiat Oncol Biol Phys 2001;51:304–10.

9. Roeske JC, Forman JD, Mesina CF, et al. Evaluation of changes in the size and location of the prostate, seminal vesicles, bladder, and rectum during a course of external beam radiation therapy. Int J Radiat Oncol Biol Phys 1995;33:1321–9.

10. Dawson LA, Mah K, Franssen E, et al. Target position variability throughout prostate radiotherapy. Int J Radiat Oncol Biol Phys 1998;42:1155–61.

11. Zellars RC, Roberson PL, Strawderman M, et al. Prostate position late in the course of external beam therapy: patterns and predictors. Int J Radiat Oncol Biol Phys 2000;47:655–60.

12. Seppenwoolde Y, Shirato H, Kitamura K, et al. Precise and real-time measurement of 3D tumor motion in lung due to breathing and heartbeat, measured during radiotherapy. Int J Radiat Oncol Biol Phys 2002;53:822–34.

13. Hamlet S, Ezzell G, Aref A. Larynx motion associated with swallowing during radiation therapy. Int J Radiat Oncol Biol Phys 1994;28:467–70.

14. van Asselen B, Raaijmakers CP, Lagendijk JJ, et al. Intrafraction motions of the larynx during radiotherapy. Int J Radiat Oncol Biol Phys 2003;56:384–90.

15. Zelefsky MJ, Happersett L, Leibel SA, et al. The effect of treatment positioning on normal tissue dose in patients with prostate cancer treated with three-dimensional conformal radiotherapy. Int J Radiat Oncol Biol Phys 1997;37:13–9.

16. Stroom JC, Koper PC, Korevaar GA, et al. Internal organ motion in prostate cancer patients treated in prone and supine treatment position. Radiother Oncol 1999;51:237–48.

17. Weber DC, Nouet P, Rouzaud M, et al. Patient positioning in prostate radiotherapy: is prone better than supine? Int J Radiat Oncol Biol Phys 2000;47:365–71.

18. Chen QS, Weinhous MS, Deibel FC, et al. Fluoroscopic study of tumor motion due to breathing: facilitating precise radiation therapy for lung cancer patients. Med Phys 2001;28:1850–6.

19. Dawson LA, Balter JM. Interventions to reduce organ motion effects in radiation delivery. Semin Radiat Oncol 2004;14:76–80.

20. Kutcher GJ, Mageras GS, Liebel SA. Control, correction, and modeling of setup errors and organ motion. Semin Radiat Oncol 1995;5:134–45.

21. Schewe JE, Balter JM, Lam KL, et al. Measurement of patient setup errors using port films and a computer-aided graphical alignment tool. Med Dosim 1996;21:97–104.

22. Killoran JH, Kooy HM, Gladstone DJ, et al. A numerical simulation of organ motion and daily setup uncertainties:

implications for radiation therapy. Int J Radiat Oncol Biol Phys 1997;37:213–21.

23. Johnson LS, Milliken BD, Hadley SW, et al. Initial clinical experience with a video-based patient positioning system. Int J Radiat Oncol Biol Phys 1999;45:205–13.

24. Pisani L, Lockman D, Jaffray D, et al. Setup error in radiotherapy: on-line correction using electronic kilovoltage and megavoltage radiographs. Int J Radiat Oncol Biol Phys 2000;47:825–39.

25. Jaffray DA, Siewerdsen JH. Cone-beam computed tomography with a flat-panel imager: initial performance characterization. Med Phys 2000;27:1311–23.

26. Ford EC, Mageras GS, Yorke E, et al. Evaluation of respiratory movement during gated radiotherapy using film and electronic portal imaging. Int J Radiat Oncol Biol Phys 2002;52:522–31.

27. Balter JM, Brock KK, Litzenberg DW, et al. Daily targeting of intrahepatic tumors for radiotherapy. Int J Radiat Oncol Biol Phys 2002;52:266–71.

28. Litzenberg D, Dawson LA, Sandler H, et al. Daily prostate targeting using implanted radiopaque markers. Int J Radiat Oncol Biol Phys 2002;52:699–703.

29. Stroom JC, Heijmen BJ. Geometrical uncertainties, radiotherapy planning margins, and the ICRU-62 report. Radiother Oncol 2002;64:75–83.

30. Lujan AE, Larsen EW, Balter JM, et al. A method for incorporating organ motion due to breathing into 3D dose calculations. Med Phys 1999;26:715–20.

31. Beckham WA, Keall PJ, Siebers JV. A fluence-convolution method to calculate radiation therapy dose distributions that incorporate random set-up error. Phys Med Biol 2002;47:3465–73.

32. Chetty IJ, Rosu M, Tyagi N, et al. A fluence convolution method to account for respiratory motion in 3D dose calculations of the liver. Med Phys 2003;30:1776–80.

33. Fontenla E, Pelizzari CA, Roeske JC, et al. Using serial imaging data to model variabilities in organ position and shape during radiotherapy. Phys Med Biol 2001;46:2317–36.

34. Fontenla E, Pelizzari CA, Roeske JC, et al. Numerical analysis of a model of organ motion using serial imaging measurements from prostate radiotherapy. Phys Med Biol 2001;46:2337–58.

35. McCullough E, Holmes T. Acceptance testing computerized radiation therapy treatment planning systems: direct utilization of CT scan data. Med Phys 1985;12:237–42.

36. Sherouse G, Novins K, Chaney E. Computation of digitally reconstructed radiographs for use in radiotherapy treatment design. Int J Radiat Oncol Biol Phys 1990;18:651–8.

37. Pan T, Lee TY, Rietzel E, et al. 4D-CT imaging of a volume influenced by respiratory motion on multi-slice CT. Med Phys 2004;31:333–40.

38. Balter J, Lam K, Technical note: acquisition of CT models for radiotherapy applications with reduced tube heating. Med Phys 2001;28:590–2.

39. Kessler ML, Pitluck S, Petti P, et al. Integration of multimodality imaging data for radiotherapy treatment planning. Int J Radiat Oncol Biol Phys 1991;21:1653–67.

40. Thornton AF, Sandler HM, Ten Haken RK, et al. The clinical utility of magnetic resonance imaging in 3-dimensional treatment planning of brain neoplasms. Int J Radiat Oncol Biol Phys 1992;24:767–75.

41. Shukla H, Vaisanen P, Steckner M. Distortion corrected MRI for radiotherapy. Int J Radiat Oncol Biol Phys 2002;54 Suppl 1:83–4.

42. Mah D, Steckner M, Palacio E, et al. Characteristics and quality assurance of a dedicated open 0.23 T MRI for radiation therapy simulation. Med Phys 2002;29:2541–7.

43. Levin-Plotnik D, Hamilton RJ. Optimization of tumour control probability for heterogeneous tumours in fractionated radiotherapy treatment protocols. Phys Med Biol 2004;49:407–24.

44. Ling C, Humm J, Larson S, et al. Towards multidimensional radiotherapy (MD-CRT): biological imaging and biological conformality. Int J Radiat Oncol Biol Phys 2000;47:551–60.

45. Tepper J. Form and function: the integration of physics and biology. Int J Radiat Oncol Biol Phys 2000;47:547–8.

46. Marks L, Spencer D, Bentel G, et al. The utility of SPECT lung perfusion scans in minimizing and assessing the physiologic consequences of thoracic irradiation. Int J Radiat Oncol Biol Phys 1993;26:659–68.

47. Boersma L, Damen E, de Boer R, et al. A new method to determine dose-effect relations for local lung-function changes using correlated SPECT and CT data. Radiother Oncol 1993;29:110–6.

48. Marks L, Munley M, Spencer D, et al. Quantification of radiation-induced regional lung injury with perfusion imaging. Int J Radiat Oncol Biol Phys 1997;38:399–409.

49. Belliveau J, Kennedy D Jr, McKinstry R, et al. Functional mapping of the human visual cortex by magnetic resonance imaging. Science 1991;254:716–9.

50. Hamilton RJ, Sweeney PJ, Pelizzari CA, et al. Functional imaging in treatment planning of brain lesions. Int J Radiat Oncol Biol Phys 1997;37:181–8.

51. Cha S, Knopp E, Johnson G, et al. Intracranial mass lesions: dynamic contrast-enhanced susceptibility-weighted echoplanar perfusion MR imaging. Radiology 2002;223:11–29.

52. Tien R, Felsberg G, Friedman H, et al. MR imaging of high-grade gliomas: value of diffusion-weighted echoplanar pulse sequences. AJR Am J Roentgenol 1994;162:671–7.

53. Scheidler J, Hricak H, Vigneron D, et al. Prostate cancer: localization with three-dimensional proton MR spectroscopic imaging—clinicopathologic study. Radiology 1999;213:473–80.

54. Pickett B, Vigneault E, Kurhanewicz J, et al. Static field intensity modulation to treat a dominant intra-prostatic lesion to 90 Gy compared to seven field 3-dimensional radiotherapy. Int J Radiat Oncol Biol Phys 1999;44:921–29.

55. ACR-NEMA. Digital Imaging and Communications in Medicine (DICOM), version 1.0. ACR-NEMA Standards Publication No.: 300-1985. Rosslyn (VA): National Electrical Manufacturers Association; 1985.

56. ACR-NEMA. Digital Imaging and Communications in Medicine (DICOM), version 2.0.ACR-NEMA Standards Publication No.: 300-1988. Rosslyn (VA): National Electrical Manufacturers Association; 1988.

57. ACR-NEMA. Digital Imaging and Communications in Medicine (DICOM), version 3.0. Rosslyn (VA): National Electrical Manufacturers Association; 2003.

58. Maurer C, Fitzpatrick J. A review of medical image registration. In: Maciunas RJ, editor. Interactive image-guided

neurosurgery. Park Ridge (IL): American Association of Neurosurgeons; 1993. p. 17–44.

59. van den Elsen P, Pol E, Viergever M. Medical image matching—a review with classification. IEEE Eng Med Biol 1993;12:26–39.

60. Maintz J, Viergever M. A survey of medical image registration. Med Image Anal 1998;2:1–36.

61. Phillips MH, Kessler ML, Chuang FYS, et al. Image correlation of MRI and CT in treatment planning for radiosurgery of intracranial vascular malformations. Int J Radiat Oncol Biol Phys 1991;20:881–9.

62. Sailer S, Rosenman J, Soltys M, et al. Improving treatment planning accuracy through multimodality imaging. Int J Radiat Oncol Biol Phys 1996;35:117–24.

63. Maguire GQJ, Noz ME, Lee EM, et al. Correlation methods for tomographic images using two and three dimensional techniques. In: Bacharach SL, editor. Information processing in medical imaging. Boston: Martinus Nijhoff; 1986. p. 266–79.

64. Pelizzari CA, Chen GTY, Halpern H, et al. Three dimensional correlation of PET, CT and MRI images. J Nucl Med 1987;28:683.

65. Pelizzari CA, Chen GTY, Spelbring DR, et al. Accurate three-dimensional registration of PET, CT and MR images of the brain. J Comp Assist Tomogr 1989;13:20–7.

66. Schad LR, Boesecke R, Schlegel W, et al. Three dimensional image correlation of CT, MR, and PET studies in radiotherapy treatment planning of brain tumors. J Comput Assist Tomogr 1987;11:948–54.

67. Levin DN, Hu XP, Tan KK, et al. The brain: integrated three-dimensional display of MR and PET images. Radiology 1989;172:783–9.

68. Bajcsy R, Kovacic S. Multiresolution elastic matching. Computer Vision, Graphics and Image Processing 1989; 1: 1–21.

69. Holman BL, Zimmerman RE, Carvalho PA, et al. Computer-assisted superimposition of magnetic resonance and high resolution Tc-99m HMPAO and TL-201 SPECT images of the brain. J Nucl Med 1991;32:1478–84.

70. Roeske JC, Pelizzari CA, Spelbring D et al. Registration of SPECT and CT images for radiolabeled antibody biodistribution analysis [abstract]. Med Phys 1991;18:649.

71. Roeske J, Lujan A, Rotmensch J, et al. Intensity-modulated whole pelvic radiation therapy in patients with gynecologic malignancies. Int J Radiat Oncol Biol Phys 2000;48:1613–21.

72. Mundt A, Lujan A, Rotmensch J, et al. Intensity-modulated whole pelvic radiotherapy in women with gynecologic malignancies. Int J Radiat Oncol Biol Phys 2002;52:1330–7.

73. Brixey C, Roeske J, Lujan A, et al. Impact of intensity-modulated radiotherapy on acute hematologic toxicity in women with gynecologic malignancies. Int J Radiat Oncol Biol Phys 2002;54:1388–96.

74. Bookstein FL. Thin-plate splines and the atlas problem for biomedical images. In: Colchester ACF, Hawkes D, editors. Information processing in medical imaging. Berlin: Springer; 1991. p. 326–42.

75. Schad L, Lott S, Schmitt F, et al. Correction of spatial distortion in MR imaging: a prerequisite for accurate stereotaxy. J Comput Assist Tomogr 1987;11:499–505.

76. Dong S, Fitzpatrick J, Maciunas R. Rectification of distortion in MRI for stereotaxy. In: Fifth IEEE Symposium on Computer-Based Medical Systems. Durham (NC): IEEE; 1992. p. 181–9.

77. Sumanaweera T, Glover G, Hemler P, et al. MR geometric distortion correction for improved frame-based stereotaxic target localization accuracy. Magn Reson Med 1995;34:106–13.

78. Kooy H, van Herk M, Barnes P, et al. Image fusion for stereotactic radiotherapy and radiosurgery treatment planning. Int J Radiat Oncol Biol Phys 1994;30:1229–34.

79. van Herk M, Gilhuis K, Holupka E, et al. A new method for automatic three-dimensional image correlation. Med Phys 1992;19:1134.

80. Maes F, Collignon A, Vandermeulen D, et al. Multimodality image registration by maximization of mutual information. IEEE Trans Med Imaging 1997;16:187–98.

81. Viola PD. Alignment by maximization of mutual information (PhD Dissertation). Available in: Artificial Intelligence Laboratory Technical Report 1548. Cambridge (MA): Massachusetts Institute of Technology; 1995.

82. Wells WM, Viola P, Kikinis R. Multi-modal volume registration by maximization of mutual information. In: Second Annual International Symposium on Medical Robotics and Computer Assisted Surgery. New York: John Wiley & Sons; 1995. p. 52–62

83. Kessler M, Archer P, Meyer C, et al. Routine clinical use of mutual information for automated 3D registration of anatomic and functional image data. Int J Radiat Oncol Biol Phys 2002;54:84.

84. West J, Fitzpatrick JM, Wang MY, et al. Comparison and evaluation of retrospective intermodality brain image registration techniques. J Comput Assist Tomogr 1997;21:554–66.

85. Jolesz F. Image-guided tumor targeting for diagnosis and therapy in oncology. In: Bragg D, Rubin P, Hricak H, editors. Oncologic imaging. Philadelphia: WB Saunders; 2002. p. 55–68.

86. Udupa J. 3D imaging: principles and approaches. In: Udupa J, Herman G, editors. 3D imaging in medicine. Boca Raton (FL): CRC Press; 2000. p. 1–73.

87. Tracton GS, Chaney EL, Rosenman JG, et al. Medical anatomy segmentation kit: combining 2D and 3D segmentation methods to enhance functionality. In: Bookstein FL, Duncan JS, Lange N, Wilson DC, editors. Mathematical methods in medical imaging. Bellingham, WA: Society of Photo-optical and Instrumentation Engineers, 1994. p. 98–109.

88. Kass M, Witkin A, Terzopoulos D. Snakes: active contour models. Int J Comput Vis 1988;1:321–31.

89. Staib L, Duncan J. Boundary finding with parametrically deformable models. IEEE Trans Patt Anal Mach Intell 1992;14:1061–75.

90. Cootes T, Hill A, Taylor C, et al. The use of active shape models for locating structures in medical images. In: Barrett H, Gmitro A, editors. Information processing in medical imaging. Berlin: Springer-Verlag; 1993. p. 33–47.

91. Székely G, Kelemen A, Brechbühler C, et al. Segmentation of 2-D and 3-D objects from MRI volume data using constrained elastic deformations of flexible Fourier contour and surface models. Med Image Anal 1996;1:19–34.

92. Bae K, Giger M, Chen C, et al. Automatic segmentation of liver structure in CT images. Med Phys 1993;20:71–8.

93. Boes J, Bland P, Weymouth T, et al. Generating a normalized

geometric liver model using warping. Invest Radiol 1994;29:281–6.

94. Collins D, Holmes C, Peters T, et al. Automatic 3-D model-based neuroanatomical segmentation. Hum Brain Map 1995;3:190–208.

95. Andreasen N, Rajarethinam R, Cizadlo T, et al. Automatic atlas-based volume estimation of human brain regions from MR images. J Comput Assist Tomogr 1996;20:98–106.

96. Davatzikos C. Spatial normalization of 3D brain images using deformable models. J Comput Assist Tomogr 1996;20:656–65.

97. Aboutanos G, Dawant B. Automatic brain segmentation and validation: image-based versus atlas-based deformable models. SPIE Proc Med Imaging 1997;3034:299–310.

98. Thompson P, Toga A. Detection, visualization and animation of abnormal anatomic structure with a deformable probabilistic brain atlas based on random vector field transformations. Med Image Anal 1997;1:271–94.

99. Dawant B, Hartmann S, Pan S, et al. Brain atlas deformation in the presence of small and large space-occupying tumors. Comput Aided Surg 2002;7:1–10.

100. Joshi S, Pizer S, Fletcher PT, et al. Multiscale deformable model segmentation and statistical shape analysis using medial descriptions. IEEE Trans Med Imaging 2002;21:538–50.

101. Fletcher P, Joshi S, Gash A, et al. Pablo: clinical prototype software for automatic image segmentation of normal anatomical structures using medially based deformable models. Int J Radiat Oncol Biol Phys 2002;54:81.

102. Chen J, Tracton G, Rao M, et al. Comparison of automatic and human segmentation of kidneys from CT images. Int J Radiat Oncol Biol Phys 2002;54:82.

103. Lorensen W, Cline H. Marching cubes: a high resolution 3D surface reconstruction algorithm. Computer Graphics (SIGGRAPH '87) 1987;21:163–9.

104. Cline HE, Lorensen WE, Kikinis R, et al. Three-dimensional segmentation of MR images of the head using probability and connectivity. J Comput Assist Tomogr 1990;14:1037–45.

105. Ashton E, Takahashi C, Berg M, et al. Accuracy and reproducibility of manual and semiautomated quantification of MS lesions by MRI. J Magn Reson Imaging 2003;17:300–8.

106. Pham D, Xu C, Prince J. Current methods in medical image segmentation. Annu Rev Biomed Eng 2000;2:315–37.

107. Austin-Seymour M, Kalet I, McDonald J, et al. Three dimensional planning target volumes: a model and a software tool. Int J Radiat Oncol Biol Phys 1995;33:1073–80.

108. Ketting C, Austin-Seymour M, Kalet I, et al. Automated planning target volume generation: an evaluation pitting a computer-based tool against human experts. Int J Radiat Oncol Biol Phys 1997;37:697–704.

109. Kalet I, Whipple M, Pessah S, et al. A rule-based model for local and regional tumor spread. In: Kohane IS, editor. Proceedings of the 2002 American Medical Informatics Association Symposium. Bethesda, MD: Hanley and Belfus, 2002. p. 360–4.

110. Li A, Bluemke D. Cancer diagnosis: imaging - magnetic resonance imaging. In: DeVita V, Hellman S, Rosenberg S, editors. Cancer: principles and practice of oncology. 6th ed. Philadelphia: Lippincott Williams and Williams; 2001. Chapter 27.

Chapter 8

PET-CT in IMRT Planning

Jeffrey T. Yap, PhD, David W. Townsend, PhD, Nathan C. Hall, MD, PhD

Historically, radiation therapy (RT) has relied on medical imaging to identify both the malignancies to be irradiated and the normal tissues to be avoided. Recent advances in instrumentation, computing, and algorithms now enable the design and delivery of intensity-modulated radiation therapy (IMRT), conforming the high dose to the tumor, thereby sparing surrounding normal tissue. Additionally, IMRT provides the unprecedented ability to deliver nonuniform doses to subvolumes within the gross tumor volume (GTV), raising the question of where and how to boost the radiation dose. Such a refinement in treatment delivery increases the need for anatomically precise and biologically relevant imaging.

The field of medical imaging has also experienced unprecedented growth. Improvements in image acquisition hardware, software algorithms, and computing allow rapid acquisition, reconstruction, and display of high-resolution three-dimensional anatomic and functional images. Computed tomography (CT) is the most widely used imaging modality for tumor diagnosis and staging. CT has also been used extensively in RT planning, providing three-dimensional anatomic boundaries for contouring and electron density information for dosimetric calculations.

More recently, positron emission tomography (PET) has been adopted for diagnosis and staging of many tumors because of its improved sensitivity and specificity. In 1998, the first hybrid PET-CT scanner was introduced, combining anatomic and functional imaging in a single device, and has rapidly gained widespread clinical acceptance and commercial production. This chapter describes the evolution of clinical PET and recent advances in the development of PET-CT and discusses the role of PET-CT in RT treatment planning.

Computed Tomography

Advances in helical CT have enabled cost-effective body imaging that is widely used in the diagnosis and staging of cancer. More recently, the development of CT scanners with multiple detector rows has brought about rapid volumetric scanning with the capability of isotropic spatial resolution. CT has been used extensively in RT, both indirectly, by providing diagnostic and staging information prior to treatment planning, and directly, by performing CT-based virtual simulation.

CT simulators have been in clinical use for over 10 to 15 years.[1] Early systems used modifications to existing simulators.[2,3] Later designs focused on adapting existing diagnostic CT scanners for virtual simulation.[4,5] An important modification was the development of a large-bore single-slice CT scanner with an 85 cm diameter to accommodate the demands of imaging in the treatment position without compromising image quality.[6] Most CT scanners used for virtual simulation today are single-slice units. However, a large 82 cm bore 16-slice CT scanner is now commercially available (Siemens Sensation-16 Open, Siemens Medical Solutions, Forcheim, Germany) that will bring the latest advances in diagnostic imaging to RT simulation, such as speed and isotropic resolution.

Although widely used, CT has a number of important limitations. First, it provides an anatomic snapshot of the end result of disease that may have begun months or even years previously. As a result, CT is not sensitive for detecting the early development of disease. An additional limitation is its inability to distinguish between active malignancy and benign tissue that appears to be abnormal owing to previous intervention, such as surgery or RT.

Positron Emission Tomography

PET is a highly sensitive molecular imaging modality capable of detecting picomolar concentrations of positron-emitting radiotracers. Unlike conventional nuclear imaging with single-photon emitters, PET measures the coincident detection of dual opposing photons produced from the annihilation of a positron. This allows the linear path of the two coincident photons to be determined with electronic collimation, leading to a major improvement in sensitivity over single-photon emission computed tomography (SPECT), which uses physical lead collimation. Another advantage of PET is the ability to perform absolute quantification by correcting for the effects of detector sensitivity and photon scatter and attenuation.

The high specificity of PET is derived from its ability to image particular molecular interactions by using the relevant radiolabeled compounds. A variety of biochemical and physiologic processes can be studied in vivo with PET by measuring the distribution and concentration of different injected radiotracers in the human body.

^{18}F-Labeled Fluorodeoxyglucose PET

The most widely used clinical radiotracer in PET is ^{18}F-labeled fluorodeoxyglucose (^{18}FDG), an analog of glucose that is transported from plasma into tissue and phosphorylated by hexokinase. However, unlike glucose, ^{18}FDG is trapped in tissue and not further metabolized. This property is the basis for the accumulation of ^{18}FDG in metabolic tissue, enabling the calculation of the metabolic rate of glucose (MRGLc) from the measured ^{18}FDG concentrations in plasma and tissue with blood sampling and PET imaging, respectively.

Over 25 years ago, a compartmental model for quantifying the cerebral MRGLc was developed using ^{14}C-labeled deoxyglucose.[7,8] This was later adapted to ^{18}FDG and has been used extensively in a variety of normal and diseased states.[9–11] By measuring the time course of ^{18}FDG in plasma with multiple blood sampling and in tissue with dynamic PET imaging, nonlinear curve fitting can be performed to estimate the MRGLc. Simplifications have been made to the original nonlinear model, including a graphical approach and methods that do not require blood sampling.[12,13] However, clinical PET studies are typically performed as static acquisitions at a single time point after sufficient uptake, such as 1 hour after injection, and it is not possible to calculate the MRGLc.

^{18}FDG PET in Oncology

Many tumors have increased glucose metabolism, making ^{18}FDG an ideal tumor imaging agent.[14–17] ^{18}FDG uptake has been shown in vitro to correlate with the number of viable tumor cells.[18] This property substantiates the use of ^{18}FDG PET not only for detecting tumors but also for determining disease extent. An important simplification for routine clinical use of ^{18}FDG PET is the quantification of the standardized uptake value (SUV). The SUV adjusts for the effects of injected radioactivity and body weight or size, providing a normalized uptake measure that can be compared between patients.[19] The ^{18}FDG SUV has been shown to correlate with the MRGLc[20] and tumor doubling time.[21] Although the SUV is a semiquantitative parameter that does not directly measure a physiologic property such as the MRGLc, higher SUVs are associated with a greater likelihood of malignancy. Furthermore, SUVs can

be used in serial imaging of the same patient to study relative changes in metabolism owing to therapy.

Although there is variability in the SUVs for different tumor types and patients, the SUVs of individual tumors in the same patient are highly reproducible. In patients scanned with ^{18}FDG-PET twice in 7 to 10 days without therapeutic intervention, Weber and colleagues measured a 10% standard deviation of the mean percentage difference in SUV.[22] Nakamoto and colleagues found a similar range of reproducibility in 10 patients with lung cancer imaged twice with FDG-PET within a week of no treatment.[23] Therefore, the metabolic response to therapy can be reliably determined with SUV changes of 20% and greater. Additional parameters can be calculated based on the SUV that may be more relevant in RT.[24] For example, Humm and colleagues found that the total ^{18}FDG uptake, defined as the product of tumor volume and ^{18}FDG activity, was the best prognostic indicator of response to fractionated RT in rodent tumor xenografts.[25]

Clinical Reimbursement for ^{18}FDG PET

The health care benefits of ^{18}FDG PET have been documented in numerous publications.[26] Early studies have shown that it improves the staging of many cancers compared with anatomic imaging, such as CT and magnetic resonance imaging (MRI),[27,28] and may impact on the selection of treatment.[29]

Widespread use of ^{18}FDG PET has been realized only in the last 5 years. In 1998, the Centers for Medicare and Medicaid Services (CMS) first approved coverage of PET in the characterization of solitary pulmonary nodules and staging of non–small cell lung cancer. Subsequently, approval expanded to the diagnosis, staging, and restaging of colorectal cancer, esophageal cancer, head and neck cancers (excluding the central nervous system and thyroid), lymphoma, and melanoma. More recently, it has been approved for staging and restaging of breast cancer.

The coverage of breast cancer also included the first use of ^{18}FDG PET for the monitoring of tumor response to treatment for women with locally advanced and metastatic disease when a change in therapy is anticipated.[30–32] The use of ^{18}FDG for monitoring early response to therapy has tremendous potential for terminating ineffective treatment and/or modifying treatments. Most recently, restaging of thyroid cancer has been approved, and additional indications are currently under review, including gynecologic malignancies.[33–35] Some private insurance providers have expanded PET coverage beyond the current CMS-approved indications (see Chapter 16, "Billing and Reimbursement").

Limitations of ^{18}FDG PET

Although extremely effective, ^{18}FDG PET has some important limitations. Because many nonmalignant processes use glucose metabolism, ^{18}FDG uptake occurs in normal tissues, and increased glucose metabolism can also be associated with muscle activity, inflammation, wound healing, and infection. This can confound the diagnostic interpretation of increased focal [18]FDG uptake, raising the need for strategies to identify normal and benign variants.[36] Some tumor types are also not hypermetabolic in comparison with surrounding tissues. One strategy to eliminate both of these limitations is the development of radiotracers that are more specific than [18]FDG to such malignancies.

There are also some general limitations with the PET process itself. One is the lack of anatomic information, which can make the diagnostic interpretation of uptake patterns difficult. In the case of therapeutic planning, it is equally important to know the precise localization of tumors in addition to merely detecting their presence. Another limitation is the relatively poor spatial resolution of PET compared with CT or MRI. The typical PET spatial resolution achieved ranges from several millimeters to a centimeter or greater. Poor spatial resolution can limit the detection and quantification of small lesions owing to the partial volume effect.

PET-CT

The combination of information and visual correlation of different imaging modalities is useful for the diagnosis of disease and patient management. In the case of [18]FDG PET, spatial co-registration and fusion with CT or MRI images allow focal uptake to be accurately localized within an anatomic framework. Image fusion compensates for some of the limitations of [18]FDG PET by reducing false-positive findings in areas with known physiologic uptake. It also increases confidence in reporting positive lesions with moderate uptake localized in suspected areas of recurrence or metastases, such as lymph nodes.

Software-Based Multimodality Image Registration

For over a decade, software methods have facilitated multimodality image registration in the brain. One of the earliest attempts to match anatomic localization with functional brain images used a stereotactic atlas.[37] An important advance in multimodality image registration techniques was the development of a semiautomated method based on surface matching.[38] An early application of this method was multimodality RT planning.[39] Later methods used similarities in image intensities to perform fully automated co-registration in the brain without the need to identify landmarks or external contours.[40–44]

Although these methods are useful in the brain, image registration in other sites is much more challenging. In the body, a rigid transformation is generally not sufficient to address the deformations of internal organs and differences in patient positioning. A number of deformable models have been developed to address these limitations.[45] Most recently, deformable methods have been developed

for co-registering PET and CT lung images from separate scanners, which typically require nonlinear transformations to account for differences in breathing protocols for the two acquisition procedures.[46,47] Whereas diagnostic CT is sufficiently rapid to be performed with breath-holding, PET acquisitions are on the order of minutes and require free breathing during the examination.

Clinical Benefits of PET-CT Software Registration

It has been shown that fusion of [18]FDG PET images with CT or MRI using software registration improves the anatomic localization of hypermetabolic foci, providing additional information that may improve patient management.[48,49] The Leuven Lung Cancer Group found in a group of 56 patients with non–small cell lung cancer that simple visual correlation of [18]FDG PET and CT images improves the accuracy of staging with PET.[50] Similarly, Magnani and colleagues imaged 28 patients with non–small cell lung cancer with PET and CT prior to surgical treatment and found that the correct identification of mediastinal lymph nodes was made in 21 patients with CT alone, 22 patients with PET alone, 24 patients with visual correlation of PET and CT, and 25 patients with fused PET and CT.[51] In a comparison of 45 patients with surgical pathologic findings, Aquino and colleagues found that staging with co-registered PET-CT was more accurate than staging with CT and PET scans interpreted independently or side by and side.[52] Clearly, the most obvious tumors can be correctly identified with PET or CT alone. However, the subtle false-negative cases that are not detected in CT or PET alone may require accurate co-registration and possibly even the use of fused images to be correctly identified. Similarly, some hypermetabolic foci may be ruled out as malignancy based on the accurate localization within areas of physiologic [18]FDG uptake.

Combined PET-CT Scanner

The first combined PET-CT scanner was developed to provide an automated hardware solution to the need for co-registered anatomic and functional images.[53] The simple concept of the combined PET-CT scanner is to merge independent PET and CT scanners into a single gantry to acquire sequential CT and PET images in the same imaging session with the patient in the same position. This eliminates the need for separate PET and CT imaging sessions while providing intrinsic co-registration. The first prototype PET-CT scanner was physically integrated with the CT and PET detectors mounted together on the same rotating gantry.[53] Today, commercial designs are based on separate and independently functioning PET and CT scanners mounted back to back.

Although some research-oriented centers have had success with PET and CT software registration, the automatic co-registration provided by combined PET-CT scanners has greatly facilitated the routine clinical use of PET-CT imaging. An accurate and precise rigid transformation for co-registering the CT and PET images is determined by carefully aligning the two scanners during installation and measuring their physical offset. This eliminates one of the major limitations of software registration approaches by providing a constant spatial transformation between PET and CT images that is known beforehand and is independent of patient positioning. The underlying assumption is that the patient does not move during the procedure. The accuracy of software-based registration methods are typically on the order of the voxel size of the modality with the lowest spatial resolution. In the case of PET and CT co-registration, this typically corresponds to 4 to 5 mm.[54] In contrast, the intrinsic registration accuracy of a combined PET-CT scanner is submillimeter.

CT-Based Attenuation Correction

Accurate PET requires the correction for photon attenuation that occurs in the body of the patient. Traditional PET scanners accomplish this by measuring the attenuation of the body using a transmission scan with an external positron-emitting radiation source such as germanium-68 (^{68}Ge).[55] An important step in the development of PET-CT was the transformation of CT information for performing attenuation correction. Although some manufacturers still provide positron or single-photon transmission sources for attenuation correction, the traditional PET transmission scan can be eliminated by using the CT images for attenuation correction. This reduces the PET-CT scanning time by up to 50% compared with PET alone. Furthermore, given that CT has a much higher photon flux than traditional PET transmission sources, essentially noise-free photon attenuation maps can be generated. However, CT x-ray energies range from 40 to 140 keV and are much lower than the 511 keV photons measured with PET. To use the CT images for attenuation correction, the measured attenuation values must be scaled to appropriate values for 511 keV photons.[56] Most commercial systems implement a bilinear interpolation scheme to account for differences in the ratio of CT to PET attenuation coefficients in tissue and cortical bone.[57] Attenuation correction using CT versus ^{68}Ge was evaluated in a clinical study of 32 patients in whom there were no significant differences.[58] Similarly, Nakamoto and colleagues compared CT versus ^{68}Ge attenuation correction in 28 patients and found that the quantitative radioactivity values were generally comparable, although the CT-based attenuation correction yielded slightly higher concentrations.[59]

Clinical Benefits of PET-CT

Imaging with a combined PET-CT scanner improves the diagnosis and staging of cancer, as was demonstrated with early studies using multimodality software registration. Promising results were demonstrated with the first prototype PET-CT scanner, showing improved identification of physiologic ^{18}FDG uptake and anatomic localization of neoplastic lesions.[60,61] The additional findings in PET-CT led to a change in patient management approximately 30% of the time.[62] The promising findings of the prototype hybrid PET-CT scanner and the body of literature demonstrating the benefits of multimodality software registration stimulated the rapid commercial development of PET-CT. The first commercial PET-CT scanner was introduced in 2001; today, all major PET tomograph vendors, including CTI Molecular Imaging, Siemens Medical Solutions, GE Healthcare, and Philips Medical Systems, sell combined PET-CT scanners.[63] Hundreds of PET-CT scanners have already been sold, and current trends suggest that combined PET-CT scanners will ultimately replace PET-only scanners.

Numerous studies have been published demonstrating the clinical benefits of PET-CT. Clinical PET-CT scanners are currently being used to accurately localize focal FDG uptake and improve the detection of tumors.[64,65] A common occurrence in PET-CT is the detection of metastatic disease based on focal uptake in lymph nodes that are too small to be found positive on CT, for example, less than 1 cm (Figure 8-1). Such lesions may also be undetected with PET alone owing to apparent localization in areas associated with physiologic uptake or diffuse uptake owing to the partial volume effect. However, the combination of increased ^{18}FDG uptake and accurate localization in a potential site of metastasis allows confident decisions to be made in challenging cases. For example, in a study of 45 patients with colorectal cancer, Cohade and colleagues found that the use of PET-CT reduced the frequency of lesions characterized as equivocal and probable by 50% compared with PET while increasing the frequency of definite lesion characterizations by 30%.[66] As a result, staging and restaging improved to 89% with PET-CT compared with 78% with PET alone. Based on the promising findings being reported at numerous centers, PET-CT is likely to replace CT or PET alone for cancer imaging in areas such as the head and neck, lung, abdomen, and pelvis.[67,68]

Potential PET-CT Attenuation Artifacts

Currently, the CT-based attenuation correction algorithms used in commercial PET-CT scanners do not account for attenuation of materials other than soft tissue and bone. A variety of artificial materials may be present in the body, which could lead to errors in attenuation correction and produce artifacts. Metallic objects such as dental implants, prostheses, and pacemakers can cause artifacts of apparent increased uptake that is due to overcorrection.[69–72] If the resulting attenuation-corrected PET images were reviewed without the use of the CT or uncorrected PET images, these focal areas of apparent increased activity could be misread as false-positive hypermetabolic tumors. However, the hyperintense focus seen on the attenuation-corrected PET image can be interpreted correctly by observing the corresponding hypodense object in the uncorrected PET images and/or the obvious

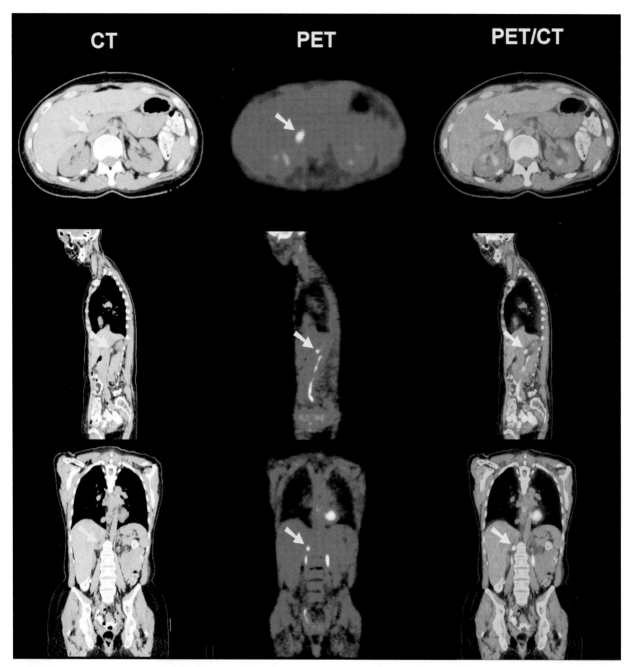

FIGURE 8-1. ^{18}F-labeled fluorodeoxyglucose positron emission tomography–computed tomography ([18]FDG PET-CT) scan of a patient with ovarian cancer with suspected recurrence. [18]FDG PET-CT identified two positive hypermetabolic pericaval lymph nodes, which were negative on CT with sizes of 4 and 9 mm (pictured). Note the lack of respiration artifacts and excellent co-registration achieved with the fast imaging performed on the 16-slice PET-CT scanner. (To view a color version of this image, please refer to the CD-ROM.)

source of the artifact in the CT image (Figure 8-2).

Some centers perform the combined PET-CT procedure with a low-dose CT examination to provide anatomic localization. However, standard diagnostic CT protocols can be performed as part of the PET-CT procedure to provide diagnostic CT images, which are clinically reviewed in addition to the PET and fused PET-CT images. As is the case with conventional CT, intravenous and oral contrast media can be used with PET-CT to improve the image quality and

diagnostic use of the CT images.[73] Similar to metal objects, high-density intravenous and oral contrast media, such as iodine and barium, are not accounted for in standard CT-based attenuation correction methods and can lead to artifacts of increased uptake.[74–77] However, there is also evidence that the use of some CT contrast agents can be of additional value in detecting tumors with little or no increase in [18]FDG uptake.[78,79] One method for avoiding PET-CT contrast artifacts is the use of water as a negative contrast

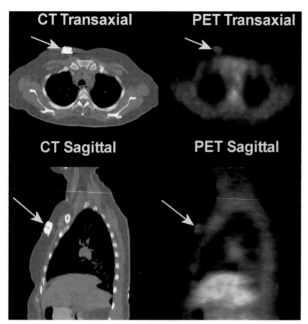

FIGURE 8-2. Attenuation artifact generated from a chemotherapy port. The overcorrection for attenuation of metal results in an apparent focus of increased ^{18}F-labeled fluorodeoxyglucose uptake. However, the artifact is easily identified and correctly interpreted by review of the computed tomography (CT) image. (To view a color version of this image, please refer to the CD-ROM.)

agent.[80] Segmentation methods are also being developed to identify contrast media in PET-CT images and appropriately correct for attenuation in the segmented voxels.[81,82]

Despite the potential artifacts caused by overcorrection for attenuation of artificial materials, most PET-CT images can be interpreted reliably in conjunction with the CT images, uncorrected PET images, and/or a thorough clinical history of the patient. Similar to the evolution of CT and MRI, appropriate education of PET-CT uptake patterns and potential artifacts will minimize the misinterpretation of diagnostic findings.

Motion Artifacts and Four-Dimensional Imaging

Although combined PET-CT scanners have an intrinsic submillimeter co-registration of PET and CT images, this precision is achieved only in clinical imaging in the absence of patient motion. Gross patient movement can be reduced with the use of immobilization devices and shorter scanning times. In addition, advances in multislice CT and three-dimensional PET have dramatically shortened scanning times, making imaging more tolerable to the patient, with less voluntary motion. Involuntary motion, such as breathing and beating of the heart, remains a challenge for both preserving image quality of the individual modalities and maintaining accurate and precise co-registration between CT and PET.

Respiration can create artifacts owing to spatial misregistration of the CT images used for attenuation correction and the PET emission images.[83–85] The PET image represents an average position of the lungs and other organs acquired over many breathing cycles, whereas typical breath-hold CT produces a snapshot at a single time point in the respiratory cycle. This results in a mismatch between the CT and PET images, which can produce spatial misregistration and result in attenuation correction artifacts. Although it is infrequent, misregistration of lesions can result in clinically significant misinterpretations.[86] Modification of the breathing protocols used during the CT portion of the PET-CT examination can improve the match between the PET and CT images. For example, co-registration is improved, and there are fewer artifacts when CT is acquired with breath-hold during normal expiration.[87,88] The rapid scanning achieved with multislice CT scanners also enables CT imaging during free breathing without the resulting motion artifacts associated with single-slice CT scanners (see Figure 8-1).

An important development to address the issues of respiratory artifacts is gating of CT and or PET images. PET gating has been performed with a camera-based patient monitoring system and has shown a volume reduction of tumors by as much as 34% and an increase in the SUV as large as 159%.[89] The same method of patient monitoring has also been used to perform gated RT of liver tumors.[90] Respiratory gating is currently being developed for PET-CT and initial studies suggest improvements in both the detection and quantification of small lesions in the lungs or upper abdomen.[91] In addition to the diagnostic benefits, gated PET-CT imaging is likely to provide the ultimate complementary imaging for gated IMRT.

PET-CT Operational Considerations

Dedicated PET-CT scanners are rapidly becoming established in a wide range of environments, ranging from hospitals, university medical centers, and private stand-alone imaging centers. Although research-oriented institutions may have on-site cyclotrons for producing short-lived radiotracers, most clinical facilities in the United States do not have them and receive [18]FDG from the existing networks of commercial distribution sites. In addition, there is a growing market of mobile PET-CT systems for centers that either cannot afford the capital investment or do not have the patient population to sustain daily scanning. For sites planning on purchasing combined PET-CT over traditional PET scanners, there are additional considerations in site preparation and facilities management. Hybrid PET-CT tomographs require a larger scanner room compared with either PET or CT alone to accommodate the greater dimensions of the PET-CT scanner, allow for longer travel of the patient bed through both the CT and PET imaging devices, and enable servicing of either the PET or the CT scanner. In addition, PET-CT systems with high-performance multi-slice CT scanners may also require additional space for the CT water cooler and additional computers.

Radiation shielding requirements of the PET-CT scanning room are an important element of site preparation that will vary according to the local regulations for both the PET and CT exposures. The daily room exposures owing to the CT component of a PET-CT scanner are less than with a stand-alone CT scanner owing to a lower scanning volume and/or lower CT dose used in some PET-CT protocols. However, the overall daily exposures associated with the [18]FDG PET portion of the PET-CT procedure are typically higher than with a PET scanner alone owing to the higher patient throughput made possible with faster scanning. An additional consideration in high-throughput PET-CT is the need for additional patient [18]FDG uptake rooms and/or additional room shielding. Given that the imaging times are significantly shorter than the typical [18]FDG uptake period, there is a need to have multiple patients injected and waiting in the [18]FDG uptake phase to maximize the scanning throughput.

The multimodality nature of PET-CT places new demands on staffing requirements. Some centers perform only low-dose CT procedures for attenuation correction and improved localization of PET images. In this case, PET-CT procedures are typically performed by nuclear medicine technologists and the images are read by PET-trained nuclear medicine physicians. However, other centers perform standard diagnostic CT protocols as part of the PET-CT procedure to obtain diagnostic quality CT images. In this case, an x-ray/CT technologist may be required to perform the CT component of the examination and a radiologist performs the reading of the CT images. In the use of PET-CT for RT planning, it is also important to include the RT staff to establish appropriate patient positioning and immobilization. Owing to the multidisciplinary nature of PET-CT, discussions are ongoing with various organizations regarding cross-training and certification programs for both technologists and physicians.

IMRT Planning with PET-CT

PET-CT will have an increasing role in IMRT planning in which there is a need for advanced biologic imaging. PET-CT is perhaps the ideal match for IMRT planning because of its ability to provide the CT information needed for identifying anatomic structures and performing dose calculations, as well as the intrinsically co-registered PET functional information for delineating biologic target volumes (BTVs). Biologic tissue characterization from PET-CT is important to identify normal tissue and the complete extent of active malignancy for target volume contouring. The same biologic information may also be useful for predicting the sensitivity to radiation and the resulting response to therapy.

PET-CT Simulation

PET-CT scanners can be optionally configured and used for RT simulation in addition to standard diagnostic imaging (Figure 8-3). It is important to recognize that PET and CT images from the combined PET-CT scanner are intrinsically co-registered independently of patient positioning. However, PET-CT simulation requires that the patient be imaged in the same position as used in treatment. This is done with the attachment of a carbon fiber flat-panel tabletop insert with an indexed patient positioning system, as is commonly used with CT simulators (MED-TEC, Inc., Orange City, IA). Standard immobilization devices can be attached to the tabletop to ensure that the patient is placed and maintained in the correct treatment position. An important decision in the development of the first commercial PET-CT system was the extension of the scanner bore diameter to 70 cm for both the PET and CT gantry.[54] Dedicated PET scanners typically have a bore diameter of 55 to 60 cm, which is not sufficient when used with a flat tabletop and immobilization devices. The 70 cm continuous patient port of the PET-CT scanner enables imaging most patients in the treatment position and diagnostic imaging of larger patients excluded by the smaller patient port of PET. It is also important to install external room lasers (LAP of America L.C., Boca Raton, FL) in the PET-CT scanner room to properly position patients and match the simulation and treatment isocenters.

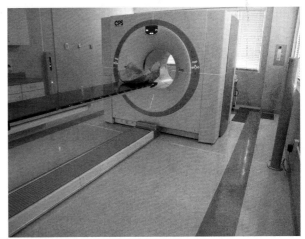

FIGURE 8-3. Sixteen-slice LSO HI-REZ positron emission tomography–computed tomography (PET-CT) scanner (CPS Innovations, Knoxville, TN) installed at the University of Tennessee Medical Center. The PET-CT scanner is configured for radiation therapy simulation with the use of a flat-panel tabletop (MED-TEC, Inc., Orange City, IA) and external room lasers (LAP of America L.C., Boca Raton, FL). The 70 cm large-diameter bore allows most patients to be imaged in the treatment position with the use of immobilization devices and provides access to diagnostic imaging for larger patients. (To view a color version of this image, please refer to the CD-ROM.)

Software Functionality Requirements

Hybrid PET-CT scanners produce separate PET and CT images in formats specified by the Digital Imaging and Communications in Medicine (DICOM) standards. The DICOM image format and communications standards were developed by the American College of Radiology and the National Electrical Manufacturers Association to promote an open standard for vendor-independent exchange of multimodality images. Important extensions to the original DICOM standard were the addition of a PET image format and DICOM RT objects.[92,93] Although some older RT planning systems do not support DICOM images, the current release of virtually all planning software packages support both CT and PET DICOM image formats and hence can import native images from combined PET-CT scanners. A common misunderstanding of PET-CT is the notion that there is a single fused PET-CT image for a given transaxial plane. In fact, a fused PET-CT image is merely the display of a superimposed CT and PET image with user-defined color tables, window contrast settings, and opacity (alpha blending) (see Figure 8-1). Hence, there is no DICOM standard for fused PET-CT images, although one can save a fused PET-CT image as a true-color snapshot (DICOM secondary capture). Such images are often useful for conveying succinct clinically relevant findings but are not sufficient for RT planning, quantitative CT and PET information is required. The important functionality requirements for planning software used with PET-CT simulation are the ability to (1) import PET and CT DICOM images, (2) interpret and apply intrinsic image coregistration of PET and CT, and (3) provide fusion display tools for multimodality contouring. Most vendors have reacted to these requirements, and relevant tools are either in development or are available in their current software releases. However, it is important for centers planning to engage in PET-CT–based IMRT to investigate the functionality of software provided by both their PET-CT vendor and their RT planning software vendor.

Tumor and Target Volume Delineation

PET-CT enables the use of biochemical and physiologic information measured in tumors and surrounding normal tissue to be incorporated into so-called BTVs.[94] It is important to recognize that the BTV is not merely a replacement for the traditional CT-based GTV. The process of using a BTV to define a planning target volume (PTV) and the associated prescribed dose is fundamentally different than with conventional GTVs. Although some authors have used the convention of reporting CT-based GTVs in comparison with PET-based GTVs, it is important to consider the biologic properties measured by the particular PET radiotracer and the resulting image intensities when using biologic information to design treatment plans. For example, the BTV determined from a PET radiotracer for metabolism

might be considered to encompass the viable tumor cells and therefore be used for determining a minimum dose, whereas a BTV resulting from a PET radiotracer for hypoxia would encompass a smaller tumor subvolume that could be used to define the maximum tumor dose (Figure 8-4).

Several studies have already shown that the improved staging with [18]FDG PET can be used to improve patient management and significantly impact RT planning.[95,96] The metabolic tumor volume information from [18]FDG PET can affect the PTV in two major ways. In the first case, [18]FDG PET may detect more extensive locoregional disease and/or distant metastasis. This can result in an increase in the PTV where possible, or, in the extreme case, a termination of therapy or a change in treatment modality. In the second case, [18]FDG PET may identify a smaller volume of viable tumor compared with the CT-based GTV, allowing for a reduction in the PTV to exclude abnormal benign tissue, for example, owing to necrosis or atelectasis.

A recent survey of the published findings show that treatment volumes are significantly altered 30 to 60% of the time with the addition of [18]FDG PET.[97] In a study of 11 patients compared with CT- and PET-based PTVs, Erdi and colleagues found that 7 of 11 patients had an increased PTV (average of 19%), whereas 4 of 11 patients had a decreased PTV (average of 18%).[98] Similarly, a retrospective study by Schmidt and colleagues found a change in RT portals in 15 of 39 patients when using [18]FDG PET in addition to CT.[99]

One should note that the direct use of PET images in RT planning will always result in different contours compared with CT and that the clinical impact of subtle and presumed insignificant changes in PTVs is not known. In a prospective study comparing CT and [18]FDG PET, Schmucking and colleagues reported that the use of metabolic information with [18]FDG PET led to a 3 to 21% reduction in PTVs in 25 of 27 patients and an increase in the PTV in only 2 of 27 patients.[100]

Combined PET-CT scanners have greatly improved the accessibility to tumor metabolic information for use in IMRT planning. Promising results with [18]FDG PET-CT scanners are now emerging with findings similar to those of previously reported studies using [18]FDG PET with software registration.[101,102] Long-term prospective studies are now needed to fully evaluate the impact of PET-CT–based IMRT on tumor control, normal tissue toxicity, and clinical outcome.

Dose Optimization

In addition to improving the definition of PTVs, PET-CT may also provide biologically relevant information for determining the optimal dose to deliver at the voxel level. For example, Alber and colleagues proposed a method for transforming a biologic image such as PET into a dose efficiency distribution to determine a prescribed maximum boost factor.[103] Brahme suggested that PET-CT could be

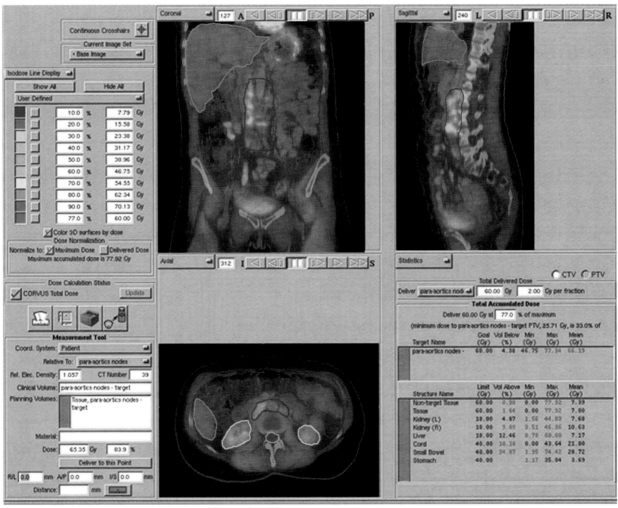

FIGURE 8-4. Positron emission tomography–computed tomography (PET-CT)–based intensity-modulated radiation therapy plan for a patient with cervical cancer with recurrent metastases in the para-aortic lymph nodes. Although abnormal lymph nodes were also identified on CT, the PET-CT–based target volume extended 14 mm axially compared with the CT-based plan owing to the detection of additional disease that was not seen on CT images. CTV = clinical target volume; PTV = planning target volume. (To view a color version of this image, please refer to the CD-ROM.)

used for adaptive RT by measuring the mean dose delivery during the early part of the treatment and the tumor response during the first week or two of therapy to revise the treatment plan.[104] The clinical impact of using PET-CT to escalate the dose in metabolically active tumor cells is speculative at this time, and further clinical studies are needed. However, the ability of PET-CT to accurately localize and quantify metabolism or other important processes in tumor cells at the voxel level holds great promise for biologic optimization of dose delivery.

Assessment of Tumor Response

[18]FDG PET is a useful tool for evaluating the response to RT by distinguishing radiation necrosis from recurrent tumor.[105–107] In preclinical studies, it has been shown that dose-dependent reductions in [18]FDG uptake correspond to effective inhibition of tumor growth.[108] Clinically, [18]FDG PET has been shown to be more effective in identifying early tumor response and recurrence than anatomic imaging, such as CT or MRI.[109,110] Several studies have shown that reduced SUVs measured with [18]FDG PET after RT have corresponded to response in therapy and are a good prognostic indicator.[111,112] Compared with CT, follow-up scanning with [18]FDG PET is a better predictor of response to radical RT in lung cancer.[110] Assessment of response using combined [18]FDG PET–CT has the added benefit of accurately localizing metabolic changes that occur as a response to therapy. Today, the simplest and most common method of assessing response to therapy is visual comparison of pre- and post-therapy images (Figure 8-5). Ultimately, the improvement of software-based co-registration of serial PET-CT studies could enable quantitative comparison of functional parameters, such as SUVs, before and after therapy at the voxel level.

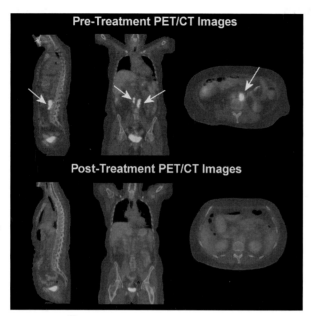

FIGURE 8-5. ^{18}F-labeled fluorodeoxyglucose–positron emission tomography–computed tomography ([18]FDG PET-CT) images of a patient with ovarian cancer before (*top row*) and 5 months after intensity-modulated radiation therapy (*bottom row*). The hypermetabolic para-aortic lymph nodes seen in the pretreatment [18]FDG PET-CT images are completely resolved in the post-treatment images, indicating a response to therapy. (To view a color version of this image, please refer to the CD-ROM.)

Timing Issues with Measuring [18]FDG Response

The timing of post-therapy PET scanning is a critical factor in assessing response with [18]FDG. Typically, a response to therapy is indicated by a decrease in glucose metabolism following therapy. However, the early effects of RT may actually increase the glucose metabolism in a responding tumor owing to the metabolic processes of inflammation, macrophage activity, radiation repair, and apoptosis. In vitro studies by Higashi and colleagues demonstrated nearly 10-fold increases in [18]FDG uptake in an ovarian cancer cell line (HTB77IP3) following 30 Gy of cobalt-60 irradiation.[113] In contrast, there was a sixfold decrease in the number of viable cells. The increase in metabolism early after RT may be associated with radiation damage, whereas a decrease in metabolism at a later time could reflect the resulting reduction in viable tumor cells. In a clinical study of four patients receiving stereotactic RT, Rozental and colleagues found that the ratio of the MRGLc in irradiated tumor to contralateral white matter increased by 25 to 42% at 1 day post-RT, whereas there was a 10 to 12% decrease at 7 days post-RT.[114]

Although early increases in [18]FDG uptake following therapy may confound traditional assessment of response associated with decreased metabolism, the early increase in metabolism after RT could also be predictive of response. In a study of 14 patients with glioma, Spence and colleagues reported that an increase in glucose metabolism measured with PET at 2 weeks post-RT compared with pretreatment correlated with longer survival.[115] Erdi and colleagues stud-

ied two patients with seven to eight serial PET scans during the entire course of RT.[24] As expected, the general trend was a decrease in metabolism for the responding patient and a constant or increased metabolism in the nonresponding patient. However, at one time point approximately 3 weeks after the initiating therapy, the responding patient showed an increase in SUV, whereas the nonresponding patient showed a decrease in SUV at a similar time.

Future of Multitracer PET-CT

Combined PET-CT is a technology that is immediately upgradable with the use of other radiotracers. Although [18]FDG has been the most successful general purpose radiotracer for clinical oncology, a need remains for more specific radiotracers to address the clinical indications and treatments where glucose metabolism is not the most relevant biologic property. There is a rich history of radiotracer development in PET and a wide range of molecular imaging probes that have been used for PET oncology research.[116,117] The use of these radiotracers as an alternative or in addition to [18]FDG imaging could greatly improve the scope and effectiveness of PET-CT in IMRT planning and assessment of response to therapy.

A number of tumor types are not well detected by [18]FDG owing to a lack of increased metabolism relative to surrounding tissues. Diagnosis, staging, and clinical management of patients with such tumors could be improved with the use of alternative radiotracers that are more effective than [18]FDG. It is also important to consider alternative radiotracers in monitoring radiation response. Comparison of multiple radiotracers shows that radiation response will be different for different mechanisms measured with PET. For example, Kubota and colleagues studied the effects of RT on [18]FDG, ^{18}F-deoxyuridine, ^{14}C-methionine, ^{3}H-thymidine, and ^{67}Ga-citrate. Although [18]FDG showed a large change in uptake and steady response to RT, ^{3}H-thymidine and ^{14}C-methionine showed a rapid response to irradiation and a high sensitivity for monitoring RT.[118]

Protein Synthesis

Normal brain has a very high glucose metabolism, which makes some brain tumors difficult to detect above the high background of surrounding tissue. Protein synthesis measured with ^{11}C-methionine has been studied as an alternative mechanism for detecting brain tumors. In a study of 45 patients with brain lesions, Chung and colleagues found that 31 of 35 brain tumors showed increased ^{11}C-methionine uptake despite uniform or decreased uptake with [18]FDG.[119] In contrast, all 10 benign lesions showed decreased or normal ^{11}C-methionine uptake. In addition to the improved detection of brain tumors, Sato and colleagues demonstrated that ^{11}C-methionine uptake correlates with proliferating cell nuclear antigen staining and can be used to distinguish between high- and low-grade gliomas.[120] Nuutinen and colleagues used ^{11}C-methionine PET for RT planning of patients with glioma, and it appears to have prognostic value.[121]

Hormone Receptors

16alpha-[^{18}F]Fluoro-17beta-estradiol ([18]FES) is a radioligand that binds to estrogen receptors and has been shown to correlate with estrogen receptor status.[122] In addition to showing promise as a diagnostic indicator of breast tumors expressing estrogen receptors, [18]FES can be used to determine response to hormone therapy, such as tamoxifen.[123] Similarly, androgen receptor radioligands have been developed to potentially detect and monitor prostate cancer.[124,125]

Hypoxia

Hypoxia is an important prognostic indicator in RT owing to well-documented radioresistance of tumor cells at low oxygen tension levels.[126] For this reason, there have been considerable efforts to develop and validate PET radiotracers for hypoxia, such as ^{18}F-labeled fluoromisonidazole (^{18}F-MISO). Early studies demonstrated that ^{18}F-MISO is metabolically trapped in hypoxic tissue and that its retention is dependent on oxygen concentration.[127,128] In human studies, ^{18}F-MISO appears to be useful for measuring hypoxia in a variety of tumors, including gliomas and prostate, head and neck, and non–small cell lung cancer.[129–131]

Cu(II)-diacetyl-bis(N(4)-methylthiosemicarbazone) (Cu-ATSM) is another hypoxia imaging radiotracer that has shown tumor uptake dependent on oxygen concentration (oxygen partial pressure [pO_2]).[132] In a 9L gliosarcoma rat model, Lewis and colleagues found a correlation between increased [60]Cu-ATSM uptake and low pO_2 measured directly with a needle oxygen electrode.[133] [60]Cu-ATSM has also been used to identify and dose-escalate hypoxic tumor subvolumes with IMRT while sparing normal tissue in the parotid glands and spinal cord,[134] (see Chapter 18.6, "Functional Imaging in Head and Neck Cancer: Emerging Technology"). Dehdashti and colleagues reported that [60]Cu-ATSM uptake is inversely related to survival in patients with cervical cancer and is predictive of a response in patients with non–small cell lung cancer.[135,136]

Cellular Proliferation

[11]C-Thymidine was developed as a marker of proliferation, and kinetic models similar to the compartmental models for [18]FDG have been developed to quantify cellular proliferation.[137,138] An important improvement in the imaging of proliferation was the development of ^{18}F-labeled thymidine ([18]FLT), which is more amenable to clinical use.[139] In a group of 30 patients with solitary pulmonary nodules, Buck and colleagues showed that the SUV measured with [18]FLT PET correlates with proliferation measured by Ki-67 immunostaining.[140] Compared with [18]FDG, [18]FLT has fewer false-positive results and better correlation with ex vivo indices of proliferation.[141] The use of [18]FLT for mon-

itoring the response to RT may eliminate some of the confounding effects of increased tumor metabolism early after treatment. Reinhardt and colleagues showed in fractionated RT of AH109A tumor-burdened rats that [18]FLT uptake decreased as a result of effective therapy, whereas [18]FDG uptake remained elevated even after eight doses, corresponding to a 100% tumor cell kill.[142]

Pharmacokinetics and Pharmacodynamics of Chemotherapy Agents

Normal tissue and tumor pharmacokinetics of chemotherapy agents can be measured by imaging radiolabeled analogs of cancer drugs with PET.[143,144] For example, standard chemotherapy agents, such as cisplatin, fluorouracil, tamoxifen, and paclitaxel, have been radiolabeled with positron-emitting isotopes and studied in humans with PET.[145–149] The pharmacodynamic effects of chemotherapy agents can also be studied by performing PET scans before and after chemotherapy with an appropriate biomarker. Although [18]FDG has been the most widely used PET radiotracer for evaluating the effects of chemotherapy, novel targeted therapies have required the use of more specific radiotracers that can measure the specific mechanism of action of the drug. For example, PET blood volume and blood flow imaging with ^{15}O-water and ^{15}O-carbon dioxide have been used to evaluate the pharmacodynamic response to novel anti-angiogenic and antivascular chemotherapy agents.[150,151]

Conclusion

The emergence of PET-CT has firmly established a new era of routine accessibility to one-stop multimodality oncologic imaging. Recent clinical studies have already demonstrated the added benefit of [18]FDG PET-CT for diagnosis and staging of cancer, and combined PET-CT is poised to replace separate imaging with conventional CT and PET. The accurate localization and characterization of tumors using PET-CT complement the precise three-dimensional design and delivery of radiation dose using IMRT. Delineation of biologic target volumes using PET-CT images should improve the therapeutic outcome of IMRT. Serial PET-CT imaging before and after IMRT may allow the characterization of dose effects, prediction of response to therapy, and, ultimately, the optimization of therapy.

Acknowledgments

We would like to thank Gwen King, MS, at the Institute for Radiation Therapy, Riverdale, Georgia, and Dwight Heron, MD, and Kristina Gerszten, MD, at the University of Pittsburgh Medical Center, Pittsburgh, PA, for discussions regarding the clinical implementation of PET-CT–based IMRT. The development of the prototype PET-CT scanner was supported by the National Cancer Institute (grants CA 65856 and CA 74135).

References

1. Nagata Y, Nishidai T, Abe M, et al. CT simulator: a new 3-D planning and simulating system for radiotherapy: part 2. Clinical application. Int J Radiat Oncol Biol Phys 1990;18:505–13.

2. Kotre CJ, Harrison RM, Ross WM. A simulator-based CT system for radiotherapy treatment planning. Br J Radiol 1984;57:631–5.

3. Leach MO, Webb S, Bentley RE. An x-ray detector system and modified simulator providing CT images for radiotherapy dosimetry planning. Phys Med Biol 1985;30:303–11.

4. Nishidai T, Nagata Y, Takahashi M, et al. CT simulator: a new 3-D planning and simulating system for radiotherapy: part 1. Description of system. Int J Radiat Oncol Biol Phys 1990;18:499–504.

5. Conway J, Robinson MH. CT virtual simulation. Br J Radiol 1997;70:S106–18.

6. Garcia-Ramirez JL, Mutic S, Dempsey JF, et al. Performance evaluation of an 85-cm-bore X-ray computed tomography scanner designed for radiation oncology and comparison with current diagnostic CT scanners. Int J Radiat Oncol Biol Phys 2002;52:1123–31.

7. Sokoloff L. [1-14C]-2-Deoxy-D-glucose method for measuring local cerebral glucose utilization. Mathematical analysis and determination of the "lumped" constants. Neurosci Res Program Bull 1976;14:466–8.

8. Sokoloff L, Reivich M, Kennedy C, et al. The [14C]deoxyglucose method for the measurement of local cerebral glucose utilization: theory, procedure, and normal values in the conscious and anesthetized albino rat. J Neurochem 1977;28:897–916.

9. Reivich M, Kuhl D, Wolf A, et al. Measurement of local cerebral glucose metabolism in man with 18F-2-fluoro-2-deoxy-D-glucose. Acta Neurol Scand Suppl 1977;64:190–1.

10. Reivich M, Kuhl D, Wolf A, et al. The [18F]fluorodeoxyglucose method for the measurement of local cerebral glucose utilization in man. Circ Res 1979;44:127–37.

11. Sokoloff L. The deoxyglucose method: theory and practice. Eur Neurol 1981;20:137–45.

12. Patlak CS, Blasberg RG, Fenstermacher JD. Graphical evaluation of blood-to-brain transfer constants from multiple-time uptake data. J Cereb Blood Flow Metab 1983;3:1–7.

13. Patlak CS, Blasberg RG. Graphical evaluation of blood-to-brain transfer constants from multiple-time uptake data. Generalizations. J Cereb Blood Flow Metab 1985;5:584–90.

14. Som P, Atkins HL, Bandoypadhyay D, et al. A fluorinated glucose analog, 2-fluoro-2-deoxy-D-glucose (F-18): nontoxic tracer for rapid tumor detection. J Nucl Med 1980;21:670–5.

15. Larson SM, Grunbaum Z, Rasey JS. Positron imaging feasibility studies: selective tumor concentration of 3H-thymidine, 3H-uridine, and 14C-2-deoxyglucose. Radiology 1980;134:771–3.

16. Di Chiro G, DeLaPaz RL, Brooks RA, et al. Glucose utilization of cerebral gliomas measured by [18F] fluorodeoxyglucose and positron emission tomography. Neurology 1982;32:1323–9.

17. Yonekura Y, Benua RS, Brill AB, et al. Increased accumulation of 2-deoxy-2-[18F]fluoro-D-glucose in liver metastases from colon carcinoma. J Nucl Med 1982;23:1133–7.

18. Higashi K, Clavo AC, Wahl RL. Does FDG uptake measure proliferative activity of human cancer cells? In vitro comparison with DNA flow cytometry and tritiated thymidine uptake? J Nucl Med 1993;34:414–9.

19. Zasadny KR, Wahl RL. Standardized uptake values of normal tissues at PET with 2-[fluorine-18]-fluoro-2-deoxy-D-glucose: variations with body weight and a method for correction. Radiology 1993;189:847–50.

20. Suhonen-Polvi H, Ruotsalainen U, Kinnala A, et al. FDG-PET in early infancy: simplified quantification methods to measure cerebral glucose utilization. J Nucl Med 1995;36:1249–54.

21. Duhaylongsod FG, Lowe VJ, Patz EF Jr, et al. Lung tumor growth correlates with glucose metabolism measured by fluoride-18 fluorodeoxyglucose positron emission tomography. Ann Thorac Surg 1995;60:1348–52.

22. Weber WA, Ziegler SI, Thodtmann R, et al. Reproducibility of metabolic measurements in malignant tumors using FDG PET. J Nucl Med 1999;40:1771–7.

23. Nakamoto Y, Zasadny KR, Minn H, et al. Reproducibility of common semi-quantitative parameters for evaluating lung cancer glucose metabolism with positron emission tomography using 2-deoxy-2-[18F]fluoro-D-glucose. Mol Imaging Biol 2002;4:171–8.

24. Erdi YE, Macapinlac H, Rosenzweig KE, et al. Use of PET to monitor the response of lung cancer to radiation treatment. Eur J Nucl Med 2000;27:861–6.

25. Humm JL, Lee J, O'Donoghue JA, et al. Changes in FDG tumor uptake during and after fractionated radiation therapy in a rodent tumor xenograft. Clin Positron Imaging 1999;2:289–96.

26. Gambhir SS, Czernin J, Schwimmer J, et al. A tabulated summary of the FDG PET literature. J Nucl Med 2001;42:1S–93S.

27. Wahl RL, Quint LE, Greenough RL, et al. Staging of mediastinal non-small cell lung cancer with FDG PET, CT, and fusion images: preliminary prospective evaluation. Radiology 1994;191:371–7.

28. von Haag DW, Follette DM, Roberts PF, et al. Advantages of positron emission tomography over computed tomography in mediastinal staging of non-small cell lung cancer. J Surg Res 2002;103:160–4.

29. Zhao DS, Valdivia AY, Li Y, et al. 18F-Fluorodeoxyglucose positron emission tomography in small-cell lung cancer. Semin Nucl Med 2002;32:272–5.

30. Wahl RL, Zasadny K, Helvie M, et al. Metabolic monitoring of breast cancer chemohormonotherapy using positron emission tomography: initial evaluation. J Clin Oncol 1993;11:2101–11.

31. Bassa P, Kim EE, Inoue T, et al. Evaluation of preoperative chemotherapy using PET with fluorine-18-fluorodeoxyglucose in breast cancer. J Nucl Med 1996;37:931–8.

32. Gennari A, Donati S, Salvadori B, et al. Role of 2-[18F]-fluorodeoxyglucose (FDG) positron emission tomography (PET) in the early assessment of response to chemotherapy in metastatic breast cancer patients. Clin Breast Cancer 2000;1:156–61; discussion 162–3.

33. Kim EE. Whole-body positron emission tomography and positron emission tomography/computed tomography in gynecologic oncology. Int J Gynecol Cancer 2004;14:12–22.

34. Patel PV, Cohade C, Chin BB. PET-CT localizes previously undetectable metastatic lesions in recurrent fallopian tube carcinoma. Gynecol Oncol 2002;87:323–6.

35. Pannu HK, Cohade C, Bristow RE, et al. PET-CT detection of abdominal recurrence of ovarian cancer: radiologic-surgical correlation. Abdom Imaging 2004.

36. Shreve PD, Anzai Y, Wahl RL. Pitfalls in oncologic diagnosis with FDG PET imaging: physiologic and benign variants. Radiographics 1999;19:61–77; quiz 150–1.

37. Fox PT, Perlmutter JS, Raichle ME. A stereotactic method of anatomical localization for positron emission tomography. J Comput Assist Tomogr 1985;9:141–53.

38. Pelizzari CA, Chen GT, Spelbring DR, et al. Accurate three-dimensional registration of CT, PET, and/or MR images of the brain. J Comput Assist Tomogr 1989;13:20–6.

39. Chen GT, Pelizzari CA. Image correlation techniques in radiation therapy treatment planning. Comput Med Imaging Graph 1989;13:235–40.

40. Studholme C, Hill DL, Hawkes DJ. Automated 3-D registration of MR and CT images of the head. Med Image Anal 1996;1:163–75.

41. Maes F, Collignon A, Vandermeulen D, et al. Multimodality image registration by maximization of mutual information. IEEE Trans Med Imaging 1997;16:187–98.

42. Studholme C, Hill DL, Hawkes DJ. Automated three-dimensional registration of magnetic resonance and positron emission tomography brain images by multiresolution optimization of voxel similarity measures. Med Phys 1997;24:25–35.

43. Woods RP, Grafton ST, Holmes CJ, et al. Automated image registration: I. General methods and intrasubject, intramodality validation. J Comput Assist Tomogr 1998;22:139–52.

44. Woods RP, Grafton ST, Watson JD, et al. Automated image registration: II. Intersubject validation of linear and nonlinear models. J Comput Assist Tomogr 1998;22:153–65.

45. Meyer CR, Boes JL, Kim B, et al. Demonstration of accuracy and clinical versatility of mutual information for automatic multimodality image fusion using affine and thin-plate spline warped geometric deformations. Med Image Anal 1997;1:195–206.

46. Mattes D, Haynor DR, Vesselle H, et al. PET-CT image registration in the chest using free-form deformations. IEEE Trans Med Imaging 2003;22:120–8.

47. Slomka PJ, Dey D, Przetak C, et al. Automated 3-dimensional registration of stand-alone (18)F-FDG whole-body PET with CT. J Nucl Med 2003;44:1156–67.

48. Wahl RL, Quint LE, Cieslak RD, et al. "Anatometabolic" tumor imaging: fusion of FDG PET with CT or MRI to localize foci of increased activity. J Nucl Med 1993;34:1190–7.

49. Wong WL, Hussain K, Chevretton E, et al. Validation and clinical application of computer-combined computed tomography and positron emission tomography with 2-[18F]fluoro-2-deoxy-D-glucose head and neck images. Am J Surg 1996;172:628–32.

50. Vansteenkiste JF, Stroobants SG, Dupont PJ, et al. FDG-PET scan in potentially operable non-small cell lung cancer: do anatometabolic PET-CT fusion images improve the localisation of regional lymph node metastases? The Leuven Lung Cancer Group. Eur J Nucl Med 1998;25:1495–501.

51. Magnani P, Carretta A, Rizzo G, et al. FDG/PET and spiral CT image fusion for mediastinal lymph node assessment of non-small cell lung cancer patients. J Cardiovasc Surg 1999;40:741–8.

52. Aquino SL, Asmuth JC, Alpert NM, et al. Improved radiologic staging of lung cancer with 2-[18F]-fluoro-2-deoxy-D-glucose-positron emission tomography and computed tomography registration. J Comput Assist Tomogr 2003;27:479–84.

53. Beyer T, Townsend DW, Brun T, et al. A combined PET/CT scanner for clinical oncology. J Nucl Med 2000;41:1369–79.

54. Makhija S, Howden N, Edwards R, et al. Positron emission tomography/computed tomography imaging for the detection of recurrent ovarian and fallopian tube carcinoma: a retrospective review. Gynecol Oncol 2002;85:53–8.

55. Ostertag H, Kubler WK, Doll J, et al. Measured attenuation correction methods. Eur J Nucl Med 1989;15:722–6.

56. Kinahan PE, Townsend DW, Beyer T, et al. Attenuation correction for a combined 3D PET/CT scanner. Med Phys 1998;25:2046–53.

57. Burger C, Goerres G, Schoenes S, et al. PET attenuation coefficients from CT images: experimental evaluation of the transformation of CT into PET 511-keV attenuation coefficients. Eur J Nucl Med Mol Imaging 2002;29:922–7.

58. Chin BB, Patel PV, Nakamoto Y, et al. Quantitative evaluation of 2-deoxy-2-[18F] fluoro-D-glucose uptake in hepatic metastases with combined PET-CT: iterative reconstruction with CT attenuation correction versus filtered back projection with [68]germanium attenuation correction. Mol Imaging Biol 2002;4:399–409.

59. Nakamoto Y, Osman M, Cohade C, et al. PET/CT: comparison of quantitative tracer uptake between germanium and CT transmission attenuation-corrected images. J Nucl Med 2002;43:1137–43.

60. Charron M, Beyer T, Bohnen NN, et al. Image analysis in patients with cancer studied with a combined PET and CT scanner. Clin Nucl Med 2000;25:905–10.

61. Kluetz P, Villemagne VV, Meltzer C, et al. 20. The case for PET/CT. Experience at the University of Pittsburgh. Clin Positron Imaging 2000;3:174.

62. Kluetz PG, Meltzer CC, Villemagne VL, et al. Combined PET/CT imaging in oncology. Impact on patient management. Clin Positron Imaging 2000;3:223–30.

63. Townsend DW, Beyer T, Blodgett TM. PET/CT scanners: a hardware approach to image fusion. Semin Nucl Med 2003;33:193–204.

64. Antoch G, Stattaus J, Nemat AT, et al. Non-small cell lung cancer: dual-modality PET/CT in preoperative staging. Radiology 2003;229:526–33.

65. Schoder H, Yeung HW, Gonen M, et al. Head and neck cancer: clinical usefulness and accuracy of PET/CT image fusion. Radiology 2004;231:65–72.

66. Cohade C, Osman M, Leal J, et al. Direct comparison of (18)F-FDG PET and PET/CT in patients with colorectal carcinoma. J Nucl Med 2003;44:1797–803.

67. Goerres GW, von Schulthess GK, Steinert HC. Why most PET of lung and head-and-neck cancer will be PET/CT. J Nucl Med 2004;45 Suppl 1:66S–71S.

68. Wahl RL. Why nearly all PET of abdominal and pelvic cancers will be performed as PET/CT. J Nucl Med 2004;45 Suppl

1:82S–95S.

69. Goerres GW, Hany TF, Kamel E, et al. Head and neck imaging with PET and PET/CT: artefacts from dental metallic implants. Eur J Nucl Med Mol Imaging 2002;29:367–70.

70. Bujenovic S, Mannting F, Chakrabarti R, et al. Artifactual 2-deoxy-2-[(18)F]fluoro-D-glucose localization surrounding metallic objects in a PET/CT scanner using CT-based attenuation correction. Mol Imaging Biol 2003;5:20–2.

71. Goerres GW, Ziegler SI, Burger C, et al. Artifacts at PET and PET/CT caused by metallic hip prosthetic material. Radiology 2003;226:577–84.

72. Halpern BS, Dahlbom M, Waldherr C, et al. Cardiac pacemakers and central venous lines can induce focal artifacts on CT-corrected PET images. J Nucl Med 2004;45:290–3.

73. Antoch G, Freudenberg LS, Stattaus J, et al. Whole-body positron emission tomography-CT: optimized CT using oral and IV contrast materials. AJR Am J Roentgenol 2002;179:1555–60.

74. Antoch G, Freudenberg LS, Egelhof T, et al. Focal tracer uptake: a potential artifact in contrast-enhanced dual-modality PET/CT scans. J Nucl Med 2002;43:1339–42.

75. Antoch G, Jentzen W, Freudenberg LS, et al. Effect of oral contrast agents on computed tomography-based positron emission tomography attenuation correction in dual-modality positron emission tomography/computed tomography imaging. Invest Radiol 2003;38:784–9.

76. Cohade C, Osman M, Nakamoto Y, et al. Initial experience with oral contrast in PET/CT: phantom and clinical studies. J Nucl Med 2003;44:412–6.

77. Nakamoto Y, Chin BB, Kraitchman DL, et al. Effects of nonionic intravenous contrast agents at PET/CT imaging: phantom and canine studies. Radiology 2003;227:817–24.

78. Dizendorf EV, Treyer V, Von Schulthess GK, et al. Application of oral contrast media in coregistered positron emission tomography-CT. AJR Am J Roentgenol 2002;179:477–81.

79. Antoch G, Freudenberg LS, Beyer T, et al. To enhance or not to enhance? 18F-FDG and CT contrast agents in dual-modality 18F-FDG PET/CT. J Nucl Med 2004;45 Suppl 1:56S–65S.

80. Antoch G, Kuehl H, Kanja J, et al. Dual-modality PET/CT scanning with negative oral contrast agent to avoid artifacts: introduction and evaluation. Radiology 2004;230:879–85.

81. Nehmeh SA, Erdi YE, Kalaigian H, et al. Correction for oral contrast artifacts in CT attenuation-corrected PET images obtained by combined PET/CT. J Nucl Med 2003;44:1940–4.

82. Townsend DW, Carney JP, Yap JT, et al. PET/CT today and tomorrow. J Nucl Med 2004;45 Suppl 1:4S–14S.

83. Goerres GW, Kamel E, Heidelberg TN, et al. PET-CT image co-registration in the thorax: influence of respiration. Eur J Nucl Med Mol Imaging 2002;29:351–60.

84. Cohade C, Osman M, Marshall LN, et al. PET-CT: accuracy of PET and CT spatial registration of lung lesions. Eur J Nucl Med Mol Imaging 2003;30:721–6.

85. Nakamoto Y, Tatsumi M, Cohade C, et al. Accuracy of image fusion of normal upper abdominal organs visualized with PET/CT. Eur J Nucl Med Mol Imaging 2003;30:597–602.

86. Osman MM, Cohade C, Nakamoto Y, et al. Clinically significant inaccurate localization of lesions with PET/CT: frequency in 300 patients. J Nucl Med 2003;44:240–3.

87. Goerres GW, Kamel E, Seifert B, et al. Accuracy of image coregistration of pulmonary lesions in patients with non-small cell lung cancer using an integrated PET/CT system. J Nucl Med 2002;43:1469–75.

88. De Juan R, Seifert B, Berthold T, et al. Clinical evaluation of a breathing protocol for PET/CT. Eur Radiol 2004;14(6):1118-23.

89. Nehmeh SA, Erdi YE, Ling CC, et al. Effect of respiratory gating on quantifying PET images of lung cancer. J Nucl Med 2002;43:876–81.

90. Wagman R, Yorke E, Ford E, et al. Respiratory gating for liver tumors: use in dose escalation. Int J Radiat Oncol Biol Phys 2003;55:659–68.

91. Boucher L, Rodrigue S, Lecomte R, et al. Respiratory gating for 3-dimensional PET of the thorax: feasibility and initial results. J Nucl Med 2004;45:214–9.

92. Bidgood WD Jr, Horii SC. Modular extension of the ACR-NEMA DICOM standard to support new diagnostic imaging modalities and services. J Digit Imaging 1996;9:67–77.

93. Neumann M. DICOM—current status and future developments for radiotherapy. Z Med Phys 2002;12:171–6.

94. Ling CC, Humm J, Larson S, et al. Towards multidimensional radiotherapy (MD-CRT): biological imaging and biological conformality. Int J Radiat Oncol Biol Phys 2000;47:551–60.

95. Mac Manus MP, Hicks RJ, Ball DL, et al. F-18 fluorodeoxyglucose positron emission tomography staging in radical radiotherapy candidates with nonsmall cell lung carcinoma: powerful correlation with survival and high impact on treatment. Cancer 2001;92:886–95.

96. Vanuytsel LJ, Vansteenkiste JF, Stroobants SG, et al. The impact of (18)F-fluoro-2-deoxy-D-glucose positron emission tomography (FDG-PET) lymph node staging on the radiation treatment volumes in patients with non-small cell lung cancer. Radiother Oncol 2000;55:317–24.

97. Bradley JD, Perez CA, Dehdashti F, et al. Implementing biologic target volumes in radiation treatment planning for non-small cell lung cancer. J Nucl Med 2004;45 Suppl 1:96S–101S.

98. Erdi YE, Rosenzweig K, Erdi AK, et al. Radiotherapy treatment planning for patients with non-small cell lung cancer using positron emission tomography (PET). Radiother Oncol 2002;62:51–60.

99. Schmidt S, Nestle U, Walter K, et al. [Optimization of radiotherapy planning for non-small cell lung cancer (NSCLC) using 18FDG-PET]. Nuklearmedizin 2002;41:217–20.

100. Schmucking M, Baum RP, Griesinger F, et al. Molecular whole-body cancer staging using positron emission tomography: consequences for therapeutic management and metabolic radiation treatment planning. Recent Results Cancer Res 2003;162:195–202.

101. Ciernik IF, Dizendorf E, Baumert BG, et al. Radiation treatment planning with an integrated positron emission and computer tomography (PET/CT): a feasibility study. Int J Radiat Oncol Biol Phys 2003;57:853–63.

102. Esthappan J, Mutic S, Malyapa RS, et al. Treatment planning guidelines regarding the use of CT/PET-guided IMRT for cervical carcinoma with positive paraaortic lymph nodes. Int J Radiat Oncol Biol Phys 2004;58:1289–97.

103. Alber M, Paulsen F, Eschmann SM, et al. On biologically conformal boost dose optimization. Phys Med Biol 2003;48:N31–5.

104. Brahme A. Biologically optimized 3-dimensional in vivo

predictive assay-based radiation therapy using positron emission tomography-computerized tomography imaging. Acta Oncol 2003;42:123–36.

105. Patronas NJ, Di Chiro G, Brooks RA, et al. Work in progress: [18F] fluorodeoxyglucose and positron emission tomography in the evaluation of radiation necrosis of the brain. Radiology 1982;144:885–9.

106. Mogard J, Kihlstrom L, Ericson K, et al. Recurrent tumor vs radiation effects after gamma knife radiosurgery of intracerebral metastases: diagnosis with PET-FDG. J Comput Assist Tomogr 1994;18:177–81.

107. Greven KM, Williams DW III, Keyes JW Jr, et al. Can positron emission tomography distinguish tumor recurrence from irradiation sequelae in patients treated for larynx cancer? Cancer J Sci Am 1997;3:353–7.

108. Daemen BJ, Elsinga PH, Paans AM, et al. Radiation-induced inhibition of tumor growth as monitored by PET using L-[1-11C]tyrosine and fluorine-18-fluorodeoxyglucose. J Nucl Med 1992;33:373–9.

109. Chaiken L, Rege S, Hoh C, et al. Positron emission tomography with fluorodeoxyglucose to evaluate tumor response and control after radiation therapy. Int J Radiat Oncol Biol Phys 1993;27:455–64.

110. Mac Manus MP, Hicks RJ, Matthews JP, et al. Positron emission tomography is superior to computed tomography scanning for response-assessment after radical radiotherapy or chemoradiotherapy in patients with non-small-cell lung cancer. J Clin Oncol 2003;21:1285–92.

111. Sakamoto H, Nakai Y, Ohashi Y, et al. Monitoring of response to radiotherapy with fluorine-18 deoxyglucose PET of head and neck squamous cell carcinomas. Acta Otolaryngol Suppl (Stockh) 1998;538:254–60.

112. Oku S, Nakagawa K, Momose T, et al. FDG-PET after radiotherapy is a good prognostic indicator of rectal cancer. Ann Nucl Med 2002;16:409–16.

113. Higashi K, Clavo AC, Wahl RL. In vitro assessment of 2-fluoro-2-deoxy-D-glucose, L-methionine and thymidine as agents to monitor the early response of a human adenocarcinoma cell line to radiotherapy. J Nucl Med 1993;34:773–9.

114. Rozental JM, Levine RL, Mehta MP, et al. Early changes in tumor metabolism after treatment: the effects of stereotactic radiotherapy. Int J Radiat Oncol Biol Phys 1991;20:1053–60.

115. Spence AM, Muzi M, Graham MM, et al. 2-[(18)F]Fluoro-2-deoxyglucose and glucose uptake in malignant gliomas before and after radiotherapy: correlation with outcome. Clin Cancer Res 2002;8:971–9.

116. Varagnolo L, Stokkel MP, Mazzi U, et al. 18F-labeled radiopharmaceuticals for PET in oncology, excluding FDG. Nucl Med Biol 2000;27:103–12.

117. Gambhir SS. Molecular imaging of cancer with positron emission tomography. Nat Rev Cancer 2002;2:683–93.

118. Kubota K, Ishiwata K, Kubota R, et al. Tracer feasibility for monitoring tumor radiotherapy: a quadruple tracer study with fluorine-18-fluorodeoxyglucose or fluorine-18-fluorodeoxyuridine, L-[methyl-14C]methionine, [6-3H]thymidine, and gallium-67. J Nucl Med 1991;32:2118–23.

119. Chung JK, Kim YK, Kim SK, et al. Usefulness of 11C-methionine PET in the evaluation of brain lesions that are hypo- or isometabolic on 18F-FDG PET. Eur J Nucl Med Mol Imaging 2002;29:176–82.

120. Sato N, Suzuki M, Kuwata N, et al. Evaluation of the malignancy of glioma using 11C-methionine positron emission tomography and proliferating cell nuclear antigen staining. Neurosurg Rev 1999;22:210–4.

121. Nuutinen J, Sonninen P, Lehikoinen P, et al. Radiotherapy treatment planning and long-term follow-up with [(11)C]methionine PET in patients with low-grade astrocytoma. Int J Radiat Oncol Biol Phys 2000;48:43–52.

122. Mortimer JE, Dehdashti F, Siegel BA, et al. Positron emission tomography with 2-[18F]fluoro-2-deoxy-D-glucose and 16alpha-[18F]fluoro-17beta-estradiol in breast cancer: correlation with estrogen receptor status and response to systemic therapy. Clin Cancer Res 1996;2:933–9.

123. Dehdashti F, Flanagan FL, Mortimer JE, et al. Positron emission tomographic assessment of "metabolic flare" to predict response of metastatic breast cancer to antiestrogen therapy. Eur J Nucl Med 1999;26:51–6.

124. Bonasera TA, O'Neil JP, Xu M, et al. Preclinical evaluation of fluorine-18-labeled androgen receptor ligands in baboons. J Nucl Med 1996;37:1009–15.

125. Larson SM, Morris M, Gunther I, et al. Tumor localization of 16beta-(18)F-fluoro-5alpha-dihydrotestosterone versus (18)F-FDG in patients with progressive, metastatic prostate cancer. J Nucl Med 2004;45:366–73.

126. Chapman JD, Engelhardt EL, Stobbe CC, et al. Measuring hypoxia and predicting tumor radioresistance with nuclear medicine assays. Radiother Oncol 1998;46:229–37.

127. Rasey JS, Koh WJ, Grierson JR, et al. Radiolabelled fluoromisonidazole as an imaging agent for tumor hypoxia. Int J Radiat Oncol Biol Phys 1989;17:985–91.

128. Martin GV, Cerqueira MD, Caldwell JH, et al. Fluoromisonidazole. A metabolic marker of myocyte hypoxia. Circ Res 1990;67:240–4.

129. Valk PE, Mathis CA, Prados MD, et al. Hypoxia in human gliomas: demonstration by PET with fluorine-18-fluoromisonidazole. J Nucl Med 1992;33:2133–7.

130. Rasey JS, Koh WJ, Evans ML, et al. Quantifying regional hypoxia in human tumors with positron emission tomography of [18F]fluoromisonidazole: a pretherapy study of 37 patients. Int J Radiat Oncol Biol Phys 1996;36:417–28.

131. Yeh SH, Liu RS, Wu LC, et al. Fluorine-18 fluoromisonidazole tumour to muscle retention ratio for the detection of hypoxia in nasopharyngeal carcinoma. Eur J Nucl Med 1996;23:1378–83.

132. Lewis JS, McCarthy DW, McCarthy TJ, et al. Evaluation of 64Cu-ATSM in vitro and in vivo in a hypoxic tumor model. J Nucl Med 1999;40:177–83.

133. Lewis JS, Sharp TL, Laforest R, et al. Tumor uptake of copper-diacetyl-bis(N(4)-methylthiosemicarbazone): effect of changes in tissue oxygenation. J Nucl Med 2001;42:655–61.

134. Chao KS, Bosch WR, Mutic S, et al. A novel approach to overcome hypoxic tumor resistance: Cu-ATSM-guided intensity-modulated radiation therapy. Int J Radiat Oncol Biol Phys 2001;49:1171–82.

135. Dehdashti F, Grigsby PW, Mintun MA, et al. Assessing tumor hypoxia in cervical cancer by positron emission tomography with 60Cu-ATSM: relationship to therapeutic response—a preliminary report. Int J Radiat Oncol Biol Phys 2003;55:1233–8.

136. Dehdashti F, Mintun MA, Lewis JS, et al. In vivo assessment of tumor hypoxia in lung cancer with 60Cu-ATSM. Eur J Nucl Med Mol Imaging 2003;30:844–50.

137. Shields AF, Lim K, Grierson J, et al. Utilization of labeled thymidine in DNA synthesis: studies for PET. J Nucl Med 1990;31:337–42.

138. Mankoff DA, Shields AF, Link JM, et al. Kinetic analysis of 2-[11C]thymidine PET imaging studies: validation studies. J Nucl Med 1999;40:614–24.

139. Shields AF, Grierson JR, Dohmen BM, et al. Imaging proliferation in vivo with [F-18]FLT and positron emission tomography. Nat Med 1998;4:1334–6.

140. Buck AK, Schirrmeister H, Hetzel M, et al. 3-Deoxy-3-[(18)F]fluorothymidine-positron emission tomography for noninvasive assessment of proliferation in pulmonary nodules. Cancer Res 2002;62:3331–4.

141. Buck AK, Halter G, Schirrmeister H, et al. Imaging proliferation in lung tumors with PET: 18F-FLT versus 18F-FDG. J Nucl Med 2003;44:1426–31.

142. Reinhardt MJ, Kubota K, Yamada S, et al. Assessment of cancer recurrence in residual tumors after fractionated radiotherapy: a comparison of fluorodeoxyglucose, L-methionine and thymidine. J Nucl Med 1997;38:280–7.

143. Hutchinson OC, Collingridge DR, Barthel H, et al. Pharmacokinetics of radiolabelled anticancer drugs for positron emission tomography. Curr Pharm Des 2003;9:917–29.

144. Hammond LA, Denis L, Salman U, et al. Positron emission tomography (PET): expanding the horizons of oncology drug development. Invest New Drugs 2003;21:309–40.

145. Ginos JZ, Cooper AJ, Dhawan V, et al. [13N]Cisplatin PET to assess pharmacokinetics of intra-arterial versus intravenous chemotherapy for malignant brain tumors. J Nucl Med 1987;28:1844–52.

146. Harte RJ, Matthews JC, O'Reilly SM, et al. Tumor, normal tissue, and plasma pharmacokinetic studies of fluorouracil biomodulation with N-phosphonacetyl-L-aspartate, folinic acid, and interferon alpha. J Clin Oncol 1999;17:1580–8.

147. Saleem A, Yap J, Osman S, et al. Modulation of fluorouracil tissue pharmacokinetics by eniluracil: in-vivo imaging of drug action. Lancet 2000;355:2125–31.

148. Inoue T, Kim EE, Wallace S, et al. Positron emission tomography using [18F]fluorotamoxifen to evaluate therapeutic responses in patients with breast cancer: preliminary study. Cancer Biother Radiopharm 1996;11:235–45.

149. Kurdziel KA, Kiesewetter DO, Carson RE, et al. Biodistribution, radiation dose estimates, and in vivo Pgp modulation studies of 18F-paclitaxel in nonhuman primates. J Nucl Med 2003;44:1330–9.

150. Anderson H, Yap JT, Wells P, et al. Measurement of renal tumour and normal tissue perfusion using positron emission tomography in a phase II clinical trial of razoxane. Br J Cancer 2003;89:262–7.

151. Anderson HL, Yap JT, Miller MP, et al. Assessment of pharmacodynamic vascular response in a phase I trial of combretastatin A4 phosphate. J Clin Oncol 2003;21:2823–30.

Chapter 9

RESPIRATORY MOTION MANAGEMENT

JOHN WONG, PhD, GEOFFREY HUGO, PhD, GIKAS S. MAGERAS, PhD, ELLEN YORKE, PhD

Intensity-modulated radiation therapy (IMRT) has greatly enhanced the ability to deliver highly conformal dose distributions with rapid dose falloff. The steep dose gradient of IMRT invites the use of tight margins for dose escalation but also increases the risk of geometric misses and normal tissue injury. IMRT with reduced margins has been achieved in the treatment of tumors in the brain, head and neck, and lower abdominal regions, albeit sometimes with invasive immobilization techniques.[1] Alternatively, when intrafraction organ motions are not significant, online image guidance methods can be used to localize the target volume prior to treatment, thus allowing margin reduction.[2–5] Likewise, off-line adaptive strategies can be effective in reducing the planning target volume (PTV) when interfraction treatment variation during the course of treatment can be modeled.[6,7]

Intrafraction organ motion associated with respiration in the thorax and upper abdomen presents a different and difficult problem for radiation therapy (RT) in general and IMRT in particular. Near the diaphragm, it is not uncommon to observe respiratory motion with amplitudes exceeding 2 cm. The conventional approach is to examine under fluoroscopy the range of target motion owing to breathing such that an adequate margin can be prescribed. For more complex noncoplanar beam arrangements, the PTV needs to account for nonuniform breathing motion in three dimensions.

With IMRT, the problem is further compounded by the interplay of respiratory motion with the delivery of many small beam segments. Given that a normal breathing cycle has a period of ~ 4 seconds, organs near the diaphragm can be moving at a speed of approximately 1 cm/s, which may significantly interfere with the dosimetry of IMRT.[8] The reader can refer to standard physiology textbooks[9,10] to review the basic mechanics and control of breathing that will aid in understanding the challenges of respiratory motion in IMRT. The impact of respiratory motion on IMRT dosimetry is currently under investigation by several groups (see Chapter 19.4, "Intrafractional Organ Motion and Planning: Emerging Technology").[11–16]

IMRT and Respiratory Motion

The predominant method of IMRT currently involves the use of a multileaf collimator (MLC). In the segmental multileaf collimator (sMLC) or step-and-shoot method, the duration, that is, monitor units (MUs), of the treatment is preset and turned on only for the individual static MLC segment. In the dynamic multileaf collimator (dMLC) mode, the radiation beam is on continuously at a nominal rate while each individual leaf moves at the appropriate speed to the next prescribed position to achieve modulation. At the present time, all major medical accelerator manufacturers in the Unites States offer sMLC for IMRT, whereas only one manufacturer (Varian Medical Systems, Palo Alto, CA) also allows dMLC (see Chapter 12, "Delivery Systems"). Both methods of delivery are viable. The choice is usually a compromise of issues pertaining to treatment efficiency and quality assurance (QA).[17]

For a tumor that moves with respiration, its cyclical motion can be out of synchrony with the mechanical motion of the MLC, resulting in significant variation of the intended dose delivered with IMRT.[8,14] Two methods are presently under clinical investigation to reduce the effects of breathing motion on IMRT dosimetry. In the respiratory gating approach, an external surrogate is sent to turn the radiation on only at a specific phase and/or window of the normal breathing cycle.[13,18,19] In the breath-hold model, the patient breathing motion is explicitly suspended or immobilized temporarily, during which the beam is turned on.[20–23] Thus, in the gating method, the machine status adapts to the patient motion, whereas with breath-hold, the patient motion is controlled. A third method involves continuously tracking the tumor motion during breathing with dMLC segments,[24,25] appropriately coordinating the required MUs and motion of the IMRT segments.[26,27] The approach is an attempt primarily to improve on the efficiency of both the gating and breath-hold methods. It is, however, in the research phase and is not discussed in this chapter.

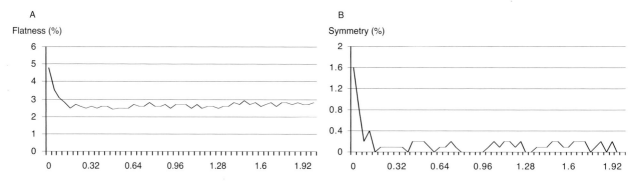

FIGURE 9-1. Characteristics of the cross-beam profile of an Elekta Precise machine in the AB cross-plane direction after beam-on (in seconds): (*A*) flatness; (*B*) symmetry.

Radiation treatment with voluntary or assisted breath-hold is typically applied at full or moderate deep inspiration.[20,22,28–31] The duration of breath-hold—thus, beam-on time—and the ensuing rest period are patient dependent. The effective duty cycle, defined as the ratio of the total beam-on time to the time for completion of delivery at one gantry angle, is approximately 25 to 30% based on the unpublished experience at William Beaumont Hospital. The longer the breath-hold period, the more efficient is the treatment. Free-breathing gating, on the other hand, is typically applied at the end of exhalation during its prolonged quiescence,[21,32] in which a gate window of 1 mm also attains a typical duty cycle of 25 to 30%.[33] A larger gate window would include the significant motion associated with the steeper phase of the breathing cycle.

There are two aspects of IMRT delivery in the presence of respiratory motion. One pertains to the performance of the linear accelerator and the MLC in delivering the correct segment dose; the other pertains to the accuracy and reproducibility of the physiologic signal driving IMRT delivery. Although the two are not entirely independent, it is useful to consider them separately.

IMRT Dosimetry Using Breath-hold and Radiation-Gated Delivery

Both breath-hold and gating methods involve many repeats of beam-on and -off time, stressing the requirement of good beam quality for short exposures. The beam needs to attain the necessary dose rate, flatness, and symmetry within a short time after the beam is on. Reassuringly, all modern accelerators provide adequate on and off beam stability. As an example, Figure 9-1 illustrates the flatness and symmetry of the in-air profile of a 20 × 20 cm in the AB cross-plane direction (defined as across the couch in its straight-on position) as a function of time after beam-on from an Elekta Precise linear accelerator (Elekta Oncology, Crawley, UK) measured with a linear array of diodes at 5 mm spacing. The beam achieves its specification of ± 3% variation in

flatness and symmetry in approximately 160 milliseconds, or 1 MU for a dose rate of 400 MU/min.

Cross-beam profiles in the AB and gun-target (defined as parallel to the couch) directions at 5 cm depth in a solid water phantom were also measured for a 10 × 10 cm field. Doses of 50, 100, and 200 cGy were delivered to the central axis with a conventional beam and two that were repeatedly interrupted to simulate a breath-hold treatment. One simulated breath-hold treatment consisted of a sequence of 7 seconds of beam-on time followed by 20 seconds of beam hold and one with 15 seconds of beam-on time and 15 seconds of beam hold. The beam-hold signal was sent via an external fiberoptic connection to interrupt the pulse repetition frequency control, as in a gated treatment. Figure 9-2 shows the beam profiles at 5 cm depth from a simulated breath-hold delivery and from a conventional beam delivery. The results for the three beam delivery schemes were similar at each of the dose levels. The maximum point-to-point deviations of the beam profiles within 80% of the

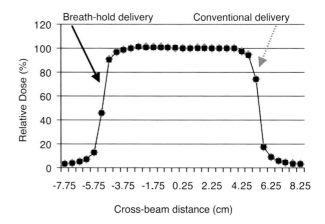

FIGURE 9-2. Sample cross-beam profiles at 5 cm depth in solid water of a breath-hold delivery with a 7-second beam-on and a 20-second beam-off sequence (*black*) and with conventional delivery (*red*) in the AB cross-plane direction. The results for 50, 100, and 200 cGy deliveries were similar.

field dimension were less than 0.6% of the central axis dose and mostly within 0.3%. The maximum deviations of central axis dose of the breath-hold deliveries were within 0.1% of the conventional delivery and mostly within 0.05%.

Varian linear accelerators (Varian Medical Systems) also produce highly desireable beam-on characterisitics. The flatness and symmetry of a 9.8 × 9.8 cm field were measured on a Novalis accelerator (BrainLab, Heimstetten, Germany) as a function of gating frequency. The comparisons of gated and nongated delivery showed no significant variation in either flatness or symmetry. Point doses were measured with an ion chamber for the gated delivery of a highly modulated sMLC field as a function of gating frequency, dose rate, and MUs delivered. The average dose difference between gated and nongated delivery was 2% of the maximum dose per field. Higher dose rates were not associated with greater delivery error than lower dose rates. In fact, the highest error was measured at the lowest dose rate and the highest gating frequency.[33] The delivery error correlated closely with the total number of gating cycles. Each delivery was very reproducible, with the average standard deviation being 0.6% of the average delivery error.

These results suggest that the repeat beam-on and beam-off sequences have insignificant impact on the dosimetry of IMRT with breath-hold or sMLC methods and a minor impact using the dMLC method. However, with dMLC delivery, an additional complexity involves coordinating the MLC motion with the respiratory gating signal. Because the command to move the MLC follows the external trigger for beam-on time, this lag-and-chase scenario can result in appreciable dosimetric variation, as observed in the delivery of wedge-shaped fields depending on the gate frequency and window.[14] Typically, a smaller gating window provides more accurate delivery.[13] However, a smaller gating window also prolongs overall treatment time. A 1 mm gating window is a reasonable choice because it provides nearly the same accuracy of delivery with a 0.5 mm window but is faster. The same compromise applies to dose rate selection, in which the lower dose rate would reduce the magnitude of motion-induced dose variation but at the expense of protracted treatment times.

It appears that the gated wedge field delivery with dMLC is a model that highlights dosimetric variations. In several planning and phantom studies with clinical nongated IMRT treatment for breast and lung tumors,[11,12,15] the presence of cyclical motion of ± 10 mm resulted in some degradation of the dose coverage. But the measurable variations for a single fraction would average out over a fractionated course of treatment, and the delivered dose was very close to the expected value. The effects of breathing motion are similar for nongated IMRT and conventional delivery. Hugo and colleagues further showed that for clinically relevant doses and MLC tolerance settings, the gated delivery of dMLC and sMLC produces similar levels of dosimetric error.[13]

Respiratory Motion Management

The studies of IMRT dosimetry in the presence of respiratory motion have been performed primarily in idealized phantoms. Simple sinusoidal functions[12,14] or more realistic motion models[33,34] have been used. Additionally, simulations of dosimetric error induced by intrafraction motion have been performed using dose-based[11,35] and fluence-based[36] convolution. Bortfeld and colleagues demonstrated that the random phase of respiratory motion at which dMLC delivery began contributed measurably to the dosimetric error, but they also argued that the error would wash out in a protracted course of treatment.[11] A planning study by Frazier and colleagues, using computed tomography (CT) scans obtained at end-inspiration and end-exhalation, demonstrated that breathing motion had minimal impact on the dosimetry of whole-breast IMRT in which the modulation was modest and much of the treatment was delivered with an open field.[16]

As discussed previously, the two principal methods to manage respiratory motion are by means of gating treatment or immobilization with breath-hold. There are pros and cons with both approaches.

Method of Gating

Radiation treatment is gated in response to a signal representative of the patient's respiration. This technique allows the patient to breathe freely and is considered more suitable for patients with compromised pulmonary status, such as those with lung cancers, who cannot sustain prolonged breath-hold. The basic components of a gating system consist of a respiration sensor whose signal is processed and evaluated by a computer for suitability to trigger, or gate, the radiation beam. The earliest experience using respiratory-gated RT is from Japan.[37,38] In the United States, Kubo and Hill reported the first technical feasibility study with a Varian 2100C accelerator (Varian Medical Systems) in 1996.[39] A variety of respiration sensors were adapted in these early studies, including a strain gauge wrapped around the trunk, a temperature sensor placed near the nose, spirometry,[40] and infrared light-emitting diodes.[38] At present, a Real-time Position Management (RPM) system is commercially available from Varian Medical Systems for automatic respiratory gating and has been employed by several investigators for evaluation and treatment.[41,42]

Respiratory Gating Simulation

The following section focuses primarily on the use of the Varian RPM system for respiratory gating at Memorial Sloan-Kettering Cancer Center (MSKCC). The RPM system is based on the breathing synchronized RT camera-based system,[43] which tracks the motion of a small plastic block with a pair of reflective markers placed on the abdomen or chest of the patient (Figure 9-3). The positions of the bottom cor-

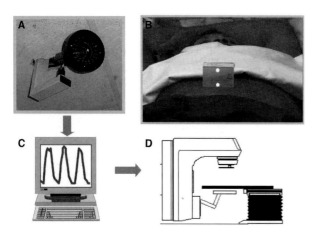

FIGURE 9-3. A pictorial schematic of the functioning of the Varian Real-time Position Management system, consisting of (*A*) a wall-mounted infrared illuminator and charge-coupled device camera; (*B*) a reflective external marker placed on the patient's abdomen or chest; (*C*) a workstation to process signals; and (*D*) a trigger to the accelerator, simulator, or CT scanner. The trigger can be based on the amplitude or phase of the respiratory signal.

ners of the marker block are tattooed on the skin for reproducible repositioning. A charge-coupled device (CCD) camera is used to capture the images of the markers illuminated by infrared light-emitting diodes. The software tracks the position of the markers, where the separation between the top and bottom markers provides a distance calibration. Figure 9-4 is a graphic representation of the marker motion displayed on the workstation. An algorithm in the RPM system monitors the waveform and determines if it is regular. It also determines the phase of the respiratory cycle, assigning phase = 0 to the waveform maximum.

In a combined immobilization and training session at a conventional simulator outfitted with the RPM system, fluoroscopy is recorded in synchrony with the external marker position. During simulation, the operator adjusts

separately the phase for the start (beam enable) and end (beam disable) of the treatment gate by inspecting the respiration waveform (see Figure 9-4) and/or by viewing the resultant anatomic motion during the gate interval with imaging. When the RPM system is used with "normal" breathing (versus breath-hold), regular and reproducible breathing is important for efficient, accurate, respiratory-gated simulation and treatment. The RPM software does not issue a beam-enable or CT trigger signal when breathing is irregular, which thus compromises the efficiency of the respiratory gating procedures. Worse, as shown in Figure 9-5, an irregular breathing pattern can potentially result in image acquisition and/or beam delivery at the wrong phase of the breathing cycle. To reduce breathing irregularity, it is advisable to set the gating thresholds around end-exhalation, that is, at functional residual capacity, for more stable lung volume and slower breathing motion. The longer quiescent period also provides a longer duty cycle. In addition, simple verbal coaching instructions ("breathe in…breathe out") have been shown to improve regularity.[41] Figure 9-6 illustrates that with verbal instructions, the patient can be coached to breathe with a higher and less variable tidal volume.

It is important to note that, at present, clinical implementation of respiratory-gated treatment delivery using the RPM system requires considerable care and patient-specific QA. With any surrogate respiratory signal, it is assumed that there is a one-to-one correspondence between the signal (the motion of the markers on the patient's chest) and the patient's internal anatomy (tumor and critical normal tissues). Figure 9-7A shows the comparison of the trace of diaphragm position measured from the recorded fluoroscopic images with that of the RPM marker. There is an apparent lag of 0.7 seconds between them.

Figure 9-7, B and C, shows the scatterplot of the positions of the diaphragm versus those of the markers before correction for a 0.7-second lag time and after correction,

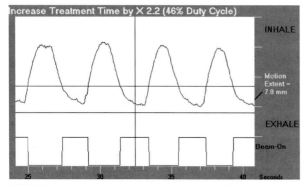

FIGURE 9-4. Example respiration trace from the Varian Real-time Position Management monitor screen for a patient treated at end-expiration. The horizontal lines specify the portion of the respiration trace within which the beam is enabled. The square-wave in the display indicates beam-enable status.

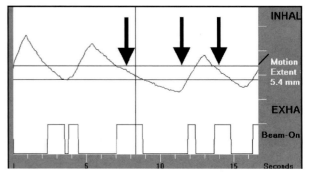

FIGURE 9-5. Irregular breathing can result in treatment or image acquisition at the wrong portion of the breathing cycle (*arrows*).

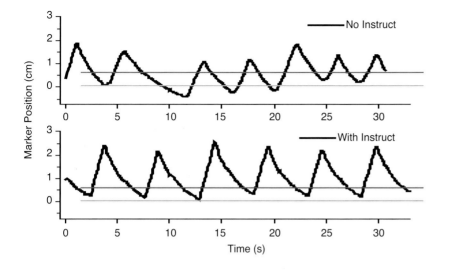

FIGURE 9-6. Comparison of the Varian Real-time Position Management traces for a free-breathing sequence (*top*) and one in which the verbal instruction is given (*bottom*). Verbal instruction improves the regularity of the breathing sequence. Reproduced with permission from Mageras GS et al.[41]

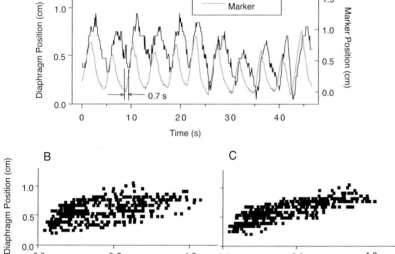

FIGURE 9-7. (*A*) Comparison of diaphragm positions measured from fluoroscopy with that of the Varian Real-time Position Management (RPM) marker, showing a lag time of 0.7 seconds. Scatterplot of the diaphragm positions versus those of the RPM marker before correction for a 0.7-second lag time (*B*) and after correction (*C*). Reproduced with permission from Mageras GS et al.[41]

respectively. The dispersion of the points is reduced after correction. These results indicate that for some patients, anatomic motion (not just the diaphragm) can be out of phase with the RPM marker trace. Given the involvement of both the diaphragm and the chest wall in ventilation, these observations are not surprising because the RPM marker block is placed in only one position on the trunk.

Three- and Four-Dimensional CT Studies

The results of Figure 9-7 indicate that with respiratory gating, it is important to examine the relationship of the surrogate respiratory signal with the patient's internal anatomy. It follows that three-dimensional CT scans are needed at the respiratory phase intended for treatment, not only for dose calculation purposes but also as repeat studies for proper design of treatment margin.

Respiratory-Triggered CT

The initial method of respiratory-triggered computed tomography (RTCT) was developed with the standard single-slice helical CT scanner in mind. The methodology is demonstrated in Figure 9-8. The RPM system is mounted to move with the CT couch. The CT scanner is triggered by the RPM system. The projection data are acquired in the stepwise axial mode with 1-second gantry rotation. Even with regular breathing, respiration-triggered image acquisition will take longer than with free breathing because only part of the breathing cycle is used. For example, if the breathing period is 5 seconds, acquiring a 60-slice study at the rate of one CT image per breathing cycle (eg, only at end-expiration) on a single-slice scanner requires 5 minutes under ideal conditions of regular breathing compared with 1 to 2 minutes for a free-breathing helical scan.

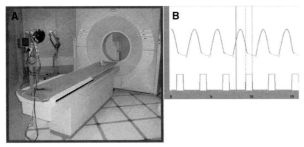

FIGURE 9-8. (*A*) A picture of the Varian Real-time Position Management (RPM) system mounted on a computed tomography (CT) scanner at the Memorial Sloan-Kettering Cancer Center. (*B*) Display of the RPM trace that was used to trigger the 1-second CT scan in the axial mode. Courtesy of G. Mageras.

Figure 9-9, A and B, illustrates the sagittal view of the patient scan acquired in the standard helical mode and one acquired with a respiratory trigger, respectively. Motion artifacts at the diaphragmatic region are clearly visible in the former but much reduced in the RTCT. However, despite vocal coaching, it is not uncommon for some irregular breathing to occur with respiratory-correlated computed tomography (RCCT), causing out-of-phase slices and motion artifacts (Figure 9-9C). At MSKCC, the "bad slices" during RTCT simulation are recorded for deletion if desired and reacquired when regular breathing resumes.

RTCT had been instrumental in demonstrating the potential gain of respiratory-gated treatment. In eight patients, end-exhalation and end-inhalation triggered scans were acquired. Shifts of the centers of the mass of the liver, right and left kidneys, and spleen and gross tumor volume were measured between the ends of the respiratory cycle and between repeat end-exhalation scans. The results are shown in Figure 9-10. On average, the shift in the superior-to-inferior direction between end-exhalation and end-inhalation scans was 12.8 mm (range 3.0–29.2 mm) and 2.0 mm (range 0.0–6.4 mm) between repeat end-exhalation scans. The larger variation observed for the spleen is not unexpected, given that this organ changes size with the cyclical wash-in and wash-out of blood.

The RTCT approach, however, has two significant limitations. First, the CT sessions tend to be long. A study of reproducibility and margin design would require repeating multiple respiration-triggered scans. The long acquisition times increase the likelihood of patient movement and irregular breathing during the CT session. Second, the respiratory phase at which the slice acquisition is triggered must be decided before the scan is performed. The appropriate phase is usually chosen by inspecting the respiration waveform or by examination of anatomic motion under fluoroscopy. There are currently no data about the three-dimensional variation of tumor and organ positions during breathing.

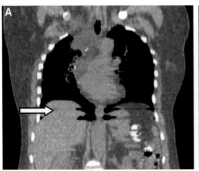
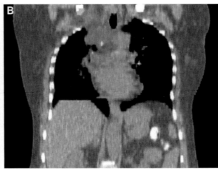
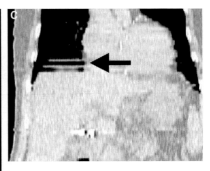

FIGURE 9-9. Sagittal views of (*A*) a helical scan acquired during free breathing with motion artifacts (*arrow*) and (*B*) a respiratory-triggered scan. (*C*) Artifacts (*arrow*) can occur for radiation therapy computed tomography if the patient's breathing is irregular. (To view a color version of this image, please refer to the CD-ROM.)

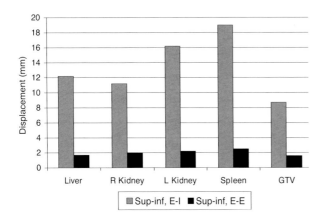

FIGURE 9-10. The displacements of the centers of the mass of different organs measured using respiratory-triggered computed tomography scans acquired at end-exhalation (E) and end-inhalation (I) and repeat end-exhalation scans. GTV = gross tumor volume. Reproduced with permission from Wagman R et al.[46]

Because of the 1-second scan time, there will also be residual motion in each RTCT. A study of repeat CT scans at the same respiratory phase has found a mean variation in diaphragm position of 3 mm, which may affect definition of the PTV.[42] A more efficient method for acquiring CT scans at different phases, that is, four-dimensional CT, is needed to provide important information in defining an appropriate PTV for respiratory-gated treatment.

Respiration-Correlated CT

The method of RCCT[32,43] is an adaptation of the technique used for cardiac imaging,[44] which allows the acquisition of complete three-dimensional image data sets at multiple phases with a single spiral CT scan. The details of the method have been published recently[32,43] and are only briefly described in this chapter.

In the RCCT procedure, there is no triggering of the spiral CT scanner by the RPM system. Instead, the x-ray signal and the corresponding spiral CT projection data are indexed with the respiration waveform from the RPM. The combined information is then used to retrospectively correlate the CT slice with the respiration phase. The principle of operation is illustrated in Figure 9-11. By setting a small pitch, that is, the ratio of table advance to the slice thickness acquired in one rotation, the table is moved slowly such that sufficient data can be acquired for CT image reconstruction over the entire respiratory cycle.

Two quantities are important in acquiring an optimal RCCT data set. They are (1) the gap between slices from successive respiratory cycles, that is, the region in which no CT data are acquired at a particular phase, and (2) the elapsed fraction of the respiratory period to acquire complete CT data for reconstructing one slice. For a 180° reconstruction algorithm and a fan beam CT geometry with the detector bank subtending an angle Φ, the data for one complete slice are acquired with a gantry rotation of $\pi + \Phi$.[32]

For RCCT acquisition using a single-slice CT scanner, such as the Philips/Marconi PQ5000 (Philips Medical Systems, Cleveland, OH), experience at MSKCC indicates that a combination of gantry rotation of 1.5 seconds and a table pitch of 0.5 offers the best compromise for temporal resolution (~ 1 second per slice) and gap width. For a slice thickness of 3 mm, the resultant resolution in couch position (including slice thickness and gap width) is between 4 and 6 mm depending on the respiratory period, comparable to 5 mm slices acquired with RTCT. Depending on the respiratory period, an RCCT will produce CT data at different respiratory phases. Because the respiratory cycle and the gantry rotation are not coordinated, the CT data for some of the reconstructed phases are not unique, meaning that the projection data might be used in adjacent slices. In theory, the number of independent phases per breathing cycle is the ratio of the respiratory period and the time that it takes to acquire a slice. In the example in which the respiratory cycle is 5 seconds, the CT gantry rotation is 1.5 seconds, and only 0.64 of the rotation is needed for a 180° reconstruction algorithm, the number of independent phases is approximately 5.

RCCT is a major advance that has supplanted the method of RTCT to study the effects of breathing motion on RT. RCCT can be used in conjunction with respiratory-gated treatment to identify the patient-specific respiratory phase of minimum tumor motion, determine residual tumor motion within the gate interval, and compare treatment plans at different phases. Equally important, RCCT provides a practical means for repeat CT studies of the patient's breathing motion during the course of treatment, which, at present, is assumed to be unchanged. Already, the quality and efficiency of RCCT have been significantly improved by replacing the single-slice helical scanner with a four-slice scanner (Discover QX/i, GE Healthcare, Waukesha, WI). Figure 9-12 shows the transverse, coronal, and sagittal views of a recent RCCT scan at the same respiratory phase (of 10)

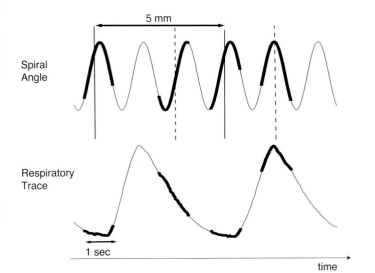

FIGURE 9-11. Schematic of the respiration-correlated computed tomography (CT) technique. The respiratory waveform (lower part of figure; actual patient data) is acquired as the table is advanced in position and the spiral progresses (upper part of the figure shows CT gantry angle vs time). Vertical lines correspond to CT slices at end-expiration (*solid line*), end-inspiration (*dot-dashed line*), and an intermediate respiratory phase (*dashed line*). In this example, the data to reconstruct a slice span an interval of 230° or approximately 1 second (*bold line segments*), and the spacing between the slices at the same respiratory phase is 5 mm. Adapted from Ford EC et al.[32]

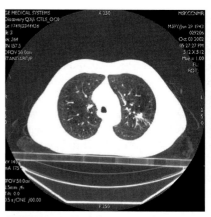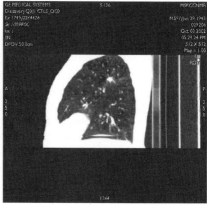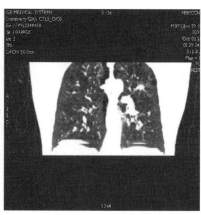

FIGURE 9-12. The (*A*) transverse, (*B*) coronal, and (*C*) sagittal views at the same respiratory phase of a respiratory-correlated computed tomography scan acquired at Memorial Sloan-Kettering Cancer Center using a four-slice scanner. Ten phases were acquired at 0.5 seconds per slice, with 2.5 cm slice spacing. Courtesy of G. Mageras.

acquired at MSKCC using a four-slice scanner. The scan length spanned 30 cm, slice spacing was 2.5 mm, and the scan period was 0.5 seconds. A variation of the method is under investigation in which a large number of CT slices is acquired at each stationary couch position to improve temporal resolution of RCCT.[45] Further improvement can be expected when the newer multislice (6–16) CT scanners find their way into radiation oncology departments.

Respiratory-Gated Treatment

At present, delivery of respiratory-gated treatment is under investigation at a few centers. The assumptions are that (1) there is a one-to-one correspondence between the external respiratory signal and internal anatomy and (2) this relationship is maintained over the entire course of treatment. However, these assumptions need to be validated before dissemination for general use in the community.

At MSKCC, the RPM system has been used for gated static and IMRT treatments of over 30 patients with lung and liver cancer.[46] RPM has been well tolerated by patients and technical staff. Clinical implementation requires considerable care and patient-specific QA. Changes in breathing pattern can occur, possibly owing to changes in the involvement of the diaphragm and chest wall or variation in the functional residual capacity from day to day. To promote breathing regularity, recorded voice instructions, customized for the individual patient, are played during treatments. Well-trained therapists are a vital component of RPM-gated treatments. They must watch the displayed motion trace and turn the beam off if they see significant irregularities or drift and then retrack the marker and/or talk to the patient before resuming the procedure. The length of the gated IMRT delivery is, by necessity, long, as dictated by ~ 30% duty cycle of gating and the compounded increase in MUs to achieve modulation.

At MSKCC, megavoltage portal images have been used for treatment QA and to determine how well the RPM signal represents internal anatomy motion. The diaphragm

is the most visible surrogate for tumor motion and has been shown to correlate well for liver tumors.[23] For some patients with lung cancer, there are also soft tissue features visible within the gross tumor volume. For each patient receiving gated treatment, anterior or posterior localization films (diaphragm films) showing the isocenter, diaphragm, and vertebral landmarks are taken in addition to the usual weekly double-exposed treatment port films. The distance between the diaphragm apex and a fixed bony landmark and the distance between the apex and the isocenter are measured. The former distance reflects the gating system performance, whereas the latter includes setup error and directly impacts the dose distribution in the patient (Figure 9-13).

Fluoroscopic studies of the first eight patients treated with RPM indicate that gated treatment is capable of reducing the patient-averaged standard deviation of the diaphragm position (ie, intrafractional motion) from 6.9 ± 2.1 mm (no gate) to 2.6 ± 1.7 mm (gated).[18] Anterior-posterior portal images (at least weekly) of these patients showed a mean deviation of the diaphragm position relative to bony anatomy (ie, interfractional variation) of 2.8 ± 1.0 mm. Figure 9-13 summarizes the results from the fluoroscopic and portal image studies.

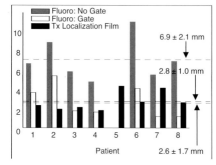

FIGURE 9-13. The comparison of diaphragm variability using gated fluoroscopy and gated localization film measurements, based on the landmark shown in the inset. Adapted from Ford EC et al.[18]

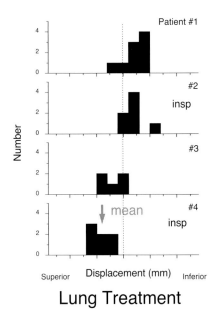

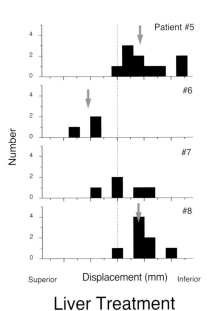

Lung Treatment

Liver Treatment

FIGURE 9-14. Analysis of the diaphragm position during the course of treatment using gated localization films. Four patients (*arrows*) exhibited systematic shifts of more than 4 mm relative to digitally reconstructed radiographs. Adapted from Ford EC et al.[18]

However, Figure 14 illustrates that for four of the eight patients, the diaphragm position on port films showed a systematic shift of more than 4 mm relative to its position on the digitally reconstructed radiograph constructed from the planning CT scan. Studies of subsequent patients confirmed these initial findings that systematic differences between the diaphragm position at simulation and at treatment occur for a significant fraction of patients. Care must be taken to detect and correct for such systematic shifts. Three diaphragm films are reviewed during each of the first 2 weeks of treatment. If no systematic differences are observed, the frequency of imaging is reduced to biweekly and then weekly. For systematic errors over 4 to 5 mm, the fields are adjusted according to the discretion of the physician. For the 30 patients treated with respiratory gating, field adjustments were made in 5 patients. Techniques for convenient visualization of tumor location throughout the course of treatment or to determine whether the diaphragm is a valid surrogate for lung tumor position would be a helpful adjunct to RPM gating or any form of gating based on an external marker.

An alternative approach to avoid the uncertainty about the one-to-one correspondence between the respiratory signal from external markers and internal anatomy with the RPM system is to trigger the radiation beam based on fluoroscopic images of a 2 mm gold marker implanted in the tumor or its vicinity.[19] Figure 9-15 shows three of the four in-room mounted fluoroscopy units, which, in pairs, allow continuous localization of the marker at 30 frames per second, regardless of gantry position. Pattern recognition software is used to detect when the marker is within a threshold window or "permitted dislocation" for triggering the radiation. Phantom studies with the marker have shown that a moving target can be irradiated with an accuracy of ± 1

mm. This approach has merits, although the validity of the single marker as a surrogate for three-dimensional motion of large tumors needs to be validated. Concerns also exist with the length of treatment and the corresponding increase of fluoroscopy dose.

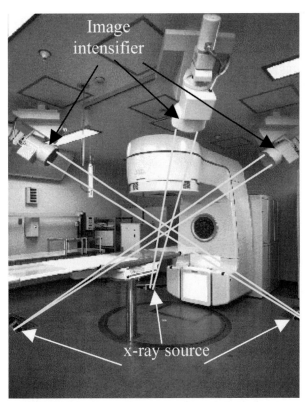

FIGURE 9-15. A picture of the in-room mounted fluoroscopy units to facilitate real-time tracking of a gold marker in the tumor for triggering radiation. (To view a color version of this image, please refer to the CD-ROM.) Reproduced with permission from Shirato H et al.[19]

It is important to note that with respiratory-gated delivery during free breathing, care must be exercised to establish sound correlation of the respiration signal and the internal target motion. The degree of organ deformation that cannot be inferred from the surrogate signal must also be examined. It is therefore imperative that the respiratory motion be analyzed in three dimensions for treatment planning. For a conventional course of fractionated treatment that might extend over a few weeks, it is equally important to monitor possible changes in the four-dimensional CT information and to generate a new plan if necessary. A recent study from M.D. Anderson Cancer Center using breath-hold scans to quantify the magnitude and position of free-breathing motion suggests that appreciable changes can occur for some patients with lung cancer during the course of treatment.[47]

Methods of Breath-hold

Breath-hold methods minimize the effects of respiratory motion on radiation treatment by means of immobilization. Breath-hold has long been used in diagnostic radiology to reduce the blurring of images. For RT, the requirement is to attain the same breath-hold position for all beams delivered during a single treatment fraction and between fractions. Reproducibility of the immobilization is based on the hypothesis that when the subject relaxes during breath-hold, the ventilation muscles go to their predisposed positions associated with the given pulmonary volume or pressure. In principle, breath-hold delivery appears to be simpler to implement than respiratory-gated methods. Achieving immobilization seems less involved than determining the margin for residual motion in gated treatment. In practice, issues such as reproducibility, patient compliance, and comfort need to be addressed, particularly in patients with compromised pulmonary status.

Although diaphragmatic contraction is the primary force driving respiration, other ventilation muscles also contribute variably during normal breathing. Tidal volumes between breaths are also variable. It is thus difficult for the patient to achieve reproducible breath-hold voluntarily during a sequence of normal breathing cycles. Instead, breath-hold methods are typically applied at maximum or moderate deep inhalation[22,48] or at the end of normal exhalation[23] to achieve better reproducibility. Deep inspiration actively recruits all ventilation muscles to expand the lungs, whereas the lung volume is at its most neutral state at the end of normal exhalation.

A breath-hold procedure typically involves applying a nose clip to the patient, preventing nose breathing (or leaking). The patient breathes through a mouthpiece connected to a digital flowmeter, which measures the ventilating lung volume. The cyclical lung volume trace is displayed for visualization by the treatment personnel outside the room or the patient for visual feedback purposes. A predefined lung volume is then used as a cue for applying breath-hold. Two approaches have been employed: voluntary deep inspiration breath-hold (DIBH) and breath-hold under active breathing control (ABC).

Voluntary DIBH

Voluntary DIBH was first implemented at MSKCC in the treatment of patients with lung cancer.[20,29] (DIBH denotes breath-hold at maximum deep inspiration for the remainder of this chapter.) Each patient was instructed to first go through a few cycles of deep breathing (ie, slow vital capacity maneuvers) to decrease the volume of carbon dioxide in the lungs and was then coached to breathe in the largest lung volume possible and hold. Breath-holding at this level of maximum inspiration capacity is expected to be reproducible because the lungs should not expand any further. For the patients with lung cancer selected for treatment, the durations of breath-hold typically would allow a beam-on time of 10 seconds. The DIBH procedure would be repeated to complete delivery of a beam if necessary or for another beam at a different gantry angle.

Figure 9-16 shows a subject in the voluntary DIBH treatment position. The reproducibility of the diaphragm position, in 1 SD, with respect to a bony landmark was examined with fluoroscopy during simulation and also with port films acquired during the course of treatment. The results for seven patients are summarized in Figure 9-16B. In general, the diaphragm position could be immobilized to within 2 mm during the same breath-hold and 3 mm between breath-holds. The port film data show larger variability but include setup variation.

Over 20 patients with lung cancer have been treated using DIBH at MSKCC since 1998.[20] As with respiratory-gated treatment, which requires CT information at the intended phase for treatment, DIBH treatment requires CT and simulation information at DIBH. Because of the limited duration of breath-hold, DIBH CT scans of any extended length would need to be acquired piecemeal. Few advantages were noted. At a large lung volume, the lung density would decrease and less lung mass would be irradiated. For some patients, as shown in Figure 9-17, deep inspiration would increase the separation of the target volume from a critical structure, such as the spinal cord, thereby making it easier to achieve normal tissue sparing. Even with keeping the same margin for free-breathing treatment, dose escalation was possible. Planning studies showed that, on average, the target dose could be increased from 69.4 to 87.9 Gy while keeping the lung normal tissue complication probability < 25%. However, the most serious disadvan-

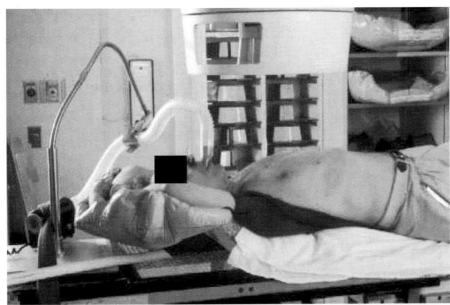

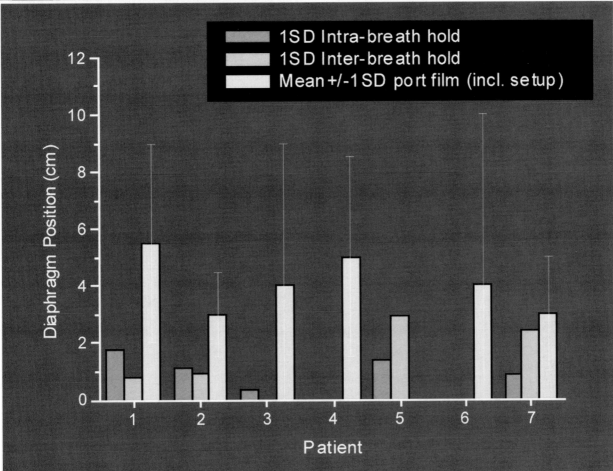

FIGURE 9-16. (*A*) A subject in the voluntary deep inspiration breath-hold treatment position. (*B*) The variation of the diaphragm position with respect to a bony landmark measured using fluoroscopy during simulation and port films during the course of treatment. (To view a color version of this image, please refer to the CD-ROM.) Adapted from Hanley J et al.[48]

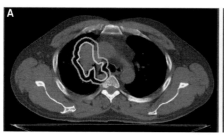
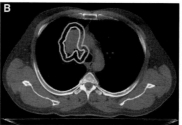

FIGURE 9-17. The separation between the planning target volume and the spinal cord in a (*A*) free-breathing plan is increased in the plan at the (*B*) deep inspiration breath-hold. (To view a color version of this image, please refer to the CD-ROM.) Courtesy of G. Mageras.

tage of DIBH is patient compliance. The procedure required significant effort, resulting in patient fatigue. At MSKCC, half of the patients could not sustain DIBH for the duration of the treatment. Although it appears that DIBH would allow appreciable margin reduction of several millimeters, patients with lung cancer need to be screened for compliance before being selected for treatment at DIBH.

Moderate DIBH with ABC

ABC is a method to facilitate reproducible breath-hold without requiring the patient to reach maximum inspiration capacity.[22,29] The ABC method, currently commercialized by Elekta Inc. (Elekta Oncology, Crawley, United Kingdom) as the Active Breathing Coordinator, is used to suspend breathing at any predetermined position in the normal respiratory cycle or at active inspiration. The device consists of a digital spirometer to measure the respiratory trace, which, in turn, is connected to a balloon valve (Figure 9-18). In an ABC procedure, the patient breathes normally through the apparatus. When an operator "activates" the system, the lung volume and the phase (ie, inhalation or exhalation) at which the balloon valve will be closed are specified and displayed. Typically, after going through two preparatory breath cycles, the patient is instructed to reach the specified lung volume. At this point, the valve is inflat-

ed within 40 milliseconds with an air compressor for a predefined duration of time, thereby "holding" the patient's breath. The breath-hold duration is patient dependent, typically 15 to 30 seconds, and should be well tolerated to allow for repeat (after a brief rest period) breath-holds without causing undue patient distress. Figure 9-19 illustrates the display of the Elekta ABC system, in which the appearance of a green color serves to indicate both the ready state of the balloon valve and the lung volume at which it will be closed to maintain breath-hold. A timer display counts down the remaining breath-hold duration in seconds.

The experience at William Beaumont Hospital and at other centers suggests that a moderate deep inspiration breath-hold (mDIBH) level set at 75% of the maximum inspiratory capacity achieves substantial and reproducible internal organ displacement while maintaining patient comfort.[29–31,49–51] With the ABC system, the intended mDIBH position is calculated from the baseline at the end of normal exhalation and is set during an initial training session for each patient. Variation of the baseline between breaths is possible. As with respiration-gated treatment delivery, verbal instructions are given to help patients achieve

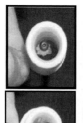
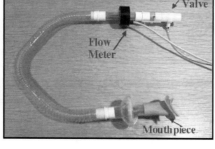

FIGURE 9-18. A picture of the mouthpiece—digital flowmeter—balloon valve connection of the active breathing control apparatus. The insets on the left show the balloon valve in the open state (*top*) and in the closed state (*bottom*) as the balloon is inflated with an air compressor. (To view a color version of this image, please refer to the CD-ROM.)

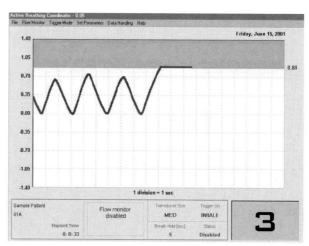

FIGURE 9-19. The screen display of the Active Breathing Coordinator system. The blue waveform is the ventilation signal converted from the digital flowmeter. The green shade indicates that the system is activated and the lung volume for breath-hold. The bottom right display counts down the remaining duration of the breath-hold in seconds. Note that this example does not show the large lung volume at the moderate deep inspiration breath-hold.

a steady breathing pattern. For each breathing cycle, the lung volume is intentionally renormalized to a zero baseline each time zero flow is detected at the end of exhalation. Renormalization occurs mostly at the beginning of a study. Once the patient achieves normal respiration in a relaxed manner, both the frequency and magnitude of the renormalization become minimal. It is from this stable baseline that three measurements of the approximate maximum inspiratory capacity are made. The mDIBH threshold is then set to 75% of the average maximum inspiration capacity. The value is recorded and used for all subsequent sessions. Given the relatively large lung volume at mDIBH, the renormalized baseline provides a sufficiently stable reference for achieving reproducible breath-holds.

It is useful to discuss the stability of the respiration signal for methods of respiratory gating and breath-hold. For the breath-hold methods, a digital spirometer is already employed to measure lung volume such that the attachment of an additional valve to assist breath-hold is inconsequential. The digital spirometer can also provide the signal for gating. However, if the desire is to have the patient breathe freely with minimal discomfort, then surface reflectors, or implanted markers, are employed. There have been some concerns as to the ability of these methods to provide robust respiration signals. Supporters of spirometry systems say that the surface reflector systems may not give an accurate portrayal of lung position because muscle relaxation can be out of phase with lung motion. This has been shown to be the case on several occasions. The varying involvement of the different muscles from breath to breath can result in variation between the surrogate signal and organ positions. Different surface marker positions may exhibit a different sensitivity and relationship with breathing motion.[52] The advocates of surface reflectors note that signal drift can occur with spirometry systems. Some flowmeters are more prone to nonlinear variation with changing flow rates, temperature, and humidity. Regardless, it needs to be stressed that, first and foremost, both surface markers and spirometers provide signals that are surrogates of tumor motion. With the present state of the science, their applications must be validated with fluoroscopic and CT imaging studies, during a signal treatment fraction and between fractions during the course of treatment.

Breath-hold Reproducibility with ABC

To develop the appropriate clinical procedures for treatment with ABC, extensive reproducibility and treatment planning studies have been performed at William Beaumont Hospital. The study protocol included the acquisition of a free-breathing CT scan for treatment planning and two mDIBH scans. The latter allowed examination of intrafraction reproducibility of the ABC procedure. In addition, a breath-hold CT scan was acquired at the end of normal inhalation and exhalation. These "end" scans provided an upper estimate of the range of organ motion in a breathing cycle, given the increased dead space of the spirometer assembly. For some patients, a repeat ABC scan at mDIBH was acquired 1 to 4 weeks later to evaluate interfraction reproducibility.

The initial studies focused mostly on patients with breast and thoracic diseases who could tolerate a breath-hold duration of > 15 seconds. For the patients with breast cancer, the CT data also allowed the study of (1) the effects of breathing motion on the dosimetry of whole-breast IMRT using "step-and-shoot" delivery[16]; (2) the use of mDIBH to reduce heart irradiation in the treatment of patients with left-sided breast cancer[30]; and (3) the use of mDIBH to facilitate locoregional treatment with wide tangents that included the internal mammary nodes.[29]

A patient setup for an ABC CT study is shown in Figure 9-20A. The ABC display can be viewed by the patient on an auxiliary monitor using prism glasses. Although all patients found verbal coaching necessary, few benefited from visual information. During a CT study session, breath-hold procedures were repeated to facilitate the acquisition of piecemeal CT scans that spanned the entire thorax region. (As with RCCT, the inconvenience of piecemeal CT scans would not be a factor with the advent of multislice CT in which a 40 cm scan length can be completed with a 10-second breath-hold.) The analysis of breath-hold reproducibility involved removing the component of setup error by registering the two mDIBH scans with respect to the vertebrae. The lungs, trachea, and first bifurcation were then contoured for each data set (Figure 9-20B). These contours were interpolated to produce 1 mm slice thickness from the original scans with 5 or 3 mm slice thickness. Three-dimensional organ surfaces were generated from the contoured organs. An in-house

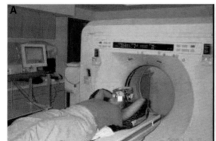 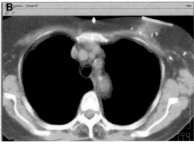

FIGURE 9-20. (*A*) A patient setup for an active breathing control (ABC) computed tomography (CT) study. (*B*) The contours of the lungs, ribs, and tracheas from two registered interfraction ABC scans at the moderate deep inspiration breath-hold are overlaid on one of the CT data. (To view a color version of this image, please refer to the CD-ROM.) Courtesy of V. Remouchamps.

algorithm was used to determine the closest distance to agreement (DTA) for each point between the two three-dimensional organ surfaces as a measure of reproducibility.

As shown in Figure 9-21, the DTA surface map provides a measure of breath-hold reproducibility in three dimensions. Data from 21 patients with breast cancer were analyzed and summarized in Table 9-1 as mean and 1 SD of the lung surface DTA distributions, divided into six regions. With the patient positioned in an alpha cradle, the mean (and standard deviation) intrafraction DTA is 1.1 (1.2) mm for the left lung and 1.0 (1.1) mm for the right lung. The corresponding values without the use of an alpha cradle are significantly higher with 1.9 (2.1) mm and 2.2 (2.2) mm for the left and right lungs, respectively ($p < .005$). These results confirm an earlier observation that breath-hold reproducibility is inherently coupled with setup variation.[22] Differences in setup position would involve the participation of different ventilation muscles during breathing. The interfraction DTA for the left and right lungs are 1.3 (1.5) mm and 1.4 (1.6) mm, respectively, similar to the intrafraction results. The results highlight the importance of minimizing setup variation for achieving effective immobilization with breath-hold.

The DTA results of the lung surface map are more pertinent for structures close to the chest wall. However, the DTA values obtained for the tracheal bifurcation in the same study were 0.9 (0.8) mm for intrafraction and 1.4 (1.0) mm for interfraction, suggesting similar reproducibility for the entire thorax. However, further studies are required to validate this hypothesis.

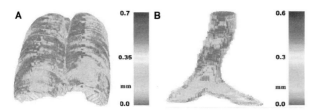

FIGURE 9-21. The distance to agreement surface maps in millimeters for the (*A*) lungs and (*B*) carina of a patient study. (To view a color version of this image, please refer to the CD-ROM.) Courtesy of V. Remouchamps.

Regional analysis demonstrates that at mDIBH with ABC, the upper two-thirds of the chest wall are better immobilized than the lower diaphragmatic region. With proper setup, a margin of 3 mm for respiratory motion would more than suffice for the upper two-thirds of the lung and 5 mm for the lower third. The reproducibility of immobilization can be dependent on the choice of lung volume at breath-hold. At mDIBH, most of the respiratory muscles are recruited, allowing better positional reproducibility. In addition, at an inflated lung volume of about 4 L or more, changes in volume of 100 to 200 cc would translate to a small positional variation (< 2 mm). The excellent reproducibility of inter- and intrafraction immobilization was recently confirmed in a similar repeat CT study at Mount Vernon Hospital in patients with lung cancer.[31] However, if breath-hold is intended at the end of normal exhalation, then one should be aware that small variations in functional residual capacity are possible between breaths and potentially larger variations can occur between days.

IMRT at mDIBH with ABC

Similar to respiratory-gated IMRT delivery, the implementation of mDIBH for IMRT treatment is also in early development. At William Beaumont Hospital, a clinical study involves patients with left-sided breast cancer who are predisposed to heart irradiation from tangential field arrangement. Figure 9-22 shows the beam's eye views on digitally reconstructed radiographs at free breathing and mDIBH. The heart, shown in the blue-shaded contour, is displaced from the beam at mDIBH. Such observations prompted the hypotheses that the implementation of ABC treatment at mDIBH will be beneficial for these patients by displacing the heart away from the fields.[29,53,54]

The sMLC method for whole-breast IMRT at William Beaumont Hospital has been used to treat over 500 patients. The step-and-shoot delivery lends itself nicely to ABC.[55] The predetermined duration of breath-hold allows appropriate allocation of sMLC segments for each breath-hold. However, combining ABC with the delivery of the tangential IMRT fields requires special care in patient preparation. The details have been published.[30] Briefly, free-breathing and mDIBH simulation and CT scanning are performed

TABLE 9-1. Mean (1 SD) of Distance to Agreement of 2 Lung Surfaces (in cm) for 2 Registered Active Breathing Control Scans Acquired at Moderate Deep Inspiration Breath-Hold

	Lung Side	Full Lung	I (Bottom 10%)	II (20%)	III (20%)	IV (20%)	V (20%)	VI (Top 10%)
No cradle (7 patients; intrafraction)	Left	0.19 (0.21)	0.43 (0.34)	0.25 (0.25)	0.15 (0.12)	0.14 (0.09)	0.14 (0.09)	0.14 (0.09)
	Right	0.22 (0.22)	0.44 (0.32)	0.35 (0.28)	0.17 (0.11)	0.14 (0.09)	0.13 (0.08)	0.15 (0.12)
Alpha cradle immobilization (14 patients; intrafraction)	Left	0.11 (0.12)	0.17 (0.15)	0.15 (0.14)	0.10 (0.09)	0.09 (0.08)	0.08 (0.08)	0.09 (0.07)
	Right	0.10 (0.11)	0.10 (0.10)	0.12 (0.13)	0.09 (0.08)	0.09 (0.08)	0.08 (0.08)	0.13 (0.09)
Alpha cradle (8 patients; interfraction)	Left	0.13 (0.15)	0.17 (0.15)	0.17 (0.20)	0.11 (0.12)	0.09 (0.09)	0.10 (0.09)	0.15 (0.10)
	Right	0.14 (0.16)	0.19 (0.18)	0.17 (0.20)	0.12 (0.09)	0.11 (0.10)	0.12 (0.11)	0.16 (0.12)

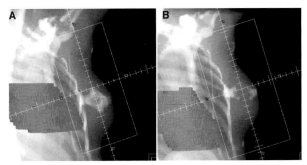

FIGURE 9-22. Beam's eye view displays showing, respectively, (A) irradiation of a portion of the heart by the tangential field arrangement with the patient breathing freely and (B) displacement of the heart from the field at the moderate deep inspiration breath-hold. Adapted from Remouchamps V et al.

for the patient. Free-breathing information is used for marking the patient for setup, whereas the mDIBH information is needed for treatment planning and delivery. The source-to-surface distances (SSDs) are checked both at free breathing and at mDIBH with a short (5–10 second) duration. Computer components (keyboard and display) in the treatment room have been useful in the operations of the ABC system. For IMRT delivery, the segments of each tangent are purposely divided into two or three separate deliveries to accommodate repeat breath-hold. Similarly, the open field segment with a significant allocation of MUs is also split into two separate deliveries. Electronic portal images acquired of these open field segments allow the examination of intra- and interfraction treatment variations that combine both breath-hold and setup.

To date, more than 35 patients at William Beaumont Hospital have been treated at mDIBH with ABC. Thirty-two were patients with left-sided breast cancer treated with IMRT, one patient had right-sided breast cancer with a significant

portion of her liver in the field, and 2 patients had lung cancer and could tolerate mDIBH for over 20 seconds. Figure 9-23A shows a patient with breast cancer in the treatment position with an electronic portal imaging device deployed for treatment verification. The treatment personnel at the control station, where a therapist (in the red box) is providing verbal instruction to the patient, are shown in Figure 9-23B. At William Beaumont Hospital, three therapists traditionally work at the treatment console. However, the ABC procedure could be managed by two therapists.

Treatments at mDIBH with the ABC system were well tolerated by all patients and treatment personnel. Twenty minutes were allocated for breath-hold treatment. With the exception of the initial five patients, all combined ABC/IMRT treatments were completed within 15 minutes. The time-trace of the lung volumes from a patient undergoing ABC treatment is shown in Figure 9-24. There is an initial short breath-hold period for setup, followed by two 20-second breath-holds for the delivery of the medial beams and two for the lateral beams. The level of mDIBH was set at 1.9 L of inspired volume or a total lung inflation of approximately 4 L. Minor volume overshoot can occur if the flow rate of the patient's inhalation exceeds the response rate of the ABC system. However, the overshoot would result in minimal positional variations owing to already large inflated lung volume at breath-hold.

For the first five patients with left-sided breast cancer treated with breath-hold, daily electronic portal images were acquired of the open field segments whenever possible. The variations of the chest wall from its reference digitally reconstructed radiograph position were quantified using an in-house template alignment tool. The analysis combines setup error and breath-hold variation. The results for 509 electronic portal images are summarized in Table 9-2.

Overall, the magnitudes of the variations are small. The larger variation in the craniocaudal direction is more indicative of setup error than breath-hold variation.

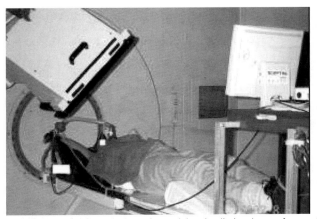
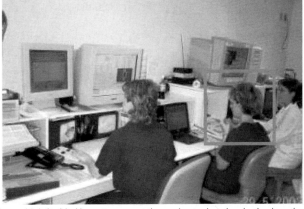

FIGURE 9-23. (A) Setup for intensity-modulated radiation therapy for a patient with left-sided breast cancer at the moderate deep inspiration breath-hold with the active breathing control (ABC) system. An electronic portal imaging device was deployed for treatment verification. (B) Therapists at the treatment console for ABC. Verbal coaching was provided by a therapist using a dedicated audio system. (To view a color version of this image, please refer to the CD-ROM.) Adapted from Remouchamps V et al.

TABLE 9-2. Combined Variations of Setup and Breath-hold (in mm) of Breast Tangent Treatments with Active Breathing Contol Measured from the 509 Daily Electronic Portal Images for the First 5 Patients

| | Medial/BH1 | Medial/BH2 | Lateral/BH1 | Lateral/BH2 |
	Mean (SD)	Mean (SD)	Mean (SD)	Mean (SD)
Transverse	1.7 (2.4)	1.2 (2.1)	1.8 (2.3)	1.8 (2.3)
Craniocaudal	2.0 (3.2)	2.1 (3.1)	3.4 (3.1)	3.2 (3.3)
Rotation	1.4 (1.0)	1.2 (1.0)	1.5 (1.0)	1.0 (1.0)

BH = breath-hold.

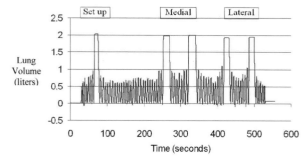

FIGURE 9-24. A time-trace of the lung volumes as recorded by the active breathing control system for a patient with left-sided breast cancer undergoing intensity-modulated radiation therapy at moderate deep inspiration breath-hold.

Conclusions

For IMRT, the already complex delivery is further compounded by the presence of respiratory motion. The unavoidable repeat beam interrupts associated with breath-hold and gated IMRT delivery necessitates stable beam-on performance for short-duration exposures. That concern appears to be well handled by the modern linear accelerator. For the sliding window delivery, there is concern about the interplay between the breathing motion of the tumor and organs and the motion of the MLC. Studies have shown that appreciable dose variations can occur owing to breathing motion.[14] On the other hand, studies with clinical IMRT fields show that the variations over a fractionated course of treatment would wash out and the mean delivered dose would closely approximate the expected dose.[11,12,15] The variations owing to breathing motion are similar for IMRT and conventional conformal RT delivery. The dosimetric differences between nongated sMLC and gated dMLC deliveries are also small. Such minimal deviation tends to suggest that the difference may be due to the less precise repeat delivery of dMLC in reference to sMLC or to measurement error. But it is important to be mindful that breathing motion perturbs the dosimetry of radiation treatment whether it is nongated or gated.

Significant advances have been made in the development of gating and breath-hold methods to manage respiratory motion in RT treatment and IMRT. Respiratory-gated delivery preserves the patient's comfort at the expense of residual breathing motion within the intended gating window. Breath-hold with ABC effectively immobilizes the patient and allows substantial margin reduction. The procedure, however, is not suitable for patients whose pulmonary status has been compromised by disease. However, it should be noted that these two approaches of managing breathing motion are not mutually exclusive. When the breath-hold signal is applied to automatically gate the machine, even for the short duration that can be maintained by the patient with lung cancer, one may achieve the optimal combination of patient immobilization and efficient operation.

At present, both gating and breath-hold methods remain investigational. Although both are commercially available and approved by the US Food and Drug Administration, great care must be exercised when applied clinically. The validity of the external respiratory signal in inferring internal anatomic position needs further in-depth evaluation. Regardless of the choice of method to manage breathing motion, the single most important factor that must be established is the reproducibility of organ position during the course of treatment. It should also be noted that the magnitude of margin reduction would likely be institution specific depending on the treatment technique and patient immobilization. The advent of RCCT and multislice CT greatly enhances the conduct of the necessary studies. Although the clinical effectiveness of gating or breath-hold radiation treatments awaits long-term evaluations, the recent experience is encouraging and suggests that the problems associated with breathing motion can be well managed. But given the current state of knowledge, we advise against margin reductions without a thorough reproducibility study.

References

1. Teh BS, McGary JE, Dong L, et al. The use of rectal balloon during the delivery of intensity modulated radiotherapy (IMRT) for prostate cancer: more than just a prostate gland immobilization device? Cancer J 2002;6:476–83.
2. Lattanzi J, McNeeley S, Pinover W, et al. A comparison of daily CT localization to a daily ultrasound-based system in prostate cancer. Int J Radiat Oncol Biol Phys 1999;43:719–25.
3. Litzenberg D, Dawson LA, Sandler H, et al. Daily prostate targeting using implanted radiopaque markers. Int J Radiat Oncol Biol Phys 2002;52:699–703.
4. Murphy MJ, Adler JR Jr, Bodduluri M, et al. Image-guided radiosurgery for the spine and pancreas. Comput Aided Surg 2000;5:278–88.
5. Meeks SL, Buatti JM, Bouchet LG, et al. Ultrasound-guided extracranial radiosurgery: technique and application. Int J Radiat Oncol Biol Phys 2003;55:1092–101.
6. Martinez AA, Yan D, Lockman D, et al. Improvement in dose escalation using the process of adaptive radiotherapy combined with three-dimensional conformal or intensity-modulated beams for prostate cancer. Int J Radiat Oncol Biol

Phys 2001;50:1226–34.

7. Jaffray DA, Yan D, Wong JW. Managing geometric uncertainty in conformal intensity-modulated radiation therapy. Semin Radiat Oncol 1999;9:4–19.

8. Yu CX, Jaffray DA, Wong JW. The effects of intra-fraction organ motion on the delivery of dynamic intensity modulation. Phys Med Biol 1998;43:91–104.

9. West JB. Respiratory physiology—the essentials. Baltimore (MD): Waverly Press, Inc.; 1974.

10. Nunn JF. Nunn's applied respiratory physiology. 4th ed. Oxford (UK): Butterworth-Heinemann; 1993.

11. Bortfeld T, Jokivarsi K, Goitein M, et al. Effects of intra-fraction motion on IMRT dose delivery: statistical analysis and simulation. Phys Med Biol 2002;47:2203–20.

12. Jiang SB, Pope C, Al Jarrah KM, et al. An experimental investigation on intra-fractional organ motion effects in lung IMRT treatments. Phys Med Biol 2003;48:1773–84.

13. Hugo GD, Agazaryan N, Solberg TD. The effects of tumor motion on planning and delivery of respiratory-gated IMRT. Med Phys 2003;30:1052–66.

14. Duan J, Shen S, Fiveash JB, et al. Dosimetric effect of respiration-gated beam on IMRT delivery. Med Phys 2003;30:2241–52.

15. Chui CS, Yorke E, Hong L. The effects of intra-fraction organ motion on the delivery of intensity-modulated field with a multileaf collimator. Med Phys 2003;30:1736–46.

16. Frazier RC, Vicini FA, Sharpe MB, et al. Impact of breathing motion on whole breast radiotherapy: a dosimetric analysis using active breathing control. Int J Radiat Oncol Biol Phys 2004;58:1041–7.

17. Boyer AL, Butler EB, DiPetrillo TA, et al. Intensity-modulated radiotherapy: current status and issues of interest. Int J Radiat Oncol Biol Phys 2001;51:880–914.

18. Ford EC, Mageras G, Yorke E, et al. Evaluation of respiratory movement during gated radiotherapy using film and electronic portal imaging. Int J Radiat Oncol Biol Phys 2002;32:522–31.

19. Shirato H, Shimizu S, Kunieda T, et al. Physical aspects of a real-time tumor-tracking system for gated radiotherapy. Int J Radiat Oncol Biol Phys 2000;48:1187–95.

20. Rosenzweig KE, Hanley J, Mah D, et al. The deep inspiration breath-hold technique in the treatment of inoperable non-small-cell lung cancer. Int J Radiat Oncol Biol Phys 2000;48:81–7.

21. Mageras GS, Yorke E. Deep inspiration breath hold and respiratory gating strategies for reducing organ motion in radiation treatment. Semin Radiat Oncol 2004;14:65–75.

22. Wong JW, Sharpe MB, Jaffray DA, et al. The use of active breathing control (ABC) to reduce margin for breathing motion. Int J Radiat Oncol Biol Phys 1999;44:911–9.

23. Dawson LA, Brock KK, Kazanjian S, et al. The reproducibility of organ position using active breathing control (ABC) during liver radiotherapy. Int J Radiat Oncol Biol Phys 2001;51:1410–21.

24. Takai Y, Mitsuya M, Nemoto K, et al. Development of real-time tumor tracking system with dMLC using dual x-ray fluoroscopy and amorphous silicon flat panel on the gantry of linear accelerator. Int J Radiat Oncol Biol Phys 2002;54 Suppl:193–4.

25. Murphy MJ, Chang SD, Gibbs IC, et al. Patterns of patient movement during frameless image-guided radiosurgery. Int J Radiat Oncol Biol Phys 2003;55:1400–8.

26. Keall PJ, Kini V, Vedam SS, et al. Motion adaptive x-ray therapy: a feasibility study. Phys Med Biol 2001;46:1–10.

27. Neicu T, Shirato H, Seppenwoolde Y, et al. Synchronized moving aperture radiation therapy (SMART): average tumour trajectory for lung patients. Phys Med Biol 2003;48:587–98.

28. Kim DJ, Murray BR, Halperin R, et al. Held-breath self-gating technique for radiotherapy of non-small-cell lung cancer: a feasibility study. Int J Radiat Oncol Biol Phys 2001;49:43–9.

29. Remouchamps V, Vicini F, Sharpe M, et al. Significant reductions in heart and lung doses using deep inspiration breath-hold with active breathing control and intensity modulated radiation therapy for patients treated with locoregional breast irradiation. Int J Radiat Oncol Biol Phys 2003;55:392–406.

30. Remouchamps V, Letts N, Vicini F, et al. Initial clinical experience with deep inspiration breath hold using an active breathing control (ABC) device in the treatment of patients with left-sided breast cancer using external beam irradiation. Int J Radiat Oncol Biol Phys 2003; 56:704–715.

31. Wilson EM, Williams FJ, Lyn BE, et al. Validation of active breathing control in patients with non-small-cell lung cancer to be treated with CHARTWEL. Int J Radiat Oncol Biol Phys 2003;57:864–74.

32. Ford EC, Mageras GS, Yorke E, et al. Respiration-correlated spiral CT: a method of measuring respiratory-induced anatomic motion for radiation treatment planning. Med Phys 2003;30:88–97.

33. Hugo GD, Agazaryan N, Solberg TD. An evaluation of gating window size, delivery method, and composite field dosimetry of respiratory-gated IMRT. Med Phys 2002;29:2517–25.

34. Lujan AE, Balter JM, Ten Haken RK. A method for incorporating organ motion due to breathing into 3D dose calculations in the liver: sensitivity to variations in motion. Med Phys 2003;30:2643–9.

35. Liang J, Yan D, Kestin LL, et al. Minimization of target margin by adapting treatment planning to target respiratory motion. Int J Radiat Oncol Biol Phys 2003;57(2 Suppl):S233–4.

36. Chetty IJ, Rosu M, Tyagi N, et al. A fluence convolution method to account for respiratory motion in three-dimensional dose calculations of the liver: a Monte Carlo study. Med Phys 2003;30:1776–80.

37. Ohara K, Okumura T, Akisada M, et al. Irradiation synchronized with respiration gate. Int J Radiat Oncol Biol Phys 1989;17:853–7.

38. Osaka Y, Kamada T, Matsuoka Y, et al. Clinical experience of heavy ion irradiation synchronous with respiration. In: Proceedings of the XIIIth International Conference on the Use of Computers in Radiation Therapy, Salt Lake City, Utah. Madison (WI): Medical Physics Publishing; 1997. p. 176–7.

39. Kubo HD, Hill BC. Respiration gated radiotherapy treatment: a technical study. Phys Med Biol 1996;41:83–91.

40. Kalender WA, Rienmuller R, Seissler W, et al. Measurement of pulmonary parenchymal attenuation: use of spirometric gating with quantitative CT. Radiology 1990;175:265–8.

41. Mageras GS, Yorke E, Rosenzweig K, et al. Fluoroscopic evaluation of diaphragmatic motion reduction with a

respiratory gated radiotherapy system. J Appl Clin Med Phys 2001;2:191–200.

42. Giraud P, Ford EC, Rosenzweig KE, et al. Reduction of organ motion in lung and liver tumors with respiratory gating. Radiother Oncol 2004. [In press]

43. Vedam SS, Keall PJ, Kini VR, et al. Determining parameters for respiration-gated radiotherapy. Med Phys 2001;28:2139–46.

44. Kachelriess M, Ulzheimer S, Kalender WA. ECG-correlated imaging of the heart with subsecond multislice spiral CT. IEEE Trans Med Imaging 2000;19:888–901.

45. Pan T, Lee TY, Rietzel E, et al. 4D-CT imaging of a volume influenced by respiratory motion on multi-slice CT. Med Phys 2004;31:333–40.

46. Wagman R, Yorke E, Ford E, et al. Respiratory gating for liver tumors: use in dose escalation. Int J Radiat Oncol Biol Phys 2003;55:659–68.

47. Forster KM, Stevens CW, Kitamura K, et al. Changes in tumor motion patterns during a course of radiation therapy for lung cancer. Int J Radiat Oncol Biol Phys 2003;57(2 Suppl):S234.

48. Hanley J, Debois MM, Mah D, et al. Deep inspiration breath-hold technique for lung tumors: the potential value of target immobilization and reduced lung density in dose escalation. Int J Radiat Oncol Biol Phys 1999;45:603–11.

49. Mah D, Hanley J, Rosenzweig KE, et al. Technical aspects of the deep inspiration breath-hold technique in the treatment of thoracic cancer. Int J Radiat Oncol Biol Phys 2000;48:1175–85.

50. Remouchamps VM, Letts N, Yan D, et al. Three dimensional evaluation of intra- and inter-fraction reproducibility of lung and chest wall immobilization using active breathing control. Int J Radiat Oncol Biol Phys 2003;57:968–78.

51. Stromberg JS, Sharpe MB, Kim LH, et al. Active breathing control (ABC) for Hodgkin's disease: reduction in normal tissue irradiation with deep inspiration and implications for treatment. Int J Radiat Oncol Biol Phys 2000;48:797–806.

52. Baroni G, Ferrigno G, Orecchia R, et al. Real-time three-dimensional motion analysis for patient positioning verification. Radiother Oncol 2000;54:21–7.

53. Sidhu K, Hong L, Yorke E, et al. Deep inspiration breath-hold technique and IMRT as methods to reduce volume of heart and liver in breast radiotherapy. Int J Radiat Oncol Biol Phys 2002;54 Suppl 1:158–9.

54. Sixel KE, Aznar MC, Ung YC. Deep inspiration breath hold to reduce irradiated heart volume in breast cancer patients. Int J Radiat Oncol Biol Phys 2001;49:199–204.

55. Vicini FA, Sharpe M, Kestin L, et al. Optimizing breast cancer treatment efficacy with intensity-modulated radiotherapy. Int J Radiat Oncol Biol Phys 2002;54:1336–44.

Chapter 10

TREATMENT PLANNING

RUSSELL J. HAMILTON, PHD, MARTIN E. LACHAINE, PHD, BENJAMIN ARMBRUSTER, BS

Treatment planning is an integral component of intensity-modulated radiation therapy (IMRT). As discussed in Chapter 2, "Physics of IMRT," there are a number of optimization algorithms for IMRT, including gradient descent, simulated annealing, iterative algebraic reconstruction, and linear optimization. Each of these algorithms requires a unique set of parameters to specify the target and normal tissue goals. Some of these parameters include the minimum or maximum dose, mean organ dose, and individual dose-volume histograms (DVHs). Likewise, there are many ways to adjust the relative importance of these parameters to create a cost function. The large number of permutations available by combining an algorithm with a particular choice of optimization parameters and a cost function has led to the emergence of a number of treatment planning systems, each with its own characteristics.

The aim of this chapter is to discuss the practical aspects of IMRT planning that are applicable to all treatment planning systems, including the selection of beam energy and orientation, planning techniques, and plan evaluation. A brief description of commercially available planning systems is provided. Lastly, a methodology is proposed to systematically investigate the characteristics of one's own planning system.

Beam Energy Selection

Once the tumor and organs at risk (OAR) are contoured, for nontomotherapy delivery techniques, the treatment planner must make a decision on the number, energy, and directions of treatment beams. It is common practice to select a fixed set of five, seven, or nine equally spaced, nonopposing coplanar beams—the class solution approach. A larger number of beams (eg, nine vs five) may produce a more conformal plan, at the expense of treatment time and complexity. Pirzkall and colleagues showed that for deep-seated targets, the dose to both planning target volume (PTV) and OAR does not depend significantly on the number of beams and/or energy.[1] Instead, the main difference

occurs in regions far from the PTV. In these regions, the dose is significantly increased for both a smaller number of beams and for lower energy. They also demonstrated that for nine beams or more, the energy dependence far from the PTV was negligible. Therefore, for a five-field plan, one may want to consider using higher-energy beams, such as 15 MV, but if one prefers to use nine fields, then a 6 MV beam could be used with the same results.

When selecting appropriate beam energies, other effects need to be considered.[2] Followill and colleagues postulated that there is an increased risk of secondary malignancies in patients treated with beam energies of > 10 MV owing to a higher neutron dose.[3] However, the degree of neutron production depends on the specific IMRT plan parameters, including the number of segments and monitor units (MUs). Moreover, the importance of considering secondary malignancies from IMRT treatments for any energy beam has been raised, especially for pediatric cases, for which IMRT may offer better dose conformity than conventional planning.[4–6] These aspects require further investigation and scrutiny.

Beam Orientation Selection

It is well known from rotational radiation therapy and stereotactic radiosurgery that the dose falloff outside the PTV is not as sharp as the penumbra of a single photon beam. The reason is that the dose gradient in the penumbra may be as high as 20%/mm, whereas photon attenuation is on the order of 2 to 3%/cm. This is also true in IMRT planning when a large number of fields are used. The dose gradient away from the PTV for a nine-field IMRT plan is less steep than is achieved with a well-designed static field (conventional) plan. The advantage of more fields, and IMRT in general, lies in the ability to better conform the high-dose region to the shape of the target. If a high gradient is required at a certain critical interface, then careful selection of beam angles is important. This phenomenon can sometimes be observed when comparing the DVH of

IMRT plans to three-dimensional conventional plans. The DVH of an IMRT plan is often better in the high-dose region owing to the high degree of dose conformity, whereas the conventional plan is often better in the low-dose region because the field placement is usually arranged specifically to cause a sharp dose falloff near a critical structure.

It is common in IMRT to use standard sets of coplanar beams. Although this is convenient, it does not always yield the best results. Price and colleagues studied the use of noncoplanar beam orientations for prostate IMRT.[7] In a typical plan, they demonstrated that the use of noncoplanar fields resulted in a 15 to 25% decrease in dose to the hottest portion of the rectum compared with coplanar field arrangements. Furthermore, a seven-field noncoplanar IMRT technique produced increased bladder sparing compared with standard field arrangements.

The optimal selection of coplanar beam arrangements has been intensely investigated, and a number of methods have emerged.[8–11] Beam orientation optimizers use a variety of parameters and cost functions, spanning a range similar to the overall problem of IMRT dose optimization. Rowbottom and colleagues developed an optimization algorithm that finds the best beam arrangement for a small number of fields and was designed to avoid orientations that pass through OAR with low radiation tolerance.[11] Das and colleagues used an unconstrained objective function based on equivalent uniform dose in combination with DVH constraints of critical OAR.[8] In a series of articles and in Chapter 2, combinations of several different parameter sets and cost functions were shown to be effective in selecting optimal beam orientations.[10,12,13] One method that combined prior geometric and dosimetric knowledge was

shown to be computationally efficient and hence is promising for eventual clinical implementation.[13] Most of the methods employed for coplanar beam orientation optimization have also been demonstrated to work for optimization of noncoplanar beams as well.

Because commercial IMRT planning systems do not offer beam orientation optimization, important practical questions remain. In particular, when should noncoplanar beams be used, and how are their directions selected? Noncoplanar beams should be considered when the path to the PTV for most coplanar beam orientations intersects critical organs. In these cases, constructing a three-dimensional conventional plan provides valuable insight into beam angle selection and also sets a standard for a potential IMRT plan to beat. Figure 10-1A shows an example of a tumor located near the optic apparatus. The best IMRT plan obtained using coplanar beams is shown in Figure 10-1B. This plan was deemed unacceptable owing to the significant amount of intermediate-dose spread into the left optic nerve. With conventional three-dimensional planning, the best approach would be to use noncoplanar beams. Although the dose distribution produced with a noncoplanar conventional plan does not provide adequate coverage owing to the OAR constraints (Figure 10-1C), it does provide a useful set of beams to be used for IMRT planning. The optimal IMRT plan was determined using the same beam directions as the noncoplanar conventional plan (Figure 10-1D). The target is fully covered, a sharp dose gradient anterior to the PTV spared the left optic nerve, and the volume of intermediate dose was small. These features were improvements on the three-dimensional conventional plan and were achieved by using the same angles determined by an experienced conventional planner.

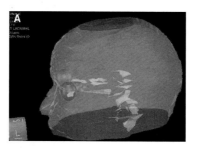
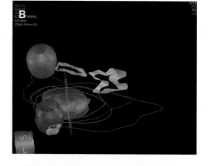
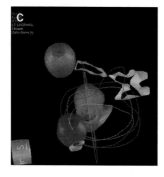
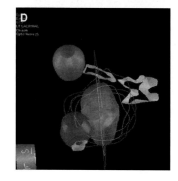

FIGURE 10-1. Illustration of the dosimetric effect of beam angle selection. (*A*) Rendering of a tumor located near the optic nerve and chiasm. (*B*) The best intensity-modulated radiation therapy (IMRT) plan generated using a coplanar beam arrangement. (*C*) Conventional plan using noncoplanar beams. (*D*) An IMRT plan using the noncoplanar beams from *C*. (To view a color version of this image, please refer to the CD-ROM).

Planning Techniques

Once the energies and beam orientations are selected, the planner must define objectives and/or constraints for the optimizer. Depending on the planning system, this could consist of dose-volume objectives, weights describing the importance of each objective, minimum and maximum target dose values, mean organ doses, or maximum OAR dose values. The problem is that although these directives can satisfy appropriate PTV coverage or keep sensitive structures to certain dose levels, it is difficult to ensure adequate dose falloff outside the PTV. In this case, the optimizer will not pay too much attention to the relatively small volume of this tissue directly surrounding the PTV unless specified in the constraints. One common solution to this problem is the use of a strategically drawn "planning structure" surrounding the PTV. Dose objectives lower than the PTV can be imposed on such a structure to guide the optimizer in producing a sharper falloff. For planning systems that permit structures to have "holes," a simple doughnut shape around the contour will suffice. Otherwise, this may be accomplished with either a horseshoe-shaped planning structure or by expanding the PTV by a known margin. For the latter option, any dose objective on the planning structure must account for the dose objective of the PTV because the PTV is inside the structure, making an appropriate selection of constraints difficult.

If dose-volume objectives are available in the planning system, one solution is to allow a fraction, $f = V_{PTV}/V_{struct}$, of the planning structure to be greater or equal to the prescription dose, whereas the objective dose is lowered for the rest of the planning structure (V_{PTV} and V_{struct} are the PTV and planning structure volumes, respectively). This technique was employed for increasing the dose gradient for the prostate cancer IMRT plan shown in Figure 10-2. The planning structure, labeled collar, was introduced around the PTV and a dose constraint was placed on it, improving the gradient in the anterior and lateral directions where the PTV is surrounded by unspecified normal tissue.

In addition to ensuring dose falloff outside the PTV, planning structures can serve a variety of purposes, for instance, to reduce hot spots in a certain region of the PTV (eg, the urethra for a prostate cancer case) or to eliminate high-dose regions appearing far from the PTV or other critical structures. Another common use of planning structures is in overlap regions, such as when the PTV overlaps the rectum in a prostate IMRT plan. In such a case, instead of setting conflicting objectives and constraints on each of the overlapping structures and having the optimizer decide on a tradeoff, the planner can create a planning structure consisting of the rectum minus the PTV, possibly with a margin between to allow for the dose gradient. This makes selection of appropriate goals and constraints manageable. It may also be useful to define another planning structure consisting of the PTV inside the rectum to reduce hot spots near the prostate-rectum interface. Two planning structures, post1 and post2, were defined for this purpose in the IMRT prostate example illustrated in Figure 10-2. Post 1 is the volume of rectum that is not in the PTV but is in the collar. Post 2 is the volume of rectum that is not in the PTV or in the collar. Separate dose-volume constraints were placed on these structures during the optimization process.

Selection Criteria

A major difference between conventional and IMRT planning is that in the former, the planner is continually evaluating the quality of a plan during its construction, whereas in the latter, control of the optimization process is governed by a computer algorithm attempting to minimize a cost function. The implication of this difference is that for IMRT, the planner must encode all of the desired components of a treatment plan into a few numbers that are used as input for the planning system. Furthermore, this must be done such that the value of the cost function computed by the IMRT planning system is lower for preferred plans.

The available parameters are planning system dependent, as are the effects of weighting and priority factors. The actual cost function is often a "black box" to the planner. Furthermore, only a limited amount of information is encapsulated in the planning parameters, and the system may ignore an obvious deficit in a plan because it was not assigned a cost. Conventional experience and intuition are

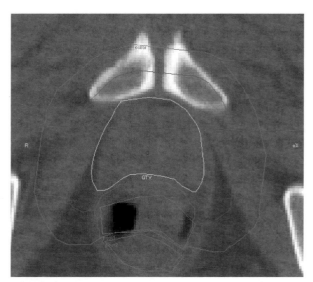

FIGURE 10-2. Illustration of the use of "planning structures." The gross tumor volume (GTV) and planning target volume (PTV) are shown in yellow and magenta, respectively. The PTV is expanded to produce a structure, denoted as "collar" (gray), which is used to conform the dose to the shape of the PTV. Other planning structures include Post 1 and Post 2 (both gray), which are used to improve the dose gradient though the rectum (red). (To view a color version of this image, please refer to the CD-ROM).

not easily transferred to IMRT planning. The phrase "a picture is worth a thousand words" aptly captures the distinction. The influence of the topology of the dose distribution, including locations of hot and cold spots, on the expected treatment outcome is easily appreciated and evaluated when a skilled dosimetrist reviews a plan. However, IMRT planning systems cannot see the big picture because they are lost in the details of the cost function. Therefore, the planner is forced to explore the solution space for various input parameters that will result in a desirable plan. The planner must make quantitative decisions that are neither intuitive nor knowledge based. For example, one may need to communicate to the planning system the relative importance of keeping the mean kidney dose to < 20 Gy versus the maximum cord dose to < 45 Gy. This is precisely why, when beginning a new IMRT program or when moving to a new treatment site, the initial time investment is large and why taking advantage of workshops focusing on a particular IMRT planning and delivery systems is warranted.

It is also essential to establish IMRT planning goals and selection criteria for each treatment site that are independent of the hardware and software. These goals may be obtained by reviewing the treatment records of patients treated with three-dimensional conventional radiation therapy at an individual center. There are now established protocols (Radiation Therapy Oncology Group [RTOG] H-0022 and 0225) and peer-reviewed articles on IMRT that may also provide starting points for establishing goals. These goals may include the maximum acceptable dose delivered to an organ and the fraction (or absolute volume) of that organ receiving a particular dose. The goals must also include values for the PTV, clinical target volume, and gross tumor volume.

Establishing general plan selection criteria that are universally applicable is difficult, even for a single treatment site. This is because the medical history of patients often has a significant impact on their care. However, site-specific guidelines are useful to structure the planning process. Developing criteria is relatively straightforward for sites with a limited number of planning goals. In the treatment of prostate cancer, for example, the planning goals may involve the percentage of the PTV receiving the prescription dose, the maximum rectal dose, the volume of bladder receiving a certain dose, and the magnitude of any hot spots outside these structures. Thus, ranking the importance of these goals may be enumerated in a few statements. For complex regions, such as the head and neck, the number of organs is increased and different dose-volume relationships are involved, so that enumerating all possibilities is not productive a priori because it is not known what is achievable by the planning system. In these cases, although the specification of only a few key criteria may be possible, it is still useful.

To meet the often stringent dosimetric goals and constraints imposed by the user, the optimizer may use field segments, which are either very small in aperture area or

have a very low number of MUs. This may create discrepancies between doses planned and actually delivered. Some planning systems have the ability to set minimum values for these parameters. The appropriate values vary depending on the linear accelerator used; therefore, accelerator-specific values should be determined experimentally.

Another issue that takes even more importance when planning IMRT is the review of the isodose lines of a candidate plan. In three-dimensional conventional planning, the high-dose volume is confined to the geometric intersection of the beams. In IMRT, the strong variation of fluence across fields can create unexpected volumes of high dose far outside the general area of beam intersections. For this reason, it is advisable to carefully examine the dose distribution on every slice of the planning scan. One instance in which the generation of unexpected hot spots can become of particular importance is when part of the PTV is very superficial. Forcing the optimizer to completely cover the PTV will likely produce extremely heavily weighted segments. In this situation, regions near the surface (< 5 mm depth) may receive a high dose. However, many dose calculation algorithms are not reliable at shallow depths. If PTV coverage is truly indicated, a better solution may be to apply a bolus.

Finally, based on the selection criteria, an IMRT plan should be better than a conventional plan before it is used. The comparison must be made using identical volume definitions for all structures. For example, it is not permissible to use tighter margins between the clinical target volume and the PTV for IMRT planning than are used in conventional planning, unless the immobilization and localization process is different between the two. Thus, a conventional plan should be constructed for each case, unless experience clearly dictates that IMRT is warranted.

Commercial Planning Systems

Listed below is a brief description of the commercially available IMRT planning systems as provided by the individual manufacturers. A summary of these planning systems is also provided in Table 10-1.

BrainLAB

BrainLAB (Heimstetten, Germany) IMRT is a component of the *BrainSCAN* treatment planning system (Figure 10-3). Planning begins after the user has defined all of the targets and relevant OAR. The planning goals are entered in the form of dose-volume constraints (ie, DVHs) for the PTVs and OAR. Other user-defined options include a variable calculation grid size, selection between dynamic or static delivery, resolution of the IMRT fluence map, optimization of the tongue-and-groove effect, and relative importance weighting between at-risk organs. In addition, normal tissue around the PTV can be easily defined as an OAR for which a constraint can be set. This will reduce the high-dose areas around the PTV.

TABLE 10-1. Intensity-Modulated Radiation Therapy Planning Systems

Company (Web Site)	Product	Input Parameters	Dose Calculation	Optimization	Plan Evaluation	Unique Features
BrainLAB (www.brainlab.com)	BrainSCAN	DVH constraints	Pencil beam algorithm	Dynamically penalized likelihood	Isodose distributions, DVHs	4 plans calculated simultaneously
CMS Inc. (www.cmsrtp.com)	XiO IMRT	Dose, dose-volume constraints	Pencil beam algorithm	Conjugate gradient	Isodose distributions, DVHs; review MLC segments	Ability to generate compensator files
Elekta Inc. (www.elekta.com)	PrecisePlan	DVH objectives and priorities	Modified Clarkson algorithm	Cimmino algorithm	Isodose distributions, DVHs; review of beams, segments	Delivery optimized with automatic segment ordering
North American Scientific, NOMOS Radiation Oncology Division (www.nasmedical.com)	CORVUS	DVH constraints, tissue types	Pencil beam or Monte Carlo algorithm	Gradient, discrete and continuous annealing	Isodose distributions, DVHs	Ability to modify isodose distribution interactively
Philips Medical Systems (www.medical.philips.com)	Pinnacle-PRO	Minimum and maximum doses, penalties	Collapsed cone convolution superposition	Sequential quadratic programming for nonlinear problems	Isodose distributions, DVHs	Includes biologic optimization
Prowess Inc. (www.prowess.com)	Panther DAO IMRT	DVH constraints, number of apertures/beam	Convolution, superposition	Simulated annealing	Isodose distributions, DVHs	Can produce intensity-modulated fields using jaws only
RAHD Oncology Products (www.rahd.com)	3-D/Pro, KonRad	DVHs, penalty factors	Multikernel pencil beam algorithm	Gradient algorithm	Isodose distributions, DVHs	Leaf sequencing incorporated into inverse planning
Siemens Medical Solutions (www.siemens.com/oncology)	KonRad	Dose-volume constraints and limits	Multikernel pencil beam algorithm	Gradient algorithm	Isodose distributions, DVHs, plan statistics	IMRT-specific report feature
TomoTherapy, Inc. (www.tomotherapy.com)	Hi-ART	DVHs, user-defined treatment variables	Convolution, superposition	Iterative least squares	Isodose distributions, DVHs	CT acquired at time of treatment and daily plan modification
Varian Medical Systems (www.varian.com)	Eclipse	DVH constraints	Pencil beam convolution	Gradient optimization	Isodose distributions, DVHs	Interactive planning

Adapted from Palacio M. IMRT treatment planning systems. Adv Imaging Oncol Admin 2004;14(4):56–9.

CT = computed tomography; DVH = dose-volume histogram; MLC = multileaf collimators.

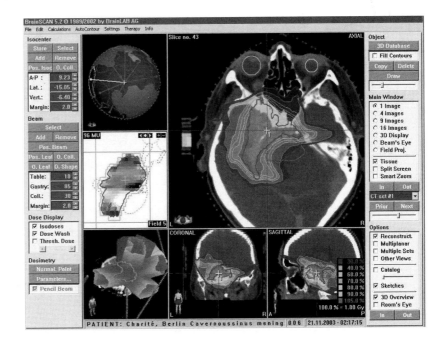

FIGURE 10-3. The BrainSCAN treatment planning environment. (To view a color version of this image, please refer to the CD-ROM). Courtesy of Franz Gum, BrainLAB.

BrainSCAN's optimization algorithm is known as the dynamically penalized likelihood (DPL) estimator. The DPL evolved from the well-known maximum likelihood estimator with dynamically changing penalization terms. Based on statistical estimation theory, the minimization of errors between desired and delivered doses is equivalent to a least squares minimization, except that the DPL yields only nonnegative beamlets and does not get trapped in local minima of the cost function (ie, it always converges to an optimal solution). Through this algorithm, beam delivery conditions imposed by the MLC and avoidance of hot spots in normal tissues are optimized inside the inversion loop.

The *BrainSCAN* pencil beam (PB) algorithm is based on the assumption that the photon scatter is implicit to the beam data measurements and does not vary significantly with the depth in a medium. The algorithm is a further development of the work of Mohan and colleagues.[14] The incident beam is divided into many small beamlets, for which an individual radiologic path length correction is performed to take tissue inhomogeneities into account. These polyenergetic PB kernels are transformed to momentum space by fast Fourier transformation (FFT) for a two-dimensional convolution with the fluence distribution of the beam.

The *BrainSCAN* leaf-sequencing algorithm is based on the algorithm published by Bortfeld and colleagues.[15] Dynamic multileaf collimator (MLC) IMRT has been implemented as an extension of the published algorithm. This implementation additionally accounts for the MLC transmission and minimizes the leakage between opposing and neighboring leaves. The dosimetric problem associated with the tongue-and-groove design of the MLC is also addressed, and the synchronization is achieved without increased beam-on time.

BrainSCAN's IMRT system provides the automatic and simultaneous calculation of four different plans for immediate plan comparison. This allows the clinician to be able to choose the best plan for the particular patient without time-consuming recalculations should the plan not suit all requirements. The four plans differ by having a different importance weighting of PTV and OAR constraints. Plan evaluation tools include isodose distributions overlaid on computed tomography (CT) slices and DVHs.

Computerized Medical Systems Inc.

Computerized Medical Systems (CMS) Inc.'s (St. Louis, MO) *XiO* is a three-dimensional treatment planning system that incorporates modern dose calculation algorithms with an intuitive user interface driven by icons and "drop-down" menus. *XiO* can be used for a variety of planning tasks, ranging from simple point dose calculations to three-dimensional conformal and complex IMRT plans (Figure 10-4).

In *XiO* IMRT, which uses a conjugate gradient optimizer, the cost function is composed of the sum of objective functions. Each objective function, or simply "objective," is an anatomy-specific function that establishes dose goals (eg, the PTV should receive at least 60 Gy and no more than 66 Gy, and the spinal cord should receive no more than 45 Gy) or dose-volume goals (eg, no more than 40% of the liver should receive more than 50 Gy). IMRT dose constraints are entered either through a spreadsheet or an interactive graph. Minimum, maximum, and goal dose constraints can be entered for target volumes. Maximum, dose-volume, and dose-threshold constraints can be entered for OAR. Importance weights and penalty powers can be specified for each dose minimum, maximum, and volume constraint.

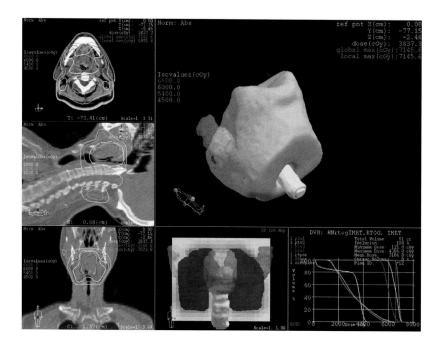

FIGURE 10-4. The XiO IMRT planning interface. (To view a color version of this image, please refer to the CD-ROM). Courtesy of Therese Munger, CMS Inc.

Beamlet doses are calculated using a variation on the PB algorithm. The total energy released per unit mass (TERMA) is computed as is normally done for convolution-based algorithms. This TERMA is then convolved with a simple two-dimensional analytic formula shown to produce self-consistent PB profiles.[16] These "fast" PBs are then corrected so that they yield the same summed result as the original, unmodulated field dose calculation. Dose is calculated using a very accurate fast Fourier transformation, superposition, or fast superposition algorithm (user selected). Therefore, the *XiO* PB calculation has the favorable property that it reproduces the characteristics of its base photon calculation. Existing dose (eg, when using IMRT for a boost to a three-dimensional conventional plan) may also be accounted for during the optimization process (the user controls this), and the original beams are unaffected by the optimizer. Tradeoffs between optimization speed and plan accuracy are made by specifying the resolution of the optimization grid, the scatter extents of the beamlets, and the size of the beamlets.

The resulting intensity maps can be displayed, edited, made discrete, and exported. Changes in the optimized intensity map, either through manual editing or discretization, are reflected in the updated isodose distribution. Optimized intensity maps can be automatically extended to account for tissue swelling and respiratory motion (useful for breast or head and neck IMRT plans). The user can control the minimum size of MLC segments and the number of intensity levels onto which the intensity map is discretized prior to segmentation. At the end of the final dose calculation, the user has the option of sending the beams (with the actual segments) back to the optimizer to fine-tune the beam weights.

Plan evaluation tools offer the ability to compare the optimized dose with the final dose; view, print, and edit intensity and fluence maps; and review MLC segments (with the ability to delete unwanted segments and view and print the leaf positions of any or all segments), as well as a plan summary, which includes the beam setup, dose calculation parameters, IMRT prescription, and MU information. MLC segments are sent to the record and verify system via DICOM (Digital Imaging and Communication in Medicine). Milling machine files can also be generated for compensating filters.

Elekta Inc.

Elekta Inc.'s (Norcross, GA) *PrecisePLAN* uses an aperture-based inverse planning method for IMRT optimization that incorporates human intuition into the planning process (Figure 10-5). This technique is a natural extension to existing three-dimensional conformal practices and yields a relatively small number of beam segments. The user specifies DVH objectives and priorities for the PTV and normal tissues. The apertures are then created in two phases. In the initial phase, the system automatically creates geometric segments using user-directed preferences for structure inclusion or exclusion. After running the optimizer (Cimmino algorithm), a second set of segments is created that targets residual low-dose regions. The optimizer is run again, after which more dose-based apertures can be drawn if desired.

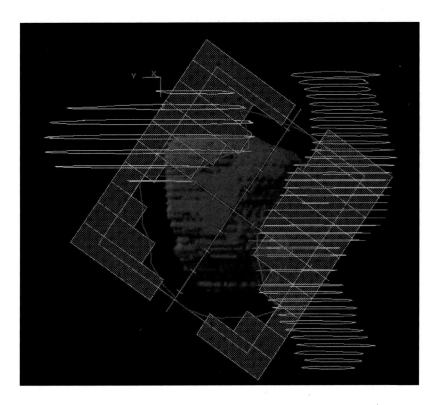

FIGURE 10-5. Example of aperture optimization using the PrecisePLAN system. (To view a color version of this image, please refer to the CD-ROM). Courtesy of Timothy Prosser, Elekta Inc.

The collimator is free to rotate between segments so that the MLC leaves may optimally conform to the requested MLC shape in either phase of segment creation.

IMRT is an extension of existing practice, and many daily cases may be non-IMRT; some patients may have part IMRT, part non-IMRT. Often a patient's treatment may start with a three-dimensional conformal plan, and then a boost plan will be done using IMRT. For patient safety and convenience, these are maintained as a single composite plan within *PrecisePLAN*. With the "fraction groups" feature, such a composite plan can be easily calculated, and the dose contribution associated with each treatment phase is maintained independently. The optimizer considers the dose to previously irradiated structures together with boost plan constraints as it calculates the composite plan. Fraction groups enable beams to be grouped together for different phases of treatment, such as initial treatment and boost. Having these fraction groups available enables composite plans using IMRT to be quickly and easily created.

During optimization, the planner is able to interact with the optimizer, view intermediate results, make adjustments when necessary, and observe the DVH approach dose objectives. Optimization continues until the rate of change drops beneath the threshold or a fixed number of iterations is reached. It may, however, be stopped at any time if a lack of progress indicates that the input segments need to be improved or the objectives reconsidered. The optimizer retains all progress and, once changes are made, resumes calculating where it paused. Dose is calculated using a modified Clarkson integration algorithm. Plan evaluation tools include image review of the beams or segments using digitally reconstructed radiographs, DVH comparison, and simultaneous, multiple-plane isodose evaluation.

North American Scientific (NOMOS)

North American Scientific, NOMOS Radiation Oncology Division (Cranberry Township, PA) pioneered IMRT with the introduction of the *CORVUS* inverse treatment planning system in 1994. Originally, *CORVUS* was used as part of the *PEACOCK* system, NOMOS's tomotherapy planning and delivery system. Shortly thereafter, *CORVUS* added capability to plan IMRT treatments using conventional static and dynamic multileaf collimation (Figure 10-6).

In the *CORVUS* planning system, the user prescribes objectives that are presented as a cumulative DVH. For each target, the user specifies the minimum and maximum allowable dose, the goal dose, and a percentage of the volume that the user will tolerate receiving less than the goal dose. For each OAR, the user specifies the maximum allowable dose, the limit dose, and a percentage of the volume that the user will tolerate receiving more than the limit dose. Also, for each OAR, the user specifies a minimum dose, below which the organ receives no detrimental damage.

The user also specifies the tissue type of each target or OAR. The type selected influences the objective function parameters that will be used for evaluating the fitness of the planned dose distribution. In the case of targets, *CORVUS* provides for specialized target types intended for intensity-modulated radiosurgery, highly uniform dose distributions (homogeneous), targets that surround other targets (surround), targets that should be ignored (reference), and standard targets (basic). In the case of OAR, *CORVUS* provides for specialized tissue types intended for parallel organs (BU), critical organs (critical), organs that should be ignored (reference), organs that are expendable to meet the target objective (expendable), and standard OAR (basic).

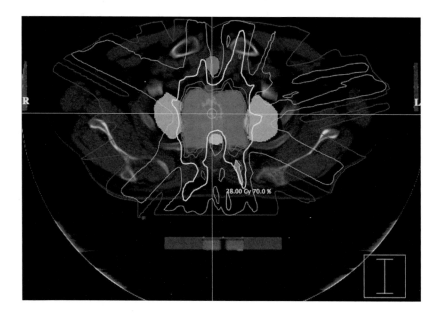

FIGURE 10-6. Modification of the 70% isodose line using ActiveRx in the CORVUS planning system. The user adjusts the 70% isodose line extending into normal tissue by "dragging" the dose toward the PTV. The fluence maps are automatically modified in this process. (To view a color version of this image, please refer to the CD-ROM). Courtesy of Robert Hill, North American Scientific, NOMOS Radiation Oncology Division.

CORVUS supports multiple optimization algorithms, which can be selected by the user. A gradient algorithm can be employed, which produces smoother intensity distributions that require fewer MUs and segments but produces a less conformal dose distribution. A discrete annealing algorithm is also available, which results in slightly more complex plans than gradient algorithms but with improved dose conformity. Lastly, the system supports a continuous annealing algorithm, which produces highly conformal and complex treatment plans.

The user may specify a tradeoff between delivery complexity and dose conformity using a number of controls and methods. For example, the *FAST IMRT* delivery control includes a term in the objective function that causes plans with higher delivery complexities to be penalized when compared with plans with lower delivery complexities. In the case of tomotherapy treatments, *FAST IMRT* allows the user to control the number of MUs used in the plan. For static or dynamic multileaf collimation, *FAST IMRT* allows the user to reduce the segment count as low as one segment per beam, should that be desired.

CORVUS uses advanced PB dose calculation software specially designed to improve dosimetric agreement over the range of field sizes used in IMRT treatments. In addition, *CORVUS* has integrated support for *PEREGRINE*, North American Scientific's Monte Carlo–based dose calculation system. *PEREGRINE* can be used as a replacement for the *CORVUS* PB dose calculation software or as a quality assurance tool to verify that the dose distribution calculated by *CORVUS* is correct.

After the plan is optimized, leaf sequencing commences. *CORVUS* includes several leaf sequencing algorithms, each specifically tuned to maximize the quality of the plan for each delivery system. Leaf sequencing includes corrections for the tongue-and-groove effect, differences between the light and radiation field, and partial transmission through MLC leaves, to create a treatment plan that matches the optimized intensity distribution to the maximal possible extent.

A number of plan evaluation tools are available, including two- and three-dimensional isodose displays, DVHs, statistical outputs, digitally reconstructed radiographs, and treatment plan summaries. At this point, the user must decide if the plan is acceptable as is or if changes are required. If changes are required, *CORVUS* includes *ActiveRx*, which allows real-time modification of the optimized treatment plan by sculpting or dragging isodose lines, erasing hot or cold spots, dragging DVHs, or constraining minimum or maximum doses to targets or OAR. *ActiveRx* uses advanced plan sampling and optimization techniques to provide treatment plan optimization to modify the plan based on a user request in just a few seconds and immediately provides feedback to the user by automatically updating dose distributions, statistics, and cumulative DVHs.

After arriving at an acceptable treatment plan, *CORVUS* allows the user to specify one or more systems to which

plan information can be transferred, including record and verify systems, various delivery systems, and image-guided therapy systems, such as North American Scientific's *BAT* (B-mode acquisition and targeting) system. The transport mechanism may use a DICOM network transfer, a variety of other network protocols, or a floppy disk as directed by the user.

Philips Medical Systems

The *Pinnacle³* treatment planning system from Philips Medical Systems (Andover, MA) provides integrated three-dimensional planning, CT simulation, and IMRT inverse planning (Figure 10-7). Inverse planning is performed using the *P³IMRT* software module developed in partnership with RaySearch Laboratories AB in Stockholm, Sweden.

For targets, the clinical objectives for an optimized plan are expressed in terms of minimum dose, maximum dose, minimum dose to a given volume, maximum dose to a given volume, and uniform dose. For OAR, any combination of maximum dose and maximum dose to a given volume may be used. A weight or penalty factor is assigned to each objective to reflect its importance in the overall treatment objective. *P³IMRT* also allows for the use of constraints (objectives that must not be violated) during optimization. Any dose-based objective can be specified as a constraint except the uniform dose objective, but a uniformity constraint can be used to force the dose within the volume to vary by less than a specified percentage. A biologic optimization and review module adds the ability to combine generalized equivalent uniform dose objectives with dose-based objectives and constraints.

The optimization algorithm divides the beam's eye view of the targets for each beam into a series of finite-sized beamlets. The corresponding weights of the beamlets are optimized to produce a fluence or intensity map for each beam. During optimization, the Delta Pixel Beam dose computation is used to determine the dose from the intensity-modulated beam.[17] The quality of the plan is scored based on the predefined treatment goals to achieve a balance between adequate target coverage and sparing OAR. In addition to intensity modulation optimization, beam weight and segment weight optimization are also available.

The *P³IMRT* optimization engine uses NPSOL, a sequential quadratic programming algorithm for solving general nonlinear optimization problems.[18,19] The generated fluence map is a transmission filter expressed as the relative intensity between the intensity-modulated beam and the open beam exiting the treatment head. Each fluence map is discretized over a grid (typically 5 mm resolution). The weight of the corresponding beam elements (pixels) constitutes the optimization variables.

Pinnacle³ uses a collapsed cone convolution superposition (CCCS) computation to determine the dose distribution from external photon beams. The CCCS dose model is a true three-dimensional dose computation that intrin-

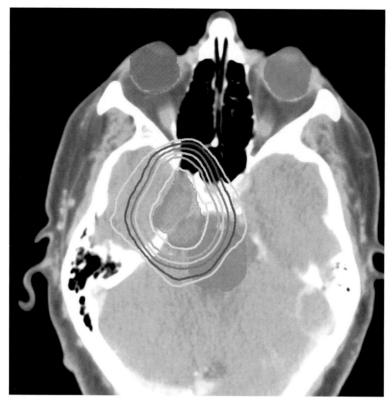

FIGURE 10-7. A treatment plan produced using the P³IMRT planning system. (To view a color version of this image, please refer to the CD-ROM). Courtesy of Todd McNutt, Philips Radiation Oncology Systems.

sically handles the effects of patient heterogeneities on both primary and secondary scattered radiation. This computation method is inherently able to account for dose distributions in areas in which electronic equilibrium is perturbed, such as tissue-air interfaces and tissue-bone interfaces. Because IMRT requires both fast and accurate dose calculation, a hybrid dose calculation of the CCCS and a finite PB technique, Delta Pixel Beam, are used to maintain CCCS accuracy while providing speed for IMRT optimization.

P³IMRT allows for both step-and-shoot and sliding window conversions. A direct machine parameter optimization module provides the ability to directly optimize MLC leaf positions and segment weights during the optimization process. This offers the potential to produce step-and-shoot plans with a minimum number of segments and total MUs. *Pinnacle³* offers a number of plan evaluation tools, including DVHs for single or multiple plans, side-by-side isodose comparison between competing plans, tumor control probabilities, and normal tissue complication probabilities.

Prowess Inc.

Prowess, Inc. (Chico, CA), in cooperation with the University of Maryland, has developed direct aperture optimization and incorporated the technology into its two Prowess *Panther IMRT* treatment planning products (Figure 10-8).

One product, *DAO IMRT*, uses an MLC, whereas the other, *Jaws-Only IMRT*, requires only the jaws of the linear accelerator to shape the beams.

The user prespecifies the number of apertures to deliver from each beam direction. Input parameters include DVH constraints for target volumes, critical volumes, the number of beams, the number of apertures per beam, and the prescribed dose. The physical limitations of the MLC are also taken into account during the optimization process, so the constraints are machine specific rather than generic. Using a simulated annealing algorithm, a technique is used that simultaneously optimizes the leaf positions and weights of the apertures rather than the relative weights of the PBs. Leaf sequencing is eliminated, and the resulting plans have significantly fewer segments. The objective function can be in the form of a dose, DVHs, or a biologic function.

DAO IMRT uses a convolution and superposition dose calculation engine that takes into account the effects of radiation scattered from surrounding tissue and provides results reasonably close to those of Monte Carlo calculations, in much less time. Plan evaluation tools include isodose overlays and DVHs.

RAHD Oncology Products

RAHD Oncology Products (St. Louis, MO) has integrated the *KonRad* inverse calculation engine into the *RAHD 3D/Pro*

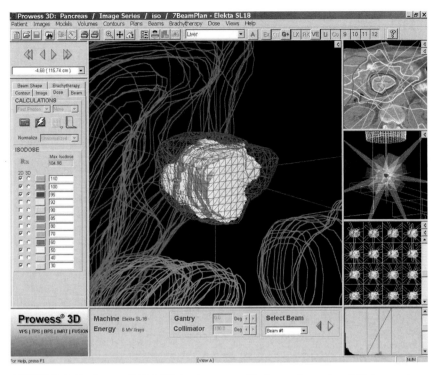

FIGURE 10-8. The Prowess DAO IMRT planning system. (To view a color version of this image, please refer to the CD-ROM). Courtesy of Brian Horvath, Prowess Inc.

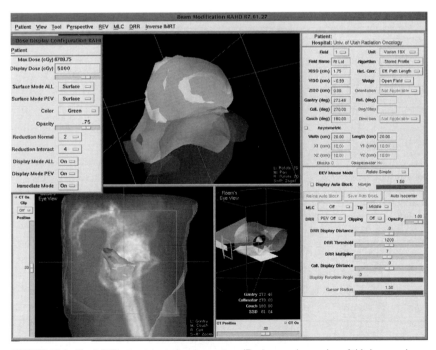

FIGURE 10-9. The 3-D/Pro treatment planning system. (To view a color version of this image, please refer to the CD-ROM). Courtesy of Mark Russell, RAHD Oncology Products.

conformal planning system desktop (Figure 10-9). Using the *RAHD 3D/Pro* virtual simulation tools, targets, structures, and regions of interest are created for either forward, conformal, or inverse planning. Plans can be developed with either approach using a common virtual patient. Once the dose is calculated, it can be evaluated, combined in a composite plan, or compared with other plans for analysis of the best solution. Many valuable variations are available from within this spectrum of tools. Inverse planning integrated with progressive three-dimensional conformal planning allows complicated problems to be evaluated using both a three-dimensional conformal plan and an IMRT plan. The planner can select between these plans or combine them.

The use of a slider-bar weighting tool dynamically assigns a relative dose value to a prescription point and is variable by individual beam or by group. In both cases, when adjusting the weight of one beam or group, the remaining beams are adjusted proportionally to maintain the prescription dose at the prescription point. The dose for any beam or group can be locked, allowing the weighting parameters to be proportionally distributed to the unlocked beams.

The efficient use of forward-planning IMRT requires simplified MLC beam design. Beam shapes for target volumes can be automatically defined with user-selected margins applied dynamically while adjusting the geometry of the setup. Importing dose volumes from three-dimensional radiation therapy or IMRT conformal plans allows field shaping around dose volumes to boost cold spots or block hot spots, improving the dose uniformity by use of multiple segments. Exporting plans to any of the record and verification systems automates the communication of plan delivery parameters to the linear accelerator.

Siemens Medical Solutions

Siemens Medical Solutions (Malvern, PA) uses the *KonRad* (MRC Systems GmbH, Heidelberg, Germany) inverse planning software for IMRT planning (Figure 10-10). By means of dose-volume constraints and/or absolute dose limits for overdosage of OAR and for underdosage and overdosage of the tumor, the oncologist provides the objectives of the optimization (gradient algorithm). Penalty factors allow for an additional ranking of these dose limits and can therefore incorporate their clinical importance. Parallel organs may be modeled using dose-volume constraints by assigning higher-tolerance doses to volume fractions of the organ if a higher dose to the tumor can be achieved. However, serial organs may be better modeled using restrictive maximum dose constraints. As its inverse planning algorithm, the system uses the weighted quadratic difference of prescribed and calculated dose distributions, which is the most common type of dose-based objective function.

Dose is calculated using the multikernel PB algorithm and full three-dimensional ray-tracing. Inhomogeneity corrections are included as part of the planning system. The leaf sequencer is used to convert an optimized fluence into a deliverable sequence of MLC segments. It takes into account machine limitations and constraints, such as the transmission through the primary and secondary collimators or through the rounded leaf-ends of some MLC. *KonRad*'s sequencer can create deliverable fluences for both

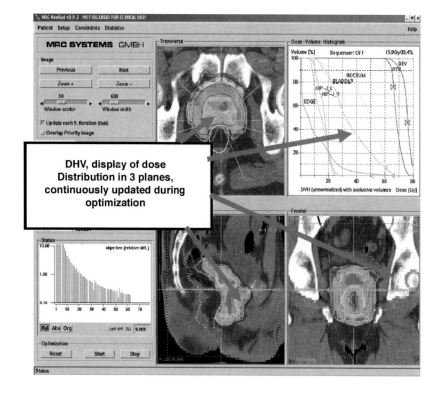

FIGURE 10-10. The Siemens IMRT planning system. DHV = dose-volume histogram. (To view a color version of this image, please refer to the CD-ROM). Courtesy of Sandi Lotter, Siemens Medical Solutions.

static or dynamic MLC modes. In addition, *KonRad* provides the user with intensity filtering features, which can significantly improve the deliverability of optimized fluences. Plans are evaluated using side-by-side comparisons of dose distribution and DVHs. Additionally, plans are summarized in tabular form to compare statistical quantities.

TomoTherapy Inc.

TomoTherapy (Madison, WI) is a unique delivery system that combines the capabilities of a helical CT scanner with those of a linear accelerator. Unlike linear accelator–based IMRT planning, there are no beam angles to define. Rather, the optimizer relies on the user to define the prescription based on regions of interests, which are divided into two categories: tumor and region at risk. If two structures are overlapping, the user may choose which structure the shared voxels belong to for optimization. The user also selects which of the contoured structures are to be used for optimization (Figure 10-11).

The helical delivery is emulated by calculating 51 projections per rotation. The planning process is typically accomplished in two phases: a relatively passive phase, in which the beamlets are precalculated, and an interactive optimization phase, in which the final plan is rapidly developed. The number of beamlets used in any particular case depends on a number of user-defined parameters. It may vary from approximately 4,500 beamlets for a prostate IMRT plan to over 100,000 beamlets for a craniospinal plan.

The *TomoTherapy* planning system uses an inverse treatment planning process based on iterative least squares minimization of an objective function. The optimization is driven by several user-defined parameters. The pitch determines the amount of beam overlap, at the machine isocenter, between gantry rotations. It is defined as the distance traveled by the couch during one complete rotation, divided by the field width. Pitch settings of less than 1 will provide more overlap between the rotations to allow for uniformity in the dose distribution. The fan beam width of the beam is defined in CT terms. It is the superior or inferior dimension of the fan beam (range 10–50 mm). The modulation factor determines the range of intensity values that are allowed in the optimized plan. The modulation factor is calculated from the leaf sinogram and is defined as the greatest leaf intensity, divided by the average intensity for all nonzero leaves. The importance factor indicates the relative weight of the selected structure compared with other structures (tumor and region at risk) included in the optimization plan. Relative importance applies to meeting the goals of the minimum and maximum doses for the selected structure (as well as the DVH dose for regions at risk) and is rated on an arbitrary scale. Lastly, the prescription is defined as the dose (Gy) to be delivered to a percentage of the tumor volume. Minimum and maximum doses are defined by the user with the appropriate "penalties" to the structure, along with a dose or volume penalty for regions at risk.

Once the beamlets are calculated, each optimization iteration takes approximately 4 seconds to calculate using full convolution or the superposition dose, which compares the results with the prescribed dose. This algorithm provides accurate results in the presence of inhomogeneities, high gradient regions, and electronic nonequilibrium situations. Optimization is an interactive process through

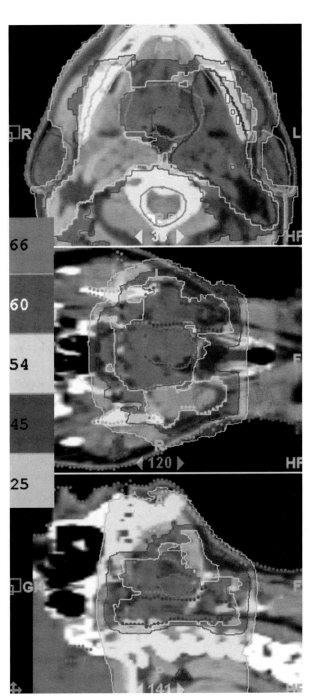

FIGURE 10-11. A head and neck intensity-modulated radiation therapy plan produced by the Hi-ART planning system. (To view a color version of this image, please refer to the CD-ROM). Courtesy of Sam Jeswani, TomoTherapy Inc.

which the user may modify the outcome of the plan. Plans are evaluated using a variety of tools, including isodose lines and clouds, as well as DVHs.

On the day of treatment, a megavoltage CT scan (*TomoImage*) of the region of interest is acquired. This image set is then aligned to the reference (planning) CT scan. Based on the difference in position between the two scans, the dose distribution can be adjusted to take into account the daily patient position.

Varian Medical Systems

Varian Medical Systems' (Palo Alto, CA) *Eclipse* treatment planning system has a full complement of capabilities that support photon, electron, and proton therapy (Figure 10-12). *Eclipse* employs interactive IMRT planning. The user specifies planning constraints in the form of DVHs, and IMRT plans are generated using a gradient optimization algorithm. The user is able to observe the progress of optimization and to modify dose objectives in real time, while the plan is optimized. This capability guarantees that desired results are achieved quickly and shortens the IMRT learning curve. *Eclipse's* interactive planning gives users the ability to make clinical tradeoffs as the plan evolves, thereby allowing the planner to create the best plan for each patient. *Eclipse* is part of Varian's *SmartBeam IMRT* solution and supports both high-resolution dynamic IMRT and segmental IMRT of any resolution.

Eclipse uses a PB convolution for photon dose calculations. Beam data configuration requires depth-dose data, beam profiles, and output factors. Blocks, MLC, enhanced dynamic wedges, motorized wedges, and virtual wedges are fully supported in *Eclipse*.

Plan evaluation in *Eclipse* allows the user to customize the display of the dose distributions in both two- and three-dimensional views. Isodose lines or colorwash can be used to view dose distributions. Users can create and modify

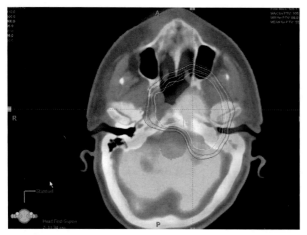

FIGURE 10-12. A computed tomography–positron emission tomography image dataset used to create an intensity-modulated radiation therapy plan in Eclipse. (To view a color version of this image, please refer to the CD-ROM). Courtesy of L. Scott Johnson, Varian Medical Systems.

templates that store isodose line values and colors. Hard copy reports include beam's eye view plots, isodose plots, flexible plan reports, and numerous other plan evaluation plots. Electronic plan approval in *Eclipse* is password protected. Approved plans cannot be modified.

Planning Methodology

Most IMRT planning systems provide a general description of their dose optimization algorithm. However, the cost function is often not specified, and the planner is given little or no guidance on how varying a single input parameter will affect the overall quality of a treatment plan. This type of knowledge can be gained only through trial and error. A systematic approach used in many clinics involves beginning with a single dose constraint (such as the PTV dose) and adding constraints one by one until an acceptable plan is achieved. This approach provides valuable insight into the cost function and the complex interplay between input parameters. Once a set of input parameters is determined, the class solution approach can be employed whereby the same input parameters are used for a given disease site (ie, prostate), and minor "tweaking" of these parameters is performed for each individual patient. Our systematic approach is illustrated in the next section using our research software to illustrate the type of results encountered.[20] Although the results are specific to our planning system, the approach can be generalized to any system.

Prostate Case Example

In this section, a prostate case is used to illustrate the thought process used in producing a clinically acceptable IMRT plan. After obtaining a CT scan, the prostate, seminal vesicles, bladder, rectum, and femoral heads were outlined. In this example, the prostate is the gross tumor volume, and a 1 cm expansion is used to generate the PTV. Starting with an anterior beam and proceeding clockwise, nine beams spaced 40º apart, all with a beamlet size of 0.5 cm, are used to generate each plan.

Iteration 1

The initial goal is to deliver a uniform dose to the PTV. The minimum PTV dose is set equal to the prescription dose, and heterogeneity is minimized. The resulting maximum PTV dose is within 1% of the prescription dose, but there is no normal tissue sparing (Figure 10-13A).

Iteration 2

The PTV dose constraints are relaxed. An additional goal of minimizing the maximum dose to the rectum outside the PTV (rectum dose – PTV dose) is added. The optimization met the planning goals in the PTV, and the maximum dose in the rectum outside the PTV is 59% of the prescription dose; however, an unanticipated result is obtained (Figure 10-13B).

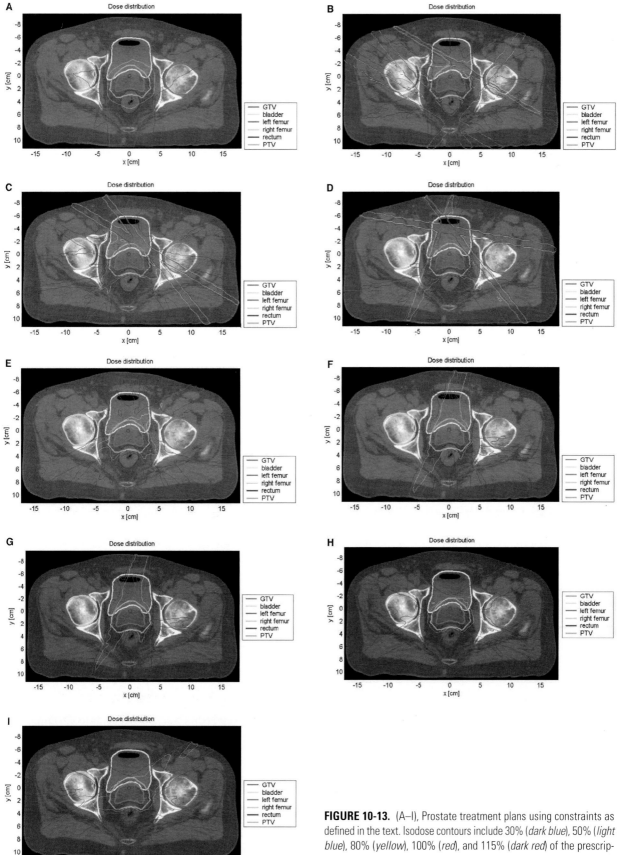

FIGURE 10-13. (A–I), Prostate treatment plans using constraints as defined in the text. Isodose contours include 30% (*dark blue*), 50% (*light blue*), 80% (*yellow*), 100% (*red*), and 115% (*dark red*) of the prescription dose. GTV = gross tumor volume; PTV = planning target volume. (To view a color version of this image, please refer to the CD-ROM).

Iteration 3

Instead of minimizing the maximum rectum dose (as above), a constraint is added to minimize the mean rectum – PTV dose. In this plan, the PTV goals were achieved, and the mean rectum – PTV dose is 15% of the prescription dose. The isodoses conform to the posterior edge of the PTV, but unacceptable hot regions and streaks remain (Figure 10-13C). Note that doses in unconstrained tissues are high because they are not penalized in the cost function.

Iteration 4

In addition to the previous constraints, an upper bound of 25% of the prescription dose is set for the femoral heads. In this case, the PTV and femoral goals are achieved, and the mean rectum – PTV dose is 30% of the prescription dose. The isodoses conform to the posterior edge of the PTV, but unacceptable hot streaks remain, and there is no significant improvement in the overall plan quality (Figure 10-13D).

Iteration 5

Building on the previous iteration, an upper bound of 33% of the prescription dose is placed on the mean rectum – PTV dose, and the mean bladder dose is minimized. The plan is significantly improved. PTV, rectal, and femur goals are achieved, and the mean bladder dose is 54% of the prescription dose. Only a few hot spots remain (Figure 10-13E). The only remaining volume to place constraints on is tissue within the external contour (skin).

Iteration 6

Small modifications are made on previous input parameters. In particular, upper bounds of 37.5%, 50%, and 71% of the prescription dose are set for the femurs, mean rectum – PTV dose, and mean bladder dose, respectively. In addition, the mean external dose is minimized (excluding all other structures). All goals are achieved, and the mean external dose is 17% of the prescription dose. However, several hot spots remain (Figure 10-13F).

Iteration 7

In the last iteration, pixels near the edge of the PTV are penalized by the external goal. Thus, a collar is added to the PTV, permitting the exclusion of this region from consideration in the minimization. The collar is 6 pixels wide (5.625 mm). The mean external dose to be minimized now represents the volume enclosed by the external contour, excluding the PTV + collar and all other structures. The goals are achieved, and the mean external dose is 17% of the prescription dose (Figure 10-13G). The most striking feature of the dose distribution is the hot spot in the bladder.

Iteration 8

The mean external dose is relaxed and set to an upper bound of 26% of the prescription dose. The mean bladder dose is added as a parameter to be minimized. In this example, the goals are achieved, and the mean bladder dose is 37% of the prescription dose (Figure 10-13H). A few regions of medium dose persist.

Iteration 9

An upper bound of the external dose is set to 80% of the prescription dose. All other parameters remain the same. All goals are achieved, and the mean bladder dose is 39% of the prescription dose (Figure 10-13I). The plan is now acceptable. Further improvement may be possible by lowering the doses of the constraint upper bounds.

Summary

Many options are available for IMRT planning. The selection of a particular planning system is limited by the IMRT delivery hardware. However, there are still several choices for most hardware platforms. Rather than converging to a smaller number, it appears that the number of options will further increase once beam orientation becomes part of the optimization engine. Thus, IMRT treatment plan optimization will become more automated, requiring careful scrutiny of the influence of the optimization parameters on the final result.

This chapter has presented several important planning considerations for IMRT. Consensus positions have also provided such a description for the entire IMRT process.[21,22] These works are useful because they provide a framework for comparison of the wide variety of methods that are available in practice. For detailed guidance on IMRT planning specific to a particular hardware or software configuration, it is becoming essential to attend workshops and participate in user groups. The topics discussed in this chapter will inevitably confront the clinician. Although the resolution of the issues will depend on the particular IMRT software, careful consideration of them is expected to lead to better patient care.

Acknowledgments

The authors and editors acknowledge the contributions of Franz Gum (BrainLAB), Robert Hill (North American Scientific, NOMOS Radiation Oncology Division), Brian Horvath (Prowess Inc.), Sam Jeswani (TomoTherapy Inc.), L. Scott Johnson (Varian Medical Systems), Sandi Lotter (Siemens Medical Solutions), Todd McNutt (Philips Medical Systems), Therese Munger (CMS Inc.), Timothy Prosser (Elekta Inc.), and Mark Russell (RAHD Oncology Products).

References

1. Pirzkall A, Carol MP, Pickett B, et al. The effect of beam energy and number of fields on photon-based IMRT for deep-seated targets. Int J Radiat Oncol Biol Phys 2002;53:434–42.

2. Schneider U, Lomax A, Lombriser N. Comparative treatment planning using secondary cancer mortality calculations. Phys Med Biol 2001;17:97–9.

3. Followill D, Geis P, Boyer A. Estimates of whole-body dose equivalent produced by beam intensity modulated conformal therapy. Int J Radiat Oncol Biol Phys 1997;38:667–72.

4. Verellen D, Vanhavere F. Risk assessment of radiation-induced malignancies based on whole-body equivalent dose estimates for IMRT treatment in the head and neck region. Radiother Oncol 1999;53:199–203.

5. Glatstein E. Intensity-modulated radiation therapy: the inverse, the converse, and the perverse. Semin Radiat Oncol 2002;12:272–81.

6. Hall EJ, Wu CS. Radiation-induced second cancers: the impact of 3D-CRT and IMRT. Int J Radiat Oncol Biol Phys 2003;56:83–8.

7. Price RA, Hanks GE, McNeeley SW, et al. Advantages of using noncoplanar vs. axial beam arrangements when treating prostate cancer with intensity-modulated radiation therapy and the step-and-shoot delivery method. Int J Radiat Oncol Biol Phys 2002;53:236–43.

8. Das S, Cullip T, Tracton G, et al. Beam orientation selection for intensity-modulated radiation therapy based on target equivalent uniform dose maximization. Int J Radiat Oncol Biol Phys 2003;55:215–24.

9. Djajaputra D, Wu Q, Wu Y, et al. Algorithm and performance of a clinical IMRT beam-angle optimization system. Phys Med Biol 2003;48:3191–212.

10. Pugachev A, Xing L. Incorporating prior knowledge into beam orientation optimization in IMRT. Int J Radiat Oncol Biol Phys 2002;54:1565–74.

11. Rowbottom CG, Nutting CM, Webb S. Beam-orientation optimization of intensity-modulated radiotherapy: clinical application to parotid gland tumours. Radiother Oncol 2001;59:169–77.

12. Pugachev A, Xing L. Computer-assisted selection of coplanar beam orientations in intensity-modulated radiation therapy. Phys Med Biol 2001;46:2467–76.

13. Pugachev AB, Boyer AL, Xing L. Beam orientation optimization in intensity-modulated radiation treatment planning. Med Phys 2000;27:1238–45.

14. Mohan R, Chui C, Lidofsky L. Differential pencil beam dose computation model for photons. Med Phys 1986;13:64–73.

15. Bortfeld T, Boyer AL, Schlegel W, Kahler DL, Waldron TJ. Realization and verification of three-dimensional conformal radiotherapy with modulated fields. Int J Radiat Oncol Biol Phys. 1994;30:899-908.

16. Alber ML. A concept for the optimization of radiotherapy [thesis].Tübingen (Germany): University of Tübingen; 2001.

17. McNutt T. Dose calculations: collapsed cone convolution superposition and Delta Pixel Beam. Pinnacle³. 2002. White Paper No. 4535 983 02474.

18. Löf J. Development of a general framework for optimization of radiation therapy [thesis]. Stockholm: Stockholm University; 2000.

19. Gill PE, Murray W, Saunders MA, et al. User's guide for NPSOL: a Fortran package for nonlinear programming. 1992. Report No.: Systems Operation Lab (SOL) 86-2.

20. Armbruster B, Lachaine ME, Hamilton RJ, et al. LP formulations for optimizing radiation treatment strategies. In: Institute of Industrial Engineering (IIE) 2004 Annual Conference Proceedings (in press).

21. Ezzell GA, Galvin JM, Low D, et al. Guidance document on delivery, treatment planning, and clinical implementation of IMRT: report of the IMRT Subcommittee of the AAPM Radiation Therapy Committee. Med Phys 2003;30:2089–115.

22. Intensity Modulated Radiation Therapy Collaborative Working Group. Intensity-modulated radiotherapy: current status and issues of interest. Int J Radiat Oncol Biol Phys 2001;51:880–914.

Chapter 11

PLAN EVALUATION

TODD PAWLICKI, PHD, QUYNH-THU LE, MD, CHRISTOPHER KING, MD, PHD

Intensity-modulated radiation therapy (IMRT) represents a novel approach to the planning and delivery of radiation therapy. Physicians and physicists implementing IMRT are thus faced with learning a number of new approaches and techniques, for example, target delineation and quality assurance. These issues have received considerable attention in the literature and are discussed in other chapters in this text.

One aspect of IMRT, however, that has received surprisingly little attention is plan evaluation. A common misconception regarding IMRT is that the treatment planning computer generates the optimal plan, which is then used for treatment. In reality, the computer generates a number of optimized plans based on specified input parameters. The physician and physicist must evaluate these various plans and select the best one to be used in treatment. In some cases, however, all of the plans may be rejected and the optimization process repeated with modified input parameters.

The purpose of this chapter is to provide an overview of the plan evaluation process from a clinical viewpoint. More theoretic considerations, such as biologic modeling of tissue structures, tumor control and tissue complication probabilities, decision making by artificial neural networks, or any of the many other score functions or figures of merit, are beyond the scope of this chapter and are not discussed. Instead, attention is focused on the various plan evaluation tools provided by the major inverse planning systems, such as cumulative dose-volume histograms (DVHs), two-dimensional dose distribution display, three-dimensional dose distribution display, and structure minimum, maximum, and mean dose values. In addition, the impact of various aspects of IMRT planning (eg, patient selection, target delineation, beam selection, field matching) on plan evaluation is also discussed.

IMRT Treatment Planning

A major clinical indication for IMRT is the need to conform a high dose to the target while keeping adjacent normal tissues within tolerance. This section is devoted to discussing the goals of IMRT planning and how those goals may differ from conventional three-dimensional conformal radiation therapy (3DCRT) treatment planning. Users of IMRT expect something different from that provided by 3DCRT techniques, namely, better target coverage and/or better normal tissue sparing. Effective and efficient IMRT plan evaluation is based, in part, on those expectations and differences. The advantages and disadvantages of IMRT in comparison with 3DCRT and some guidelines to determine the optimal patient and tumor characteristics for IMRT are outlined below.

Is IMRT Always Better than 3DCRT?

Whether IMRT is better than 3DCRT depends, in part, on the treatment goals. With IMRT, there are larger volumes of normal tissues receiving low doses, increased monitor units needed for delivery, and verification port film requirements. These can result in an increase in patient exposure from head leakage, neutron production, and scatter.[1–3] This may increase the risk of secondary malignancies in long-term survivors[4] and the probability of pneumonitis in thoracic cancer patients, in whom large volumes of the lungs may receive moderate radiation doses. IMRT also requires significant patient cooperation and more precise immobilization than 3DCRT. However, these drawbacks may be considered acceptable if a more conformal dose distribution is achieved with IMRT.

Target and Normal Tissue Contouring

Tissue contouring impacts plan evaluation. Targets must be drawn carefully, and a marginal miss is a concern in IMRT. It is important to contour not only the gross tumor volume (GTV) but also the clinical target volume (CTV), which includes tissues at risk of microscopic disease involvement. Surrounding normal tissues should also be identified for treatment avoidance. It is best to use the International Commission on Radiation Units and Measurements (ICRU) Report 50[5] or the more current ICRU Report 62[6] definitions and available anatomic atlases or publications to facilitate the accuracy and consistency of contouring.[7–9] Accurate volume delineation will result in optimal IMRT planning and lower the risk of geographic misses.

In situations in which target volumes overlap with normal tissue structures, a priority must be assigned to these overlapping structures, and clinical consideration must be taken into account for these priorities. It is our practice to assign a higher priority to the GTV than surrounding normal tissues and a higher priority to critical neural tissues (ie, optic chiasm, brainstem, and spinal cord) than the adjacent planning target volume (PTV). When it is difficult to achieve a good IMRT plan, an apparently easy solution is to modify the target to conform to the isodose lines. However, such maneuvers limit the efficacy of IMRT and may result in increased risk of treatment failure. It is preferable to loosen the dose constraints and accept increased heterogeneity within the target.

Normal tissue contouring must also be performed carefully. One should avoid contouring the skin as part of the CTV, unless it is explicitly involved. Inclusion of the skin can lead to an unacceptably high skin dose, especially when immobilization materials act as a bolus.[10] Lastly, it is important to define not only what are truly GTV and CTV but also a physically realistic target for the optimization algorithm. Figure 11-1 illustrates a case in which the target was drawn

outside the skin. It is better to draw the target inside the skin and use a bolus to increase the skin dose if necessary.

IMRT versus 3DCRT Treatment Plans

In general, IMRT allows for smaller margins and is better for concave-shaped targets. In addition, IMRT planning is less dependent on beam energy than 3DCRT.[11] The best IMRT plan may require beam directions that are counterintuitive. For example, a beam direction directly through a critical structure may result in the best plan, whereas with conventional planning techniques, beams rarely enter through a critical structure that is not in or directly adjacent to the treatment volume. Guided by appropriate dose-volume constraints, optimization algorithms can limit the dose within parts of the beam, avoiding overdosage of a critical structure.

Figure 11-2 illustrates such a situation for an IMRT prostate cone-down plan. Figure 11-2A shows an axial computed tomography (CT) slice through the prostate for a six-field

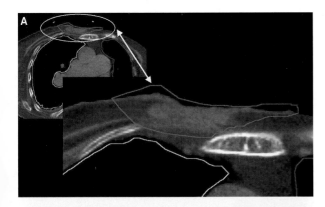

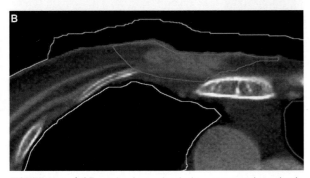

FIGURE 11-1. (*A*) Example of a carelessly drawn target volume that is outside the patient's skin. This can limit the quality of the intensity-modulated radiation therapy plan by requiring that the dose be delivered to the surrounding air. (*B*) A better approach is to draw the target volume carefully and add bolus to increase the dose to the skin. (To view a color version of this image, please refer to the CD-ROM).

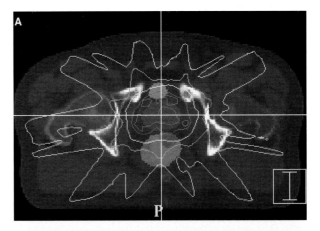

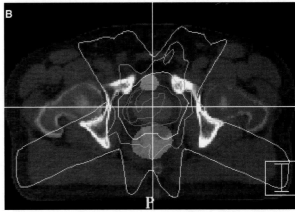

FIGURE 11-2. Two intensity-modulated radiation therapy (IMRT) plans for a 24.0 Gy prostate boost that demonstrates nonstandard beam directions in IMRT planning. The isodose curves are 24.8 Gy (*dark blue*), 24.0 Gy (*purple*), 22.7 Gy (*red*), 16.8 Gy (*yellow*), 12.0 Gy (*green*), and 7.2 Gy (*cyan*). (*A*) Six-field IMRT plan avoiding the rectum. The maximum dose in this plan is 25.7 Gy. (*B*) Five-field IMRT plan with a posterior – anterior beam directly through the rectum. The maximum dose in this plan is 25.3 Gy. (To view a color version of this image, please refer to the CD-ROM).

IMRT plan with beam directions of left posterior oblique (one), left anterior oblique (two), right anterior oblique (two), and right posterior oblique (one). Figure 11-2B shows the corresponding CT slice for a five-field plan with beam orientations as left posterior oblique (one), left anterior oblique (one), right anterior oblique (one), and right posterior oblique (one) and a direct posterior – anterior (one) beam through the rectum. The plans are similar, but the five-field plan has slightly more homogeneous dose coverage of the prostate and smaller hot spots. The minimum dose to the prostate for the five-field plan is 2.0% higher than that produced by the six-field plan. Moreover, the maximum dose to the prostate for the five-field plan is 1.6% lower than that for the six-field plan. The maximum dose to the rectum is only slightly different between the two plans (< 1%). The improvement of the five-field plan over the six-field plan is marginal, but this case demonstrates that counterintuitive beams play a role in IMRT planning. In addition, fewer beams imply a more efficient delivery. Thus, treatment time is a criterion to judge the quality of an IMRT plan. It is easier for patients to hold still in the treatment position for short treatment times. Furthermore, long delivery times may have a negative effect on tumor control.[12]

Another issue one must address is field abutment. For example, with head and neck IMRT, the question arises regarding how to treat the supraclavicular lymph nodes. The physician and planner must decide if these nodes are to be included in the IMRT fields or within a conventional anterior field. Unlike conventional approaches in which the dose at the field edge is sharp and easily identified, the dose at IMRT field edges is often jagged and not well delineated. Figure 11-3 demonstrates the different cases for a conventionally planned supraclavicular field and an IMRT planned target in the head. It is best to avoid matching IMRT treatment fields to one another or IMRT fields with conventional fields because it can be difficult to achieve a homogeneous dose at the junction. A consistent policy should be estab-

lished in situations in which field matching is used. Approaches for optimal field junctioning have been published.[13,14] Readers are strongly encouraged to evaluate these approaches in detail to identify a method that best fits with their clinical scenario and treatment planning system.

An additional consideration is the spatial differences between 3DCRT and IMRT dose distributions, as highlighted in Figure 11-4. 3DCRT dose distributions are very intuitive and predictable compared with IMRT dose distributions. In 3DCRT, the physician and planner know what to expect in terms of dose gradients at field boundaries, regions of high dose and their location, and the low-dose volume. In contrast, IMRT dose distributions have somewhat randomly located hot and cold spots. The conformity of an IMRT dose distribution comes at the expense of spreading a low dose to a larger volume of the patient. Notice that in Figure 11-4, even though the treatment volume is much larger for the 3DCRT plan, the low-dose region in the IMRT plan covers an area similar to that of the 3DCRT plan. It is important to remember that in IMRT planning, it is very difficult to adjust an isodose line by a few millimeters to avoid a critical structure or increase target coverage. IMRT is not like 3DCRT, in which one can change a block edge by a finite amount and subsequently shift an isodose curve by a similar amount. One should not try to force IMRT to "behave" like 3DCRT. IMRT is a completely different treatment technique. To reap the benefits of IMRT, one must also accept its limitations. The following sections elaborate on these points.

Other Considerations

Another issue that should be considered is that IMRT planning is a time-consuming process with extensive quality assurance procedures. It takes time to generate a good IMRT plan, more so than with 3DCRT. It thus may not be optimal to use IMRT in situations that require rapid plan generation, for example, in patients requiring emergency

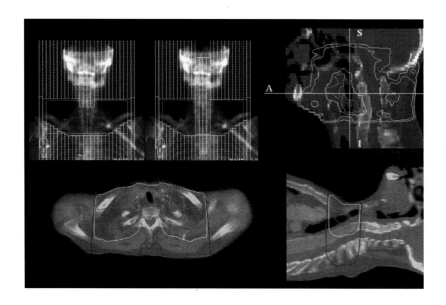

FIGURE 11-3. A picture of a conventionally planned supraclavicular field and an intensity-modulated radiation therapy (IMRT) plan in which the two plans were abutted for treatment. The green isodose line in the IMRT plan (*upper right*) is the 50% isodose line. The supraclavicular field (*upper left and bottom panels*) is matched at 3 mm inferior to the 50% isodose line in the IMRT plan. This gap significantly reduces the chance for unwanted hot spots at the match line, but this approach should not be used where positive nodes exist in the neck. A = anterior view. S = superior view. (To view a color version of this image, please refer to the CD-ROM).

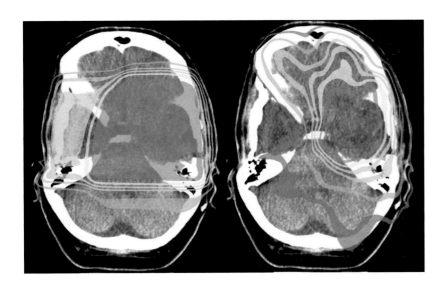

FIGURE 11-4. This figure demonstrates the differences between three-dimensional conformal radiation therapy (3DCRT) and intensity-modulated radiation therapy (IMRT) dose distributions. The 3DCRT plan was treated to 20 Gy, and IMRT was used to treat the clinical target volume plus the margin for another 28 Gy. The isodose bands (± 2%) shown are 100%, 90%, 80%, 70%, and 50% of the prescription dose (the IMRT plan also shows the 30% isoband). (To view a color version of this image, please refer to the CD-ROM).

treatment or with rapidly growing tumors. One option is to start with 3DCRT for a few fractions to allow time for generating and implementing the IMRT plan. Judicious use of this option is warranted. One must remember that, at present, an IMRT plan requires 1 to 4 hours of physics and dosimetry time to prepare for treatment and perform the necessary quality assurance procedures. Furthermore, it is best to use this option only if your IMRT planning system allows for optimization on the 3DCRT dose distribution that was already delivered to the patient. This will reduce the concern of overlapping hot spots in the two plans.

As previously mentioned, ease of treatment delivery (eg, coplanar vs noncoplanar beams) and delivery time (eg, number of beam and/or segments) are also important. The best IMRT plan is not optimal if it takes too long to deliver. The duration of treatment depends on the delivery method and the vendor to some extent, and these must be considered in the planning process. Beam directions are also important because it is not ideal to treat through immobilization devices that attenuate the beam. There are also cases in which 3DCRT seems to be the best choice, but, after consideration, IMRT is the better treatment option. Figure 11-5 shows a 3DCRT plan

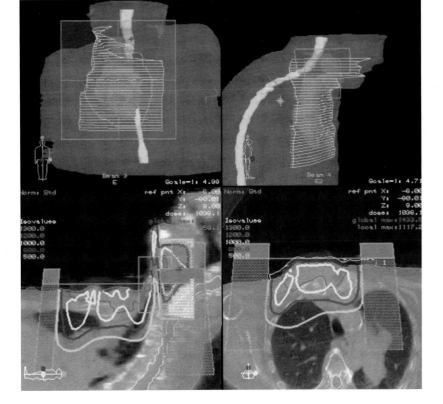

FIGURE 11-5. Three-dimensional conformal radiation therapy plan for a superficial target. The plan consisted of four fields: three photon fields and one abutting electron field with 1 cm of bolus. Note that not all fields are shown in the upper panel. The isodose curves are 60 Gy (*magenta*), 50 Gy (*yellow*), 45 Gy (*purple*), and 25 Gy (*cyan*). The maximum dose in the plan is 71.5 Gy. (To view a color version of this image, please refer to the CD-ROM).

for a case in which the patient was unable to lie flat. The patient was immobilized in a thermoplastic mask on an incline board. The best 3DCRT plan shown in Figure 11-5 consists of combined photon and electron beams. Bolus was also used to increase the surface dose. Because the patient tolerated immobilization well, an IMRT plan was attempted. Figure 11-6 shows the resultant six-field IMRT plan that can be delivered in one treatment time slot. With the 3DCRT plan in Figure 11-5, therapists would have to enter the treatment room to apply the electron applicator for the electron fields, and there would also be the uncertain dosimetry issues of abutting electron and photon fields. The IMRT plan obviates these concerns.

It has been shown that dose calculation plays a role in the extent of optimization.[15,16] The accuracy of beamlet dose distributions impacts IMRT plan optimization, and one will get a better optimized plan when accurate dose calculation models are used. Also, because IMRT plans can

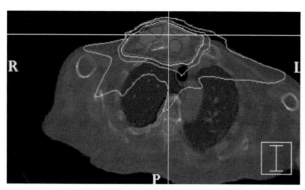

Axial Slice

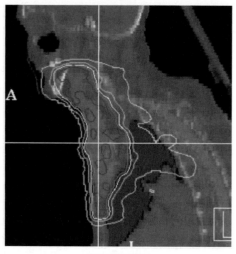

Sagittal Slice

FIGURE 11-6. Six-field intensity-modulated radiation therapy plan for a superficial target with 1 cm of bolus to treat the same target as shown in Figure 11-5. The isodose curves are 55 Gy (*blue*), 50 Gy (*purple*), 45 Gy (*yellow*), 35 Gy (*green*), and 15 Gy (*cyan*). The maximum dose in the plan is 61.7 Gy. R = right view. L = Left view. A = anterior view. P = posterior view. (To view a color version of this image, please refer to the CD-ROM).

have nonstandard beam directions, clinical experience based on uncorrected 3DCRT treatments with conventional beam directions may not translate to IMRT. Although the issues related to dose calculation are usually transparent to the IMRT user, it is recommended that heterogeneity corrections are used for IMRT planning,[17] especially in head and neck or thoracic tumors. Organ motion and setup uncertainty are important considerations when treating with IMRT.[18–26] In contrast to 3DCRT, an IMRT field consists of many subfields, and each subfield treats only part of the target at any give time. There can be significant dosimetric problems if the patient or target moves during delivery of the IMRT treatment. For patients with tumors that move owing to respiration, IMRT should be attempted only with some method to account for intrafraction motion, such as active breathing control, respiratory gating, four-dimensional tumor tracking, or a breath-holding technique.

Optimal Candidates for IMRT Treatment

IMRT candidates are patients with immobilizable tumors that are often irregularly shaped and located adjacent to critical structures, whose functions may be compromised by standard radiation treatment or dose escalation. Ideal IMRT patients should also be cooperative and can withstand prolonged immobilization without excessive discomfort or pain during treatment. Morbidly obese patients with poor immobilization, agitated patients, or those with resting tremors are not ideal candidates for IMRT. Some claustrophobic patients are also poor candidates for IMRT for head and neck cancers unless they receive adequate sedation during treatment. In general, an uncomfortable patient makes a poor IMRT candidate.

Aspects of IMRT Plan Evaluation

Before embarking on generating an IMRT plan, issues that should be considered and communicated with the IMRT planning systems are definitions of the target and avoidance structures, definition of the objectives and constraints for optimization (ie, what is the exact treatment plan), and dose prescriptions (simultaneous integrated boost vs sequential cone-down plans).

IMRT plan evaluation is a compromising process, requiring considerable time and attention. One cannot ask for an impossible goal such as zero dose to the critical tissue adjacent to the target volume. One has to define the problem sufficiently as to what is absolutely necessary and what can be compromised, a process similar to that with 3DCRT planning. One has to understand that the IMRT product may not be exactly as desired but may be adequate for the treatment purpose. In some situations, a comparison between an IMRT and a 3DCRT plan may be necessary to identify the best approach. However, overuse of comparison plans is strongly discouraged because it can significantly tax physics and dosimetric resources.

Target Coverage

As previously mentioned, in IMRT plans, there are routinely regions of high dose (hot spots) and regions of low dose (cold spots). Hot spots are volumes of tissues that receive doses greater than the prescribed dose, and cold spots are those that receive doses less than the prescribed dose. Important issues to consider for these hot and cold spots are magnitude, volume, and location. At present, there is no accepted consensus regarding the magnitude and the volumes for these spots for most tumor types. In head and neck cancer, we recommend the Radiation Therapy Oncology Group (RTOG) H-0222 trial guidelines, namely, that 95% of the PTV should be covered by the prescribed isodose line. The hot spots (defined in this study as regions receiving a dose > 110% of the prescribed dose) should cover < 20% of the PTV and < 1% of tissues outside the PTV. Such spots should be within the CTV (ideally within the GTV), not in the overlapping normal tissues. Similar constraints can be used for IMRT of tumors located elsewhere. For example, investigators from the University of Chicago limit 15% or less of the PTV volume to receive the dose at the 110% level and 1% or less to receive the dose at the 115% level for gynecologic patients undergoing intensity-modulated pelvic irradiation.[27]

RTOG H-0222 defines cold spots as regions within the PTV receiving doses < 93% of the prescribed dose. The total volume of cold spots should be < 1% of the PTV; however, this constraint may need to be relaxed if more conformity is desired. The location of cold spots is important. They should not be located within the GTV and ideally should be at the periphery of the PTV, as far from the GTV as possible.

It is also worth noting that it is easier to get a good conformal treatment plan on smaller target volumes than on larger ones.[28] In our experience, one can achieve a better IMRT plan with a simultaneous integrated boost than with a sequential cone-down approach.

Target coverage in IMRT treatment plans is different than in 3DCRT. Some hallmark aspects of an IMRT dose distribution distinguish it from conventional approaches. First, IMRT isodose curves are wavier than in 3DCRT (see Figure 11-4). Second, target coverage is more heterogeneous. Thus, one can also expect a more pronounced shoulder and usually a small high-dose tail associated with the DVH of the PTV. These high- and low-dose regions must be accounted for in the evaluation of the treatment plans because they may affect toxicity and tumor control probability.

A simple case will demonstrate these points. Figure 11-7 shows a 3DCRT plan, and Figure 11-8 shows a corresponding IMRT plan for partial breast irradiation. The conformal nature of the IMRT plan comes at the expense of dose heterogeneity within the target. The prescription dose for these plans was 34 Gy. Note that the IMRT plan has hot spots within or near the target of 112%, whereas the 3DCRT has a maximum hot spot in the patient of only 107%. An evaluation of

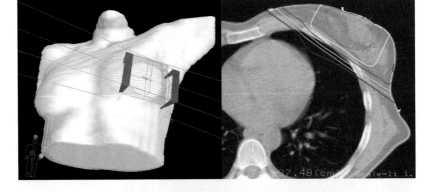

FIGURE 11-7. A conformal partial breast treatment plan consisting of tangential photon beams with an en face electron beam. One centimeter of bolus is used. The isodose curves are 34 Gy (*yellow*), 30 Gy (*purple*), 20 Gy (*cyan*), 10 Gy (*white*), and 5 Gy (*blue*). The maximum dose in this plan is 36.4 Gy. (To view a color version of this image, please refer to the CD-ROM).

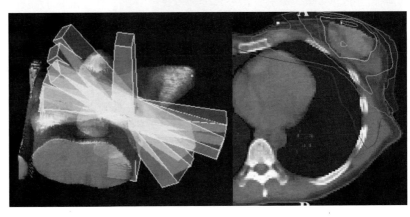

FIGURE 11-8. A seven-field noncoplanar intensity-modulated radiation therapy partial breast treatment plan. One centimeter of bolus is used. The isodose curves are 38 Gy (*orange*), 34 Gy (*yellow*), 30 Gy (*purple*), 20 Gy (*cyan*), 10 Gy (*white*), and 5 Gy (*blue*). The maximum dose in this plan is 39.5 Gy. (To view a color version of this image, please refer to the CD-ROM).

the DVHs in Figure 11-9 shows this information. What is clear from the DVHs is that there is an underdosage of the PTV in the IMRT plan compared with 3DCRT. Both the hot spots and the cold spots must be investigated on a slice-by-slice basis to determine whether they are acceptable. This is almost always a clinical decision that must be made by the physician. Difficult decisions are routinely required concerning the balance between target coverage and critical structure sparing.[29] Figure 11-10 demonstrates this for a case in which

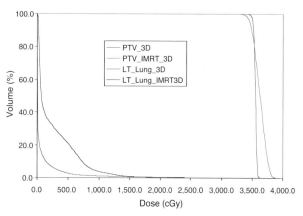

FIGURE 11-9. Dose-volume histograms for the treatment plans in Figures 11-7 and 11-8. IMRT = intensity-modulated radiation therapy; PTV = planning target volume.

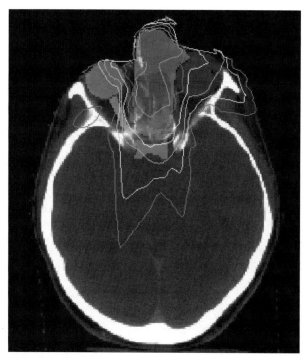

FIGURE 11-10. This figure demonstrates the trade-off between target coverage and critical structure (optic chiasm) sparing. The isodose lines are 66 Gy (*orange*), 60 Gy (*red*), 50 Gy (*yellow*), 40 Gy (*green*), 30 Gy (*light blue*), and 20 Gy (*blue*). (To view a color version of this image, please refer to the CD-ROM).

the CTV may be slightly underdosed to spare the critical structure. Such compromises are common because IMRT is not ideal for every case that cannot be adequately treated with 3DCRT.

An important principle regarding target coverage in IMRT is the trade-off between conformity and dose heterogeneity. Requirements for increased conformity will result in decreased dose uniformity. If the priority is conformity, one must accept increased inhomogeneity and vice versa. In addition, dose uniformity can also be affected by increased target concavity and decreased beam number. These considerations should be taken into account during evaluation of target coverage. It is absolutely critical to evaluate IMRT plans slice by slice on the planning computer because one has little control of the location of hot or cold spots. For our slice-by-slice plan evaluation, we typically normalize the plan to the maximum dose in the plan. We then evaluate the following isodose lines: the prescribed doses for the GTV and CTV, 5% less than the prescribed doses for the GTV and CTV, and 95%, 90%, 50%, and 30% of the maximum dose in the plan. Detailed evaluation of isodose coverage allows for accurate determination of plan conformity and location of the hot and cold spots.

Normal Tissue Sparing

Unfortunately, there are few data regarding partial organ tolerance at present; therefore, most guidelines for normal tissue tolerances are based on previously published whole organ data. Table 11-1 shows a partial list of the dose limits that have been published regarding whole and partial organ tolerance with radiation alone. We generally follow these dose limits for both IMRT and 3DCRT planning. Lowering these limits by 10% when concurrent chemotherapy is used may be appropriate. In cases of the mandible or larynx in which the mean dose may be as important as the maximum dose, we also restrict the mean dose to less than 35 to 45 Gy for the mandible and less than 25 to 30 Gy for the larynx. These constraints are not "set in stone" and may be relaxed or tightened on a case-by-case basis.

On occasion, an IMRT plan may produce a maximal point dose that exceeds the so-called tolerance of a critical structure. It is important to review the DVH to determine how much of the critical structure actually receives doses exceeding the specified limit. In many cases, it may correlate to only a few voxels and thus may be acceptable. However, this decision should be individualized based on other clinical considerations, such as prior treatments (radiation or surgery), comorbidities, and the use of concurrent chemotherapy. A rule of thumb is that < 5% of the contoured normal structure should receive doses exceeding the limits. For the brain and spinal cord in which the entire structure is often not delineated, the volume in cubic centimeters is more important, and we usually require that < 1 cc of contoured volumes receives doses exceeding the limits. If there is concern about exceeding dose tolerance for adjacent critical structures based

TABLE 11-1. Dose Limits Related to Whole Organ and Partial Organ Tolerance with Radiation Alone

Tissue	Maximal Dose*, Gy	Mean Dose, Gy	Other Volume Doses, Gy	Reference
Brain	60			30
Brainstem	54			30
Optic chiasm/nerves	54			30
Retina	45			30
Lens	12			30
Parotid gland	70	26		31
Larynx	70	≤ 25†		
Mandible	65	≤ 35–45†		
Spinal cord	45			30
Lung		20	V20 < 35% radiation therapy alone; V20 < 20% with chemotherapy	32
Esophagus			V45 < 30%	33
Small bowel	50			30
Rectum			V50 < 66%	34
Bladder			V47 < 53%	35

*Maximal dose limits should be decreased by 10% when concurrent chemotherapy is used.
†Additional dose specifications used at Stanford University for head and neck cancer intensity-modulated radiation therapy.

on maximum doses, one should also evaluate the isodose lines that correspond to or are within a couple of percentage points of this maximum dose to determine the volume and location of critical structures that receive a higher dose than previously constrained. A situation such as this is shown in Figure 11-11. If the maximum spinal cord dose is constrained at 45 Gy and the plan showed the maximal achievable dose of 46 Gy, one should also look at the 46 Gy isodose line to determine the location and volume of the cord covered within these isodose lines and whether it is clinically acceptable.

What are achievable normal structure doses with present-day IMRT planning systems? This is a seminal question in IMRT planning. Tables 11-2 and 11-3 give some of our results for achievable dosimetry. Table 11-2 presents our data for localized prostate treatment, and Table 11-3 presents our data for head and neck treatment. The results shown are an average of 10 cases per site. The minimum dose and maximum dose for all 10 cases are given in brackets. Although the dose to structures in IMRT depends strongly on each specific case, these data give an indication

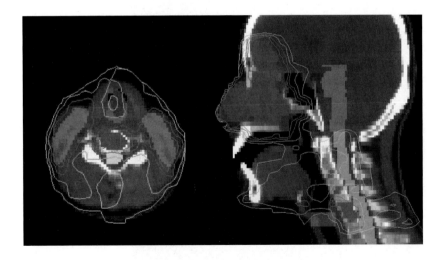

FIGURE 11-11. A case showing high dose near the spinal cord (C4–C5). The maximum dose to the spinal cord as tabulated in the plan statistics is 46.4 Gy. The isodose lines are 58.4 Gy (*dark blue*), 50.4 Gy (*purple*), 45.0 Gy (*red*), 35.0 Gy (*green*), 25.0 Gy (*cyan*), 30.0 Gy (*light blue*), and 20.0 Gy (*blue*). The magnitude of setup uncertainty associated with immobilization and the amount of spinal cord receiving > 45.0 Gy must both be considered when determining if this plan is acceptable for treatment. (To view a color version of this image, please refer to the CD-ROM).

TABLE 11-2. Achievable Dose Levels for Structures in Prostate Intensity-Modulated Radiation Therapy

Structure	Volume, cc	Dose at 100% Volume, Gy	Mean Dose, Gy	Dose at 1% Volume, Gy
Prostate	80.4 ± 1.3 (78.7, 82.7)	70.8 ± 1.0 (69.4, 72.9)	75.3 ± 0.4 (74.9, 76.1)	79.0 ± 0.8 (77.8, 80.3)

Structure Name	Volume, cc	Dose at 25% Volume, Gy	Dose at 5% Volume, Gy	Maximum Dose, Gy
Rectum	67.5 ± 28.1 (41.3, 122.8)	57.3 ± 2.2 (55.1, 61.0)	71.6 ± 1.4 (69.2, 73.3)	77.4 ± 1.7 (75.2, 80.0)

Listed are the mean values for 10 cases and the standard deviations. Minimum and maximum doses for each structure are in brackets. For the 10 cases, the average maximum value in the dose distribution is 80.4 Gy ± 1.3 Gy (78.7 Gy, 82.7 Gy).

TABLE 11-3. Dose Statistics for Head and Neck Intensity-Modulated Radiation Therapy

Structure	Volume, cc	Minimum Dose, Gy	Mean Dose, Gy	Maximum Dose, Gy
Gross tumor volume	82.4 ± 49.1 (20.2, 195.8)	54.2 ± 11.8 (24.3, 63.6)	70.6 ± 0.8 (69.9, 72.4)	78.4 ± 2.6 (74.6, 82.5)
Nodes	423.3 ± 163.9 (258.2, 710.3)	26.0 ± 7.2 (14.0, 35.7)	62.0 ± 2.3 (56.1, 64.3)	77.8 ± 2.2 (74.2, 80.5)
Spinal cord*	17.7 ± 5.4 (7.1, 24.1)	1.6 ± 2.3 (0.4, 7.8)	19.2 ± 4.7 (11.6, 26.6)	34.3 ± 7.7 (13.9, 40.5)
Brainstem*	27.4 ± 3.1 (22.5, 33.3)	7.3 ± 5.5 (1.9, 16.7)	22.1 ± 8.4 (6.5, 33.0)	39.9 ± 7.0 (26.8, 48.9)
Ipsilateral parotid gland	22.0 ± 10.6 (10.9, 42.5)	15.4 ± 9.2 (7.1, 35.7)	34.7 ± 13.0 (18.0, 61.1)	61.2 ± 8.2 (45.0, 74.5)
Contralateral parotid gland	25.4 ± 10.2 (10.5, 47.1)	8.8 ± 2.6 (3.4, 12.3)	21.6 ± 4.9 (13.3, 27.9)	49.5 ± 8.4 (31.4, 56.9)
Mandible	66.6 ± 16.7 (40.8, 85.6)	11.8 ± 5.7 (3.8, 20.2)	43.3 ± 3.3 (39.4, 49.9)	66.7 ± 5.1 (58.0, 73.5)
Larynx	9.8 ± 6.3 (3.7, 23.4)	9.9 ± 6.6 (2.9, 24.7)	18.2 ± 9.4 (7.5, 40.7)	42.1 ± 11.4 (30.9, 68.0)

These are the mean values for 10 cases and the standard deviations. Minimum and maximum doses are in the brackets. On average, the maximum value in the dose distribution is 79.3 Gy ± 2.6 Gy (75.0 Gy, 82.5 Gy).

*The maximum dose to the spinal cord and brainstem is given as the maximum dose to 1 cc of that tissue. The difference between the maximum dose to 1 cc of tissue and the maximum dose as reported by the dose distribution statistics (ie, the single voxel dose value) is 10.6% for the spinal cord (38.4 Gy ± 8.3 Gy [16.1 Gy, 45.0 Gy]) and 13.4% for the brainstem (46.1 Gy ± 7.4 Gy [31.8 Gy, 55.5 Gy]).

of what is achievable. These cases were planned on the *CORVUS* inverse planning system, version 4.0 (North American Scientific, NOMOS Radiation Oncology Division, Cranberry Township, PA), with 1 × 1 cm^2 beamlets and segmented with 10 intensity levels for step-and-shoot IMRT delivery on a Varian C-series linear accelerator (Varian Medical Systems, Palo Alto, CA).

On occasion, hot spots can be found in normal tissue outside the target tissues. Figure 11-12 shows a head and

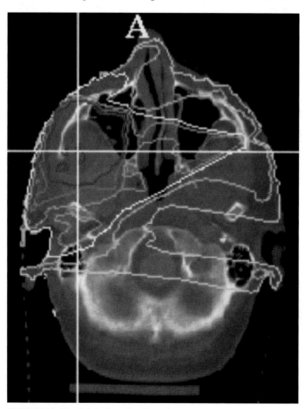

FIGURE 11-12. Axial slice showing a hot spot in normal tissue and a region of low dose through the brainstem. The isodose curves shown in this figure are 63.0 Gy (*dark blue*), 60.2 Gy (*purple*), 55.0 Gy (*orange*), 45.0 Gy (*light green*), 35.0 Gy (*green*), and 25.0 Gy (*light blue*). (To view a color version of this image, please refer to the CD-ROM).

neck IMRT treatment that covers the tumor adequately but deposits a hot spot (63 Gy) in the contralateral uninvolved side. In addition, the 25 Gy isodose line streaks across the skull base through the brainstem to the opposite side. This would not be seen in 3DCRT treatment planning but is typical in IMRT owing to unconventional beam arrangements used to improve dose conformity. The hot spot in normal tissue and low-dose streaks can be modified by the use of a "tuning structure." Figure 11-13A shows the addition of such a structure to reduce unwanted dose outside the target volume, as shown in Figure 11-13B. No change was made in the beam directions. This is a useful tool to modify the IMRT dose distribution specifically when one desires the same beam directions to avoid physical constraints (eg, not wanting to direct a beam through part of the treatment couch or immobilization device). The hot spots and low dose in Figure 11-13 are reduced at the expense of increased heterogeneity within the target (see Figure 11-13B). In summary, the beam directions in 3DCRT are very important in achieving a conformal target dose and adequate normal tissue sparing. However, with IMRT, the beam directions are not as critical. Other tools are used in IMRT planning to achieve planning goals, such as dose-volume constraints and tuning structures.

New IMRT users or experienced users on a new system need to be aware of unexpected consequences when planning IMRT. For example, a CyberKnife (Accuray Inc, Sunnyvale, CA) treatment plan generated to treat the prostate in Figure 11-14 results in streaking doses over the right femoral head. This appeared with identical dose constraints on the left and right femoral heads. This anomaly was due to unforeseen limitations in the optimization algorithm that have since been corrected. Figure 11-14 highlights the point that IMRT planning is significantly different from 3DCRT planning. An IMRT plan can have unexpected results in the dose distribution, and each plan should be considered carefully.

DVHs provide a global view of whether the plan meets the specified goals and constraints. One can extract data on the underdosed volumes for the GTV, CTV, and PTV and

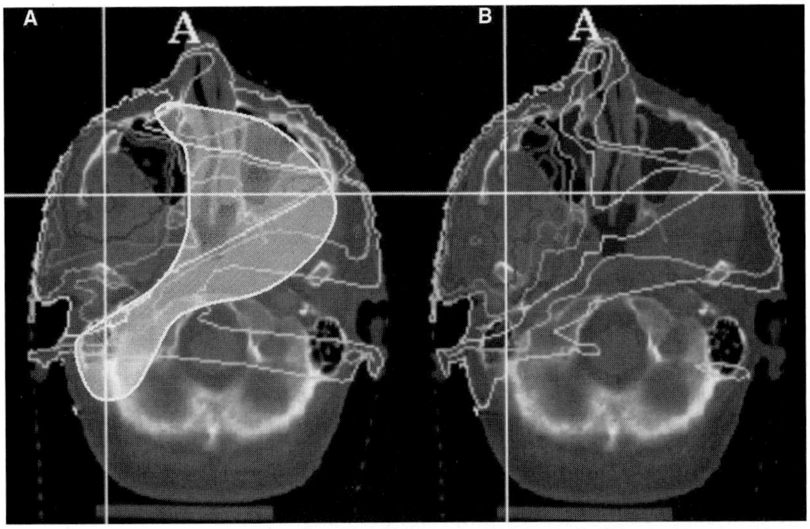

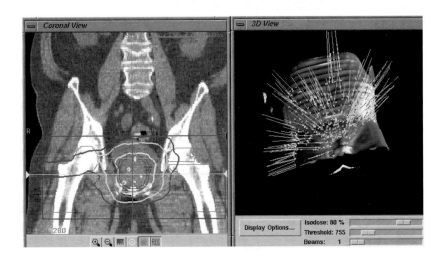

FIGURE 11-13. This figure shows the effect of a tuning structure in improving the dose distribution. (*A*) The plan (see Figure 11-12) was optimized without a tuning structure and, (*B*) the plan was optimized with a tuning structure (*yellow*). The isodose curves shown in this figure are 63 Gy (*dark blue*), 60.2 Gy (*purple*), 55 Gy (*orange*), 45 Gy (*light green*), 35 Gy (*green*), and 25 Gy (*light blue*). (To view a color version of this image, please refer to the CD-ROM).

FIGURE 11-14. A CyberKnife treatment plan showing the dose distribution in the coronal plane (*left*) and the individual beams (*right*). (To view a color version of this image, please refer to the CD-ROM).

the overdose volumes for each normal structure. In general, we evaluate the DVH to ensure that at least 95% of the target receives the prescribed dose. In addition, the DVH provides data on mean and partial volume doses, which can be used to determine partial volume tolerances in the future. Another method to evaluate a treatment plan is to use a three-dimensional dose display. This type of display complements the DVHs by showing where hot or cold spots exist relative to other tissues. Figure 11-15 illustrates a three-dimensional display for a head and neck IMRT plan, showing the location of hot spots outside the target. Although this type of display provides qualitative information only, it gives a huge amount of information quickly and may assist in rapidly evaluating multiple plan iterations.

Final Comments on IMRT Planning

The goal of treatment planning is to maximize the therapeutic ratio. This may be difficult to achieve in real life. The planner must understand what the physician will accept as a dose limit to critical structures and, at the same time, must attempt to achieve those limits within the constraints of the prescription dose for the target. Often, when planning IMRT, the physician and planner will unnecessarily go in circles, without a satisfactory solution, because neither party knows what can be achieved. Hopefully, what to expect from IMRT has been demonstrated in this chapter. The remaining burden falls on treating physicians to determine exactly what they will accept in terms of target coverage and normal tissue sparing. It is essential to be realistic in the expectations of IMRT. Unfortunately, IMRT cannot produce miracles because its dose distributions are bound by physical principles. It is also essential to be prepared to accept some of the dose to critical structures (but keeping them below tolerance) to obtain more conformal target coverage than with 3DCRT. In many cases, a small volume of the critical structures will receive more of the dose than it would with 3DCRT, but the IMRT plan will show better dose conformity. If this trade-off is unacceptable, then IMRT may not be the best treatment techique.

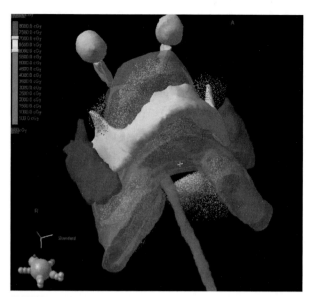

FIGURE 11-15. A three-dimensional dose display showing the dose distribution between 60 and 70 Gy (*yellow-red-green*). Two high-dose regions are evident. One is near the mandible and the other is in the posterior neck, outside the contour of the neck nodes (*cyan*). Another intensity-modulated radiation therapy plan should be attempted to remove or reduce these hot spots outside the target. The gross tumor volume is shown in red wire mesh within the clinical target volume. (To view a color version of this image, please refer to the CD-ROM).

The physician and planner need a method to achieve their planning goals. We have used an approach that is helpful for those new to IMRT planning and even for experienced IMRT users when treating new sites. The first step is to ask the physician to make a difficult decision. If one had to choose between treating the target (ie, push normal tissue to near tolerance dose) or spare critical structures (ie, underdose part of the target), what would be more important for this patient? This question will help guide the planner's focus during the planning process. Next, it is important to understand what the physician will absolutely not accept in terms of dose to a structure. Whether or not it is expressed explicitly, every physician has a dose limit in mind. The job of the IMRT planner is to understand what those limits are for each physician and for each case. Another aspect of IMRT planning is that the goals of sparing critical structures may change during the planning process. It may be decided by the physician that a structure can take a large fraction of the dose, but once the planning begins, the planner may realize that the achievable dose may be much lower. In IMRT treatment planning, slight modification of the planning goals should be expected until the physician and planner have gained a considerable amount of experience.

As can be seen from the discussion above, good physician and planner communication is essential for successful IMRT planning. This is partly due to the fact that IMRT is a relatively new technology with minimal long-term outcome data.

The development of IMRT plans usually takes several iterations. Even for experienced IMRT users, the physician and planner do not always know a priori the quality of plan that can be achieved. The ability to define treatment goals at the outset and communicate them to both the planner and the treatment planning system is part of the IMRT learning process, which will hopefully become easier with clinical experience and available outcome data.

References

1. Followill D, Geis P, Boyer A. Estimates of whole-body dose equivalent produced by beam intensity modulated conformal therapy. Int J Radiat Oncol Biol Phys 1997;38:667–72.
2. Williams PO, Hounsell AR. X-ray leakage considerations for IMRT. Br J Radiol 2001;74:98–100.
3. Waller EJ. Neutron production associated with radiotherapy linear accelerators using intensity modulated radiation therapy mode. Health Phys 2003;85(5 Suppl):S75–7.
4. Hall EJ, Wuu CS. Radiation-induced second cancers: the impact of 3D-CRT and IMRT. Int J Radiat Oncol Biol Phys 2003;56:83–8.
5. International Commission on Radiation Units and Measurements (ICRU). Prescribing, recording, and reporting photon beam therapy. ICRU report 50. Bethesda (MD), 1993.
6. International Commission on Radiation Units and Measurements (ICRU). Prescribing, recording, and reporting photon beam therapy (supplement to ICRU report 50). ICRU report 62. Bethesda (MD), 1999.
7. Martinez-Monge R, Fernandes PS, Gupta N, et al. Cross-sectional nodal atlas: a tool for the definition of clinical target volumes in three-dimensional radiation therapy planning. Radiology 1999;211:815–28.
8. Grégoire V, Coche E, Cosnard G, et al. Selection and delineation of lymph node target volumes in head and neck conformal radiotherapy. Proposal for standardizing terminology and procedure based on the surgical experience. Radiother Oncol 2000;56:135–50.
9. Levendag P, Braaksma M, Coche E, et al. Rotterdam and Brussels CT-based neck nodal delineation compared with the surgical levels as defined by the American Academy of Otolaryngology-Head and Neck Surgery. Int J Radiat Oncol Biol Phys 2004;58:113–23.
10. Lee N, Chuang C, Quivey JM, et al. Skin toxicity due to intensity-modulated radiotherapy for head-and-neck carcinoma. Int J Radiat Oncol Biol Phys 2002;53:630–7.
11. Pirzkall A, Carol MP, Pickett B, et al. The effect of beam energy and number of fields on photon-based IMRT for deep-seated targets. Int J Radiat Oncol Biol Phys 2002;53:434–42.
12. Wang JZ, Li XA, D'Souza WD, et al. Impact of prolonged fraction delivery times on tumor control: a note of caution for intensity-modulated radiation therapy (IMRT). Int J Radiat Oncol Biol Phys 2003;57:543–52.
13. Sethi A, Leybovich L, Dogan N, et al. Matching tomographic IMRT fields with static photon fields. Med Phys 2001;28:2459–65.
14. Dogan N, Leybovich LB, Sethi A, et al. Automatic feathering of split fields for step-and-shoot intensity modulated radiation

therapy. Phys Med Biol 2003;48:1133–40.

15. Laub W, Alber M, Birkner M, et al. Monte Carlo dose computation for IMRT optimization. Phys Med Biol 2000;45:1741–54.

16. Jeraj R, Keall PJ, Siebers JV. The effect of dose calculation accuracy on inverse treatment planning. Phys Med Biol 2002;47:391–407.

17. Intensity Modulated Radiation Therapy Collaborative Working Group. Intensity-modulated radiotherapy: current status and issues of interest. Int J Radiat Oncol Biol Phys 2001;51:880–914.

18. Yu CX, Jaffray DA, Wong JW. The effects of intra-fraction organ motion on the delivery of dynamic intensity modulation. Phys Med Biol 1998;43:91–104.

19. Keall PJ, Kini VR, Vedam SS, et al. Motion adaptive x-ray therapy: a feasibility study. Phys Med Biol 2001;46:1–10.

20. Manning MA, Wu Q, Cardinale RM, et al. The effect of setup uncertainty on normal tissue sparing with IMRT for head-and-neck cancer. Int J Radiat Oncol Biol Phys 2001;51:1400–9.

21. Bortfeld T, Jokivarsi K, Goitein M, et al. Effects of intra-fraction motion on IMRT dose delivery: statistical analysis and simulation. Phys Med Biol 2002;47:2203–20.

22. Chui CS, Yorke E, Hong L. The effects of intra-fraction organ motion on the delivery of intensity-modulated field with a multileaf collimator. Med Phys 2003;30:1736–46.

23. George R, Keall PJ, Kini VR, et al. Quantifying the effect of intrafraction motion during breast IMRT planning and dose delivery. Med Phys 2003;30:552–62.

24. Samuelsson A, Mercke C, Johansson KA. Systematic set-up errors for IMRT in the head and neck region: effect on dose distribution. Radiother Oncol 2003;66:303–11.

25. Duan J, Shen S, Fiveash JB, et al. Dosimetric effect of respiration-gated beam on IMRT delivery. Med Phys 2003;30:2241–52.

26. Hugo GD, Agazaryan N, Solberg TD. The effects of tumor motion on planning and delivery of respiratory-gated IMRT. Med Phys 2003;30:1052–66.

27. Mundt AJ, Mell LK, Roeske JC. Preliminary analysis of chronic gastrointestinal toxicity in gynecology patients treated with intensity-modulated whole pelvic radiation therapy. Int J Radiat Oncol Biol Phys 2003;56:1354–60.

28. Mohan R, Wang X, Jackson A, et al. The potential and limitations of the inverse radiotherapy technique. Radiother Oncol 1994;32:232–48.

29. Tsien C, Eisbruch A, McShan D, et al. Intensity-modulated radiation therapy (IMRT) for locally advanced paranasal sinus tumors: incorporating clinical decisions in the optimization process. Int J Radiat Oncol Biol Phys 2003;55:776–84.

30. Emami B, Lyman J, Brown A, et al. Tolerance of normal tissue to therapeutic irradiation. Int J Radiat Oncol Biol Phys 1991;21:109–22.

31. Eisbruch A, Ship JA, Dawson LA, et al. Salivary gland sparing and improved target irradiation by conformal and intensity modulated irradiation of head and neck cancer. World J Surg 2003;27:832–7.

32. Tsujino K, Hirota S, Endo M, et al. Predictive value of dose-volume histogram parameters for predicting radiation pneumonitis after concurrent chemoradiation for lung cancer. Int J Radiat Oncol Biol Phys 2003;55:110–15.

33. Hirota S, Tsujino K, Endo M, et al. Dosimetric predictors of radiation esophagitis in patients treated for non-small-cell lung cancer with carboplatin/paclitaxel/radiotherapy. Int J Radiat Oncol Biol Phys 2001;51:291–5.

34. Fiorino C, Sanguineti G, Cozzarini C, et al. Rectal dose-volume constraints in high-dose radiotherapy of localized prostate cancer. Int J Radiat Oncol Biol Phys 2003;57:953–62.

35. Zelefsky MJ, Fuks Z, Leibel SA. Intensity-modulated radiation therapy for prostate cancer. Semin Radiat Oncol 2002;12:229–37.

Chapter 12

Delivery Systems

Cheng B. Saw, PhD, Komanduri M. Ayyangar, PhD, Komanduri V. Krsihna, PhD,
Andrew Wu, PhD, Shalom Kalnicki, MD

Intensity-modulated radiation therapy (IMRT) is a method of radiation treatment planning and delivery that conforms the high-dose region to the shape of the target volume.[1–5] An essential component of any IMRT delivery system is the beam intensity modulator. There are three general categories of intensity modulators: physical modulators, binary beam modulators, and multileaf collimators (MLCs). Physical intensity modulators are similar to compensators used in conventional radiation therapy and hence are inserted manually. Binary beam modulators are computer-controlled modulators that can operate automatically. These are either "open" or "closed." The last type of modulator is the conventional MLC, which is a component of the modern linear accelerator. Given that linear accelerators are readily accessible,[6] the MLC is the most common delivery system for IMRT. The goal of this chapter is to review the beam delivery systems used in IMRT. The physical characteristics (Table 12-1) and system integration issues are discussed using examples from the major manufacturers. Quality assurance on these systems is discussed in Chapter 13, "Commissioning and Dosimetric Quality Assurance."

Physical Beam Modulators

The simplest method of performing IMRT is through the use of physical beam intensity modulators.[7,8] A physical modulator is similar to a compensator except that the former is used to modulate the radiation beam intensity

TABLE 12-1. Summary of Commercially Available Delivery Systems

Vendor (Web Site)	Type	Delivery	No. of Leaves	Resolution, mm	Thickness, cm	Transmission, %	Focus	Maximum Field Size, cm	Overtravel, cm	Speed
BrainLAB <www.brainlab.com>	Micro-MLC	Static or dynamic	52	3–5	6.4	2	Single; rounded ends	10 × 10	5	1 cm/s
Elekta Inc. <www.elekta.com>	MLC	Static	80	10	7.5	1.8–2.5	Single; rounded ends	40 × 40	12.5	2 cm/s
North American Scientific (Nomos) <www.nasmedical.com>	Binary	Tomotherapy	40	4, 8, or 16	8	0.5	Double	20 × 30	NA	50 cm/s
Southeastern Radiation Products <www.seradiation.com>	Compensator	NA	NA	Based on planning system	5.1 aluminum or brass	~ 65 aluminum; ~ 84 brass	NA	40 × 40	NA	NA
Siemens Medical Systems <www.siemens.com>	MLC	Static	82	10	7.5	0.9–1.25	Double; flat ends	40 × 40	10	2 cm/s
TomoTherapy Inc. <www.tomotherapy.com>	Binary	Tomotherapy	64	6.25	10	0.4	Double	160 (long) × 40 (diameter)	NA	< 40 msec transit time
Varian Medical Systems <www.varian.com>	MLC	Static or dynamic	120	5–10	6	1.6–1.9	Single; rounded ends	40 × 40	17	3 cm/s

MLC = multileaf collimator; NA = not available.

instead of compensating for missing tissue. Use of these modulators requires mechanical fabrication. During treatment, each physical modulator must be manually inserted into the tray mount of the linear accelerator. Entering the treatment room and inserting these modulators is laborious, especially when multiple gantry angles are used. A recent technical development by Yoda and Aoki reported the introduction of an automatic tray mount that can hold up to six physical modulators, allowing autoinsertion prior to treatment of a given beam.[9] The number of monitor units (MUs) is significantly less with a physical modulator compared with MLC-based modulation. However, a potential disadvantage of physical modulators is the increase in photon scatter outside the portal, which can produce a higher skin dose.

Southeastern Radiation Products

Southeastern Radiation Products (Sanford, FL) markets the .decimal system for the remote fabrication of physical modulators. The ordering facility creates the filter specification file from the treatment planning software and then either e-mails this file or uses a Web site directly linked to the manufacturing process to upload the files. These file specifications can be in the proprietary .decimal file format or any other modulator file format from the various treatment planning systems. Once the filter specifications are received, the device is automatically produced to the customer's specifications. Customized software enables the order to be processed and ready for shipment in an average of 1.5 hours or less.

The filters (Figure 12-1) are manufactured using industrial (Mazak, Florence, KY) machining centers that mill the IMRT modulators out of solid blanks of aluminum or brass. This process thereby eliminates all porosity issues associated with pouring individual molds. In addition, it enables inspection of the filter while on the Mazak CNC milling machine using five-axis "touch probe" technology. A hard copy quality control report is sent with each filter. The tolerance of each filter is ± 0.25 mm. Southeastern Radiation Products also provides traceability of the alloy, thereby providing customers with a consistent attenuation factor (eg, for a 6 MV linear accelerator, the attenuation coefficient is 0.112/cm for aluminum and 0.359/cm for brass).

Binary Beam Modulators

The first commercially available system that used a binary beam modulator was the *PEACOCK* System (North American Scientific, NOMOS Radiation Oncology Division, Cranberry Township, PA) introduced in 1996. This system employs a slice-by-slice beam delivery method and hence is referred to as serial tomotherapy.[10–14] Stacking a series of slices through a target constitutes a complete single-fraction treatment. In principle, such a beam delivery technique can be used to treat a target of any length. The

thickness of the slice is defined by the leaf size of the specially designed beam-modulating delivery system, referred to as the multileaf intensity-modulating collimator (MIMiC). The MIMiC is mounted on the gantry of an existing linear accelerator.

Another commercially available binary system is the TomoTherapy system (TomoTherapy Inc., Madison, WI). Many of the dosimetric features were derived based on the assessment of the MIMiC delivery system.[15–17] From the outside, the TomoTherapy Hi-Art machine looks like a computed tomography scanner. This unit performs IMRT with a helical (or spiral) dose delivery pattern. A 6 MV linear accelerator is mounted onto the gantry ring and directed toward the center of the gantry. Using slip-ring technology, this device is capable of continuously rotating around a couch, enabling a smooth dose delivery.

NOMOS MIMIC

The MIMiC is a binary beam modulator that has 40 leaves (or vanes) divided onto two banks (Figure 12-2).[10,11] Each leaf projects a beam length of 0.8 cm at the isocenter in the 1 cm treatment mode and a 1.6 cm beam length in the 2 cm treatment mode. The thickness of each leaf is approximately 8 cm, resulting in a transmission of ~ 0.5%. Because the MIMiC has two banks, the nominal treatment slice length is double the leaf size to either 1.6 or 3.3 cm. IMRT delivery is achieved by rotating the gantry (equipped with the MIMiC) around the patient while the beam is on. During the rotation, the binary modulator opens and closes via electropneumatic actions according to the instructions prescribed by the planning system. The add-on

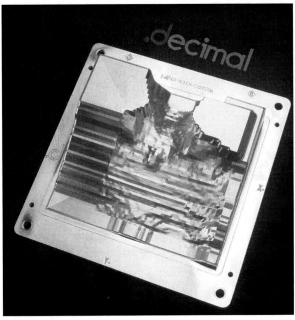

FIGURE 12-1. An aluminum filter constructed to produce an intensity-modulated anterior right lung/supraclavicular port. Courtesy of Richard Sweat, Southeastern Radiation Products, Inc.

components for this delivery system are the MIMiC, a controller, a dual-computer system for control and continuous monitoring of the MIMiC, a radiotherapy table adapter device for patient immobilization, and a NOMOS CRANE II (North American Scientific) for indexing the treatment couch.

The treatment planning system *CORVUS* (originally called *PEACOCK PLAN*) was developed to support the MIMiC beam delivery system. The *CORVUS* system uses an inverse planning algorithm for optimization.[10,11] Beam delivery instructions are transferred via a floppy disk from CORVUS to a controller connected to the MIMiC. The controller automatically directs the modulation of the leaves as the gantry of the linear accelerator rotates around the patient to produce a narrow highly varying field of 1.6 × 20 cm or 3.3 × 20 cm. The dose and gantry rotation rates are kept constant during the delivery. The controller senses faults based on gantry position and halts treatment if necessary. Because this delivery system supports the slice-by-slice treatment paradigm, the abutment of contiguous slices must be precise to minimize dose nonuniformity at the slice junction.[13,14]

The NOMOS CRANE II is used to position the treatment couch to within 0.1 mm accuracy (a tolerance that is typically not available on a linear accelerator couch). This device is attached to the side of the treatment couch and latched to the handrail. A crank controls the movement of the treatment couch. During actual dose delivery, the therapist must enter the room after each treatment slice to reposition or advance the couch to the next index. More recently, the AutoCrane has been introduced as a method of providing remote, automated table positioning (Figure 12-3).

TomoTherapy

The TomoTherapy Hi-Art system (Figure 12-4) uses a binary modulator that has 64 interdigitated tungsten leaves that move in a steel guide. The leaves are 10 cm thick in the beam direction. The tongue and the groove dimensions are both 0.30 (± 0.03) mm, with a nominal overlap of 0.15 (± 0.03) mm. This results in an interleaf leakage of 0.5% and an intraleaf leakage of 0.3%. Each leaf projects a 0.625 cm width at the center of the gantry (85 cm from the source) and is capable of opening from 0 to > 5 cm. The leaves are pneumatically controlled by individual air values so that each leaf can open and close quickly. The length of opening or closing of each leaf modulates the intensity of the beam. The transit time (opening or closing of each leaf) is less than 40 milliseconds. The length of the treatment beam can be as long as 160 cm, and the fan beam width can vary from 0.6 to 5.0 cm.

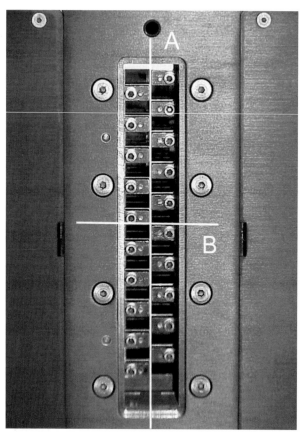

FIGURE 12-2. The multileaf intensity-modulating collimator (MIMiC) delivery system. This binary modulator consists of two banks, each with 20 leaves. Reproduced with permission.

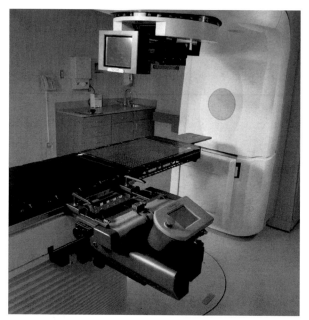

FIGURE 12-3. Attachment of the multileaf intensity-modulating collimator (MIMiC), AutoCrane, and radiotherapy table adapter to a linear accelerator. The AutoCrane provides a remote, automated table positioning for serial tomotherapy. The treatment table can be repositioned from outside the treatment room, eliminating the time associated with entering the room for manual indexing. (To view a color version of this image, please refer to the CD-ROM.) Courtesy of Tim Biertempfel, North American Scientific, NOMOS Radiation Oncology Division.

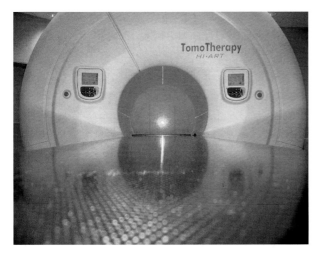

FIGURE 12-4. The TomoTherapy Hi-Art system. Treatment is delivered as the couch advances through the gantry and the beam rotates continuously around the patient. Courtesy of Sam Jeswani, TomoTherapy, Inc.

The TomoTherapy unit uses a compact linear accelerator for both imaging and treatment. The bremsstrahlung target has a unique design: a button of tungsten that is free to rotate in a stream of water. The photon beam is unflattened with a maximum dose rate of 8.5 Gy/min at the central axis. The primary collimator and jaw pair, which define the fan beam width, are immediately downstream from the target. In the forward direction, the total shielding thickness of the primary collimator and jaw is 23 cm of 94% purity tungsten. This shielding reduces the leakage radiation for helical IMRT to levels much lower than those of conventional IMRT.

Treatment is delivered as beam rotation is synchronized with the continuous longitudinal movement of the couch through the bore of the gantry, forming a helical beam pattern (sinogram) from the patient's point of view. Simultaneously, the set of binary collimator leaves rapidly transitions between open (leaf retracted) and closed (leaf blocking) states according to the treatment plan.

MLC-Based Delivery

Originally, the MLC was introduced as an autofield shaping device to replace custom blocks. As such, MLCs were designed with specifications for purposes other than IMRT. All MLC systems consist of a series of collimating blocks, vanes, or leaves arranged side by side, as shown in Figure 12-5. These leaves are separated into two banks, and each leaf is driven independently using microprocessors to facilitate autofield beam shaping. The movement of the leaves is limited to one dimension, either in or out.

Currently, there are two mechanisms of modulating beam intensity using an MLC. The first mechanism is termed "segmental IMRT," in which the collimator's shape is constant during irradiation and changes while the beam is "off."[5] This mechanism is also called the "step-and-shoot" technique or static multileaf collimation (sMLC). The planned intensity-modulated beam at each gantry angle is deconvolved into a series of segments (subfields) that are delivered by the MLC system of a linear accelerator. This process, known as leaf sequencing, is carried out by a computer algorithm.[18,19] By superimposing a series of segments, each with a uniform intensity (but a unique number of monitor units), a nonuniform fluence pattern is produced. The linear accelerators from the manufacturers discussed below (BrainLAB, Elekta, Siemens, and Varian) all support the sMLC dose delivery mechanism.

The second mechanism of dose delivery is termed "dynamic IMRT," in which the collimator's shape changes during irradiation.[5] This is different from sMLC, in which the collimator's shape remains stationary during irradiation. This mechanism is also called the "sliding window" technique or dynamic multileaf collimation. In this technique, each MLC leaf pair defines a gap or section of a field shape that moves unidirectionally. The leaves move with various velocities as a function of time to create the nonuniform intensity field. A fast-moving gap creates a low-intensity region, whereas a slow-moving gap produces a high-intensity region.

FIGURE 12-5. Side view (*A*) and a beam's-eye-view (*B*) of a Siemens' multileaf collimator (MLC). In general, MLCs are constructed with two banks of leaves. Each leaf has its own motor, allowing it to move independently.

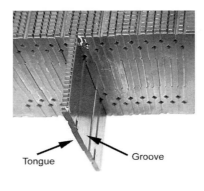

Tongue   Groove

A

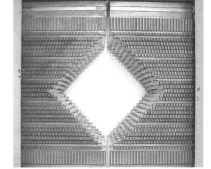

B

MLC designs differ from one manufacturer to another. Thus, leaf sequencing algorithms must take into consideration the design and mechanical limitations of each MLC system. As an example, one such design characteristic is known as interdigitation. This is the property whereby the tips of neighboring leaves on opposed MLC banks are allowed to pass one another. Figure 12-6 shows interdigitation limits based on existing MLC designs. Depending on the MLC design, full interdigitation, no interdigitation, or no interdigitation with a gap may be allowed. Consequently, a deliverable segment for one MLC may not be deliverable on a different manufacturer's MLC. Other features, such as leaf width, leaf divergence, leaf motion, leaf travel, and tongue-and-groove design, are also different for each MLC. Each vendor has provided its MLC design specification to the treatment planning systems so that these characteristics can be modeled during the planning process.

The design and dosimetric characteristics of three commercially available conventional MLCs are described by Xia and Verhey and Arnfield and colleagues.[19,20] These MLCs and a specialized micro–multileaf collimator (mMLC)[21] for stereotactic radiosurgery (SRS) are briefly presented here.

BrainLAB

The Novalis dedicated Shaped Beam Surgery System (BrainLAB, Heimstetten, Germany) is a megavoltage treatment unit (Figure 12-7). It has a single 6 MV photon beam with an output range of 0.3 to 20 cGy/deg (arc mode) and up to 800 cGy/min (fixed mode). This allows efficient delivery of a high-dose single fraction and conventional fractionation schemes. The maximum field size of the unit is 10 × 10 cm. An mMLC is installed under the primary collimators as an integrated component of the treatment unit. The m3 mMLC is also available as an add-on system, which can be adapted to an existing linear accelerator There are 26 pairs of leaves: 14 pairs with a leaf width of 3 mm at the isocenter, 6 pairs with a leaf width of 4.5 mm at the isocenter, and 6 pairs with a leaf width of 5.5 mm at the isocenter. The single-focused mMLC has a special tongue-and-groove design, full over-center travel, a low leakage of (1.5–2%), and a maximum speed of 1 cm/s.[21] The leaves have rounded ends to minimize the penumbra size. Circular cones with different diameters can also be mounted below the mMLC.

Novalis can operate in different treatment modes, including conventional circular arc SRS, conformal SRS (multiple static shaped beams), dynamic conformal arc SRS (arc delivery combined with mMLC field shaping that continuously conforms to the beam's eye view projection of the target), and dynamic or step-and-shoot IMRT. The primary components of the system—linac, MLC, treatment planning system, infrared and x-ray tracking and positioning system—are fully integrated through a record and verify system, which is a patient information management system. All treatment planning parameters, including the gantry, couch, collimator position, monitor units, and leaf position, are automatically transferred from the treatment planning system to Novalis through this information management system.

Elekta

The Elekta Precise (Elekta, Stockholm, Sweden) MLC delivery system replaces the upper movable jaws inside the linear accelerator head (Figure 12-8). The close proximity to the target results in a minimal range of motion required for

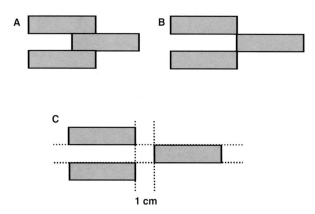

FIGURE 12-6. Schematic diagram illustrating the interdigitation restrictions for various multileaf collimators (MLCs) based on their design specifications. (A) Full interdigitation is allowed; (B) leaf tips from opposing MLC banks are allowed to meet, but not pass, each other; (C) leaf tips from opposing leaf banks must remain 1 cm apart. Adapted from Xia P and Verhey LJ.[19]

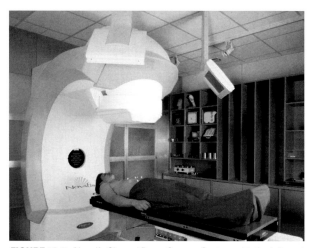

FIGURE 12-7. Novalis Shaped Beam Surgery System with the infrared and x-ray tracking and positoning system. (To view a color version of this image, please refer to the CD-ROM.) Courtesy of Franz Gum, BrainLAB.

precise field shaping. There are several benefits to this design, placing less wear and tear on the leaf positioning mechanism, and it allows the head size to be very compact at only 62 cm in diameter. A smaller head size reduces the potential for gantry and table collisions when noncoplanar beams are used. The system is capable of delivering a dose at 0.1 MU resolution, allowing for the accurate delivery of small-dose segments common to IMRT prescriptions.

The Elekta MLC consists of 40 pairs of tungsten alloy leaves with a 7.5 cm thickness and each leaf projecting a 1.0 cm width at the isocenter. The average leakage through the MLC system is 1.8 to 2.5%.[20] Transmission is reduced to less than 0.5% by 3 cm thick backup jaws directly underneath the leaves. Because of the integrated nature of Elekta's design, the same computer controls the MLC, the leaves, and the backup jaws. Therefore, the backup jaws automatically follow to the edge position of the outermost withdrawn leaf. Each leaf has a length of 32.5 cm at the isocenter and is single focus, with a rounded end. The maximum field size for conventional treatment is 40 × 40 cm. Each leaf can travel 12.5 cm over the beam central axis, allowing an IMRT field of 25 × 40 cm. The maximum leaf speed is 2.0 cm/s, defined at the isocenter. IMRT is delivered using the step-and-shoot technique. The Precise linear accelerator is capable of delivering each segment automatically through an autofield sequencer available either with the *PreciseBEAM* software or an external record and verification system.

Elekta's PreciseBEAM IMRT interface adheres to an open-systems philosophy using the Digitial Imaging and Communication in Medicine (DICOM) radiation therapy standard for communications with other systems, allowing an interface to all major record and verification systems. Unique to Elekta's PreciseBEAM IMRT design is the option to receive prescriptions directly from the treatment planning system without passing through an external record and verification system. Elekta's MLC provides real-time

display of leaf position via charge injection device camera technology on color monitors in both the treatment room and the control room. It also offers beam's eye view verification of the actual leaf setup, with the precision of the individual leaf position being ± 0.6 mm.

Siemens Medical Solutions

In the Siemens (Siemens Medical Solutions, Malvern, PA) PRIMUS and ONCOR linear accelerators, the MLC delivery system replaces the lower movable jaws inside the linear accelerator head (Figure 12-9). The OPTIFOCUS MLC for the ONCOR linear accelerators has 39 pairs of inner leaves with a 1.0 cm width and two pairs of outer leaves with a 0.5 cm width. This provides coverage of a full 40 cm IMRT field length. The three-dimensional MLC on the PRIMUS linear accelerators consists of 27 pairs of inner leaves with a 1.0 cm width at the isocenter and two pairs of outer leaves with a 6.5 cm width. The leaf length for both systems is 31 cm at the isocenter, with a straight edge facing toward the center of the beam. A double-focus leaf design follows the beam divergence so that the end and side of the leaves follow the beam divergence in both directions

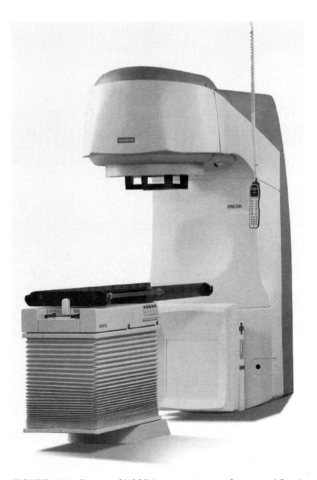

FIGURE 12-9. Siemens ONCOR linear accelerator. Courtesy of Sandi Lotter, Siemens Medical Solutions.

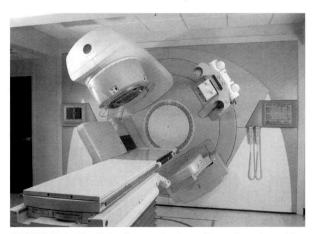

FIGURE 12-8. The Elekta Synergy (registered) uses Cone-beam kilovoltage computed tomography (KVCT) to guide IMRT treatments. (To view a color version of this image, please refer to the CD-ROM.) Courtesy of Timothy Prosser, Elekta.

(along and perpendicular to the leaf motion). This configuration produces a relatively narrow beam penumbra. Because of the complex design for an arc trajectory, the leaf position is accurate only to within 2 mm.

The average leakage through the Siemens MLC is 0.9 to 1.25%.[20] Each leaf can travel a maximum distance of 15 cm over the beam central axis, which may limit the IMRT field width in some cases to 27 cm. The maximum speed of the leaf is 2 cm/s, defined at the isocenter. The upper jaws must be positioned no more than 0.5 cm beyond the boundary of the MLC shape. Siemens linear accelerators provide a maximum field size for conventional treatment of 40 × 40 cm.

The MLC-based IMRT is designed for the automated segmental treatment technique, also known as CINEMATIC IMRT. Siemens linear accelerators are capable of delivering each segment automatically through an autofield sequencer available on the LANTIS record and verification system. To efficiently deliver IMRT, a delivery module known as SIMTEC (Siemens Intensity Modulation Technology) has been developed. This delivery module contains an autofield sequencer that automatically delivers all fields without human intervention provided that all fields are coplanar. In addition, *IM-MAXX* is a software package from Siemens designed for efficient IMRT dose delivery. These optimization tools can provide the user with faster IMRT delivery times, keeping all of the verification elements intact.

Varian Medical Systems

The Varian (Varian Medical Systems, Palo Alto, CA) Clinac MLC delivery system is a tertiary system mounted below the lower movable jaws inside the linear accelerator head (Figure 12-10). The MLC consists of 26, 40, or 60 pairs of tungsten alloy leaves with 6 cm thickness and each projecting a 0.5 or 1.0 cm width at the isocenter. For the newer delivery system, the Millennium 120 MLC, there are 40 inner pairs of leaves, with each leaf projecting a 0.5 cm width, and 20 outer pairs of leaves, with a 1.0 cm width at the isocenter. The average leakage through the Varian MLC is 1.6 to 1.9%.[20] Each leaf has a length of 16 cm measured at the isocenter and is single focus, with a rounded end. In the single-focused MLC, the leaf motion is along a straight line in a plane perpendicular to the beam central axis. The mechanical design is therefore simpler, with a leaf positional accuracy of 1 mm at the isocenter. The rounded end is used to ensure that leaf end transmission is nearly independent of the leaf position. The maximum leaf speed is 3 cm/s.

With two MLC leaf carriages, the maximum conventional field size is 40 × 40 (26) cm, depending on the number of leaf pairs available on the MLC. The travel range of each leaf is 15 cm from the end of the carriage.[22] The carriage can be retracted up to 20 cm from the beam axis and can travel up to 2 cm beyond the axis. Therefore, the leaf positions can vary between 20 cm away from the isocen-

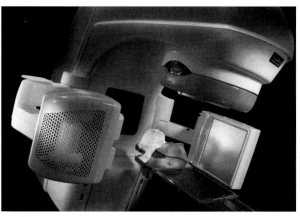

FIGURE 12-10. Varian Clinac with On-Board Imager. The On-Board Imager is used to fine-tune patient setups before delivery of intensity-modulated radiation therapy begins. (To view a color version of this image, please refer to the CD-ROM.) Courtesy of L. Scott Johnson, Varian Medical Systems.

ter to 17 cm beyond the isocenter as long as multiple carriage positions are used. There is no restriction in the upper and lower movable jaw location relative to the MLC shape. However, the recommended jaw position is 0.5 cm distal to the boundary of the MLC shape for conventional treatment. Because the leaf length is 16 cm, the distance between the most leading and the most retracted leaves from the same bank is limited to 14.5 cm to avoid radiation leakage through the tail of the most leading leaf or the tip of the most retracted leaf.[22] The MLC system supports all types of IMRT delivery: segmental, dynamic, combined dynamic and segmental in the same field, and conformal arc.

The dynamic IMRT delivery module is called the dose mode in the Varian system. In this mode, an intensity-modulated MLC file is executed, consisting of a sequence of all leaf positions as a function of a dose index, starting from 0.0 to 1.0. This dose index is a percentage of the total MU for this intensity-modulated field. During the delivery, the MLC leaf positions are controlled by the MLC control computer, whereas the total MU is controlled by console computer. The MLC control computer and the MU console computer communicate with each other every 50 milliseconds to establish the correspondence between the leaf position and the cumulative MU, as described in the intensity-modulated file.[23]

Summary

The intensity beam modulator is the primary component of the treatment machine that allows for the delivery of IMRT. Each of the modulation systems described here has its advantages and disadvantages. The choice of a particular manufacturer's system depends on a number of factors, including available hardware and software, the scope of the IMRT program, and cost. IMRT delivery systems are continually evolving. Future systems will improve on the features of existing technologies by reducing radiation transmission, providing improved integration with accelerator hardware, and increasing delivery efficiency to reduce overall treatment times.

Acknowledgments

The authors and editors wish to thank the following individuals for contributing to this chapter: Tim Biertempfel (North American Scientific, Nomos Radiation Oncology Division), Franz Gum (BrainLAB), Sam Jeswani (TomoTherapy Inc.), L. Scott Johnson (Varian Medical Systems), Sandi Lotter (Siemens Medical Solutions), Timothy Prosser (Elekta), and Richard Sweat (Southeastern Radiation Productions).

References

1. Purdy JA. Intensity-modulated radiation therapy [editorial]. Int J Radiat Oncol Biol Phys 1996;35:845–6.
2. Saw CB, Zhen W, Ayyangar KM, et al. Clinical aspects of IMRT—part III. Med Dosim 2002;27:75–7.
3. Saw CB, Ayyangar KM, Enke CA. MLC-based IMRT—part II. Med Dosim 2001;26:111–2.
4. Saw CB, Ayyangar KM, Enke CA. MIMiC-based IMRT—part I. Med Dosim 2001;26:1.
5. Intensity Modulated Radiation Therapy Collaborative Working Group. Intensity modulated radiotherapy: current status and issues of interest. Int J Radiat Oncol Biol Phys 2001;51:880–914.
6. Yang CCJ, Raben A, Carlson D. IMRT: high-definition radiation therapy in a community hospital. Med Dosim 2001;26:215–26.
7. Chang SX, Cullip TJ, Deschesne KM. Intensity modulation delivery technique: "step & shoot" MLC auto-sequence versus the use of a modulator. Med Phys 2000;27:948–59.
8. Bakai A, Laub WU, Nusslin F. Compensators for IMRT—an investigation in quality assurance. Z Med Phys 2001;11:15–22.
9. Yoda K, Aoki Y. A multiportal compensator system for IMRT delivery. Med Phys 2003;30:880–6.
10. Curran B. "Where goest the peacock?" Med Dosim 2001;26:3–9.
11. Saw CB, Ayyangar KM, Thompson RB, et al. Commissioning of Peacock system for intensity-modulated radiation therapy. Med Dosim 2001;26:55–64.
12. Salter BJ. Nomos Peacock IMRT utilizing the BEAK post collimation device. Med Dosim 2001;26:37–45.
13. Low DA, Mutic S, Dempsey JF, et al. Abutment dosimetry for serial tomotherapy. Med Dosim 2001;26:79–82.
14. Salter BJ, Helvezi JM, et al. An oblique arc capable positioning system for sequential tomotherapy. Med Phys 2001;28:2475–88.
15. Balog JP, Mackie TR, Reckwerdt P, et al. Characterization of the output for helical delivery of intensity modulated beams. Med Phys 1999;26:55–64.
16. Kapatoes JM, Olivera GH, Ruchala KJ, et al. A feasible method for clinical delivery verification and dose reconstruction in tomotherapy. Med Phys 2001;28:528–42.
17. Yang JN, Mackie TR, Reckwerdt P, et al. An investigation of tomotherapy beam delivery. Med Phys 1997;24:425–36.
18. Saw CB, Siochi RA, Ayyangar KM, et al. Leaf sequencing techniques for MLC-based IMRT. Med Dosim 2001;26:199–204.
19. Xia P, Verhey LJ. Delivery systems of intensity-modulated radiotherapy using conventional multileaf collimators. Med Dosim 2001;26:169–77.
20. Arnfield MR, Wu Q, Tong S, et al. Dosimetric validation for multileaf collimator-based intensity modulated radiotherapy: a review. Med Dosim 2001;26:179–88.
21. Xia P, Geis P, Xing L, et al. Physical characteristics of a miniature multileaf collimator. Med Phys 1999;26:65–70.
22. LoSasso TL, Chui CS, Ling CC. Physical and dosimetric aspects of a multileaf collimation system used in the dynamic mode for implementing intensity modulated radiotherapy. Med Phys 198;25:1919–27.
23. Xia P, Chuang CF, Verhey LJ. Communication and sampling rate limitations in IMRT delivery with a dynamic multileaf collimator system. Med Phys 2002;29:412–23.

Chapter 13

COMMISSIONING AND DOSIMETRIC QUALITY ASSURANCE

JOSEPH TING, PHD

The highly conformal dose distributions produced by intensity-modulated radiation therapy (IMRT) offer a means of reducing the volume of normal tissue irradiated and potentially allowing for dose escalation. However, IMRT is a complex process, involving patient selection, immobilization, simulation, target and tissue delineation, treatment planning, plan evaluation, and treatment delivery.[1] As such, a comprehensive quality assurance (QA) program is essential to the safe and accurate delivery of IMRT treatment fields. This chapter discusses specific QA requirements for linear accelerators and multileaf collimators (MLCs) delivering IMRT, initial IMRT commissioning, patient-specific QA (Figure 13-1), and the regulatory requirements of IMRT QA. Although there are many other clinical aspects of IMRT QA, this chapter concentrates only on the physics component.

The focus of this chapter is on the practical aspects of these topics. It is written from the perspective of a clinical physicist with experience in implementing IMRT programs in both the university and the community setting. For a broader perspective on IMRT QA, the reader is referred to Chapter 2, "Physics of IMRT," and the individual case studies. The future direction of IMRT QA is discussed in Chapter 14, "Quality Assurance Processes and Future Directions." Interested readers should also refer to task group reports and articles associated with IMRT commissioning and QA.[1–14]

Linear Accelerator and MLC Quality Assurance

To achieve dose conformity, IMRT makes use of highly nonuniform treatment fields. Typically, an IMRT field is composed of many beamlets, with dimensions as small as 0.5×0.5 cm^2. Within a given field, these beamlets have a wide range of intensity values (0–100%). Such intensity variation is the result of a set of complex software routines

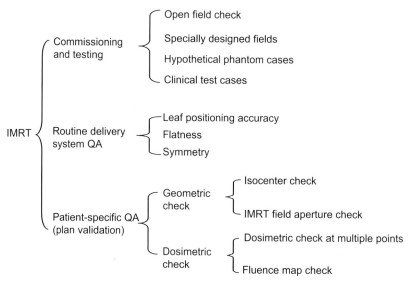

FIGURE 13-1. Major components associated with intensity-modulated radiation therapy (IMRT) commissioning and patient-specific quality assurance (QA). Courtesy of Lei Xing, PhD.

that compute the ideal radiation intensity to achieve an optimized dose distribution for a particular target geometry. A separate program then converts the ideal intensity map to a deliverable intensity map by taking into consideration the characteristics of the linear accelerator and the MLC. Two methods are commonly used for such conversion.[14–17] In segmental IMRT (also known as "step and shoot"), the MLC shape is constant during irradiation and changes only when the beam is "off." For dynamic IMRT, the leaf positions change while the beam is "on." In both cases, the positions of each leaf are constantly monitored, and a feedback mechanism is used to ensure that the leaves are at their predetermined locations as a function of the monitor units (MUs) delivered.

Each of these delivery mechanisms places additional requirements on the linear accelerator. For example, in segmental IMRT, the beam-on characteristics influence the accuracy of the intensity levels within each beamlet.[4,6,18] Highly conformal treatment plans typically have a large number of beam segments. The majority of these segments deliver < 5 MUs, and a significant fraction may deliver < 1 MU. As such, the dose/MU should be validated over the range of clinically delivered values. Additionally, field flatness and symmetry should also be checked over the same range of MUs (Figure 13-2). A fast film, such as Kodak TL (Eastman Kodak, Rochester, NY), should be used for such tests, although multiple exposures for a standard film (such as XV) may be used to produce a suitable optical density.

The accuracy of the delivered dose/MU is also affected by the communication between the linear accelerator and the MLC controller software.[4,6,11,18,19] For example, the Varian MLC controller (Varian Medical Systems, Palo Alto, CA) communicates with the linear accelerator console every 65 milliseconds. Such a delay leads to an overshoot phenomenon whereby the first segment delivers a slightly larger dose, whereas the last segment delivers a slightly smaller dose than expected. The effects are generally compensatory for the intermediary segments, and these receive the correct dose. In general, the communication lag introduces a small error that can be minimized by using a lower dose rate (MU/min). However, given that MLC controllers differ from one vendor to another, a systematic understanding of this effect on one's linear accelerator is essential.

A thorough linear accelerator QA program should be in place before IMRT is implemented. The American Association of Physicists in Medicine (AAPM) Task Group (TG) 40 has published a comprehensive description of linear accelerator QA.[2] The details of the TG 40 report are beyond the scope of this chapter; however, relevant linear accelerator QA tests are summarized in Table 13-1, and the interested reader is referred to the TG report. It is important to note that the TG 40 report was prepared prior to the widespread implementation of IMRT. As such, many of the tolerances, although adequate for conventional radiation therapy, may need to be modified to meet the stringent requirements of IMRT. Palta and colleagues provide

TABLE 13-1. Photon Beam Quality Assurance Tests for a Linear Accelerator

Frequency	Procedure	Tolerance
Daily	X-ray output constancy	3%
	Localizing lasers	2 mm
	Distance indicator	2 mm
	Door interlock	Functional
	Audiovisual monitor	Functional
Monthly	X-ray output constancy	2%
	Backup monitor constancy	2%
	X-ray central axis dosimetry	2%
	Flatness constancy	2%
	Symmetry	3%
	Emergency off switches	Functional
	Light/radiation field	2 mm or 1% on a side
	Gantry/collimator angle indicators	1°
	Field size indicators	2 mm
	Crosshair centering	2 mm diameter
	Treatment couch position indicators	2 mm/1°
	Jaw symmetry	2 mm
	Field light intensity	Functional
Annually	X-ray output constancy	2%
	Field size dependence of x-ray constancy	2%
	Central axis parameter constancy	2%
	Off-axis factor constancy	2%
	X-ray output constancy vs gantry angle	2%
	Monitor chamber linearity	1%
	Off-axis constancy vs gantry angle	2%
	Arc mode	Manufacturer's specifications
	Safety interlocks	Functional
	Collimator rotation isocenter	2 mm diameter
	Gantry rotation isocenter	2 mm diameter
	Couch rotation isocenter	2 mm diameter
	Coincidence of collimator, gantry, couch axes	2 mm diameter
	Coincidence of radiation and mechanical isocenters	2 mm diameter
	Tabletop sag	2 mm
	Vertical travel of table	2 mm

Adapted from Kutcher GJ et al.[2]

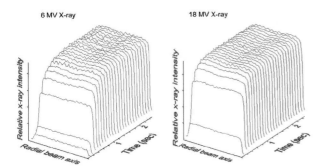

FIGURE 13-2. Example of the beam-on stability of a linear accelerator. These two sets of time sequence graphs show that this linear accelerator is in good calibration and the radiation field flatness and symmetry circuits function properly immediately after the beam is turned on.

a proposed set of tolerances, summarized in Table 13-2, based on the type of delivery method used.[12] The level of action for each of these tests is set to twice the tolerance value.

In addition to the requirements placed on the linear accelerator, IMRT demands accurate positioning of the MLC leaves. A detailed description of the characteristics of individual MLCs is provided in Chapter 12, "Delivery Systems." Table 13-3 lists a series of tests that should be conducted on an MLC to validate its use in both static cases and IMRT delivery.[10] Many of these tests are performed at the time of commissioning or when an MLC upgrade occurs. Two QA tests that are used on a weekly basis in our clinic to validate leaf positioning accuracy are the MLC positioning test and the MLC dose delivery test. Each of these is described below.

MLC Positioning Test

MLC positioning tests should be done with a film located in a reproducible position (independent of gantry angle) on the linear accelerator. For example, one option involves taping the film to the blocktray of the linear accelerator.

TABLE 13-2. Machine Tolerances for Intensity-Modulated Radiation Therapy Delivery

Items to Be Checked	Segmental	Dynamic
Multileaf collimator		
Leaf position accuracy	1 mm	0.5 mm
Leaf position reproducibility	0.2 mm	0.5 mm
Gap width reproducibility	0.2 mm	0.2 mm
Leaf speed	NA	± 0.1 mm/s
Gantry, MLC, and table isocenter	0.75 mm radius	0.75 mm radius
Beam output stability		
Low MU (< 2 MU)	2%	3%
Symmetry (< 2 MU)	2%	2%

Adapted from Palta JR et al.[12]
MLC = multileaf collimator; MU = monitor unit; NA = not applicable.

TABLE 13-3. Multileaf Collimator Tests for Static and Intensity-Modulated Radiation Therapy Delivery

Static MLC tests
  Carriage skew
  Physical gaps between carriages
  Lead position offset/radiation vs light field
  Leaf positioning reproducibility and accuracy
  Leaf transmission
IMRT tests
  Leaf speed
  Dose rate evaluation
  Leaf position tolerance and reproducibility
  Leaf acceleration
  Rounded tip transmission
  Beam stability for low MUs
  Treatment interruption

Adapted from Moran JM.[10]
IMRT = intensity-modulated radiation therapy; MLC = multileaf collimator; MU = monitor unit.

The test is then performed as follows. The gantry is set at 90° or 270° on alternate weeks, and the collimator is set to 0° (Figure 13-3). With this configuration, the MLC leaf travel is under the maximum influence of the earth's gravitational force.

A number of MLC test patterns are available for these tests. One such test, known as the "picket fence," is shown in Figure 13-4. In this example, the leaves from opposing banks form a small gap (0.25 cm). The beam is then turned

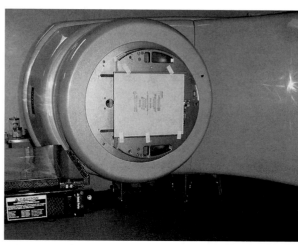

FIGURE 13-3. Routine intensity-modulated radiation therapy quality assurance (QA) film mounted on a linear accelerator. Weekly dynamic multileaf collimation QA is performed with a film mounted on the accessory tray of the linear accelerator. In this configuration, the multileaf collimator travels against gravity. (To view a color version of this image, please refer to the CD-ROM.)

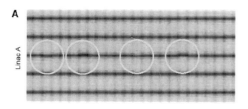

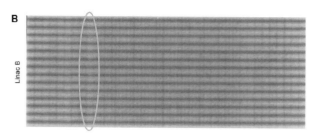

FIGURE 13-4. Examples of the "picket fence" test using (A) an electronic portal imaging device and (B) standard verification film (Kodak RP/V). The dark regions represent the gaps formed between opposing multileaf collimators. The highlighted regions indicate leaves that deviate from the expected positions. Linac = linear accelerator. (To view a color version of this image, please refer to the CD-ROM.)

"on," and the film is irradiated for a preset number of MUs. After irradiation, the leaves are then shifted by 0.75 cm. The same gap is formed by the MLC, and the film is again irradiated. This test pattern is automatically repeated 14 times across a 14 cm–wide field. Alternative tests can be designed that test both travel extremes of the MLC leaves instead of only the central displacements of the MLC.

It is important that these tests use the same dose rate as is used clinically. At our center, a dose rate of 400 MU/min is used for this test. Leaf deviations as small as 0.2 mm can be visually detected using this approach. These test images can also be analyzed using a number of commercially available QA programs. Using these programs, leaf travel and positional deviations can be tracked on a regular basis and compared with baseline values. Additionally, this MLC positional accuracy test can also be performed using an electronic portal imaging device (EPID).

MLC Dose Delivery Test

The radiation dose delivery constancy check using the MLC is performed with two separate MLC test patterns depending on the type of delivery mechanism, segmental or dynamic. For segmental delivery, the MLC is set to deliver a 10 × 10 cm^2 field with the first segment and a narrow slit for the second segment (Figure 13-5). An ionization chamber positioned in a solid water phantom is used to measure the radiation dose after the delivery of the first segment (the second segment is ignored). This reading is compared with a static 10 × 10 cm^2 field reading using the collimator jaws while MLC leaves are fully retracted. These two readings should agree to within 1.0%. If differences between these two readings exceed 2.0%, this may indicate a communication problem with the MLC and the linear accelerator controllers. In this case, IMRT treatments on this linear accelerator should be discontinued.

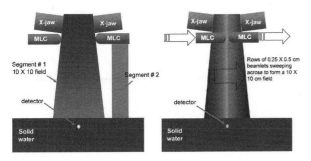

QA using segmental delivery method   QA using dynamic delivery method

FIGURE 13-5. Measurement setup for a routine intensity-modulated radiation therapy (IMRT) dose delivery check. It is necessary to measure the IMRT dose delivery on a weekly basis. The measured output using an ion chamber is compared with a standard 10 × 10 cm^2 field output using the collimator jaws only. MLC = multileaf collimator; QA = quality assurance. (To view a color version of this image, please refer to the CD-ROM.)

For dynamic delivery, the leaf speed constancy and transmission test sweeps the MLC leaves from one edge of the field to the opposite edge. For example, the leaves may move from –6 cm to +6 cm, with varying gaps between leaves on the right and left sides. In our implementation of this test, seven measurement points (ionization chamber measurements) in a solid water phantom are taken along the direction of the MLC travel. The measured values are logged and compared with values from the treatment planning system. The constancy of these values provides an indication of leaf travel speed, transmission, and leakage as a performance history of this particular MLC. If any of these values differ from the initial acceptance values by more than 1.0%, engineering services on the MLC and/or the linear accelerator may be required.

Commissioning

Prior to commissioning an IMRT planning system, the physicist and a representative from the planning system will perform acceptance testing to confirm that the planning system performs according to the manufacturer's specifications. TG 53 divides acceptance testing into three major categories: computer hardware, software function and features, and benchmark tests.[3] In many cases, these tests will be functional (yes or no), whereas some tests may be quantitative and based on the manufacturer's tolerances. A summary of the acceptance tests for a typical IMRT planning system is listed in Table 13-4.[3]

Commissioning of the IMRT portion of the treatment planning package should be done after the conventional treatment planning tasks have been fully completed and accepted into clinical service. AAPM TGs 40 and 53 have produced guidelines for commissioning a conventional treatment planning system.[2,3] Several reports have also described the commissioning of an IMRT planning system.[7–9,13] Xing and colleagues outlined a methodology for commissioning an IMRT planning system using open fields (nonmodulated) and progressing through more complex treatments that ultimately simulate an IMRT treatment.[8] The suggested tests in Table 13-5 serve as a basis for commissioning and accepting an IMRT planning system.[8] Although the exact implementation of these tests will vary by institution, general recommendations on the type of phantom and measurement devices are described below. Other considerations, such as user-modified planning parameters and data transfer issues, are also discussed.

Phantom and Dosimetric Requirements

It is not necessary to acquire a specialized phantom for IMRT commissioning. However, to commission the IMRT portion of the treatment planning system, one needs to create a phantom that can also be incorporated into the planning system. For example, a typical solid water phantom with dimensions of 30 (width) × 20 (height) × 30 cm (depth

TABLE 13-4. Acceptance Testing for an Intensity-Modulated Radiation Therapy Planning System

Component	Functionality of
Computer hardware	Printer
	Hard disk drive
	Monitor
	Mouse
	Keyboard
	Floppy disk drive
	Magnetic tape drive
Software features and function	Data transfer
	Contouring
	Selection of treatment machine
	Axial, sagittal, and coronal views
	Dose calculation
	Dose statistics
	Dose-volume histograms
	Report printout
	Monitor unit calculations
	Transfer plan to MLC controller
	MLC load treatment plan
	MLC leaves move according to plan
Benchmark test	Scan phantom and transfer to system
	Plan phantom
	Transfer to MLC controller
	Irradiate phantom
	Compare film and ion chamber measurements

Adapted from Fraas BK et al.[3]
MLC = multileaf collimator.

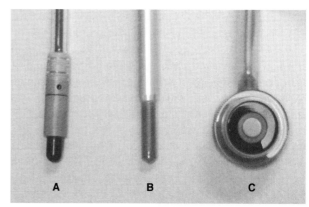

FIGURE 13-6. Types of ionization chambers suitable for commissioning and patient-specific intensity-modulated radiation therapy quality assurance (QA). Chambers A and B (cylindrical chambers) are useful for commissioning, whereas chamber C (parallel plate chamber) is used in the patient-specific QA procedure described in the text.

or length) can be used. The simplest way to input the phantom geometry into the planning system is to obtain a computed tomography (CT) scan. Using this approach, one can also validate the integrity of data transfer between the CT scanner and the treatment planning computer. Note that the phantom should be scanned with the ion chamber that will be used for commissioning in place.

The selection of an ionization chamber for IMRT QA is crucial.[20,21] Typical ionization chambers used for QA are shown in Figure 13-6. A chamber with a large active volume (eg, 0.6 cc Farmer-type ionization chambers [MEDTEC, Orange City, IA]) will integrate over a relatively large region, and its reading will represent an average value. Ionization chambers with very small active volumes (eg, 0.01 cm^3 radiosurgery chambers) have a poor signal-to-noise ratio and in an IMRT delivery may yield erroneous results. Based on our experience, a suitable ionization chamber should have an active volume of $\sim 0.1 \text{ cm}^3$. To obtain reproducible results with an ionization chamber, one should perform the measurement in a region with a low dose gradient. Otherwise, small differences in the relative position of the measurement point within the IMRT field can cause significant errors in the measured values, regardless of how small the measurement volume of the detector may be.

Once the phantom is scanned and transferred to the planning system, a target is created within the virtual phantom.

In the example shown in Figure 13-7, a cylindrical target with a diameter of 8.5 cm and a length of 6 cm was created. The planning system is then used to generate a series of plans, as described in Table 13-5. For example, one may design fields to deliver a uniform target dose of 2.0 Gy to the cylindrical target volume, as shown in Figure 13-7. It is also useful to contour the active volume of the ionization chamber and obtain a dose-volume histogram for this structure. The mean dose and standard deviation can be obtained and compared with measured values. By examining the relative deviation (standard deviation divided by mean value), one can quantitatively determine if the point of measurement is in a high dose gradient. If the relative deviation exceeds 5%, it may be useful to choose a different measurement point because small uncertainties in the setup may lead to measurements that are difficult to interpret. It is also important to maintain a record of measurements obtained during commissioning because these will serve as a baseline for future patient-specific measurements.

Film dosimetry is used to validate the spatial dose distribution and is an important component of IMRT commissioning. Depending on the phantom design, film may be placed in either the axial, coronal, or sagittal plane.

TABLE 13-5. Intensity-Modulated Radiation Therapy Treatment Planning Commissioning

Open fields	Square fields: output factors, depth dose, profiles
	Rectangular fields: output factors, depth dose, profiles
Offset fields	Small fields offset from isocenter: output factors
	Large fields offset from isocenter: output factors
Irregular fields	Output factors, depth dose
IMRT fields	Output factors, depth dose, profiles
IMRT treatment	Output factors, isodose distributions

Adapted from Xing L et al.[8]
IMRT = intensity-modulated radiation therapy.

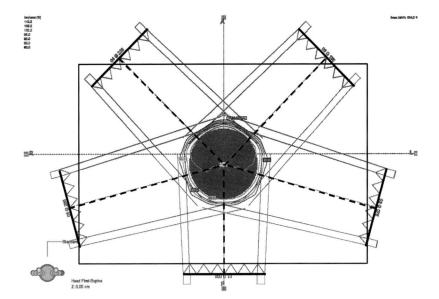

FIGURE 13-7. Test phantom configuration used to commission an intensity-modulated radiation therapy planning system. This test phantom consists of a solid water phantom that was scanned and transferred to the treatment planning system. For initial testing, the dose inside the planning target volume is purposely made uniform such that the measurement point is in a low dose gradient. (To view a color version of this image, please refer to the CD-ROM.)

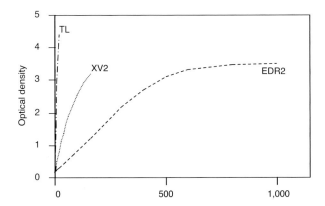

FIGURE 13-8. Film responses of some commonly used Kodak films. EDR film has an extended dose range in which the response is linear, making it desirable for intensity-modulated radiation therapy commissioning and patient-specific quality assurance.

Additionally, the film may be irradiated with or without the ionization chamber in place. At our clinic, Kodak EDR film is used because of its extended dose range (Figure 13-8).[22,23] However, EDR films are more sensitive to processor conditions, such as temperature, chemistry, and workload. If one chooses to use EDR film for IMRT QA, rigid processor control protocols should be followed.[22,23]

In performing film dosimetry, a Hunter-Driffield (H-D) curve, which relates the optical density to the absorbed dose, should be obtained.[24] The simplest method of producing such a curve is to irradiate a series of films to a known set of doses. For example, one may choose to irradiate film using a 10×10 cm^2 film in a solid water phantom under calibration conditions. The film should be exposed to doses ranging from zero (background + fog) to the maximum

dose expected by the treatment plan. It is important to note that the film response will depend on the processor conditions. Therefore, an H-D curve should be obtained each day on which film dosimetry is performed. Recently, a technique was described whereby the MLC is used to automatically define the different exposure regions on a single film to produce the H-D curve.[25] Not only is this method efficient, it can also be used as a test of leaf positioning accuracy. With careful film dosimetric calibration and with good film processor QA, the dose measured on the film should be consistent with the ionization chamber value. Therefore, the ionization chamber measurement serves as a double check of the film dosimetry system. A sample output from a film dosimetry system is shown in Figure 13-9.

Measured and calculated dose distributions are compared using dose differences or distances to agreement criteria. Commonly accepted values are 3% dose differences or 3 mm distance to agreement.[26] Recently, these two parameters have been combined into a single factor called the Gamma index.[26] Regions in which $\gamma > 1$ indicate that the calculation and measured values do not meet the acceptance criteria.

EPIDs have been in clinical use for over 10 years. However, the use of EPIDs as a dosimetry device has not been widespread, although there are many articles on the subject.[27–37] With the availability of image analysis software, initial IMRT QA can be accomplished by using an EPID, thus resulting in a significant time reduction. EPIDs can also be used to acquire either segmental or dynamic IMRT delivery methods, as shown in Figure 13-10.

The EPID should be set up and calibrated according to the manufacturer's protocol.[30,31] The EPID is then exposed to the IMRT field without any phantom material or treatment couch in front of the device. Similar to film analysis,

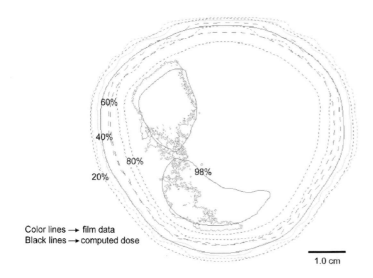

Color lines → film data
Black lines → computed dose

1.0 cm

FIGURE 13-9. Comparison of film measurements and the corresponding isodose distribution produced by the treatment planning system. (To view a color version of this image, please refer to the CD-ROM.)

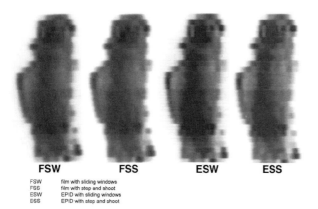

| FSW | FSS | ESW | ESS |

FSW   film with sliding windows
FSS   film with step and shoot
ESW   EPID with sliding windows
ESS   EPID with step and shoot

FIGURE 13-10. Comparison of intensity-modulated radiation therapy (IMRT) images captured on film and on an electronic portal imaging device (EPID). As illustrated in these images, the film and the EPID produce similar images for both segmental and dynamic IMRT.

EPID and treatment planning computer results are compared with dose differences or distances to agreement criteria. However, EPID dosimetry is in its infancy and needs to be refined before it can be used to measure doses reliably.[35,36] Of note, unlike film, EPIDs can be exposed only to a radiation beam perpendicular to the imaging panel. Therefore, the EPID cannot be used to obtain composite planar dose distributions, as can be done with film.

It is important to point out that all of the phantom measurements should be done using the record and verification software as if a patient were to be treated. This provides a system check, including data transfer between the treatment planning system, record and verification software, linear accelerator, and MLC controller. One should not perform IMRT QA measurements in the "service mode" or any other nonclinical mode of the linear accelerator.

IMRT Modeling Parameters

Depending on the inverse planning system, certain user-adjustable modeling parameters may need to be modified during commissioning to bring calculated and measured values into agreement. For example, the leading-edge penumbra of the MLC leaf is modeled by a parameter called the dosimetric leaf gap, and the transmission through the MLC leaf is modeled by another parameter, called leaf transmission. Although both of these parameters can be measured with a high degree of accuracy,[38] an alternative approach is to start with default values provided by the treatment planning system and to quantify the agreement between measured and calculated doses. Often the default values will produce an agreement of better than 3% between calculated and measured values. If the error is greater than 3%, the conventional planning portion of the system should be checked for proper commissioning and correct data entry (eg, output factors, percentage depth doses, beam profiles). If these data appear to be correct, then direct measurement and modification of these parameters may be necessary.

Data Transfer Issues

During the initial acceptance process, physicists should verify the integrity of data transfer through the entire system (CT, treatment planning, record and verify, and linear accelerator controller). In addition, treatment machine parameters and coordinate conventions should also be verified. As part of the initial commissioning process, one should scan a solid water phantom, transfer it to the planning computer, generate inverse plans, pass the treatment data to the record and verification system, schedule this phantom for treatment, and, finally, deliver the treatment plan to the test phantom in full clinical mode.

Patient-Specific QA

Although there is some debate regarding the need for patient-specific QA, the fact remains that IMRT fields are unique to an individual patient's anatomy, field arrangements, and dose prescription. Unlike conventional treatments, IMRT treatment fields cannot be periodically checked by simple tests or routinely scheduled calibrations. Our policy is that each field for every IMRT patient must be verified before the start of actual treatment. Below is a description of a QA procedure developed at our center. It is simple to implement and provides direct verification of an individual patient's treatment fields.

Dosimetric Verification

A requirement of patient-specific QA is that the setup must be simple, easy to handle, and reproducible. Our QA setup

aims to ensure that the delivered fluence maps are in agreement with the computed ones. This setup is not designed to test other aspects of the treatment planning system because this was done during the commissioning phase. An effective method for patient-specific QA is described as follows. The solid water phantom used during commissioning is placed on the treatment table. The surface of the phantom is set at a 95.0 cm source-to-skin distance. A film is placed at a 5.0 cm depth from the phantom surface and is located at the isocenter, or 100 cm from the radiation source. An ionization chamber is then placed at a 10.0 cm depth from the phantom surface (105.0 cm from the radiation source). This setup is shown in Figure 13-11. In this configuration, all IMRT fields are delivered with the gantry set to 0° (gantry pointing vertically downward toward the phantom surface). Within the treatment planning computer, a phantom plan is created and the individual patient fields are projected onto the phantom using the same beam arrangement (all beams at gantry = 0 degrees). Measurements obtained using this geometry are then compared with those produced by the planning system.

An ideal ionization chamber for dose measurement using this setup is a parallel plate ionization chamber with a 0.1 cc collection volume. A parallel plate ionization chamber provides symmetry along and perpendicular to the direction of MLC leaf travel.[21] An example of such an ionization chamber is shown in Figure 13-6. In this setup, the ionization chamber measurement is taken together with the film exposure using the same MUs as for the actual treatment of the patient. The electrometer readings are not "reset" between each field. Based on 5 years of IMRT measurements (over 1,500 patients), our ionization chamber data show a gaussian distribution with a mean at −1.1% and a standard deviation of 0.5% from the calculated data. Figure 13-12 shows a comparison of measured and calculated doses of a newly commissioned IMRT program in a small community hospital.

To simplify and aid the registration process of the film image and the computed dose matrix, either a 15 × 15 cm^2 or a 20 × 20 cm^2 field is added to the IMRT exposure. This is done in both the treatment planning system and actual

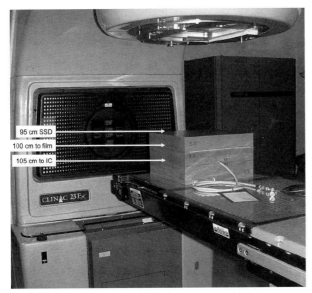

FIGURE 13-11. Phantom and irradiation geometry used during patient-specific quality assurance. To minimize the time required on the linear accelerator, the film and ionization chamber are exposed to all intensity-modulated radiation therapy fields simultaneously with the gantry in the home position. SSD = source-to-skin distance. (To view a color version of this image, please refer to the CD-ROM.)

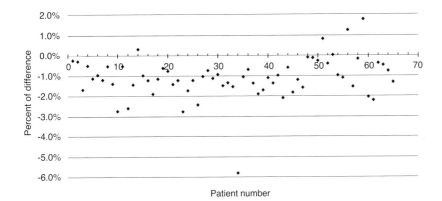

FIGURE 13-12. Comparison of measured versus calculated doses for patient-specific intensity-modulated radiation therapy (IMRT) quality assurance. This chart shows a newly commissioned IMRT program at a small community radiation oncology clinic. The average disparity is −1.1%.

film irradiation. The actual IMRT patient treatment fields are not altered. This added dose is computed and accounted for in both cases. An example is shown in Figure 13-13. This film is analyzed with a commercially available software package. Based on the dose gradient, either percent deviation on individual points or distance to agreement is used for evaluation. Figure 13-14 shows two clinical examples of superimposing of film data and the computed dose matrix.

Patient-specific QA for IMRT patients can be reliably accomplished using film dosimetry if proper film calibration and processor control are done. As described previously, a "control film" exposed to a known dose is processed at the same time as the IMRT QA films. This will account for film processor temperature and chemical variations, which have a dramatic effect on the reproducibility of film dosimetry.[22,23]

It is important to use the identical monitor units from the actual patient treatment in the IMRT patient QA test. Otherwise, errors resulting from leaf transmission, interleaf gap, and beam-on and beam-off delays may enter into the QA process. Thus, the QA results may become invalid.

EPIDs can also be used for dosimetric evaluation of patient IMRT fields.[22,28,29,32] They can be used to analyze IMRT field shapes and fluence maps (Figure 13-15). However, at present, calibrating the EPID for the purpose of absolute dosimetry presents a challenge because of the strong energy dependence of the device, improper buildup material, the lack of backscatter material, and the lack of constancy check on the imaging matrix.[30,31]

For relative IMRT dosimetry and documentation of field shapes, using the EPID can significantly reduce the time required for IMRT QA. Because of the efficient database management, the acquired images can be directly com-

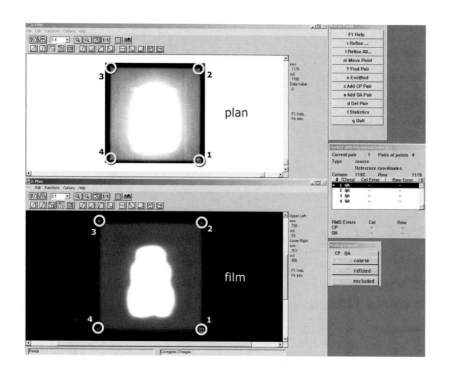

FIGURE 13-13. An open field (15 × 15 cm²) is added onto the composite intensity-modulated radiation therapy fields in both the calculated dose and the actual film exposure. The corners of this standard field size are used to align the computed dose matrix and the exposed film image.

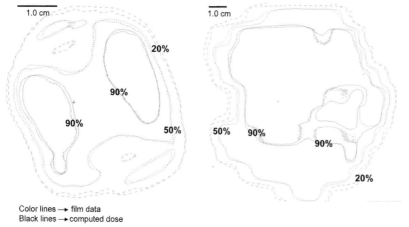

Color lines → film data
Black lines → computed dose

FIGURE 13-14. Examples of film data compared with computed dose matrices. Agreement shown here is within clinically acceptable criteria of 3% or 3 mm. (To view a color version of this image, please refer to the CD-ROM.)

pared with the output from the treatment planning system (see Figure 13-15). With EPID, patient-specific IMRT QA can be streamlined and integrated with the record and verification system. Additionally, patient-specific QA results are automatically documented for future reviews and audits.

Other Approaches

Currently, there is no standard procedure for performing patient-specific QA. Rather, each institution must implement its own program based on available equipment and personnel. Many centers use the phantom plan approach in which each field is delivered at the gantry angle corresponding to the treatment plan. Briefly, a CT scan is first obtained of the phantom. The individual fluence maps for a given patient plan are then cast onto the phantom scan, and the dose is calculated. At the treatment machine, the phantom is treated in the same manner as the patient is. Ion chambers, film, and/or thermoluminescent dosimeter measurements are then compared with calculated doses. For a more detailed description, see individual case studies.

In using this approach, it is important to choose a phantom that mimics the patient. Solid water slabs provide a reasonable approximation for many adult disease sites. However, in pediatric cases, the dimensions are much smaller, and the tumor may be only slightly deeper than the buildup depth. In these cases, a phantom that is comparable to the size of the patient may be necessary. Chapter 26.3, "Rhabdomyosarcoma: Case Study," describes a special phantom that was used to validate an IMRT plan that was delivered to the leg of an infant. Another case that requires special consideration is when inhomogeneity corrections are used. Chapter 25.1, "Paraspinal Soft Tissue Sarcoma: Case Study," describes the use of a phantom with

a lung inhomogeneity to validate the dose calculated near the lung-tissue interface.

Many centers are also using independent calculations to validate the MUs computed by the treatment planning system. One such commercially available product is *RadCalc* (Lifeline Software, Inc., Tyler, TX). *RadCalc* uses a modified Clarkson integration technique to calculate the dose contribution from each IMRT field to the point of interest.[39] Studies comparing *RadCalc* with the *CORVUS* system (North American Scientific, NOMOS Radiation Oncology Division, Cranberry Township, PA) indicate an average disparity of 1.4% with a standard deviation of 1.2%.[40] Values outside the average disparity, ± 2 SD, can be used to alert the physicist to a problem prior to measurement. Moreover, unlike phantom measurements, *RadCalc* uses the actual patient depths and thus provides an additional level of patient-specific QA. Details on the use of an MU verification program are provided in Chapters 18.5, "Pyriform Sinus Cancer: Case Study"; 22.4, "ProstaScint-Guided IMRT: Case Study"; and 26.3.

Lastly, patient-specific verification can also be performed using leaf positions as recorded by the MLC controller. Litzenberg and colleagues described a program to evaluate the delivered fluence of segmental and dynamic MLC fields using the dynamic log files produced by a Varian 2100EX (Varian Medical Systems).[41] This file reports the expected and actual position for each leaf and the dose fraction every 0.055 seconds. Leaf trajectories are calculated from these data, and the expected and actual fluence can be compared. Recently, this analysis tool has become commercially available as part of the Argus system from Varian Medical Systems.

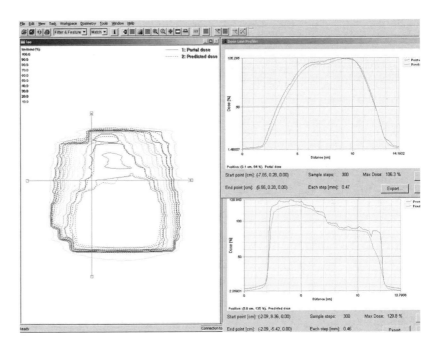

FIGURE 13-15. Comparison of measurements obtained using an electronic portal imaging device with a calculated dose distribution. (To view a color version of this image, please refer to the CD-ROM.)

Geometric Verification

As in conventional radiation therapy, it is essential that the location of the isocenter is radiographically verified. This is most commonly done by comparing anterior and lateral portal images with digitally reconstructed radiographs or simulation films. Others have described a technique whereby the leaves are set to the maximum extent of the treatment field and portal images are acquired for each treatment field.[42] A double-exposure technique is used so that the field boundary can be visualized relative to the patient's anatomy. A simulation film using the MLC boundary as the radiation field is also produced for comparison. An example of this technique is shown in Figure 2-25 of Chapter 2.

The frequency of isocenter verification should be, at a minimum, once per week. However, many institutions obtain verification images twice per week in patients receiving IMRT. New IMRT programs may want to verify the isocenter position on a daily basis during the first week of treatment and then twice per week thereafter.

Necessity and Regulatory Requirements

One may eventually ask the question, "When will there be enough QA: after 100 IMRT patients, after 500 IMRT patients, or after 1,500 IMRT patients?" What should one do to ensure the safety of our patients? Given that IMRT is increasingly used, is it safe? Of course, every treatment delivery system is "safe" until the first accident occurs. Because every IMRT patient is treated with customized field intensities, every intensity map should be checked to ensure that the delivered intensity maps agree reasonably well with those generated by the treatment planning computer.

Some believe that the additional effort spent for each patient is redundant and has little value beyond the initial commissioning of the IMRT package. Others may believe that "proper" initial commissioning of the IMRT package can uncover all potential errors and there will be no need to "duplicate" efforts in performing patient-specific IMRT QA for each patient. Unfortunately, an accident with IMRT delivery may eventually serve to alert the clinical staff that the "proper" initial commissioning of the IMRT package may not be adequate. However, by this time, some patients or a group of patients may have been injured by the undiscovered problem associated with an IMRT delivery system.

Although IMRT has been in clinical use since the mid-1990s by a few large institutions, widespread use of this new treatment delivery technology in community hospitals has only just begun. IMRT technology is still in its infancy. The complex computer networks, inverse planning algorithms, MLC leaf sequencing software routines, dynamic MLC controller software, and MLC hardware systems dictate that patient IMRT QA should be done to ensure

that delivered dose distribution agrees with that produced by the treatment planning computer. At present, patient-specific QA is time consuming and resource intensive. However, with recent advances in EPID dosimetry, IMRT QA may eventually be accomplished in less than 15 minutes.

Aside from the clinical necessity of validating patient IMRT plans, an elaborate set of regulations exists for proper submission of billing charges to various insurance organizations. To date, most of these billing codes follow the recommendations of the American College of Radiology, which clearly specify the need to verify data. The economics and billing aspects of IMRT are discussed in Chapter 16, "Billing and Reimbursement." Although billing codes are subject to future changes, at this time, they state that patient-specific IMRT QA must be completed prior to the start of IMRT for each patient. Therefore, patient-specific QA is not only a clinical necessity but also a regulatory requirement.

The future of IMRT QA is subject to speculation. Computational approaches are gaining more acceptance and are likely to compete with direct measurement.[39–41] An independent dose calculation system that computes and compares the dose distribution with that produced by the treatment planning system will make the process of patient-specific QA both easier and more thorough than the current practice. The use of computational approaches in the IMRT process is discussed in Chapter 14.

References

1. Xia P, Chuang C. Patient-specific quality assurance in IMRT. In: Palta JR, Mackie TR, editors. Intensity-modulated radiation therapy: the state of the art. Colorado Springs (CO): Medical Physics Publishing; 2003. p. 495–514.
2. Kutcher GJ, Coia L, Gillin M, et al. Comprehensive QA for radiation oncology: report of AAPM Radiation Therapy Committee Task Group 40. Med Phys 1994;21:581–618.
3. Fraass BK, Doppke K, Hunt G, et. al. American Association of Physicists in Medicine Radiation Therapy Committee Task Group 53: quality assurance for clinical radiotherapy treatment planning. Med Phys 1998;25:1773–829.
4. Intensity Modulated Radiation Therapy Collaborative Working Group. Intensity modulated radiotherapy: current status and issues of interest. Int J Radiat Oncol Biol Phys 2001;51:880–914.
5. Galvin JM, Ezzell G, Eisruch A, et al. Implementing IMRT in clinical practice: a joint document of the American Society for Therapeutic Radiology and Oncology and the American Association of Physicists in Medicine. Int J Radiat Oncol Biol Phys 2004;58:1616–34.
6. Ezzell GA, Galvin JM, Low D, et al. Guidance document on delivery, treatment planning, and clinical implementation of IMRT. Report of the IMRT Subcommittee of the AAPM Radiation Therapy Committee. Med Phys 2003;30:2089–115.
7. Sharpe MB. Commissioning and quality assurance for IMRT treatment planning. In: Palta JR, Mackie TR, editors. Intensity-modulated radiation therapy: the state of the art. Colorado

Springs (CO): Medical Physics Publishing; 2003. p. 495–514.

8. Xing L, Curran B, Hill R, et al. Dosimetric verification of a commercial inverse treatment planning system. Phys Med Biol 1999;44:463–78.

9. Essers M, deLangen M, Dirkx MLP, et al. Commissioning of a commercially available system for intensity-modulated radiotherapy dose delivery with dynamic multileaf collimation. Radiother Oncol 2001;60:215–24.

10. Moran JM. Dosimetry metrology for IMRT. In: Palta JR, Mackie TR, editors. Intensity-modulated radiation therapy: the state of the art. Colorado Springs (CO): Medical Physics Publishing; 2003. p. 415–37.

11. LoSasso TJ. IMRT delivery system QA. In: Palta JR, Mackie TR, editors. Intensity-modulated radiation therapy: the state of the art. Colorado Springs (CO): Medical Physics Publishing; 2003. p. 561–91.

12. Palta JR, Kim S, Li JG, et al. Tolerance limits and action levels for planning and delivery of IMRT. In: Palta JR, Mackie TR, editors. Intensity-modulated radiation therapy: the state of the art. Colorado Springs (CO): Medical Physics Publishing; 2003. p. 593–612.

13. Low DA, Mutic S, Dempsey JF, et al. Quantitative dosimetric verification of an IMRT planning and delivery system. Radiother Oncol 1998;49:305–16.

14. Burman C, Chui CS, Kutcher G, et al. Planning, delivery, and quality assurance of intensity-modulated radiotherapy using dynamic multileaf collimator: a strategy for large-scale implementation for the treatment of carcinoma of the prostate. Int J Radiat Oncol Biol Phys 1997;39:863–73.

15. Mott JH, Hounsell AR, Budgell GJ, et al. Customized compensation using intensity modulated beams delivered by dynamic multileaf collimation. Radiother Oncol 1997;53:59–65.

16. Convery DJ, Webb S. Generation of discrete beam-intensity modulation by dynamic multileaf collimation under minimum leaf separation constraints. Phys Med Biol 1998;43:2521–38.

17. Spirou S, Chui CS. Generation of arbitrary intensity profiles by dynamic jaws or multi-leaf collimators. Med Phys 1994;21:1031–41.

18. Hensen VN, Evans PM, Budgell GJ, et al. Quality assurance of the dose delivered by small radiation segments. Phys Med Biol 1998;43:2665–75.

19. Xia P, Chuang C, Verhey L. Communication and sampling rate limitations in IMRT delivery with a dynamic multileaf collimator system. Med Phys 2002;29:412–23.

20. Martens C, DeWagter C, DeNeve W. The value of the PinPoint ion chamber for characterization of small field segments used in intensity-modulated radiotherapy. Phys Med Biol 2000;45:2519–30.

21. Lee HR, Pankuch M, Chu JC, et. al. Evaluation and characterization of parallel plate microchamber's functionalities in small beam dosimetry. Med Phys 2002;29:2489–96.

22. Dogan N, Leybovich LB, Sethi A. Comparative evaluation of Kodak EDR2 and XV2 films for verification of intensity modulated radiation therapy. Phys Med Biol 2002;47:4121–30.

23. Zhu XR, Jursinic PA, Grimm DF, et al. Evaluation of Kodak EDR2 film for dose verification of intensity modulated radiation therapy delivered by a static multileaf collimator. Med Phys 2002;29:1687–92.

24. Williamson JF, Khan FM, Sharma SC. Film dosimetry of megavoltage photon beams: a practical method of isodensity-to-isodose curve conversion. Med Phys 1981;8:94.

25. Childress NL, Dong L, Rosen II. Rapid radiographic film calibration for IMRT verification using automated MLC fields. Med Phys 2002;29:2384–90.

26. Low DA, Harms WB, Mutic S, et. al. A technique for the quantitative evaluation of dose distributions. Med Phys 1998;25:660–1.

27. Partridge M, Evans F, Mosleh-Shirazi A, et al. Independent verification using portal imaging of intensity-modulated beam delivery by the dynamic MLC technique. Med Phys 1998;25:1872–9.

28. Pasma KL, Kroonwijk M, Quint S, et al. Transit dosimetry with an electronic portal imaging device (EPID) for 115 prostate cancer patients. Int J Radiat Oncol Biol Phys 1999;45:1297–303.

29. Kroonwijk M, Pasma KL, Quint S, et al. In vivo dosimetry for prostate cancer patients using an electronic portal imaging device (EPID): demonstration of internal organ motion. Radiother Oncol 1998;49:125–32.

30. Moran JM, Nurushev TS, Litzenberg DL, et al. Commissioning of an a:Si active matrix flat panel dosimeter for IMRT quality assurance. Med Phys 2002;29:1367.

31. Antonuk LE, El-Mohri I, Yorkston J, et al. Initial performance evaluation of an indirect-detector, active-matrix, flat-panel imager (AMFPI) prototype for megavoltage imaging. Int J Radiat Biol Phys 1998;42:437–54.

32. Nederveen AJ, Lagendijk JJ, Hofman P. Feasibility of automatic marker detection with an a-Si flat-panel imager. Phys Med Biol 2001;46:1219–30.

33. Pasma KL, Kroonwijk M, de Boer JC, et al. Accurate portal dose measurement with a fluoroscopic electronic portal imaging device (EPID) for open and wedged beams and dynamic multileaf collimation. Phys Med Biol 1998;43:2047–60.

34. Siewerdsen JH, Jaffray DA. Cone-beam computed tomography with a flat-panel imager: magnitude and effects of x-ray scatter. Med Phys 2001;28:220–31.

35. Liu G, Van Doorn T, Bezak E. Evaluation of the mechanical alignment of a linear accelerator with an electronic portal imaging device (EPID). Aust Phys Eng Sci Med 2000;23:74–80.

36. El-Mohri Y, Antonuk LE, Yorkston J, et al. Relative dosimetry using active matrix flat-panel imager (AMFPI) technology. Med Phys 1999;26:1530–41.

37. Kirby M, Williams PC. The use of an electronic portal imaging device for exit dosimetry and quality control measurements. Int J Radiat Oncol Biol Phys 1995;31:593–603.

38. Arnfield MR, Siebers JV, Kim JO, et al. A method for determining multileaf collimator transmission and scatter for dynamic intensity modulated radiotherapy. Med Phys 2000;27:2231–41.

39. Kung JH, Chen GTY, Kuchnir KT. A monitor unit verification calculation in intensity modulated radiotherapy as a dosimetry quality assurance. Med Phys 2000;27:2226–30.

40. Haslam JJ, Bonta DV, Lujan AE, et al. Comparison of dose calculated by an intensity modulated radiotherapy treatment planning system and an independent monitor unit verification program. J Appl Clin Med Phys 2003;4:224–30.

41. Litzenberg DW, Moran JM, Fraass BA. Verification of dynamic and segmental IMRT delivery by dynamic log file analysis. J Appl Clin Med Phys 2002;3:63–72.

42. Chen Y, Xing L, Luxton G, et al. A multi-purpose quality assurance tool for MLC-based IMRT [abstract]. ICCR, Heidelberg, Germany, May 2000.

Chapter 14

Quality Assurance Processes and Future Directions

Daniel A. Low, PhD, Eric E. Klein, MS

Intensity-modulated radiation therapy (IMRT) is a complex form of conformal therapy. The process of delivering the highly conformal dose distribution uses nonstandard field shapes and sizes, overlapping and abutting fields, and often uses dynamic delivery that is substantially different from the established delivery of conventional three-dimensional conformal radiation therapy (3DCRT). Although IMRT can deliver extremely conformal dose distributions, it requires a reliance on the treatment planning system software, its data and algorithms, the information transfer process, and the linear accelerator calibration and operation that is unprecedented in radiation therapy. Errors anywhere in the process can lead to catastrophic mistakes in dose delivery that may be detected first by their clinical consequences.

Before continuing, it is important to distinguish commissioning-level quality assurance (QA) from patient-specific QA. The process of commissioning a planning system or new implementation (eg, upgrade) typically requires significantly more manpower than routine patient-specific QA. Most of the QA procedures described in Chapter 13, "Commissioning and Dosimetric Quality Assurance," are well suited to commissioning. The fact that they are relatively inefficient is balanced against the relative infrequency of their implementation. The main advances in efficiency and thoroughness will come in patient-specific and more routine QA processes. Thus, the majority of this chapter is dedicated to this topic.

One would expect that the thoroughness of the QA process would mirror the complexity and potential hazards of IMRT. However, medical physicists are limited to the available technology for conducting their quality QA procedures. An accurate, thorough evaluation of the delivered dose distribution is not possible, so compromises are required. Typically, these involve the use of direct phantom measurements using the patient's treatment delivery parameters, such as monitor units and beam energy. This process can provide a lot of dose information that may be compared against the results of the treatment planning system, but QA guidelines are not yet available to aid the physicist in determining whether discrepancies between the measurement and calculation are acceptable.

Patient-Specific QA

The direct measurement of the IMRT dose distribution is currently the only widely available method for checking the delivered dose distribution against the calculation. The process usually involves the preparation of a special "phantom plan" by the treatment planning system. This treatment plan uses the beam fluences and energies, monitor units, gantry angles, and other delivery parameters that were selected for the patient plan and calculates the dose to the computed tomography (CT) scan of the phantom. The phantom is subsequently irradiated, and the measured dose is compared against the calculated dose distribution. The thoroughness of this process is limited by the available dosimetry systems, reasonable manpower use, and differences between the phantom and patient geometries.

There are three categories of measurement-based QA processes, which will be described as categories I through III. Categories I and II involve the placement of a phantom and dosimeter near the isocenter, whereas category III may have a phantom, but the dosimeter is distal to the isocenter (eg, a portal imager).

Category I Measurements

Category I uses the same gantry angles as those used in the patient's treatment to irradiate a phantom placed near the isocenter. The measurements are conducted for the entire irradiation, and the doses can be considered "composite" in that they reflect the contribution from all of the beams. The thoroughness of category I measurements is a function of the dosimeters used. Ionization chambers are used because their dosimetric response is well understood. Their chief limitations are that they provide only one data point for each irradiation and that the measurement needs to be considered as an average throughout the chamber's active volume. Assuming that the user identifies and locates the ionization chamber in a low dose-gradient region, volume averaging does not appear to yield significant errors, even for relatively large chambers.[1] However, although a single point measurement provides quantitative data that can be used to identify if the overall dose normalization is correct, it does not yield sufficient information to evaluate the dose throughout the target or critical structures.

Thermoluminescent dosimeters (TLDs) have been used for multiple point measurements for IMRT QA,[2,3] but they require significant preparation and postirradiation time to obtain the data. Before irradiation, each TLD chip must be either selected for a uniform response or independently calibrated such that its response relative to a collection of TLDs can be determined. This calibration process typically requires repeated irradiations to a common dose, readout, and annealing to determine the relative calibration with a statistical precision of a few percentages. The readout is greatly assisted by automation, but even with this, the preparation of the phantom (placing the TLDs within the phantom) and subsequent data analysis (selecting the points within the phantom plan) make the use of TLDs for routine patient QA inefficient.

Radiographic film yields dose information at a significantly higher spatial density than either TLDs or ionization chambers, but quantitative information is possible only if care is taken when using film. Radiographic film uses silver halide as its active ingredient. Recently, there has been some debate as to the accuracy of radiographic film owing to its expected uneven energy sensitivity to low-energy photons because of the silver in the emulsion.[4–8] This would, in theory, lead to overresponse in the beam penumbra (where a significant dose is delivered using Compton-scattered x-rays) with respect to the beam center (where the film calibration is conducted) or at deep depths with respect to shallow depths. In principle, the variations in sensitivity would cause problems with IMRT dose distribution measurements because much of the dose to a point is delivered by penumbra from neighboring beam segments. Some investigators have seen little or no significant errors in dose measurements for megavoltage beams when measuring depth doses or beam profiles.

Chetty and Charland evaluated the response of Kodak EDR-2 film (Eastman Kodak, Rochester, NY) as a function of depth and field size for two megavoltage beam energies (6 and 18 MV).[5] Note that this film has a relatively linear response up to 300 cGy. They found that the film optical density normalized to a 10×10 cm^2 field and 5 cm depth varied by less than 3% for 3×3 cm^2 and 10×10 cm^2 fields at 3, 5, and 15 cm depths. When compared against a 25×25 cm^2 field, however, variations of almost 5% were observed. Esthappan and colleagues found comparable agreement (approximately 4%) with a similar evaluation using 6 and 18 MV fields between 4×4 cm^2 and 15×15 cm^2.[6] Dogan and colleagues conducted similar experiments, extending

the energy range down to ^{60}Co.[4] They developed a depth-dependent characteristic curve measurement using films oriented parallel to the radiation beam central axis. Application of the depth-dependent characteristic curve improved the depth response considerably, and an example of the improved correspondence between measurement and calculation was shown for an IMRT measurement. Currently, the physicist has to decide how important quantitative information from film is to their own QA program and provide sufficient processes in place to ensure this.

Some clinics use radiographic film only for its ability to localize the radiation dose distribution using the location of the steep dose gradients. As an example, they may irradiate the film and, after processing it, compare the film with a printout of the phantom plan dose distribution side by side using a light box. This may detect catastrophic errors such as the wrong patient treatment being selected (if the user is sufficiently careful to mark and preserve the film orientation), but it will not determine the accuracy of dose delivered to a critical structure. Qualitative film measurements, for example, without a sensitometric curve measurement, have similar utility as a manual check. However, it is a relatively straightforward step to add the sensitometric film measurements and obtain quantitative results.

Even when quantitative results are obtained using film, there are still some significant limitations to its use. As with any direct dose measurements, it requires significant time to prepare, acquire, and analyze the resulting data. Although the experiments will yield a large amount of data, they are still essentially two-dimensional. This means that multiple films are required to sample the irradiated volume, especially if that volume is to include all of the specified normal structures.

Dosimetry measurements are not limited to two dimensions. Polyacrylamide gels offer the potential for three-dimensional dose measurements and read-out using either magnetic resonance imaging[9] or optical CT.[10–14] There are still some issues regarding stability and sensitivity variations from sample to sample, and validation of the quantitative nature of the optical readout process has not yet been completed.

Even with thorough film or three-dimensional dose distribution measurements, the use of phantom plan irradiation has some significant limitations. In particular, the locations of critical structures are not typically identified on the phantom plan, so dose errors cannot be directly correlated with anatomic location. Additionally, although the irradiated fluence may be the same, the dose distribution is not the same as in the patient owing to the difference between the patient and phantom geometries. Therefore, absolute, and perhaps even relative, dose errors detected in the phantom measurement may not be directly related to dose errors in the patient. Decisions on whether measured discrepancies are clinically relevant will be made more difficult owing to the differences between the patient and phantom geometries.

Category II Measurements

Category II phantom QA methods use a single gantry angle. Each radiation beam is aimed independently at the dosimeter from the vertical direction. Thus, validation is conducted on a beam-by-beam basis, and the doses are compared independently for each beam. There are more dosimetry options available when using this method, but the results are more difficult to evaluate and are even more removed from the patient treatment than category I measurements. Because the measurements are conducted using a single gantry angle, the phantom design is typically very simple, consisting of a uniform thickness of plastic (eg, water-equivalent plastic) with the dosimeters at a uniform depth and followed by backscatter material. Like category I validation, ionization chambers and radiographic films are often used to measure the single-beam irradiations. Comparisons against calculation are made similar to category I measurements, but discrepancies are more difficult to quantify. For example, if there is a 5% discrepancy for one field, how will that translate to an error in the composite treatment plan? Will it wash out or be isolated within the patient? Also, identification of a discrepancy with a specific critical structure is currently impossible. Although it would be possible to engineer a process that takes the measurement calculation discrepancies and recompute the dose within the patient, this has not been implemented commercially. In fact, the validation of individual beams is so disconnected from the total composite dose that development of quantitative acceptance criteria has not been done. Users have to develop their own in-house criteria for accepting the results from category II measurement.

Even with perfect agreement of category II measurements, there is still the possibility that the total dose computed within the patient is in error owing to a mishandling of the dose summation by the planning system. Therefore, when relying on category II measurement, the user would be wise to ensure during commissioning that the beam summation process works correctly by conducting sufficient composite beam validation.

One important consideration of categories I and II is that they do not validate some important potential sources of error. For example, although an error in the patient surface contour could yield a large treatment error, the treatment planning system recomputes the dose to the phantom. Consequently, the measured dose may agree with the phantom while the error goes undetected. Currently, the best method for detecting these sources of error is careful review of the treatment plan and direct physical measurements of the patient geometry at the linear accelerator (eg, source-to-surface distances).

Category III Measurements

Category III measurements involve the placement of the dosimeter beyond the phantom or the patient or simply placed beyond the isocenter when there is no intervening phantom. The detectors include portal imagers using optical,[15] liquid scintillator,[16,17] or amorphous silicon[18–21] and radiographic film. There are two approaches to using the measured dose distribution from the portal imager. One is to compute the dose within the patient (or phantom) and compare the dose with the treatment planning system,[22–28] and the other is to have the treatment planning system compute the dose within the imager for comparison.[15,29,30] Assuming that the accurate dose or fluence calculation is provided by the treatment planning system, the comparison of portal dose will provide information similar to category II. If the dose is computed within the phantom, this provides information similar to category I measurements. However, if the patient is present during the measurements, discrepancies between calculated and measured doses may be caused by variations in patient positioning rather than the treatment plan or delivery.

An advantage of quantitative category I to III measurement-based validation is that because it involves irradiating, it checks the operation and calibration of the linear accelerator multileaf collimator (MLC). However, one difficulty with this approach is that it makes the process of determining the source of discrepancies more difficult. For example, if a discrepancy between calculation and measurement is detected, the following question arises: Was it due to the MLC or a problem with the treatment planning system?

Proposed Methodology

It is clear that the measurement-based dose validation is time-consuming and may not present a thorough determination of the dose to the patient. A relatively efficient process has been developed for traditional conformal therapy treatments, namely, that the processes of validating the linear accelerator operation, patient positioning, and treatment plan accuracy are separated and each has formalized programs. With some software development, this philosophy could be applied to IMRT.[31] The processes that would be employed are described below.

Linear Accelerator

The operation of the linear accelerator would be checked using a series of standardized tests. These would provide validation of the leaf position calibration and positioning accuracy, monitor unit delivery, and dynamic multileaf operation. The frequency of these tests would be a function of the perceived risk of failure and the staff necessary to conduct the test. For example, a relatively simple multileaf sequence that uses abutting narrow radiation fields can be used to check multileaf positioning accuracy (Figure 14-1).[32] The cost of conducting this test includes the time to get the film and phantom, set it up, and irradiate, process, and review the film (~ 10 minutes). However, modern films

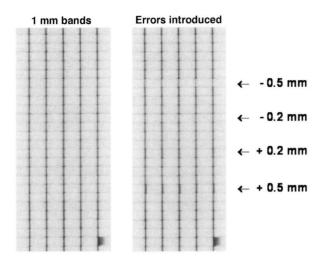

Figure 14-1. Multileaf collimator test film for validating leaf positioning accuracy. The field on the right has intentionally introduced positioning errors to highlight the sensitivity of this simple test. Reproduced with permission from Memorial Sloan-Kettering Cancer Center.[32]

typically are not large enough to subtend the entire multi-leaf bank. Also, some linear accelerators cannot deliver radiation throughout the entire field using a single irradiation but must subdivide large fields into two or more irradiations, further extending the delivery time.

Patient Positioning

In the past, validation of patient positioning consisted of manual evaluation of each portal film and comparison against a diagnostic film obtained using a conventional simulator. With the advent of 3DCRT, more fields began to be used, as well as an increased use of noncoplanar fields. Validation of patient positioning using noncoplanar fields was typically difficult and often did not provide the physician with quantitative patient alignment information. Therefore, the concept was developed that patient positioning verification and portal outline verification did not have to be conducted simultaneously. For many tumor sites, the most useful patient positioning information typically came from anterior-posterior and lateral fields. This further led to the concept of developing fields for the purpose of position validation. For example, if the treatment beams did not include a lateral portal, a lateral beam was added just for portal verification. A similar concept could be applied to IMRT QA. Portals selected by the treatment planner, or eventually by the optimization software, do not necessarily provide the optimal beam geometry for patient positioning verification. Thus, independent positioning portals should be used. This becomes even more useful for IMRT, in which there is no longer a single irradiation portal for each beam; thus, a single film does not provide the same portal shape information as it did for 3DCRT.

A logical extension of this is the advent of on-board kilovoltage imaging, in which a diagnostic x-ray unit is attached to the linear accelerator gantry (Figure 14-2).[33–39] The imaging unit can provide kilovoltage positioning verification images that have higher contrast than megavoltage images. The potential also exists for generating a cone-beam CT image dataset that would enable the user to image and treat the tumor at the unique position and orientation for each setup.

Dose Calculation and Data Transfer

The validation of the dose calculation, including the transfer of MLC settings, monitor units, beam energy, and gantry geometry, is currently checked by visual verification and direct measurement. However, this does not quantify the dose distribution to the patient, nor does it tell the physician what the doses are to the targets or critical structures. The most thorough and time-efficient method for validating the treatment plan dose would be to have an independent, fully three-dimensional computation of the dose distribution. Figure 14-3 shows a sketch of the proposed process. The treatment plan dose distribution, CT scan, contours, dose-volume histograms (DVHs), and beam isocenters would be sent from the clinical IMRT treatment planning system to the independent dose calculation system (plan parameters in Figure 14-3). Because an error could be made in transferring the MLC motion instructions or other parameters to the linear accelerator, the record

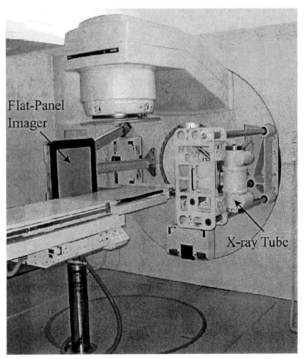

Figure 14-2. Prototype on-board kilovoltage imaging system that can be used to validate patient positioning with high image contrast. Reproduced with permission from Jaffray DA et al.[35]

and verify system that stores these data for use in the treatment would send these values to the independent dose calculation system (treatment parameters in Figure 14-3).

The independent system, with its own dose calculation algorithm and implementation, would use the CT scan, beam isocenters, and linear accelerator parameters to compute the three-dimensional dose. It would then compute DVHs and compare these against the treatment planning system's calculation. Additional methods would be provided to compare the two dose distributions and allow an evaluation of the differences between the two calculations. One important consideration would be dose distribution differences that are caused not by an error but by differences in the calculational algorithms or modeling of the linear accelerator operation. For example, if the treatment planning system uses a convolution-superposition algorithm, whereas the independent system uses Monte Carlo calculation, one would expect differences in the dose calculated in the lung and lung tumors. Similar differences might be seen near the patient's surface at depths at which secondary electronic equilibrium has not been established. The identification of these differences as caused by the algorithm, rather than an error in implementation, would be a challenge. However, it would be expected that reasonably sophisticated dose calculation algorithms applied to other sites would produce relatively small dose differences that would cause a minor change in the DVHs.

In such a model, category III measurements would still be an important component because they have the ability to check the chain of data transfer that is used to treat the patient. An error in the treatment that is caused by software that operates independently of the multileaf settings and data export used by the independent dose calculation software could cause an undetected dose delivery error. The only method for detecting these errors is to conduct in vivo dosimetry measurements. For 3DCRT patient treatments, these are conducted using diodes or TLDs, but owing to the large dose gradients, they are impractical for use in IMRT. Instead, transmission dosimetry measurements might prove useful in ensuring that the treatment was delivered correctly. As with the previous discussion, development of action-level criteria will be required to make this type of check useful.

Summary

The process of IMRT QA has matured significantly since the mid-1990s, when IMRT was first clinically introduced. One of the most time-consuming aspects of the QA process is patient-specific QA, which still relies in large part on individual dose measurements. Limitations with the dosimeters and staff cause these measurements to be insufficient to completely characterize the IMRT dose distributions. Significant systematic errors may take place and not be detected using the current protocols. An independent, sophisticated dose calculation system that computes and compares the dose distribution against the clinically approved distribution will make the process of patient-specific QA both easier and more thorough than the current practice.

On-board imaging has the potential to provide periodic validation of the delivered MLC leaf sequence and validate the patient's relative position. However, broad integration of on-board imaging will take considerable time to implement.

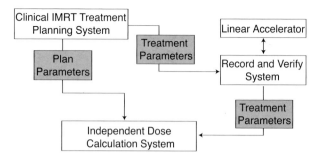

Figure 14-3. Proposed patient-specific quality assurance process using an independent dose calculation system. The gray boxes indicate the types of data that are transferred. IMRT = intensity-modulated radiation therapy.

References

1. Low DA, Parikh P, Dempsey JF, et al. Ionization chamber volume averaging effects in dynamic intensity modulated radiation therapy beams. Med Phys 2003;30:1706–11.

2. Van Esch A, Bohsung J, Sorvari P, et al. Acceptance tests and quality control (QC) procedures for the clinical implementation of intensity modulated radiotherapy (IMRT) using inverse planning and the sliding window technique: experience from five radiotherapy departments. Radiother Oncol 2002;65:53–70.

3. Low DA, Mutic S, Dempsey JF, et al. Quantitative dosimetric verification of an IMRT planning and delivery system. Radiother Oncol 1998;49:305–16.

4. Dogan N, Leybovich LB, Sethi A. Comparative evaluation of Kodak EDR2 and XV2 films for verification of intensity modulated radiation therapy. Phys Med Biol 2002;47:4121–30.

5. Chetty IJ, Charland PM. Investigation of Kodak extended dose range (EDR) film for megavoltage photon beam dosimetry. Phys Med Biol 2002;47:3629–41.

6. Esthappan J, Mutic S, Harms WB, et al. Dosimetry of therapeutic photon beams using an extended dose range film. Med Phys 2002;29:2438–45.

7. Olch AJ. Dosimetric performance of an enhanced dose range radiographic film for intensity-modulated radiation therapy quality assurance. Med Phys 2002;29:2159–68.

8. Zhu XR, Jursinic PA, Grimm DF, et al. Evaluation of Kodak EDR2 film for dose verification of intensity modulated radiation therapy delivered by a static multileaf collimator. Med Phys 2002;29:1687–92.

9. McJury M, Oldham M, Cosgrove VP, et al. Radiation dosimetry using polymer gels: methods and applications. Br J Radiol 2000;73:919–29.

10. Islam KT, Dempsey JF, Ranade MK, et al. Initial evaluation of commercial optical CT-based 3D gel dosimeter. Med Phys 2003;30:2159–68.

11. Doran SJ, Koerkamp KK, Bero MA, et al. A CCD-based optical CT scanner for high-resolution 3D imaging of radiation dose distributions: equipment specifications, optical simulations and preliminary results. Phys Med Biol 2001;46:3191–213.

12. Kelly BG, Jordan KJ, Battista JJ. Optical CT reconstruction of 3D dose distributions using the ferrous-benzoic-xylenol (FBX) gel dosimeter. Med Phys 1998;25:1741–50.

13. Gore JC, Ranade M, Maryanski MJ, et al. Radiation dose distributions in three dimensions from tomographic optical density scanning of polymer gels: I. Development of an optical scanner. Phys Med Biol 1996;41:2695–704.

14. Oldham M, Baustert I, Lord C, et al. An investigation into the dosimetry of a nine-field tomotherapy irradiation using BANG-gel dosimetry. Phys Med Biol 1998;43:1113–32.

15. Pasma KL, Kroonwijk M, de Boer JC, et al. Accurate portal dose measurement with a fluoroscopic electronic portal imaging device (EPID) for open and wedged beams and dynamic multileaf collimation. Phys Med Biol 1998;43:2047–60.

16. Chang J, Mageras GS, Ling CC. Evaluation of rapid dose map acquisition of a scanning liquid-filled ionization chamber electronic portal imaging device. Int J Radiat Oncol Biol Phys 2003;55:1432–45.

17. Parsaei H, el Khatib E, Rajapakshe R. The use of an electronic portal imaging system to measure portal dose and portal dose profiles. Med Phys 1998;25:1903–9.

18. McDermott LN, Louwe RJ, Sonke JJ, et al. Dose-response and ghosting effects of an amorphous silicon electronic portal imaging device. Med Phys 2004;31:285–95.

19. Norrlinger B, Islam MK, Heaton R, et al. Relative dosimetry using an amorphous silicon electronic portal imaging device for the quality assurance of dynamic intensity modulated radiation therapy. Int J Radiat Oncol Biol Phys 2003;57:S423.

20. Grein EE, Lee R, Luchka K. An investigation of a new amorphous silicon electronic portal imaging device for transit dosimetry. Med Phys 2002;29:2262–8.

21. El Mohri Y, Antonuk LE, Yorkston J, et al. Relative dosimetry using active matrix flat-panel imager (AMFPI) technology. Med Phys 1999;26:1530–41.

22. Partridge M, Ebert M, Hesse BM. IMRT verification by three-dimensional dose reconstruction from portal beam measurements. Med Phys 2002;29:1847–58.

23. Boellaard R, Essers M, van Herk M, et al. New method to obtain the midplane dose using portal in vivo dosimetry. Int J Radiat Oncol Biol Phys 1998;41:465–74.

24. Boellaard R, van Herk M, Uiterwaal H, et al. Two-dimensional exit dosimetry using a liquid-filled electronic portal imaging device and a convolution model. Radiother Oncol 1997;44:149–57.

25. Boellaard R, van Herk M, Mijnheer BJ. A convolution model to convert transmission dose images to exit dose distributions. Med Phys 1997;24:189–99.

26. Hansen VN, Evans PM, Swindell W. The application of transit dosimetry to precision radiotherapy. Med Phys 1996;23:713–21.

27. McNutt TR, Mackie TR, Reckwerdt P, et al. Modeling dose distributions from portal dose images using the convolution/superposition method. Med Phys 1996;23:1381–92.

28. Ying XG, Geer LY, Wong JW. Portal dose images. II: Patient dose estimation. Int J Radiat Oncol Biol Phys 1990;18:1465–75.

29. Vieira SC, Dirkx ML, Pasma KL, et al. Dosimetric verification of x-ray fields with steep dose gradients using an electronic portal imaging device. Phys Med Biol 2003;48:157–66.

30. Pasma KL, Vieira SC, Heijmen BJ. Portal dose image prediction for dosimetric treatment verification in radiotherapy. II. An algorithm for wedged beams. Med Phys 2002;29:925–31.

31. Ezzell GA. Quality assurance: when and what is enough for IMRT? In: Palta JR, Mackie TR, editors. Intensity modulated radiation therapy: the state of the art. Colorado Springs (CO): Medical Physics Publishing; 2003. p. 613–6.

32. MSKCC. A practical guide to intensity-modulated radiation therapy. Colorado Springs (CO): Medical Physics Publishing; 2003.

33. Letourneau D, Watt L, Gulam M, et al. Implementation of an on-board kilovoltage cone-beam CT imaging system for clinical applications. Int J Radiat Oncol Biol Phys 2003;57:S185.

34. Siewerdsen JH, Cunningham IA, Jaffray DA. A framework for noise-power spectrum analysis of multidimensional images. Med Phys 2002;29:2655–71.

35. Jaffray DA, Siewerdsen JH, Wong JW, et al. Flat-panel cone-beam computed tomography for image-guided radiation therapy. Int J Radiat Oncol Biol Phys 2002;53:1337–49.

36. Groh BA, Siewerdsen JH, Drake DG, et al. A performance comparison of flat-panel imager-based MV and kV cone-beam CT. Med Phys 2002;29:967–75.

37. Siewerdsen JH, Jaffray DA. Cone-beam computed tomography with a flat-panel imager: magnitude and effects of x-ray scatter. Med Phys 2001;28:220–31.

38. Siewerdsen JH, Jaffray DA. Optimization of x-ray imaging geometry (with specific application to flat-panel cone-beam computed tomography). Med Phys 2000;27:1903–14.

39. Jaffray DA, Siewerdsen JH. Cone-beam computed tomography with a flat-panel imager: initial performance characterization. Med Phys 2000;27:1311–23.

Chapter 15

IMRT IN THE COMMUNITY SETTING

NORMAN LEHTO, MS, BRENT MURPHY, MS, PETER LAI, MD, PHD

Tremendous enthusiasm exists for the use of intensity-modulated radiation therapy (IMRT) in the radiation oncology community. Many studies have documented reductions in normal tissue volumes irradiated through the use of the highly conformal IMRT planning. Moreover, in certain disease sites, IMRT may be able to provide higher than conventional doses to the tumor, improving patient outcome.

Despite this enthusiasm, many reasons exist for not performing IMRT outside an academic setting: (1) IMRT requires target delineation to a degree that is beyond the training level of many community-based radiation oncologists; (2) physics manpower required to implement and oversee an IMRT program is often not present at these centers; and (3) IMRT is still experimental and therefore should be limited to academic centers.

These arguments should not be dismissed lightly. A community center must determine how the challenges of implementing a new complex program such as IMRT will be met. Administrators, physicians, and physicists must come to a common agreement as to if, when, and how an IMRT program will be implemented. If one of the above-mentioned groups is not aware of what is required to realize IMRT, implementation will be inevitably delayed. Moreover, the entire radiation oncology team must be willing to acquire the additional training necessary to correctly use IMRT.

One factor that cannot be ignored or underestimated is the market pressure to adopt IMRT that exists in some areas. The increase in direct to consumer (DTC) marketing of health care that has occurred in recent years has been commented on by others.[1] With patients having more information available via the Internet and DTC, some centers are forced to implement IMRT or lose a nontrivial percentage of their patients to competing centers that have IMRT. Medicine is a product in the United States, and market pressures influence product development.

Aside from the market pressure to implement IMRT, community physicians need to evaluate what their goals are for an IMRT program. Goals for IMRT in a community setting include normal tissue sparing, dose escalation, and a reduction in overall treatment time by using a concomitant boost. Most of the time, community centers are not going to originate research, but instead follow the lead of academic centers. Community physicians must carefully evaluate which patients they will treat with IMRT so that the staffing and financial impact of implementing IMRT can be evaluated. More importantly, the physician must access how IMRT will benefit the patient. Although it is true that IMRT outcome data are not as mature as one would like, a growing number of studies are being published showing the benefits from sparing critical structures with IMRT.[2–6] If dose escalation is a goal, one must consider the potential hazards.[7] If a protocol from an academic center is going to be followed, one must consider much more than time, dose, and fractionation. Patient selection, immobilization, positioning, targets or organs at risk (OAR), contouring details, and daily patient setup and treatment issues must all be considered if the results reported by an academic institution are to be reproduced. One final consideration when starting an IMRT program is the financial benefit that IMRT provides over three-dimensional conformal radiation therapy (3DCRT).[8] The increased revenue from IMRT may cover the cost of upgrading equipment.

Misconceptions

One encounters a number of common misconceptions when visiting community centers planning to implement an IMRT program. A major misconception is that if a linear accelerator is capable of delivering intensity-modulated beams, then IMRT can be easily done. Having a machine that can deliver an IMRT treatment is only the final step in a complicated process that starts at simulation and involves all members of the radiation oncology team. The entire process must be considered. It is strongly suggested that a team be assembled early in the planning process that includes representatives for physicians, physicists, dosimetrists, therapists, nurses, and information services. A process is only as good as its weakest link.

Another mistaken belief is that dose escalation is the main goal of IMRT. Although dose escalation is one potential goal of an IMRT program, it should not be the first goal in a community setting. As previously stated, community centers generally follow the path of academic centers. Although more data regarding dose escalation are becoming available, much of the follow-up remains relatively short and needs to mature. It should be noted that in an IMRT plan, it is not uncommon for two-thirds of the planning target volume (PTV) to be 5% above the prescribed dose. The dose heterogeneity found in most IMRT plans leads to an inherent dose escalation when switching to IMRT, even when prescribing the same dose used in 3DCRT.

Referring physicians are sensitive to patient complaints about side effects. The ability of IMRT to spare critical structures may therefore be the primary goal of IMRT in the community setting. In sparing critical structures, physicians must use caution so as not to spare a structure at the expense of local control.

Within the radiation therapy community, some have the notion that the inverse planning algorithm generates the plan automatically. Although these algorithms iterate to find an optimum dose distribution, much user input is still required. When generating a plan, the sequence of events after adding the contours and beams consists of adding dose constraints, optimizing, segmenting, evaluating, modifying constraints and contours, optimizing, segmenting, evaluating, and repeating the process until the plan is acceptable. As a rule, IMRT planning takes 2 to 6 hours longer than conventional 3DCRT planning.

A final misconception is that IMRT is appropriate only for small targets. The target for most head and neck tumors is definitely not small. Indeed, elective targets for head and neck IMRT treatments are typically 25 cm long (including the supraclavicular nodes). IMRT techniques for the treatment of abdominal and pelvic tumors have also been described.[9–11] One final observation regarding this misconception is that it has been shown that for small- and intermediate-sized brain lesions, stereotactic radiosurgery (Gamma Knife, Elekta Inc., Norcross, GA) provided better normal tissue sparing.[12]

Early in the planning process, it is recommended that the IMRT planning team review the IMRT guidance document published by the American Association of Physicists in Medicine IMRT Subcommittee.[13] This document covers a range of issues that a center must consider both during IMRT implementation and on an ongoing basis. Two other helpful documents are "Intensity-Modulated Radiation Therapy: The Current Status and Issues of Interest," by the Intensity-Modulated Radiation Therapy Collaborative Working Group,[14] and the American College of Radiology's "Practice Guidelines for Intensity-Modulated Radiation Therapy."[15]

Equipment

An area that must be addressed when implementing an IMRT program is equipment. Starting a new program such as IMRT offers the opportunity to get needed equipment into the budget. One should remember that equipment that is specified as optional on a budget is often cut. So if an item is desired, it should be listed as required to start the program. The revenue generated by IMRT provides the opportunity to include items into the budget that it might otherwise not be possible to include. Time should be taken to ensure that the equipment list is complete because it is difficult to go back and ask for more once the budget for a project is set. A community center planning to implement IMRT should ensure that a suitable linear accelerator is available. Decisions that need to be made include whether IMRT will be delivered using a multileaf collimator or with compensators. Mechanical accuracy and treatment delivery times are also important considerations in the type of hardware that will be used.

Shielding of the accelerator vault is often overlooked. Several authors have published on the requirements of shielding for IMRT.[13,14,16,17] Secondary barriers should be evaluated because the high monitor unit settings associated with IMRT lead to greater leakage. Neutron shielding may also be an issue if higher-energy beams are used.

As an extension of 3DCRT, IMRT is image intensive. Targets and OAR contours are used by the planning system. If there are inaccuracies in simulation, they will be propagated throughout the entire IMRT process. A computed tomography (CT) simulator located in the radiation oncology department allows better control over scheduling and quality assurance (QA). At our center, the treatment isocenter is marked at the time of simulation to avoid potential errors in shifting the patient on the treatment table. Access to images from other imaging modalities and fusion capability are also desirable to aid in structure delineation. The selection of software that can handle these imaging modalities is paramount to the success of an IMRT program.

Although most centers addressed the issue of immobilization when they implemented 3DCRT, IMRT implementation presents a good opportunity to re-evaluate patient immobilization. Treatment times can be significantly longer for IMRT than for 3DCRT. Therefore, it is important that immobilization devices ensure that the patient remain in the same position throughout the treatment as well as aid in positioning of the patient from day to day. Vendors have developed a large array of immobilization products for IMRT. Community centers rarely have the staff or tools to conduct a thorough evaluation of setup error and intrafraction motion. Studies on setup reproducibility from academic institutions should be used when available, but, at a minimum, a community center should try any device under evaluation on a few patients to see how it works for the staff who will use it. Sales demonstrations alone should not be the basis for a purchase.

A number of systems are now available to localize the target on a daily basis. The community center should keep in mind the possibility of current or future image guidance systems when specifying equipment. A number of articles have been published on the accuracy of the various systems currently available.[18–23] As stated earlier, community centers often do not perform setup error studies, and vendors will often present published accuracy data for their system. However, several of these systems are user dependent, and the published accuracy may not be achieved. Proper training and supervision by the physician and physicist are critical. Establishing a trigger level for the size of the shift above which the physician must be called to check the setup is recommended.

Lastly, some important considerations are treatment planning software and a record and verify system that is compatible with the method of IMRT delivery selected. Physics equipment is also an important consideration. The appropriate equipment must be available both for initial commissioning and for ongoing QA. A more detailed description of required equipment and QA recommendations is provided in Chapter 13, "Commissioning and Dosimetric Quality Assurance."

Staffing

Staffing and time requirements are another area that must be considered when planning IMRT implementation. Management must be aware of the impact that IMRT will have on the workload of various members of the radiation oncology staff. Gillin estimated that the time increase relative to a 3DCRT case for IMRT was 100% for physicians, 200% for physicists, 200% for dosimetrists, and 200% for therapists.[8]

Physicists are involved in the planning and implementation of IMRT from the beginning. At community centers, physicists are often responsible for gathering information on new technologies. It is important for them to "do their homework" up front. Attending seminars and reading publications are a good start, but one should also speak to others who have already implemented an IMRT program. Getting experience either at a "hands-on" course or an academic institution can save time in the process. Physicists should not only research the technical aspects of IMRT, they should also become experienced with all aspects of IMRT planning and clinical use. IMRT planning is considerably different than conventional planning, and the physicist should be a resource for the dosimetrists and physicians in the department. The time required to implement an IMRT program can vary greatly depending on the existing clinical workload for physicists, their level of expertise, and the availability of the necessary equipment in the

department. Typical IMRT implementation tasks for the physicist include gathering information on IMRT for the rest of the department, assessing equipment needs, and commissioning and validating the selected system.

A number of consulting groups specialize in IMRT implementation. By using a consulting IMRT implementation team, a community center can implement IMRT faster, benefit from the knowledge of individuals who have already implemented IMRT, and prevent the in-house physics staff from being overwhelmed.

Once the IMRT program is implemented, ongoing tasks for a physicist may include treatment planning, plan review, and verification QA (2–3 hours per plan). Community centers that treat 40 to 50 patients per day need an additional 0.5 full-time equivalent physicist once they begin doing IMRT (more if the physicist does the planning).

IMRT also places an additional burden on the dosimetrists. Planning time is typically 2 to 6 hours per plan more than 3DCRT. At smaller centers, dosimetrists may also assist with the patient-specific QA. Dosimetrists must be willing to seek out training and have a thorough understanding of their treatment planning system. This training can come through formalized courses provided by vendors or through user groups. In addition, IMRT planning is often counterintuitive. Sometimes, better plans may be achieved by relaxing planning constraints. Dosimetrists need time to "experiment" with their planning system.

Community center physicians have to determine how they are going to use this new tool. This is probably one of the most difficult tasks for a center starting IMRT. There are still many unknowns, and the physician must carefully access all of the options that IMRT offers. One issue is contouring (Figure 15-1). For 3DCRT, a structure is contoured only if

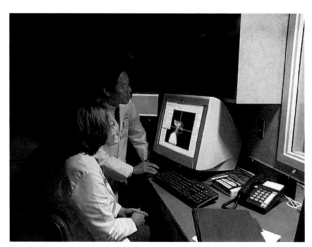

FIGURE 15-1. Owing to the increased time required for contouring, dedicated contouring workstations are used to delineate structures, thereby eliminating the need to use valuable time on a treatment planning workstation. Radiation oncologists often consult with diagnostic radiologists to define the target volume. (To view a color version of this image, please refer to the CD-ROM.)

one wants a dose-volume histogram for that structure or if one wants to see a soft tissue structure on a digitally reconstructed radiograph. IMRT often requires structures that would not be considered at risk for a 3DCRT treatment to be contoured. Contours are taken literally by the inverse planning algorithm, so one must be more careful about what is defined as a target and what is defined as normal tissue. The target definition guidelines found in the International Commission on Radiation Units and Measurements (ICRU) Reports 50 and 62 are recommended.[24,25]

Owing to the large number of contours that are found in IMRT anatomic data sets, a center should develop a consistent naming convention to avoid confusion. It is helpful to enter predefined structure names into the treatment planning system or contouring software. When starting IMRT for a new site, one of the items that should be specified is which structures are to be routinely contoured for that site, how those structures are to be contoured, and who will be responsible for contouring specific structures.

An IMRT prescription must be more detailed than a 3DCRT prescription. In addition to the standard items listed in a prescription (site, fields, energy, prescription reference, dose/fraction, total dose), the physician must specify dose constraints for all targets and all OAR.[26] The physician, in consultation with a physicist, must also define the PTVs. This is commonly accomplished by specifying an expansion of a gross tumor volume and/or the clinical target volume that the physician contoured. One may also specify an expansion around OAR to allow for setup and organ motion uncertainties. Figure 15-2 shows a sample IMRT prescription form that is used in addition to the standard prescription in the treatment chart. Such a form can be customized with default values for specific sites to reduce the time required for the physician to complete it.

Plan review for IMRT is much more complex than for 3DCRT. The planner and physician should review all IMRT plans on a workstation. The plan should be analyzed slice

---

Treatment Site:

Diagnosis: Stage:

Statement of Medical Necessity:

- o The target is irregularly shaped and in close proximity to critical structures.

- o IMRT is the only option to cover the volume of interest with narrow margins and protect immediately adjacent structures.

- o An immediately adjacent area has been previously treated and abutting portals must be established with extreme precision.

- o IMRT is the only option when additional precautions at reducing the GTV, CTV, or PTV margins, such as gating, are used.

- o Only IMRT can produce an acceptable dose distribution due to an extremely concave target geometry.

Planning Goals:_____

_____

_____

_____

Physician:_____   Date:_____

FIGURE 15-2. Example intensity-modulated radiation therapy (IMRT) prescription form. The physician states the medical necessity and provides a brief statement of the planning goals. CTV = clinical target volume; GTV = gross tumor volume; OAR = organ at risk; PTV = planning target volume.

Planning Goals

PTV$_1$ Expansion of GTV to form PTV

Uniform:_____ cm

Nonuniform

Anterior:	cm	Right:	cm	Superior:	cm
Posterior:	cm	Left:	cm	Inferior:	cm

PTV$_2$ Expansion of GTV to form PTV

Uniform:_____ cm

Nonuniform

Anterior:	cm	Right:	cm	Superior:	cm
Posterior:	cm	Left:	cm	Inferior:	cm

PTV$_3$ Expansion of GTV to form PTV

Uniform:_____ cm

Nonuniform

Anterior:	cm	Right:	cm	Superior:	cm
Posterior:	cm	Left:	cm	Inferior:	cm

Target Dose Specification

Beam Energy:_____   Fractions/week:_____

	Total Dose	Dose/fraction	Coverage Goal	
PTV$_1$			% of goal dose covers	% of volume
PTV$_2$			% of goal dose covers	% of volume
PTV$_3$			% of goal dose covers	% of volume

Organs at Risk Dose Specification

	Name	Goal
OAR$_1$		
OAR$_2$		
OAR$_3$		
OAR$_4$		
OAR$_5$		

Physician: _____   Date:_____

FIGURE 15-2 Continued

by slice because IMRT planning systems can sometimes produce unexpected dose distributions. Organs sometimes not considered at risk can receive doses beyond their tolerance. One such example is the skin toxicity that has been reported for head and neck IMRT.[27] Dose-volume information should also be analyzed to ensure that prescription constraints have been met. Figure 15-3 shows a plan review form used at our center.

Date	Treatment Site
Patient Name	Total Dose
Patient ID	Dose/Fraction

Plan Review

Specified PTV goals accomplished

    ◦ Yes

    ◦ No

    Explain:_____

    _____

    _____

Dose @ ICRU ref pt_____cGy Mean PTV dose_____cGy

Specific normal structure goals accomplished?

    ◦ Yes

    ◦ No

    Explain:_____

    _____

    _____

Isocenter Location:_____

	Yes	No
Total Dose_____ Correct?	_____	_____
# Fractions_____ Correct?	_____	_____
Min. MU/seg_____ Acceptable?	_____	_____
Final calculation with 2 mm grid?	_____	_____

Comments_____

_____

_____

_____

QA Plan

Phantom	
Configuration	
Gantry Angles	
Chamber Location	
Film Location	
Signature	Date:

FIGURE 15-3. Example intensity-modulated radiation therapy (IMRT) plan summary form. ICRU = International Commission on Radiation Units and Measurements; MU = monitor unit; PTV = planning target volume; QA = quality assurance.

IMRT also affects radiation therapists, requiring an additional 5 to 10 minutes/treatment than 3DCRT. At many centers, the move toward IMRT is accompanied by a new linear accelerator or upgraded controller software. Therapists may be confronted with learning the operation of new equipment and delivery procedures at the same time. In addition, educating the patient regarding positioning is also an important role of therapists. Because accurate patient positioning is paramount to the success of IMRT (see Chapter 6, "Immobilization and Localization"),

A

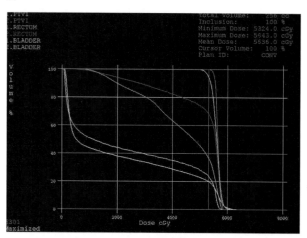

B

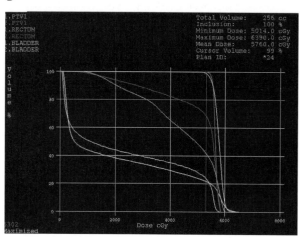

FIGURE 15-4. Using a three-dimensional conformal radiation therapy (3DCRT) plan as a baseline for comparison can give the physician information about what is being gained with intensity-modulated radiation therapy (IMRT). (*A*) shows a dose-volume histogram (DVH) comparison between an IMRT plan (plan 1) and a 3DCRT plan (plan 2). Before comparisons are made, the IMRT plan is adjusted to achieve the minimum planning target volume (PTV) coverage that is acceptable. (*B*) shows the DVH comparison again after the IMRT plan was adjusted to meet the minimum PTV coverage criteria (in this case, the 95% isodose line was to cover 99% of the PTV). Only after the minimum coverage criteria are met can evaluation of the volume of the hot spot (volume above 110% of the prescribed dose), the critical structure DVHs, and the comparison with the 3DCRT plan be performed. (To view a color version of this image, please refer to the CD-ROM.)

immobilization devices will work better if patients are aware of what they need to do to help the process.

Nurses work closely with patients, so they should have a general knowledge of IMRT. In addition, nurses should collect data on how patients tolerate the IMRT during treatment and during follow-up visits.

Lastly, IMRT is data intensive and often involves establishing communication between equipment from several vendors. Information services departments in community hospitals are often short-staffed, so giving them ample notice of the impending implementation is crucial to getting the system up and running in a timely manner.

Implementation

The transition to IMRT should be an evolution, not a revolution. First, it is ideal if one is experienced in 3DCRT before implementing IMRT. The staff and physicians should be comfortable with acquiring and working with three-dimensional image sets and defining structures on those images. When evaluating an IMRT plan, one should remember what was important when a 3DCRT plan was evaluated. Centers should run competing 3DCRT plans as a basis of comparison when they are starting IMRT (Figure 15-4). Physicians should pay particularly close attention to the target that is treated with IMRT relative to the target that was treated in the past with 3DCRT. Target definition is critical because the IMRT planning system will not treat areas not defined as a target. In the head and neck, target definition is particularly daunting, and academic institutions have gone to considerable effort to analyze failure patterns relative to target definition.[28–32] Chao and colleagues go as far as to state that although CT and magnetic resonance imaging have created a virtual operative suite, "these technologies require training and expertise available only at a handful of academic institutions."[30]

Often it is difficult to identify the target, but it is easy to visualize the critical structures one wants to avoid. By defining the PTV based on the volume of tissue that would have been treated with 3DCRT and simply avoiding the critical structures that are not at risk of disease, one reduces the amount of difference between what was treated in the past and what is treated with IMRT. It has been shown that using such a "conformal avoidance" technique reduces the amount of time it takes the physician to contour for head and neck IMRT, and it has been proposed that conformal avoidance may be a practical way to implement head and neck IMRT in the community center.[33]

Again, the emphasis is evolution, not revolution. One should treat the volume that one has clinical experience treating rather than tightly define a new target. Figure 15-5 shows the blocks from the conventional field a physician defined being projected onto transverse CT images on a virtual simulation system. The projection of the blocks serves as a guide for definition of the PTV. Physicians should take

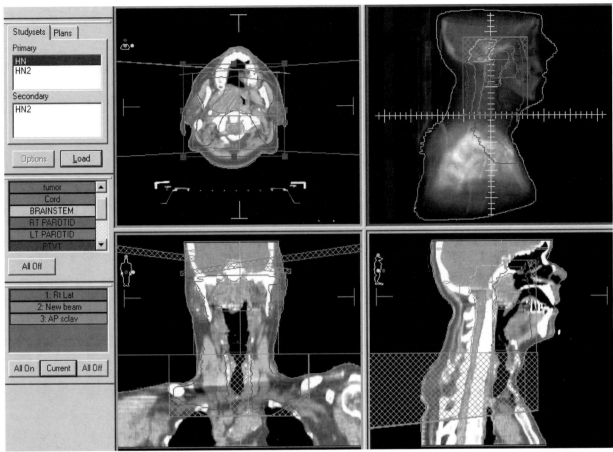

FIGURE 15-5. To define the conformal avoidance target, the physician draws the traditional blocks on a digitally reconstructed radiograph. The blocks are then projected onto the axial computed tomography images and serve as a guide to define the volume that would have been treated traditionally. Critical structures that are to be spared, such as the cord and bilateral parotid glands in this case, are avoided when defining the target. Also, tissue that is clearly not at risk, such as the posterior neck, can be avoided. The physician must take into consideration that block edges represent the 50% isodose line for the traditional plan and the target being defined will be covered by a dose near the prescribed dose. Alternatively, at least one particular treatment planning system allows the user to convert an isodose line to a structure. The physician can therefore pick an isodose line from a three-dimensional conformal radiation therapy plan to serve as the planning target volume for the intensity-modulated radiation therapy plan. Some editing of the converted isodose line is often necessary. (To view a color version of this image, please refer to the CD-ROM.)

into account the fact that the block edge has an associated penumbra. In addition, physicians can use their knowledge of tissues at risk to eliminate some areas, such as the posterior neck, from the PTV. Figure 15-6 illustrates an IMRT dose distribution for a conformal avoidance head and neck plan. The principle of conformal avoidance can be used for other sites for which the target is not clearly visible. For example, conformal avoidance is useful in the abdomen.

When initiating IMRT for a new treatment site, it is recommended that centers define a protocol that can be easily followed. Items to be specified in the protocol include the patient position or immobilization to be used, imaging protocol, structures to be contoured, dose-volume constraints for targets and OAR, dose/fraction, total target dose, and the time from when the physician contouring is complete to when the patient will start treatment.

When planning IMRT, one should always start with modest constraints on critical structures to generate a plan that has acceptable PTV coverage. Once the target coverage is acceptable, one may increase the constraints on critical structures as much as possible while still maintaining acceptable PTV dose coverage. It is important to realize that the constraints one enters into a planning system are not the physician's prescription but, rather, are a planning tool that is used to achieve a final plan that meets the physician's prescription constraints. The physician must set realistic constraints. For example, we generally find that it is not possible to achieve a gradient of greater than 5% per millimeter. One will note that as OAR are spared more, the dose-volume histogram for the PTV will degrade. IMRT planning involves finding a compromise between PTV coverage or dose heterogeneity and OAR sparing.

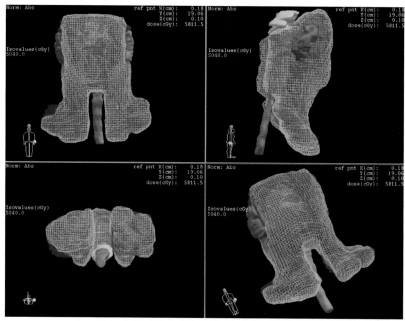

FIGURE 15-6. An isodose distribution from a conformal avoidance planning target volume. (To view a color version of this image, please refer to the CD-ROM.)

Conclusions

IMRT represents a new technology that allows for an unprecedented level of dose conformity around the target volume. Owing to market pressures and the interest in doing what is best for the patient, community physicians are under tremendous pressure to implement IMRT. However, IMRT should be implemented in the community setting only after careful consideration of the goals for an IMRT program and an assessment of staffing and equipment. The radiation oncology team must work together to ensure the safe and accurate delivery of this modality.

References

1. Glatstein E. The return of the snake oil salesmen. Int J Radiat Oncol Biol Phys 2003;55:561–2.

2. Eisbruch A, Kim HM, Terrell J, et al. Xerostomia and its predictors following parotid-sparing irradiation of head-and-neck cancer. Int J Radiat Oncol Biol Phys 2001;50:695–704.

3. Mundt AJ, Roeske JC, Lujan AE. Intensity-modulated radiation therapy in gynecologic malignancies. Med Dosim 2002;27:131–6.

4. Mundt AJ, Mell LK, Roeske JC. Preliminary analysis of chronic gastrointestinal toxicity in gynecology patients treated with intensity-modulated whole pelvic radiation therapy. Int J Radiat Oncol Biol Phys 2003;56:1354–60.

5. Kwong DL, Pow E, McMillan A, et al. Intensity-modulated radiotherapy for early stage nasopharyngeal carcinoma: preliminary results on parotid sparing. Int J Radiat Oncol Biol Phys 2003;57(2 Suppl 1):303.

6. Pollack A, Zagars GK, Starkschall G, et al. Prostate cancer radiation dose response: results of the M. D. Anderson phase III randomized trial. Int J Radiat Oncol Biol Phys 2002;53:1097–105.

7. Kuban D, Pollack A, Huang E, et al. Hazards of dose escalation in prostate cancer radiotherapy. Int J Radiat Oncol Biol Phys 2003;57:1260–8.

8. Gillin MT. Socio-economic issues of intensity-modulated radiation therapy. In: Palta JR, Mackie TR, editors. Intensity-modulated radiation therapy, the state of the art. Madison (WI): Medical Physics Publishing; 2003. p. 829–40.

9. Roeske JC, Lujan A, Rotmensch J, et al. Intensity-modulated whole pelvic radiation therapy in patients with gynecologic malignancies. Int J Radiat Oncol Biol Phys 2000;48:1613–21.

10. Hong L, Alektiar K, Chui C, et al. IMRT of large fields: whole-abdomen irradiation. Int J Radiat Oncol Biol Phys 2002;54:278–89.

11. Duthoy W, De Gersem W, Vergote K, et al. Whole abdominopelvic radiotherapy (WAPRT) using intensity-modulated arc therapy (IMAT): first clinical experience. Int J Radiat Oncol Biol Phys 2003;57:1019–32.

12. Ma L, Xia P, Verhey L, et al. A dosimetric comparision of fan-beam intensity modulated radiotherapy with Gamma Knife stereotactic radiosurgery for treating intermediate intracranial lesions. Int J Radiat Oncol Biol Phys 1999;45:1325–30.

13. Ezzell GA, Galvin JM, Low DA, et al. Guidance document on delivery, treatment planning, and clinical implementation of IMRT: report of the IMRT Subcommittee of the AAPM Radiation Therapy Committee. 2003;30:2089–115.

14. Intensity Modulated Radiation Therapy Collaborative Working Group. Intensity-modulated radiation therapy: current

status and issues of interest. Int J Radiat Oncol Biol Phys 2001;51:880–914.

15. American College of Radiology. ACR practice guidelines for intensity-modulated radiation therapy. 2002.

16. Mutic S, Low DA, Klein EE, et al. Room shielding for intensity-modulated radiation therapy treatment facilities. Int J Radiat Oncol Biol Phys 2001;50:239–46.

17. Low DA. Radiation shielding for IMRT. In: Palta JR, Mackie TR, editors. Intensity-modulated radiation therapy, the state of the art. Madison (WI): Medical Physics Publishing; 2003. p. 401–14.

18. Meeks SL, Buatti JM, Bouchet LG, et al. Ultrasound-guided extracranial radiosurgery: technique and application. Int J Radiat Oncol Biol Phys 2003;55:1092–101.

19. Tome WA, Meeks SL, McNutt TR, et al. Optically guided intensity modulated radiotherapy. Radiother Oncol 2001;61:33–44.

20. Chandra A, Dong L, Huang E, et al. Experience of ultrasound-based daily prostate localization. Int J Radiat Oncol Biol Phys 2003;56:436–47.

21. Litzenberg D, Dawson LA, Sandler H, et al. Daily prostate targeting using implanted radiopaque markers. Int J Radiat Oncol Biol Phys 2002;52:699–703.

22. Herman MG, Pisansky TM, Kruse JJ, et al. Technical aspects of daily online positioning of the prostate for three-dimensional conformal radiotherapy using an electronic portal imaging device. Int J Radiat Oncol Biol Phys 2003;57:1131–40.

23. Wong JR, Grimm SL, Oren R, Uematsu M. Image-guided radiation therapy of primary prostate cancer by a CT-linac combination: prostate movements and dosimetric considerations. Int J Radiat Oncol Biol Phys 2003;57(2 Suppl):S334–5.

24. International Commission on Radiation Units and Measurements. Prescribing, recording and reporting photon beam therapy. Report 50. Washington (DC): International Commission on Radiation Units and Measurements; 1993.

25. International Commission on Radiation Units and Measurements. Prescribing, recording and reporting photon beam therapy. Report 62. Supplement to ICRU Report 50. Washington (DC): International Commission on Radiation Units and Measurements; 1999.

26. American College of Radiology. ACR standard for radiation oncology. 1999.

27. Lee N, Chuang C, Quivey JM, et al. Skin toxicity due to intensity-modulated radiotherapy for head-and-neck carcinoma. Int J Radiat Oncol Biol Phys 2002;53:630–7.

28. Lee N, Xia P, Fischbein NJ, et al. Intensity-modulated radiation therapy for head-and-neck cancer: the UCSF experience focusing on target volume delineation. Int J Radiat Oncol Biol Phys 2003;57:49–60.

29. Chao KSC, Ozyigit G, Tran BN, et al. Patterns of failure in patients receiving definitive and postoperative IMRT for head-and-neck cancer. Int J Radiat Oncol Biol Phys 2003;55:312–21.

30. Chao KSC, Wippold II FJ, Ozyigit G, et al. Determination and delineation of nodal target volumes for head-and-neck cancer based on patterns of failure in patients receiving definitive and postoperative IMRT. Int J Radiat Oncol Biol Phys 2002;53:1174–84.

31. Lin A, Marsh L, Dawson LA, Eisburch A. Local-regional (LR) recurrences near the base of the skull following IMRT of head and neck (HN) cancer: implications for target delineation in the high neck and for the parotid sparing. Int J Radiat Oncol Biol Phys 2003;57(2 Suppl):S155.

32. Yau J, Lieskovsky YC, Horst K, et al. An evaluation of patterns of failure and subjective salivary function in patients treated with intensity modulated radiotherapy for head and neck cancers. Int. J Radiat Oncol Biol Phys 2003;57(2 Suppl):S156.

33. Song S, Tome WA, Mehta MP, Harari PM. Emphasizing conformal avoidance versus target definition for IMRT planning in H&N cancer. Int J Radiat Oncol Biol Phys 2003;57(2 Suppl):S299–300.

Chapter 16

BILLING AND REIMBURSEMENT

CHET SZERLAG, MBA, FACHE, CMPE, LUIS CANOVAS, CPC

Intensity-modulated radiation therapy (IMRT) represents a technologically advanced approach to the planning and delivery of radiation therapy (RT) treatments. Consequently, all members of the radiation oncology team are faced with learning new approaches and techniques. This is true not only for radiation oncologists and physicists but also for the radiation oncology administrative team, which must ensure the economic soundness and financial payback for such new technology.

The purpose of this chapter is to review how the domestic health care market is structured in the United States, examine the duality of the payment policies for health care services under the Medicare program, and analyze the specific reimbursement provisions of those federal policies for IMRT services. This chapter does not cover payment mechanisms for centrally planned health care systems such as those in Canada, Europe, and Asia. In those systems, the accounting and financial emphasis is typically placed on cost and productivity management instead of on billing methodologies and systems.

US Health Care Market Sector

Payment for health care services in the United States is a mixture of private and public funding sources. In addition to federal health care programs (eg, Medicare, Medicaid, Veterans' Administration), there are approximately 1,500 commercial, for-profit companies in the private marketplace, ranging from large national corporations (eg, Blue Cross/Blue Shield) to small, local, self-insured organizations.

The major sources for health care coverage and payment in the US marketplace are the private employer-sponsored insurance plans for the working population and federal programs for retired, indigent, and disabled individuals. The health coverage market is further segmented into people under 65 and people over 65 years of age.

For 2004, the Census Office data indicate that there are approximately 285 million individuals living in the United States. Data from the Centers for Medicare and Medicaid

Services (CMS) indicate that the segment of the population over 65 years of age comprises approximately 35 million (12% of the population). The segment under 65 years of age totals approximately 250 million, and in that segment, individuals with private insurance coverage comprise ~ 70%. Individuals without insurance average 16 to 17%, whereas those covered by Medicaid comprise 9 to 11%.

Medicare as a Key Payor of Oncology Services

Medicare is a major insurer of health care services for cancer patients. The program is composed of two major policy and legislative sections, known as "Part A" and "Part B." Part A covers payments for hospital or facility services, whereas Part B covers payments for physician services. These systems are independent of each other, with each having a unique regulatory structure and payment framework. When developing an IMRT business model, one must take into account these different payment systems. The common denominator of both is their reliance on "fixed fee" payments, which are based on vastly different calculation methodologies (Table 16-1).

Ambulatory payment classifications (APCs) represent the first major reform of Medicare reimbursement for hospital-based outpatient services since the inception of Medicare in 1965. The APC Final Rule had an effective date of August 1, 2000. For freestanding centers, Medicare approved global billing through Part B effective January 2002. In some states, freestanding centers are also allowed to bill a facility charge to Part A.

APC payment rates are applicable to hospital outpatient departments. Of note, the APCs do not apply to the 10 cancer centers that are legislatively exempt from inpatient

TABLE 16-1. US Health Care Payment Methodologies

Service Type	Payment Calculation Methodology
Inpatient hospital	Diagnosis-related group payment rates
Outpatient hospital	Ambulatory payment classifications
Physician's services	Resource-based relative value system

reimbursement based on the diagnosis-related group (DRG) methodology. Those facilities are reimbursed under pre-existing Part A cost reimbursement policies.

Prior to 2000, hospital outpatient services were reimbursed by Medicare using an institution-specific formula that blended costs and charges, unique to each hospital's individual economic structure. Prospective payment for Medicare inpatient services was implemented in 1983 with the DRG methodology.

Adoption Curve for IMRT Technology

When IMRT reimbursement was approved by CMS in 2000, there were a limited number of published clinical studies. As Figure 16-1 illustrates, reimbursement economics were the primary fuel igniting growth in IMRT linear accelerator sales. Medicare's APC payment rate for IMRT treatments was pegged at approximately $407 versus $95 for conventional non-IMRT payments, a fourfold differential (payment rate is for Medicare Locale 16).

Figure 16-1 illustrates the rapid specialty-wide "adoption rate" for IMRT by radiation oncology providers, which strengthened the ongoing research and development efforts of the linear accelerator manufacturers for this technology. The capital investment required to establish IMRT capability is quite significant. A fully configured, IMRT-ready linear accelerator with planning software may cost upward of 2 million dollars. Such costs significantly raise the capital equipment payback period and increase the risk for providers and medical practices. However, through its facility payment differential, Medicare recognized the clinical utility of IMRT as well as its greater capital investment costs. This fostered IMRT's rapid adoption, reducing the market risk while stimulating provider demand. The net result is that the installed linear accelerator base grew from 2,600 to nearly 3,000 units in the United States during the 5-year period from 1998 to 2002.

Figure 16-2 illustrates a different facet of the growth trend: despite an increasing acquisition of multileaf collimators (MLCs) with new linear accelerators, many of these advanced MLC-equipped systems were not being used for IMRT. Instead, these units are being used to deliver conventional treatments, an expensive underutilization of advanced technology. This seemingly paradoxical trend reflects the steep learning curve and time-intensive nature of commissioning and implementing IMRT. Many community-based practices do not have adequate physics resources for launching IMRT capability in addition to performing the normal daily clinical duties.

Evolution of IMRT Reimbursement

IMRT procedures were clinically introduced in the mid-1990s, but health insurers did not immediately recognize and establish a higher payment differential for this new procedure, despite the significantly higher level of capital investment required. Coincidentally, in the late 1990s, the Medicare program began development of its new hospital outpatient prospective payment system (HOPPS). Federal policy makers included a payment differential mechanism in the HOPPS system for encouraging introduction of new technology, thereby creating an incentive to adopt cutting-edge technology to improve quality of care, reduce health care costs, and recoup capital costs. Thus, through this explicit federal policy mechanism encouraging "early adopters," IMRT came to have a higher reimbursement rate than conventional treatment.

IMRT is a classic example of how federal payment policy can foster new technology and raise standards of care. It is also an illustration of how federal health care payment policies can stimulate or retard technology adoption. In the case of IMRT, Medicare coverage and payment policies clearly stimulated its rapid adoption. Despite its early clinical adoption in the mid-1990s, it was not until the introduction of the HOPPS that Medicare established specific reimbursement rates for IMRT treatments.

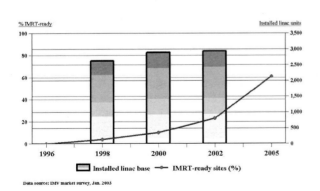

FIGURE 16-1. IMRT adoption curve (1996–2005) (as a percentage of 1,860 US sites offering radiation therapy services) for the radiation oncology specialty as a whole. Linac = linear accelerator.

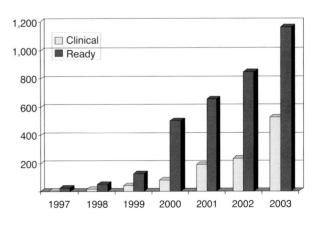

FIGURE 16-2. Intensity-modulated radiation therapy (IMRT)-ready linear accelerators versus IMRT clinical implementation among the Varian Medical Systems customer base.

A specific "facility payment rate" for IMRT treatments was made effective for Medicare's 2000 fiscal year, but only for hospital-based practices. In 2002, the policy was expanded to include freestanding centers. The initial Medicare billing code was a "temporary code" (G0174), followed in 2001 by the formal assignment of current procedural terminology (CPT) code 77418. Initially, the Medicare payment rate for an IMRT treatment represented a payment multiple that was four times that for conventional treatments ($407 vs $95). However, by 2004, this facility payment differential was reduced to $294 owing to federal budgetary pressures.

Prior to the availability of IMRT technology, there was no strong rationale for hospital-based providers to upgrade perfectly functional, but aging, linear accelerators because basic linear accelerator technology had not significantly evolved over the prior decade. In fact, at the beginning of the 1990s, the average age of linear accelerators was 11 to 15 years according to industry data analyses by Varian Medical Systems (Palo Alto, CA). By the end of the 1990s, the average age of linear accelerators had dropped to less than 5 years as providers rapidly acquired IMRT-ready machines. Fueled by the Medicare payment differential, one can see how federal policies act as a powerful stimulant for technology demand. This scenario repeated itself in 2001 when Medicare approved reimbursement for positron emission tomography (PET) scans, stimulating a new commercial market for PET technology.

Payment Policy Framework

Health care reimbursement policies are ever-changing. Ongoing Medicare policy changes often result from political and market pressures, feedback from physician and hospital providers, and evolving medical practice.

Over the years, federal payment policy formulations for the Medicare program have become the de facto policy standard setter. Many private insurers now follow federal health coverage policies, and some even design their payment systems along Medicare's lines. This should not be too surprising because the government routinely contracts with private health insurers to serve as Medicare fiscal intermediaries and carriers.

The complexity of health care technology and the pace of innovation have greatly accelerated in recent years. The ability of insurers to evaluate health care trends has outstripped their internal resources and expertise; thus, many health insurers informally rely on Medicare's policy-making bureaucracy to determine which technological innovations should be reimbursable. Although this promotes standardization and timely policy making, it also serves to propagate federal reimbursement policies throughout the private sector, driving down provider payment levels.

Understanding the Medicare Coverage Database

The Medicare Coverage Database (MCD) is an important reference source for determining current Medicare service coverages and is available on-line at http://www.cms.hhs.gov/mcd. This database describes health care services eligible for reimbursement under the Medicare program. Health benefit coverage can be national and/or local in scope, and the database helps identify covered services. It is a useful resource for determining if a specific health care service is eligible for Medicare reimbursement and whether formal policy statements are available for reference.

Medicare's policy formulations and payment information are not unified or consistent between Parts A and B. One must research and gather information from several places to pull together the total reimbursement picture for a given clinical procedure such as IMRT.

Professional versus Facility Billing

With respect to payment policy and reimbursement in the US health care market, there are two major policy frameworks. These frameworks cover hospital (or facility) payments and physician payments. The hospital-based radiation oncology service delivery model is an excellent example of how these two frameworks are organized.

Hospital-based radiation oncology services have two billable components: a professional fee and a facility fee. Freestanding facilities often bill a global fee, which combines the professional and technical components into one fee per given CPT procedure. Professional billing (also known as pro fees or physician fees) represents the physician component of the service. The facility billing (also referred to as the technical fee or hospital outpatient fee) represents the costs associated with the capital acquisition of the equipment, facilities, utilities, staff, etc. Taken together, they represent the total price of the service. Payment mechanisms for each component are complex and vary according to the insurer. There are also instances in which the practice incurs the capital costs of the equipment and facilities. In these instances, the billing methodology follows the global fee approach.

When reviewing Medicare billing and reimbursement policies, it is important to differentiate between facility and pro fee billing systems because they use different payment methodologies. Some private insurance payment systems are organized along similar dual systems. For example, in the Blue Cross/Blue Shield system, Blue Cross handles the facility payment and Blue Shield handles the physician payment. In freestanding clinics, where a facility bills a "global" fee, the overall reimbursement payment for the global fee is the same as if the billing for each component were done separately.

The CMS has outsourced the management and administration of the Medicare Part A and Part B programs to fiscal intermediaries and carriers, respectively. These fiscal intermediaries are private health insurers under contract to administer the Part A facility payment system. Carriers are also private health insurers under contract to administer the Part B physician payment system. There are more than 40 separate fiscal intermediaries and carriers administering the Part A and Part B programs throughout the US. The government has traditionally outsourced the day-to-day administration of Medicare to private insurers responsible for regionalized claims processing and medical policy administration.

Medicare Policy Statements for Payment of the Facility Component of IMRT

The higher payment rate for IMRT is found only in the Medicare Part A program. HOPPS has established a higher APC payment rate for IMRT delivery than for conventional treatments. (There is no comparable differential for physician payments for IMRT in the resource-based relative value system [RBRVS] for physician services.) The weekly physician management payment rate (CPT code 77427) does not differentiate between IMRT and non-IMRT. It is only through the higher facility payment rate that Medicare recognizes the significant capital investment incurred.

More than 25 Part A fiscal intermediaries are under contract to Medicare, each with their own set of policies and procedures. These policies and procedures are not 100% uniform across the country, but the only policies and procedures that matter are those followed by the fiscal intermediary responsible for *your* state or region. The Web site http://www.cms.hhs.gov/medlearn/tollnums.asp contains a complete listing of carriers and fiscal intermediaries.

A prototypical example of a Medicare Part A policy statement on the facility component of IMRT is posted on the AdminaStar Federal (Indianapolis, Indiana) Web site (www.adminastar.com/providers/intermediary/medicalpolicy /currentlmrps.cfm), the fiscal intermediary for the state of Illinois. This policy statement is known as a local coverage determination (LCD). Similar Part B policy statements are referred to as a local medical review policy (LMRP).

It is instructive to read the actual language and understand the range of information contained in such policy statements. The format and content follow a standard outline used for many, if not all, LCD and LMRP formulations, and this specific policy is applicable to all providers performing facility billing in the states assigned to the AdminaStar Federal fiscal intermediary. Actual APC payment rates are published and updated separately from policy formulations. One must remember to refer to the fiscal intermediary covering one's state for policies specifically applicable to one's facility. It should be noted that there are also national coverage decisions that emanate from CMS headquarters and are applicable nationwide. So whenever one is researching a particular policy or coverage issue, one must be sure to check both the local and the national policy statements.

Professional Billing and Reimbursement for IMRT

Physicians performing IMRT bill the same weekly management fee (CPT 77427) as they would for conventional RT. As mentioned previously, Medicare Part B policies also apply to billing by freestanding centers. A representative Medicare Part B policy statement on billing for the physician component of IMRT is available at www.wpsic.com/medicare/policies/illinois/rad14.shtml.

As has been noted, the format and content of such policy statement follow a typical content outline used for all LMRP and LCD formulations. This policy is applicable to all providers performing physician billing in the states of Illinois, Wisconsin, Michigan, and Wisconsin. For policy information that may be applicable for any other states or localities, consult the appropriate carrier for that area. Actual RBRVS payment rates are published annually by CMS in the *Federal Register* and updated separately from carrier-specific LMRP policy formulations.

Differences between Facility and Physician Payment Policies

First, one should pay attention only to those policies and procedures originating from the carrier and/or intermediary in one's region. See www.cms.hhs.gov/contacts/incardir.asp for a complete listing of Part B carriers and Part A fiscal intermediaries throughout the United States. As of 2004, 19 Part B carriers and 23 Part A intermediaries operate as Medicare contractors.

The Medicare program publishes national and local policies for both hospital outpatient and physician services. National policies come from CMS headquarters, whereas local policies come from the regional intermediaries and carriers. Although one can expect national policies to be uniformly interpreted, local policies are just that and can vary among carriers and intermediaries. Local policy statements are applicable only in the regions for which intermediaries and carriers serve as Medicare program contractors.

Second, be sure that you understand whether a given policy statement is intended for facilities or physicians. Policy statements on the same issue or topic will vary, depending on the point of view from which they are written (ie, hospital vs physician provider). They may also use different terminology or nomenclature for the same concept. Care must be exercised if one is trying to read and interpret policies side by side because there may be language incongruity. In addition, the billing forms and payment systems used to process hospital outpatient and pro fee claims are distinct from each other.

So, for example, if one is a provider in Illinois, one would rely on AdminaStar Federal for claims policy and payment processing guidance for hospital (facility) outpatient billing and Wisconsin Physician Service (Milwaukee, Wisconsin) for pro fee (physician) claims policy and payment processing guidance. Then, of course, many private health insurers have unique payment policies that bear no resemblance to federal policies! When in doubt, one should call the patient's health insurer directly for answers to policy and payment questions.

Third, these policy statements change periodically, so it is important to check for the latest policy statements. In the case of Medicare, all policy statements are published in the *Federal Register* and are often available on-line. Web sites for your regional carrier or intermediary should be consulted for the latest policies and guidelines.

Inpatient versus Outpatient Services under Medicare

Another key concept and important billing distinction that must be kept in mind is the setting in which services are rendered. RT services are most commonly provided in an outpatient setting. But inpatients can also receive RT services.

Since 1983, Medicare has used a prospective payment system (PPS) for reimbursing inpatient hospital operating costs, based on DRG coding schema. The DRG system replaced the retrospective cost reimbursement system whereby interim rates were paid on each bill and end-of-year adjustments were made based on information contained in hospitals' annual cost report filings. With the DRG system, hospitals are paid a fixed amount, determined in advance, for the operating costs of each patient hospitalization, based on the assignment of one of 523 DRGs. Approximately 70% of hospitals in the United States are included in the PPS system for inpatient services; the remaining 30% of hospitals are exempt, including the following 10 academic cancer centers (Memorial Sloan-Kettering Cancer Center, M. D. Anderson Cancer Center, Dana-Farber Cancer Institute, Roswell Park Cancer Institute, Fox Chase Cancer Center, Hutchinson Cancer Center, James Cancer Hospital, University of Miami Hospital, City of Hope Medical Center, and University of Southern California/Norris Comprehensive Cancer Center and Hospital).

Under the inpatient PPS system, a patient discharge is assigned a DRG based on diagnosis, surgery, age, discharge destination, and sex. Each DRG has a weight based on billing

and cost data, reflecting the relative cost, across all hospitals, of treating cases classified in that DRG.

Reimbursement for RT services under the DRG system is folded into the overall payment for a given DRG code. Generally speaking, from the hospital perspective, it is preferable to provide RT services on an outpatient basis so that the DRG payment is optimized. Of the 523 DRG codes, one code (409) is listed as "radiotherapy." DRG 409 is used when concomitant chemo-RT is administered or when an inpatient admission is coded as V58.0, which groups to DRG 409.

Understanding and Correlating APC and CPT Coding for IMRT Services

It requires considerable effort to understand both the facility and the physician payment systems used by Medicare. Most billing professionals specialize in only one system or the other. However, knowing how both systems work will give health care managers and physicians a complete picture of IMRT economics and the associated income streams, which is vital when developing capital funding requests and business plan justifications.

Within the Medicare program, even though the facility and physician payment systems are independently administered, a common CPT/Healthcare Common Procedure Coding System coding schema is used. Table 16-2 provides a cross-reference between APC and CPT coding for facility and physician IMRT services, respectively. Applying the payment rate in the table, one can see that 30 fractions of IMRT would result in an APC reimbursement of $8,823 ($294.11 × 30) minus the patient copayment. Thirty fractions of conventional RT would yield a payment of only $3,493 (116.43 × 30) minus the copayment. In either case, the physician payment for the weekly management would stay the same, that is, $1,076 (179.41 × 6) minus the copayment. Interested readers can refer to http://www.cms. hhs.gov/providers/hopps/fr2004.asp for a full listing of 2004 APC payment rates. The proposed HOPPS policy changes for FY 2005 can be viewed at http://www.cms.hhs.gov/ providers/hopps/2005p/1427p.asp.

TABLE 16-2. Facility versus Physician Payment Rates for Intensity-Modulated Radiation Therapy for Illinois (Medicare Locale 16)

CPT Code with Modifer	Description	2003 APC Payment Rate, $	2004 APC Payment Rate, $	2004 RBRVS Payment Rate, $	New APC No.	Old APC No.
77301	IMRT plan New Technology–Level X	875	850		1510	0712
77301-26	IMRT plan			425.29		
77418	IMRT treatment per fraction	400	294.11		0412	0710
77427	Physician treatment management, per 5 fractions			181.49		

APC = ambulatory payment classification; CPT = current procedural terminology; IMRT = intensity-modulated radiation therapy; RBRVS = resource-based relative value system.

The remaining sections in this chapter provide more detail on each payment system.

Billing and Reimbursement for the Facility Service Component (Medicare Part A)

Medicare Part A (also known as Hospital Insurance) covers both inpatient and outpatient care in hospitals. The payment made by the Part A program is for the facility component and does not include the pro fee billed by physicians. Unlike Part B, most individuals do not pay a monthly premium for coverage because they (or a spouse) have paid Medicare taxes through their employer's payroll deductions. Even if one did not pay Medicare taxes, one may still be eligible for coverage.

Medicare Part A is the funding source for payment of facility claims submissions, both inpatient and outpatient. Inpatient facility billings are processed through the DRG system, whereas the outpatient facility claims submissions are processed by the HOPPS system using APC payment rates. Payment of all physician charges is from Medicare Part B. All physician payments (for both inpatient and outpatient claims submissions) are adjudicated and processed using the Resource-Based Relative Value System payment rates. Freestanding centers are a unique exception, with their "global" billings processed exclusively through the Part B system. A "global charge" includes both the technical and professional charge in one fee amount per CPT code.

Radiation oncology treatments are delivered primarily on an outpatient basis. However, in academic medical centers, outpatient therapy can be as low as 75% of the patient mix due to the prevalence of experimental clinical protocols. Conversely, in the community setting, 95 to 100% of patients are treated as outpatients. When inpatient treatment is delivered, payment is included as part of the DRG for the primary diagnosis.

APC System Used for Payment of Outpatient Facility Claims

HOPPS was first proposed as part of the Balanced Budget Act of 1997. The final regulation was published in the *Federal Register* on April 7, 2000. The APC system is the methodology used to make payments in the HOPPS system. Prior to HOPPS, Medicare payment for services performed in the hospital outpatient setting was primarily cost based. Hospitals were paid under a number of different payment methods, including fee schedules. For most other services, payments were based on costs.

The Balanced Budget Act required CMS to replace the cost-based system with the HOPPS, which pays at specific predetermined payment rates (based on APCs) for outpatient services. This law also changed the way in which beneficiary coinsurance is determined for services. Generally, under HOPPS, coinsurance amounts are based on 20% of the national median charge. The Balanced Budget Refinement Act of 1999 contained a number of major provisions affecting HOPPS. Special "pass through" payments for new technologies were established to foster their introduction. IMRT was one such new technology given a special payment rate.

HOPPS includes most hospital outpatient services and Medicare Part B services furnished to hospital inpatients who do not have Part A coverage. The APC system classifies all outpatient services into approximately 660 individual payment rates, including APC codes for handling "new technology," such as IMRT treatment planning (APC 1510). Theoretically, the services within each group are clinically similar and consume comparable resources.

Each APC is assigned a relative payment weight based on the median cost of the services within the APC. The payment rates are initially determined on a national basis. The rates actually paid to hospitals vary, depending on the area wage level. To adjust for wage differences across geographic areas, the labor-related portion of the payment rate (60%) is adjusted, using an individual hospital's wage index. Some incidental items and services are packaged into the APC payment for the services. A hospital may furnish a number of services to a beneficiary on the same day and receive an APC payment for each service.

In December 2003, CMS issued an interim final rule for 2004 revising payment policies for hospital outpatient services to Medicare beneficiaries. Under this rule, the "IMRT treatment planning" code continues to be listed as APC 1510 (New Technology–Level X in the APC range), allowing for continuing payment and tracking of service utilization data. Medicare policy makers felt that the cost data for the IMRT planning code were flawed due to miscoding errors. This resulted in the $875 payment rate for 2003 declining only slightly to $850 for 2004. The final rule was published in the January 6, 2004 *Federal Register*. APC payment rates for IMRT (as of January 2004) are shown in Table 16-3.

Billing and Reimbursement for the Physician Service Component (Medicare Part B)

Medicare Part B pays for physician services. It also pays for other medical services such as laboratory tests, physical therapy, radiotherapy, and other cancer care services. The Medicare Part B premium is currently $45.50 per month for individuals. Unlike Part A, enrolment is voluntary.

As previously mentioned, Medicare Part A and B carriers periodically issue policy statements clarifying practices and procedures, known as LMRP and LCD policies. These two concepts are becoming increasingly interchangeable, with LMRPs being converted to LCDs, so be sure to determine if the policy is intended to provide facility or physician guidance.

TABLE 16-3. APC Payment Rates

APC	Group Title IMRT Services	Status Indicator	Relative Weights	2004 Payment Rate, $	2004 National Unadjusted Copayment, $	2005 Proposed Payment Rate, $
1510	New Technology–Level X (IMRT Plan)	S	6.0369	850.00	170.00	812.00
0412	IMRT Treatment Delivery	S	5.3904	294.11	58.82	308.00

APC = ambulatory payment classification; IMRT = intensity-modulated radiation therapy.

RBRVS System Used for Payment of Physician Claims

For the physician component of IMRT, there was no additional reimbursement established for the weekly physician management code (77427) under the RBRVS system. This means that for IMRT, any incremental revenues on the physician side are the result of increased volume of procedures per case (per patient utilization) rather than through higher payment rates.

In 2003, CMS added a feature to its Web site that makes it possible for physicians to determine in advance what they will be paid for a particular service. The Medicare Physician Fee Schedule Look-up provides both the unadjusted payment rates and the payment rates by geographic location (http://www.cms.hhs.gov/providers/pufdownload/default.asp#pfspayment).

Coding Nomenclatures

No discussion of billing and payment systems would be complete without a review of the several coding schemas used to describe and adjudicate claims submissions. Both Part A and Part B programs employ complex, automated claim review and payment processing systems to adjudicate and administer the payment policy provisions legislated by Congress. Each payment system also uses a computerized editing system known as the National Correct Coding Initiative (NCCI), which screens each claim submission to determine whether the reported CPT code(s) and ICD-9CM diagnosis are payable. Due to the complexity and patient specificity of RT, the NCCI edits can generate numerous rejections and payment denials for radiation oncology practices. NCCI edits are discussed in greater detail in the following section of this chapter.

The primary "language" of health care claims processing is based on application of two coding systems: the HCPCS/CPT procedure codes and the diagnoses codes contained in the *International Classification of Diseases*, 9th Edition, Clinical Modification (ICD-9CM) coding guidebook. These codes are used on claims submissions to describe and itemize the services provided. HCPCS is currently a two-level coding system. Level I is synonymous with the CPT coding system used for codifying claim submissions for physician services and is a five-digit numeric

system. Level II is a system used for codifying claims for the facility component of health care services. CMS updates this system on an annual basis.

CPT is a set of descriptive terms and identifying codes used for reporting medical services and procedures performed by physicians. As stated above, CPT can also be referred to as HCPCS level I codes. The CPT nomenclature was originally developed in 1966 and undergoes annual revisions. Its purpose is to provide a uniform language to describe medical, surgical, and diagnostic services, providing an effective communication tool for physicians, patients, and insurance programs. The CPT nomenclature is copyrighted by the American Medical Association (AMA).

HCPCS/CPT and the ICD-9CM are important coding systems mandated by CMS in coding and preparing all Medicare facility and physician claims. The nomenclature used by these two systems must be understood to codify IMRT services. To ensure accuracy and completeness, it is recommended that professionally certified coders (eg, Certified Professional Coder, Certified Professional Coder-Hospital, Certified Coding Specialist, Certified Coding Specialist-Physician) be employed by radiation oncology practices and hospital departments to prepare and submit claims. The certification examinations for the CPC and CPC-H credentials are offered by the American Academy of Professional Coders. The certification examinations for CCS and CCS-P credentials are offered by the American Health Information Management Association.

The following are the 2004 CPT definitions for IMRT:

77301 Intensity modulated radiotherapy plan, including dose-volume histograms for target and critical structure partial tolerance specifications. (Dose plan is optimized using inverse or forward planning technique for modulated beam delivery (e.g. binary, dynamic MLC) to create highly conformal dose distribution. Computer plan distribution must be verified for positional accuracy based on dosimetric verification of the intensity map with verification of treatment set up and interpretation of verification methodology.)

77418 Intensity modulated treatment delivery, single or multiple fields/arcs, via narrow spatially and temporally modulated beams (eg binary, dynamic MLC), per treatment session.

ICD9-CM Codes

The ICD9-CM is designated by the CMS as the primary diagnosis coding schema for all IMRT claims. Virtually all insurers use this system. ICD9-CM nomenclature is used for reporting both physician and facility services on all claim forms.

Most ICD9-CM codes used for radiation oncology are under the "neoplasm" section. Given the number of neoplastic codes, one should employ a professionally certified coder to ensure that proper coding is performed, thus minimizing and/or avoiding claim denials and payment delays.

NCCI Edits

Medicare's payment system edits (NCCI edits) are a major source of confusion and misinterpretation among providers The edits use dates of service to determine which procedures are payable. Many pairs of CPT codes are deemed nonpayable if billed on the same date of service. Conversely, these same pairs of codes are usually payable if the dates are not identical or if CPT code modifiers are appropriately used to define and quantify services performed. Table 16-4 illustrates the correct usage of CPT code modifiers for IMRT claim submissions.

The NCCI edits work as a filtering tool and are used by all fiscal intermediaries and carriers nationwide that have contracted with the federal government to process and pay Medicare claims. The edits for physician CPT codes were first made available on the CMS Web site (http://cms.hhs.gov/physicians/cciedits/default.asp) in September 2003. In January 2004, the CMS posted edits for facility providers at http://www.cms.hhs.gov/providers/hopps/cciedits/.

The NCCI schema includes two types of edits. The "comprehensive/component" edits identify code pairs that should not be billed together because one service inherently includes the other. The "mutually exclusive" edits identify code pairs that, for clinical reasons, are unlikely to be performed on the same day.

The NCCI edits are posted on the CMS Web site in a spreadsheet format, allowing one to sort by procedural code and effective date. A "find" feature allows one to search for a specific code. The edit files are indexed by procedural code ranges, and the Web site includes links to helpful reference materials, including the *NCCI Policy Manual for Part B Medicare Carriers*, the *Medicare Carriers Manual*, and the NCCI Question and Answer page.

TABLE 16-4. CPT Coding Schema Illustrating Use of Modifier Codes for Billing of Intensity-Modulated Radiation Therapy Services

Description	Technical			Professional			Comments
	Units	CPT Code	Modifier(s)	Units	CPT Code	Modifier(s)	
Consultation	1	99245		1	99245		Code initial patient visit appropriately, CPT 99201–99245
Physician treatment planning, complex		NA		1	77263		Pro fee only
Simulation, complex	1	77290	TC	1	77290	26	Billing date is date of simulation
CT planning slices acquisition	1	76370	TC		NA		Technical only; pro fee is included in 77290
Treatment devices, complex	1	77334	TC	1	77334	26	Positioning devices (alpha cradle)
Special treatment procedure	1	77470	TC	1	77470	26	If applicable
IMRT plan	1	77301	TC	1	77301	26	Billing date is date of physician approval (signature)
Basic dosimetry calculation	7	77300	TC	5	77300	26	Only 5 per line allowed
				2	77300	26-76	76 overrides duplicate edit
Treatment devices, complex	1	77334	TC-59	1	77334	26-59	
	1	77334	TC-59-76	1	77334	26-59-76	
	1	77334	TC-59-76	1	77334	26-59-76	MLC, per port (gantry angle)
	1	77334	TC-59-76	1	77334	26-59-76	59 overrides CCI edit
	1	77334	TC-59-76	1	77334	26-59-76	76 overrides duplicate edit
	1	77334	TC-59-76	1	77334	26-59-76	
	1	77334	TC-59-76	1	77334	26-59-76	
IMRT treatment delivery	1	77418			NA		For IMRT twice daily, add modifier 59 to second treatment
Simulation, simple	1	77280	TC	1	77280	26	Verification simulation, if necessary
Continuing physics consultation (weekly)	1	77336			NA		Each 5 fractions
Port film	1	77417			NA		Each 5 fractions, one charge
Physician treatment management		NA		1	77427		Each 5 fractions. Billing date is first date of each 5. May be billed if 3 or more fractions at end

CCI = correct coding initiative; CPT = current procedural terminology; CT = computed tomography; IMRT = intensity-modulated radiation therapy; MLC = multileaf collimator; NA = not available; TC = technical component.

The NCCI coding policies are based on a range of coding conventions as defined by the AMA CPT manual; national and local Medicare policies and edits; coding guidelines developed by national medical specialty societies, such as the American Society of Therapeutic Radiology and Oncology, the American College of Radiology, and the American College of Radiation Oncology; analysis of standard medical and surgical practice; and review of current coding practice. The NCCI edits are updated quarterly, but there is little explanatory narrative available on how the edits really work.

Impact of NCCI Edits on IMRT

Date of service is the key variable in understanding the mechanics of the NCCI edits. Services *are* payable when performed on other dates and are not specifically excluded. The NCCI edits require that health care providers and billing personnel have an in-depth understanding of claim form modifiers because, in many instances, use of the appropriate modifiers (such as modifier 59, separate and distinct procedural service) renders services payable when provided on the "same day, same patient." Providers should appeal wrongful denials if they believe that the clinical and medical circumstances justify providing multiple services on the same date of service. It is very important to review all claim rejections for coding errors and resubmit as appropriate. This is best done by radiation oncology practices employing certified coding professionals. Do not solely rely on your billing service to get this done. When in doubt on how to resubmit and appeal rejected claims, you can also seek professional advice on correct coding. A number of skilled and expert consulting firms can help with this.

IMRT Revenue Modeling and Business Planning

The first step in modeling the revenue for a new service is adopting a sound methodology. Revenue modeling should be thought of as a multidisciplinary process including clinical, physics, and financial personnel. This process usually culminates in a written business plan that incorporates revenue and expense forecasts and projects bottom-line profitability for the new service or procedure. When developing a business plan for a specific health care service or procedure, the following 10-step process can be used:

1. Define the scope of the proposed service.
2. Determine if the proposed service has both a facility and a technical component. Table 16-5 illustrates this framework for radiation oncology.
3. Assign CPT codes to each discrete service wherever possible.
4. Determine if the service is currently offered as covered benefits under one's current health insurance programs and managed care contracts
5. If it is not covered, develop a rationale as to why it should be. Typically, covered benefit and payment decisions are made by the medical directors of private sector health insurers, based on research and discussion or consultation with specialty societies. For requesting and obtaining reimbursement for new procedures in the Medicare program, there is the American Medical Association's Specialty Society Relative Value Scale Update Committee (RUC committee), which reviews and recommends new services for reimbursement.

TABLE 16-5. Radiation Oncology Intensity-Modulated Radiation Therapy Billing Policy Framework

Category of Service	Fee		Comments
	Professional	Facility	
Physician consultation (evaluation and management) CPT 99241–99275 and 99201–99215	Yes	Yes	
Clinical treatment planning CPT 77261–77263	Yes	No	Pro fee only
Simulation CPT 77280–77299	.Yes	Yes	
Radiation physics CPT 77300–77399	Yes	Yes	Note the pro fee exceptions below for 77336 and 77370
Dosimetry CPT 77300–77399	Yes	Yes	
Radiation physics			
Continuing consultation CPT 77336	No	Yes	Facility fee only
Special consultation CPT 77370	No	Yes	Facility fee only
Treatment delivery—port films CPT 77417	No	Yes	Facility fee only
Treatment devices CPT 77332–77334	Yes	Yes	
Treatment delivery CPT 77401–77418	No	Yes	Daily treatments are technical only
Physician treatment management CPT 77427–77499	Yes	No	Weekly management is pro fee only
Other services, such as diagnostic radiology, laboratory services, injections. Facility billing for CT simulation (76370), BAT (76950) procedures also fall into this category	Yes/no*	Yes/no*	The fees from these procedures may not all directly accrue to radiation oncology, but they are an important revenue driver for the overall organization and should be included in the overall revenue model because this will help support capital equipment justification

BAT = B-mode acquisition and targeting; CPT = current procedural terminology; CT = computed tomography.

*Indicates that, in some instances, there is a radiation oncology facility charge, whereas in other instances, the procedures may be billed by the ancillary departments.

6. If this is an established procedure with existing payment rates, identify the technical and professional payment rates used by one's private sector and federal insurers. This usually requires use of multiple techniques, which include a review of Medicare RBRVS and APC payment files and individual managed care contracts. In some cases, existing payment rates may be kept confidential by private insurers for competitive reasons, and analysis of reimbursement and payment check vouchers may be the only means to determine payment rates.

7. Develop a gross charge or fee for the procedure. Several fees can be market based, pegged to a multiple of payment rates(eg. 3× the reimbursement rate), cost plus a markup percentage, or the fee can be fully cost determined through classic time study and cost accounting techniques.

8. Use spreadsheet software to set up the data elements of the model, including technical and/or professional payment rates and expected unit volumes, payor mix percentages, and charges. The payment data are then multiplied by the unit volume to obtain estimated net revenues. This analysis can be refined by applying payor mix ratios to obtain specific revenue projections by payor, as illustrated in Table 16-6.

9. The estimated direct expenses are then subtracted from projected net revenues to determine overall profitability (contribution margin) and breakeven points.

10. Finally, assess profitability. If profitability is calculated to be negative, readjust expense and revenue variables to determine at what volume and pricing levels one can achieve a breakeven or positive margin (using a "what if" scenario to test out various expense and revenue data points). If profitability cannot be achieved owing to low volume, poor payor mix, or high operating costs, opportunities for cross-subsidy must be identified. The proposed procedure should not be implemented if it is a money loser. The alternative may be to charge the patient directly for such services, but a review of the Medicare regulations is recommended to ensure that there are no regulatory compliance or policy issues with the decision to charge the patient.

TABLE 16-6. Intensity-Modulated Radiation Therapy Pro Forma Revenue Model Using Medicare Payment Rates

CPT Code	Description	Professional Fee Unit Quantity	Payment Rates, $	Expected Part B Payments, $	Example of Pro Fee Gross Charge, $	Facility Fee Unit Quantity	APC Payment Rates, $	Expected Part A Payments, $	Example of Facility Gross Charge, $
99245	Consultation, outpatient	1	195	195	597	1	76	76	226
77263	Treatment planning, complex	1	177	177	1,074	NA	NA		NA
77290	Simulation, complex	1	84	84	408	1	201	201	1,212
76370	CT planning data acquisition		NA		NA	1	87	87	234
77334	Treatment devices, alpha cradle	1	67	67	529	1	157	157	234
77334	Treatment devices, MLC (primary plan)	7	67	473	529	1	157	157	475
77334	Treatment devices, MLC (boost plan)	7	67	473	529	1	157	157	475
77470	Special treatment procedure	1	114	114	408	1	314	314	1,000
77301	IMRT plan, primary plan	1	425	425	1,372	1	850	850	3,745
77301	IMRT plan, boost plan	1	425	425	1,372	1	850	850	3,745
77300	Basic dosimetry calculation (primary plan)	7	34	243	182	7	NA	NA	266
77300	Basic dosimetry calculation (boost plan)	7	34	243	182	7	NA	NA	266
77418	IMRT treatment delivery		NA		NA	38	294	11,172	2,140
77280	Simulation, simple	38	0	203	0	91	0	533
77336	Continuing physics consultation (weekly)		NA		NA	8	91	728	266
77417	Port film verification		NA		NA	7	43	301	85
77315	Isodose plan	1	84	84	390	1	201	201	808
77280	Simulation, simple	0	38	0	203	0	91	0	533
77370	Special physics consultation		NA		NA	0	201	0	567
77427	Weekly physician management	8	181	1,267	1,113	NA	NA	NA	NA
76950	BAT localization		NA		NA	38	71	2,698	193
	Total expected payments	32		4,270		114		17,949	
	Gross charges				23,895				107,255
	Collection rate (Medicare billings)			18%				17%	

APC = ambulatory payment classification; BAT = B-mode acquisition and targeting; CPT = current procedural terminology; CT = computed tomography; IMRT = intensity-modulated radiation therapy; MLC = multileaf collimator; NA = not applicable; RBRVS = resource-based relative value system.
In this example, the patient was treated with an initial dose of 50 Gy (in 2 Gy daily fractions) followed by a boost of 26 Gy to the prostate (total dose 76 Gy). Seven gantry angles and the BAT system were used daily. The patient was treated on a Varian Medical Systems linear accelerator equipped with a 120 multileaf collimator and electronic portal imaging. Medicare rates are rounded off to the nearest dollar. Because these rates change annually and vary by region, it is necessary to check with one's local carrier and fiscal intermediary for payment rates in different regions.

Radiation Oncology Billing and Reimbursement under the Medicare Program

Within the Medicare program, each medical specialty has a payment methodology reflecting past practices and conventions. Radiation oncology is no different. Some services have both components payable, whereas other services have only one.

For IMRT, there is a daily facility-only fee for IMRT treatment delivery, but for the pro fee component, Medicare's weekly physician management fee (77427) does not differentiate between conventional and IMRT treatments. In effect, the Medicare policy framework recognizes an incremental value for the facility component costs but not for the physician component.

As illustrated in Table 16-7, the format of one's spreadsheet-based revenue model should be organized by CPT code and provide a clear outline of both sides of the IMRT reimbursement model (facility and professional revenues). The model should include market-based charge levels and expected net payments from the Medicare program. When the utilization volume (unit quantity) per CPT code is added (see Table 16-6), the spreadsheet model will allow one to capture the detailed cash flow estimates that are used to build up the overall revenue stream and develop concrete business plans. Medicare payments are often used as a proxy for estimating a baseline of revenues across all payors.

By establishing a unit quantity (frequency) estimate for each charge code, the payment matrix can be used to estimate expected cash revenues by CPT code, by diagnostic

TABLE 16-7. Intensity-Modulated Radiation Therapy Payment Matrix

Charge Code	CPT Code	Description	Professional		Technical		Comments
			Medicare RBRVS 2004, $	Gross Charge (Typical), $	Medicare APC 2004, $	Gross Charge (Typical), $	
Prior to IMRT planning							
11291	99245	Consultation	194.82	597.00	82.00	$226.00	Code initial patient visit appropriately, CPT 99201–99245
11129	77263	Treatment planning, complex	177.13	1,074.00	NA	NA	Pro fee only
11136	77290	Simulation, complex	84.64	408.00	201.00	1,212.00	
11773	76370	CT planning slices acquisition	NA	NA	92.00	234.00	Technical only
11341	77334	Treatment devices, complex	67.60	237.00	157.00	475.00	Positioning devices (alpha cradle); only 1 pro fee allowed
11328	77470	Special treatment procedure	114.65	408.00	314.00	1,000.00	
IMRT planning charges							
11755	77301	IMRT plan	425.29	1,372.00	850.00	3,745.00	Includes isodose plan (77315); this is also APC 1510
11220	77300	Basic dosimetry calculation	34.69	182.00	91.00	266.00	Per field
11183	77334	Treatment devices, complex	67.60	237.00	157.00	475.00	Per gantry angle
IMRT treatment charges							
11756	77418	IMRT treatment delivery	NA	NA	294.11	2,140.00	For IMRT twice daily, add modifier 59 to second treatment; this is also APC 0412
11134	77280	Simulation, simple	38.57	203.00	91.00	533.00	Verification simulation, if necessary
11264	77336	Continuing physics consultation (weekly)	NA	NA	91.00	266.00	Each 5 fractions
11418	77417	Port film	NA	NA	43.00	85.00	Each 5 fractions, per port
IMRT boost charges							
11223	77315	Isodose plan	84.64	390.00	201.00	808.00	
11220	77300	Basic dosimetry calculation	34.69	182.00	91.00	266.00	Per field
11134	77280	Simulation, simple	38.57	203.00	91.00	533.00	Verification simulation, if necessary
11183	77334	Treatment devices, complex	67.60	237.00	157.00	475.00	Per gantry angle
Only when medically appropriate							
11272	77370	Special physics consultation	NA	NA	201.00	567.00	With physician request
11728	77427	Treatment management	181.49	1,113.00	NA	NA	Weekly physician management, per 5 fractions

APC = ambulatory payment classification; CPT = current procedural terminology; CT = computed tomography; IMRT = intensity-modulated radiation therapy; NA = not applicable; RBRVS = resource-based relative value system.
See Table 16-5 for patient and treatment details.

case mix, or by the total number of treatment courses. The hypothetical revenue model in Table 16-6 illustrates the specific payment rates that can be expected from Medicare for both facility (Part A) and physician (Part B) services. Taken together, the individual payment rates and unit volumes enable one to determine an overall average cash flow per case, which can be plugged into a larger business plan to determine the needed caseloads and cash flows for breakeven profitability, projecting incremental profitability by payor class and validating one's capital equipment justification. Freestanding centers would use both revenue streams to build their business plan projections.

Tables 16-6 and 16-7 are a good illustration of how the Medicare program fragments its reimbursement and payment policies for radiation oncology in general and for IMRT in particular. In developing a complete revenue model, such policy "patchworks" must be understood by both clinicians and the billing staff. Table 16-7 outlines the major service categories for a course of treatment, and Table 16-5 outlines whether Medicare policy allows a pro fee or technical fee to be billed. Revenue differences exist between the freestanding and outpatient hospital settings in terms of billing and reimbursement. Table 16-8 highlights several of these differences.

Table 16-6 can be extended into a full revenue model simply by adding payment rates for all of the nonfederal health insurers comprising one's payor mix and extending the per-case revenue estimates using present and expected future caseload volumes. However, use of Medicare rates

is a good proxy for establishing a conservative revenue estimate. The addition of other payors into the model usually improves the overall collection rate, but that depends heavily on one's referral base. Covering the underpayments from Medicare and the underinsured by making up the difference from billings to commercial insurers (commonly referred to as cost shifting) is largely a strategy of the past, given the growth in the fixed-rate reimbursement environment brought on by managed care contracting.

What can we conclude about the "bottom-line" revenue differential between IMRT and conventional treatments? Using the 2004 Medicare APC rates for facility payments, the average cash revenue per case for non-IMRT and IMRT is $10,000 to $12,000 and $18,000 to $20,000, respectively. The APC facility payment rate for IMRT treatment was cut nearly 30%, from $407 to $294 (in Medicare Locale 16) with the implementation of the 2004 rates.

In the health care industry, the "retail charges" listed on fee schedules and hospital chargemasters do not function in the same way as prices in other business sectors owing to the distorting and insulating effect of third-party insurance coverage. Health insurers routinely negotiate discounted fee payments with providers, and when combined with the fixed rates that Medicare pays, the true "market rate" for health care services is significantly less than published "sticker" prices.

Chargemasters do serve a useful purpose as a master reference for clinical services and are usually the starting point

TABLE 16-8. Comparison of Freestanding vs Outpatient Hospital Reimbursement

		Freestanding Center Setting				Outpatient Hospital Setting		
CPT Code	Description	Medicare Part B 2004 26, $	Medicare Part B 2004 TC, $	Part B Global, $	CPT	Physician Part B 26, $	Facility Part A APC, $	Total, $*
Prior to IMRT planning								
99245	Consultation	194.82	—	194.82	99245	194.82	82.00	276.82
77263	Treatment planning, complex	177.13	—	177.13	77263	177.13	—	177.13
77290	Simulation, complex	84.64	290.18	374.82	77290	84.64	201.00	285.64
76370	CT planning slices acquisition	Bundled	131.63	131.63	76370	—	92.00	92.00
77334	Treatment devices, complex	67.60	144.55	212.15	77334	67.60	157.00	224.60
77470	Special treatment procedure	114.65	496.60	611.25	77470	114.65	314.00	428.65
IMRT planning charges								
77301	IMRT plan	425.29	1,244.09	1,669.38	77301	425.29	850.00	1,275.29
77300	Basic dosimetry calculation	34.69	59.83	94.52	77300	34.69	91.00	125.69
77334	Treatment devices, complex	67.60	144.55	212.15	77334	67.60	157.00	224.60
IMRT treatment charges								
77418	IMRT treatment delivery	—	744.83	744.83	77418	—	294.11	294.11
77280	Simulation, simple	38.57	154.20	192.77	77280	38.57	91.00	129.57
77336	Continuing physics consultation (weekly)	—	132.85	132.85	77336	—	91.00	91.00
77417	Port film	—	26.79	26.79	77417	—	43.00	43.00
77427	Treatment management	181.49	—	181.49	77427	181.49	—	181.49

APC = ambulatory payment classification; CPT = current procedural terminology; CT = computed tomography; IMRT = intensity-modulated radiation therapy.
*Note that the total is an artificial number, useful for comparison purposes only. Reimbursement is always paid separately to physicians and facility.

for any price negotiations with payors. The chargemaster can be developed in several ways, depending on accounting methodologies and business traditions in your organization. Ideally, individual procedure prices ought to be developed through detailed analyses of the cost inputs for delivering a given procedure such as labor, supplies, equipment, facility expense, and overhead. However, a more common short-hand approach to setting charges is a ratio formula based on cost to charges or as a ratio of the Medicare rate. With the latter approach, retail charges are set at a multiple of the APC rate. A "markup" ratio of 3:1 is not uncommon. An informal market survey can also be performed to determine price levels in your market. One such recent survey revealed the price range for IMRT delivery (CPT code 77418) to be $1,500 to $2,600 gross charge/fraction. For IMRT planning (CPT code 77301), the gross charge range was $3,500 to $4,500.

Regardless of the approach used, one's prices should reflect a rational methodology because many managed care contracts use a discounted percentage off the charge (ie, 90% of gross hospital charge) or a percentage of the fixed payment rate (ie, 150% of Medicare RBRVS) as their payment model. In these circumstances, the "retail" or gross charge pricing structure does matter. The retail price also matters for organizations that still do Medicare cost reporting because cost-to-charge ratios determine payments.

Because charge-based payors are becoming increasingly rare, hospitals can no longer "cost-shift" their uncompensated care or underpayment deficits onto charge-based payors. In a fixed rate environment, the only effective revenue strategy is to create volume and operational scale so that costs can be spread broadly. IMRT and other specialized services can help do that by shifting referral patterns in your marketplace.

As is often the case, "the devil is in the detail"; hence, the monitoring and management of billing data by skilled coding and practice management professionals are essential and pay for themselves many times over. Coding and practice management specialists are trained in the idiosyncrasies of payment policies and procedures for a given medical specialty, and they know how to get the right answers to billing policy questions. At the "front end" of the charge capture and accounting process, they ensure that the right codes are used with the right quantity in the right format and will also audit medical chart documentation for completeness and regulatory compliance. At the "back end" of the accounting cycle, these professionals perform focused follow-up for incomplete payments and nonpayments, ensuring that charges are not incorrectly or prematurely written off and that the payors followed correct payment policies and contractual terms when issuing reimbursement. The important auditing and control functions performed by these professionals help ensure that payments and collection rates are optimized. Table 16-4 illustrates how the CPT coding and use of CPT modifiers would typically look in a claim submission for IMRT services.

"Gray Areas" in Medicare Billing Policy

When implementing new procedures such as IMRT, one must re-analyze how existing billing and payment policies prospectively apply to such new technology, especially as it relates to understanding the application of the NCCI edit system to billing. Additionally, in certain categories such as "treatment devices," the CPT codes have multiple, mutually exclusive definitions. A good example of this is the treatment device category (77332-34), which has only three CPT codes, but these codes must be used for vastly dissimilar services that include cerrobend block fabrication, patient immobilization aids, and computer-controlled MLC use.

How does one clarify "gray areas" in billing policy? In the first instance, it is important to have a solid understanding of the commonly accepted billing practices in one's specialty and to follow them. Knowledge of the published regulations is vital; reading of federal payment regulations can be supplemented by attendance at billing and coding seminars and awareness of how colleagues interpret and apply published billing policies. The following are some common areas of confusion and ambiguity with existing CPT codes when used for IMRT billing:

1. CPT 76370: Facility charge for computed tomography simulation. Per a local policy interpretation from the medical director at AdminaStar Federal in Indianapolis, CPT 76370-TC is not included with 77295 or 77301 (three-dimensional or IMRT planning) and is therefore billable separately as a facility charge. The professional component is bundled and not separately billable.

2. CPT 77263: Physician clinical treatment planning. This is not bundled into 77301 when billed on a different date of service than 77301. Otherwise, it is bundled, per the NCCI edits.

3. CPT 77300: Basic dosimetry calculations. Per the *CPT Assistant* guidebook (October 97:1), use of CPT 77300 is as follows: "This code may be reported any time during a course of RT in which a calculation is done, as many times as necessary. Each procedure should have the appropriate documentation in the chart."

   Note that the AMA description states "as many times as necessary." CMS also has no stated limit on the number of calculations because this is determined by medical necessity. Many payors are not sufficiently informed about requirements for IMRT. Given that this technology requires more treatment portals and each field requires a calculation, there will be a higher number of units per patient. Often the billing for 77300 looks like duplicate submissions to payors due to the repetitive "series billing" nature of treatment. As a result, RT providers should expect to get frequent requests for documentation to verify that services were provided.

4. CPT 77301: IMRT physics plan. Bill one plan per treatment course and again whenever the treatment volume changes significantly.

5. CPT 77334: Complex treatment device (MLC). This code reflects the use of an MLC as a treatment device during IMRT and is billed per gantry angle. For IMRT, it is not uncommon to have as many as nine gantry angles. So an MLC device charge (77334) can be billed for each angle, in addition to the other services (eg, immobilization).

Readers are reminded again that LMRP and LCD policy statements will vary from one carrier to another, sowing confusion and creating "gray areas" if one is trying to compare billing and payment practices among different regions.

Rejection of IMRT Claims Submissions for "Excessive Charges"

IMRT services normally generate a larger unit quantity of billed services (and charges) due to their increased complexity. This higher frequency of units billed may trigger a billing inquiry or rejection from the fiscal intermediary because their computerized payment systems look for statistical variations in billing patterns. The wording for such a claim rejection may take the following form:

> ….The claim is being returned to you for verification because some or all of the charges appear to be excessive. Review the line item and total charges to determine if an error was made.
>
> A. If an error was made and charges are incorrect, correct the line and total charges claim page 2.
>
> B. If an error was not made and the charges are correct, in the remarks field enter the statement "charges verified….

In such situations, it is important to provide a complete explanation of the IMRT course of therapy; complete, legible and accurate medical chart documentation becomes invaluable in appealing the rejection and getting correctly paid for the services provided.

Capital Investment Decisions

Radiation oncology is among the most expensive of all medical equipment purchases, with modern computer-controlled linear accelerators and their related software systems exceeding $2 million in purchase price. The consequences of poor capital decision making are significant, both on the organization and the individual manager. There are several methodologies one can use (eg, payback method, net present value, internal rate of return, and weighted cost of capital) to evaluate whether a specific capital decision should be made. This final section suggests using the net present value (NPV) methodology as a "best practices" tool for management to analyze and choose among competing capital equipment purchase proposals. Familiarity with the NPV model will help one speak the same language that financial professionals often use when evaluating whether large-dollar capital proposals should be approved for purchase.

If one plans to finance capital acquisition rather than make an outright purchase, a monthly "cash flow budget" is also prepared showing the effect of the capital purchase project on net revenues, confirming that the monthly loan payments can be met.

Payback Analysis

Payback analysis is the simplest method for evaluating one or more capital project proposals. It tells one how long it will take to earn back the capital dollars spent on the project or equipment purchase. The formula is

Payback period = Cost of project/Annual cash inflow (1)

To understand how payback analysis works, consider the purchase of a new digital linear accelerator with MLC and electronic portal imaging costing a total of $2 million. Such equipment is expected to return $1 million net cash per year for 10 years ($10 million total cash inflow). It is important to note that assumptions about average patient caseload, payor mix, and collection rates are key variables in correctly estimating the annual cash inflow figure to use. In this simple example the payback period would be $2 million divided by $1 million, or 2 years. Often the net cash inflows vary from year to year, so in that situation, one can simply add up the expected annual cash inflows for each succeeding year until one arrives at the point at which cash inflows equal or exceed the initial purchase cost, which is known as the breakeven or payback period.

Under the payback analysis method, capital purchases with shorter payback periods will be more attractive than those with longer paybacks, all other things being equal. The thought here is that projects with shorter paybacks are more liquid (and perhaps less risky), allowing one to recoup the capital investment sooner. With a shorter payback period, there is less chance that market conditions, interest rates, payor mix, collection rates, referral patterns, or other factors will markedly change. For example, when APCs were implemented, hospital-based IMRT treatments were reimbursed at $407 per fraction. Today, these treatments are down to $294 per fraction. This payment rate reduction results in a marked difference in computing the payback period. Clearly, early adopters of IMRT technology realized a shorter payback period than late adopters.

What is the ideal benchmark for payback periods? Generally, the shorter the better! For capital equipment purchases in a health care setting, typically, a payback period of 2 to 3 years is not unreasonable. However, much can change in 2 to 3 years! With many capital projects, especially in the ever-changing health care reimbursement environment, many variables will get less certain or knowable as the payback horizon is extended into the future.

Are there any limitations to using the payback method? The major drawback is that it ignores the "time value of money." A dollar received today is worth more than a dollar received in the future because the dollar received today can be invested and thus earn interest. To overcome this limitation in the payback analysis, one should also consider calculating the NPV of the capital purchase or project and its internal rate of return.

NPV Model as a Tool for Capital Decision Making

The NPV method for capital equipment decision analysis is considered by many to be a "best practice" because it factors in the time value of money (in today's dollars) and the future cash flow streams from the investment, which can then be compared with the amount of money required to make the capital purchase or invest in a project. The NPV formula is given by the following equation:

$$\text{Present Value} = CF_0 \frac{CF_1}{(1+r)^1} + \frac{CF_2}{(1+r)^2} + \frac{CF_3}{(1+r)^3} + \frac{CF_n}{(1+r)^n} \quad (2)$$

where CF_x = cash flow in the period x, n = the number of periods, and r = the interest rate, also known as the discount rate. (This percentage is normally the organization's average cost of borrowing based on its credit rating.)

If the NPV exceeds the cost of the equipment purchase, that capital investment will be profitable. If a decision has to be made between several capital investment projects, by computing the NPV of each project, the one with the greatest difference between NPV and cost (profitability) will be preferred if all other variables are equal. Clearly, the key variable in this model is the accuracy of estimated cash flows.

Example NPV Calculation

In the above example, the digital linear accelerator equipped with an MLC and an electronic portal imaging device costs $2 million. This equipment would be expected to return $1 million in net cash collections per year for 10 years, or $10 million in total. With the payback method, the capital equipment purchase would pay for itself in 2 years. Using an NPV analysis and a discount rate of 5% to evaluate the purchase on the basis of the "time value of money (NPV)," the expected total $10 million cash return over 10 years would be $5,107,820 in today's dollars. In other words, this project has a very positive NPV of $5,107,820 (profit), flowing from an initial capital investment of $2 million. Because the NPV exceeds the $2 million cost of the capital equipment and is profitable to the organization, this investment decision should be approved. Likewise, if the NPV were determined to be a negative value (ie, an NPV less than the $2 million investment cost in the equipment), it would be an unprofitable capital investment decision and should not be approved.

The above analysis may seem complex, but a good financial calculator will have the NPV formula embedded as one of its standard functions. Also, a free Web-based NPV tool is available on-line (http://www.toolkit.cch.com/text/P06_6530.asp).

Revenue Modeling in IMRT Equipment Justification and Purchase

The estimation of net revenues through spreadsheet modeling techniques is an important first step in developing a business plan that supports capital equipment justification and purchase. Accurate estimation of net revenues is central to capital allocation and spending decisions. The following methodology outlines the thought processes for formulating an economic justification for capital equipment such as MLC-equipped linear accelerators for IMRT treatment delivery. These steps comprise the generic process of developing a capital budget justification:

- *Step 1: Estimate cash flows through revenue modeling.* Use actual cash payment reimbursement rates from one's insurance payor mix to determine average net revenue per case. The revenue model for IMRT should assume a higher level of service intensity or procedure utilization than for non-IMRT. Not all disease sites are suitable candidates for IMRT. Assumptions can also reflect estimates of growth in market share owing to IMRT introduction.
- *Step 2: Review direct expenses versus fee schedule.* Every organization's cost structure is unique, so financial ratios can be highly variable from one organization to another. Academic medical centers are more typically found with ratios on the lower end of the range, such as a 4:1 ratio for charges versus direct expenses. Conversely, community hospitals have ratios nearer the high end, such as 10:1.
- *Step 3: Review indirect or overhead expenses for facility component.* This will vary widely by the type of organization, but a good starting point is a ratio of 1:1.
- *Step 4: Identify capital costs of equipment and software needed to perform IMRT treatments.* Linear accelerator system and IMRT software packages can run from $2 to 2.5 million. Facility renovations and infrastructure upgrades can run from $400 to 600 per square foot. IMRT software typically would have a 5-year depreciation cycle, whereas linear accelerator systems have a 10-year cycle.
- *Step 5: Apply the NPV model to determine if the proposed capital purchase of IMRT technology meets or exceeds the organization's financing decision rules or "hurdle" rates for the rate of return on its capital.* From the many investment choices that organizations face, the NPV formula helps identify which choice provides the best positive return on the organization's capital.
- *Step 6: Compare financial decision criteria against nonfinancial criteria.* Financial decision criteria are solution sets derived from application of the NPV formula. Nonfinancial decision criteria include market share, strate-

gic goals, and competitive position. This comparison is used to determine how the proposed technology investment in IMRT fits the organization's overall goals and strategic market objectives.

Capital dollars are a finite resource, and there are never enough dollars to meet all needs. The above steps will help hospital and departmental management make smart capital decisions and selections from among competing investment alternatives or purchase choices.

Conclusion

In the US marketplace, the first step toward understanding reimbursement issues is knowledge of the fundamentals of Medicare Part A and Part B payment policies and procedures. For most hospital providers, the RT center is a profitable patient care center, and it is not uncommon for hospital management to use income from RT to cross-subsidize other, less-profitable patient care services. With Medicare's higher facility payment rate for IMRT, departmental profitability significantly improves when the appropriate technology investments are made.

This chapter presented an overview of several important concepts and methodologies underlying the Medicare program and their application to billing and payment of IMRT services The Medicare program has increasingly become a policy and payment benchmark and a financial driver for many private sector health insurers operating in the US marketplace. It is not uncommon to find oneself in managed care contract negotiations that peg payments to formulas using Medicare payment rates. This is an indirect but deliberate form of price control.

On a global basis, RT and cancer care are increasingly important elements of the health care delivery system in the industrialized countries of Europe and Asia due to the increasing cancer incidence among aging populations. Quality of care and treatment outcomes are no less important in centrally planned health care economies than in free-market economies, but in centralized economies, the challenge is to prioritize and allocate technology resources, balancing larger societal needs with the reality of a lower per capita health care spending. All high-technology health care services require systematic reinvestment in the medical equipment and systems that enable those services so as to preserve and protect their income-generating potential. In both competitive marketplaces and centrally planned ones, IMRT technology helps to differentiate providers and foster competition on the basis of quality of care and medical outcomes.

Finally, what is written in this chapter reflects what is true in 2004. Much of the detailed payment information presented here will change annually and become obsolete over time. But with an understanding of the Medicare policy framework and the strong likelihood that the methodology underlying the APC and RBRVS payment systems will not change anytime soon, one's basic knowledge of billing and payment policies will not become outdated.

Chapter 17

CENTRAL NERVOUS SYSTEM TUMORS OVERVIEW

VOLKER W. STIEBER, MD, MICHAEL T. MUNLEY, PhD

The treatment of central nervous system (CNS) tumors involves two aspects, which, theoretically, may benefit from the use of intensity-modulated radiation therapy (IMRT). First, given that multiple critical structures are located within the narrow confinement of the intracranial vault, one may reason that improved dose distributions should allow a reduction in dose to these sensitive structures, thereby decreasing the risk of treatment sequelae. Second, given that high-grade gliomas typically recur within their original treatment volumes, IMRT should allow the exploration of dose escalation in these tumors, potentially improving tumor control.

The purpose of this chapter is to provide an overview of the limitations of conventional radiation therapy (RT) in CNS tumors, based on both biology and anatomy; to discuss the appropriate designation of treatment volumes for the purposes of IMRT treatment planning; to review the published data in this field; and to discuss future directions for the exploration of IMRT in the treatment of CNS tumors.

Rationale
Improved Dose Delivery

In selected CNS cases, IMRT should improve dose delivery to the target tissues. If the biology of the tumor is suggestive of a homogeneous cell population, such as is the case with a benign meningioma, IMRT may allow for more homogeneous dose delivery with decreased dose to normal surrounding tissues, especially in irregularly shaped lesions. Conversely, a glioblastoma multiforme is typically composed of heterogeneous cell populations, and dose escalation with increased dose per fraction to areas of gross tumor compared with the surrounding areas of microscopic infiltration is quite feasible using IMRT. Furthermore, when treating the craniospinal axis, IMRT may improve homogeneous dose delivery to the contents of the spinal canal and allow improved conformity of any boost volumes.

Normal Tissue Sparing

IMRT is ideally suited for sparing normal organs in patients with CNS tumors. Dose-limiting structures within the cranium include the optic chiasm, optic nerves, bilateral globes, brainstem, inner ears, area postrema, and uninvolved normal brain, especially the optic cortex and bilateral temporal lobes.[1]

The decision to use IMRT in a patient with a CNS tumor should involve an assessment of which dose-limiting structures are uninvolved by tumor and therefore do not need to receive a clinically significant dose. If conventional RT planning suggests unacceptable dose delivery (high dose per fraction, excessive total dose, or both) to any of the above critical structures, IMRT should be considered. This decision should include an assessment as to the patient's expected life span because many potential chronic toxicities will not become manifest until 6 months or more after treatment. Patients with Radiation Therapy Oncology Group (RTOG) recursive partitioning analysis class V and VI high-grade glioma and class III brain metastasis, for example, are unlikely to survive long enough to benefit from such organ-sparing approaches.[2,3] A possible exception may be to spare the area postrema to reduce the incidence of treatment-related nausea.[1]

Based on anatomic location of the treatment volumes, one may imagine several examples in which IMRT could be beneficial. Patients with a concave or otherwise irregularly shaped target in a frontal lobe may benefit from sparing of the adjacent eye and uninvolved optic apparatus. In patients with well-lateralized tumors, sparing of the contralateral hemisphere is a desirable goal. Patients with infiltrative gliomas traditionally have large margins placed around the treatment volumes, and these often encompass uninvolved normal structures (usually the optic chiasm and the brainstem). In these cases, IMRT may allow nonuniform reduction of the treatment volume around these structures. Patients with large, well-circumscribed lesions near the base of the skull (eg, meningiomas, acoustic neuromas, chordomas, and chondrosarcomas) should also be considered for IMRT to minimize the dose to the brainstem, inner ear, and posterior fossa. In the setting of retreatment (eg, previous whole-brain RT for brain metastases), IMRT may be considered if the clinical situation suggests that these patients may be long-term survivors with aggressive treatment.

Issues and Challenges
Imaging Studies

For both benign and malignant CNS tumors undergoing IMRT planning, magnetic resonance imaging (MRI) with and without contrast remains the gold standard imaging approach.[4] The preferred slice thickness is ≤ 5 mm. T_1-weighted images with contrast allow excellent visualization of contrast-enhancing tumors, such as meningioma and glioblastoma multiforme. T_2-weighted images demonstrate areas of edema, which are often involved by infiltrating high-grade gliomas; in addition, T_1-weighted fluid-attenuated inversion recovery (FLAIR) images are useful in differentiating brain infiltrated by malignant gliomas from edema caused by mass effect, as well as allowing delineation of otherwise nonenhancing tumors, such as grade 2 gliomas. Magnetic resonance fusion with the planning computed tomography (CT) scan should be used for target definition. The integration of magnetic resonance spectroscopy and positron emission tomography (PET) is a current topic of research.[5–7]

Target Volume Definitions

Critical to the ability to perform treatment planning is the accurate description of multiple volumes of interest. Based on the International Commission on Radiation Units and Measurements (ICRU) Reports 50 and 62, the gross tumor volume (GTV) represents grossly visible disease.[8,9] Typically, this is the T_1-enhancing abnormality on MRIs or nonenhancing tumor on T_1-weighted FLAIR images. If there is no residual abnormality after surgical resection, the tumor cavity may be defined as the GTV. Surrounding edema should not be considered part of the GTV. The clinical target volume (CTV) is the T_2 or FLAIR abnormality (which includes edema) on MRI.[9]

The planning target volume (PTV) in high-grade tumors typically consists of two components and is defined as follows: PTV_1 is the CTV plus a dosimetric margin.[9] The smaller PTV_2 includes the GTV plus a dosimetric margin. The dosimetric margin of the PTV takes into consideration two additional margins.[8] The internal margin is defined to take into account variations in the size, shape, and position of the CTV in relation to anatomic reference points. The setup margin is added to account for uncertainties in patient positioning. Segregating the internal and setup margins

reflects the differences in the source of uncertainties. The internal margin is due mainly to physiologic variations that are difficult or impossible to control, such as (potential) fluctuations in the mass effect from cerebral edema, which may occur over the course of treatment. In contrast, the setup margin is added because of uncertainties related mainly to technical factors that can be reduced by more accurate positioning and immobilization of the patient (such as stereotactic positioning), as well as improved mechanical stability of the treatment machine.

The addition of uniform margins that take into account all types of uncertainties would generally lead to an excessively large PTV, potentially exceeding normal tissue tolerances. Clearly, a balance between disease control and the risk of complications when selecting such margins requires considerable experience and judgment on the part of the clinician. The PTV_2 margin may therefore be reduced in areas near critical structures. Moreover, dosimetric margins as low as 3 to 5 mm may be acceptable with appropriate immobilization devices.

Dose Specification

In general, the PTV is usually considered to be appropriately treated if enclosed within the 95% isodose line. For plans emphasizing homogeneous dose delivery, typically no more than 20% of the PTV should exceed 110% of the prescribed dose. The New Approaches to Brain Tumor Therapy Consortium Radiation Therapy Subcommittee recently embarked on the task of standardizing the definitions of these volumes in the treatment of glioblastoma multiforme with IMRT (John Fiveash, MD, personal communication, November 2003).

Recommendations contained in ICRU Report 50 for dose specification reporting are maintained in ICRU Report 62.[8] First, the absorbed dose at the ICRU reference point should be reported. Second, the maximum and the minimum PTV doses should be recorded. Any additional relevant information should be given when available, for example, dose-volume histograms (DVHs). Absorbed doses to the normal tissues should also be given. When reporting doses in a series of patients, the treatment prescription should be described in detail, including treatment volumes, absorbed dose levels, and fractionation. The treatments should be reported following the above recommendations, and the deviations from the prescription should be stated. In particular, the proportion of patients in whom the dose variation is less than ± 5%, ± 5 to 10%, and more than ± 10% of the prescribed dose at the ICRU reference point should be reported.

Normal Tissues

Organs at risk (OAR) are defined as critical normal structures at risk of toxicity in the judgment of the treating physician. Such OAR are normal tissues whose radiosensitivity and proximity to the PTV may significantly influence the

prescribed dose and the treatment planning strategy. When possible to do so without compromising target coverage, attempts should be made to limit the maximum dose to the following normal structures as follows: optic chiasm (54 Gy); optic nerves (60 Gy); optic globes, including the retina (50 Gy); brainstem, including the midbrain, pons, and medulla (54 Gy); pituitary gland (50 Gy); and spinal cord (50 Gy).

ICRU Report 62 describes the concept of the planning organ at risk volume (PRV).[8] The relationship between the PRV and the OAR is analogous to that between the PTV and the CTV. For reporting, the description of the PRV (like that of the PTV) should include the extent of the margins in all directions. The PTV and the PRV may overlap and often do so, which requires a compromise, as discussed above, when determining the maximum allowable dose. For each OAR, when part of or the whole organ is irradiated above the accepted tolerance level, the maximum dose should be reported.[9] The volume receiving more than the maximum allowable dose should be evaluated using the corresponding DVH.

Preclinical Data

A comprehensive search of published data on the use of IMRT in the treatment of CNS lesions (including skull base and spinal tumors) yielded 30 research articles.[10] These studies can be grouped into three categories: immobilization and localization techniques,[11–13] physics and dosimetry issues,[14–29] and clinical IMRT outcomes.[30–40] Figure 17-1 illustrates the number of publications by topic and year. Studies in the first two categories are described below. Clinical outcome reports are included in the following section.

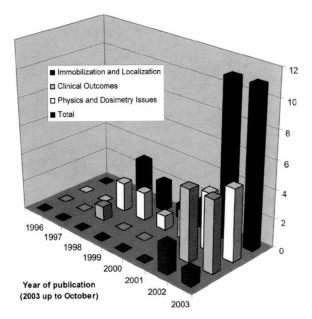

FIGURE 17-1. Number of publications on central nervous system intensity-modulated radiation therapy by year and topic.

Immobilization and Localization

Leybovich and colleagues described a noninvasive immobilization and localization technique for both stereotactic radiation therapy (SRT) and IMRT in intracranial tumors.[12] Immobilization was based on a commercially available Gill-Thomas-Cossman relocatable frame. A stereotactic localization frame with the attached localization device (CT pointer) was used during the planning CT scan so that CT slices contained fiducial marks for both IMRT and SRT. Because all treatment plans used the same contour set, the accuracy of competing plans could be compared. A modified and lighter IMRT target box compatible with the localization frame was fabricated so that the SRT immobilization system could be used for IMRT delivery. This IMRT target box was attached to the SRT localization frame, replacing the IMRT CT pointer. Day-to-day reproducibility of the patient setup was evaluated using an SRT depth helmet and was found to be 1.0 ± 0.3 mm.

Yin and colleagues evaluated the feasibility of using an image-guided intensity-modulated stereotactic radiosurgery (IM-SRS) procedure for spinal stereotactic radiosurgery (SRS) using a micro–multileaf collimator (mMLC) with a single 6 MV photon beam.[11] Each patient was CT-simulated with infrared sensitive markers for localization. A variety of different treatment plans were generated, most commonly with seven coplanar intensity-modulated beams. An automatic localization device based on infrared and video cameras was used to guide the initial patient setup, and 2 keV x-ray imaging systems were used to identify potential deviations from the planned isocenter. Twenty-five patients with spinal tumors were treated using this procedure with a single fraction dose ranging from 6 to 12 Gy. The final verification images indicated that the average deviation from the planned isocenter was ≤ 2 mm. The phantom verification of isocenter doses indicated that the average deviation of measured isocenter doses from the planned isocenter doses for all patients treated with IMRT was < 2%. Film dosimetry measurements in a phantom study demonstrated good agreement of the 50% isodose lines between the planned and measured results. This approach is described in detail in Chapter 27.2, "Recurrent Nasopharyngeal Cancer: Case Study."

Yenice and colleagues described a noninvasive stereotactic immobilization technique using a stereotactic body frame (SBF) and daily CT image-guided positioning to treat patients with paraspinal lesions.[13] The authors also quantified the systematic and random patient setup errors by means of phantom studies. Seven patients with thoracic and lumbar spine lesions were immobilized with the SBF and positioned for 33 treatment fractions using daily CT scans. For all seven patients, the daily setup errors, as assessed from the daily CT scans, were corrected prior to each treatment fraction. A retrospective analysis was performed to assess what the impact on patient treatment would have

been without the CT-based corrections (ie, if patient setup had been performed only with the SBF). The average magnitude of systematic and random errors from uncorrected patient setups using the SBF was approximately 2 and 1.5 mm (1 SD), respectively. For fixed phantom targets, the system accuracy for the SBF localization and treatment was shown to be within 1 mm in any direction (1 SD). DVHs of lumbar spine lesions for the IMRT plans incorporating these uncertainties were generated, and the effects on the DVHs were studied. The authors demonstrated that for highly conformal paraspinal treatments, uncorrected systematic and random setup errors of 2 mm in magnitude could result in a significantly greater (> 100%) dose to the spinal cord than planned, even though the planned target coverage did not always change substantially. Daily CT guidance using the SBF ensured that the maximal spinal cord dose was within 10 to 15% of the planned value.

Physics and Dosimetry Studies

Investigators at the University of Alabama examined the physical radiation dose differences between two multileaf collimator (MLC) leaf widths in the treatment of CNS and head/neck tumors with IMRT.[18] Three patients with CNS tumors were planned with two different leaf sizes, 5 and 10 mm, representing 120- and 80-leaf MLCs, respectively, and using dynamic MLC delivery. Two sets of IMRT plans were generated. The goal of the first was three-dimensional dose conformity. The goal of the second was avoidance of a nearby critical structure while maintaining adequate target coverage. Beam parameters and optimization (cost function) parameters were identical for the 5 and 10 mm plans. For all cases, beam number, gantry angles, and table positions were taken from clinically treated three-dimensional conformal radiation therapy (3DCRT) plans. Conformity was assessed by the ratio of the planning isodose volume to the target volume. Organ avoidance was measured by the volume of the critical structure receiving greater than 90% of the prescribed dose (V_{90}).

Conformity improved in all three cases for the 5 mm plans compared with the 10 mm plans. For the organ avoidance plans, V_{90} also improved in two cases when the 5 mm leaf width was used for IMRT delivery. In the third case, both the 5 and 10 mm plans were able to spare the critical structure, with none of the structure receiving > 90% of the prescribed dose, but in the moderate-dose range, less dose was delivered to the critical structure with the 5 mm plan.

Gabriele and colleagues evaluated the use of dynamic IMRT in the treatment of advanced cervical chordoma.[24] A single patient with an incompletely resected chordoma surrounding C2–C3 was irradiated with a dose of 58 Gy (ICRU point) in 2 Gy daily fractions. The beam arrangement consisted of seven nonopposed 6 MV beams. Treatment was delivered with a 120-leaf MLC in the sliding window mode. To verify the daily setup, orthogonal portal image pairs were compared with the simulation images before treatment delivery (manual matching) and after treatment delivery (automatic anatomy matching). The mean PTV dose was 57.6 ± 2.1 Gy, covering 95% of the PTV. The dose covering 99% of the PTV was 53.6 Gy in the overlapping area between the PTV and the spinal cord PRV. The spinal cord and spinal cord PRV (8 mm margin) doses were 42.2 Gy and 53.7 Gy, respectively. The average deviation in setup was −1.1 ± 2.5 mm (anterior-posterior), 2.4 ± 1.3 mm (laterolateral), 0.7 ± 0.9 mm (craniocaudal), and −0.43 ± 1° (rotation).

Investigators at the German Cancer Research Center presented an IMRT technique delivering a simultaneous integrated boost (SIB) to the macroscopic tumor volume in the treatment of high-grade gliomas.[26] The authors compared stereotactic conformal radiation therapy (SCRT) and IMRT with regard to their suitability for SIB delivery. In 20 patients treated with conventional RT, an additional treatment plan (for the SIB) with seven noncoplanar beams using IMRT and SCRT was compared. PTV_1 consisted of the T_1-enhancing lesion plus a 1 mm margin owing to setup errors and received 75 Gy; PTV_2 was defined as edema plus a 15 mm margin owing to microscopic spread and setup error and received 60 Gy. The part of PTV_2 irradiated with > 107% of the prescribed dose was 14% for IMRT and 31% for SCRT. Dose coverage of PTV_2 (volume > 95% of the prescribed dose) was improved with IMRT (88% vs 75% with SCRT). Dose coverage of PTV_1 was slightly higher with SCRT (94% vs 88% with IMRT), but the conformity to the boost shape was improved by IMRT (conformity index = 0.85 vs 0.69 with SCRT). Additionally, the brain volume receiving > 50 Gy was reduced from 60 to 33 cm^3 with IMRT. The authors concluded that IMRT was suitable for local dose escalation in the enhancing lesion while simultaneously delivering a homogeneous dose to the PTV_2 outside the PTV_1.

Benedict and colleagues at the Medical College of Virginia explored how dynamic leaf motion on an mMLC system for IM-SRS affected tumor coverage and normal tissue sparing for small cranial tumors relative to plans based on multiple fixed uniform-intensity beams or traditional circular collimator arc-based SRS techniques.[19] Four cases were analyzed, representing a variety of target shapes, number of targets, and adjacent critical areas. Plans generated for these comparisons included standard arcs with multiple circular collimators and fixed noncoplanar static fields with uniform-intensity beams and IM-SRS. Parameters used for evaluation of the plans included the percentage of irradiated volume to tumor volume, normal tissue DVHs, and dose homogeneity ratios. For all cases, the IM-SRS plans showed a high degree of conformity of the dose distribution with the target shape. For all cases, the IM-SRS plans also provided either a smaller volume of normal tissue irradiated to significant dose levels (generally taken as doses > 50% of the prescription) and/or a lower dose to an important adjacent critical organ. The

reduction in volume of normal tissue irradiated in the IM-SRS plans ranged from 10 to 50% relative to the circular collimated arc and uniform fixed-field plans. A more complete discussion is provided in Chapter 17.4, "Intensity-Modulated Radiosurgery: Emerging Technology."

Kulik and colleagues used normal tissue dose constraints to optimize mMLC IMRT parameters and compared the results with those for circular collimator linear accelerator SRS or Gamma Knife (GK) (Elekta Inc., Norcross, GA) radiosurgery.[14] mMLC protocols were optimized in two stages. The orientation of the fields, delineated by a beam's eye view technique, was determined using a genetic algorithm method. The weighting of the fields and subfields when using intensity modulation and the position of the leaves were optimized using a simulated annealing method. The authors compared the results obtained for eight clinical cases using five IMRT fields with those obtained using the two SRS techniques. The comparison indexes were those defined by the RTOG.[41] The coverage indexes were all practically identical and equal to 1 because of the choice of the optimization process made, so that the comparison could be made while taking into account solely the target dose homogeneity and conformity indexes and the different ratios of volumes irradiated to the target volume values.

In the case of the smaller target volumes, SRS enabled better conformity than the GK, to the detriment of the homogeneity index, but conformity and homogeneity were better using IMRT than with either of the other two methods, although the volume of normal tissue irradiated at high doses was greater. For target volumes ≥ 3 cm³, whereas the GK gave better conformity and better homogeneity than did SRS, IMRT yielded results better than or equivalent to those of the other techniques for all of the irradiation quality parameters. The results of this study demonstrated the possibility of using intensity modulation for the optimization of small field conformity indexes, although normal peripheral tissues were less exposed to dose with SRS.

Sankaranarayanan and colleagues compared the dosimetric parameters of IMRT and SRS in CNS tumors.[15] Six patients treated with SRS were replanned and evaluated with an IMRT planning system. Contouring of all structures, including the target volume, was performed on the IMRT system to match the SRS system. Various parameters, such as conformity index, homogeneity index, target volume coverage, nontarget tissue, and brainstem doses, were calculated and compared between the IMRT and SRS plans. Patient data were divided into two groups based on the complexity of the lesion and the number of SRS isocenters used. Superior conformity and homogeneous dose distributions were observed for the multiple-isocenter IMRT cases. In addition, critical structure volumes receiving 50%, 70%, and 90% of the prescribed dose were lower for IMRT planning compared with SRS. However, other normal tissue regions not specified as critical areas of avoidance received significantly higher doses with IMRT.

Investigators at the University of California, San Francisco performed a dosimetric comparison of IMRT and GK SRS in the treatment of medium-sized intracranial lesions (range 4–25 cm³).[17] Plans were evaluated using DVHs, tissue-volume ratios, and maximum dose to the prescribed dose ratios. The investigators evaluated both simulated targets and clinical targets with irregular shapes and in different locations. The maximum dose to the prescribed dose ratios were significantly greater for the GK compared with fan-beam IMRT. GK plans produced equivalent tissue-volume ratio values to the IMRT plans. Based on the DVH comparison, the fan-beam IMRT delivered significantly more dose to the normal brain tissue, regardless of target location.

Borden and colleagues developed a quality factor (QF) to compare the dosimetry of GK SRS and IMRT quantitatively as a function of target volume and shape.[22] The QF related the percentage of target covered (PTC) by the prescription isodose, the target volume (VT), and the tissue volume receiving more than a particular dose (VX): QF = PTC × VT/VX. The authors also investigated target shape independent of volume in predicting SRS complications. Plastic targets of defined volumes (0.2, 0.5, 1.5, and 10 cm³) and four increasingly complex shapes (spherical, ellipsoid, simulated arteriovenous malformation, and horseshoe) were created and analyzed. Corresponding treatment plans were then generated. For larger targets, the GK and IMRT plans showed similar conformity (QF assuming 15 Gy volume [QF15]). For small and round targets, the GK plan quality was significantly higher (QF assuming 12 Gy volume [QF12]). As VT and complexity increased, the IMRT QF12 approached that of the GK. The QF12 of GK dosimetry had an inverse correlation with target shape complexity independent of VT. At a prescribed dose of 15 Gy to the target margin, the QF15 was a conformity index. The 12 Gy volume (volume receiving at least 12 Gy) was used to estimate the SRS normal tissue complication rate for arteriovenous malformations. When the target was well covered, the QF12 was inversely proportional to the complication risk and was felt to be a useful measure of plan quality.

Nakamura and colleagues quantitatively compared IM-SRS using 3 mm mMLC to GK SRS for irregularly shaped skull base lesions.[28] Ten challenging skull base lesions treated with GK were selected for comparison with IM-SRS using inverse planning and the step-and-shoot delivery. The lesions ranged in volume from 1.6 to 32 cm³ and were treated with 9 to 20 GK isocenters (mean 13). The IM-SRS plans were designed with the intent to, at a minimum, match the GK plans with regard to OAR sparing and target coverage. For each case, IM-SRS plans were generated using 9 coplanar, 11 equally spaced noncoplanar, and 11 OAR-avoidant noncoplanar beams. The best approach was selected for comparison with the original GK plan with respect to target conformity, OAR sparing, and target coverage. Assuming no patient motion or setup error,

IM-SRS provided comparable target coverage and OAR sparing and an improved conformity index at the prescription isodose contour. However, IM-SRS displayed less conformity at lower isodoses compared with the GK. Moreover, IM-SRS plans were associated with less dose heterogeneity and shorter estimated treatment times.

Kramer and colleagues performed a dosimetric comparison of SRS and IMRT for an irregularly shaped, moderate-sized target.[29] A treatment plan was selected from 109 single fraction SRS cases having had multiple noncoplanar arc therapy using a 6 MV linear accelerator fitted with circular tertiary collimators 1 to 4 cm in diameter at the isocenter. The CT scan, with delineated regions of interest, was then entered into an IMRT planning system. Optimized dose distributions using a back-projection technique for dynamic MLC delivery were generated with a simulated annealing algorithm. DVHs, homogeneity indices, conformity indices, minimum and maximum doses to surrounding highly sensitive intracranial structures, and the volume of tissue treated to > 80%, 50%, and 20% of the prescribed dose from the IMRT plan were compared with those from the single-isocenter SRS plan used and to a hypothetical three-isocenter SRS plan. For an irregularly shaped target, the IMRT plan produced a homogeneity index of 1.1 and a conformity index of 1.5 compared with 1.8 and 4.4, respectively, for the single-isocenter SRS plan (SRS_1) and 3.3 and 3.4 for the three-isocenter SRS plan (SRS_3). The maximum and minimum doses to surrounding critical structures were less for the IMRT plan. However, the volume of nontarget tissue treated to > 80%, 50%, and 20% of the prescribed dose with the IMRT plan was 137%, 170%, and 163%, respectively, of that treated with the SRS_1 plan and 85%, 100%, and 123%, respectively, of the volume when compared with the SRS_3 plan. The IMRT system provided more conformal target doses than were provided by the single-isocenter or three-isocenter SRS plans. IMRT delivered less dose to critical normal tissues and provided increased homogeneity within the target volume for a moderate-sized irregularly shaped target, at the cost of larger penumbra.

Zabel and colleagues compared inversely planned IMRT dose distributions in the treatment of esthesioneuroblastoma to forward planned 3DCRT.[16] Thirteen patients were planned both with IMRT and 3DCRT using complete three-dimensional data sets to a total dose of 60 Gy. Although target coverage was similar, the dose distribution was more conformal using IMRT. Moreover, IMRT was associated with lower mean and maximum doses to the brainstem, chiasm, optic nerves, and orbits. The additional sparing by IMRT was positively correlated to the size of the target volume, which was clearly evident with target volumes > 200 cm^3. Treatment time was approximately 20 minutes per fraction for IMRT versus 15 minutes per fraction for 3DCRT.

Investigators at the Medical College of Virginia performed a comparison of three stereotactic RT techniques: arcs, noncoplanar fixed fields, and IMRT.[20] Dose conformity and normal brain dose characteristics were compared for various nonspherical target shapes. Three intracranial test targets were constructed using a three-dimensional planning system. Targets included an ellipsoid (major axis dimensions of 4.0, 2.0, and 2.0 cm), a hemisphere (a diameter of 4.0 cm), and an irregularly shaped tumor (maximum dimension of 5.3 cm). The following stereotactic techniques were compared for each target: (1) five arcs as used in traditional linear accelerator SRS (noncoplanar arcs [ARCS]), (2) six fixed noncoplanar custom blocked fields (three dimensions), and (3) IMRT using six noncoplanar beams and an mMLC. For the ellipsoidal lesion, dose conformity was similar for all three techniques, and normal brain isodose distributions were more favorable with the ARCS plan. For the hemisphere and irregular tumor geometries, target dose conformity and normal brain DVHs were more favorable with IMRT. Overall, IMRT resulted in improved dose conformity and decreased dose to nontarget brain in the high- and low-dose regions compared with the ARCS or three-dimensional techniques for the nonellipsoidal targets.

A dosimetric comparison of 3DCRT, stereotactic radiosurgery arc therapy (SRS/T), IMRT, and proton RT was presented by Bolsi and colleagues.[21] CT-based plans for five acoustic neuromas, five meningiomas, and two pituitary adenomas were generated for each method. Protons were shown to be superior to all photon approaches in the treatment of small brain lesions in terms of target dose uniformity and conformity and in terms of sparing normal tissues. No major differences were observed between the results of the photon techniques. Minimum target doses ranged from 81% with SRS/T to 93% with IMRT. The volume receiving > 95% of the dose ranged from 95% (SRS/T) to 99% (protons). No clear patterns of coverage dependence on target shape were observed.

Khoo and colleagues at the Royal Marsden Hospital compared IMRT tomotherapy with 3DCRT for patients with medium-sized, convex-shaped brain tumors.[23] Five patients originally planned with 3DCRT were replanned with IMRT. The PTV and OAR were assessed using dose statistics, DVHs, and RTOG SRS criteria.[41] The PTV homogeneity achieved with IMRT was 12% compared with 14% with 3DCRT. Using RTOG guidelines, IMRT provided acceptable PTV coverage for all plans compared with minor coverage deviations in four of the five 3DCRT plans. Both techniques resulted in an acceptable homogeneity (5.1 each) index and comparable conformity indices (1.4 each). As a consequence of the transaxial tomotherapy delivery method, the optic nerves received mean and maximum doses that were 11 to 12% and 10 to 15% higher, respectively, using IMRT planning. The maximum optic lens and brainstem doses were 3 to 5% higher and 1% lower, respectively, with IMRT. However, all doses remained below the tolerance thresholds.

Thilmann and colleagues presented a comparison of IMRT and 3DCRT in a case of partially resected sacral chordoma.[25] The PTV received 60 Gy and the GTV received 72 Gy using inversely planned IMRT. IMRT resulted in improved dose homogeneity within regions of the PTV outside the GTV and allowed simultaneous dose escalation within the GTV. The volume of bowel receiving a dose higher than 40 Gy was reduced from 400 cm^3 with 3DCRT to 220 cm^3 with IMRT.

Baumert and colleagues compared intensity-modulated stereotactic radiation therapy (IM-SRT) and 3DCRT in the treatment of meningiomas.[27] Ten patients (seven with a skull base meningioma) planned for routine 3DCRT were replanned with IM-SRT. For 3DCRT, OAR sparing was achieved by conformal avoidance using five to six fields. The IM-SRT inverse planning process used optimized OAR sparing through user-defined dose constraints. Doses to the PTV and OAR were assessed by DVHs, maximum dose, two conformity indices, and volumes of relevant isodose clouds. The conformity index was consistently higher for IM-SRT, the largest improvement being for multifocal and irregular cases ($n = 10$). Volumes of the 90% and 80% isodoses were smaller for IM-SRT, whereas the volumes of the 30% isodoses were larger for six IM-SRT cases. The maximum dose was consistently higher for IM-SRT (mean values 102% and 108% for 3DCRT and IM-SRT, respectively). Sparing of OAR was better with IM-SRT, especially for those OAR situated in or near a concave PTV.

Clinical Outcome Data

Animal Studies

Kippenes and colleagues performed a randomized trial to determine the clinical significance of improved spatial accuracy of fractionated IMRT in canine paraspinal RT.[40] The goal of this study was to determine if a method of dynamic IMRT could be used to deliver a high dose to a concave-shaped target around the cervical spine. Fifteen adult dogs were randomly divided into two groups. A dose of 84 Gy in 4 Gy fractions was delivered with a conventional four-field technique (group A) and with dynamic IMRT to a C-shaped target close to the cervical spinal cord (group B). Neurologic status, MRI results, and histopathologic changes were compared between the two groups. Group A developed myelomalacia with a latency period of 65 ± 9 days. Group B did not have any histologic changes in the cervical spinal cord when euthanasia was performed at 12 months following RT.

Human Studies

Pirzkall and colleagues reported the clinical outcomes of IMRT treatment in complex-shaped benign meningiomas of the skull base.[30] Twenty patients with benign skull base meningiomas (16 histopathologically proven) underwent IMRT. Each tumor was complex in shape and adherent to or encompassed various OAR (cranial nerves, optic apparatus, and/or brainstem). All patients immobilized in a customized head mask integrated into a stereotactic system were planned on an inverse treatment planning system using five or seven coplanar, equidistant beams with five intensity levels. Each plan was verified extensively before treatment. Follow-up MRI and clinical examination were performed at 6 and 18 weeks and every 6 months thereafter. Target volumes ranged from 27 to 278 cc (median 108 cc). The mean dose delivered in 32 fractions ranged from 55.8 to 58.2 Gy.

At a median follow-up of 36 months (range 31–43 months), preexisting neurologic symptoms improved in 12 patients (60%), remained stable in 7 (35%), and worsened in 1 (5%). Radiographic follow-up revealed significant tumor response 6 weeks post-IMRT in two patients and a partial remission in three more patients at 9 to 17 months; other tumors remained stable. There was no RT-induced edema or new neurologic deficits. Transient, acute sequelae included nausea and vomiting and single occurrences of conjunctivitis or increased tearing and serous tympanitis. A case study is presented in Chapter 17.1, "Meningioma: Case Study."

Grant and Cain reported the results of IMRT treatment in two patients with CNS tumors.[31] One had an optic sheath meningioma; the other had a craniopharyngioma surrounding the optic chiasm. The meningioma received 50 Gy in 25 fractions using two IMRT arcs. The total setup and delivery treatment time was < 15 minutes. Planning and quality assurance required approximately 3 days. The patient with meningioma had complete restoration of all visual fields, and the tumor remained stable at 3 years of follow-up. In the other patient, 50.4 Gy in 28 fractions was prescribed, and the optic chiasm dose was limited to 45 Gy. The treatment required three IMRT arcs; the total treatment time was < 20 minutes. The tumor remained stable 15 months post-therapy.

Fuss and colleagues reported the clinical outcomes of eight patients with acoustic neuroma treated using IMRT.[32] The method incorporated high-precision invasive fixation, obliquely oriented tomotherapy arcs, and reduced-dimension pencil beams. Total prescribed doses were 54 Gy in 1.8 Gy daily fractions. The results showed that the median PTV (GTV plus 2 mm) was 2.5 cm^3 (range 1.6–17 cm^3) and that the median conformity and homogeneity indices were 1.7 and 1.1, respectively. Average mean and maximum brainstem doses were 13 Gy and 54 Gy, respectively. At a median follow-up of 18.5 months, all eight tumors remained locally controlled and all patients had preservation of their hearing. No impairment of the facial or trigeminal nerves was observed.

Investigators at the Baylor College of Medicine evaluated the impact of sparing of the auditory apparatus (cochlea and cranial nerve VIII) with IMRT in pediatric patients with medulloblastoma undergoing chemotherapy.[33] Twenty-six cases were retrospectively divided into two groups that received either conventional RT or IMRT. One hundred thirteen pure-tone audiograms were performed, and hearing function was graded on a scale of 0 to 4 according to Pediatric Oncology Group toxicity criteria. When compared with conventional RT, IMRT delivered a lower mean dose to the auditory apparatus (36.7 vs 54.2 Gy) compared with conventional RT. Mean decibel hearing thresholds of the IMRT group were lower at every frequency compared with those of the conventional RT group, although patients who underwent conventional RT received a higher cumulative dose of cisplatin. Overall, 13% of the IMRT group developed grade ≥ 3 ototoxicity compared with 64% of the conventional RT group ($p < .014$) (see Chapter 26, "Pediatric Tumors: Overview").

Milker-Zabel and colleagues at the German Cancer Research Center evaluated local control, pain relief, neurologic improvement, side effects, and survival rates after fractionated 3DCRT or IMRT of patients with recurrent spinal metastases.[34] Eighteen patients with 19 radiologic manifestations were retreated using 3DCRT ($n = 5$) or IMRT ($n = 14$). All had previously undergone conventional RT (median dose 38 Gy). Indications for reirradiation were tumor progression associated with pain ($n = 16$) or neurologic symptoms alone ($n = 12$). The median time from initial treatment to recurrence was 17.7 months. The median prescribed dose for reirradiation was 39.6 Gy. The overall local control rate was 95% at a median follow-up of 12 months. Of 16 patients with pain, 13 experienced significant relief. Neurologic improvements were noted in 5 of 12 patients. Tumor size remained unchanged in 84% of lesions irradiated. A partial response was seen in two patients, and one patient experienced local progression 9.5 months after reirradiation. Six patients received chemotherapy after reirradiation because of progressive distant metastases. Twelve patients died (10.5 months median) after repeat irradiation. No clinically significant late toxicity was seen in follow-up. An example case is presented in Chapter 27.1, "Recurrent Spinal Metastasis: Case Study."

Investigators at Kinki University reported the clinical outcomes of a feasibility study of an SIB approach in malignant gliomas using IMRT.[36] Six patients with malignant gliomas received 70 Gy in 28 fractions (2.5 Gy daily) to the GTV and 56 Gy in 28 fractions (2.0 Gy daily) to the surrounding edema, defined as the CTV annulus. No delay owing to acute RT-related toxicity was observed in any patient. In the patients with glioblastoma, the tumor recurred locally in five of the six patients: in two patients during RT and in three at 5.4, 4.0, and 7.0 months after IMRT. Sites of recurrence or progression were local (within the GTV) in four patients; one patient developed subependymal dissemination. Three patients, two with glioblastoma and one with anaplastic astrocytoma, died of the disease at 4, 16, and 7 months, respectively. The details

of their approach can be found in Chapter 17.3, "Glioblastoma Multiforme: Case Study."

Voynov and colleagues reported on the outcome of 10 patients with recurrent malignant gliomas treated with IMRT.[37] Initial tumor histologies included one low-grade glioma (upgraded to anaplastic astrocytoma at recurrence), four anaplastic astrocytomas, and four glioblastomas. Before recurrence, all patients had undergone conventional RT (median dose 59.7 Gy). Recurrences were confirmed by repeat surgery (five patients) or by imaging (five patients). The median tumor volume was 35 cm^3. Treatment was delivered on a 10 MV linear accelerator with an mMLC. The dose was 30 Gy in 5 Gy fractions, prescribed at the 71 to 93% isodose line. The median overall survival time was 10.1 months from IMRT, with 1- and 2-year survival rates of 50% and 33%, respectively.

Investigators at the Baylor College of Medicine reported on the safety and efficacy of IMRT in the treatment of meningioma.[39] Forty patients with intracranial meningioma (excluding optic nerve sheath tumors) underwent IMRT, 25 patients after surgery (as adjuvant or salvage) and 15 patients without surgery. Thirty-two had skull base lesions. The median prescribed dose was 50.4 Gy (range 40–56 Gy) in 1.71 to 2 Gy fractions, and the median target volume was 20 cm^3 (range 1.6–325 cm^3). The median dose to the target was 53 Gy (range 44–60 Gy). Follow-up ranged from 6 to 71 months (median 30 months).

The 5-year actuarial local control, progression-free survival, and overall survival rates of the entire group were 93%, 88%, and 89%, respectively. Two patients progressed, one locally and one distantly. Each was treated with IMRT after multiple recurrences. Both were found to have malignant tumors at the time of relapse. The most common acute toxicity was mild headache, which was usually relieved with steroids. One patient experienced RTOG grade 3 acute toxicity, and two patients experienced ≥ grade 3 late toxicity, with one possible treatment-related death. No toxicity was observed with mean doses to the optic nerve or chiasm up to 47 Gy and maximum doses up to 55 Gy.

Kuo and colleagues reported the outcomes of eight patients who received 10 courses of IMRT for primary or metastatic disease of the spine.[35] Tumors irradiated included lung and renal metastases, adrenocortical cancers, primary sarcomas, and a giant cell tumor. Five cases had six courses given for reirradiation of symptomatic disease, and three cases had four courses of IMRT as primary management. Although three courses were given postoperatively, these were for gross residual disease. For patients who underwent reirradiation, the mean follow-up interval was 4 months and the local control rate was 14%. Of patients treated with primary intent, the mean follow-up was 9 months and the local control rate was 75%. No patients developed spinal cord complications.

Ryu and colleagues reported on an IM-SRS boost technique in patients with spinal metastases.[38] Treatment was performed with an image-guided IMRT approach using mMLC. Immobilization was accomplished with a noninvasive, frameless positioning device using infrared, passive marker technology together with corroborative image fusion of the digitally reconstructed images from CT simulation and orthogonal x-ray imagery in the treatment position. The patients were treated with fractionated external beam RT followed by a single-dose IM-SRS boost (6–8 Gy) to the most involved portion of the spine or to the site of spinal cord compression. Setup accuracy at the isocenter ranged from 0.1 to 1.4 mm.

Following IM-SRS, the majority of patients had prompt pain relief within 2 to 4 weeks of treatment. Complete and partial recovery of motor function was achieved in patients with spinal cord compression. The maximum radiation dose delivered to the anterior edge of the spinal cord within a transverse section was, on average, 50% of the prescribed dose. There was no acute RT-related toxicity detected at a mean follow-up of 6 months.

Future Directions

Future applications of IMRT in treating CNS tumors should focus on demonstrating that the theoretical benefit of IMRT is a clinical reality. To this end, investigators must first determine what level of evidence they seek to demonstrate to design the appropriate studies. The National Cancer Institute has established standards for levels of evidence ranging from 1 to 3 (strongest to weakest).[42] For any given therapy, the results are ranked on each of the following two scales: strength of the study design and strength of the end points. A formal description of the level of evidence provides a uniform framework for the data, leading to specific recommendations (Table 17-1). Of all of the publications referenced in the section on

published data, only one provides level 1 clinical evidence (the sole animal study).[40] All of the human studies provide only level 3 evidence.

In addition, use factors, such as cost and equipment time, must be considered, along with issues of safety and efficacy. This requires a careful evaluation of the technology in the context of its clinical application. The Agency for Healthcare Research and Quality, which provides technology assessments for the Centers for Medicare and Medicaid Services, in partnership with Evidence-Based Practice Centers, has developed a toolkit of Technology Evaluation Center (TEC) criteria that can be used to evaluate the effectiveness of new technology (Table 17-2).[43,44] These guidelines may be adapted by clinicians seeking to develop IMRT studies that demonstrate level 1 or 2 evidence. The TEC assessment format permits determination of whether the quality of the body of evidence permits conclusions to be drawn regarding the effectiveness of IMRT, whether IMRT improves clinically significant outcomes, and whether the benefits of IMRT outweigh its risks. Such an analysis suggests that IMRT may decrease late side effects by allowing avoidance of dose-limiting structures but has not yet shown any improvements in tumor control.

Integration of biologic data (eg, magnetic resonance spectroscopy and/or PET scans) into the planning process may allow further optimization based on biologic parameters. Munley and colleagues proposed that it is possible to

TABLE 17-1. Physican Data Query Levels of Evidence for Adult Cancer Treatment Studies

Strength of study design (ranked in descending order of strength)
1. Randomized controlled clinical trial(s)
   - Double-blinded
   - Nonblinded (allocation schema or treatment delivery)
2. Nonrandomized controlled clinical trial(s)
3. Case series
   - Population-based, consecutive series
   - Consecutive cases (not population based)
   - Nonconsecutive cases

Strength of end points (ranked in descending order of strength)
1. Total mortality (or overall survival from a defined point in time)
2. Cause-specific mortality (or cause-specific mortality from a defined point in time)
3. Carefully assessed quality of life
4. Indirect surrogates
   - Disease-free survival
   - Progression-free survival
   - Tumor response rate

Adapted from Agency for Healthcare Research and Quality.[43]

TABLE 17-2. Technology Evaluation Criteria Developed in Partnership with the Agency for Healthcare Research and Quality

1. The technology must have final approval from the appropriate governmental regulatory bodies.
2. The scientific evidence must permit conclusions concerning the effect of the technology on health outcomes.
   - The evidence should consist of well-designed and well-conducted investigations published in peer-reviewed journals. The quality of the body of studies and the consistency of the results are considered in evaluating the evidence.
   - The evidence should demonstrate that the technology can measure or alter the physiologic changes related to a disease, injury, illness, or condition. In addition, there should be evidence or a convincing argument based on established medical facts that such measurement or alteration affects health outcomes.
   - Opinions and evaluations by national medical associations, consensus panels, or other technology evaluation bodies are evaluated according to the scientific quality of the supporting evidence and rationale.
3. The technology must improve the net health outcome.
4. The technology must be as beneficial as any established alternatives.
   - The technology should improve the net health outcome as much as or more than established alternatives.
5. The improvement must be attainable outside the investigational settings.
   - When used under the usual conditions of medical practice, the technology should be reasonably expected to satisfy TEC criteria 3 and 4.

Adapted from Blue Cross Blue Shield Technology Evaluation Center.[44]
TEC = Technology Evaluation Center.

simultaneously use functional (biologic) and physical (anatomic) data during IMRT planning optimization and evaluation.[7] Three cases were simulated using lung, prostate, and brain geometries. Physical and functional imaging distributions were defined for each lesion. Initially, an IMRT plan was calculated for each based only on anatomic objectives (using DVHs). Another set of IMRT plans was then calculated using both DVH and dose-function histogram (DFH) objectives. DFHs, which display the relative function of a structure versus the dose, were calculated using the functional imaging distributions. The incorporation of the DFH into the inverse planning process was achieved and could be used concurrently with DVH data. The DFH, when used with the appropriate DVH objectives, provided the additional data needed to obtain and/or evaluate the desired heterogeneous dose distributions. The dose could be conformed either directly or inversely proportional to the biologic properties of a target and/or normal tissues depending on what information the corresponding functional imaging set represented for a particular structure.

Summary

Overall, IMRT is a promising approach in the treatment of CNS tumors. Improved coverage of irregularly shaped targets is possible, but it is not known how this affects clinical outcomes, especially because it may come at the cost of increased volumes of normal tissues receiving low doses of radiation. A small database suggests that sparing of normal tissues is both clinically feasible and significant. Bioanatomic treatment planning appears to be possible using IMRT but is still in its infancy. As in any disease, appropriate matching of the treatment modality to the patient will require thoughtful evaluation of the individual case by the clinician.

References

1. Miller AD, Leslie RA. The area postrema and vomiting. Front Neuroendocrinol 1994;15:301–20.
2. Shaw EG, Seiferheld W, Scott C, et al. Reexamining the Radiation Therapy Oncology Group (RTOG) recursive partitioning analysis (RPA) for glioblastoma multiforme (GBM) patients. Int J Radiat Oncol Biol Phys 2003;57:S135–6.
3. Gaspar LE, Scott C, Murray K, et al. Validation of the RTOG recursive partitioning analysis (RPA) classification for brain metastases. Int J Radiat Oncol Biol Phys 2000;47:1001–6.
4. Ricci PE, Dungan DH. Imaging of low- and intermediate-grade gliomas. Semin Radiat Oncol 2001;11:103–12.
5. Pirzkall A, Larson DA, McKnight TR, et al. MR-spectroscopy results in improved target delineation for high-grade gliomas. Int J Radiat Oncol Biol Phys 2000;48:115–21.
6. Nuutinen J, Sonninen P, Lehikoinen P, et al. Radiotherapy treatment planning and long-term follow-up with [C-11]methionine PET in patients with low-grade astrocytoma. Int J Radiat Oncol Biol Phys 2000;48:43–52.
7. Munley MT, Kearns WT, Hinson WH, et al. Bio-anatomic IMRT treatment planning with dose function histograms. Int J Radiat Oncol Biol Phys 2002;54:126–31.
8. International Commission on Radiation Units and Measurements. Prescribing, recording and reporting photon beam therapy. Report 62. Supplement to ICRU Report 50. Bethesda (MD): Nuclear Technology Publishing; 1999.
9. International Commission on Radiation Units and Measurements. Prescribing, recording, and reporting photon beam therapy. Report 50. Bethesda (MD): Nuclear Technology Publishing; 1993.
10. National Institutes of Health, NCBI National Library of Medicine. Available at: http://www.ncbi.nlm.nih.gov/entrez/query.fcgi (accessed Oct 30, 2003).
11. Yin FF, Ryu S, Ajlouni M, et al. A technique of intensity-modulated radiosurgery (IMRS) for spinal tumors. Med Phys 2002;29:2815–22.
12. Leybovich LB, Sethi A, Dogan N, et al. An immobilization and localization technique for SRT and IMRT of intracranial tumors. J Appl Clin Med Phys 2002;3:317–22.
13. Yenice KM, Lovelock DM, Hunt MA, et al. CT image-guided intensity-modulated therapy for paraspinal tumors using stereotactic immobilization. Int J Radiat Oncol Biol Phys 2003;55:583–93.
14. Kulik C, Caudrelier JM, Vermandel M, et al. Conformal radiotherapy optimization with micromultileaf collimators: comparison with radiosurgery techniques. Int J Radiat Oncol Biol Phys 2002;53:1038–50.
15. Sankaranarayanan V, Ganesan S, Oommen S, et al. Study on dosimetric parameters for stereotactic radiosurgery and intensity-modulated radiotherapy. Med Dosim 2003;28:85–90.
16. Zabel A, Thilmann C, Zuna I, et al. Comparison of forward planned conformal radiation therapy and inverse planned intensity modulated radiation therapy for esthesioneuroblastoma. Br J Radiol 2002;75:356–61.
17. Ma L, Xia P, Verhey LJ, et al. A dosimetric comparison of fan-beam intensity modulated radiotherapy with Gamma Knife stereotactic radiosurgery for treating intermediate intracranial lesions. Int J Radiat Oncol Biol Phys 1999;45:1325–30.
18. Fiveash JB, Murshed H, Duan J, et al. Effect of multileaf collimator leaf width on physical dose distributions in the treatment of CNS and head and neck neoplasms with intensity modulated radiation therapy. Med Phys 2002;29:1116–9.
19. Benedict SH, Cardinale RM, Wu Q, et al. Intensity-modulated stereotactic radiosurgery using dynamic micromultileaf collimation. Int J Radiat Oncol Biol Phys 2001;50:751–8.
20. Cardinale RM, Benedict SH, Wu Q, et al. A comparison of three stereotactic radiotherapy techniques: ARCS vs. noncoplanar fixed fields vs. intensity modulation. Int J Radiat Oncol Biol Phys 1998;42:431–6.
21. Bolsi A, Fogliata A, Cozzi L. Radiotherapy of small intracranial tumours with different advanced techniques using photon and proton beams: a treatment planning study. Radiother Oncol 2003;68:1–14.
22. Borden JA, Mahajan A, Tsai JS. A quality factor to compare the dosimetry of Gamma Knife radiosurgery and intensity-

modulated radiation therapy quantitatively as a function of target volume and shape. Technical note. J Neurosurg 2000;93 Suppl 3:228–32.

23. Khoo VS, Oldham M, Adams EJ, et al. Comparison of intensity-modulated tomotherapy with stereotactically guided conformal radiotherapy for brain tumors. Int J Radiat Oncol Biol Phys 1999;45:415–25.

24. Gabriele P, Macias V, Stasi M, et al. Feasibility of intensity-modulated radiation therapy in the treatment of advanced cervical chordoma. Tumori 2003;89:298–304.

25. Thilmann C, Schulz-Ertner D, Zabel A, et al. Intensity-modulated radiotherapy of sacral chordoma—a case report and a comparison with stereotactic conformal radiotherapy. Acta Oncol 2002;41:395–9.

26. Thilmann C, Zabel A, Grosser KH, et al. Intensity-modulated radiotherapy with an integrated boost to the macroscopic tumor volume in the treatment of high-grade gliomas. Int J Cancer 2001;96:341–9.

27. Baumert BG, Norton IA, Davis JB. Intensity-modulated stereotactic radiotherapy vs. stereotactic conformal radiotherapy for the treatment of meningioma located predominantly in the skull base. Int J Radiat Oncol Biol Phys 2003;57:580–92.

28. Nakamura JL, Pirzkall A, Carol MP, et al. Comparison of intensity-modulated radiosurgery with Gamma Knife radiosurgery for challenging skull base lesions. Int J Radiat Oncol Biol Phys 2003;55:99–109.

29. Kramer BA, Wazer DE, Engler MJ, et al. Dosimetric comparison of stereotactic radiosurgery to intensity modulated radiotherapy. Radiat Oncol Invest 1998;6:18–25.

30. Pirzkall A, Debus J, Haering P, et al. Intensity modulated radiotherapy (IMRT) for recurrent, residual, or untreated skull-base meningiomas: preliminary clinical experience. Int J Radiat Oncol Biol Phys 2003;55:362–72.

31. Grant W III, Cain RB. Intensity modulated conformal therapy for intracranial lesions. Med Dosim 1998;23:237–41.

32. Fuss M, Salter BJ, Sadeghi A, et al. Fractionated stereotactic intensity-modulated radiotherapy (FS-IMRT) for small acoustic neuromas. Med Dosim 2002;27:147–54.

33. Huang E, Teh BS, Strother DR, et al. Intensity-modulated radiation therapy for pediatric medulloblastoma: early report on the reduction of ototoxicity. Int J Radiat Oncol Biol Phys 2002;52:599–605.

34. Milker-Zabel S, Zabel A, Thilmann C, et al. Clinical results of retreatment of vertebral bone metastases by stereotactic conformal radiotherapy and intensity-modulated radiotherapy. Int J Radiat Oncol Biol Phys 2003;55:162–7.

35. Kuo JV, Cabebe E, Al Ghazi M, et al. Intensity-modulated radiation therapy for the spine at the University of California, Irvine. Med Dosim 2002;27:137–45.

36. Suzuki M, Nakamatsu K, Kanamori S, et al. Feasibility study of the simultaneous integrated boost (SIB) method for malignant gliomas using intensity-modulated radiotherapy (IMRT). Jpn J Clin Oncol 2003;33:271–7.

37. Voynov G, Kaufman S, Hong T, et al. Treatment of recurrent malignant gliomas with stereotactic intensity modulated radiation therapy. Am J Clin Oncol 2002;25:606–11.

38. Ryu S, Yin FF, Rock J, et al. Image-guided and intensity-modulated radiosurgery for patients with spinal metastasis. Cancer 2003;97:2013–8.

39. Uy NW, Woo SY, Teh BS, et al. Intensity-modulated radiation therapy (IMRT) for meningioma. Int J Radiat Oncol Biol Phys 2002;53:1265–70.

40. Kippenes H, Gavin PR, Parsaei H, et al. Spatial accuracy of fractionated IMRT delivery studies in canine paraspinal irradiation. Vet Radiol Ultrasound 2003;44:360–6.

41. Shaw E, Kline R, Gillin M, et al. Radiation Therapy Oncology Group: radiosurgery quality assurance guidelines. Int J Radiat Oncol Biol Phys 1993;27:1231–9.

42. National Cancer Institute cancer.gov. Levels of evidence for adult cancer treatment studies. Available at: http://www.cancer.gov/ cancerinfo/pdq/levels-evidence-adult-treatment (accessed Oct 30, 2003).

43. Agency for Healthcare Research and Quality. Technology assessments. Available at: http://www.ahrq.gov/clinic/techix.htm (accessed Oct 30, 2003).

44. Blue Cross Blue Shield Technology Evaluation Center. Available at: http://www.bcbs.com/tec/index.html (accessed Oct 30, 2003).

MENINGIOMA CASE STUDY

ANDREA PIRZKALL, MD

Patient History

A 63-year-old female presented with right-sided ptosis and double vision. Magnetic resonance imaging (MRI) of the head revealed a brightly enhancing mass on the contrast-enhanced T_1-weighted images without significant edema evident on T_2-weighted images. The lesion extended laterally to the cavernous sinus and along the right sphenoid wing, inferiorly along the clivus and the sella turcica, superiorly to the optic chiasm, and posteriorly (with an evident dural tail) along the tentorium (Figure 17.1-1). In addition, an arachnoid cyst in the anterior aspect of the temporal lobe was noted. A repeat MRI 2 months later revealed no significant change.

Radiographically, the tumor was consistent with a benign meningioma. Owing to significant cardiac comorbidity, however, resection (or even a biopsy) was not recommended. The patient was thus referred for definitive radiation therapy (RT). To spare the surrounding normal tissues, particularly the optic apparatus, and to deliver a conformal dose distribution encompassing the entire tumor, including the dural tail, intensity-modulated radiation therapy (IMRT) was administered in this patient. Treatment was delivered at the German Cancer Research Center (DKFZ) in Heidelberg, Germany.

Simulation

The patient was immobilized using a customized head mask (Scotch-Cast, 3M, St. Paul-Minneapolis, MN) attached to a stereotactic frame. In patients with intracranial lesions treated at the DKFZ, this immobilization device has been shown to provide a repositioning accuracy of better than 2 mm.[1]

For the purpose of treatment planning, a computed tomography (CT) and a MRI of the entire head with 3 mm slices were obtained. Intravenous contrast was administered for both studies. All imaging data sets were acquired with the patient immobilized in the customized mask with an attached stereotactic localizer. This localizer consists of

four triangular plates that contain metal wire (for CT) or Gadolinium-filled pipes (for MRI). The center of the frame represents the origin of the stereotactic coordinate system. Because the CT and MRI localizers have the same geometry, image registration is efficiently and accurately accomplished using the external markers.[2]

Target and Tissue Delineation

Target and normal tissue delineation was performed on coregistered CT and MRI data sets in order to take advantage of the superior soft tissue contrast on MRI. The clinical target volume (CTV) consisted of the contrast-enhancing lesion on the T_1-weighted MRI, modified to include hyperostotic changes evident on the CT scan. A margin of 1 to 2 mm was added to account for setup uncertainty generating a planning target volume (PTV). The resultant PTV in this patient was 94 cc.

The organs at risk (OAR) outlined in this patient included the optic nerves, optic chiasm, orbits, lenses, lacrimal glands, brainstem, and brain. Representative axial slices on the planning CT scan illustrating the target and normal tissues are shown in Figure 17.1-1.

Treatment Planning

Inverse planning was performed using the *CORVUS* treatment planning system, version 3.0 (North American Scientific, NOMOS Radiation Oncology Division, Cranberry Township, PA), which uses entered partial volume data to drive a multifaceted cost function that controls a simulated annealing algorithm The *CORVUS* prescription process involves setting goals and limits for the target(s) and structures. The *CORVUS* optimizer then attempts to find a solution that best meets these goals and limits. In practice, trade-offs are required because these constraints create mutually exclusive situations. The trade-offs are based on cost functions programmed into the system that prioritize goals and limits based on an importance

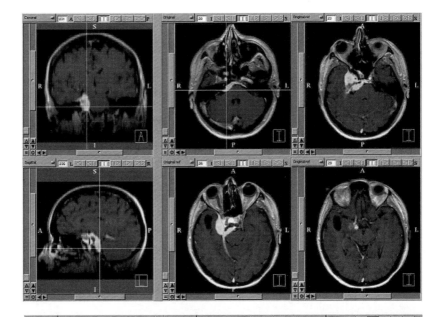

FIGURE 17.1-1. Axial T₁-weighted postcontrast magnetic resonance images of a patient with right-sided sphenoid wing meningioma also involving the cavernous sinus. The lower image set shows the treatment planning computed tomography slices with the target and critical structures outlined (red = target; green shades = right and left optic nerves and optic chiasm; purple shades = right and left eyes; orange shades = right and left lenses; blue = brainstem; the lacrimal gland was not outlined in this case but is present in slice 26). (To view a color version of this image, please refer to the CD-ROM.)

designation (ie, choice of target or structure type) assigned to the target and normal tissues. Unlike the "hard constraints" used by some planning systems that cannot be exceeded, all of the *CORVUS* goals and limits are "soft constraints." Soft limits or goals can be violated; however, the cost associated with such violation increases in a manner proportional to the amount of the violation.

The prescription process for the patient is summarized in Table 17.1-1. A total dose of 52 Gy was prescribed (goal) to the PTV (type Basic) in 32 fractions based on our prior experience with three-dimensional conformal RT.[3] Although some institutions have experience in prescribing 54 Gy, the increased inhomogeneity seen in most IMRT plans has led us to prescribe a slightly lower total dose. Minimum (95% of prescribed dose) and maximum (110% of prescribed dose) doses were chosen per the recommendations pro-

TABLE 17.1-1. Input Parameters

Target	Type	Goal, Gy	Volume below Goal, %	Minimum Dose, Gy	Maximum Dose, Gy
Meningioma	Basic	52.0	5	49.0	57.0

Structure	Type	Limit, Gy	Volume above Limit, %	Minimum Dose, Gy	Maximum Dose, Gy
Optic chiasm	Basic	50	50	40	54
Optic nerve (R)	Basic	50	33	40	54
Optic nerve (L)	Basic	50	33	40	54
Orbit (R)	Basic	30	25	10	45
Orbit (L)	Basic	30	25	10	45
Lens (R)	Basic	8	30	1	10
Lens (L)	Basic	8	30	1	10
Brainstem	Basic	52	10	40	56
Spinal cord	Basic	36	10	20	40

vided by *CORVUS*. Based on our clinical experience, the OAR were given the following prescription values: maximum doses of 54 Gy for the optic apparatus, 32 Gy for the lacrimal glands, 10 Gy for the lenses, and 54 Gy for the brainstem (< 1 cc receiving 56 Gy).

The three-dimensional shape of the PTV must be taken into account when selecting the treatment planning constraints. For example, if the PTV abuts the optic nerve(s) and/or chiasm and if the target goal is 52 Gy, then prescribing a lower maximum dose for the optic apparatus in an attempt to protect it will result in a conflict for the planning system. Either the minimum PTV dose must be lowered or the maximum dose to the optic apparatus must be raised to allow the optimizer the best chance of finding an optimal solution. However, if the neurologic function of an organ or structure is already compromised (eg, only bright or dark distinction or even blindness in one eye) owing to tumor growth or prior surgery, target coverage can be improved by setting a high limit to the respective structure(s) or even by designating it as expendable. This is even more apparent when a higher target dose is prescribed, for example, in patients with malignant brain tumors. Discussion with the patient prior to the planning process as to the desired outcome, should a trade-off have to made, is critical.

A specific OAR worth mentioning is the lens. In skull base meningiomas, and even more so in malignant skull base tumors, it is impossible to deliver the desired dose and guarantee preservation of lens function. This is especially true for IMRT because there is usually an increase in scatter dose due to an increase in the number of monitor units (MUs) required to deliver the treatment. It does not make sense to force the optimizer to limit the dose to the lens to 2 Gy while trying to deliver a minimum of 52 Gy to the tumor (and even higher for malignant cases). Therefore, prior to treatment, one should discuss with the patient the possible complication of cataracts and the need for post-treatment implantation of an artificial lens.

Seven equally spaced beam angles and five intensity levels were chosen for this case based on a theoretical comparison study that demonstrated the superiority of seven coplanar beams over noncoplanar beam arrangements in skull base lesions.[4] Additionally, our experience has taught us to avoid beam directions that enter near the eyes. Thirteen of 20 patients experienced increased tearing toward the end of their treatment lasting for 1 to 3 weeks. This side effect was most likely due to the coplanar, equidistant beam arrangements, with some portion of the beam entering through the eye or lacrimal gland even though the dose limits for these sensitive structures were met. Consequently, we now spread the equidistant beam arrangement so that no or only a portion of a beam passes directly through the eye or lacrimal gland. Noncoplanar beams can be added but are usually not necessary for skull base meningiomas. In this patient, the following beam arrangement was chosen: couch fixed at 0 degrees and seven coplanar beams at 0, 75, 120, 155, 205, 240, and 290 degrees.

Figure 17.1-2 illustrates the dose distribution overlaid on axial CT slices. Dose-volume histograms for this case are shown in Figure 17.1-3. This patient received the prescribed dose of 52 Gy, which covered 96.8% of the target. The mean dose was 56 Gy. Maximum and minimum doses to 1 cc of the target were 60.5 Gy and 48.6 Gy, respectively. The maximum dose was well within the target. Only 0.3 cc of nontarget tissue received ≥ 52 Gy. The tolerance doses to the surrounding OAR were respected in all cases; maximum doses to the OAR are summarized in Table 17.1-2.

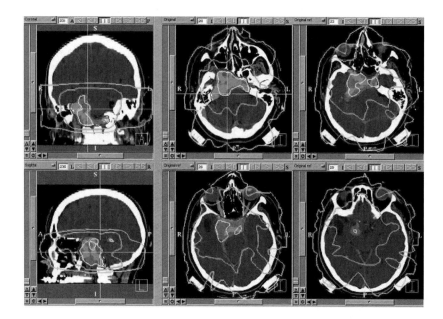

FIGURE 17.1-2. Dose distribution for the treated case. Isodose lines are as follows: 56 Gy (*yellow*), 52 Gy (prescription isodose line, *blue*), 30 Gy (*green*), and 10 Gy (*turquoise*). (To view a color version of this image, please refer to the CD-ROM.)

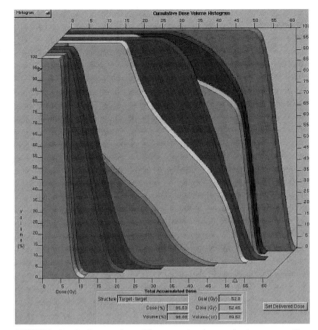

FIGURE 17.1-3. Dose-volume histogram for the meningioma case. The different colors represent the following structures: red = target; dark green = optic chiasm; bright green = right optic nerve; yellow-green = left optic nerve; two purple shades = both orbits; two orange shades = both lenses; dark blue = brainstem; bright blue = spinal cord. (To view a color version of this image, please refer to the CD-ROM.)

TABLE 17.1-2. Maximum Doses to Organs at Risk

	Maximum Point Dose Gy	Maximum Dose to 0.5 cc Gy
Target	61.3	60.5
Optic chiasm	53.9	50.4
Optic nerve (R)	52.4	51.3
Optic nerve (L)	51.2	48.5
Orbit (R)	29.7	25.2
Orbit (L)	19.9	17.5
Lens (R)	10.7	7.2
Lens (L)	10.7	6.8
Brainstem	55.5	51.8
Spinal cord	43.6	39.7

The patient was then aligned to the "zero position" on the coordinate system using the room lasers. Next, the patient was moved to the isocenter coordinates derived from the treatment plan. The stereotactic target point (isocenter) was verified with a double-exposure portal image and then marked on the patient's mask to allow for faster setup on subsequent treatment days.

The treatment table and/or gantry were moved in position for the first treatment portal. The accuracy of the couch and gantry angles, as well as the light field for the first subfield, was checked. The actual delivery of all segments for each gantry angle was monitored with the Beam View Plus System (Siemens Oncology Systems), allowing the treated field to be compared with the intensity map generated by the planning system.

Treatment Delivery and Quality Assurance

Treatment was delivered using a 6 MV KD2 linear accelerator (Siemens Oncology Systems, Concord, CA) equipped with automated delivery capability (*SIMTEC*). The integrated multileaf collimator was driven in the "step-and-shoot" mode.[5] The segments for each subfield were created through a customized segmentation algorithm embedded in the inverse treatment planning program. The total time required for treatment of this patient using seven gantry angles divided into 63 segments was 16 minutes (total 707 MU).

Dose verification was carried out extensively for each of our first patients with meningioma prior to treatment. A phantom plan was created whereby the intensity patterns of the approved plan were cast onto a CT-scanned water-equivalent phantom within the planning system. The plan was then delivered to the phantom, in which ion chambers and film had been inserted, to measure absolute and compare relative dose distributions, respectively. Dose verification revealed a deviation of the measured from the calculated dose of 1 to 8% by film dosimetry and less than 5% by ionization chamber (absolute dose).[6] In addition, each subfield for each treatment field was checked for orientation and shape prior to delivery using the accelerator light field.

Prior to the initial treatment, the patient was set up in the customized mask and attached to the stereotactic frame.

Clinical Outcome

Significant clinical improvement was observed at the time of her first follow-up examination. The preexisting right-sided oculomotor palsy and double vision had improved significantly within 6 weeks after completion of IMRT and showed a complete recovery on subsequent follow-up (see also Figure 5 in our clinical article[6]).

At the DKFZ, skull base meningiomas have been treated with IMRT since June 1998. Of 20 patients in our published report, 5 were irradiated after a subtotal resection and 11 were treated for recurrence.[6] Four did not have histologic confirmation owing to significant medical comorbidities. After treatment, preexisting neurologic symptoms improved in 12 of 20 (60%) patients, remained stable in 7 of 20 (35%) patients, and worsened in 1 (5%) patient. Radiographic follow-up revealed significant tumor shrinkage 6 weeks after treatment in two patients and partial remission in three more patients at 9 to 17 months, whereas other tumors remained stable. There was no radiation-induced peritumoral edema, increase in tumor size, or onset of new neurologic deficits. Acute treatment side effects remained transient and included nausea and vomiting and single occurrences of conjunctivitis, increased tearing, and serous tympanitis.

References

1. Schlegel W, Pastyr O, Bortfeld T, et al. Stereotactically guided fractionated radiotherapy: technical aspects. Radiother Oncol 1993;29:197–204.

2. Schad LR, Gademann G, Knopp M, et al. Radiotherapy treatment planning of basal meningiomas: improved tumor localization by correlation of CT and MR imaging data. Radiother Oncol 1992;25:56–62.

3. Debus J, Wuendrich M, Pirzkall A, et al. High efficacy of fractionated stereotactic radiotherapy of large base-of-skull meningiomas: long-term results. J Clin Oncol 2001;19:3547–53.

4. Pirzkall A, Carol M, Lohr F, et al. Comparison of intensity-modulated radiotherapy with conventional conformal radiotherapy for complex-shaped tumors. Int J Radiat Oncol Biol Phys 2000;48:1371–80.

5. Keller-Reichenbecher MA, Bortfeld T, Levegrün S, et al. Intensity modulation with the "step and shoot" technique using a commercial MLC: a planning study. Multileaf collimator. Int J Radiat Oncol Biol Phys 1999;45:1315–24.

6. Pirzkall A, Debus J, Haering P, et al. Intensity modulated radiotherapy (IMRT) for recurrent, residual, or untreated skull-base meningiomas: preliminary clinical experience. Int J Radiat Oncol Biol Phys 2003;55:362–72.

BASE OF SKULL TUMOR CASE STUDY

MARC W. MÜNTER, MD, JÜRGEN DEBUS, MD, PHD

Patient History

A 63-year-old male presented with a 6-month history of reduced visual acuity of the right eye. Furthermore, the patient had developed amaurosis, right eye proptosis, reduced nasal breathing, and recurrent right-sided epistaxis. Examination in the ear, nose, and throat (ENT) department revealed a tumor in the nasal cavity with a visible invasion to the oral cavity. Biopsy of the maxillary bone was consistent with a well-differentiated adenoid cystic carcinoma.

Radiographic studies included both magnetic resonance imaging (MRI) and computed tomography (CT). MRI revealed invasion of the base of the skull by the lesion with infiltration of the right maxillary sinus, right nasal cavity, sphenoid sinus, and right orbit. In addition, the tumor involved the cavernous sinus and infratemporal fossa. The CT scan demonstrated destruction of the bones in this anatomic region. Additionally, CT (as well as ultrasonography of the neck) revealed no suspicious cervical lymph nodes. A bone scan, a sonogram of the abdominal region, and a chest radiograph were negative for metastatic spread. Therefore, the patient was staged as cT4cN0cM0, Grade 1 (GI).

Owing to the location and size of the tumor, a resection was felt by the neurosurgeons and ENT surgeons not to be possible. The patient was thus transferred to the department of radiation oncology for definitive treatment with intensity-modulated radiation therapy (IMRT). Before initiation of therapy, the patient underwent a full dental evaluation and necessary dental extractions.

Simulation

Patient immobilization is an important aspect of IMRT treatment. At our institution, a customized immobilization device is fabricated for all patients undergoing IMRT based on the site irradiated. For lesions of the brain or skull base, a customized wrap-around headmask is fabricated (Scotch-Cast, 3M Corporation, St Paul, MN) with the patient in the supine position. The entire head (including the mandible) is immobilized by the mask, with only the nose remaining

visible. Fabrication of the mask requires approximately 15 minutes. This device can be attached to a stereotactic head and neck localization system, allowing stereotactic imaging with CT, MRI, positron emission tomography (PET) or single-photon emission computed tomography (SPECT). Our approach has a setup accuracy of ~ 1 mm, particularly in tumors of the base of skull region.

The extent of the planning CT scan in an individual patient is based on the tumor site and stage. For tumors of the head and neck region, it may be necessary to irradiate different cervical lymph node levels. Therefore, before performing the planning CT, a diagnostic CT scan and a sonogram of the neck should be obtained. Additionally, the radiation oncologist should decide whether noncoplanar beams are required to achieve an adequate dose distribution. If noncoplanar beams are used, the planning CT scan should include the entire head.

In the patient presented here, the planning CT scan was obtained with 3 mm slices. The uppermost extent was 5 cm superior to the base of the skull and lesion. The inferiormost extent included cervical node levels I to III. The patient received intravenous contrast according to our in-house protocol. Additionally, a contrast-enhanced MRI was obtained with the patient immobilized in the treatment position. The isocenter of the IMRT treatment is defined stereotactically at our institution in all cases.

Target and Tissue Delineation

The target volume and critical structures were defined for all axial slices on the treatment planning CT using the *VIRTOUS* (developed at our institution) three-dimensional planning system. For a more accurate definition of the critical normal structures and the target volume, an image fusion of the treatment planning CT scan and MRI was performed (Figure 17.2-1).

The gross tumor volume (GTV) consisted of the visible tumor from the imaging studies with a 3 mm margin (Figure 17.2-2). The clinical target volume (CTV) includ-

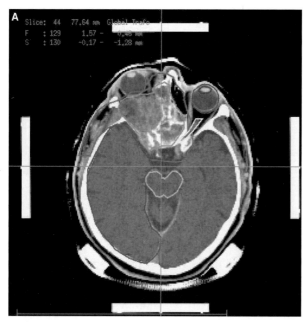
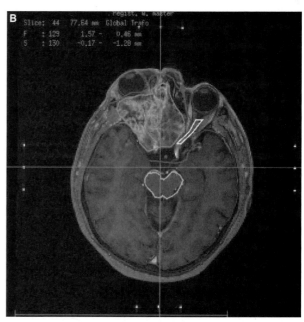

FIGURE 17.2-1. Comparison of the stereotactic matching between a computed tomography scan (*A*) and a magnetic resonance image (*B*) for the definition of the target volume (*light blue*: gross tumor volume; *red*: clinical target volume). (To view a color version of this image, please refer to the CD-ROM).

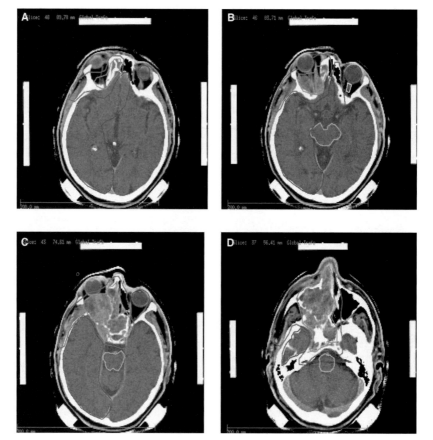

FIGURE 17.2-2. Definition of the target volumes and the organs at risk in different slices of the treatment planning computed tomography (CT) (*light blue*: gross tumor volume; *red*: clinical target volume; *blue*: left lens; *yellow*: left optic nerve; *green*: brainstem; *dark blue*: temporal lobe). (To view a color version of this image, please refer to the CD-ROM).

ed the GTV plus a 5 mm margin, depending on the the anatomic relationship of adjacent structures and potential microscopic spread (see Figure 17.2-2). Owing to the propensity of adenoid cystic tumors to spread along nerves, these were included in the CTV. At our institution, level II to III neck nodes are included bilaterally in the CTV in all patients with adenoid cystic carcinoma, even when these nodes are clinically negative (as in this patient). No additional margins around the target volumes (GTV and CTV) were added in the inverse treatment planning process of this patient.

All surrounding critical normal structures were contoured on each axial slice. Organs at risk (OAR) included the spinal cord, brainstem, optic chiasm, optic nerve, and temporomandibular joint.

Treatment Planning

At the German Cancer Research Center, inverse planning is performed using *KonRad* (MRC System GmbH, Heidelberg, Germany), a system developed at our institution. *KonRad* is linked to the *VIRTOUS* three-dimensional planning system to calculate and display three-dimensional dose distributions.

To initiate the optimization process using the *KonRad* system, the treatment planner must define maximum and minimum dose constraints for both the target volumes and the critical normal structures. Furthermore, penalties must be specified, defining the relative importance of each constraint. Based on these constraints and penalties, the *KonRad* system uses an iterative algorithm (gradient technique) to optimize the three-dimensional dose distribution by minimizing the objective function. The optimum solution is reached if the value of the objective function does not change by more than a prespecified threshold between subsequent iterations.

In addition to dose specifications, the user can select the couch, gantry, and collimator angles and the number of intensity levels (representing the complexity of the beam modulation). During the optimization process of the case presented here, treatment plans with five, seven, or nine

equidistant gantry angles, with a coplanar couch position (angle 0°), were evaluated to determine the beam arrangement with the best target coverage and maximal sparing of critical normal structures. To deliver this plan, the intensity patterns were converted into a leaf sequence using the methodology described by Bortfeld and colleagues.[1] Approximately four to eight nonzero intensity levels were used to define the fluence maps at each gantry angle.

An integrated boost technique was used in the treatment of this patient.[2] This technique allows the treatment of different target volumes simultaneously with different daily fraction sizes. The total doses for all target volumes were prescribed to the median of the target volume (50% of the target volume receiving 100% of dose). At our institution, the dose of all IMRT treatment plans is prescribed to the median, which allows a good comparison of the different plans. Levegrün and colleagues concluded that the median dose is a significant predictor for the clinical outcome in conformal radiation therapy.[3]

The maximum doses of the spinal cord, brainstem, and optic nerve and chiasm were limited to 45, 54, and 54 Gy, respectively. Dose-volume histograms for all critical structures were generated (Figure 17.2-3). Specific values of the target volumes and OAR are also displayed in Table 17.2-1. For the different target volumes, 90% dose coverage was defined as the fraction of the target volume that was covered with ≥ 90% of the prescribed dose.

The final treatment plan consisted of seven coplanar equidistant beams. The predefined constraints for the OAR were satisfied. Using the integrated boost technique, a daily fraction size of 2.2 Gy to the GTV was delivered to a median total dose of 66 Gy in 30 fractions. The CTV received 1.86 Gy per fraction to a total dose of 55.8 Gy in the same number of fractions. The optimized treatment plan for this patient is shown in Figure 17.2-4.

Treatment Delivery and Quality Assurance

A Primus linear accelerator (Siemens AG, Munich, Germany) with 6 and 15 MV photons and an integrated

TABLE 17.2-1 Dosage of the Target Volumes and Organs at Risk

Target Volume/Organ at Risk	Maximum Dose, Gy	Minimum Dose, Gy	Mean Dose, Gy	< 90% of the Prescribed Dose, %
Gross tumor volume	75.9	50.8	66.0	4.6
Clinical target volume	68.6	30.8	55.9	5.0
Brainstem	54.0	1.0	30.7	
Optic chiasm	53.2	31.7	41.0	
Left eye	45.1	9.9	24.3	
Left optic nerve	54.2	29.8	48.2	
Left lens	15.1	10.4	12.6	
Left temporomandibular joint	30.2	21.0	26.3	
Right temporomandibular joint	58.7	51.3	53.2	
Temporal lobe	67.9	5.3	32.1	

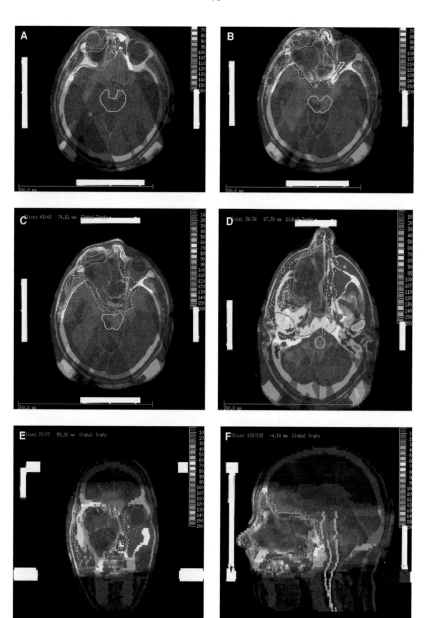

FIGURE 17.2-3. Dose distribution on axial (*A–D*), coronal (*E*), and sagittal (*F*) slices. The red line represents the 90% isodose line, and the yellow dotted line encompasses the 80% isodose line. (To view a color version of this image, please refer to the CD-ROM).

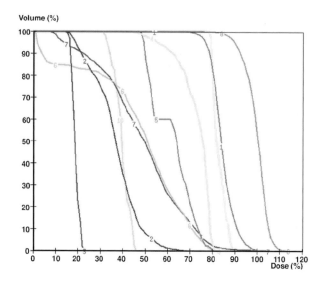

FIGURE 17.2-4. Dose-volume histogram of the treatment plan: 1, clinical target volume; 2, left eye; 3, left lens; 4, left optic nerve; 5, optic chiasm; 6, brainstem; 7, temporal lobe; 8, gross tumor volume; 9, right temporomandibular joint; 10, left temporomandibular joint.

motorized multileaf collimator was used to deliver the IMRT plan in the step-and-shoot mode. The leaf sequences were delivered automatically. The treatment plan consisted of 97 subsegments. By using 15 MV photons, 6.5 subsegments could be delivered over 1 minute. The actual treatment time was ~ 15 minutes. Patient immobilization and positioning required ~ 5 minutes/d.

An important aspect of IMRT delivery is the verification process. Currently, film dosimetry is the primary form of verification at our institution. Initially, the intensity patterns of the treated plan are recalculated onto a solid water head and neck phantom. This phantom has the same approximate dimensions as a patient and is adaptable to the stereotactic system. Next, the treatment plan is delivered on the linear accelerator to the phantom with film placed at several locations (EDR2, Eastman Kodak, Rochester, NY). Accurate dosimetry (± 2%) is made possible by the use of a stereotactic coordinate system defined for the phantom, detector, and verification film.

After treatment delivery, the films were developed and scanned into the computer using the PTW Lumniscan 50 laser densitometer (PTW, Freiburg, Germany). In-house software was used to evaluate the calculated dose distribution of the phantom plan and the measured verification films. Both data sets were automatically matched using the stereotactic coordinates. Treatment will be initiated only if the absolute difference between calculated and measured values is less than 3%. This condition was satisfied in this patient.

Clinical Outcome

The patient tolerated treatment well without any significant acute side effects. By the end of treatment, the proptosis of the right eye was improved. The patient experienced complete loss of both taste and smell, as well as a dryness of the nasal mucosa. Even though the parotid glands were not entered as avoidance structures in the inverse planning process, the patient did not develop xerostomia. Only slight erythema of the skin (Radiation Therapy Oncology Group grade 2) was noted. No weight loss occurred. Treatment was completed as planned without any therapy-related interruptions.

Eighteen months after completion of therapy, a near-complete response was noted on follow-up MRI (Figure 17.2-5). Proptosis of the right eye resolved completely, and the patient remains free of untoward treatment-related chronic sequelae.

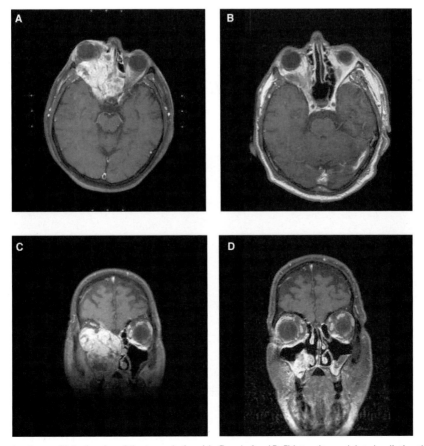

FIGURE 17.2-5. Treatment outcome. Note the size of the tumor before (*A, C*) and after (*B, D*) intensity-modulated radiation therapy.

References

1. Bortfeld TR, Kahler DL, Waldron TJ, et al. X-ray field compensation with multileaf collimators. Int J Radiat Oncol Biol Phys 1994;28:723–30.

2. Thilmann C, Zabel A, Grosser KH, et al. Intensity-modulated radiotherapy with an integrated boost to the macroscopic tumor volume in the treatment of high-grade gliomas. Int J Cancer 2001;96:341–9.

3. Levegrun S, Jackson A, Zelefsky MJ, et al. Analysis of biopsy outcome after three-dimensional conformal radiation therapy of prostate cancer using dose-distribution variables and tumor control probability models. Int J Radiat Oncol Biol Phys 2000;47:1245–60.

Glioblastoma Multiforme

Case Study

Minoru Suzuki, MD, PhD, Masahiko Okumura, MP, Yasumasa Nishimura, MD, PhD

Patient History

A 71-year-old man presented with a 1-month history of headache, nausea, and vomiting. On physical examination, mild left-sided weakness was noted in the upper and lower extremities. Workup included magnetic resonance imaging (MRI), which revealed an enhancing mass in the right temporal lobe with surrounding edema (Figure 17.3-1). Three years previously, the patient had been diagnosed with a low-grade glioma of the right temporal lobe. No treatment was administered at that time.

Surgery was recommended, and the patient underwent a partial resection of the enhancing mass. The pathology was consistent with a glioblastoma multiforme. Adjuvant radiation therapy was recommended following surgery.

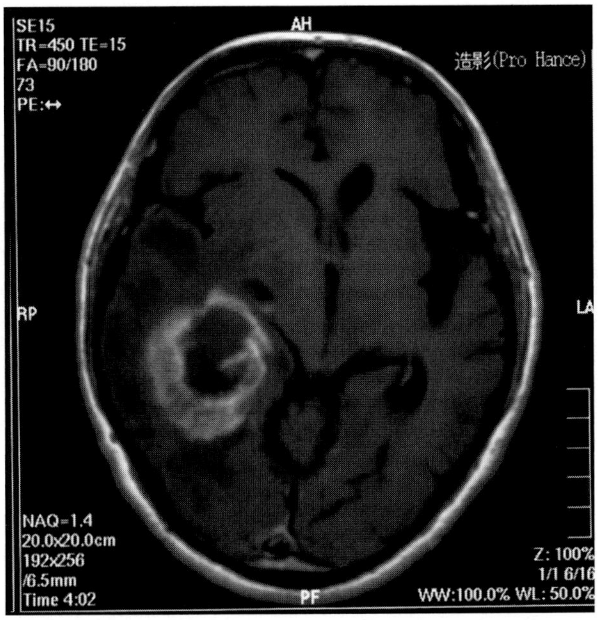

FIGURE 17.3-1. Gadolinium-enhanced T$_1$-weighted magnetic resonance image demonstrating the enhanced brain tumor in the right temporal lobe.

Intensity-modulated radiation therapy (IMRT) was used to allow the delivery of a simultaneous integrated boost (SIB), allowing the overall treatment time to be shortened and a higher than conventional dose to be delivered.

Simulation

The patient was simulated in the supine position. A thermoplastic mask was fabricated for immobilization covering the head, neck, and shoulders (Uni-frame form, MED-TEC, Orange City, IA). A planning computed tomography (CT) scan (Aquilion, Toshiba Medical Systems Corporation, Tokyo, Japan) was performed from the vertex of the head to the clavicles with 5 mm slice intervals. Intravenous contrast was administered prior to the scan.

Target and Tissue Delineation

Gross tumor volume (GTV) was delineated on the axial slices of the planning CT scan. The GTV consisted of the contrast-enhanced residual tumor. In patients who have undergone complete resection, the area in which the tumor was present on the preoperative MRI is designated as the GTV. Fusion of the preoperative MRI and planning CT was not performed in this case, although the MRI was used to help delineate the GTV.

The clinical target volume (CTV) consisted of the GTV plus a 2 cm margin. This margin was expanded where necessary to encompass areas of edema extending beyond 2 cm from the GTV. In addition, it was decreased in regions that serve as anatomic barriers, such as the intracerebral fissures or tentorium cerebelli.

At Kinki University, the surrounding edema at risk of microscopic invasion is defined as a clinical target volume–annulus (CTV-A) and consists of the CTV excluding the GTV. Figure 17.3-2 illustrates the target volumes in this patient. The following normal tissues were defined as organs at risk (OAR): brain, brainstem, eye (retina), optic nerves, lens, and pituitary gland.

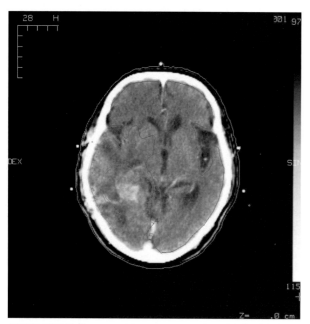

FIGURE 17.3-2. Contours of the gross tumor volume (*pink*), clinical target volume–annulus (*red*), and normal brain (*blue*). (To view a color version of this image, please refer to the CD-ROM).

Treatment Planning

In this patient, three separate planning target volumes (PTVs) were defined. PTV-G consisted of the GTV plus a 0.5 cm margin. The PTV-C was defined as the CTV plus a 0.5 cm margin to account for setup errors. The planning target volume–annulus (PTV-A) was delineated by subtracting the PTV-G from the PTV-C. Figure 17.3-3 shows the relationships among the three PTVs.

Inverse treatment planning was performed using Helios Cadplan, version 6.01 (Varian Medical Systems, Palo Alto,

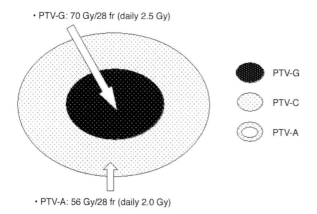

• PTV-G: 70 Gy/28 fr (daily 2.5 Gy)

PTV-G
PTV-C
PTV-A

• PTV-A: 56 Gy/28 fr (daily 2.0 Gy)

FIGURE 17.3-3. Schematic illustration of the three planning target volumes (PTVs) defined in the present case. The planning target volume–annulus (PTV-A) was delineated by subtracting the gross tumor volume plus a 0.5 cm margin (PTV-G) from the clinical target volume plus a 0.5 cm margin (PTV-C). Adapted from Suzuki M et al.[1]

CA). As noted above, a SIB approach was used in this patient. In this approach, the prescribed doses to PTV-G and PTV-A were 70 Gy in 2.5 Gy daily fractions and 56 Gy in 2 Gy daily fractions, respectively. In these patients, our treatment goals are as follows:

1. The dose delivered to 95% of the volume (D_{95}) of PTV-G and PTV-A should be greater than the prescribed doses.
2. The dose delivered to 5% of the volume (D_{05}) of PTV-G should be < 77 Gy, that is, 110% of the prescribed dose to PTV-G.
3. D_{05} of PTV-A should be less than the prescribed dose to the PTV-G (70 Gy).

Table 17.3-1 summarizes the IMRT input parameters used in this case. The treatment plan generated in this patient consisted of five equally spaced coplanar beams at 72°, 20°, 92°, 164°, 236°, and 308° intervals. All beams had a nominal energy of 4 MV.

Table 17.3-2 summarizes the treatment volumes, D_{95}, D_{90} (dose delivered to 90% of the volume), D_{05}, %V_{110} (percentage of the volume receiving greater than 110% of the prescribed dose), and mean doses for PTV-G and PTV-A. In this particular case, the treatment plan was normalized to deliver the prescribed dose (70.0 Gy) to 90% volume of the PTV-G ($D_{90} = 70.0$ Gy). The mean doses to PTV-G and PTV-A were 73.0 and 60.6 Gy, respectively. The value of %V_{110} for PTV-G was 0.6%. This high homogeneity was achieved by setting the maximum and minimum dose constraints for PTV-G within a very narrow range, namely, within ± 2% of the prescribed dose to the GTV with a strict

TABLE 17.3-1. Input Parameters

Target/OAR	Dose Constraints and Penalties	
	Maximum, Gy/Penalty	Minimum, Gy/Penalty
PTV-G	71.4/100	68.6/100
PTV-A	67.2/100	53.2/100
Brain[†]	Maximum = 54/80	
	V_{33} = 45/80	
	V_{66} = 40/80	
Brainstem[†]	Maximum = 54/80	
	V_{33} = 42/80	
	V_{66} = 38/80	
Eye (retina)	40/90	
Optic nerve	40/90	
Lens	6/90	
Pituitary gland	30/90	

CTV = clinical target volume; CTV-A = clinical target volume–annulus; GTV = gross tumor volume; OAR = organs at risk; PTV-A = planning target volume–annulus; PTV-G = gross tumor volume plus a 0.5 cm margin; V_{33} = 33% of volume; V_{66} = 66% of volume.
*Variable maximum dose constraints for the clinical target volume or clinical target volume–annulus were analyzed.
[†]Dose-volume constraints were set for the brain and brainstem.

penalty (100). On the other hand, we set the minimum and maximum dose constraints for PTV-A at a wider range, 53.2 and 65.8 Gy, respectively. This setting of the dose constraints led to a more inhomogeneous dose distribution within PTV-A than that within PTV-G. However, this dose

inhomogeneity appears to be favorable from the clinical point of view because greater microscopic invasion will be expected within the region closer to PTV-G. The value of $\%V_{110}$ for PTV-A was 40.7%. Table 17.3-3 summarizes the maximum and mean doses for the normal tissues. Isodose distribution curves and DVHs are shown in Figures 17.3-4 and 17.3-5, respectively.

TABLE 17.3-2. Summary of Dose-Volume Histogram Analysis for PTV-G and PTV-A

Targets	Volume, cm^3	Maximum, Gy	D_{95}, Gy	D_{90}, Gy	Mean, Gy	D_{05}, Gy	$\%V_{110}$
PTV-G	63.4	78.0	68.0	70.0*	73.0	76.0	0.6
PTV-A	172.2	72.7	55.0	56.2	60.6	67.0	40.7

D_{95} = dose delivered to 95% of the volume; D_{90} = dose delivered to 90% of the volume; D_{05} = dose delivered to 5% of the volume; PTV-A = planning target volume–annulus; PTV-G = gross tumor volume plus a 0.5 cm margin; $\%V_{110}$ = percentage of the volume receiving greater than 110% of the prescribed dose. *Prescribed dose for PTV-G.

TABLE 17.3-3. Summary of the Dose-Volume Histogram Analysis for Normal Tissues

Organs	Maximum, Gy	D_{05}, Gy	Mean, Gy
Brain	70.6	46.9	19.9
Brainstem	59.4	54.1	42.6
Right eye (retina and optic nerve)	45.8	21.2	9.6
Right lens	6.7		5.4
Left lens	6.3		5.1

D_{05} = dose delivered to 5% of the volume.

Treatment Delivery and Quality Assurance

Treatment was delivered on a Clinac-600C accelerator (Varian Medical Systems) equipped with an 80-leaf dynamic multileaf collimator. The treatment time was approximately 15 to 20 minutes.

Careful quality assurance was performed prior to and throughout the course of treatment. The ability of the MLC to position individual leaves accurately was verified on a weekly basis by exposing film to a test pattern. A 0.1×40 cm^2 slit beam intermittently irradiated the film at 1 cm intervals, yielding narrow, dark lines. A leaf position error > 0.2 mm could be easily detected by viewing the film on a light box. On a daily basis (prior to the start of IMRT treatments), the beam profile through the isocenter was also verified using a diode array (Profiler, Sun Nuclear, Melbourne, FL).

Patient-specific quality assurance involved verification of the intensity maps on portal films for each beam. The identity of the intensity maps from the patients and the phantom was verified by visual inspection. All beams were assessed on the first day of treatment. For verification of the treatment isocenter, lateral and anterior-posterior portal films were taken every day for the first week and weekly thereafter.

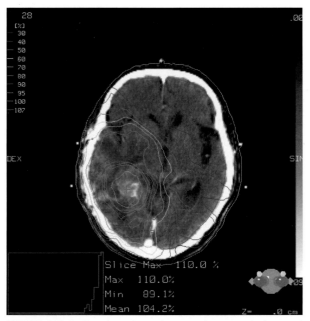

FIGURE 17.3-4. Contrast-enhanced computed tomography image of the treatment plan illustrating the isodose distribution. (To view a color version of this image, please refer to the CD-ROM).

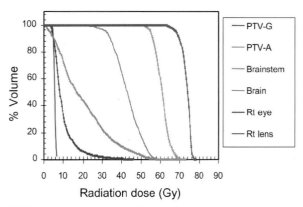

FIGURE 17.3-5. Dose-volume histograms for the target volumes and normal tissues. PTV-A = planning target volume–annulus; PTV-G = gross tumor volume plus a 0.5 cm margin.

Clinical Outcome

The patient tolerated treatment well without any acute or late radiation therapy–related toxicity. Unfortunately, the patient developed progressive disease within the GTV at 5.4 months following treatment. He ultimately died of the disease progression at 16 months after the start of IMRT.

The results of our pilot trial of the SIB technique in patients with malignant glioma undergoing IMRT were recently published.[1] Between December 2000 and November 2002, six patients with malignant gliomas were enrolled in this study. No treatment delays were seen owing to acute toxicity. The tumor recurred locoregionally in five of the six patients. Sites of recurrence were local (within the GTV) in four patients, and in one patient, subependy-mal dissemination was observed. Three patients, two with glioblastoma multiforme and one with anaplastic astro-cytoma, died of the disease at 4, 16, and 7 months after the start of IMRT, respectively.

Based on these results, we recently initiated a phase I clinical trial using SIB IMRT in these patients. The initial dose level consists of 77.5 Gy in 2.5 Gy daily fractions to the PTV-G and 58.9 Gy in 1.9 Gy daily fractions to the PTV-A.

Reference

1. Suzuki M, Nakamatsu K, Kanamori S, et al. Feasibility study of the simultaneous integrated boost (SIB) method for malignant gliomas using intensity-modulated radiotherapy (IMRT). Jpn J Clin Oncol 2003;33:271–7.

Intensity-Modulated Radiosurgery Emerging Technology

Stanley H. Benedict, PhD, Robert M. Cardinale, MD, Danny Song, MD

Stereotactic radiosurgery (SRS) involves the precise delivery of high doses of ionizing radiation to intracranial targets. Because of the importance of neurologic structures and their radiosensitivity, normal tissue sparing is a key goal of the SRS procedure. There have been numerous publications on the development of linear accelerator–based SRS techniques, from arc-based approaches with circular collimators[1] to fixed-field arrangements and dynamic SRS.[2,3] Several investigators have also explored the use of dynamic field shaping of arc-based treatment systems to generate improved isodose distributions for nonspherical targets.[3,4] Others have shown a benefit to noncoplanar fixed fields in terms of dose conformity and dose-volume histogram analysis for selected intracranial targets compared with arc-based treatment.[5,6]

One can now extend these analyses to improve dose conformity with intensity-modulated radiation therapy (IMRT). Recent studies have quantified the advantages of combining the precision of stereotactic positioning with the dose-delivery capabilities of IMRT in the treatment of small critically located targets. In this chapter, the reader is introduced to the (1) dedicated hardware necessary to deliver intensity-modulated stereotactic radiosurgery (IM-SRS), (2) clinical cases demonstrating the potential for improving dose conformity with IM-SRS, and (3) a discussion on forward and inverse planning and optimization of IM-SRS.

Mini–Multileaf Collimators

Provisions for conventional SRS include rigorous requirements for patient fixation, immobilization, repositioning, and relocalization, in addition to high precision requirements for the mechanics of the linear accelerator.[7] The accepted limit for accurate dose delivery for a linear accelerator used in SRS is 1 mm for all gantry, couch, and collimator angles. The mechanical isocenter accuracy for these accelerators is also in the range of ± 1 mm. Any inaccuracy with the mechanics of the linear accelerator is primarily due to gantry sag and alignment of the couch rotation axis.

This tolerance requirement places a very tight accuracy on any design for a multileaf collimator (MLC) system used for SRS delivery. It is important to note that most commercially available MLCs have a leaf positioning accuracy of 1 mm and thus are not acceptable for SRS in which submillimeter precision is required. However, these MLCs may be perfectly acceptable for standard fractionated radiation therapy. Therefore, to deliver IM-SRS and satisfy the stringent requirements for high precision delivery with small treatment fields, substantial hardware development was required to develop "mini and micro" MLC technology.

The primary requirements of an MLC used for SRS include precision and a steep dose gradient (dose falloff). Both features are necessary to protect normal brain tissue (conformity) and adjacent critical structures (avoiding adjacent organs at risk [OAR]) from the high doses. The penumbra is the important parameter in determining how sharply the dose gradient extends beyond the target boundary. The physical characteristics of these mini-MLC devices, specifically the leaf tips, have been designed to satisfy the rigorous requirements for IM-SRS. Although conventional MLCs have penumbra widths between 6 and 8 mm (measured from 80 to 20%), for mini-MLCs, the penumbra widths are on the order of 2.5 to 3.5 mm. Four micro–multileaf collimators (mMLCs) are now commercially available for SRS beam shaping using fixed static fields, dynamic conformal arcing, and IMRT. The specific features of these devices for IM-SRS are presented below and summarized in Table 17.4-1.

NOMOS MIMiC

The MIMiC (North American Scientific, NOMOS Radiation Oncology Division, Cranberry Township, PA)

TABLE 17.4-1. Mini–Multileaf Collimator Technical Specifications and Features

Mini-MLC Manufacturer	North American Scientific MIMiC BEAK	BrainLAB m3	Radionics MMLC	3D-LINE DMLC
Field size at isocenter, cm	0.8 × 20	10.0 × 10.0	10 × 12	10.8 × 12
Number of leaves (pairs)	40 (20)	52 (26)	62 (31)	48 (24)
Leaf width at isocenter	1 cm	14 pairs at 0.3 cm, 6 pairs at 0.45 cm 6 pairs at 0.55 cm	4.0 mm	4.2 mm
Leaf material	Tungsten	Coated tungsten	Tungsten	Tungsten, dual-focused
Leaf transmission, %	1	< 2	< 1	0.2
Interleaf leakage, %	< 1	< 2	< 2	0.5
Maximum leaf speed, cm/s	50	1.0	2.5	2.0
Maximum overcenter travel, cm	Not applicable	5	5	3
Weight, kg	22.7	30	38	32
Treatment planning system	CORVUS	BrainSCAN	X-Knife	ERGO

MLC = multileaf collimator.

is a mini-MLC driven by the *CORVUS* inverse treatment planning software component of the PEACOCK system (North American Scientific). The MIMiC provides a 40-leaf binary temporal modulator specifically designed for the delivery of sequential tomotherapy and was the first MLC developed to deliver IMRT. The device directs thousands of pencil-thin beams at a tumor target, which may be varied in intensity as the gantry rotates. MIMiC can be used with a wide range of linear accelerators to deliver highly conformal dose distributions. In addition, an attachment to the MIMiC, the BEAK slit collimator, fine-tunes the delivery beam further to enhance MIMiC's potential for SRS applications (Figure 17.4-1) (T. Biertempfel, personal communication, 2004). North American Scientific's STAT RS complete SRS package combines MIMiC and BEAK with an immobilization and table indexing system, ensuring the highest level of conformity and steep dose gradients.

BrainLAB m3

The BrainLAB m3 MLC (BrainLAB AG, Heimstetten, Germany) was designed specifically for SRS with 3 mm–thick center leaves, for an effective penumbra of < 3.0 mm for all SRS field sizes (Figure 17.4-2). Over the total field size of 10 × 10 cm, the m3 leaves are of variable width, including 14 pairs of 0.3 cm, 6 pairs of 0.45 cm, and 6 pairs of 0.55 cm leaves. The characteristics of this system have been described.[8,9] Full integration and interlocks with Varian Medical Systems (Palo Alto, CA) and Siemens Medical Solutions (Malvern, PA) linear accelerators allow dynamic treatments in which leaf positioning is continually verified by two independent readouts. The m3 high-resolution mini-MLC can be attached to linear accelerators with or without a standard MLC and can be integrated with most commonly used accelerator types. With the help of a storage trolley, the m3 is quickly attached and removed

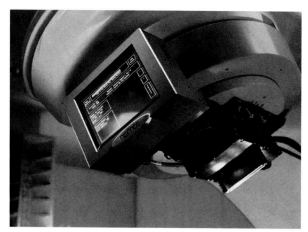

Figure 17.4-1. The NOMOS mini–multileaf collimator system for intensity-modulated stereotactic radiosurgery (includes the MIMiC with the attachment of the BEAKslit collimator system). (To view a color version of this image, please refer to the CD-ROM.)

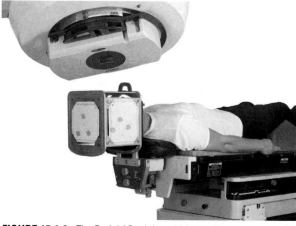

FIGURE 17.4-2. The BrainLAB mini–multi-leaf collimator system for intensity-modulated stereotactic radiosurgery (SRS) (includes the m3, which may be removable, as shown in this photograph, or available on a dedicated SRS linear accelerator) (Novalis [BrainLAB]). (To view a color version of this image, please refer to the CD-ROM.)

from the accessory mount in less than 10 minutes. The m3 leaves move according to the dynamic conformal arc leaf sequence or inverse planning fluency map calculated by the BrainSCAN treatment planning system (D. James, personal communication, 2004).[10]

Radionics MMLC

The Radionics (Tyco Healthcare, Burlington, MA) mini-MLC is called the MMLC and has 31 pairs of 4 mm leaves, with a total field size of 10 × 12 cm and a leaf height of 7 cm of tungsten (Figure 17.4-3). The leaf geometry of the MMLC is divergent lock and key, to minimize leakage and transmission characteristics critical for IMRT. Planning for the MMLC is performed with the *XKnife* (Radionics) software (Z. H. Leber, personal communication, 2004).[11]

3DLINE DMLC

The mMLC manufactured by 3DLINE USA Inc. (Reston, VA) is called the DMLC (dynamic multileaf collimator) and is an autocontrolled dual-focused system (Figure 17.4-4). The DMLC is designed as an accessory for all models of accelerators and consists of 24 tungsten leaf pairs, providing a maximum field size of 10.8 × 12 cm. The dual-focused characteristic of the DMLC is a unique feature, providing a penumbra that is independent of field size. The DMLC is capable of delivering dynamic conformal arcs and IMRT for SRS treatments (C. Azevedo, personal communication, 2004).

Treatment Planning Studies

Traditionally, linear accelerator–based SRS has been delivered with circular collimators using noncoplanar arcs. Several authors have compared this early technique with fixed conformal fields (with blocks or mini-MLC) and even IMRT.[12–15] Cardinale and colleagues demonstrated the dosimetric advantages of IMRT applied to intracranial targets, which were relatively large (9.6–36.7 cm³) and of various geometric shapes, such as an ellipsoid and a hemisphere.[17] Using target volumes derived from actual patients, Benedict and colleagues demonstrated that IMRT using a set of fixed fields and delivered with dynamic mMLC is associated with improved dose distributions for small lesions (1.2–3.5 cm³) when compared with multiple arcs or fixed uniform-intensity fields.[14] These studies demonstrate that circular collimation with arcs is optimal for small spherical lesions. For irregularly shaped lesions, however, substantial improvements are achieved with fixed conformal fields, and a further incremental improvement is achieved with the addition of IMRT. To demonstrate the potential benefits of IMRT applied to SRS, two treatment planning studies are presented below.

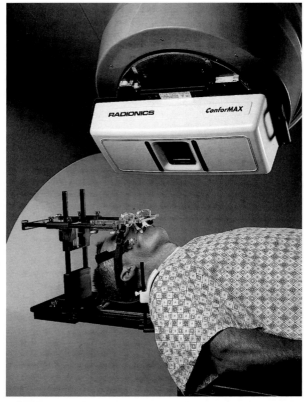

FIGURE 17.4-3. The Radionics mini–multi-leaf collimator system for intensity-modulated stereotactic radiosurgery (includes the MMLC attachment). (To view a color version of this image, please refer to the CD-ROM.)

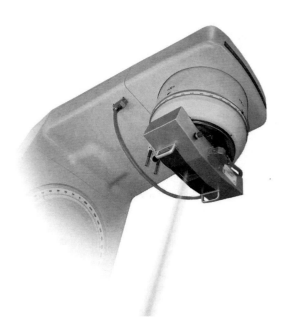

FIGURE 17.4-4. The 3D-LINE mini–multileaf collimator system for intensity-modulated stereotactic radiosurgery (includes the DMLC attachment). (To view a color version of this image, please refer to the CD-ROM.)

Recurrent Ependymoma

In this case, the patient had a recurrent posterior fossa ependymoma adjacent to the brainstem. Multiple plans based on noncoplanar static, uniform-intensity beams defined by the mMLC (BrainLAB m3) were generated. The plans were optimized to provide a minimum percentage of irradiated volume to tumor volume ratio (PITV) and minimal normal tissue irradiation at high dose levels. The PITV and dose-volume histograms of adjacent critical organs were then compared with those from corresponding IM-SRS plans. IM-SRS plans were generated using an institutionally developed IMRT optimization program with varying beam configurations.[16] For all plans, the dose homogeneity within the planning target volume (PTV) was assigned a low priority relative to target conformity and minimization of dose to adjacent structures. The Philips Pinnacle[3] (Philips Pinnacle[3] Systems, Milpitas, CA) treatment planning system, which uses an adaptive convolution calculation algorithm, was used for all dose calculations. For comparison purposes, all plans were prescribed to a dose of 10 Gy, with the requirement that 99% of the target volume receive the prescription dose or greater. The PTV was assigned the same volume as the gross tumor volume (GTV).

For the fixed-field arrangement, an initial beam geometry of 15 fields was used for each plan. The design of the initial fixed-field arrangement was established to incorporate three fields each along five planes of the patient's skull, providing approximately 2π steradian solid-angle coverage. Once the template of 15 fields was scripted to the patient, manual adjustments of 6° to 10° were made in each of the couch and gantry orientations to minimize the dose to critical areas. Beam weights were also optimized by trial and error to provide the prescribed target coverage while minimizing dose contributions to adjacent areas. Block margins for these beams were optimized to yield a minimum PITV and were typically 0.0 to 0.3 cm. Block margin optimization for fixed fields has been previously reported.[13] The BrainLAB m3 collimator angle was optimized to minimize the effects of the leaf trajectories and to provide for increased conformity around the PTV. Simply put, this optimization of collimator angle was chosen such that the sum of the unblocked field areas (external to the optimal block margin owing to the leaf shapes) and the blocked areas internal to the margin was minimized, typically at a value of < 0.5 cm².

The objective function for optimizing intensity distributions in these calculations was specified in terms of dose-volume limits. The criteria used included the requirement that 99% of the target volume should be enclosed in the prescription isodose surface. Penalties for dose inhomogeneity within the target were marginalized relative to those assigned to the conformity index. It is important to note that in the absence of any strong data demonstrating the importance of dose homogeneity in these cases, hot spots within the target volume were assigned a low priority. The dose to normal tissue was constrained to limit the volume allowed to receive a dose higher than a chosen limit without a high penalty.

Figure 17.4-5 illustrates a transverse computed tomography (CT) slice through the center of the tumor. The IMRT plan is derived from many plans produced, and multiple plans were generated for different beam configurations and for a range of values of the objective function parameters. Note that the PTV and the brainstem are positioned very closely. The isodose curves from the multiple fixed fields and IMRT plan for doses of 11, 10, 9, 8, and 5 Gy are overlaid on the transverse CT slice. It is evident that the fixed static field plan is less conformal to the target volume than the IMRT plan. Moreover, the IMRT plan provides a modest additional degree of critical organ avoidance along the border with the brainstem. The advantages realized from the improved conformity achieved with IMRT are demonstrated in the reduced PITV shown in Table 17.4-2. The dose-volume (including target) data in Table 17.4-2 further

TABLE 17.4-2. Intensity-Modulated Stereotactic Radiosurgery and Static Fixed-Field Intercomparison for a Recurrent Ependymoma (Benedict[14])

Plan Type	PITV	Volume 9.0 Gy	Volume 8.0 Gy	Volume 5.0 Gy	Brainstem 9.0 Gy	Brainstem 5.0 Gy
IMRT	1.79	6.14	6.76	15.55	0.89	2.42
Fixed fields	2.12	6.84	8.44	17.39	0.95	2.41

IMRT = intensity-modulated radiation therapy; PITV = percentage of irradiated volume to tumor volume; PTV = planning target volume.
All plans prescribe 10 Gy to 99% of planning target volume; volume of lesion 2.6 cm³. All volumes have units of cm³.

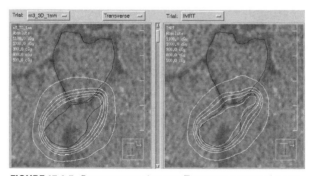

FIGURE 17.4-5. Recurrent ependymoma. Transverse computed tomography scan of dose distributions on a section through the planning target volume (PTV), comparing a plan with 15 fixed-gantry uniform-intensity fields (*left*) and the same fixed-field arrangement with intensity modulation (*right*). All plans were normalized to deliver 10 Gy to 99% of the PTV. The lesion and brainstem are the dark contours, and the dose lines surrounding the lesion are 11, 10, 9, 8, and 5 Gy, respectively. IMRT = intensity-modulated radiation therapy. (To view a color version of this image, please refer to the CD-ROM.)

confirm the sparing of normal tissue with the IMRT technique, showing a reduction of about 20% in the volume of normal tissue treated at the 9 Gy level. Improved sparing of the brainstem is also seen.

This case demonstrates the potential benefit of thin-leafed, dynamic MLC–based IMRT (IM-SRS) for stereotactic irradiation of small lesions. In particular, the IM-SRS plans showed that an additional measure of conformity and reduction to adjacent critical areas could be achieved when IMRT was applied to static fixed fields.

Skull-Based Lesions

Nakamura and colleagues compared gamma-knife SRS to IMRT using an mMLC for several complex skull-based lesions.[17] Given that these lesions are typically irregular in shape, they demonstrate the full capabilities of each system to produce a highly conformal isodose distribution.

The IM-SRS treatment plans were created using a commercial inverse treatment planning system (*CORVUS*, version 4.0), a stand-alone IMRT planning system that uses partial volume data to drive a multifaceted cost function controlling a simulated annealing algorithm.[18] Beam delivery was performed with a simulated 3 mm mMLC (beam delivery characteristics based on the BrainLAB m3 MLC, BrainLAB, Heimstetten, Germany) operating in the step-and-shoot delivery mode.

Gamma-Knife SRS and IM-SRS were compared using a series of indexes, including coverage (ratio of the target volume within the prescribed isodose surface to the total target volume), standard conformity index (ratio of the prescription volume to the target volume), and dose to OAR. Additionally, a new conformity index, as described by Paddick,[19] which takes into account the location of the prescription volume with respect to the target volume, was used. This new conformity index is defined as the ratio of the prescription volume to the target volume within the prescribed isodose surface divided by the coverage. Differences in the Gamma-Knife and IM-SRS plans at lower isodoses were also evaluated by examining the conformity index at 50% of the prescribed dose (defined as the ratio of the volume of tissue receiving 50% of the prescribed dose to the target volume).

The results of this comparison for all 10 patients are summarized in Table 17.4-3. In all cases, IM-SRS plans had better conformity indexes at the level of the prescription isodose, with a mean improvement in the new

conformity index of 20.3% (range 12–31%). The mean conformity index was 1.53 versus 1.25, and the mean new conformity index was 1.73 versus 1.36 for Gamma-Knife SRS versus IM-SRS, respectively.

However, at 50% of the prescribed dose, Gamma-Knife plans were slightly better; in 6 of 10 cases, Gamma-Knife SRS plans demonstrated better conformity. In all cases, IM-SRS plans produced less inhomogeneity within the target compared with Gamma-Knife SRS plans (this may not be clinically relevant, however), reflecting the higher isodose contours to which IM-SRS plans are typically prescribed.

Theoretically, improved conformity at lower isodose contours should improve OAR sparing, yet the IM-SRS plans generally matched the Gamma-Knife doses delivered to OAR. Moreover, all IM-SRS plans made it possible to prescribe to a significantly higher isodose contour than the Gamma-Knife SRS plans, a finding observed in comparisons of linear accelerator–based SRS with Gamma Knife SRS,[20] as well as to multiisocentric linear accelerator SRS.[21]

An additional comparison was the evaluation of overall treatment delivery times for the selected IM-SRS plan and the estimated treatment times with the latest Gamma-Knife model (Model C, Elekta Inc., Norcross, GA), which uses automatic repositioning.[22] The mean delivery time for IM-SRS (averaged over 10 patients) was 44 minutes, whereas the mean Gamma-Knife delivery time was 123 minutes. The nonautomated Gamma Knife required a mean treatment time of 149 minutes. Treatment time is of growing importance, not only from a practical and patient comfort standpoint but also in terms of the reduced biologic effectiveness that may potentially occur when treatment times and delivery are protracted. Treatment variations for extensive and prolonged deliveries have not been routinely corrected to provide equivalent biologic effectiveness, although variations for SRS treatment options requiring minutes versus hours have been demonstrated.[23] The biologic impact of prolonged treatment time is discussed in Chapter 18.9, "Impact of Prolonged Treatment Times: Emerging Technology." This study clearly indicates that this aspect of treatment duration variability should be further investigated.

Forward versus Inverse Planning

In general, many believe that the optimal method of IMRT planning is inverse planning. However, a recent discussion

TABLE 17.4-3. Conformity Indexes (CI) for Gamma-Knife Radiosurgery and Intensity-Modulated Stereotactic Radiosurgery

Lesion	GK Coverage (%)	IM-SRS Coverage (%)	GK CI	IM-SRS CI	GK New CI	IM-SRS New CI	GK CI 50% PD	IM-SRS CI 50% PD
Mean	95.5	95.5	1.53	1.25	1.73	1.36	4.48	4.93

Adapted from Nakamura JL et al.[17]

CI = conformity index; GK = gamma knife; IM-SRS = intensity-modulated stereotactic radiosurgery; PD = prescription dose.

by Hacker and Low suggests that inverse planning may be unnecessary for IM-SRS and that satisfactory results can be obtained by a conventional forward planning approach.[24] Moreover, owing to the simplicity inherent in forward planning IMRT, these IM-SRS treatments may be faster to plan, easier to verify, and more reliable to deliver.

Hacker and colleagues described a forward planning IM-SRS technique whereby initial beam approaches and apertures are set based on conventional beam's eye view SRS planning.[25] Using an iterative process, the isodose distributions are assessed, field apertures are modified, and a small number of subfields are added to a subset of field approaches. This technique was compared with inverse planned IMRT using dynamic mMLC delivery and was evaluated for normal tissue involvement, target coverage, dose homogeneity, and OAR sparing. For all categories, the two approaches result in comparable performance.

Although there is little dosimetric difference between forward and inverse IMRT, there are substantial practical advantages to forward planning, most notably a reduction in the required quality assurance. Given that forward planning uses a few relatively large subfields, standard hand calculation models can be used to verify the dose. This is in contrast to inverse planning, in which the complex fluence maps must be verified with patient-specific phantom measurements, typically requiring a minimum of 2 to 3 hours. This time can be of critical importance in SRS in which a rigid and invasive head frame is used, and patients need to be treated within hours of simulation. Forward planning should also be less prone to delivery errors caused by small errors in mMLC characterization and calibration. Given these practical advantages to forward planning and the lack of any compelling dosimetric advantage for either, this approach may clearly be the preferable choice for IM-SRS.

An additional consideration is the optimization of beam orientation. Although fluence modulation may improve dose conformity for larger volumes, Kulik and colleagues demonstrated that for small target volumes, the selection of beam orientations is more important.[23] Moreover, this study demonstrated that beam orientation optimization improves doses to normal structures relative to larger numbers of preselected orientations. Thus, the process of optimizing beam directions, which can be easily performed by an experienced SRS planner, is more complex compared with fluence modulation because the influence of reorienting beams on the dose distribution is highly nonlinear.

However, there are limitations inherent in the use of manual SRS planning techniques to consider all or at least a large number of possible delivery combinations. Therefore, this method will, at some point, be replaced by automated techniques. Indeed, as the sophistication of both the treatment planner and commercial systems expands, the benefits of inverse planning will ideally be exploited for the patient's benefit. Additionally, quality assurance of inverse planning dose delivery, now requiring a significant workforce, will become more convenient, ultimately using automated calculation–based verification methods.

Future Directions

The potential for further improvement in IM-SRS planning is possible using dynamic micro–multileaf collimation. IM-SRS has been shown to provide dosimetric improvements for small, highly irregularly shaped lesions of the brain when compared with complex, multiisocenter linear accelerator–based stereotactic arc plans or with uniform-intensity fixed static field plans. In addition to improved dose conformity and minimization of dose outside the PTV, IM-SRS provides an additional option for prioritizing dose minimization to adjacent critical areas. IM-SRS with an mMLC has the potential for superior treatment planning relative to uniform-intensity, fixed-field, arc-based methods with circular collimators and even the gamma knife.

A future direction in IM-SRS is the explicit consideration and avoidance of critical structures that surround the target. These subregions may be manually defined or located using functional imaging modalities.[24,26] As the technology of functional brain mapping improves, one may be able to use this information to limit the dose to specific areas of the brain in an attempt to retain specific brain functions. Given these new developments, IM-SRS will be instrumental in the treatment planning of these patients.

References

1. Lutz W, Winston KR, Maleki N. A system for stereotactic radiosurgery with a linear accelerator. Int J Radiat Oncol Biol Phys 1988;14:373–81.

2. Podgorsak EB, Olivier A, Pla M, et al. Dynamic stereotactic radiosurgery. Int J Radiat Oncol Biol Phys 1988;14:115–26.

3. Leavitt DD, Gibbs FA, Heilbrun MP, et al. Dynamic field shaping to optimize stereotactic radiosurgery. Int J Radiat Oncol Biol Phys 1991;21:1247–55.

4. Nedzi LA, Kooy HM, Alexander E, et al. Dynamic field shaping for stereotactic radiosurgery: a modeling study. Int J Radiat Oncol Biol Phys 1993;25:859–69.

5. Bourland JD, McCollough KP. Static field conformal stereotactic radiosurgery: physical techniques. Int J Radiat Oncol Biol Phys 1993;28:471–9.

6. Marks LB, Sherouse GW, Das S, et al. Conformal radiation therapy with fixed shaped coplanar or noncoplanar radiation beam boquets: a possible alternative to radiosurgery. Int J Radiat Oncol Biol Phys 1995;33:1209–19.

7. Schell MC, Bova FJ, Larson DA, et al. Stereotactic radiosurgery. AAPM Report No.: 54. Woodbury (NY): American Institute of Physics Inc.; 1995.

8. Xia P, Geis P, Xing L, et al. Physical characteristics of a miniature multileaf collimator. Med Phys 1999;26:65–70.

9. Cosgrove VP, Jahn U, Pfaender M, et al. Commissioning of a micro multi-leaf collimator and planning system for stereotactic radiosurgery. Radiother Oncol 1999;50:325–36.

10. Solberg TD, Boedeker KL, Fogg R, et al. Dynamic arc radiosurgery field shaping: a comparison with static field conformal and noncoplanar circular arcs. Int J Radiat Oncol Biol Phys 2001;49:1481–91.

11. Shiu AS, Kooy HM, Ewton JR, et al. Comparison of miniature multileaf collimation (mMLC) with circular collimation for stereotactic treatment. Int J Radiat Oncol Biol Phys 1997;37:679–88.

12. Woo SY, Grant WH, Bellezza D, et al. A comparison of intensity modulated conformal therapy with a conventional external beam stereotactic radiosurgery system for the treatment of single and multiple intracranial lesions. Int J Radiat Oncol Biol Phys 1996;35:593–7.

13. Cardinale RM, Benedict SH, Wu Q, et al. A comparison of three stereotactic radiotherapy techniques: arcs vs. non-coplanar fixed fields vs. intensity modulation. Int J Radiat Oncol Biol Phys 1998;42:431–6.

14. Benedict SH, Cardinale RM, Wu Q, et al. Intensity-modulated stereotactic radiosurgery using dynamic micro-multileaf collimation. Int J Radiat Oncol Biol Phys 2001;50:751–8.

15. Kulik C, Caudrelier J-M, Vermandel M, et al. Conformal radiotherapy optimization with micromultileaf collimators: comparison with radiosurgery techniques. Int J Radiat Oncol Biol Phys 2002;53:1038–50.

16. Wu Q, Mohan R. Algorithms and functionality of an IMRT optimization system. Med Phys 2000;27:701–11.

17. Nakamura JL, Pirzkall, A, Carol, MP, et al. Comparison of intensity-modulated radiosurgery with gamma knife radiosurgery for challenging skull base lesions. Int J Radiat Oncol Biol Phys 2003;55:99–109.

18. Carol MP, Nash R, Campbell R, et al. DVH-based inverse treatment planning: partial volume prescription and area cost function. Med Phys 1997;24:1078.

19. Paddick I. A simple scoring ratio to index the conformity of plans. J Neurosurg 2000;93 Suppl 3:219–22.

20. Ma L, Xia P, Verhey LJ, et al. A dosimetric comparison of fan-beam intensity modulated radiotherapy with gamma knife radiosurgery for treating intermediate intracranial lesions. Int J Radiat Oncol Biol Phys 1999;45:1325–30.

21. Shiu AS, Kooy HM, Ewton JR, et al. Comparison of miniature multileaf collimation (MMLC) with circular collimation for stereotactic treatment. Int J Radiat Oncol Biol Phys 1997; 37:679–88.

22. Horstmann GA, Schopgens H, van Eck AT, et al. First clinical experience with the automatic positioning system and Leksell gamma knife model C: technical note. J Neurosurg 2000;93:193–7.

23. Benedict SH, Lin P-S, Zwicker RD, et al. The biological effectiveness of intermittent irradiation as a function of overall treatment time: development of correction factors for linac-based stereotactic radiotherapy. Int J Radiat Oncol Biol Phys 1997;37:765–9.

24. Hacker F, Low D. Point/counterpoint: compared with inverse-planning, forward planning is preferred for IMRT stereotactic radiosurgery. Med Phys 2003;30:731–4.

25. Hacker F, Zygmanski P, Ramakrishna N. A comparison of forward planned IMRT to inverse planned IMRT for stereotactic radiotherapy. Med Phys 2002;29:1367.

26. Hamilton R, Sweeney PJ, Pelizzari CA, et al. Functional imaging in treatment planning of brain lesions. Int J Radiat Oncol Biol Phys 1997;37:181–8.

Chapter 18

HEAD AND NECK CANCER

OVERVIEW

AVRAHAM EISBRUCH, MD

Advancements in computer technology and imaging in the late 1980s introduced methods to identify the targets for irradiation of head and neck cancer on computed tomography (CT) scans and display the radiation beams in three dimensions relative to the anatomy. The introduction of multileaf collimators (MLCs) facilitated an increase in the number of beams that could be delivered without a large extension of treatment time, and methods to evaluate and compare rival plans using dose-volume histograms (DVHs) became available. Treatment could now be delivered from multiple angles, including noncoplanar directions, when required. The result was the emergence of three-dimensional conformal radiotherapy (3DCRT), which allowed better precision of irradiation delivery to image-based targets, and some improvements in the sparing of noninvolved critical tissue. Early studies of the utility of 3DCRT in head and neck cancer examined cancers of the larynx, nasopharynx, hypopharynx, and paranasal sinus.[1–4] These studies demonstrated a significant benefit from 3DCRT in better coverage of the tumors and reduced doses to critical tissue compared with standard techniques. In the community, 3DCRT became increasingly used, essentially using the traditional arrangement of three fields while using beam's eye views to ensure adequate coverage of the targets (standard radiation therapy [RT]).

The use of three-dimensional technology has been applied mostly to the boost phase of treatment. An analysis of the results of 3DCRT of nasopharyngeal cancer at Memorial Sloan-Kettering Cancer Center showed no difference in the outcome of patients treated with standard techniques compared with more recent patients whose boost phase was delivered with 3DCRT.[5] These authors concluded that further benefit could be gained if highly conformal doses were delivered throughout therapy, not just during the boost. More advanced techniques would be required for this end. Intensity-modulated radiation therapy (IMRT) facilitates a higher degree of dose conformity and offers opportunities for additional clinical gains.

Rationale

The anatomy of the neck is complex, with many critical and radiation-sensitive organs in close proximity to the targets. Tight dose gradients around the targets that limit the doses to the noninvolved tissue, features characteristic of IMRT, are desirable and offer the potential for therapeutic gains. Noninvolved tissues whose sparing may offer tangible gains include the major salivary glands, the minor salivary glands dispersed within the oral cavity, and the mandible. In cases of nasopharyngeal and paranasal sinus cancer, critical normal tissue that may be partly spared using IMRT includes the inner and middle ears, temporomandibular joints, temporal brain lobes, and optic pathways.

In addition to noninvolved tissue sparing, IMRT offers the potential for improved tumor control by reducing the constraints on the tumor dose owing to critical organs (eg, the spinal cord, brainstem, and optic pathways) that may limit the tumor boost doses in conventional RT (Figure 18-1). This is achieved by specifying a maximum dose to the critical organs and a high penalty in the optimization process if that dose is exceeded. In addition, IMRT eliminates the need for posterior neck electron fields, which are commonly used in conventional RT, and their associated dose deficiencies. IMRT in the head and neck is more feasible than in other sites because organ motion is practically absent. The only factor that has to be taken into account is patient setup uncertainties. This can be addressed by using adequate immobilization and by assessing the resulting setup variations.

Patient Selection

Head and neck IMRT is labor intensive and lengthens treatment time. Not every patient is expected to benefit. Those who would benefit the most are patients with paranasal sinus or advanced nasopharyngeal cancer in whom the targets are near the optic pathways, patients with oropharyngeal or nasopharyngeal cancer in whom standard RT fields would encompass most of the salivary glands, and, similarly, patients with laryngeal cancer who present with advanced nodal disease.

In many patients with locally advanced head and neck tumors, standard techniques would require a compromise in the tumor dose owing to the proximity of the tumor to the spinal cord or to the brainstem. In these cases, the advantage of IMRT, through its ability to produce concave dose distributions, is obvious (see Figure 18-1). Patients with laryngeal cancer and clinically noninvolved cervical lymph nodes receiving treatment to the larynx alone or requiring irradiation of the neck encompassing the jugulodigastric nodes but not extending to the base of the skull may not benefit from IMRT compared with simpler techniques. The same applies to patients requiring irradiation to the ipsilateral neck alone.

Additional concerns relate to the doses delivered to the oral cavity in cases of oral cavity or oropharyngeal cancer, in which IMRT may have an advantage over standard RT in partial sparing of the oral cavity, especially where the primary tumor is lateralized. Such sparing is expected to reduce the extent of acute mucositis and improve long-term xerostomia through the reduction in the volume of the minor salivary glands exposed to high radiation doses.

Immobilization

Head and neck immobilization is typically performed using a thermoplastic mask with several attachment points to the treatment table and a head support. Several commercial systems are available. Typically, immobilization with these systems results in daily setup errors of a few millimeters.[6] These errors require an extension of the targets by 3 to 5 mm to ensure adequate irradiation (see "Planning Target Volumes").

If the targets in the lower neck and the supraclavicular nodes are included in the IMRT plans, it is important to extend the mask to include the lower neck and shoulders, such that the lower neck is immobilized. This may enhance skin reactions in the low-lateral neck owing to a bolus effect of the mask, which increases the dose to the skin delivered by beams, which are tangential to the skin. In our experience, cutting holes in the low-lateral parts of the mask, bilaterally, reduces the skin effects remarkably (Figure 18-2).

An alternative used in many institutions is to treat the lower neck with an anterior field. This field matches to the IMRT fields treating the primary tumor and the upper neck using a split-beam technique. In these cases, the head and upper neck alone need to be immobilized. Skin effects are expected to be less severe using this method, and the time required for target delineation is reduced. However, in these cases, the targets in the low neck are not expected to receive the full prescribed doses. This approach is justified when the risk of subclinical disease in the low neck is small, such as in patients with no or minimal clinical evidence of upper neck disease.

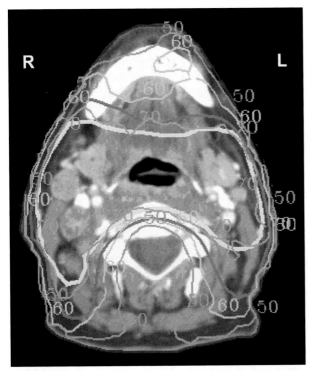

FIGURE 18-1. Isodose distributions of an intensity-modulated radiation therapy plan for posterior pharyngeal wall cancer. The concave shapes of the planning target volumes (PTVs) of the tumor and lymph node metastases (*yellow*) and the PTV of subclinical disease (*blue*) are well covered by the prescribed isodoses (70 and 60 Gy, respectively). In contrast, it is apparent that a standard radiation therapy plan would underdose the PTVs had off-cord lateral beams and abutted posterior neck electrons been used after delivering the initial 44 to 46 Gy by wide lateral beams. (To view a color version of this image, please refer to the CD-ROM.)

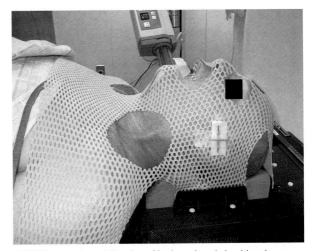

FIGURE 18-2. Immobilization of both neck and shoulders is necessary if the targets in the low neck are included in the intensity-modulated radiation therapy plans. Cutting holes in the mask in the low neck, bilaterally, reduces skin reactions. (To view a color version of this image, please refer to the CD-ROM.)

Imaging

The simulation contrast-enhanced CT is, in most cases, the only imaging modality required for the delineation of the targets. Magnetic resonance imaging (MRI) is limited by its sensitivity to artifacts, difficulty in interpretation, long examination time, and cost. MRI is a necessary adjunct to CT for tumors close to the base of the skull, that is, nasopharyngeal and paranasal sinus cancer, in which it provides better details of tumor extension and better details of the parapharyngeal and retropharyngeal spaces compared with CT (Figure 18-3).[7] MRI is therefore essential for delineating the targets in these cases (see Chapter 18.1, "Nasopharyngeal Cancer: Case Study").

[18]Fluorodeoxyglucose positron emission tomography ([18]FDG-PET) has recently been found to add significantly to the staging information gained from CT regarding the tumor extent in lung cancer.[8] It was anticipated that similar benefit would be demonstrated in head and neck cancer. However, a series of head and neck cancer in which CT, MRI, and [18]FDG-PET were obtained, and surgery was then performed to validate the primary tumor extent and lymph node involvement, reported a rather limited benefit of [18]FDG-PET compared with CT or MRI.[9] (See Chapter 18.6, "Functional Imaging in Head and Neck Cancer: Emerging Technology") Thus, [18]FDG-PET remains, for the time being, a research tool for defining the extent of the target (an exception is defining the target in recurrent cancer, in which [18]FDG-PET has demonstrated a higher utility than CT or

MRI). We use [18]FDG-PET in cases in which the demonstration of [18]FDG avidity would change target delineation, for example, where borderline enlarged nodes are noted on the CT scan in a neck level that has been judged to be at low risk of metastases. In all cases, the findings of a careful clinical examination, including direct endoscopy under anesthesia, form the basis for assessing the extent of the primary tumor.

Target Selection and Delineation

A major potential pitfall of IMRT is the failure to select and delineate the targets accurately. This is especially relevant in head and neck cancer, in which a high risk of subclinical local and nodal disease exists and adequate irradiation of the lymph nodes at risk is crucial for local-regional control and survival. For example, in standard three-field RT of oropharyngeal cancer, the first echelon and the retropharyngeal nodes are treated when the primary tumor is targeted. In contrast, these nodes will not be adequately irradiated by IMRT if they are not specified as targets on the planning CT.

The gross tumor volumes (GTVs) consist of the primary tumor and of lymph nodes with apparent or suspected metastasis. Lymph node GTVs include nodes with radiologic criteria of involvement: diameter > 1 cm (in the case of the jugulodigastric nodes, > 1.1–1.5 cm), smaller nodes with spherical rather than ellipsoid shape, nodes containing inhomogeneities suggestive of necrotic centers, or a

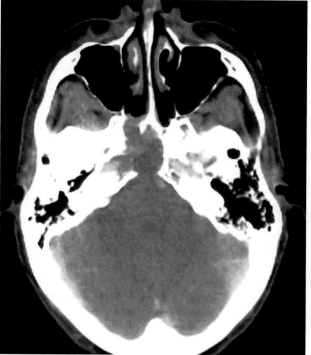
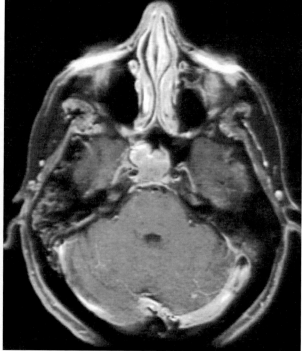

FIGURE 18-3. Computed tomography and magnetic resonance images at comparable levels in a case of locally advanced nasopharyngeal cancer. The extent of the primary tumor near the base of the skull is better appreciated in the magnetic resonance image.

cluster of three or more borderline nodes, or PET-positive nodes.[10] The clinical target volume (CTV) surrounding the primary tumor consists of tissue perceived to contain a microscopic, subclinical tumor extension. In addition to the primary tumor CTV, the lymphatic CTVs consist of nodal areas that are at risk of metastatic disease but do not match the radiologic criteria of involved nodes.

Primary Tumor CTV Delineation

Factors used for assessing the extent of the CTV margins in each case include tumor site, size, stage, differentiation, and morphology (exophytic vs ulcerative, infiltrative vs pushing front). Rather than expand the GTV uniformly, we recommend outlining the CTV on the planning CT on a slice-by-slice basis. A knowledge of the anatomic and clinical patterns of tumor extension, clinical judgment, and a familiarity with head and neck imaging are necessary for accurate estimation of the CTV margins around the tumor. Specific recommendations for each tumor site have been detailed elsewhere.[11]

Lymphatic CTV Selection and Delineation

Our knowledge of the pattern and risk of lymphatic drainage from different head and neck sites is based on the classic anatomic work of Rouviere,[12] reviewed recently[13]; the assessment of the location and prevalence of clinical neck metastasis by Lindberg[14]; and the large experience with elective neck dissections providing information about microscopic metastases, reported by Byers and colleagues and Shah.[15,16] A division of the neck to six levels has been developed by surgeons from Memorial Sloan-Kettering Hospital and revised by Robbins and colleagues, allowing standardized and improved reporting of the nodal involvement and surgical therapy of the neck.[17,18]

Adoption of this system for identification and outlining of the nodal CTVs for IMRT is highly recommended. It should be emphasized that the retropharyngeal nodes, which are not routinely dissected surgically, are not considered in the classification of surgical neck levels but are important targets in the irradiation of nasopharyngeal and other advanced head and neck cancer. Reviews of the risk of metastases to each neck level and of the neck levels at risk for each tumor site and stage were published recently.[11,19]

Several publications are recommended for identifying the neck levels on the planning CT scans. An imaging-based nodal classification, using CT- or MRI-based criteria that correspond to the surgical anatomic landmarks, has been developed by head and neck radiologists.[20] In addition, several recent articles have been published by radiation oncologists demonstrating how to outline the lymph node neck levels as CTVs on the planning CT scans[19,21–23] or axial MRIs.[19] A recent consensus about the delineation of the target in the N0 neck has been reached by major cooperative radiotherapy groups. Details of this consensus and a detailed atlas that shows the CTVs in each axial slice of a head and neck CT scan are available on the Radiation Therapy Oncology Group (RTOG) Web site.[24] We have found this atlas to be highly practical.

In the node-positive neck, it is important to take into account "upstream" and "downstream" extension of metastases owing to lymphatic obstruction and higher risk of metastatic disease in neighboring neck levels that would be at low risk had the neck been negative or minimally involved. For example, in cases of oropharyngeal cancer, level IB and V and the retropharyngeal nodes are at risk in the neck side in which level II is involved and should therefore be defined as targets. Had level II been clinically noninvolved in these cases, nodal levels IB and V would be at very low risk.

Details about the selection of lymphatic CTVs for each head and neck site are provided elsewhere[11] and in the site-specific chapters of this book. An example of the delineation of the targets, as practiced at the University of Michigan, is provided in Figure 18-4. Several general principles are suggested:

1. In cases of lateralized cancers in which only the ipsilateral neck would ordinarily require therapy, contralateral neck treatment is always added when the ipsilateral neck nodal stage is greater than N1.

2. Level II (upper jugular) neck nodes are the most frequent metastatic site for tumors originating in most mucosal sites. These nodes can be divided into the subdigastric (jugulodigastric) nodes, located below the level at which the posterior belly of the digastric muscle crosses the jugular vein (see Figure 18-4C), and more cranially located nodes below the base of the skull ("junctional" nodes according to Million and colleagues, corresponding to the upper level IIB[25]). The subdigastric nodes are the main nodes involved when contralateral metastasis occurs, whereas the more cephalad nodes are at risk bilaterally in cases of nasopharyngeal cancer and in the neck side that contains gross level II to III metastasis. At the University of Michigan, the subdigastric nodes are defined as the cranial (superior)-most targets in the clinically N0 neck that is contralateral to the primary tumor in non-nasopharyngeal cases.

3. Level IB (submandibular) and IV (low jugular) nodes are treated in all cases in the neck side with clinical involvement of levels II or III.

4. Level V (posterior neck) nodes are treated in the neck side with involvement of levels II to IV, in all cases.

5. The retropharyngeal nodes are treated bilaterally in all cases of oropharyngeal and hypopharyngeal cancer with clinical involvement of levels II to IV (in cases of early lateralized oropharyngeal tumors with small N1 disease, they are outlined ipsilaterally).

6. Level VI (prelaryngeal and pretracheal) nodes are treated in all cases with clinical involvement of level IV nodes.

7. In cases in which there is radiographic evidence of extracapsular lymph node metastatic spread, a large part of the involved muscle is included in the CTV (see Figure 18-4D).

In postoperative cases, the surgical specimens provide information that helps in determining the neck levels at risk. Neck dissection disrupts some of the anatomic landmarks used to define the borders between the levels. On the other hand, the surgical bed is apparent on the CT scan and should be encompassed entirely within the CTV. It is often impossible to distinguish between the primary tumor resection

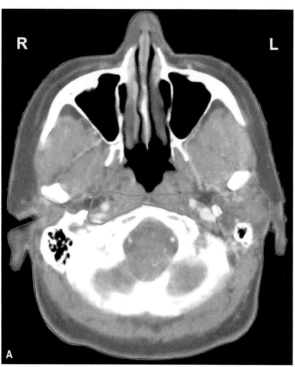

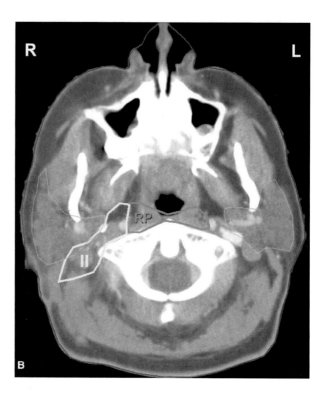

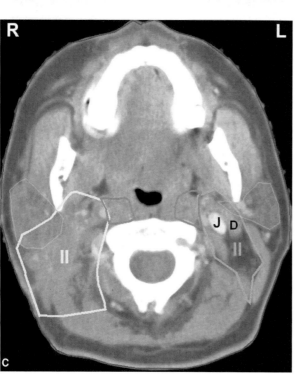

FIGURE 18-4. Delineation of neck nodal clinical target volumes (CTVs) in a case of oropharyngeal cancer metastatic to the right neck. The CTVs of each neck level were outlined separately. In clinical practice, levels that receive the same dose are encompassed by one CTV line. All of the CTVs need to be expanded uniformly by 3 to 5 mm to yield the corresponding planning target volumes. Green: parotid glands. *(A)*, The retropharyngeal nodal CTV is outlined bilaterally. Ipsilateral to the tumor (*right*), the CTV also encompasses the jugular vein and carotid artery. *(B)*, At a lower (caudal) cut, level II is outlined in the ipsilateral (right) side of the neck, whereas the retropharyngeal nodes (RP) are outlined bilaterally. *(C)* On the axial computed tomography (CT) image in which the posterior belly of the digastric muscle (D) crosses the jugular vein (J), level II is outlined as a target in the left side of the neck, which was contralateral to the primary tumor and did not contain gross metastases. The lateral retropharyngeal nodes (*blue*) are outlined bilaterally, medial to the carotid arteries. (To view a color version of this image, please refer to the CD-ROM.) *Continued on next page.*

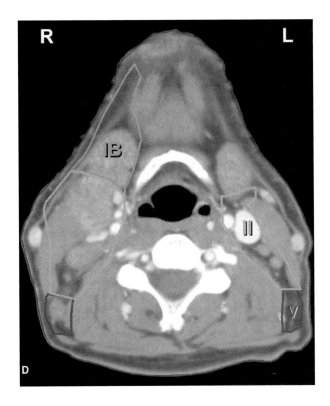

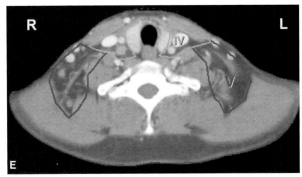

FIGURE 18-4 Continued. *(D)* Gross metastatic disease is apparent in right levels II and V. Level IB is therefore included in the right neck targets (but not in the left side of the neck). The nodal metastasis in right level II shows gross extracapsular invasion. Therefore, most or all of the sternocleidomastoid muscle is encompassed within level II CTV. In contrast, only the fatty tissue containing lymph nodes is encompassed within the CTVs in the left side of the neck, where nodal extracapsular extension is not suspected. *(E)* In the lower neck, several metastases are seen in right level V. The distribution of these metastases corresponds to distribution of the transverse cervical veins, which are also seen in this CT image and illustrate how wide and posterior in the neck level V should be outlined. It is clear that using an anterior low-neck field and prescribing its dose to 3 cm depth would underdose large volumes of level V. (To view a color version of this image, please refer to the CD-ROM.)

bed and the adjacent neck dissection bed. Thus, these are encompassed within a unified CTV (Figure 18-5). Neck levels in which microscopic extracapsular lymph node extension has been found are considered high-risk CTVs. Chao and colleagues recommended extension of the delineation of these targets to the skin.[23] At the University of Michigan, the CTVs in the neck levels with extracapsular lymph node extension are assigned a higher dose (see below).

Planning Target Volumes

After the GTVs and the CTVs are delineated on the axial CT images, a uniform expansion of these targets is performed to obtain the planning target volumes (PTVs) that accommodate setup uncertainties (typically by 3–5 mm). Doses are prescribed to the PTVs or to comparable "growth" areas in some commercial planning systems. When the targets are close to the skin, as may occur in postoperative cases, the PTV may extend beyond the surface. In such cases, the PTV should be "edited" back to the surface. If the PTV extends to the skin, but the skin is not at high risk, the external body contour may be defined as a noninvolved organ for the optimization system. This may facilitate avoiding excessive dosing to the skin.[26]

Similar to the expansion of the targets to yield the PTVs, there is a need to accommodate uncertainties regarding the critical normal organs, especially the spinal cord, brainstem, and optic pathways, that may lie in regions of steep

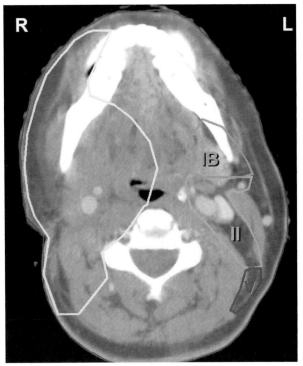

Figure 18-5. Clinical target volume (CTV) outlined in a postoperative case. Right neck dissection and excision of right oral cancer were performed. The CTV in the right neck includes all of the surgical bed (*yellow*). This encompasses the neck levels at risk and the primary tumor surgical bed. (To view a color version of this image, please refer to the CD-ROM.)

dose falloff near the targets. This can be accomplished by expanding these organs uniformly, yielding the planning risk volumes (PRVs).[27] At the University of Michigan, the spinal cord is expanded by 0.5 cm to yield the spinal cord PRV. The maximal accepted doses are 45 Gy to the spinal cord and 50 Gy to the PRV. Similarly, the optic nerves and chiasm are expanded by 3 to 5 mm for treatment plans of nasopharynx or paranasal sinus tumors.

No margins are usually given to accommodate potential organ motion in head and neck IMRT. In a study of intrafraction motion of the larynx during RT, it was found that the incidence and duration of swallowing were very low; therefore, they need not be taken into account. However, the tip of the epiglottis was found to move within a range of 7 mm.[28] This may have implications for the expansion of the primary target in cases of supraglottic larynx cancer.

Prescription and Normal Tissue Dose Constraints

The delivery of a single treatment plan throughout the course of treatment provides better dose conformity compared with several consecutive plans[29] and is therefore typical of IMRT. This deviates substantially from the practice of standard RT for head and neck cancer. When a single plan is prescribed, the gross tumor PTV receives both a higher total dose and a higher dose per fraction than the PTVs representing subclinical disease. Owing to the differences in the daily fraction doses, a correction of the total dose to yield the normalized total dose (NTD) for a 2 Gy fraction regimen is required when the fraction dose is substantially different from standard fractionation. An extensive discussion of this issue is provided by Mohan and colleagues.[29] (See Chapter 18.7, "Simultaneous Integrated Boost: Emerging Technology.")

Dose prescription modes for head and neck IMRT can be divided into two general approaches. The first would be the prescription of total dose and treatment duration that deliver a standard fraction dose of 2 Gy to the gross disease PTV, for example, 70 Gy over 35 fractions, whereas lower-than-standard fraction doses are prescribed to the subclinical disease PTVs. For example, a total prescribed dose of 64 Gy to high-risk subclinical PTVs (tissue at risk near the primary tumor, tumor resection bed, first echelon nodes) and 60 Gy to lesser-risk elective target PTVs would deliver (over 35 treatments) daily fraction doses of 1.8 Gy and 1.7 Gy, respectively. These would yield NTDs of 60 and 56 Gy, respectively (the NTDs are calculated for late-reacting tissue, assuming $\alpha/\beta = 3$ Gy). When used for advanced disease, this schedule should be delivered concurrently with chemotherapy. This approach is used at the University of Michigan for stage III to IV head and neck cancer, and the chemotherapy agents delivered concurrently with IMRT consist of combinations of cisplatin or carboplatin and paclitaxel.

The second strategy is to deliver a higher-than-standard fraction dose to the gross disease PTV, adjusting the total dose to yield NTD near 70 Gy, and standard fraction doses to the elective target PTVs. Such a strategy was adopted by the RTOG study of IMRT for oropharyngeal cancer (RTOG study H-0022). In this study, the gross disease PTV receives a total of 66 Gy in 30 fractions, yielding 2.2 Gy/fraction. PTVs of high-risk subclinical disease receive 60 Gy, and low-risk PTVs receive 54 Gy, yielding 2.0 and 1.8 Gy/fraction, respectively. This results in the gross disease PTV receiving an NTD of 70 Gy over 6 weeks, similar to the total time and dose delivered by an accelerated RT regimen.[30]

More aggressive reported regimens rely on the high conformity achieved by IMRT to deliver higher than standard NTDs to the gross disease PTVs. Investigators at Baylor College of Medicine reported a regimen with a total of 60 Gy in 25 fractions (2.4 Gy/fraction) to the gross disease and 50 Gy (2.0 Gy/fraction) to electively treated volumes. This treatment course yields an NTD of 66 Gy delivered over 5 weeks, representing an aggressive accelerated course.[31] If one accounts for the relatively large target dose inhomogeneity produced by IMRT, it is apparent that large tissue volumes within the targets receive even higher doses per fraction and thus a higher NTD. Lee and colleagues reported the University of California at San Francisco (UCSF) experience, in which a prescribed GTV dose of 70 Gy was delivered at 2.12 to 2.25 Gy/fraction over 31 to 33 fractions.[32] The prescribed dose was close to the minimal dose encompassing the target to avoid target underdosing. This yielded a mean GTV dose of 74.5 Gy and mean GTV dose per fraction of 2.24 to 2.4 Gy. The resulting NTD (calculated for late-responding tissue) approaches 80 Gy.

A phase I dose escalation study is currently being conducted at the Medical College of Virginia in which the fraction size and the total dose to the gross disease PTVs are escalated from 68.1 to 73.8 Gy over 6 weeks, whereas the doses to subclinical PTVs are kept constant at 54 to 60 Gy over the same period.[33,34] It is postulated that limiting the high-dose volume to the target alone by IMRT may reduce the risk of late complications arising from large fraction doses.[31,33] However, critical normal tissues at risk in the head and neck (eg, nerves, noninvolved mucosa, blood vessels, bone) are embedded within the targets and are thus at risk of late toxicity. These schemes, therefore, should be performed only within a well-defined clinical trial. As yet, the follow-up periods of published head and neck cancer IMRT series are not yet sufficient to assess the risk of late complications arising from such an approach.[31,32]

Dose and dose/volume specifications are made to impose constraints on the DVHs of the targets, noninvolved tissue of interest, and nonspecified tissue outside the targets. RTOG protocol H-0022 (IMRT of early-stage oropharyngeal cancer) specifies the prescription dose as the dose that encompasses at least 95% of the PTV. No more than 20% of the PTV can receive > 110%, and no more than 1% of the PTV can receive < 93% of the prescribed dose. To limit hot spots outside the targets, the protocol specifies that no more than 1% of the tissue outside the PTVs can receive > 110% of the prescribed dose. These goals can be accomplished by adding a dose constraint for all nonspecified tissue (all tissue outside the targets and the specified organs) to prevent volumes of high dose outside the targets.

Dose constraints regarding critical organs are usually stated in terms of the maximal dose. Commonly applied constraints in the head and neck are maximal doses of 45 Gy to the spinal cord, 54 Gy to the brainstem, 70 Gy to the mandible, and 50 to 55 Gy to the optic pathway. These constraints were derived from standard irradiation, in which the organs at risk typically receive irradiation at a standard daily fraction dose for part of the therapy course and are then fully shielded. In contrast, IMRT delivers lower daily fraction doses to these organs throughout therapy. In addition, the maximal dose derived from the DVH represents only a small organ volume, whereas standard RT delivers the specified doses homogeneously to relatively large volumes. Therefore, in most instances, the same dose constraints are much more conservative when applied to IMRT compared with standard RT.

On the other hand, steep dose falloff near the critical organs may increase the risk of inadvertent overdosage to these organs owing to motion and setup uncertainties. This issue can be addressed by a uniform expansion of the critical organs to yield the PRVs, as discussed above. Organs with parallel functional architecture require specification of the mean dose or partial organ volume dose rather than the maximum dose. Examples are the specification in RTOG protocol H-0022 of the maximal mean dose to the parotid salivary glands at 26 Gy or limiting the dose to at least 50% of the gland volume to < 30 Gy and constraining the dose to two-thirds of the larynx at < 50 Gy.

Beam Number and Orientation

IMRT using MLCs requires one to choose the number and orientation of the treatment beams. It was suggested early on that if the number of segments (or beamlets) is large enough, the direction of the beams is not important, and coplanar beams arranged at equidistance around the patient's head and neck would achieve satisfactory results. Most investigations of IMRT of the head and neck with MLCs use this approach.

The beam number should be odd to prevent opposed beams, which would increase hot spots near their entrance to the neck. Nine beams arranged at equidistance (40° apart) were found to be optimal; they provided better dose distributions than five or seven beams, whereas 15 beams did not seem to improve the plans.[33] Optimization of the beam angles was found to be unnecessary by some authors,[34] whereas others reported an improvement in head and neck plans when optimized, noncoplanar beam angles were

used.[35] This issue continues to be a subject to research, whereas the current recommended field arrangement for IMRT of head and neck cancer with MLCs is nine equidistant coplanar fields (Figure 18-6).

At the University of Michigan, complex cases such as nasopharyngeal cancer or advanced tumors in other sites, or cases with clinical evidence of bilateral neck disease, are planned using nine equidistant beams. In less advanced cases in which the neck requires treatment bilaterally, five or seven equidistant beams may achieve satisfactory results. Choosing the lowest number of beams that achieves the planning objectives is expected to reduce treatment time and increase efficiency.

Plan Optimization

The PTVs and noninvolved organs lie in close vicinity or may overlap with each other. It is necessary to assign weighting factors (or penalty or importance factors) to each target and organ that determine the relative importance of fulfilling their dose specifications or constraints. These weighting factors are derived following an iterative trial-and-error process, which requires refinement for each patient to produce an optimal plan. These factors differ among the various optimization systems. Examples of penalty factors for head and neck cancer plans have been provided by several authors.[35–37]

It was noted that because normal structure doses are penalized during optimization only if they exceed the limits set by the user, the constraints need to be more stringent than the clinical criteria.[37] At the University of Michigan, the optimization system uses a cost function that strives to

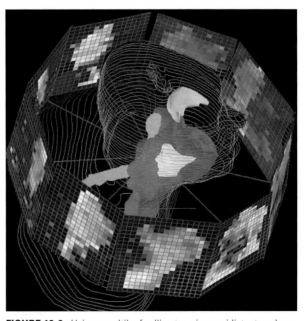

FIGURE 18-6. Using a multileaf collimator, nine equidistant coplanar beams are recommended for advanced cases.

minimize the dose to some noninvolved structures, in addition to setting a maximal dose constraint, facilitating a reduction of the doses to these organs.[38] For example, in the case of doses to the spinal cord, the system would assign both an allowed maximal dose, which would result in a high penalty if exceeded, and a low-penalty cost function striving to reduce the dose to the spinal cord as much as possible. Also, using a combination of linear and high-power objective functions (in addition to the quadratic objective function used in most commercial systems), strict head and neck target dose homogeneity can be achieved.[38]

In addition to the physical dose and dose/volume optimization criteria, several investigators examined the utility of biologic or clinical criteria as a basis for optimization in the head and neck. These investigations include optimization using the probability of uncomplicated tumor control,[39] tumor control probability and normal tissue complication probability,[40] and the equivalent uniform dose (EUD) concept. EUD is defined as the biologically equivalent dose that, if given uniformly, will lead to the same cell kill in the tumor volume as the actual nonuniform dose distribution.[41] The latter investigators found that optimizing using EUD as the cost function for head and neck cancer IMRT was superior to optimization using dose or dose volume.

Work at the University of Michigan comparing various biologic factors and dose or dose/volume as the bases for optimization for head and neck IMRT found that the balancing of power and weights, rather than the specific cost function, is the determining factor for the optimization results.[42] Biologic cost functions are expected to be superior to dose-based functions when the parameters of the biologic models, derived from clinical dose-response and dose-complication data, are known with greater confidence. An example is the optimization of advanced paranasal sinus cancer plans, in which optic pathway normal tissue complication probabilities derived from patient complication data were used for the critical organ cost function.[43]

Clinical Results
Tumor Control

The clinical results of tumor control rates were still quite limited at the time this chapter was written. Reported clinical series are either very heterogeneous regarding tumor sites and stages[44–47] and have small patient numbers[31,48] or patient selection factors.[32] All series suffer from relatively short follow-up periods. These factors prevent meaningful direct comparisons of tumor control rates with similar series of standard RT. The series cited above reported local-regional tumor control rates ranging between 81 and 97%. These rates seem to be better than most series of standard RT for similar tumors, suggesting that there is no compromise in tumor control rates following head and neck IMRT. Additional data are expected to be accumulated

rapidly in the near future, providing an opportunity to assess whether tumor control rates are indeed superior to those achieved following standard RT. A randomized study comparing IMRT with standard RT for head and neck cancer was recently started in Europe (C. Nutting, MD, personal communication, December 2003). The results of this study will help clarify this issue.

Lacking a well-controlled comparison between standard RT and IMRT, the most reliable current information from clinical series of IMRT for head and neck cancer relates to the pattern of tumor recurrences relative to the targets and the locally delivered doses. These data allow an assessment of the adequacy of target selection and delineation. In all reported cases, it seems that careful selection and delineation of the targets resulted in very few or no marginal or out-of-field recurrences. Lee and colleagues reported that all recurrences in their series were in-field.[46] Chao and colleagues reported that most marginal recurrences occurred in the lower neck, which was treated with an anterior field that was matched to the IMRT-treated upper neck.[45]

The pattern of local-regional tumor recurrence following IMRT of head and neck cancer at the University of Michigan, where the majority of patients had oropharyngeal cancer, has been reported.[44] Almost all recurrences occurred in-field, in high-risk volumes that had received the full prescribed doses. An update of this study included 133 patients treated with primary (63 patients) or postoperative (70 patients) multisegmental static IMRT.[47] At a median follow-up of 32 months (range 6–106 months), 21 local-regional failures (16%) occurred. Of these, 17 recurred in-field and 4 were marginal recurrences, of which less than 95% of the tissue volume harboring the recurrent tumor had received the prescribed dose. Of note, no marginal recurrence occurred in the contralateral high neck where the cranial-most target included the subdigastric nodes (all patients had a contralateral N0 neck that was judged to be at high risk of subclinical disease). Two marginal recurrences were noted in the retropharyngeal nodes, in which the cranial-most extent of the targets was defined at the top of C1, according to Rouviere's observations of the locations of the lateral retropharyngeal nodes.[12] Following these observations, we currently define the retropharyngeal nodes through the base of the skull.

In addition to the two marginal recurrences near the base of the skull, another case of marginal recurrence in our series included a patient with a past history of neck surgery for oral cancer who was treated with RT for tumor recurrence. Tumor subsequently recurred in unpredicted lymph nodes and subcutaneous tissue. This case highlights the unpredictability of the lymphatic drainage in patients with a past history (more than a year) of surgery, who therefore may not be suitable candidates for IMRT. Careful examination and reporting of the pattern of local-regional recurrence by radiation oncologists treating head and neck cancer with IMRT are essential to further understand and improve it.

Treatment Sequelae

In general, apart from xerostomia (discussed below), the rates of acute side effects seem to be similar to the rates observed during standard RT in the series that employed total doses and fractionation schemes that were close biologically to standard RT schemes. The rate of late sequelae, however, cannot yet be adequately assessed in these series owing to insufficient follow-up intervals.

Noninvolved Organ Sparing

Several clinical studies assessed the utility of IMRT in parotid salivary gland sparing and in reducing xerostomia. At the University of Michigan, the partial parotid gland doses and volumes following multisegmental IMRT were correlated with selective salivary output from each parotid gland.[49] It was found that the output related to the mean doses to the glands. The large majority of the glands receiving a mean dose of more than 26 Gy did not produce measurable saliva and did not recover, whereas glands receiving lower mean doses produced variable salivary output that increased over time. One year after RT, parotid glands receiving a moderate dose (mean dose of 17–26 Gy) recovered, on average, to the pre-RT salivary production levels (Figure 18-7).[50] When the doses to the parotid glands were very low, as in cases of unilateral neck RT in which the contralateral glands received mean doses < 10 Gy, an "overcompensation" of the damage of the ipsilateral glands was noted in the second post-therapy year. In particular, the salivary flow rates from the contralateral glands exceeded, on average, their preradiation flow rates (see Figure 18-7).

These data support an effort to reduce the mean doses to the parotid glands as much as possible without underdosing the targets. A correlation of the salivary output with the mean doses to the parotid glands was also found by Chao and colleagues.[51] They examined whole-mouth salivary output and found that this output dropped by 4% for each increase in the mean dose by 1 Gy. Some differences exist among different series in the relationships between the mean doses received by the parotid glands and the reduction in salivary output. These differences may be related to methodologic differences in the salivary output measurements and to the models used, but they are also likely to be related to differences in the spatial dose distributions produced by different techniques.[52] This issue merits further research.

An analysis at the University of Michigan of a validated patient-reported xerostomia questionnaire demonstrated that xerostomia improved significantly over time, in tandem with the increase in saliva production.[50] Two years following irradiation, xerostomia reported by patients receiving parotid-sparing bilateral neck radiation was only slightly worse than in patients receiving unilateral neck RT. Statistically significant predictors of patient-reported xerostomia included the mean dose to the major salivary glands and the mean dose to the oral cavity (representing radiation received by the minor salivary glands).[50] An improvement to mild or no xerostomia during the second year was also reported by investigators at UCSF using the RTOG toxicity scale, following IMRT for nasopharyngeal cancer.[32] A significant correlation between xerostomia and the doses to the major salivary glands was also reported by Chao and colleagues and Amosson and colleagues.[51,53] It is apparent from all of these studies that the partial sparing of the salivary glands, made possible by IMRT, achieves tangible gains both in the retention of the salivary production and in the symptoms of xerostomia.

Additional potential functional gains from IMRT compared with conventional RT include swallowing and speech measures following aggressive chemoirradiation, reported to be superior using IMRT compared with standard RT.[54] These potential benefits may translate into improvements in broad aspects of quality of life.[55] Thus, IMRT of head and neck cancer may achieve broad improvements in quality of life rather than be limited to improvements in xerostomia alone.

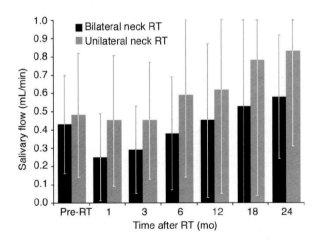

FIGURE 18-7. Stimulated salivary flow rates from contralateral parotid glands that were partially spared using static multisegmental intensity-modulated radiation therapy. Glands in patients treated with bilateral neck radiation therapy (RT) received mean doses of 17 to 26 Gy. On average, the salivary output from these glands recovered to the pre-RT levels 1 year after RT. Glands in patients treated with unilateral neck RT received mean doses < 10 Gy. Two years after RT, these glands produced saliva flow rates that were higher than pre-RT.[50]

Future Directions

The combination of radiation protectors, such as amifostine (Ethyol, MedImmune Inc., Gaithersburg, MD), or salivary production stimulants, such as pilocarpine, and IMRT is expected to further improve xerostomia. For example, Roesink and colleagues found that increasing the compensatory potential of the nondamaged parotid gland in irradiated rats explains, at least in part, the protective effect of pilocarpine.[56] Thus, reducing the volume of the irradiated salivary glands by IMRT may enhance the effect of salivary protectors and/or stimulators, and combining the two strategies may provide an additive or even synergistic effect. This concept requires clinical testing.

Current studies of dose escalation in head and neck cancer using IMRT are being undertaken, notably the study from the MCV.[33,34] The rationale for these studies is the limited tissue volume receiving a high dose. To gain any measure of confidence in these studies, they need to include patient numbers that are large enough to detect potential differences in toxicity among different tumor sites and sizes, as well as long follow-up periods to detect potential severe late complications. An alternative to radiation dose escalation is intensification of concurrent chemotherapy while keeping radiation dose constant. Whether IMRT and aggressive concurrent chemotherapy may reduce the rate of severe complications compared with the combination of standard RT and the same chemotherapy is not clear.[57]

The physical limitations posed by current IMRT techniques using photon beams may improve marginally as technology improves. A significant leap will be achieved by the use of protons. The combination of the physical properties of protons and IMRT is expected to yield better dose conformity and to reduce low-dose distributions in non-involved tissue. If proton RT becomes less expensive and complex, it may prove to be a promising improvement in head and neck IMRT.

References

1. Coia L, Galvin J, Sontag M, et al. Three dimensional photon treatment planning in carcinoma of the larynx. Int J Radiat Oncol Biol Phys 1991;21:183–92.
2. Leibel S, Kutcher G, Harrison L, et al. Improved dose distributions for 3D conformal boost treatment in carcinoma of the nasopharynx. Int J Radiat Oncol Biol Phys 1991;20:823–33.
3. Esik O, Schlegel W, Boesecke R, et al. Three dimensional radiotherapy planning for laryngeal and hypopharyngeal cancer. Radiother Oncol 1991;20:238–44.
4. Roa WH, Hazuka MB, Sandler HM, et al. Results of primary and adjuvant CT-based 3-dimensional radiotherapy for malignant tumors of the paranasal sinuses. Int J Radiat Oncol Biol Phys 1994;28:857–65.
5. Wolden SL, Zelefsky MJ, Hunt MA, et al. Failure of a 3D conformal boost to improve radiotherapy for nasopharyngeal carcinoma. Int J Radiat Oncol Biol Phys 2001;49:1229–34.
6. Gilbeau L, Octave-Prignot M, Renard L, et al. Comparison of setup accuracy of three different thermoplastic masks for the treatment of brain and head and neck tumors. Radiother Oncol 2001;58:155–66.
7. Som PM. The present controversy over the imaging method of choice for evaluating the soft tissues of the neck. AJNR Am J Neuroradiol 1997;18:1869–72.
8. Pieterman RM, van Putten JW, Meuzelaar JJ, et al. Preoperative staging of non-small cell lung cancer with positron-emission tomography. N Engl J Med 2000;343:254–61.
9. Schechter NR, Gillenwater AM, Byers RM, et al. Can positron emission tomography improve the quality of care for head and neck cancer patients? Int J Radiat Oncol Biol Phys 2001;51:4–9.
10. Brekel van den NWM, Stel HV, Castelijns JA, et al. Cervical lymph node metastasis: assessment of radiologic criteria. Radiology 1990;177:379–84.
11. Eisbruch A, Foote RL, O'Sullivan B, et al. IMRT of head and neck cancer: emphasis on the selection and delineation of the targets. Semin Radiat Oncol 2002;12:238–49.
12. Rouviere H. Lymphatic systems of the head and neck. Ann Arbor (MI): Edwards Brothers; 1938.
13. Mukherji SK, Armao D, Joshi VM. Cervical nodal metastases in squamous cell carcinoma of the head and neck: what to expect. Head Neck 2001;23:995–1005.
14. Lindberg RD. Distribution of cervical lymph node metastases from squamous cell carcinoma of the upper respiratory and digestive tracts. Cancer 1972;29:1446–49.
15. Byers RM, Wolf PF, Ballantyne AJ. Rationale for elective modified neck dissection. Head Neck Surg 1988;10:160–7.
16. Shah JP. Patterns of cervical lymph node metastasis from squamous carcinomas of the upper aerodigestive tract. Am J Surg 1990;160:405–9.
17. Robbins KT, Medina JE, Wolfe GT, et al. Standardizing neck dissection terminology. Official report of the Academy's committee for head and neck surgery and oncology. Arch Otolaryngol Head Neck Surg 1991;117:601–5.
18. Robbins KT. Integrating radiological criteria into the classification of cervical lymph node disease. Arch Otolaryngol Head Neck Surg 1999;125:385–7.
19. Gregoire V, Coche E, Cosnard G, et al. Selection and delineation of lymph node target volumes in head and neck conformal radiotherapy. Proposal for standardizing terminology and procedure based on the surgical experience. Radiother Oncol 2000;56:135–50.
20. Som PM, Curtin HD, Mancuso AA. An image-based classification for the cervical nodes designed as an adjunct to recent clinically based nodal classification. Arch Otolaryngol Head Neck Surg 1999;125:388–96.
21. Nowak PJ, Wijers OB, Lagerwaard FJ, Levendag PC. A three-dimensional CT-based target definition for elective irradiation of the neck. Int J Radiat Oncol Biol Phys 1999;45:33–9.
22. Wijers OB, Levendag PC, Tan T, et al. A simplified CT-based definition of the lymph node levels in the node negative neck. Radiother Oncol 1999;52:35–42.
23. Chao KSC, Wippold FJ, Ozygit G, et al. Determination and delineation of nodal target volumes for head and neck cancer based on patterns of failure in patients receiving definitive and postoperative IMRT. Int J Radiat Oncol Biol Phys 2002;53:1174–84.
24. Gregoire V, Levendag P, Ang KK, et al. CT-based delineation of lymph node levels in the node negative neck: consensus guidelines. Available at: www.rtog.org/hnatlas/main.htm (accessed 2003).
25. Million RR, Cassisi NJ, Mancuso AAA, et al. Management of the neck for squamous cell carcinoma. In: Million RR, Cassisi NJ, editors. Management of head and neck cancer: a multidisciplinary approach. 2nd ed. Philadelphia: JB Lippincott; 1994. p. 75–142.
26. Lee N, Chuang C, Quivey JM, et al. Skin toxicity due to intensity-modulated radiotherapy for head and neck carcinoma. Int J Radiat Oncol Biol Phys 2002;53:630–7.

27. Purdy JA. Dose-volume specification: new challenges with intensity-modulated radiation therapy. Semin Radiat Oncol 2002;12:199–209.

28. Van Asselen B, Raaijmakers CPJ, Lagendijk JJW, et al. Intrafraction motion of the larynx during radiotherapy. Int J Radiat Oncol Biol Phys 2003;56:384–90.

29. Mohan R, Wu Q, Manning M, Schmidt-Ullrich R. Radiobiological considerations in the design of fractionation strategies for intensity modulated radiation therapy of the head and neck. Int J Radiat Oncol Biol Phys 2000;46:619–30.

30. Fu KK, Pajak TF, Trotti A, et al. RTOG phase III randomized study to compare hyperfractionation and two variants of accelerated fractionation to standard fractionation radiotherapy for head and neck squamous cell carcinomas: first report of RTOG 9003. Int J Radiat Oncol Biol Phys 2000; 48:7–16.

31. Butler EB, Teh BS, Grant WS, et al. SMART (simultaneous modulated accelerated radiation therapy) boost: a new accelerated fractionation schedule for the treatment of head and neck cancer with intensity modulated radiotherapy. Int J Radiat Oncol Biol Phys 1999;45:21–32.

32. Lee N, Xia P, Akazawa P, et al. Intensity modulated radiotherapy in the treatment of nasopharyngeal carcinoma: an update of the UCSF experience. Int J Radiat Oncol Biol Phys 2002;53:12–21.

33. Wu Q, Manning M, Schmidt-Ullrich R, Mohan R. The potential for sparing of parotids and escalation of biologically equivalent dose with intensity modulated radiation treatments of head and neck cancers: a treatment design study. Int J Radiat Oncol Biol Phys 2000;46:195–205.

34. Wu Q, Mohan R, Morris M, et al. Simultaneous integrated boost intensity-modulated radiotherapy for locally advanced head and neck squamous cell carcinomas. I. Dosimetric results. Int J Radiat Oncol Biol Phys 2003;56:573–85.

35. Pugachev A, Li JG, Boyer AL, et al. Role of beam orientation optimization in intensity modulated radiation therapy. Int J Radiat Oncol Biol Phys 2001;50:551–60.

36. Chao KSC, Low D, Perez CA, Purdy JA. Intensity-modulated radiation therapy in head and neck cancer: the Mallincrodt experience. Int J Cancer 2000;90:92–103.

37. Hunt MA, Zelefsky MJ, Wolden S, et al. Treatment planning and delivery of intensity-modulated radiation therapy for primary nasopharyngeal cancer. Int J Radiat Oncol Biol Phys 2001;49:623–32.

38. Vineberg KA, Eisbruch A, Kessler ML, et al. Is uniform target dose possible in IMRT plans for head and neck cancer? Int J Radiat Oncol Biol Phys 2002;52:.1159–72.

39. Agren AK, Brahme A, Turesson I. Optimization of uncomplicated control for head and neck tumors. Int J Radiat Oncol Biol Phys 1990;19:1077–85.

40. De Neve W, De Gersem W, Derycke S. Clinical delivery of IMRT for relapsed or second-primary head and neck cancer using a multileaf collimator with dynamic control. Radiother Oncol 1999;50:301–14.

41. Wu Q, Mohan R, Niemierko A. IMRT optimization based on the generalized equivalent uniform dose (EUD). Int J Radiat Oncol Biol Phys 2002;52:224–35.

42. Vineberg KA, McShan DL, Kessler ML, et al. Comparison of dose, dose-volume, and biologically-based cost functions for IMRT plan optimization [abstract]. Int J Radiat Oncol Biol Phys 2001;51 Suppl 1:71.

43. Tsien C, Eisbruch A, McShan R, Fraas B. IMRT for locally advanced paranasal sinus cancer: application of clinical decisions in the planning process [abstract]. Int J Radiat Oncol Biol Phys 2001;51 Suppl 1:123.

44. Dawson LA, Anzai Y, Marsh L, et al. Local-regional recurrence pattern following conformal and intensity modulated RT for head and neck cancer. Int J Radiat Oncol Biol Phys 2000;46:1117–26.

45. Chao KS, Ozygit G, Tran BN, et al. Pattern of failure in patients receiving definitive and postoperative IMRT for head and neck cancer. Int J Radiat Oncol Biol Phys 2003;56:312–21.

46. Lee N, Xia P, Fischbain NJ, et al. Intensity-modulated radiation therapy for head and neck cancer: the UCSF experience focusing on target volume delineation. Int J Radiat Oncol Biol Phys 2003;57:49–60.

47. Eisbruch A, Marsh LH, Dawson LA, et al. Recurrences near the base of skull following IMRT of head and neck cancer: implications for target delineation in the high neck and for parotid gland sparing. Int J Radiat Oncol Biol Phys 2004;59:28–42.

48. Chao KSC, Majhail N, Huang C, et al. Intensity-modulated radiation therapy reduces late salivary toxicity without compromising tumor control in patients with oropharyngeal carcinoma: a comparison with conventional techniques. Radiother Oncol 2001;61:275–80.

49. Eisbruch A, Ten Haken R, Kim HM, et al. Dose, volume and function relationships in parotid glands following conformal and intensity modulated irradiation of head and neck cancer. Int J Radiat Oncol Biol Phys 1999;45:577–87.

50. Eisbruch A, Kim HM, Terrell JE, et al. Xerostomia and its predictors following parotid-sparing irradiation of head and neck cancer. Int J Radiat Oncol Biol Phys 2001;50:695–704.

51. Chao KSC, Deasy JO, Markman J, et al. A prospective study of salivary function sparing in patients with head and neck cancers receiving intensity-modulated or three-dimensional radiation therapy: initial results. Int J Radiat Oncol Biol Phys 2001;49:907–16.

52. Eisbruch A, Rhodus N, Rosenthal D, et al. How should we measure and report xerostomia? Semin Radiat Oncol 2003;13:226–34.

53. Amosson CM, Teh BS, Van TJ, et al. Dosimetric predictors of xerostomia for head and neck cancer patients treated with simultaneous modulated accelerated radiation therapy boost technique. Int J Radiat Oncol Biol Phys 2003;56:136–44.

54. Mittal B, Kepka A, Mahadevan A, et al. Use of IMRT to reduce toxicity from concomitant radiation and chemotherapy for advanced head and neck cancer [abstract]. Int J Radiat Oncol Biol Phys 2001;51 Suppl 1:82.

55. Lin A, Kim HM, Terrell JE, et al. Quality of life following parotid-sparing IMRT of head and neck cancer: a prospective longitudinal study. Int J Radiat Oncol Biol Phys 2003;57:61–70.

56. Roesink JM, Konings AW, Terhaard CH, et al. Preservation of the rat parotid gland function after radiation by prophylactic pilocarpine treatment: radiation dose dependency and compensatory mechanisms. Int J Radiat Oncol Biol Phys 1999;45:483–9.

57. Milano MT, Vokes EE, Witt ME, et al. Retrospective comparison of IMRT and conventional three-dimensional RT in advanced head and neck patients treated with definitive chemoradiation [abstract]. Proc Am Soc Clin Oncol 2003;22:499.

NASOPHARYNGEAL CANCER

CASE STUDY

WILLIAM W. CHOU, MD, NANCY Y. LEE, MD

Patient History

A 67-year-old Cantonese male presented with a 3-month history of left otalgia. Fiberoptic nasopharyngoscopy revealed a left nasopharyngeal mass arising from the fossa of Rosenmüller extending toward the midline with involvement of the torus tubarius and eustachian tube orifice. No cranial nerve deficits were noted on physical examination.

A magnetic resonance image (MRI) was obtained and revealed an expansile soft tissue mass emanating from the left posterolateral nasopharynx extending into the left parapharyngeal fat (Figure 18.1-1). No lymphadenopathy was noted within the neck or the superior mediastinum. A biopsy of the nasopharyngeal mass demonstrated a poorly differentiated squamous cell carcinoma. The remainder of his workup revealed no evidence of metastatic disease. The tumor was staged as T2bN0M0.

The patient was treated with concurrent chemotherapy with cisplatin (100 mg/m^2) and radiation therapy followed by adjuvant chemotherapy with cisplatin (80 mg/m^2) and 5-fluorouracil (1,000 mg/m^2).[1,2] Intensity-modulated radiation therapy (IMRT) was used to improve tumor coverage and spare surrounding normal tissues.[3] Prior to the initiation of treatment, a baseline audiogram was performed, a complete dental evaluation was initiated, and prophylaxis was instituted.

Simulation

The patient was simulated in the supine position with his head hyperextended. Immobilization consisted of an Aquaplastic mask (Aquaplast, Wycoff Heights, NJ) extending from the vertex of the scalp to the shoulders and attached to a headboard (Timo S-type, MED-TEC, Orange City, IA) (Figure 18.1-2). A planning computed tomography (CT) scan was performed with the patient in the treatment position on a PQ5000 CT simulator (Philips Medical Systems, Andover, MA) extending from 5 to 10 cm superior to the tumor to below the clavicles. The slice thickness was 5 mm, except in the region of the nasopharynx, where 3 mm slices were obtained.

To aid in target delineation, MRIs and positron emission tomography (PET) scans were obtained and fused to the planning CT scan. Owing to the size of the head rest and immobilization setup, diagnostic MRI with the head coil could not be performed. However, an MRI with a body coil setup accommodated the immobilization devices, allowing for duplication of the CT simulation process with good image resolution.

It was elected to treat the primary tumor and upper neck with IMRT and the lower neck with a conventional

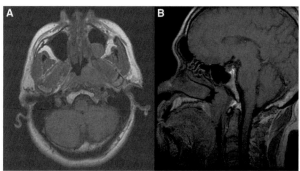
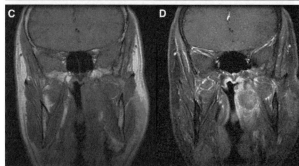

FIGURE 18.1-1. (*A*) A sagittal T$_1$-weighted magnetic resonance image (MRI) demonstrating abnormal soft tissue in the upper nasopharynx. No invasion of the high signal intensity marrow of the clivus is noted. (*B*) An axial T$_1$-weighted MRI showed parapharyngeal expansion. (*C*) A coronal T$_1$-weighted MRI revealed a mass obliterating the parapharyngeal fat space but with limited signal intensity difference from surrounding normal tissues. (*D*) A coronal postcontrast T$_2$-weighted image with fat saturation.

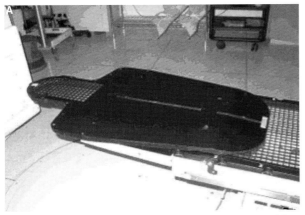

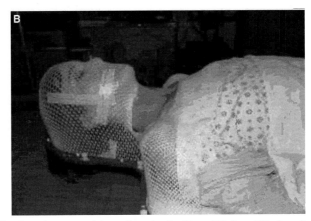

FIGURE 18.1-2. Headboard (*A*) and thermoplastic mask system (*B*) extending from the vertex of the scalp to the shoulders aid in immobilization of the patient. (Image courtesy of Ping Xia, PhD.)

anterior field. An isocenter was chosen for the IMRT field based on the patient's anatomy and tumor extent. The IMRT and conventional fields were matched using a slit-beam technique, with the match line set above the vocal cords (Figure 18.1-3). Multiple radiation therapy techniques and IMRT methods in defining the isocenter and match line have been described.[4]

Target and Tissue Delineation

The ability to precisely delineate both the tumor and normal structures is crucial in IMRT treatment planning of nasopharyngeal cancers.[5-7] Fusion of MRI and the planning CT scan improves the delineation of the primary tumor and surrounding normal tissues (Figure 18.1-4). As suggested by others,[8] PET can further supplement MRI findings (Figure 18.1-5).

Target volumes were delineated slice by slice on the treatment CT axial images in conjunction with

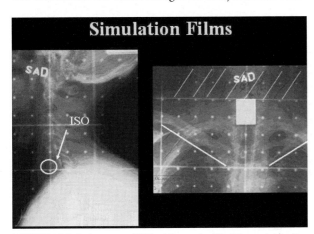

FIGURE 18.1-3. Isocenter (ISO) with matched half-beam intensity-modulated radiation therapy field and conventional anterior field. Anterior field of lower jugular and supraclavicular lymph nodes with the isocenter at match line and the cord block is shown. Source to axis distance (SAD) = 100 cm. (Image courtesy of Ping Xia, PhD.)

a neuroradiologist (Figure 18.1-6). The gross tumor volume (GTV) was defined as all known gross disease determined from clinical information, endoscopic findings, and imaging studies. This included the nasopharyngeal primary tumor with local extension. In patients with more advanced disease, the GTV should include all gross retropharyngeal lymphadenopathy and all lymph nodes > 1 cm in size or with a necrotic center. Close attention should be paid to the retropharyngeal region to detect any abnormal lymph nodes. When in doubt, nodes in this region should be included within the GTV.

The clinical target volume (CTV) was defined as the GTV plus all areas of potential microscopic disease. Three different CTVs were defined in this patient, namely, a CTV1 for the GTV, CTV2 for high-risk nodal regions and adjacent soft tissues, and CTV3 for low-risk nodal regions (Table 18.1-1). In this patient, a 5 mm margin was placed around the GTV to generate the CTV1. This margin can be reduced to 1 mm in patients with clivus infiltration, in whom the GTV is adjacent to the brainstem.

At-risk adjacent tissues as defined by CTV2 included the entire nasopharynx, clivus, skull base, retropharyngeal nodal regions, pterygoid fossae, parapharyngeal space, sphenoid sinus, and the posterior third of the maxillary sinus and posterior half of the nasal cavity. High-risk lymph node groups included the upper deep jugular (junctional, parapharyngeal), subdigastric (jugulodigastric), midjugular, posterior cervical, retropharyngeal lymph nodes and submandibular lymph nodes.[9,10] Elective treatment of all cervical lymph nodes was performed owing to the high likelihood of cervical metastases, even in clinically N0 patients. A failure rate of 40% has been previously reported for a clinically negative neck not electively treated.[11] At the discretion of the treating physician, coverage of level 1 nodes can be excluded in patients with stage T1N0 cancer. Lower-risk lymph node groups, such as lower neck and supraclavicular lymph nodes bilaterally, were included in CTV3 and irradiated with the conventional anterior low neck field.

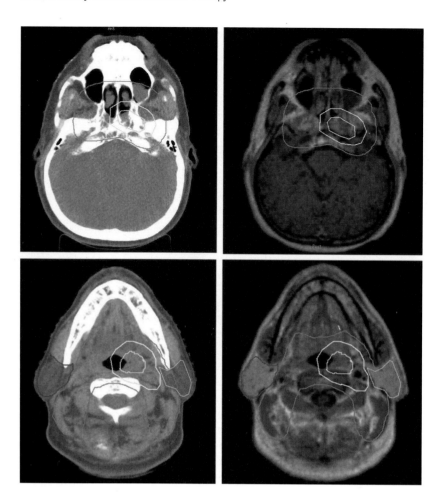

FIGURE 18.1-4. Computed tomography delineation of the tumor volume correlated with magnetic resonance images: gross tumor volume (*light blue*), planning target volume 1 (*yellow*), planning target volume 2 (*red*), right parotid gland (*dark blue*), and left parotid gland (*orange*). (To view a color version of this image, please refer to the CD-ROM).

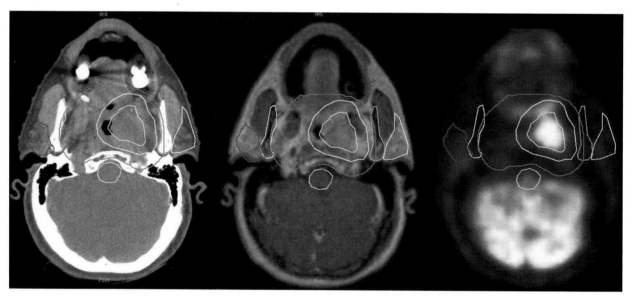

FIGURE 18.1-5. Computed tomography (CT) and magnetic resonance (MR) imaging supplemented by positron emission tomography (PET) information: gross tumor volume (*light blue*), planning target volume 1 (*yellow*), planning target volume 2 (*red*), right parotid gland (*dark blue*), and left parotid gland (*orange*). (To view a color version of this image, please refer to the CD-ROM).

As shown in Table 18.1-1, a planning target volume (PTV) was generated for each CTV, accounting for internal organ motion and setup uncertainty. Studies should be performed by each institution to define the appropriate CTV to PTV expansion. At our center, a 5 mm expansion around the CTV is used. This is reduced to 1 mm in patients in whom the CTV is adjacent to the brainstem. Figure 18.1-6 illustrates serial GTV, PTV1, and PTV2 axial delineation in this patient.

Critical normal structures delineated included the brainstem, spinal cord, optic nerves, optic chiasm, temporomandibular joints, mandible, and brain and were outlined in three dimensions. The spinal cord contours were 5 mm larger in the radial dimension than the spinal cord. The brainstem and chiasm were defined as 1 mm larger in all directions than the corresponding structure. Important but less critical normal structures, such as the parotid gland,

eyes, lens, middle and inner ears, tongue, and glottic larynx, were also included.

Treatment Planning

The number of fields was determined by the treatment planner to produce the most conformal plan. In this patient, seven coplanar beams were used. The following beam angles were used: 90, 120, 150, 180, 210, 240, and 270 degrees. The energy of all beams was 6 MV. Inverse planning was performed using in-house IMRT planning software developed at the Memorial Sloan-Kettering Cancer Center.

A total dose of 70 Gy in 33 fractions at 2.12 Gy per fraction was prescribed to the PTV1. PTV2 received 59.4 Gy in 33 fractions at 1.8 Gy per fraction. No more than 20% of the PTV1 received ≥ 110% of the prescribed dose, and no more than 1% of the PTV1 and PTV2 received < 93% of the prescribed dose. A dose > 110% of 70 Gy was limited to ≤ 1% or 1 cc of the tissue outside the PTVs. As noted above, the lower neck and supraclavicular region (PTV3) was treated with a conventional field. A total dose of 50.4 Gy in 28 fractions of 1.8 Gy per fraction was prescribed to a depth of 3 cm from the anterior surface.

This dose distribution (dose painting) may allow for a differential radiobiologic advantage. The GTV receives a higher dose per fraction when compared with the CTV, and all surrounding normal tissues may potentially benefit from a greater radiobiologic effect. Other investigators have reported encouraging results from the differential dose delivery and minimization of toxicity.[12,13]

As noted above, we elected to treat this patient with a combination of IMRT and a conventional anterior low neck field. The dose uncertainty at the match line has led to the use of extended-field IMRT, which treats the primary tumor with all of the regional lymph nodes, including the supraclavicular nodes. Head, neck, and shoulder immobilization must be used in these situations. In those cases in which the dose per fraction in PTV3 is 1.64 Gy, to compensate for the lower than conventional fractionation of 1.8 Gy, the low neck and supraclavicular fields should be treated to a higher total dose of 54.0 Gy. A third alternative is to plan to treat the low neck in the IMRT plan, define the low neck and supraclavicular fossae as PTV2, and, after 28 fractions, close these fields and do another IMRT plan to complete the remainder of the treatments.

Conforming to the critical normal structure constraints and prescription goals were the most important treatment planning priorities. Other planning goals included a low mean dose to the parotid glands, a reduced dose to the submandibular glands and oral cavity, and meeting dose constraints for other normal structures. Dose constraints for the critical normal structures are summarized in Table 18.1-2. In cases in which constraints to critical structures lead to underdosing the target tissues, these limits can be exceeded at the discretion of the physician, but the patients should

TABLE 18.1-1. Target Volumes and Margins

Target	Definition	Margin (Prescription Dose)
GTV	CTV1 = nasopharyngeal primary and gross nodal disease + at least 5 mm margin (see CTV2: CTV1 should be encompassed by CTV2) except in areas adjacent to critical structure, ie brainstem, where margin can be as small as 1 mm	PTV1 (70 Gy)* = 5 mm in all directions from CTV1 except for areas adjacent to critical structures, ie, brainstem, where margin can be as small as 1 mm *GTV will have 1 cm margin in all directions except for regions near critical structures
High-risk subclinical disease	CTV2 = adjacent soft tissue/ structures, ie, entire nasopharynx, clivus, skull base, retropharyngeal nodal regions, pterygoid fossae, parapharyngeal space, sphenoid sinus, and posterior third of maxillary sinus and up to posterior half of nasal cavity (CTV2 should encompass CTV1) High-risk nodal groups a. Upper deep jugular b. Subdigastric c. Midjugular d. Posterior cervical e. Retropharyngeal f. Submandibular (may omit at discretion of treating physician if T1N0)	PTV2 (59.4 Gy)† = 5 mm in all directions of CTV2 except when near brainstem, where margin can be as small as 1 mm
Low-risk subclinical disease	CTV3 = lower jugular nodes, supraclavicular lymph nodes	PTV3 (50.4 Gy) = low anterior field. Alternatively, if PTV3 is encompassed in the IMRT field and there is no low anterior field, the prescription for PTV3 should be 54 Gy (see text).

CTV = clinical target volume; GTV = gross tumor volume; IMRT = intensity-modulated radiation therapy; PTV = planning target volume.
†PTV2 should encompass PTV1 in all directions.

TABLE 18.1-2. Normal Tissue Dose Constraints

Normal Structure	Dose Constraints
Brainstem	≤ 54 Gy or 1 cc vol ≤ 60 Gy
Optic chiasm/optic nerves	≤ 54 Gy or 1 cc vol ≤ 60 Gy
Spinal cord	≤ 45 Gy or 1 cc vol ≤ 50 Gy
Mandible/TM joint	≤ 70 Gy or 1 cc vol ≤ 75 Gy
Temporal lobes	≤ 60 Gy or 1% vol ≤ 65 Gy

TM = temporomandibular.

be fully consented for the anticipated injury risk to these normal structures. Dose constraints for other normal structures, including the tongue, inner and middle ear, eyes, and glottic larynx, were of lower priority and did not compromise the GTV or CTV coverage. Table 18.1-3 lists the recommended doses for these lower-priority normal structures.

The optimized IMRT plan delivered in this patient is shown in Figure 18.1-7. Dose-volume histograms were generated

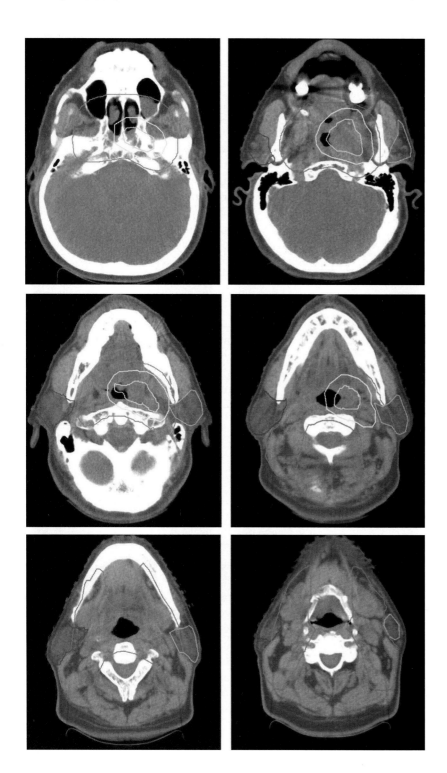

FIGURE 18.1-6. Clinical target volume delineation for a T2bN0M0 nasopharyngeal carcinoma receiving definitive intensity-modulated radiation therapy: gross tumor volume (*light blue*), planning target volume 2 (*red*), right parotid gland (*dark blue*), and left parotid gland (orange). (To view a color version of this image, please refer to the CD-ROM).

TABLE 18.1-3. Lower-Priority Normal Tissue Dose Limits

Normal Structure	Dose Constraints
Parotid glands	Mean dose ≤ 26 Gy in at least one gland or 20 cc of both ≤ 20 Gy
Tongue	≤ 55 Gy or 1% volume ≤ 65 Gy
Inner/middle ear	Mean dose ≤ 50 Gy
Eyes	Mean dose ≤ 35 Gy
Lens	As low as possible
Glottic larynx	Mean dose ≤ 45 Gy

for all target volumes, critical normal structures, and the unspecified tissues (Figure 18.1-8). No more than 5% of the nontarget tissue received more than 70 Gy, and this included all transmitted and scattered doses.

In this patient, the mean dose to the left parotid gland was 24.6 Gy and the contralateral (right) parotid gland received 23.8 Gy. For the parotid glands, a mean dose of 26 Gy should be achieved in at least one gland or at least 20 cc of the combined volume for both parotid glands

should receive less than 20 Gy. The degree of xerostomia is largely dependent on the radiation dose and the volume of the salivary gland that is irradiated. Salivary flow is markedly reduced following 10 to 15 Gy of radiation delivered to most of the gland. Recovery of salivary function is possible over time with doses up to 40 to 50 Gy, although irreversible xerostomia occurs with higher doses.[14–16] Doses to the submandibular and sublingual glands were reduced to the lowest possible.

Treatment Delivery and Quality Assurance

Treatment was delivered once daily for a total of five fractions per week on a Varian 2100C linear accelerator (Varian Medical Systems, Palo Alto, CA) equipped with a multileaf collimator (MLC) consisting of 26 pairs of leaves (52 total), 1 cm side at the center. All targets were treated simultaneously except for the supraclavicular area, which was stopped after 28 fractions. During the treatment, port films were taken for each field on a weekly basis. The accuracy of the

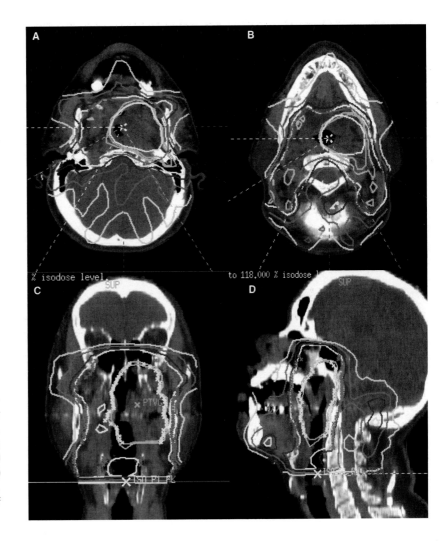

FIGURE 18.1-7. Intensity-modulated radiation therapy dose distribution. (*A*) Superior axial. (*B*) Inferior axial. (*C*) Coronal. (*D*) Sagittal. Planning target volume 1 (*yellow*); planning target volume 2 (*red*); 118% isodose line (70 Gy) (*green*), 114% (*orange*), 100% (59.4 Gy) (*yellow*), 90% (*dark blue*), 70% (*magenta*), 50% (*light blue*). (To view a color version of this image, please refer to the CD-ROM).

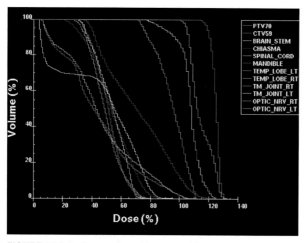 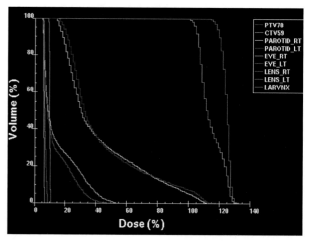

FIGURE 18.1-8. Dose-volume histogram: (*A*) critical normal structures, and (*B*) lower-priority normal structures. CTV = clinical target volume; NRV = nerve; PTV = planning target volume; TEMP = temporal lobe; TM = temporomandibular. (To view a color version of this image, please refer to the CD-ROM).

patient's position and MLC aperture was monitored by weekly verification films.

For pretreatment patient-specific quality assurance, a thorough plan check and independent monitor unit (MU) calculations were performed similarly to conventional treatments. During radiation delivery, we monitored accelerator MLC position readout and the record and verify system to verify the start and stop leaf positions of each field for the daily treatments. Routine film dosimetry for pretreatment delivery verification has been eliminated owing to long-term comparison between film and calculation, which consistently demonstrated agreement to within 2%. Film dosimetry is now reserved for new treatment sites, unusual intensity profiles, or MU verification checks with discrepancies in excess of 3%.

Clinical Outcome

The patient tolerated IMRT and concurrent chemotherapy well, with minimal side effects. He reported grade 1 xerostomia, mucositis, and skin acute toxicities during treatment. He was examined 4 months following completion of IMRT and continues to experience grade 1 skin and subcutaneous tissue fibrosis and grade 1 xerostomia. He currently remains without evidence of disease 6 months following completion of chemotherapy and IMRT.

Our experience treating 67 patients with nasopharyngeal cancer with IMRT at the University of California at San Francisco was published earlier.[4] Disease stages were stage I (8), II (12), III (22), and IV (25). Fifty patients received concomitant and adjuvant chemotherapy, and 26 received an intracavitary brachytherapy boost. The prescribed dose was 65 to 70 Gy to the GTV and positive neck nodes, 60 Gy to the CTV, 50 to 60 Gy to the clinically neg-

ative neck, and 5 to 7 Gy in two fractions for the brachytherapy boost. With a median follow-up of 31 months, the 4-year actuarial local progression-free, locoregional progression-free, and distant metastases–free survival rates were 97%, 98%, and 66%, respectively. The worst acute toxicities were grade 1 to 2 in 51 patients, grade 3 in 15 patients, and grade 4 in 1 patient. At 3 months post-IMRT, grades 0, 1, and 2 xerostomia were seen in 8%, 28%, and 64%, respectively. Of note, xerostomia decreased with time. At 24 months, only 1 of the 41 evaluable patients had grade 2, 32% had grade 1, and 66% had grade 0 xerostomia.

References

1. Al-Sarraf M, Leblanc M, Giri PG. Superiority of chemoradiotherapy (CT-RT) vs radiotherapy (RT) in patients with locally advanced nasopharyngeal cancer (NPC). Preliminary results of Intergroup (0099) (SWOG 8892, RTOG 8817, ECOG 2388) randomized study [abstract]. Proc Am Soc Clin Oncol 1996;15:313.
2. Cooper JS, Lee H, Torrey M, et al. Improved outcome secondary to concurrent chemoradiotherapy for advanced carcinoma of the nasopharynx: preliminary corroboration of the intergroup experience. Int J Radiat Oncol Biol Phys 2000;47:861–6.
3. Xia P, Fu KK, Wong GW, et al. Comparison of treatment plans involving intensity-modulated radiotherapy for nasopharyngeal carcinoma. Int J Radiat Oncol Biol Phys 2000;48:329–37.
4. Lee N, Xia P, Quivey JM, et al. Intensity-modulated radiotherapy in the treatment of nasopharyngeal carcinoma: an update of the UCSF experience. Int J Radiat Oncol Biol Phys 2002;53:12–22.
5. Chao KS, Wippold FJ, Ozyigit G, et al. Determination and delineation of nodal target volumes for head-and-neck cancer based on patterns of failure in patients receiving definitive and postoperative IMRT. Int J Radiat Oncol Biol Phys 2002;53:1174–84.
6. Lee N, Xia P, Fischbein NJ, et al. Intensity-modulated radiation therapy for head-and-neck cancer: the UCSF experience focusing

on target volume delineation. Int J Radiat Oncol Biol Phys 2003;57:49–60.

7. Eisbruch A, Foote RL, O'Sullivan B, et al. Intensity-modulated radiation therapy for head and neck cancer: emphasis on the selection and delineation of the targets. Semin Radiat Oncol 2002;12:238–49.

8. Rahn AN, Baum RP, Adamietz IA, et al. [Value of 18F fluoro-deoxyglucose positron emission tomography in radiotherapy planning of head-neck tumors]. Strahlenther Onkol 1998;174: 358–64.

9. Som PM, Curtin HD, Mancuso AA. Imaging-based nodal classification for evaluation of neck metastatic adenopathy. AJR Am J Roentgenol 2000;174:837–44.

10. Nowak PJ, Wijers OB, Lagerwaard FJ, et al. A three-dimensional CT-based target definition for elective irradiation of the neck. Int J Radiat Oncol Biol Phys 1999;45:33–9.

11. Lee AW, Poon YF, Foo W, et al. Retrospective analysis of 5037 patients with nasopharyngeal carcinoma treated during 1976-1985: overall survival and patterns of failure. Int J Radiat Oncol Biol Phys 1992;23:261–70.

12. Butler EB, Teh BS, Grant WH III, et al. Smart (simultaneous modulated accelerated radiation therapy) boost: a new accelerated fractionation schedule for the treatment of head and neck cancer with intensity modulated radiotherapy. Int J Radiat Oncol Biol Phys 1999;45:21–32.

13. Mohan R, Wu Q, Manning M, et al. Radiobiological considerations in the design of fractionation strategies for intensity-modulated radiation therapy of head and neck cancers. Int J Radiat Oncol Biol Phys 2000;46:619–30.

14. Leslie MD, Dische S. The early changes in salivary gland function during and after radiotherapy given for head and neck cancer. Radiother Oncol 1994;30:26–32.

15. Eisbruch A, Ten Haken RK, Kim HM, et al. Dose, volume, and function relationships in parotid salivary glands following conformal and intensity-modulated irradiation of head and neck cancer. Int J Radiat Oncol Biol Phys 1999;45:577–87.

16. Roesink JM, Moerland MA, Battermann JJ, et al. Quantitative dose-volume response analysis of changes in parotid gland function after radiotherapy in the head-and-neck region. Int J Radiat Oncol Biol Phys 2001;51:938–46.

ETHMOID SINUS CANCER

CASE STUDY

FILIP CLAUS, MD, PhD, WIM DUTHOY, MD, WILFRIED DE NEVE, MD, PhD

Patient History

A 67-year-old male presented with nasal obstruction, headache, and a mucopurulent postnasal drip. Rhinoscopy demonstrated mucosal congestion, and rigid nasal endoscopy revealed purulent crusts. A computed tomography (CT) scan was ordered and demonstrated a polypoid mass in the right ethmoidal air cells with remodeling of the right lamina papyracea, opacification of the ethmoidal and right frontal sinuses, and mucosal thickening of the maxillary and sphenoidal sinuses. No pathologically enlarged lymph nodes were noted. The remainder of the workup was negative.

Using a combined transfacial and neurosurgical approach, a gross total resection was performed, and the pathology was consistent with adenocarcinoma. The tumor was staged as pT4cN0M0, and the patient was referred for postoperative radiation therapy. Owing to the close proximity of the optic pathways and lacrimal apparatus to the target volume, the patient was treated with intensity-modulated radiation therapy (IMRT).

Simulation

The patient was simulated in the supine position. A custom-made thermoplastic head cast was fabricated for immobilization, and a knee cushion was used for patient comfort. A planning CT scan was obtained on a Somatom Plus 4 scanner (Siemens Medical Systems, Munich, Germany). The planning CT scan extended from the vertex of the head to the sternoclavicular junction. Over the region of the paranasal sinuses, a CT slice thickness of 2 mm was used. Outside this region, 5 mm slices were obtained. No contrast was administered. The dataset consisted of 105 transverse slices (pixel resolution 512 × 512). A magnetic resonance image (MRI) (slice thickness 1 mm) was also obtained and registered with the planning CT scan to aid in the delineation of the target and normal tissues.

Target and Tissue Delineation

Given the initial tumor extent and the difficulty of assessing resection margins, the entire region of the ethmoid air cells and the adjacent sinonasal cavities were felt to be at risk. A compartment-related definition of the clinical target volume (CTV) was used, that is, the region of the ethmoid sinus air cells, and the directly flanking sinonasal cavities were included. These cavities included the nasal cavity, the right maxillary sinus, and both sphenoidal sinuses (the tumor invaded the posterior ethmoidal sinus cells). A portion of the anterior cranial fossa was also included owing to the disruption of the leptomeningeal structures. A gross tumor volume (GTV) was not specified in this case in light of the gross total surgical resection. The CTV was uniformly expanded by 3 mm, generating a planning target volume (PTV) accounting for setup uncertainty. The CTV and PTV delineated in this patient are shown in Figure 18.2-1.

Organs at risk (OAR) in this case included the optic chiasm, optic nerves, retinae, lacrimal glands, pituitary gland, brainstem, brain, mandible, and both parotid glands. Delineation of the posterior aspect of the optic nerves, optic chiasm, and pituitary gland was based on the MRI dataset. The lens was not considered an OAR because cataract surgery is a minor operation with a high success rate and with almost no risk of complications. The optic pathway structures (optic chiasm, optic nerves, and both retinae) and brainstem were expanded to form planning at-risk volumes (PRVs). The optic pathway structures were expanded by 2 mm, whereas the brainstem was expanded by 3 mm. Figure 18.2-1 illustrates the OAR and corresponding PRV in this patient.

Treatment Planning

Prior to the optimization process, three nonanatomic (virtual) OAR were automatically generated by subtracting from the patient volume the PTV, the PTV expanded by 20 mm,

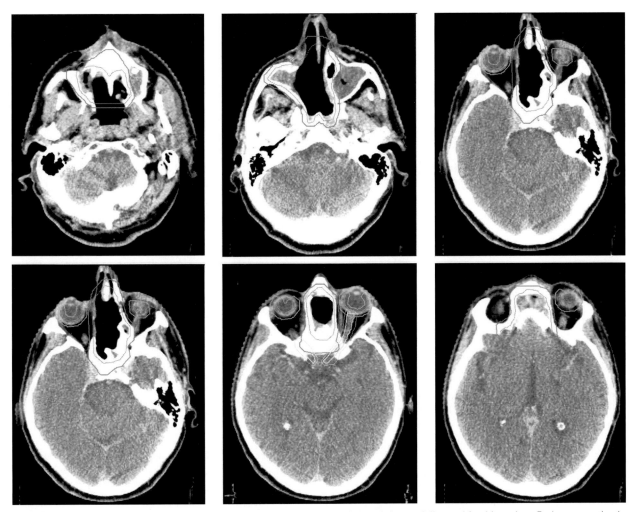

FIGURE 18.2-1. Axial computed tomography slices illustrating the target and normal tissues delineated for this patient. Each structure (optic nerve, optic chiasm, retina, clinical target volume [CTV]) is represented as two contours; the inner contour is the structure itself, and the outer contour is the expanded structure (the planning at-risk volume, and in case of the CTV, this is the planning target volume). (To view a color version of this image, please refer to the CD-ROM).

and the PTV expanded by 50 mm. For optimization purposes, two subvolumes of the PTV were created: a PTV without a buildup region (PTV-wbu), that is, the PTV without the subvolume within a range of 6 mm from the skin contour, and a PTV without buildup and without overlap with OAR (PTV-wbu-woars), that is, all points inside the PTV-wbu but not closer than 6 mm to the optic structures (optic chiasm, optic nerves, and retinae). Subvolumes inside the PTV, that is, the PTV-wbu and the PTV-wbu-woars, were used to remove conflicts during the optimization phase. When the PTV and the expanded optic structures intersect, a conflicting dose prescription is present. By prescribing 70 Gy to the PTV subvolume outside the overlap or buildup region (PTV-wbu-woars) and a maximal dose of 60 Gy inside this region, the conflict is removed.

Treatment planning was performed using in-house inverse planning software. A flow diagram of the planning process used in this patient is shown in Figure 18.2-2. Beam incidences were defined upfront by the treatment planner. A template of seven beams was used: five beams with the central axes located in the sagittal plane (table rotation angle of 90 degrees and gantry angles of 0, 30, 60, 90, and 330 degrees) and two beams with central axes in a transverse plane (table rotation angle of 0 degrees and gantry angles of 75 and 285 degrees). The isocenter of all beams was located at the xyz-midpoint of the PTV. The energy of all beams was 6 MV.

The components of our planning approach include an anatomy-based segmentation tool, which creates segments for each beam incidence.[1] The segment outlines are based on the beam's eye view of the PTV and OAR. The purpose of this tool is to create an increasing number of segments with decreasing distance to the optic structures and increasing thickness of overlying tissue. Sixty-seven segments were generated for this patient. Segment weight optimization is then performed using in-house biophysical cost function

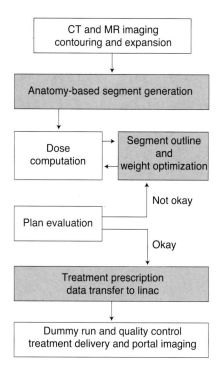

FIGURE 18.2-2. The intensity-modulated radiation therapy planning platform consists of several modular units, including tools to generate segments, compute doses, optimize plans, and generate treatment prescriptions. The units with gray background are in-house–developed software programs. CT = computed tomography; MR = magnetic resonance. Linac = linear accelerator.

software.[2] The segment outlines are further optimized using a leaf position optimization scheme.[3] This tool evaluates the effects of changing the position of each leaf within each segment on the biophysical objective function. Leaf position changes that decrease the value of the objective function are retained. After several possible positions (eg, changes of 1, 3, 5, and 10 mm) have been evaluated, an external dose engine recomputes the dose distribution, based on the adapted leaf positions and weights. Only leaf position changes that comply with the multileaf collimator (MLC) constraints of the linear accelerator are evaluated (ie, segments that can be delivered). The remaining number of segments after shape and weight optimization was 40. The segments are provided as separate MLC beams to the dose computation unit (convolution-superposition algorithm). In the last step, the segment delivery sequence is optimized to ensure the shortest possible delivery time. For a more detailed description and discussion of the treatment planning process, the reader is referred to previously published research.[4,5]

The PTV prescription dose was 70 Gy, delivered in 2 Gy daily fractions. An underdosage of more than 5% inside the PTV was accepted in the regions adjacent to or overlapping with the optic structures (PRVs), as well as in the buildup region of the 6 MV photon beams. With regard to PTV over-

dosage, the International Commission on Radiation Units and Measurements guideline of 7% was followed. The three-dimensional maximum dose was located inside the PTV.

Table 18.2-1 summarizes the dose constraints for the OAR in this case. The dose limit for the 2 mm expanded optic structures (optic chiasm, optic nerves, and retinae) was 60 Gy, that is, 5% of the volume of the structure was allowed to receive more than 60 Gy. Although this limit may seem high, the normal tissue complication probability of the optic structures using our approach is low for a number of reasons. First, the 60 Gy limit is applied to the expanded structure. Second, the use of a biologic optimization model results in an inhomogeneous irradiation of the nerves and a low mean dose. Finally, the maximum daily fraction size is 1.7 Gy. The maximum dose for the brainstem was a hard constraint of 60 Gy (applied to the PRV). No specific dose constraints were used for the lacrimal glands, pituitary gland, brain tissue, mandible, and parotid glands, although biologic constraints were used for these structures during optimization.

Figure 18.2-3 displays the isodose distributions for the optimized treatment plan (normalized to a median PTV dose of 70 Gy). Dose-volume histograms of the target and OAR are shown in Figure 18.2-4.

TABLE 18.2-1. Summary of Optimization Parameters used for IMRT Planning

Target Volumes	Physical Constraints
PTV-wbu	Median dose 70 Gy, ICRU guidelines (–5% to +7%)*
PTV-wbu-woars	ICRU guidelines (–5% to +7%)

Three-dimensional maximum dose has to be located inside the PTV

Organs at risk	Biophysical constraints
Optic chiasm (PRV)	$D_{95} \leq 60$ Gy, biologic optimization (DVH reduction scheme[†])
Optic nerve (PRV)	$D_{95} \leq 60$ Gy, biologic optimization
Retina (PRV)	$D_{95} \leq 60$ Gy, biologic optimization
Brainstem (PRV)	$D_{max} \leq 60$ Gy, biologic optimization
Brain	No physical constraints, biologic optimization
Mandible	No physical constraints, biologic optimization
Virtual organs at risk	No physical constraints, biologic optimization

D_{95} = the dose that covers 95% of the organ at risk; D_{max} = the maximum dose; DVH = dose-volume histogram; ICRU = International Commission on Radiation Units and Measurements; PRV = planning at-risk volume (ie, the expanded structure); PTV = planning target volume; PTV-wbu = planning target volume without buildup; PTV-wbu-woars = planning target volume without buildup and without overlap with an organ at risk.

*An underdosage of more than 5% inside the planning target volume was accepted in the regions adjacent to or overlapping the optic structures (planning at-risk volumes).

†The parameters for the biologic optimization were calculated according to a dose-volume histogram reduction scheme. The volume and slope parameters to calculate the normal tissue complication probability were based on published data. For the optic structures and the brainstem, the median toxic dose values were decreased to customize the plan to the protocol constraints (see Claus F et al[5] for details).

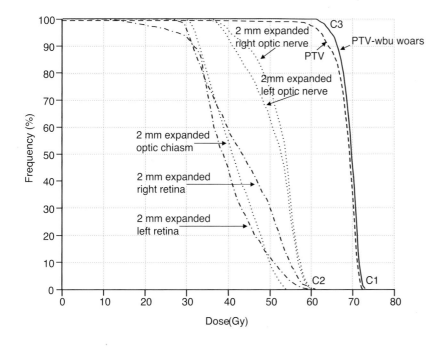

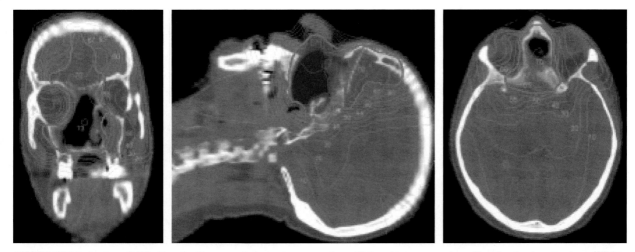

FIGURE 18.2-3. Dose-volume histograms for the target volumes and the optic structures for the presented case. A median dose of 70 Gy is prescribed to the planning target volume (PTV). Planning constraints: C1 = maximal dose in the PTV ≤ 107% of the prescribed dose; C2 = maximally 5% of the volume of the optic structures is allowed to receive ≥ 60 Gy; C3 = the maximal underdosage in the PTV without buildup and without overlap with an organ at risk (PTV-wbu-woars) is 5%.

FIGURE 18.2-4. Isodose distributions for the presented case in a coronal, sagittal, and transverse plane. The planning target volume (PTV) is shown as a red solid line. A median dose of 70 Gy is prescribed to the PTV. (To view a color version of this image, please refer to the CD-ROM).

Treatment Delivery and Quality Assurance

Treatment was delivered on an SL*i* plus linear accelerator (Elekta, Crawley, UK) equipped with the Precise MLC. This MLC replaces the upper movable jaws inside the linear accelerator head and has 40 pairs of tungsten alloy leaves that project a width of 1.0 cm at the isocenter. The treatment delivery time was completed within a 15-minute time slot (electronic portal imaging included).

Rigorous quality assurance procedures were performed to ensure accurate treatment delivery. Gel dosimetry was used before the IMRT treatments for ethmoid sinus tumors were clinically implemented. For the presented case, the patient's treatment fields were delivered to a head phantom with an ionization chamber located near the isocenter position. Daily electronic portal imaging was performed for the first five treatment fractions to reduce systematic setup errors. Weekly portal imaging was performed thereafter.

Clinical Outcome

IMRT treatment was well tolerated except for the development of grade 2 conjunctivitis (ie, symptomatic conjunctivitis, not interfering with activities of daily living). The patient also complained of fatigue. No grade 3 or 4 toxicity was seen. At his latest follow-up (14 months post-treatment), the patient remained without evidence of disease recurrence, and his only subjective ocular complaint was occasional tearing. An ophthalmologic evaluation did not reveal any difference with the pretherapeutic findings, that is, the vision and ocular pressure were not changed, the fundoscopy was normal, and there were no signs of cataracts in either eye.

Our clinical results using IMRT in patients with ethmoid sinus tumor were reported earlier.[5] Eleven patients with T1–4N0M0 ethmoid sinus cancer were treated at Ghent University between February 1999 and July 2000. Ten patients were treated postoperatively, and one was treated definitively. In 9 of 10 patients who underwent surgery, the resection was macroscopically complete. Microscopic invasion of the resection margins was observed in 1 patient. Overall, treatment was well tolerated. Light sensitivity (grade 1) was observed in 8 patients. Tearing, cornea, and lacrimalation symptoms were observed in 10 patients (5 grade 1, 5 grade 2). Pain and dryness of the eyes were reported in 8 patients (6 grade 1, 2 grade 2). None of the patients developed dry-eye syndrome.

Patient follow-up reports revealed no evidence of disease in 7 patients. Two patients died, one of a locoregional relapse and the other from distant metastases. No unilateral or bilateral visual impairment has been observed thus far.

References

1. De Gersem W, Claus F, De Wagter C, et al. An anatomy based segmentation tool for intensity modulated radiotherapy of head and neck cancer. Int J Radiat Oncol Biol Phys 2001;51:849–59.
2. Derycke W, De Gersem S, Colle C, et al. Inhomogeneous target-dose distributions: a dimension more for optimization? Int J Radiat Oncol Biol Phys 1999;44:461–8.
3. De Gersem W, Claus F, De Wagter C, et al. Leaf position optimization for step and shoot IMRT. Int J Radiat Oncol Biol Phys 2001;51:1371–88.
4. Claus F, De Gersem W, Vanhoutte I, et al. Evaluation of a leaf position optimization tool for IMRT of head and neck cancer. Radiother Oncol 2001;61:281–6.
5. Claus F, De Gersem W, De Wagter C, et al. An implementation strategy for IMRT of ethmoid sinus cancer with bilateral sparing of the optic pathways. Int J Radiat Oncol Biol Phys 2001;51:318–31.

Maxillary Sinus Cancer

Case Study

Bahman Emami, MD, Stephanie King, CMD, Anil Sethi, PhD, Guy Petruzzelli, MD, PhD

Patient History

A 72-year-old female presented with episodes of imbalance over the previous 3 to 6 months. Magnetic resonance imaging (MRI) of the head and neck revealed a 2.8 × 2.6 cm enhancing mass in the right maxillary sinus. The mass extended to the inferior and medial aspects of the right orbit, right ethmoid sinus, and nasal cavity. A biopsy was performed, and the pathology was consistent with an adenoid cystic carcinoma.

The patient subsequently underwent a right medial maxillectomy with resection of the periorbital tumor component, periorbital reconstruction, and lacrimal canalicular intubation. It was elected not to sacrifice the right eye. The tumor involved the maxillary bone and the inferior, middle, and superior turbinates. Although a gross total resection was performed, the superior, lateral, and deep periorbital margins were positive. The final pathology was consistent with an adenoid cystic carcinoma of the maxillary sinus.

Owing to her locally advanced disease and multiple positive margins, postoperative radiation therapy was recommended. Intensity-modulated radiation therapy (IMRT) was used in an effort to deliver a high dose to the target tissues while minimizing the risk of injury to the nearby eyes and optic pathway structures (optic nerves, chiasm).

Simulation

Computed tomography (CT) simulation (PQ5000, Philips Medical Systems, Andover, MA) was performed with the patient immobilized in an Alpha Cradle (Smithers Medical Products, Hudson, OH) and an aquaplast mask. The Alpha Cradle was fabricated extending from the midthigh to the top of the head, and the aquaplast mask was then attached. The planning CT scan extended from the top of the patient's head to the bottom of the clavicles, using 3 mm slices. Intravenous contrast was not used.

Target and Normal Tissue Delineation

All target volumes and normal tissues were contoured using the *AcQSim* software (Philips Medical Systems) (Figures 18.3-1 and 18.3-2). To aid in tissue delineation, an MRI was fused to the planning CT. Postoperative irradiation in patients with adenoid cystic carcinoma of the maxillary sinus requires inclusion of the second (maxillary) division of the trigeminal nerve in the clinical target volume (CTV) all the way to the cavernous sinus. Identifying and contouring this nerve pathway are a definite challenge and should be confirmed by a neuroradiologist. In this patient's case, the CTV included the tumor bed and the contents of the right bony orbit but excluded the optic nerve and chiasm. No gross tumor volume was contoured because the patient was treated postoperatively.

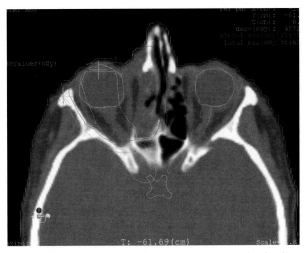

FIGURE 18.3-1. Axial computed tomography slice illustrating the planning target volume (*green*), clinical target volume (*dark blue*), right optic nerve (*magenta*), chiasm (*yellow*), and left and right eyes. The "OPTIC expand," which is used to limit the dose to the right optic nerve, is shown in light blue. (To view a color version of this image, please refer to the CD-ROM.)

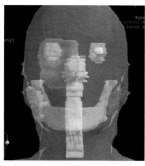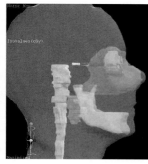

FIGURE 18.3-2. Anterior and right lateral renderings of the patient illustrating the target and normal tissues. (To view a color version of this image, please refer to the CD-ROM.)

Selected normal tissue structures were delineated by the radiation oncologist on the axial slices of the planning CT scan, including the optic nerves and chiasm (see Figures 18.3-1 and 18.3-2). The dosimetrist contoured all other structures of interest, including the spinal cord, brainstem, mandible, and parotid glands. These contours were then reviewed and approved by the treating physician.

The rigid immobilization system used in this patient allowed the CTV to be expanded uniformly by only 3 mm, creating a planning target volume (PTV). To improve target coverage, an additional 3 mm was then added to the PTV, creating a "PTV expand." The PTV expand was used by the treatment planning system in target dose optimization. A slightly higher dose (65 Gy) was assigned to the PTV expand to ensure that the PTV would be covered by the prescription dose of 60 Gy (Table 18.3-1).

Owing to the proximity of the PTV to the right optic nerve and eye, a pseudostructure called an "OPTIC expand" was created consisting of a 3 mm expansion around the right optic nerve extending from the optic chiasm to the right eye. This pseudostructure was used in treatment planning to create a "tunnel effect," allowing the full dose to be delivered to the tumor volume but limiting the optic nerve to a maximum dose of 50 Gy.

Treatment Planning

IMRT planning was performed on the Focus Treatment Planning System, version 3.1 (Computerized Medical Systems, St. Louis, MO). Six coplanar 6 MV beams were used at the following gantry angles: 0, 30, 140, 160, 200, and 345 degrees. The input parameters used in this case, including maximum doses, weights, and overlap priorities, are summarized in Table 18.3-1. In the overlap priority column, smaller numbers indicate a higher priority or importance. Note that a high priority was assigned to the right optic nerve to limit the total dose to 5,000 cGy.

The IMRT plan was evaluated by visualizing the three-dimensional dose cloud at different isodose levels (Figure 18.3-3), reviewing the isodose lines on individual CT slices through critical structures (Figure 18.3-4), and assessment of dose-volume histograms (Figure 18.3-5). The use of the pseudostructure allowed the creation of a low-dose "tunnel" through the PTV, limiting the dose to the right optic nerve. Such a treatment plan would not have been possible using conventional three-dimensional conformal planning.

Treatment Delivery and Quality Assurance

The IMRT plan was delivered on a Clinac 21EX linear accelerator (Varian Medical Systems, Palo Alto, CA) equipped with an 80-leaf collimator. Treatment was delivered in the step-and-shoot mode. The average number of segments per field was 22.

Prior to the initiation of treatment, multiple quality assurance procedures were performed. The fluence maps from the treatment plan were projected onto the CT scan of a cubic box phantom ($25 \times 25 \times 25$ cm^3). Based on examination of the resulting phantom plan, an ionization chamber was placed in a high-dose, low-gradient region and irradiated. Film (EDR2, Eastmann Kodak, Rochester, NY) was also placed in a coronal plane through the isocenter. Our quality assurance acceptance criteria are that measurement and calculation must agree within ± 2% within

TABLE 18.3-1. Input Parameters

Structure	Minimum Dose (cGy)	Maximum Dose (cGy)	Goal Dose (cGy)	Importance Weighting	Overlap Priority
PTV expand	6,100	6,600	6,500	100	3
Patient		6,600	—	3	8
Cornea		4,000	—	85	5
Left optic nerve		5,000	—	15	6
Right optic nerve		4,950	—	95	1
Optic chiasm		4,000	—	35	7
Left lens		100	—	99	4
OPTIC expand		5,100	—	87	2

PTV = planning target volume.

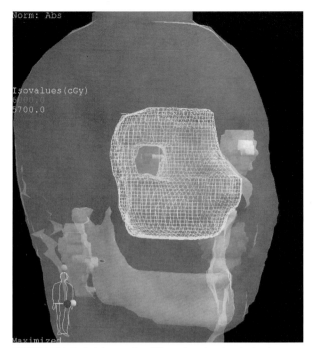

FIGURE 18.3-3. A right-anterior oblique view showing the isodose surface. Note the opening in the surface produced by limiting the right optic nerve dose to 50 Gy. (To view a color version of this image, please refer to the CD-ROM.)

the high-dose region. Isodose lines (measured and calculated) in the low-dose region must also be within 2 to 3 mm. These criteria were satisfied for this patient.

On the first treatment day, anterior and right lateral electronic portal images were obtained. These were compared with digitally reconstructed radiographs produced from the CT simulation. Throughout the course of treatment, weekly portals were obtained and compared with the digitally reconstructed radiographs. Based on these comparisons, adjustments were made as needed.

Clinical Outcome

The patient has been followed in our joint head and neck clinic. At a follow-up of 2 years, she was clinically without evidence of disease recurrence. Moreover, she had retained complete vision in both eyes. Of note, she did experience an episode of transient keratitis, which resolved with medical management. No late toxicities have thus far been observed.

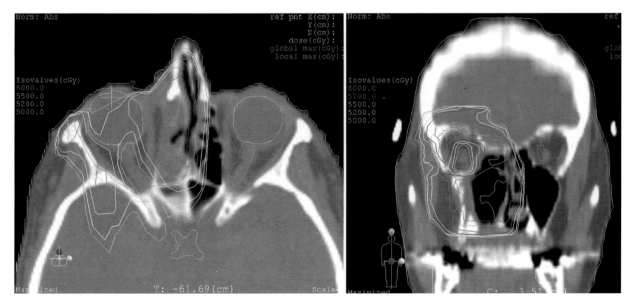

FIGURE 18.3-4. Isodose lines overlaid on the planning computed tomography scan in the axial (*left*) and coronal (*right*) planes. (To view a color version of this image, please refer to the CD-ROM.)

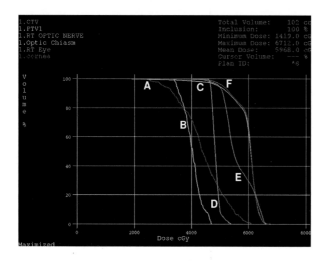

FIGURE 18.3-5. Dose-volume histograms of the planning target volume (PTV) and normal tissues for this patient. (*A*) cornea, (*B*) optic chiasm, (*C*) PTV1, (*D*) right optic nerve, (*E*) right eye, (*F*) CTV. CTV = clinical target volume. (To view a color version of this image, please refer to the CD-ROM.)

BASE OF TONGUE CANCER

CASE STUDY

QUYNH-THU LE, MD, TODD PAWLICKI, PHD

Patient History

A 52-year-old male presented with odynophagia and intermittent right-sided otalgia. On a complete head and neck evaluation, he was noted to have an exophytic right base of tongue (BOT) mass involving the glossotonsillar sulcus, pharyngoepiglottic fold, and vallecula. A head and neck magnetic resonance image (MRI) revealed a $3.8 \times 2.6 \times 2.7$ cm^3 T$_2$-weighted hyperintense lesion involving the right BOT and the right lateral oropharyngeal wall (Figure 18.4-1). There were multiple enlarged right-sided cervical nodes. In addition, there was a small node (< 10 mm in short axis) in the left level II region. Panendoscopy and biopsy of the tumor revealed moderately differentiated invasive squamous cell carcinoma. A positron emission tomography (PET) scan that was performed for staging and treatment planning confirmed increased metabolic uptake in the right BOT and right-sided cervical nodes. In addition, it showed increased metabolic uptake in a left level II neck node (Figure 18.4-2A). The patient was therefore staged as having a T2N2CM0 squamous cell carcinoma of the BOT and was recommended to receive concurrent chemoradiotherapy with the radiation delivered via an intensity-modulated radiation therapy (IMRT) approach.

Simulation

The patient was immobilized in an Aquaplastic mask (Aquaplast, Wycoff Heights, NJ). A custom-made head and neck immobilization device was used to maximize reproducibility of the head and chin position (Figure 18.4-3A; AccuForm, MED-TEC Inc., Orange City, IA). In addition, the shoulders were immobilized by having the patient hold on to two hand dowels or pegs on a customized plastic board. The location of the hand dowels can be adjusted for each patient to maximize the patient's comfort and reproducibility of the position. Figure 18.4-3B shows the patient in the treatment position. Simulation studies show that this device can immobilize the shoulders with 2 to 3 mm anterior-posterior (A-P) and left-right (L-R) maximal daily variability. The addition of an Aquaplastic shoulder immobilization system to this device does not improve the daily reproducibility and increases skin dose to the lower neck area.[1] In addition, three tattoos were placed over the shoulder and anterior chest wall to maximize daily setup reproducibility.

A computed tomography (CT) scan was obtained with the patient in the treatment position on the PQ 5000 CT scanner (Philips Medical Systems, Andover, MA). Routine

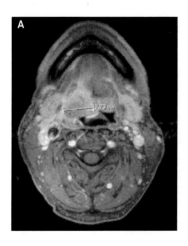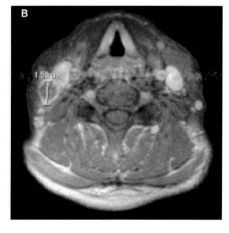

FIGURE 18.4-1. Axial images from pretreatment magnetic resonance imaging showing (*A*) a right tongue base cancer and (*B*) a necrotic right level III neck node.

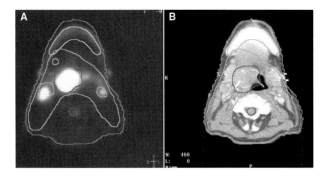

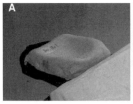
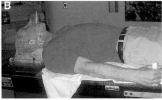

FIGURE 18.4-2. (*A*) Axial image of the staging positron emission tomography (PET) scan showing increased metabolic uptake in the right base of the tongue and right level II and left level II neck nodes. (*B*) Treatment planning computed tomography scan showing target and normal tissue contours of primary tumor gross tumor volume (*dark blue*), nodal gross tumor volume (*green*), planning target volume (*light orange*), mandible (*light blue*), skin (*dark orange*), and spinal cord (*purple*). (To view a color version of this image, please refer to the CD-ROM.)

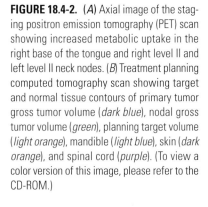

FIGURE 18.4-3. (*A*) Picture of an AccuForm custom-made head and neck support. (*B*) Patient immobilized for treatment on an institutional custom-made shoulder immobilization device using hand dowels. (To view a color version of this image, please refer to the CD-ROM.)

administration of intravenous contrast (150 cc of Visipaque [Iodixanol] in a contrast injector) is used in most patients receiving head and neck IMRT who have adequate renal function and no history of contrast allergy. Axial CT slices of 3 mm thickness were obtained from the skull base to the carina. Figure 18.4-2B illustrates a cross-sectional image through the BOT on the treatment planning CT scan.

We are presently conducting a systematic study to determine the impact of ^{18}F-fluorodeoxyglucose ([18]FDG) PET on radiation treatment planning in head and neck cancers. A fiducial-based system is used for the PET-CT fusion. As part of this protocol, three to five radiopaque fiducials are placed on the patient's mask and neck during the treatment planning CT scan. Patients then undergo a PET scan on a

GE Discovery LS PET/CT scanner (GE Healthcare, Waukesha, WI) in the same treatment planning position immobilized with the same mask and base-plate. For the PET fiducials, approximately 1 μCi of [18]FDG is mixed in 10 μL of either water or normal saline. The PET scan is then fused to the appropriate treatment planning CT using the fiducial locations and the AcQSim VoxelQ fusion tools (Philips Medical Systems). For all of the patients in the study, the primary tumor is defined using the CT scan, whereas involved neck nodes are identified based on both CT pathologic nodal criteria (lymph nodes ≥ 1 cm in short axis, spherically shaped small nodes in the draining lymphatic regions, nodes with radiographic evidence of necrosis or extracapular extension and cluster of three or more borderline-sized nodes) and [18]FDG PET criteria (all lymph nodes with increased metabolic activity, regardless of nodal size).

Target and Tissue Delineation

We usually use contrast-enhanced CT and, whenever possible, MRI-CT fusion for delineation of the primary tumor. In this case, MRI was used complementary to the treatment planning CT for tumor definition, but fusion was not performed because the MRI was obtained at an outside institution. In our experience, both CT and MRI provide excellent anatomic details for BOT cancers, with the exception of patients with metallic dental fillings, in whom MRI

FIGURE 18.4-4. Representative cross-sectional images from the treatment planning computed tomography (CT) scan showing gross tumor volume contours of the primary tumor (*bright red*), involved neck nodes (*dark red*), planning target volume (*orange*), right parotid gland (*light green*), left parotid gland (*light blue*), mandible (*light violet*), true vocal cords (*purple*), brainstem (*dark purple*), and spinal cord (*dark blue*). (To view a color version of this image, please refer to the CD-ROM.)

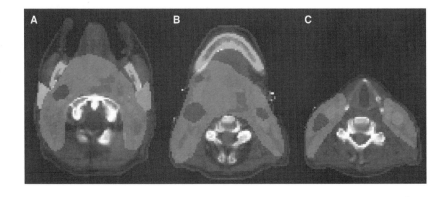

is superior to CT. [18]FDG PET, on the other hand, lacks the anatomic details for tumor definition and is not useful for defining primary tumors, except in situations of PET-CT hybrid scans or accurate PET-CT fusion. The opposite is true for nodal staging. Multiple studies have suggested that [18]FDG PET is more sensitive and specific in evaluating nodal metastasis than CT or MRI.[2–5] Emerging studies with hybrid PET-CT devices demonstrated that the fused image is superior to either image alone for the staging and management of solid tumors.[6,7] Based on the above information, we recommend using the combination of PET and CT scans for contouring involved neck nodes in head and neck cancer patients based on the criteria described previously. Figure 18.4-4 shows target definition of the primary tumor and nodal gross tumor volumes (GTVs) for this case.

In this case, the clinical target volume (CTV) for the primary tumor included the entire BOT, vallecula, ipsilateral tonsillar bed, epiglottis, and preepiglottic space. A 1 to 3 cm anterior margin was also included. The CTV for the regional nodes included ipsilateral level 1b owing to anterior tumor extension and involvement of level II nodes, bilateral level II to V nodes, and upper mediastinal nodes owing to tumor involvement of the ipsilateral level IV region. In addition, the CTV and planning target volume (PTV) of the ipsilateral level II nodes were extended to the skull base to ensure

adequate coverage of the superior retropharyngeal nodes (Figure 18.4-5A). On occasions, excessive large hot spots are noted in certain areas of the neck after generating the initial IMRT plans owing to the extensive nodal coverage in the PTV (from the skull base to the carina). These areas can be contoured as separate nodal structures. This approach provides more control over the optimization and minimizes excessive dose to these locations (Figure 18.4-6 and the PTV2 dose-volume histogram [DVH] in Figure 18.4-10).

The following normal tissues are routinely outlined for BOT cancers: the eyes, optic nerves, optic chiasm, brainstem, individual parotid glands, mandible, glottic larynx, and spinal cord. In this case, owing to extensive nodal involvement, we elected to spare only the superficial parotid lobes and therefore did not include the deep lobes when outlining the parotid glands. On occasion, excessive hot or cold spots are noted in certain regions of the PTV after generating the initial IMRT plans. Specialized structures named "tuning structures" are added for the purpose of minimizing hot spots outside the target volume(s) and generating a conformal dose distribution for head and neck IMRT plans (Figure 18.4-7).

Treatment Planning

Typical values for head and neck immobilization and setup uncertainty are A-P 1.1 ± 2.3 mm, superior–inferior 0.9 ± 2.3 mm, and L-R 0.8 mm.[8] These margins are included in our contours of the tumor and upper neck CTV to create the PTV used for treatment planning and dose evaluation. As previously mentioned, the interfraction organ setup uncertainty for our custom-made immobilization

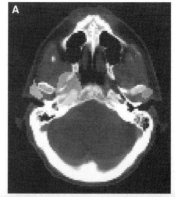
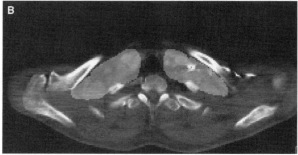

FIGURE 18.4-5. Representative cross-sectional images of the treatment planning computed tomography (CT) showing (A) planning target volume (PTV) extension into the skull base on the right side to ensure adequate coverage of the ipsilateral retropharyngeal lymph nodes and (B) PTV contours of the lower neck nodes. (To view a color version of this image, please refer to the CD-ROM.)

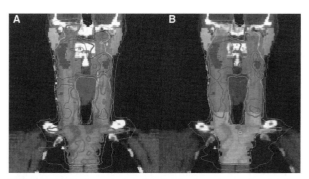

FIGURE 18.4-6. Coronal slice showing the importance of separating the planning target volume (PTV) into two parts to improve dose homogeneity. (A) The PTV contoured as one structure (red) with the 60 Gy isodose curve (red) extending superiorly into the skull base and inferiorly into the mediastinum. (B) The PTV divided into two separate structures (red and green) and a subsequent reduction in the 60 Gy isodose curve superiorly and inferiorly. Corresponding dose-volume histograms are shown in Figure 18.4-10. The isodose curves shown in this figure are 66 Gy (dark blue), 60 Gy (red), 54 Gy (yellow), and 40 Gy (green). The 60 Gy isodose curve is shown thicker to highlight the differences. (To view a color version of this image, please refer to the CD-ROM.)

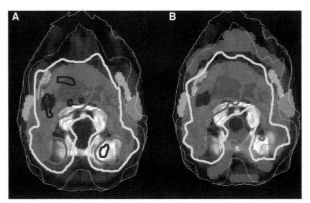

FIGURE 18.4-7. This figure shows the effect of a tuning structure in improving the dose distribution conformity. (*A*) The plan was optimized without a tuning structure, and (*B*) the plan was optimized with a tuning structure (*light purple*). The same dose constraints were used for both cases. The isodose curves shown in this figure are 73 Gy (*dark blue*), 66 Gy (*purple*), 60 Gy (*red*), 54 Gy (*yellow*), 40 Gy (*green*), and 20 Gy (*light blue*). Note the reduction in the left posterior 73 Gy hot spot in *B* while maintaining coverage of the base of tongue tumor and the involved lymph node. The 73 Gy, 66 Gy, and 54 Gy isodose curves are shown thicker to highlight the differences. (To view a color version of this image, please refer to the CD-ROM.)

device ranges from 2 to 3 mm. These margins are included in the PTV contours of the lower neck and upper mediastinum for treatment planning.

The prescription dose is 66 Gy in 30 fractions (2.2 Gy/fraction) to the GTV and 54 Gy in 30 fractions to the PTV (1.8 Gy/fraction). The planning parameters necessary to achieve this prescription are specific to the implementation of each optimization algorithm. The *CORVUS* inverse planning software version 4.0 (North American Scientific, NOMOS

Radiation Oncology Division, Cranberry Township, PA) was used to generate the IMRT plan for patient treatment. This software version uses a stochastic optimization algorithm with a pencil beam dose calculation algorithm. The IMRT treatment plans were calculated with heterogeneity correction turned on during both beamlet optimization and final dose calculation. The exact planning parameters used for this case are given in Table 18.4-1.

As previously mentioned in the target contouring section, a special arrangement of structures or tissue contours was used to produce the optimal dose distribution. Owing to the large volume of the PTV in this case (to treat all nodal regions from the skull base to the upper mediastinum), it is difficult to control the larger areas of hot spots throughout the PTV, as shown in the superior and inferior aspects of the PTV in Figure 18.4-6A. Figure 18.4-6B shows a coronal image of the contours where the PTV was split into two structures (PTV1 in orange and PTV2 in green). By breaking up the PTV volume, a more homogeneous dose coverage of the PTV is obtained. A tuning structure was placed adjacent to the target in noncontoured regions of the CT scan. The doses in Figure 18.4-7B were generated with the same optimization parameters as those in Figure 18.4-7A except that the tuning structure was added and used in the optimization procedure for Figure 18.4-7B. The use of tuning structures has proved to be an efficient method to obtain conformal dose distributions in head and neck IMRT planning using *CORVUS*.

It should be reiterated that the planning parameters shown here are specific to the *CORVUS* version 4.0 inverse planning system. Furthermore, they do not necessarily represent what is clinically required for the patient's treatment. They do, however, give the optimal isodose distribution and DVHs for treatment. The AcQSim segmentation tools

TABLE 18.4-1. Input Parameters

Structure Name	Goal/Limit, Gy	Volume below Goal/above Limit, %	Minimum, Gy	Maximum, Gy	Tissue Type
GTV	66	2	65	68	Homogeneous
Node	66	2	65	68	Homogeneous
PTV1	54	5	53	56	Homogeneous
PTV2	52	5	50	54	Homogeneous
Nontarget tissue	45	0	0	45	Homogeneous
Spinal cord	30	5	30	40	Basic structure
Mandible	40	30	20	50	Basic structure
Brainstem	45	2	40	50	Basic structure
Larynx	25	30	11	45	Basic structure
RT parotid gland	30	10	25	60	Basic structure
LT parotid gland	20	2	15	50	Basic structure
Eyes	45	5	40	50	Basic structure
Optic nerves	45	5	40	50	Basic structure
Chiasm	45	5	40	50	Basic structure
Tuning structure	40	10	35	45	Basic structure

GTV = gross tumor volume; PTV = planning target volume.

were used for tumor and normal tissue contouring. The AcQSim system has a 16-structure limit on the number of structures permitted for each patient. Hence, for this case, it was required to combine the right and left eyes and the right and left optic nerves into one structure. This did not play a significant role in the optimization process because those structures are superior to the target volume.

The patient was treated on a Varian 2100EX (Varian Medical Systems, Palo Alto, CA) dual-energy linear accelerator. The plan was created with a 6 MV photon beam and 1×1 cm^2 beamlets. On Varian accelerators, the maximum treatable field width in one beam-on time for IMRT is limited to 14.5 cm. This is due to the finite length of the Varian multileaf collimator leaves in the travel direction and the inability of collimator jaws to move during treatment. The *CORVUS* inverse planning system automatically accounts for these limitations by splitting a field into two fields if the target width exceeds the Varian field size limit in the beam's eye view. Therefore, although the treatment plan was developed with seven axial coplanar fields, the actual number of treated fixed fields was 15. The beam angles, in Varian convention, were 0 posterior-anterior (PA), 80 left posterior oblique (LPO), 120 left anterior oblique (LAO), 160 (LAO),

200 right anterior oblique (RAO), 240 (RAO), and 280 right posterior oblique (RPO) degrees.

The dose statistics for this treatment are summarized in Table 18.4-2. Isodose curves showing GTV coverage are shown in Figure 18.4-8. The maximum dose anywhere in the patient is 75.9 Gy and is located in the tumor volume. Only 1 cc of the target volume receives doses 74.0 Gy or greater. The maximum dose is located in the nodal region designated as PTV1 about 3 mm superior to the CT slice shown in Figure 18.4-8B. For nontarget tissue, only 1 cc receives doses 70.2 Gy or greater. The DVH shows that 97.7% of the GTV receives doses ≥ 66 Gy and 3.9% of the GTV receives doses > 72.6 Gy (≥ 110% of the prescription dose; Figure 18.4-10). The mean dose to the GTV was 69.4 Gy, whereas 97.2% of the involved neck nodes receives doses ≥ 66 Gy and 2.8% receives doses > 72.6 Gy.

PTV2 was defined as the nodal regions superior and inferior to the region of the tumor and the involved neck nodes. The isodose curves for PTV2 are shown in Figure 18.4-9. The dose homogeneity is particularly good in these regions. The DVHs show that 94.5% of PTV2 receives 54 Gy (prescription dose) and 6.1% receives doses > 59.4 (> 110% of the prescription dose; Figure 18.4-10). Within

TABLE 18.4-2. Dose Statistics

Structure Name	Goal/Limit, Gy	Volume below Goal/above Limit, %	Minimum, Gy	Maximum, Gy	Mean, Gy
GTV	66.0	2.2	64.1	75.5	69.4
Node	66.0	2.7	63.3	74.0	69.5
PTV1	54.0	4.3	30.3	75.9	61.5
PTV2	54.0	2.7	40.6	67.1	56.4
Nontarget tissue	45.0	7.7	0.0	72.1	13.4
Spinal cord	30.0	28.8	12.5	44.4	29.1
Mandible	40.0	71.4	14.8	69.0	45.0
Brainstem	45.0	4.4	5.7	49.7	24.8
Larynx	25.0	41.9	18.2	42.9	25.3
RT parotid gland	30.0	39.9	14.8	63.0	30.4
LT parotid gland	20.0	53.0	11.4	50.5	21.8
Eyes	45.0	0.0	1.9	3.0	2.3
Optic nerves	45.0	0.0	2.3	3.0	2.6
Chiasm	45.0	0.0	3.0	4.2	3.3

GTV = gross tumor volume; PTV = planning target volume. Maximum, minimum, and mean values reflect the final plan approved for treatment.

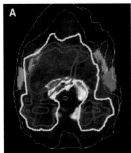
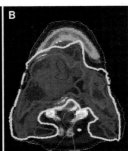
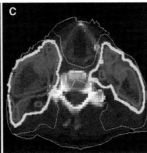

FIGURE 18.4-8. Isodose curves illustrating coverage of the gross tumor volume (GTV) and planning target volume (PTV). The isodose curves shown in this figure are 73 Gy (*dark blue*), 66 Gy (*red*), 60 Gy (*purple*), 54 Gy (*yellow*), 40 Gy (*green*), and 20 Gy (*light blue*). The prescribed doses are 66 Gy at 2.2 Gy/fraction to the GTV and 54 Gy at 1.8 Gy/fraction to the PTV. (To view a color version of this image, please refer to the CD-ROM.)

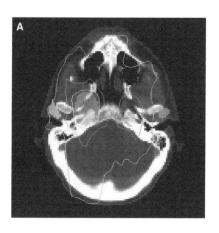

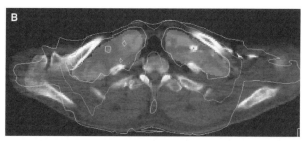

FIGURE 18.4-9. Isodose curves showing planning target volume (PTV) coverage in regions superior (*A*) and inferior (*B*) to the tumor site or involved neck nodes. The isodose curves shown in this figure are 66 Gy (*purple*), 54 Gy (*yellow*), 40 Gy (*green*), and 20 Gy (*light blue*). The prescribed dose is 54 Gy at 1.8 Gy/fraction to the PTV. (To view a color version of this image, please refer to the CD-ROM.)

the PTV1 that surrounds the BOT tumor and involved neck nodes, 95.7% receives doses ≥ 54 Gy, whereas 63.2% receives doses ≥ 110% of the prescription dose. The large volume of PTV1 receiving high doses is expected because all of the GTVs are located within this volume by definition.

The maximum brainstem dose is 49.7 Gy, whereas ≤ 1 cc of the brainstem volume receives ≥ 45.6 Gy. For the spinal cord, the maximum dose is 44.4 Gy and ≤ 1 cc of the contoured volume receives ≥ 40.0 Gy. The mean doses to the larynx, right parotid gland, and left parotid gland are 25.3, 30.4, and 21.8 Gy, respectively. The optic apparatus is located far from the treated regions, and the maximum dose to any of these structures is 4.2 Gy over 30 fractions. The DVHs for all structures are shown in Figures 18.4-10 and 18.4-11.

Treatment Delivery and Quality Assurance

Before starting treatment, all patients receiving head and neck IMRT at Stanford University undergo a verification step, during which the immobilization system is checked, the orthogonal images of the isocenter(s) are reproduced on simulation films for better visualization of bony landmarks, and the lower neck fields are defined in cases in which the lower neck is treated with conventional techniques. In this patient, the primary tumor and the entire neck were comprehensively treated with IMRT; therefore, only the IMRT isocenter location was verified. Figure 18.4-12A shows the A-P digitally reconstructed radiograph and Figure 18.4-12B shows a lateral digitally computed radiograph (DCR) of the isocenter. The DCR uses additional manipulation of the CT data to enhance the bony anatomy for better comparison with either simulation or portal films. Also note that the lateral DCR shown in Figure 18.4-12B is created using half of the patient's CT data. The image gives the impression of looking inside the cranium. This technique is useful for enhancing the skull base, sella turcica, and cervical spine processes. The simulation and portal images of the isocenter are shown in Figure 18.4-12C–F. During the active treatment period, portal images

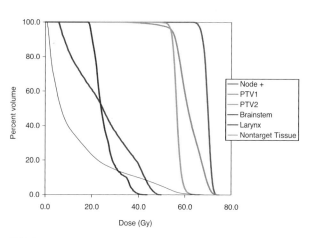

FIGURE 18.4-10. Dose-volume histograms of the involved neck nodes (Node+), planning target volumes (PTV), and selected normal tissues.

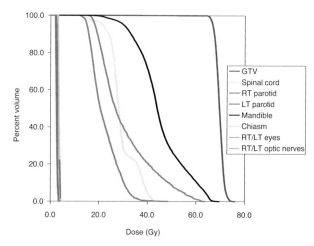

FIGURE 18.4-11. Dose-volume histograms of a primary tumor (gross tumor volume [GTV]) and selected normal tissues.

of the isocenter and the lower neck fields are taken weekly or more often if necessary. In addition, outlines of the modulated anatomic region for each beam angle are filmed at the beginning of treatment to ensure the accuracy of the isocenter location.

At our institution, all IMRT treatments are delivered using the step and shoot technique. For the 7 beam angles (and 15 total beams), approximately 18.8 minutes of beam-on time is necessary to deliver 1,763 monitor units in this case. The overall duration for each treatment session, which includes both beam-on time and patient setup, is approximately 37 minutes. Acquisition of weekly isocenter portal films typically adds 3 to 5 minutes to the entire process 1 day a week. For a conventional five-field head and neck treatment (L-R lateral opposed photon fields, L-R posterior neck electron fields, and an A-P supraclavicular field), approximately 22 minutes is required for each treatment session. Overall, the IMRT treatment time is about 15 minutes longer than conventional head and neck treatment for each session. Inverse planning systems that provide more control over field splitting should allow IMRT treatment plans to be developed with fewer beams, yet are dosimetrically comparable to the plan described here. In this case, IMRT treatment times should be comparable to conventional treatment times.

Clinical Outcome

The patient completed the radiation treatment course in 6 weeks without any interruption. He also received two cycles of cisplatin and 5-fluorouracil concurrently with radiotherapy. He did not receive the third course of chemotherapy owing to grade 4 granulocytopenia. His treatment course was complicated by protracted nausea and vomiting secondary to chemotherapy and thick mucus production, requiring frequent intravenous fluid hydration and placement of a percutaneous gastrostomy feeding tube. He lost a total of 16 lb (9.5% body weight) during active therapy. His feeding tube was removed 2 months after treatment, and a follow-up MRI at 3 months showed complete resolution of the BOT mass and bilateral neck node (Figure 18.4-13). The patient returned to work full time at approximately 1 month after completion of therapy and was disease free at 6 months with minimal (grade 1) xerostomia.

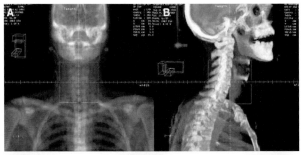
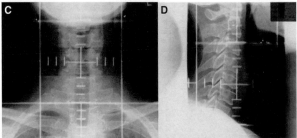
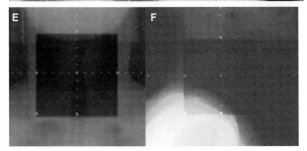

FIGURE 18.4-12. (*A*) Anterior-posterior (A-P) digitally reconstructed radiograph. (*B*) Lateral digitally computed radiograph. (*C*) A-P simulation film. (*D*) Lateral simulation film. (*E*) A-P portal image. (*F*) Lateral portal image.

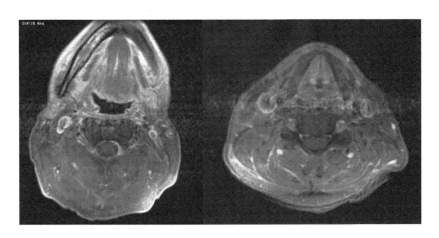

FIGURE 18.4-13. Axial images from follow-up magnetic resonance imaging at 3 months postradiotherapy. Note the complete resolution of the base of the tongue mass and bilateral neck node (see Figure 18.4-1).

References

1. Lee N, Chuang C, Quivey JM, et al. Skin toxicity due to intensity-modulated radiotherapy for head-and-neck carcinoma. Int J Radiat Oncol Biol Phys 2002;53:630–7.

2. Adams S, Baum RP, Stuckensen T, et al. Prospective comparison of 18F-FDG PET with conventional imaging modalities (CT, MRI, US) in lymph node staging of head and neck cancer. Eur J Nucl Med 1998;25:1255–60.

3. Stuckensen T, Kovacs AF, Adams S, et al. Staging of the neck in patients with oral cavity squamous cell carcinomas: a prospective comparison of PET, ultrasound, CT and MRI. J Craniomaxillofac Surg 2000;28:319–24.

4. Kao CH, Hsieh JF, Tsai SC, et al. Comparison of 18-fluoro-2-deoxyglucose positron emission tomography and computed tomography in detection of cervical lymph node metastases of nasopharyngeal carcinoma. Ann Otol Rhinol Laryngol 2000;109:1130–4.

5. Kau RJ, Alexiou C, Laubenbacher C, et al. Lymph node detection of head and neck squamous cell carcinomas by positron emission tomography with fluorodeoxyglucose F 18 in a routine clinical setting. Arch Otolaryngol Head Neck Surg 1999;125:1322–8.

6. Lardinois D, Weder W, Hany TF, et al. Staging of non-small-cell lung cancer with integrated positron-emission tomography and computed tomography. N Engl J Med 2003;348:2500–7.

7. Hany TF, Steinert HC, Goerres GW, et al. PET diagnostic accuracy: improvement with in-line PET-CT system: initial results. Radiology 2002;225:575–81.

8. Booth JT, Zavgorodni SF. Set-up error and organ motion uncertainty: a review. Australas Phys Eng Sci Med 1999;22:29–47.

Pyriform Sinus Cancer

Case Study

Michael T. Milano, MD, PhD, Wells Jackson, MS, CMD, Daniel J. Haraf, MD

Patient History

A 51-year-old female with a smoking history of 70-pack-years presented with a 1-month history of mild sore throat, left-sided otalgia, and a left neck mass. On physical examination, a 2.5 × 3.5 cm firm, nontender left juglodigastric lymph node was observed. Direct laryngoscopy revealed a bulky, predominantly submucosal tumor arising from the left pyriform sinus, involving the posterior portion of the left arytenoids but not the true vocal cords. The tumor extended to the left glossoepiglottic fold and medial and inferior portions of the tonsil and along the lateral pharyngeal wall.

A computed tomography (CT) scan of the head and neck demonstrated a 3 × 4 × 5 cm pyriform sinus mass with extension to the left supraglottic larynx and tonsillar bed. Invasion of the strap muscles was noted. In addition, a 2 × 2 cm left juglodigastric lymph node and a 1.5 cm right level II lymph node were seen. Fine-needle aspiration of the larger neck mass revealed a moderately differentiated squamous cell carcinoma. The remainder of the metastatic workup was negative.

The patient was diagnosed as having a T4N2cM0 pyriform sinus carcinoma and was enrolled in a multi-institutional phase II study. Treatment consisted of two cycles of induction carboplatin and paclitaxel, followed by concurrent chemoradiotherapy with paclitaxel, 5-fluorouracil, and hydroxyurea, in conjunction with twice-daily radiation therapy on a week-on, week-off basis.[1–3] After completion of induction chemotherapy, the patient was noted to have a partial response. As part of this protocol, patients are treated with intensity-modulated radiation therapy (IMRT) in an effort to spare the surrounding normal tissues, including the parotid glands.

Simulation

The patient was immobilized in the supine position, with her neck hyperextended and arms at her sides. The patient's headrest was securely attached to a custom-made headboard, which is indexed to the simulation and treatment tables (Varian Exact Couch, Varian Medical Systems, Palo Alto, CA). Immobilization of the head with appropriate neck extension was accomplished by securing a large custom-made "litecast" (Caraglas Ultra, Carapace, New Tazewell, TN) to the headboard. Reference radiopaque markers were placed on the litecast for treatment planning purposes. The shoulders were immobilized with adjustable straps that extend from the wrists to a board at the foot of the patient. Using the fixed side and ceiling lasers in the CT simulation room, the patient was aligned to the bore of an AcQSim CT scanner (Philips Medical Systems, Andover, MA). The planning CT scan extended from the base of the skull to the level of the carina and was performed with 3 mm slices. Scanning commenced 40 seconds after the start of the contrast injection.

To improve target delineation, all patients with advanced head and neck cancer at our institution undergo two planning CT scans (prior to and following induction chemotherapy). Intravenous contrast is used in both scans. The pre- and postinduction CT scans were aligned using the AcQSim VoxelQ fusion tools (Philips Medical Systems).

Target and Tissue Delineation

Target volumes and normal structures were contoured on the AcQSim VoxelQ workstation. A gross tumor volume (GTV), including the primary tumor and clinically involved lymph nodes, was entered using the preinduction CT scan. The GTV was then uniformly expanded by 1.2 cm to create the final boost volume, referred to as the 72 Gy planning target volume (PTV) (PTV_{72Gy}). The PTV_{72Gy} was subsequently modified in such a manner that it did not extend beyond the skin or encroach on the spinal cord. To avoid overlap with the skin, a few millimeters of skin were allowed between the PTV_{72Gy} and air. In addition, the PTV_{72Gy} contours were edited such that the vertebral body was surrounded by, but not encompassed within, the PTV_{72Gy} to avoid overdosing the spinal cord.

Two additional PTVs were then entered: PTV$_{51Gy}$ and PTV$_{36Gy}$. The PTV$_{51Gy}$ and PTV$_{36Gy}$ encompass the first echelon and first plus second echelon lymph nodes, respectively. In patients with nodal involvement (as in this patient), PTV$_{51Gy}$ extends one nodal level beyond the grossly involved nodes. PTV$_{36Gy}$ includes bilateral supraclavicular and level V lymph nodes, whereas PTV$_{51Gy}$ includes the supraclavicular and level V lymph nodes on the ipsilateral side only. Bilateral level II to IV lymph nodes are included in both PTV$_{36Gy}$ and PTV$_{51Gy}$. Given that this patient had bilateral clinical lymph node involvement, PTV$_{36Gy}$ and PTV$_{51Gy}$ were very similar.

A clinical target volume (CTV) is not routinely contoured in our patients with head and neck cancer undergoing IMRT. A PTV expansion of the CTV would require modifying the expanded PTV near the skin and spinal cord. Instead, PTVs are entered that equate to an expanded CTV. We have found that it is more time-efficient to enter the PTV directly rather than entering a CTV, expanding the CTV to generate the PTV, and then editing this volume. This approach necessitates an understanding and appreciation of how volume expansion not only affects the expansion on axial slices but also the expansion in caudal and cephalad directions. The AcQSim VoxelQ virtual fluoroscopy software allows one to visualize a projection of the PTV on digitally reconstructed anterior and lateral radiographs. Hence, the anterior and lateral dimensions of the entered PTV can be seen as the PTVs are being entered, assisting in proper target delineation.

On each axial slice, PTV$_{51Gy}$ was entered as one contiguous structure encompassing the lymph node regions, areas of suspected microscopic disease, and, if present, PTV$_{72Gy}$. This volume was then appropriately expanded by editing the PTV$_{51Gy}$ contours on each slice to create PTV$_{36Gy}$.

The organs at risk (OAR) outlined in this case included the bilateral parotid glands (superficial lobes), oral cavity anterior to the PTV, and posterior neck tissues. Entering oral cavity and posterior neck tissues allows for the inverse planning software to more effectively conform the high-dose isodose lines to the shape of the PTV. In addition, three separate regions for the spinal cord were entered: 36 Gy cord (denoted by spinal cord$_{36Gy}$), 51 Gy cord, and 72 Gy cord. Each of these regions corresponds to the portion of the spinal cord that is visible on CT slices with the corresponding PTV. Thus, spinal cord$_{36Gy}$ is located on slices containing only PTV$_{36Gy}$, whereas spinal cord$_{72Gy}$ exists on slices containing all PTVs. The rationale for splitting these volumes is that a higher dose may be delivered to spinal cord$_{36Gy}$ because it will be irradiated only during that portion of treatment (0–36 Gy). Conversely, care must be taken in limiting the dose to spinal cord$_{72Gy}$ during each of the individual plans so that cord tolerance is not reached when all plans are considered. Based on our experience, having various cord constraints in this region can lead to an improved treatment plan. Figures 18.5-1 to 18.5-2 illustrate

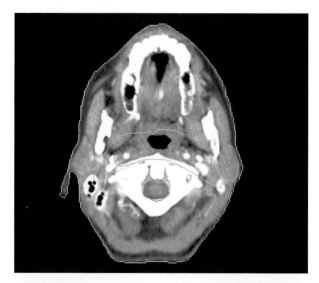

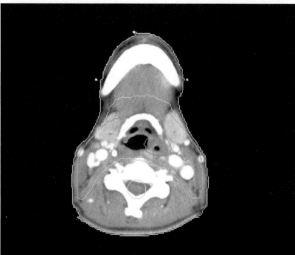

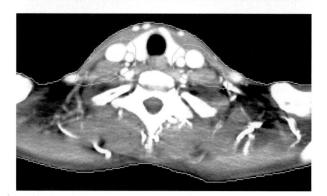

FIGURE 18.5-1. Representative axial computed tomography (CT) scan slices depicting the contoured gross tumor volume (*red*), planning target volume (PTV)$_{36Gy}$ (*light blue*), and PTV$_{51Gy}$ (*orange*). The salivary glands are shown in blue and green (the overlap of the PTV contours is also in green). The skin contour is yellow. The spinal cord traversing CT scan slices with the PTV$_{72Gy}$ (spinal cord$_{72Gy}$) is shown in light blue; using similar nomenclature, the spinal cord$_{36Gy}$ is shown in purple and the spinal cord$_{51Gy}$ is shown in dark blue. (To view a color version of this image, please refer to the CD-ROM.)

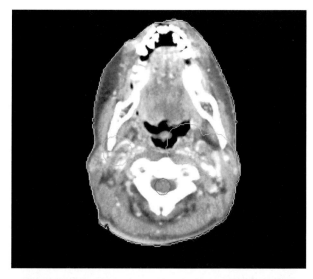

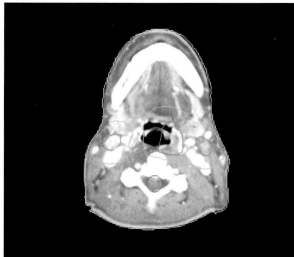

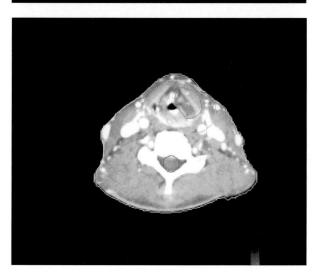

FIGURE 18.5-2. Representative axial computed tomography (CT) scan slices depicting the contoured gross tumor volume (*red*) and planning target volume at 76 Gy (*green*). The spinal cord and salivary glands are shown in purple, and the skin contour is yellow. (To view a color version of this image, please refer to the CD-ROM.)

representative axial slices highlighting the OAR in this patient and PTV$_{36Gy}$ and PTV$_{72Gy}$, respectively.

Treatment Planning

Inverse treatment planning was performed using *CORVUS*, version 4.0 (North American Scientific, NOMOS Radiation Oncology Division, Cranberry Township, PA). The *CORVUS* treatment planning system computes the optimal intensity modulation profiles using a simulating annealing algorithm. The user specifies the number of beams and their orientations, along with the target and normal tissue dose constraints. A total dose of 72 Gy was prescribed to the gross tumor and clinically involved neck nodes (PTV$_{72Gy}$) and was delivered in 1.5 Gy twice-daily fractions. As described above, the treatment volumes encompassing the tumor and first and second echelons draining lymphatics received 36 and 51 Gy, respectively (also in 1.5 Gy twice-daily fractions).

Nine equally spaced coplanar 6 MV photon beams (separated by 40°) were selected for this patient. Table 18.5-1 summarizes the input parameters for the PTVs and OAR used in the inverse planning program.

Once optimization was complete, the IMRT plan was evaluated both qualitatively (by assessing dose conformity and the presence of hot and cold spots on each axial slice) and quantitatively (by assessing the PTV and OAR dose-volume histograms [DVHs]). At our institution, cold spots are allowed only along the periphery of the PTV. Head and neck IMRT plans are considered acceptable if no volume within the PTV (ie, not at the periphery) receives < 95% and no more than 10% of the PTV receives > 105% of the prescription dose.

The output parameters of the PTVs and OAR are summarized in Table 18.5-2. We tend to place stringent limits on normal structures, such as the parotid glands and oral mucosa, but allow a relatively large volume to exceed the limit. Hence, the high-dose lines are forced away from these normal structures (as evidenced by the mean doses being lower than the limits) without compromising target coverage. The mean left and right parotid doses were approximately 40% of the prescribed dose to PTV$_{36Gy}$; the mean oral cavity dose was about 50%. For the entire 72 Gy treatment, the mean left parotid dose was 24.4 Gy and the mean right parotid dose was 20.9 Gy. Figures 18.5-3 and 18.5-4 depict the isodose curves for the 36 Gy and 72 Gy treatment plans, respectively. The DVHs for PTV$_{36Gy}$, PTV$_{51Gy}$, and PTV$_{72Gy}$ are shown in Figures 18.5-5 to 18.5-7, respectively; the DVHs for the OAR are shown as well.

Treatment Delivery and Quality Assurance

The patient was treated on a Varian 21EX linear accelerator (Varian Medical Systems) equipped with a 120-leaf multileaf collimator. Treatment was delivered in the

TABLE 18.5-1. Input Parameters

Structure	Limit (Gy)	Volume above Limit (%)	Minimum (Gy)	Maximum (Gy)
PTV$_{36Gy}$				
PTV	36	5	34.2	38.5
Left parotid gland	17	50	14	19
Right parotid gland	17	50	14	19
Oral mucosa	25	50	20	29
Posterior neck tissues	25	55	20	26
PTV$_{52Gy}$				
PTV	15	5	14.2	16.1
Left parotid gland	5.5	50	5.5	5.7
Right parotid gland	5.5	50	5.5	5.7
Oral mucosa	9.4	50	9.4	9.8
Posterior neck tissues	8.8	55	8.8	9
PTV$_{72Gy}$				
PTV	21	2	20	22.5
Left parotid gland	5	50	2.2	8
Right parotid gland	5	50	2	8
Oral mucosa	12	50	6	15
Posterior neck tissues	13	45	7	14

PTV = planning target volume.

TABLE 18.5-2. Output Parameters

Structure	Limit (Gy)	Volume below Limit (%)	Volume above Limit (%)	Minimum (Gy)	Maximum (Gy)	Mean (Gy)
PTV$_{36Gy}$						
PTV	36	15		16.2	39.1	36.7
Left parotid gland	17		38.9	7.8	29.7	15.9
Right parotid gland	17		35.7	3.9	30.5	15.4
Oral mucosa	25		13.6	1.8	36.2	17.4
Posterior neck tissues	25		79.9	5.5	35.4	30
PTV$_{51Gy}$						
PTV	15	15		12.4	16.4	15.3
Left parotid gland	5.5		56.6	1.2	12.4	5.2
Right parotid gland	5.5		79.8	1.1	11.5	4.1
Oral mucosa	9.4		79.2	1.2	14.4	7.3
Posterior neck tissues	8.8		8.6	3.5	14.3	11.4
PTV$_{72Gy}$						
PTV	21	15		17.6	22.9	21.4
Left parotid gland	5		25.1	0.6	17.1	3.3
Right parotid gland	5		0.5	0.5	7	1.4
Oral mucosa	12		26.5	2.2	19.5	10.2
Posterior neck tissues	13		65.7	3.9	19.2	13.7

PTV = planning target volume.

"step-and-shoot" mode. Together with daily setup, the total daily treatment time was approximately 15 minutes. A monitor unit verification calculation (*RadCalc*, version 4.3, Lifeline Software, Inc., Tyler, TX) was used to confirm the dose delivered to the isocenter. *RadCalc* uses a modified Clarkson integration technique to calculate the dose contribution from individual IMRT fields to a point of interest. In this particular case, the discrepancy between *CORVUS* and *RadCalc* was +0.3%, +1.1%, and +1.1% for the 36 Gy, 51 Gy, and 72 Gy plans, respectively. These discrepancies are considered acceptable.

Prior to initiating treatment, the patient underwent setup verification, at which time, orthogonal images were generated and compared with digitally reconstructed radiographs. Treatment setup films were obtained at least once per treatment cycle (once every 5 treatment days). To ensure

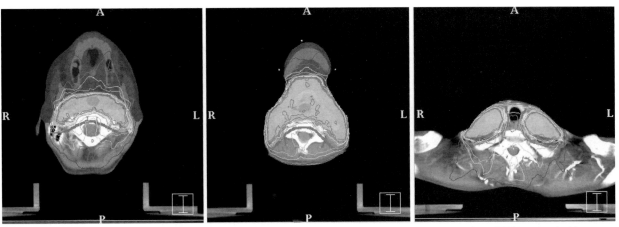

FIGURE 18.5-3. Axial sections of the 36 Gy intensity-modulated radiation therapy plan. The planning target volume (PTV) is colored with a green wash; the anterior sparing volumes are shown in a light purple wash, and a dark green line demarks the posterior sparing volume. The isodoses shown are 50% (*dark blue*), 60% (*light blue*), 70% (*lighter blue*), 80% (*blue-green*), 90% (*green-blue*), 94% (*yellow*), 98% (*red*), and 100% (*purple*). The most cephalad computed tomography slice shown demonstrates sparing of the parotid glands. The most caudal slice shows the PTV coverage of the supraclavicular lymph nodes. (To view a color version of this image, please refer to the CD-ROM.)

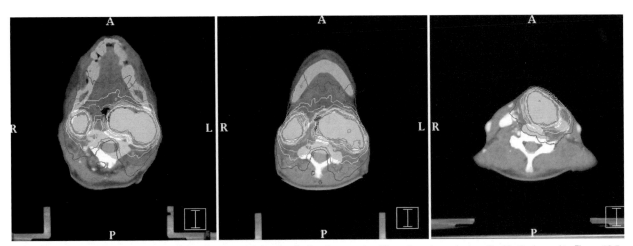

FIGURE 18.5-4. Axial sections of the 72 Gy intensity-modulated radiation therapy plan. The color scheme is described in the legend to Figure 18.5-3. The planning target volume covers the primary tumor and bilateral level II lymph nodes, all of which are present on the two more cephalad slices shown. (To view a color version of this image, please refer to the CD-ROM.)

accurate reproducibility of patient setup, a video-based positioning system developed at our institution was used with each treatment.[4] On the first day of treatment, a video image was captured with the patient aligned in the verified treatment position. On subsequent treatments, real-time images of the patient were obtained and video subtraction techniques were used to enable an interactive patient setup.

Prior to the final 72 Gy boost, the patient was resimulated to account for any weight loss and/or tumor shrinkage. Image fusion was again performed using the AcQSim VoxelQ fusion tools to align the initial (postinduction) CT scan with the midtreatment scan. Thus, when entering PTV$_{72Gy}$ onto the midtreatment scan, the originally entered PTV$_{72Gy}$ was used to facilitate target delineation.

Clinical Outcome

As with most patients treated with our aggressive chemoradiation regimen, this patient experienced confluent mucositis by her second cycle.[1–3] As a result, analgesics were required for pain, and a gastrostomy tube was placed to assist with feeding. She was able to swallow only small amounts of liquid during treatment. She also developed dry desquamation and a small area of moist desquamation on the skin of her anterior neck. Mouthwashes and antifungal agents were also used as needed for oral care.

The patient underwent a selective left neck dissection, which is commonly done in patients treated on our protocols with ≥ N2b disease,[5] and pyriform sinus biopsy 2 months

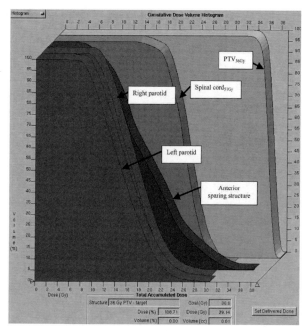

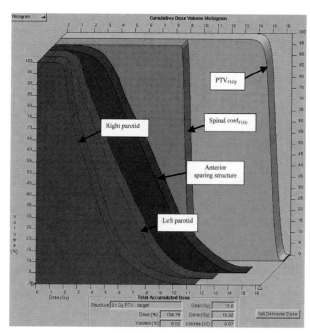

FIGURE 18.5-5. Dose-volume histograms for the 36 Gy intensity-modulated radiation therapy plan. The following structures are shown: planning target volume (PTV) (*green*), spinal cord51Gy (*olive*), anterior sparing structure (*maroon*), left parotid gland (*blue*), and right parotid gland (*blue*). The spinal cord36Gy and spinal cord72Gy are not shown. (To view a color version of this image, please refer to the CD-ROM.)

FIGURE 18.5-6. Dose-volume histograms for the 51 Gy intensity-modulated radiation therapy plan. The color scheme is described in Figure 18.5-5. The dose-volume histograms are not cumulative. The spinal cord72Gy is not shown. PTV = planning target volume. (To view a color version of this image, please refer to the CD-ROM.)

after completing treatment. There was no evidence of disease; hence, she had a pathologic complete response. At last follow-up (more than 1 year after diagnosis), the patient was alive and without evidence of disease recurrence. She was eating a diet of mostly soft foods and denied having xerostomia.

References

1. Vokes EE, Stenson K, Rosen FR, et al. Weekly carboplatin and paclitaxel followed by concomitant paclitaxel, fluorouracil, and hydroxyurea chemoradiotherapy: curative and organ-preserving therapy for advanced head and neck cancer. J Clin Oncol 2003;21:320–6.

2. Haraf DJ, Rosen F, Stenson K, et al. Induction chemotherapy followed by concomitant TFHX chemoradiotherapy with reduced dose radiation in advanced head and neck cancer. Clin Cancer Res 2003;9:5936–43.

3. Milano MT, Vokes EE, Witt ME, et al. Retrospective comparison of intensity modulated radiation therapy (IMRT) and conventional three-dimensional RT (3DCRT) in advanced head and neck patients treated with definitive chemoradiation [abstract]. Proc Am Soc Clin Oncol 2003;22:499.

4. Milliken BD, Rubin SJ, Hamilton RJ, et al. Performance of a video-image-subtraction-based patient positioning system. Int J Radiat Oncol Biol Phys 1997;38:855–66.

5. Stenson KM, Haraf DJ, Pelzer H, et al. The role of cervical lymphadenectomy after aggressive concomitant chemoradiotherapy: the feasibility of selective neck dissection. Arch Otolaryngol Head Neck Surg 2000;126:950–6.

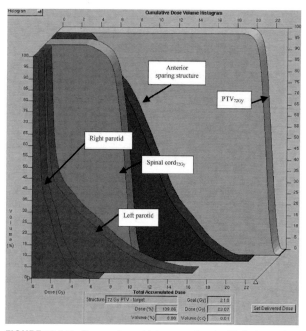

FIGURE 18.5-7. Dose-volume histograms for the 72 Gy intensity-modulated radiation therapy plan. The color scheme is described in Figure 18.5-5. The dose-volume histograms are not cumulative. The spinal cord72Gy is shown in tan. PTV = planning target volume. (To view a color version of this image, please refer to the CD-ROM.)

FUNCTIONAL IMAGING IN HEAD AND NECK CANCER

EMERGING TECHNOLOGY

THOMAS YANG, MD, K. S. CLIFFORD CHAO, MD

The twentieth century witnessed the advent and development of radiography, computed tomography (CT), and magnetic resonance imaging (MRI), all of which have enabled physicians to visualize both pathologic and normal anatomy in a way that was never before possible. Major advances have also occurred in nuclear medicine with the development of positron emission tomography (PET) and single photon emission computed tomography (SPECT). The standard radiologic images (CT, MRI) provide anatomic information, whereas biologic images (PET, SPECT) provide metabolic, physiologic, genotypic, and phenotypic data. Important to the practice of oncology have been the numerous radioisotopes that have become available. For nuclear medicine, these can provide critical information on the metabolism and function of different tumors.

Radiation oncology has been a beneficiary of the progress in imaging technology. In particular, biologic imaging has had a tremendous impact on intensity-modulated radiation therapy (IMRT) because IMRT allows the delivery of different doses of radiation to multiple targets. Important to an understanding of IMRT is the concept of the biologic target volume first proposed by Ling and colleagues (Figure 18.6-1).[1] The important advantage of IMRT is that normal tissue is spared; thus, the side effects of radiation therapy (RT) can be reduced. For obvious reasons, this capability is particularly useful in the treatment of tumors of the head and neck.

The purpose of this chapter is to discuss the current applications of functional imaging in head and neck cancer IMRT planning and the monitoring of treatment response. Future directions in functional imaging are also discussed.

Nuclear Medicine Modalities

Nuclear medicine, and in particular [18]fluorodeoxyglucose positron emission tomography ([18]FDG-PET), is the functional imaging method most commonly used in head and neck cancer. [18]FDG-PET is used both to stage patients and to monitor their therapeutic response (or the lack thereof). With the advent of hybrid PET-CT scanners, one can now combine metabolic and anatomic information in planning RT, including IMRT. The use of hybrid scanners is likely to become more widespread in medical centers throughout the United States.

In this section, the role of [18]FDG-PET and hybrid PET-CT scanners is described in detail. Alternative metabolic imaging methods are also discussed, namely, methods employing radiolabeled amino acids and nucleosides. The noninvasive imaging of tumor hypoxia is also presented. Interested readers should also refer to Chapter 8, "PET-CT in IMRT Planning."

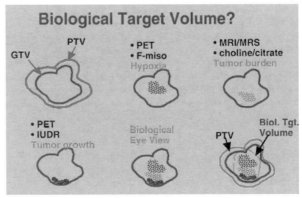

FIGURE 18.6-1. The concept of biologic target volume shown in a manner that incorporates the different aspects of functional imaging, namely, tumor hypoxia, tumor burden, and tumor growth. GTV = gross tumor volume; IUDR = Iodine 124-iododeoxyuridine; MRI = magnetic resonance imaging; MRS = magnetic resonance spectroscopy; PET = positron emission tomography; PTV = planning target volume. (To view a color version of this image, please refer to the CD-ROM.) Reproduced with permission from Ling CC et al.[1]

18FDG-PET

The long half-life of 18-fluorine (^{18}F) has made ^{18}FDG-PET the most popular metabolic imaging modality. Its popularity is also due to the fact that, because tumor growth requires energy, the marker can be used to determine the degree of tumor proliferation.

The use of ^{18}FDG-PET in RT planning has been evaluated in several studies. Rege and colleagues noted that local control and survival were improved in patients with head and neck cancer whose tumors had a metabolic rate greater than that in the cerebellum.[2] These results suggest that pretreatment ^{18}FDG-PET could be used to predict which irradiated patients will attain local control. It may also help identify which patients require combined-modality therapy or adjusted fractionation schedules.

Brun and colleagues noted that a low metabolic rate of glucose in primary and metastatic lesions was associated with local complete response in patients with squamous cell carcinoma of the head and neck undergoing RT.[3] Allal and colleagues found that patients with head and neck cancer who showed a high initial FDG uptake may require more aggressive treatment (Figure 18.6-2).[4]

In a recent Radiation Therapy Oncology Group (RTOG) symposium, the application of hybrid ^{18}FDG-PET–CT imaging to RT was highlighted.[5] An important point made at this symposium was that delineation of the gross tumor volume (GTV) is a critical step in RT treatment planning. However, the visualization of primary and abnormal lymph nodes and observer variation are key limitations when using CT alone, as shown by a study of 30 patients with non–small cell lung cancer presented at the symposium. The first goal of the study was to determine if hybrid ^{18}FDG-PET–CT improves treatment planning. The second was to determine if hybrid ^{18}FDG-PET–CT reduces interobserver variation. Three radiation oncologists contoured the GTV on the basis of CT alone; they then did GTV contouring using PET-CT data, after which separate treatment plans were generated on the basis of each GTV. Comparison of the resultant treatment plans revealed that the plans were changed in seven patients (23%) when metabolic information was incorporated. In particular, the fused images provided better target volume definition owing to the detection of lymph node involvement and distant metastases by PET not seen on CT. Hybrid ^{18}FDG-PET–CT was associated with reduced interobserver variation, as evidenced by a reduction in the mean ratio of the largest to smallest GTV from 2.31 (CT alone) to 1.56 (hybrid). It was concluded that hybrid ^{18}FDG-PET–CT more consistently defines the GTV in these patients.

To corroborate these findings, Ciernik and colleagues studied 39 patients with different solid tumors.[6] All underwent CT and FDG-PET using a hybrid scanner. Initially, the GTV was delineated by two radiation oncologists based on CT alone. The ^{18}FDG-PET information was then incorporated into the CT data, and GTV was again delineated. The GTV was modified in more than half (56%) of the patients once the ^{18}FDG-PET information was incorporated. Moreover, variability in the volumes delineated by the two radiation oncologists decreased from an average of 25.7 to 9.2 cm^3 (Figure 18.6-3).

Given that multimodality imaging is becoming more widespread, feasibility and quality assurance issues regarding the coregistration of images have been raised. To address these issues, Daisne and colleagues studied the accuracy, reproducibility, and consistency of the coregistration procedure using a phantom and four patients with pharyngolaryngeal tumors.[7] In particular, they studied the translation and rotational displacements relative to a reference CT scan and found that the coregistration accuracy ranged from 0.8 to 6.2 mm for the phantom and from 1.2 to 4.6 mm for the patients. The accuracy was only slightly worse in the z-axis, and inter- and intraobserver variations were small. These results suggest that the coregistration of anatomic (CT, MRI) and functional (PET) images is accurate in patients with head and neck cancer (Figure 18.6-4).

In addition to its utility in treatment planning, ^{18}FDG-PET has also been shown to be useful in predicting treatment response. Greven and colleagues studied 45 patients with head and neck cancer who underwent ^{18}FDG-PET and CT or MRI prior to RT.[8] Follow-up studies were obtained at 1 month (36 patients), 4 months (28 patients), 12 months (19 patients), and 24 months (15 patients). At 4 months, none of the 18 patients with a negative pretreatment ^{18}FDG-PET had persistent tumor, whereas 6 of 7 patients with positive pretreatment findings had persistent tumor and 2 of 3 with equivocal findings had positive

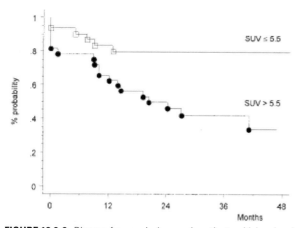

FIGURE 18.6-2. Disease-free survival curves in patients with head and neck carcinoma who showed a standardized uptake value (SUV) of ≤ 5.4 versus ≥ to 5.5 and hence the ability of the SUV to predict the outcome of radiation therapy in head and neck carcinoma. Reproduced with permission from Allal AS et al.[4]

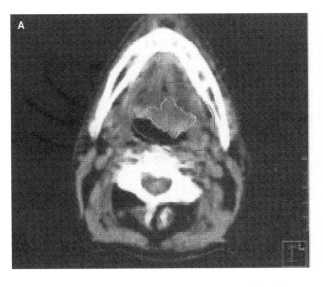
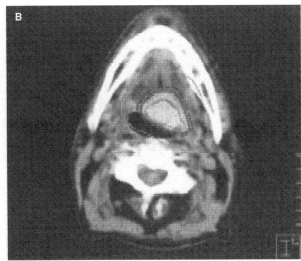
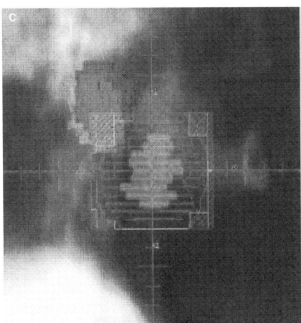
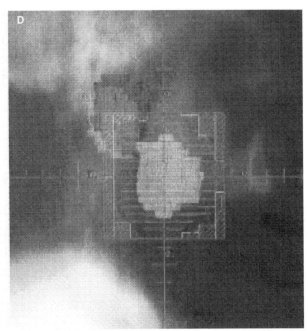

FIGURE 18.6-3. Treatment plans for a patient with supraglottic carcinoma generated based on computed tomography (CT) alone (*A*) and positron emission tomography (PET)-CT (*B*). Axial section through tumor showing gross tumor volume delineated from CT alone (*C*) and PET-CT (*D*). (To view a color version of this image, please refer to the CD-ROM.) Reproduced with permission from Ciernik IF et al.[6]

biopsy results. It was felt that PET is excellent for the initial visualization of head and neck cancers and that 4 months after RT is the best time to repeat scans to determine tumor response (Figure 18.6-5).

Terhaard and colleagues evaluated [18]FDG-PET in detecting local recurrence in irradiated patients with laryngeal and pharyngeal cancer.[9] Of 75 patients studied, local recurrence was noted in 37 on the basis of biopsy findings. All patients with recurrent tumor also had a positive [18]FDG-PET scan. The [18]FDG-PET findings were positive in the first set of scans in 34 of the 37 patients, for a sensitivity of 92%. The positive predictive value (PPV) was 71% (34 of 48

patients). [18]FDG-PET was then repeated in 27 patients (34 more scans). When scans were collectively analyzed, positive scans were found in 45 of 48 patients (94% sensitivity). The PPV was 67% (45/67). False-positive results were attributed to extensive speaking or swallowing after [18]FDG administration and to inflammation, radionecrosis, and edema. The authors concluded that [18]FDG-PET should be the first diagnostic scan when local recurrence is suspected. If the scan results are negative, no biopsy is required. However, if the results are positive, a biopsy should be performed; if the biopsy is negative and a follow-up scan shows decreased [18]FDG uptake, local recurrence is unlikely (Figure 18.6-6).

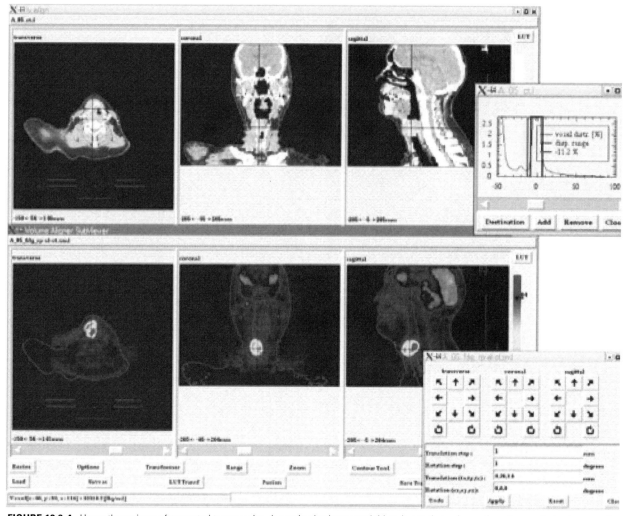

FIGURE 18.6-4. Upper three views of computed tomography–determined volume overlaid on lower three views of positron emission tomography (PET) –determined volume. Interactive translations and rotations enable fusion of the two images. (To view a color version of this image, please refer to the CD-ROM.) Reproduced with permission from Daisne JF et al.[7]

Rogers and colleagues studied the use of [18]FDG-PET in 12 irradiated patients with stage III–IV head and neck cancer who underwent [18]FDG-PET imaging before and 1 month after RT.[10] A planned neck dissection and pathologic correlation with post-RT scans were performed. The sensitivity, specificity, PPV, and negative predictive value (NPV) of [18]FDG-PET were 45%, 100%, 100%, and 14%, respectively. These results suggest that whereas positive PET findings after RT might accurately indicate the presence of residual disease, negative PET scans after RT cannot be

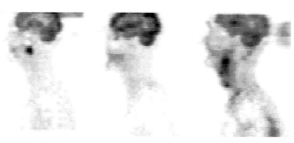

FIGURE 18.6-5. A patient with head and neck cancer who underwent pretreatment positron emission tomography (*left*), which was negative 1 month after radiotherapy (*middle*) and positive 4 months after radiotherapy (*right*). Reproduced with permission from Greven KM et al.[8]

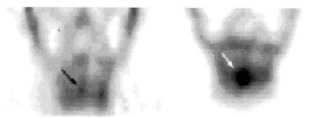

FIGURE 18.6-6. Fluorodeoxyglucose–positron emission tomography study obtained in a patient with glottic squamous cell carcinoma 19 months (*left*) and 30 months (*right*) after radiation therapy. Reproduced with permission from Terhaard CH et al.[9]

relied on to indicate absence of disease. More data are clearly necessary before [18]FDG-PET should be used as the sole basis for deciding whether to omit post-RT neck surgery.

With the increasing use of hybrid scanners, [18]FDG-PET will likely have an increasing role in the planning of IMRT. However, the two studies just described also demonstrate the utility of [18]FDG-PET in monitoring treatment response.

Radiolabeled Amino Acids

Although [18]FDG is the most commonly used metabolic imaging marker, radiolabeled amino acids have also been studied. The advantages of amino acids over [18]FDG in PET include less uptake in inflammatory tissue and that the total amino acid signal corresponds to the extent of tumor proliferation.[11]

Leskinen-Kallio and colleagues studied the efficacy of ^{11}C]-methionine (^{11}C]-MET)–PET in head and neck tumors.[12] In 46 patients evaluated, tumors were visualized by ^{11}C]-MET–PET in 42 patients. In 3 patients, the tumor was not well delineated owing to tracer accumulation in adjacent structures. Only one tumor was not visualized. These results suggest that ^{11}C]-MET may be effective in imaging malignant head and neck tumors. The disadvantages of ^{11}C]-MET include a short half-life and its tendency to accumulate in the salivary glands.

Recently, de Boer and colleagues used L-[1-^{11}C]-tyrosine (TYR)–PET to evaluate treatment response in 19 irradiated patients with laryngeal cancer.[13] These patients underwent a TYR-PET scan before RT (PET$_1$) and at 3 months (PET$_2$). Patients who had suspected recurrence on physical examination then underwent a third TYR-PET scan (PET$_3$). If recurrence was suspected, CT and biopsy were also performed. All 19 patients had a positive PET$_1$ scan. Of 15 who agreed to have the PET$_2$ scan, 7 had residual disease suspected on physical examination. Of these, 4 had a positive PET$_2$ scan and 3 had a negative PET$_2$ scan, all of which were confirmed by histologic studies. The other 8 had no residual disease on physical examination; 1 had a positive PET$_2$ scan, and the remaining 7 had a negative PET$_2$ scan, with, again, all findings confirmed by histologic studies. The sensitivity, specificity, PPV, and NPV of the PET$_2$ were all 100%. Of 6 patients with a suspected recurrence, 4 had a positive PET$_3$ scan and 2 had a negative PET$_3$ scan. These results were also verified by histologic studies. Thus, for the PET$_3$ scan, the sensitivity, specificity, PPV, and NPV were all 100%. The results of this small study suggest that TYR-PET is highly accurate in determining the response to RT in laryngeal cancer. However, larger studies are needed to further corroborate these results and to determine whether TYR-PET is predictive in other tumor sites.

Other radiolabeled amino acids that remain to be tested include L-3-iodo-a-methyltyrosine, O-(2-[^{18}F] fluoroethyl-L-tyrosine, and [^{18}F-α-methyl]-TYR. These two radioisotopes have longer half-lives than the two amino acids described above. More studies of these markers are also required to assess their predictive value in head and neck cancer.

Radiolabeled Nucleosides

Radiolabeled nucleosides may also prove useful for metabolic imaging for IMRT planning. This modality directly assesses the synthesis of deoxyribonucleic acid (DNA). Several of these radiopharmaceuticals have been studied.

[^{11}C]-Thymidine and [methyl-^{11}C]-thymidine have been found to achieve high uptake in head and neck carcinomas.[14] However, although [^{11}C]-thymidine achieved substantial uptake in patients in early studies, consistently high levels were not achieved in numerous patients.

Because of the 20-minute half-life of the [^{11}C]-thymidines, bromodeoxyuridine (BrdU), a thymidine analog, is being used instead to label cells undergoing DNA synthesis. BrdU has been labeled with [76]Br for imaging tumors in mice.[15] More work needs to be done, however, to make the uptake of this reagent more DNA specific.

High expression of thymidine phosphorylase has been associated with decreased survival in patients with head and neck cancer. An inhibitor of this enzyme, 5-chloro-6-(2-iminopyrrolidin-1-yl)methyl-2,4(1H,3H)-pyrimidinedione, has been shown to shrink tumors in mice.[16] This has prompted the use of radiolabeled analogs of this inhibitor to image tumors expressing the enzyme at high levels. Commonly used isotopes in this setting are [125,131]I and [211]At.

Recently, Cobben and colleagues compared [18]F-3′-fluoro-3′-deoxy-L-thymidine (FLT) and FDG imaging of laryngeal cancer.[17] In this study, 11 patients with suspected recurrence and 10 with histologically confirmed primary laryngeal cancer underwent biopsy after PET. Mean standardized uptake values (SUVs), maximum SUVs, and tumor to nontumor (TNT) ratios were determined. Both modalities correctly detected laryngeal cancer in 15 of 17 patients. However, the uptake values were higher for FDG. Namely, the maximum SUVs were 3.3 for [18]FDG versus 1.6 for FLT. Corresponding mean SUVs and TNT ratios were 2.7 versus 1.2 and 1.9 versus 1.5, respectively. In one patient, FLT-PET showed only faint uptake of the marker, whereas [18]FDG-PET showed intense uptake. FLT may thus not be ideal for clinically detecting laryngeal cancer and for RT treatment planning.

Although, to date, radiolabeled amino acids and nucleosides have not been used for planning IMRT in head and neck cancer, the future may see their use as alternatives to FDG.

Functional Imaging of Tumor Hypoxia

In 1955, Thomlinson and Gray first described the phenomenon of tumor hypoxia.[18] Over the next half-century, researchers established that tumor hypoxia is associated with radioresistance and hence the poor locoregional control of locally advanced cancers. This prompted efforts to visualize tumor hypoxia in a noninvasive way.

Iodinated azomycin arabinoside for SPECT and fluoromisonidazole for PET were among the first markers used to image tumor hypoxia.[19] Because of limitations in spatial resolution, however, neither gained widespread acceptance.

In 1997, Fujibayashi and colleagues reported that Cu (II) diacetyl-bis-(N^4- methylthiosemicarbazone), or ^{60}Cu-ATSM, was selectively retained in ischemic myocardial tissue but washed out of normoxic myocardium.[20] Lewis and colleagues confirmed this selective uptake in rat tumor models.[21] The partial pressure of oxygen in tissue was measured via a needle oxygen electrode. Some animals breathed 100% O_2 to mimic normoxic conditions; hydralazine was administered in others to simulate hypoxic conditions. ^{60}Cu-ATSM uptake was increased by 37% in the rats administered hydralazine.

Chao and colleagues evaluated the feasibility of this noninvasive hypoxia tumor marker in guiding head and neck cancer IMRT planning.[19] Specifically, a subvolume of hypoxic tumor within the GTV (hGTV) was determined using ^{60}Cu-ATSM-PET. This image was then fused with a corresponding CT image, and an IMRT treatment plan was generated. This process involved several steps.

First, the quality of the image fusion needed to be evaluated in terms of image integrity after transfer, spatial target alignment, image fusion accuracy, and system functionality. A custom-made head phantom with CT and PET visible targets was fabricated to determine the spatial accuracy of target volume mapping (Figure 18.6-7). The spatial accuracy was then confirmed after coregistration by containing visible targets on the CT scans and checking them on the PET image. These contours were within 2 mm of each other on the two images.

Second, ^{60}Cu-ATSM–PET and CT images were obtained and fused. Patients underwent CT scanning wearing a thermoplastic immobilization head mask, with the markers described above used to assist in image fusion. For PET scanning, the patients were first injected intravenously with 13 mCi of ^{60}Cu-ATSM. Patients then underwent 60 minutes of dynamic PET scanning in the thermoplastic masks. The respective images were sent to an imaging workstation for image segmentation and fusion using the *AcQSim* software (Philips Medical Systems, Andover, MA) (Figures 18.6-8 and 18.6-9).

Third, target determination and delineation were performed. GTV and clinical target volume (CTV) were demarcated per International Commission on Radiation Units and Measurements reports 50 and 62.[9,10] To subdelineate the hGTV, tumor volumes shown by ^{60}Cu-ATSM PET to have a minimum threshold intensity were designated as ATSM-avid. ^{60}Cu-ATSM uptakes in normoxic muscle in the contralateral neck were also examined, and this involved the calculation of the average normoxic muscle intensity. Volumes with a tumor to muscle (T:M) ratio of 2 or greater were deemed hypoxic. No normal tissues in the neck exhibited T:M ratios of 2 or greater. Thus, the volume within the GTV with a T:M of 2 or greater was considered hypoxic.

After the volumes and subvolumes were demarcated, these images were transferred to a planning computer to generate IMRT plans (Figure 18.6-10). The dose prescription strategy for hypoxia imaging-guided IMRT was modified. Dosing

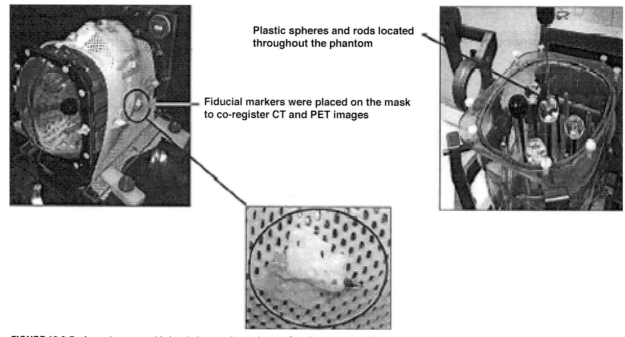

Plastic spheres and rods located throughout the phantom

Fiducial markers were placed on the mask to co-register CT and PET images

FIGURE 18.6-7. An anthropomorphic head phantom is used to confirm the accuracy of image registration and the fusion process. Plastic ampules, serving as fiducial markers, were placed to help assess the accuracy of coregistration of computed tomography (CT) and positron emission tomography (PET) images. Reproduced with permission from Chao KS et al.[19]

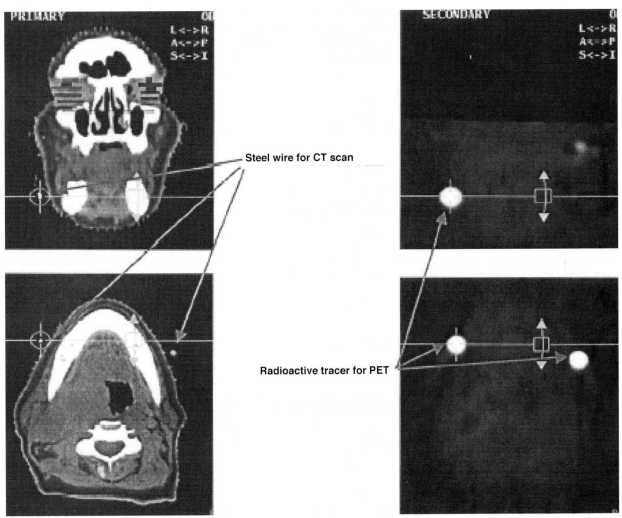

Steel wire for CT scan

Radioactive tracer for PET

FIGURE 18.6-8. Computed tomography (CT)–positron emission tomography (PET) image fusion done using fiducial markers in a patient with squamous cell carcinoma of the right tonsil and neck nodes. Reproduced with permission from Chao KS et al.[19]

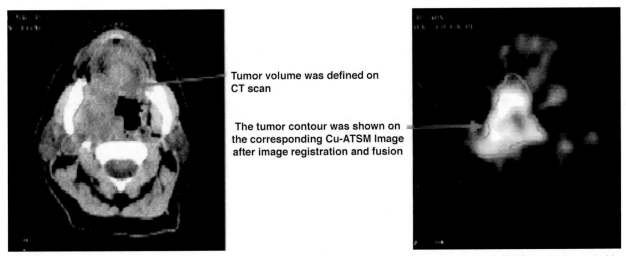

Tumor volume was defined on CT scan

The tumor contour was shown on the corresponding Cu-ATSM Image after image registration and fusion

FIGURE 18.6-9. Using the fused image shown in Figure 18.6-8, the hypoxic tumor fraction (hypoxic gross tumor volume [GTV]) is subdelineated within the GTV. CT = computed tomography; ^{60}Cu-ATSM = Cu (II) diacetyl-bis-(N^4- methylthiosemicarbazone). (To view a color version of this image, please refer to the CD-ROM.) Reproduced with permission from Chao KS et al.[19]

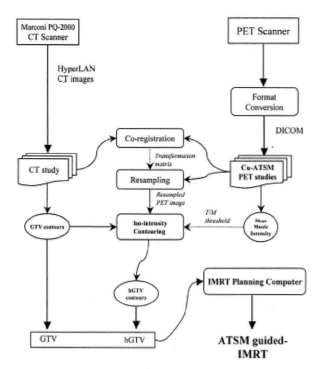

FIGURE 18.6-10. Flow chart summarizing the overall process used to coordinate hypoxia imaging-guided intensity-modulated radiation therapy (IMRT). CT = computed tomography; Cu-ATSM = Cu (II) diacetyl-bis-(N^4-methylthiosemicarbazone); DICOM = Digital Imaging and Communication in Medicine; GTV = gross tumor volume; hGTV = hypoxic gross tumor volume; PET = positron emission tomography; T/M = tumor to muscle. Reproduced with permission from Chao KS et al.[19]

was as follows: 80 Gy in 35 fractions to the hGTV, 70 Gy in 35 fractions to the GTV, 60 Gy total to the CTV, and no more than 30 Gy total to the parotid glands (Figure 18.6-11).

This study demonstrated the utility of hypoxia imaging-guided IMRT. However, several issues remain. First, the dose needed to overcome radioresistance owing to tumor hypoxia

is unclear. The relationship between ^{60}Cu-ATSM intensity and radiocurability through the correlation of pathologic and imaging findings needs to be more closely examined. In addition, the tumor target uncertainty of the hGTV within the GTV needs to be better ascertained. Last, we need to better understand tumor reoxygenation kinetics.

Magnetic Resonance Imaging
MRI Fusion

MRI is very useful in target volume delineation. Emami and colleagues evaluated eight patients with nasopharyngeal carcinoma who underwent CT with T_1- and T_2-weighted MRIs.[22] Three treatment plans were generated: (1) a three-dimensional conformal radiation therapy (3DCRT) plan based on CT, (2) a 3DCRT plan based on fused CT and MRI targets, and (3) an IMRT plan based on fused CT and MRI targets (Figure 18.6-12). The first plan achieved adequate target coverage and critical structure sparing. However, because MRI-based targets were larger and more irregularly shaped, some of the target might not have been incorporated. The second plan led to underdosing of the GTV and the exposure of critical structures to increased doses. The last plan achieved both better PTV coverage and critical structure sparing.

Quantitative Tissue Perfusion

Tissue perfusion can significantly affect tumor responsiveness to RT; thus, it is important to gauge perfusion to improve treatment planning. A noninvasive MRI spin-labeling technique has been studied to see if it could accurately show tissue prefusion.[23] Specifically, the long relaxation time T_1 was measured with segmented snapshot fast low-angle shot (FLASH) imaging. Using a two-compartment tissue model, perfusion values were determined pixelwise. Perfusion images with a slice thickness of 10 mm and an in-plane resolution of 1.9×2.8 mm^2 were acquired.

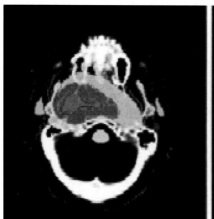
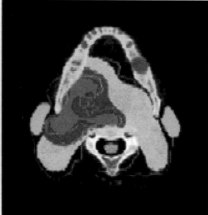
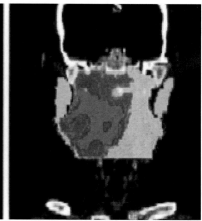

FIGURE 18.6-11. Dose distribution of hypoxia imaging-guided intensity-modulated radiation therapy. The yellow line corresponds to 80 Gy, the green line corresponds to 70 Gy, and the blue line corresponds to 50 Gy. (To view a color version of this image, please refer to the CD-ROM.) Reproduced with permission from Chao KS et al.[19]

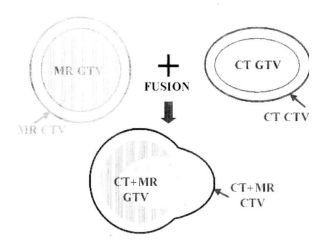

FIGURE 18.6-12. Schematic demonstrating magnetic resonance and computed tomography (CT) image fusion as part of three-dimensional conformal radiation therapy and intensity-modulated radiation therapy treatment planning in nasopharyngeal carcinoma. CT = computed tomography; CTV = clinical target volume; GTV = gross tumor volume; MR = magnetic resonance imaging. Reproduced with permission from Emami B et al.[22]

This spin-labeling technique visualizes tumor and normal tissue perfusion plus changes in perfusion during RT. However, the technique needs further refinement before it can be used for IMRT planning (Figure 18.6-13).

Future Trends in Functional Imaging
Apoptosis Assessment

Apoptosis has recently been studied as a marker of tumor response to chemotherapy[24] and is also a major form of cell death that occurs in response to RT. Researchers therefore needed to develop a technique to measure apoptosis and recognized the annexin V–phosphatidylserine complex that is expressed on the extracellular membrane when a cell undergoes apoptosis as a potentially useful marker. One resulting imaging method, technetium 99m (^{99m}Tc)-rh-annexin V PET-SPECT, has been used as a way to measure apoptosis in cancer patients undergoing chemotherapy.[24] Currently, ^{99m}Tc-rh-annexin V uptakes in human tumor after RT are also being studied.

Epidermal Growth Factor Receptor

Several studies have shown that the antagonism of growth factor receptors may promote radiosensitivity. Most attention has focused on the epidermal growth factor (EGF) pathway. The monoclonal antibody IMC-225, which blocks ligand binding and inhibits autophosphorylation and downstream intracellular signaling, has been shown to improve tumor response to RT.[25]

The in vivo visualization of the EGF receptor EGFR may thus enable clinicians to determine which patients should concurrently receive IMC-225. Several radiopharmaceuticals have been tested for this purpose. A ^{99m}Tc-labeled anti-EGF antibody has been shown to accurately gauge EGFR expression both in tumor-bearing animal models and in a patient with head and neck carcinoma.[26] Other radioisotopes being tested include ^{123}I-EGF and ^{111}In–diethylenetriamine pentaacetic acid (DTPA)-EGF.[27,28] However, more studies need to be done before these drugs can be used clinically.

Molecular Imaging and Radiobiologic Phenotyping

Several strategies are being developed that make use of molecular imaging and that may be useful in IMRT planning. These strategies use nuclear magnetic resonance or nuclear medicine techniques for the actual imaging.

FIGURE 18.6-13. A patient with head and neck carcinoma with right-sided lymph node neck metastasis. (A) Fast low-angle shot (FLASH) image before radiation therapy; enhanced perfusion values are observed at the edge of the tumor, (D) (A) FLASH image obtained after 54 Gy of treatment shows a moderate reduction in the size of the tumor with high perfusion in the center of the tumor (E); (C) and (f) show decreases in areas of poor perfusion. (To view a color version of this image, please refer to the CD-ROM.) Reproduced with permission from Schmitt P et al.[23]

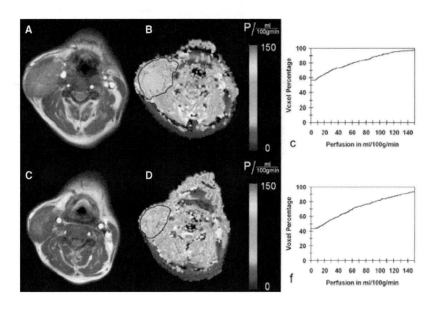

The first strategy is "indirect" or reporter gene imaging. Hackman and colleagues[29] and Blasberg and Gelovani[30] transfected W256 tumor cells with adenovirus containing the *Escherichia coli* cytosine deaminase (CD)–herpes simplex virus type 1 thymidine kinase (HSV1-tk) fusion (*CD/TK*) gene. Noninvasive imaging to monitor *CD/TK* gene expression was performed with [^{124}I]2′-fluoro-2′-deoxy-1-β-D-arabinofuranosyl-5-iodouracil (FIAU)–PET. HSV1-tk activity was monitored with [^{124}I]-FIAU–PET, and CD activity was determined by the CD enzyme assay. [^{124}I]-FIAU accumulation was found to be directly related to *CD/TK* expression. CD enzyme activity was also directly related to *CD/TK* expression. Further, a significant linear relationship between [^{124}I]-FIAU accumulation and CD enzyme activity was observed. Thus, it was concluded that individual elements of *CD/TK* gene expression can be measured by noninvasive imaging, in particular [^{124}I]-FIAU–PET.

The second strategy is "direct" imaging of endogenous molecules, such as cell surface receptors. An example of such "direct" imaging involves the use of antisense ribonucleic acid (RNA) targeting the messenger ribonucleic acid (mRNA) of key oncogenes.[31] This strategy entails the use of radiolabeled oligonucleotides (RASONs), which are small oligonucleotide sequences complementary to target mRNA or DNA. RASON probes directly image gene expression at the point of transcription. However, critical issues with RASONs are generating a sufficient amount of antisense RNA, stabilizing the antisense RNA, confirming the accessibility of the binding domain, and ensuring sufficient amounts of target mRNA.

The third strategy is "surrogate" or biomarker imaging.[30] Surrogate imaging is best defined as monitoring of the downstream events that result from molecular-genetic processes. This method may be useful in the development of biochemical pathway–specific drugs. In particular, it may be useful for monitoring the response to antiangiogenesis treatment. However, a key drawback of the method is its decreased specificity owing to the number of other molecular-genetic processes.

These molecular imaging strategies are still very new, and more work is needed to make them useful for the planning of different RT modalities.

Future Trends in Molecular Imaging

Many other novel approaches to molecular imaging that may find application in RT planning and monitoring are also being pursued. One method is to assess angiogenesis by imaging the binding motif on integrin, a proangiogenic factor that binds to numerous ligands in the extracellular matrix. This binding motif is composed of –Arg-Gly-Asp– (RGD). The imaging of cyclic RGD peptides, using ^{18}F, ^{99m}Tc, and ^{111}In, has been used to gauge angiogenesis.[32] More studies of this approach are needed.

Another molecular imaging method uses as its basis P-glycoprotein, the product of the multidrug-resistance gene *MDR1*, which belongs to a group of energy-dependent efflux transporters. Pgp is overexpressed in numerous malignant tumors. The imaging of Pgp expression to predict resistance to both chemotherapy and RT has been investigated using the myocardial perfusion agents ^{99m}Tc-tetrofosmin and ^{99m}Tc-furifosmin (Figure 18.6-14).[33] However, these SPECT agents need to be examined further in clinical settings.

Conclusions

The field of radiation oncology is at a key crossroad. Throughout the twentieth century, RT was planned based on anatomic imaging. However, with the advent of IMRT and functional imaging, the era of physical conformity is coming to an end. We are now entering the era of biologic conformity.[1] Biologic imaging, which includes imaging tumor hypoxia, tumor proliferation, and tumor burden, will enable radiation oncologists to define a "biologic target" volume. Use of the biologic target volume, in conjunction with IMRT, can vastly enhance target delineation and dose delivery. Such multidimensional RT may improve the success of cancer treatment.

Similarly, Coleman has advocated a molecular approach to RT. In this approach, radiation is viewed as an instigator of molecular events (Figure 18.6-15).[34] In short, this novel approach could enable scientists to study radiation's effects on molecular damage and molecular treatment. Such molecular profiling could be performed before and after RT and over time. Ultimately, the combination of molecular and functional imaging with molecular profiling and novel therapeutics holds great promise.

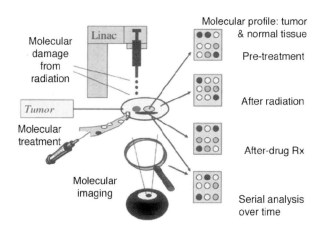

FIGURE 18.6-15. The changing view of radiation oncology as the instigator of molecular events. Molecular profiling can be performed before and after radiation therapy and after chemotherapy. Linac = linear accelerator; Rx = treatment. Reproduced with permission from Coleman CN.[34]

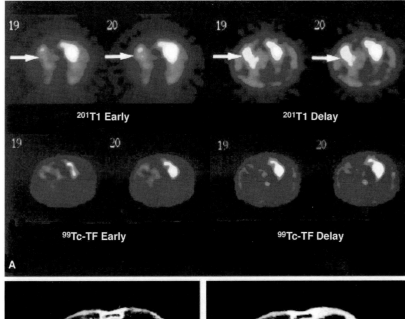

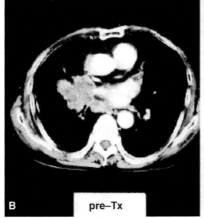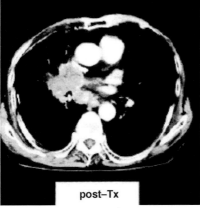

FIGURE 18.6-14. Imaging of P-glycoprotein expression with technetium 99m (^{99m}Tc)-tetrofosmin and ^{99m}Tc-furifosmin in lung cancer to predict response to radiation therapy and chemotherapy. In the future, similar modalities may be used in head and neck cancers. Tx = therapy. (To view a color version of this image, please refer to the CD-ROM.) Reproduced with permission from Fukumoto M et al.[33]

References

1. Ling CC, Humm J, Larson S, et al. Towards multidimensional radiotherapy (MD-CRT): biological imaging and biological conformality. Int J Radiat Oncol Biol Phys 2000;47:551–60.

2. Rege S, Safa AA, Chaiken L, et al. Positron emission tomography: an independent indicator of radiocurability in head and neck carcinomas. Am J Clin Oncol 2000;23:164–9.

3. Brun E, Ohlsson T, Erlandsson K, et al. Early prediction of treatment outcome in head and neck cancer with 2-18FDG PET. Acta Oncol 1997;36:741–7.

4. Allal AS, Dulguerov P, Allaoua M, et al. Standardized uptake value of 2-[(18)F] fluoro-2-deoxy-D-glucose in predicting outcome in head and neck carcinomas treated by radiotherapy with or without chemotherapy. J Clin Oncol 2002;20:1398–404.

5. Chapman JD, Bradley JD, Eary JF, et al. Molecular (functional) imaging for radiotherapy applications: an RTOG symposium. Int J Radiat Oncol Biol Phys 2003;55:294–301.

6. Ciernik IF, Dizendorf E, Baumert BG, et al. Radiation treatment planning with an integrated positron emission and computer tomography (PET/CT): a feasibility study. Int J Radiat Oncol Biol Phys 2003;57:853–63.

7. Daisne JF, Sibomana M, Bol A, et al. Evaluation of a multimodality image (CT, MRI and PET) coregistration procedure on phantom and head and neck cancer patients: accuracy, reproducibility and consistency. Radiother Oncol 2003;69:237–45.

8. Greven KM, Williams DW III, McGuirt WF Sr, et al. Serial positron emission tomography scans following radiation therapy of patients with head and neck cancer. Head Neck 2001;23:942–6.

9. Terhaard CH, Bongers V, van Rijk PP, et al. F-18-Fluoro-deoxy-glucose positron-emission tomography scanning in detection of local recurrence after radiotherapy for laryngeal/ pharyngeal cancer. Head Neck 2001;23:933–41.

10. Rogers JW, Greven KM, McGuirt WF, et al. Can post-RT neck dissection be omitted for patients with head-and-neck cancer who have a negative pet scan after definitive radiation therapy? Int J Radiat Oncol Biol Phys 2004;58:694–7.

11. Van de Wiele C, Lahorte C, et al. Nuclear medicine imaging to predict response to radiotherapy: a review. Int J Radiat Oncol Biol Phys 2003;55:5–15.

12. Leskinen-Kallio S, Lindholm P, Lapela M, et al. Imaging of head and neck tumors with positron emission tomography and [11C]methionine. Int J Radiat Oncol Biol Phys 1994;30:1195–9.

13. De Boer JR, Pruim J, Burlage F, et al. Therapy evaluation of laryngeal carcinomas by tyrosine-PET. Head Neck 2003;25:634–44.

14. Mankoff DA, Dehdashti F, Shields AF. Characterizing tumors using metabolic imaging: PET imaging of cellular proliferation and steroid receptors. Neoplasia 2000;2:71–88.

15. Ryser JE, Blauenstein P, Remy N, et al. [76Br]Bromodeoxyuridine, a potential tracer for the measurement of cell proliferation by positron emission tomography, in vitro and in vivo studies in mice. Nucl Med Biol 1999;26:673–9.

16. Fukushima M, Suzuki N, Emura T, et al. Structure and activity of specific inhibitors of thymidine phosphorylase to potentiate the function of antitumor 2{165}-deoxyribonucleosides. Biochem Pharmacol 2000;59:1227–36.

17. Cobben DC, Van Der Laan BF, Maas B, et al. 18F-FLT PET for visualization of laryngeal cancer: comparison with (18)F-FDG PET. J Nucl Med 2004;45:226–31.

18. Thomlinson RH, Gray LH. The histological structure of some human lung cancers and the possible implications for radiotherapy. Br J Cancer 1955;9:539–49.

19. Chao KS, Bosch WR, Mutic S, et al. A novel approach to overcome hypoxic tumor resistance: Cu-ATSM-guided intensity-modulated radiation therapy. Int J Radiat Oncol Biol Phys 2001;49:1171–82.

20. Fujibayashi Y, Cutler CS, Anderson CJ, et al. Comparative studies of Cu-64-ATSM and C-11-acetate in an acute myocardial infarction model: ex vivo imaging of hypoxia in rats. Nucl Med Biol 1999;26:117–21.

21. Lewis JS, McCarthy DW, McCarthy TJ, et al. Evaluation of 64Cu-ATSM in vitro and in vivo in a hypoxic tumor model. J Nucl Med 1999;40:177–83.

22. Emami B, Sethi A, Petruzzelli GJ. Influence of MRI on target volume delineation and IMRT planning in nasopharyngeal carcinoma. Int J Radiat Oncol Biol Phys 2003;57:481–8.

23. Schmitt P, Kotas M, Tobermann A, et al. Quantitative tissue perfusion measurements in head and neck carcinoma patients before and during radiation therapy with a non-invasive MR imaging spin-labeling technique. Radiother Oncol 2003;67:27–34.

24. Belhocine T, Steinmetz N, Hustinx R, et al. Increased uptake of the apoptosis-imaging agent (99m)Tc recombinant human annexin V in human tumors after one course of chemotherapy as a predictor of tumor response and patient prognosis. Clin Cancer Res 2002;8:2766–74.

25. Ciardiello F, Tortora G. A novel approach in the treatment of cancer: targeting the epidermal growth factor receptor. Clin Cancer Res 2001;7:2958–70.

26. Schechter NR, Yang DJ, Azhdarinia A, et al. Assessment of epidermal growth factor receptor with 99mTc-ethylenedicysteine-C225 monoclonal antibody. Anticancer Drugs 2003;14:49–56.

27. Senekowitsch-Schmidtke R, Steiner K, Haunschild J, et al. In vivo evaluation of epidermal growth factor (EGF) receptor density on human tumor xenografts using radiolabeled EGF and anti-(EGF receptor) mAb 425. Cancer Immunol Immunother 1996;42:108–14.

28. Reilly RM, Kiarash R, Cameron RG, et al. ^{111}In-labeled EGF is selectively radiotoxic to human breast cancer cells overexpressing EGFR. J Nucl Med 2000;41:429–38.

29. Hackman T, Doubrovin M, Balatoni J, et al. Imaging expression of cytosine deaminase-herpes virus thymidine kinase fusion gene (CD/TK) expression with [124I]FIAU and PET. Mol Imaging 2002;1:36–42.

30. Blasberg RG, Gelovani J. Molecular-genetic imaging: a nuclear medicine-based perspective. Mol Imaging 2002;1:280–300.

31. Urbain JL. Oncogenes, cancer and imaging. J Nucl Med 1999;40:498–504.

32. Britz-Cunningham SH, Adelstein SJ. Molecular targeting with radionuclides: state of the science. J Nucl Med 2003;44:1945–61.

33. Fukumoto M, Yoshida D, Hayase N, et al. Scintigraphic prediction of resistance to radiation and chemotherapy in patients with lung carcinoma: technetium 99m-tetrofosmin and thallium-201 dual single photon emission computed tomography study. Cancer 1999;86:1470–9.

34. Coleman CN. Radiation oncology-linking technology and biology in the treatment of cancer. Acta Oncol 2002;41:6–13.

Simultaneous Integrated Boost Emerging Technology

Qiuwen Wu, PhD, Radhe Mohan, PhD

Compared with the conventional three-dimensional conformal radiation therapy (3DCRT), intensity-modulated radiation therapy (IMRT) offers many potential benefits. For example, IMRT can improve dose conformity around the target volume, thereby increasing the dose differential between the target and organs at risk (OAR). This differential can permit tumor dose escalation, resulting in improved local control and reduced risk of treatment-related complications.[1,2] The ability to modulate the intensity near the target boundaries can also lead to reduced penumbra margins and thus smaller treated volumes.[3,4] IMRT has been implemented clinically for many tumor sites, as described in other chapters in this book. Early results from a few clinical studies have demonstrated the superiority of IMRT.[5–8]

Another advantage of IMRT is its ability to generate dose distributions of specific levels of nonuniformity in target volumes. This is due to the nature of inverse planning, in which the prescription dose is specified as an objective to be achieved by the planning process. Traditionally, the prescription dose is based on a point, for example, 200 cGy to the isocenter. Alternatively, one can prescribe to an isodose line, for example, 180 cGy to the 95% isodose line. In contrast, a dose prescription for IMRT uses dose-volume combinations, for example, 200 cGy to 95% of the planning target volume (PTV). Naturally, different dose levels can be prescribed to different targets or different regions of the target. An immediate application of this characteristic of IMRT is to plan and treat the boost dose together with the large field prescription dose. Simultaneous treatment of multiple targets with different prescribed doses is called the simultaneous boost (SB) technique.

The simultaneous boost technique is not a new concept.[9] In fact, it has been practiced in various clinical scenarios using 3DCRT in which large field and boost prescriptions are planned separately but delivered as two separate sets of fields in the same fraction within a short period of time (a few minutes).[10–12] What is different in the SB technique is the ability of IMRT to plan both the large field and boost doses in a single plan and deliver them as a single fraction. In the following sections, the rationale and techniques of SB as applied to head and neck squamous cell carcinomas are described and the issues related to the implementations of SB are discussed.

Rationale

Standard head and neck radiation therapy (RT) often delivers doses greater than or equal to 70 Gy to gross tumor, intermediate doses of between 50 and 70 Gy to tissues surrounding the gross tumor, and approximately 50 Gy to electively irradiated tissues such as lymph node–bearing tissues at risk of subclinical or microscopic disease. The success of curative head and neck RT depends on the principle that the entire head and neck region must be irradiated with a dose sufficient to control subclinical disease. This is normally accomplished in the first phase of a traditional RT course, during which fraction sizes of 1.8 to 2.0 Gy are used for the treatment of the tumor and the electively irradiated tissues. In the second phase, an additional dose is delivered, also at 1.8 to 2 Gy/fraction, to tissues at greater risk of a larger tumor burden, typically tissues involved with or immediately surrounding the gross tumor. Such a treatment course frequently requires times of up to 7 weeks or more. Tissues irradiated during the initial phase of RT receive a substantial unwanted additional dose during the boost phase from beams used to treat the gross tumor.

The same disadvantage exists in the accelerated RT schedules. These schedules were developed with the recognition that overall treatment time is critically associated with tumor control probability.[13–15] Such schedules commonly use twice-daily accelerated fractionation to deliver similar or higher doses in shorter overall treatment times.[16–19] Accelerated fractionation approaches have demonstrated impressive improved tumor control without significant increases in late normal tissue morbidity at some institutions.[20]

In principle, fractionation strategies similar to the conventional or accelerated ones can also be used to design IMRT plans. For example, in a strategy similar to the conventional 1.8 to 2 Gy/fraction schedule, a major portion of the dose could be delivered in the initial phase using uniform fields designed with standard 3DCRT followed by an IMRT boost. Alternatively, separate IMRT plans could be designed for both the initial large-field treatment and the boost treatment. Such strategies are termed IMRT-boost strategies. It may be intuitively obvious that, if a large portion of the dose has already been delivered using large fields, it may be very difficult to achieve a high level of dose conformation with the remaining fractions in the IMRT-boost phase.

Thus, the dose distributions of IMRT treatment plans can be expected to be significantly superior in terms of higher conformity if designed to deliver different dose levels to different tissues of the head and neck region simultaneously in a single treatment session. This permits delivery of graded dose levels to tumor-bearing tissues and tissues at risk of subclinical tumor spread, such as tissues surrounding the gross tumor and lymph node–bearing areas, and spares normal tissues to the greatest extent possible. The simultaneous integrated boost (SIB)-IMRT strategy not only produces superior dose distributions but also is an easier, more efficient, and perhaps less error-prone way of planning and delivering IMRT because it involves the use of the same plan for the entire course of treatment. Furthermore, there is no need for electron fields because the supraclavicular nodes can be included in the IMRT fields, thus avoiding the perennial problem of field matching and junctioning. Assuming that the IMRT is delivered from a set of fixed gantry positions with a multileaf collimator (MLC), a single sweep of MLC leaves across the gross disease, regional disease, and electively treated volumes can be used to deliver each of the intensity-modulated fields in such treatments.

Volume Definitions

We follow the terminology defined in the International Commission on Radiation Units and Measurements reports 50 and 62 for defining the anatomic volumes for radiation treatments.[21,22] For head and neck tumors, the gross tumor volume (GTV) includes the primary tumor and clinically involved lymph nodes, that is, those palpable or identified with sizes ≥ 1 cm on computed tomography (CT) or magnetic resonance imaging. Smaller nodes are included if contrast enhancement can be demonstrated. The clinical target volume (CTV) has several components, which are separated according to their corresponding prescription doses. CTV3 is defined the same as the GTV. CTV2 consists of the GTV plus a 1 cm margin, expanded in three dimensions. However, CTV2 excludes the area that is known to be free of suspected disease, such as outside the skin, oral cavity, bone, and other critical structures. This can be achieved either by manually editing the contours or through the use of semiautomatic tools. CTV1 consists of the uninvolved lymph node groups electively irradiated based on their risk of subclinical involvement (typically bilateral level I to VI nodes, including the supraclavicular nodes).[23–25]

For IMRT treatment planning, dosimetric reporting, and evaluation purposes, the PTVs comprise the corresponding CTVs, with appropriate margins for setup uncertainties and organ motions. These margins may vary from institution to institution because they depend on the immobilization technique and the use of setup verification imaging devices, and they are, in principle, patient dependent and not necessarily the same for all three-dimensional directions. Typical values for such margins are in the range of 3 to 5 mm.

Critical structures delineated in head and neck patients include the spinal cord, brainstem, parotid glands, larynx, optic nerves or chiasm, and globes. To further ensure sparing of the spinal cord and brainstem, a 0.5 cm circumferential margin (to account for setup uncertainty and organ motion) around each of these structures, except in the cranial-caudal direction, may be added to form the planning OAR volume.[7,22,26]

Radiobiology and Fractionation Considerations

Given that each of the target regions receives different doses per fraction in the SIB-IMRT strategy, the prescribed nominal (physical) dose and dose per fraction must be appropriately adjusted. The adjusted nominal dose and fraction size for each region depends on the number of fractions chosen. At the same time, the effect of the modified fractionation on acute and late toxicity of normal tissues both outside and within the treated volumes must be considered. One can select the conventional 2 Gy per fraction for the gross disease for an SIB strategy, but that may lead to a significantly lower dose per fraction to volumes of microscopic disease and electively treated nodes. On the other hand, one can choose to deliver 2 Gy per fraction to the lower- and intermediate-dose volumes, but this would require a high dose per fraction, as high as 2.5 Gy or more, to the gross disease. The latter scheme may have the advantage of shortening the treatment duration and a potential for improvement in local control but at an increased risk of injury to the embedded normal tissues.

The choice of an SIB fractionation strategy must take into account the clinical outcome data available from extensive experience in head and neck RT. It has been established that gross tumors should be treated to doses between 65 and 75 Gy to optimize control rates. Furthermore, the elective irradiation of subclinical disease in lymph nodes to 45 to 54 Gy results in > 90% control rates. In addition, tissues within 1 to 2 cm around the gross tumor, frequently referred to as the margin, require an intermediate dose for optimal control of subclinical extension.

To evaluate the IMRT fractionation strategies, an isoeffect relationship based on the linear-quadratic (LQ) model has been used. The parameters of the LQ model are obtained from the published results of analysis of head and neck carcinomas[13,14,27,28] and are listed in Table 18.7-1. It is recognized that there is considerable uncertainty in the available data and numerous assumptions in the LQ model and isoeffect formalism, the validity of which has not been fully established. Therefore, the application of these models and data to estimate the dependence of response of tumors and normal tissues on fractionation regimens may be questioned. However, the model parameters can be adjusted so that they produce results consistent with existing knowledge and current strategies before designing new fractionation strategies for clinical tests.

The isoeffect formalism that may be used to design SIB fractionation strategies is described briefly here. Let us define the term "normalized total dose" (NTD) as the biologically equivalent total dose, normalized to 2 Gy per fraction. We also use the term "nominal dose" (ND) to denote the actual physical dose. The parameters of the isoeffect formalism are d_{ref}, the reference fraction size, which we select to be 2 Gy/fx; SF_{dref}, the surviving fraction for the reference dose; $T_{d,a}$, the accelerated tumor clonogen doubling time; and α/β.

The tumor cell surviving fraction, when incorporating tumor repopulation, including accelerated repopulation, can be expressed as follows[29]:

$$SF = 2^{\left[\frac{T_{lag}}{T_{d,u}}+\frac{T_t-T_{lag}}{T_{d,a}}\right]} \times \left(SF_{d_{ref}}\right)^{\left\{\frac{n_f \times d_f}{d_{ref}} \times \frac{\alpha/\beta+d_f}{\alpha/\beta+d_{ref}}\right\}} \tag{1}$$

where T_t is the total treatment time in days, T_{lag} is the lag time before accelerated repopulation begins, and $T_{d,u}$ is the unperturbed doubling time. Other parameters are defined in the previous paragraph. For a given fractionation strategy in which the same dose per fraction (d_f) is used for the entire course of treatment (consisting of n_f fractions), the biologically equivalent NTD, for which the dose per fraction is equal to d_{ref}, can be expressed as

$$SF_{d_{ref}}^{n_{f,NTD}} = 2^{\left[\frac{T_t-T_{t,NTD}}{T_{d,a}}\right]} \times \left(SF_{d_{ref}}\right)^{\left\{\frac{n_f \times d_f}{d_{ref}} \times \frac{\alpha/\beta+d_f}{\alpha/\beta+d_{ref}}\right\}} \tag{2}$$

where $n_{f,NTD}$ is the number of fractions in which the NTD will be delivered in $T_{t,NTD}$ days at a rate of d_{ref}/fx. This easily leads to the expression for $n_{f,NTD}$:

$$n_{f,NTD} = \left[\frac{T_t-T_{t,NTD}}{T_{d,a}}\right] \times \left[\frac{\ln(2)}{\ln(SF_{d_{ref}})}\right] + \left\{\frac{n_f \times d_f}{d_{ref}} \times \frac{\alpha/\beta+d_f}{\alpha/\beta+d_{ref}}\right\}. \tag{3}$$

TABLE 18.7-1. Parameters Used for the Linear-Quadratic Model and Isoeffect Formalism Based on Published Values from the Literature

Parameters for tumors in LQ model	
α/β (Gy)	20.0
$T_{d,a}$ (d)	4.0
d_{ref} (Gy)	2.0
SF_{dref}	0.5
α/β values for various critical structures (Gy)	
Mucosa	10
Spinal cord	2.5
Brainstem	2.5
Bone	0.85
Muscle	3.1
Parotid gland	12

d_{ref} = reference fraction size; LQ = linear-quadratic; SF_{dref} = surviving fraction for the reference dose; $T_{d,a}$ = accelerated tumor clonogen doubling time.

There are two unknowns in the above expression: $n_{f,NTD}$ and $T_{t,NTD}$. If the treatment is delivered once per day and only on weekdays, as commonly practiced, the difference between the number of fractions is not equal to the difference in elapsed days. An iterative search can be performed to calculate $n_{f,NTD}$. Notice that the solution may not be unique. Assuming further that the treatments begin on Mondays, the corresponding elapsed time is then computed using the following algorithm:

$$T_{t,NTD} = n_{f,NTD} + Integerize\left(\frac{n_{f,ntd}}{5}\right) \times 2 - 2 \tag{4}$$

If $n_{f,NTD}$ is evenly divisible by 5, or otherwise

$$T_{t,NTD} = n_{f,NTD} + Integerize\left(\frac{n_{f,ntd}}{5}\right) \times 2 \tag{5}$$

For OAR, assuming no regeneration of tissues and no change in sensitivity as a result of treatment, $n_{f,NTD}$ becomes

$$^n f_{,NTD} = \frac{n_f \times d_f}{d_{ref}} \times \frac{\alpha/\beta+d_f}{\alpha/\beta+d_{ref}}. \tag{6}$$

The NTD then becomes

$$NTD = n_{f,NTD} \cdot d_{ref} \tag{7}$$

The isoeffect models may be used to design SIB-IMRT strategies for head and neck carcinomas for a fixed number of fractions (eg, 30), with escalating NTDs to the gross disease (PTV3), same 60 Gy to the microscopic extensions (PTV2), and same 50 Gy to the electively treated regions (PTV1). Typically, these values are converted into the corresponding

TABLE 18.7-2. Dose Levels for Several SIB-IMRT Fractionation Schemes Based on the Isoeffect Formalism and LQ Models

Structure/Quantity	Conventional 3DCRT	SIB1	SIB2	SIB3	SIB RTOG
PTV1					
NTD (Gy)	50	50	—	—	—
ND (Gy)	50/54	54	—	—	—
No. of fractions	25/30	30	—	—	—
Dose/fraction (Gy)	2.0/1.8	1.8	—	—	—
PTV2					
NTD (Gy)	60	60.0	—	—	—
ND (Gy)	60	60.0	—	—	—
No. of fractions	30	30	—	—	—
Dose/fraction (Gy)	2.0	2.0	—	—	—
PTV3					
NTD (Gy)	70	74.4	78.4	84.4	70.0
ND (Gy)	70	68.1	70.8	73.8	66.0
No. of fractions	35	30	—	—	—
Dose/fraction (Gy)	2.0	2.27	2.36	2.46	2.2
Bone NTD (Gy)	70	74.6	79.7	85.7	70.4
Muscle NTD (Gy)	70	71.7	75.8	80.5	68.4
Mucosa NTD (Gy)	70	69.6	72.9	76.6	67.0

3DCRT = three-dimensional conformal radiation therapy; IMRT = intensity-modulated radiation therapy; LQ = linear-quadratic; ND = nominal dose; NTD = normalized total dose; PTV = planning target volume; RTOG = Radiation Therapy Oncology Group; SIB = simultaneous integrated boost. Cells marked with "—" mean that they have the same value as in the previous column.
Listed values are for different target volumes and those normal tissues embedded in the gross tumor volume.
For reference, the dose levels in Radiation Therapy Oncology Group protocol H-0022[30] are also listed in the last column.

ND values, which are then used to design IMRT plans. Normal tissue constraints are also specified in terms of ND.

Table 18.7-2 compares several SIB-IMRT fractionation schemes with the conventional fractionation at different dose levels for PTVs and normal tissues embedded in the GTV. The doses to PTV2 and PTV1 are maintained the same as the conventional treatments. For PTV1, a dose of 50 Gy in 25 fractions is considered equivalent to 54 Gy in 30 fractions because both are practiced in the clinic. The dose escalation components apply only to PTV3, that is, where the gross tumor is. The number of fractions for different SIB-IMRT strategies in Table 18.7-2 is set at 30, so treatment can be finished in 6 weeks, resulting in a total of 40 days if the treatment starts on Monday and there are no breaks during the treatment. The NTDs for other OAR are not listed, but they all should be lower than their NDs.

Treatment Planning

The IMRT system for head and neck SIB planning should be able to handle a complex set of objectives and criteria, typically expressed in terms of dose-volume relationships. Normally, a number (eg, nine) of 6 MV coplanar photon beams at equally spaced gantry angles may be used for the planning and delivery.[31] The number of beams needed for the head and neck IMRT planning is usually high compared with other sites. This is due to the complexity of

the anatomy in the head and neck region and the various surrounding OAR. Previous planning studies for head and neck IMRT show that the dose distribution improves as the number of beams increases. However, minimal gains are observed when more than nine coplanar beams are used.[26] Although noncoplanar beams may provide some additional benefit, they are not typically included for reasons of simplicity and delivery efficiency. The noncoplanar beam setup requires changing the couch angle, which, for most treatment machines, cannot be executed without entering the treatment room and thus prolonging the overall treatment time substantially. Table 18.7-3 shows the planning requirement for SIB-IMRT. An IMRT plan is considered acceptable only when all of the objectives listed in Table 18.7-3 are met. In the treatment of head and neck cancer, it is often desirable to have a uniform dose distribution in the target,

TABLE 18.7-3. SIB-IMRT Planning Goals

Volume of Interest	Planning Requirements
PTV3	D_{99} = Rx; $D_1 < 110\% \times D_{99}$
PTV2	D_{95} = Rx = 60 Gy
PTV1	D_{90} = Rx = 54 Gy
Spinal cord	$D_1 < 45$ Gy
Brainstem	$D_1 < 55$ Gy

D_{99}, D_{95}, and D_1 = doses given to 99%, 95%, or 1% volume of the concerned region; IMRT = intensity-modulated radiation therapy; PTV = planning target volume; Rx = prescription dose; SIB = simultaneous integrated boost.

thus necessitating that the homogeneity index of the PTV3 be less than 10%, that is, D_1 (dose given to 1% volume of the concerned region) is within 10% of the D_{99} (dose given to 99% volume of the concerned region).

As described in other chapters of this book, the treatment objectives of various targets and OAR are often in conflict, and not all constraints can be met for all structures owing to the limitations of the planning system or because of the laws of physics of radiation transport. In such situations, the priority or relative importance of anatomic structures may need to be established. Although this should be considered on a case-by-case basis, in general, the following guidelines, in descending order of importance, may be considered: the sparing of serial critical structures such as the spinal cord and brainstem; the coverage of PTV3, PTV2, and PTV1; and the sparing of parallel critical structures, such as salivary glands.

The final result of IMRT optimization is usually a compromise among the various competing requirements. Therefore, planning parameters are not the same as treatment objectives, and they should be adjusted in an iterative fashion to obtain improved results. Parameters for different patients may vary substantially in an effort to generate optimized plans for each patient. It is quite possible that a better plan may exist for a different set of parameters and can be achieved with additional trial and error. Continued research may lead to automated methods of defining these parameters. The optimized intensities are subsequently converted to MLC leaf control sequences for delivery. The intensity patterns generated from these leaf control sequences (which are usually slightly different from the original optimized ones) are used for the final plan dose calculation and subsequent plan evaluation by attending physicians.

Sample planning results to demonstrate the ability of the SIB-IMRT to spare the parotid gland and still meet the treatment goals are shown in Figures 18.7-1 and 18.7-2. Depending on the locations of the GTV, attempts were made to spare either one parotid gland or both glands.

Early clinical results of SIB-IMRT of head and neck cancer patients were analyzed for 20 patients treated under an institutional dose escalation protocol at Virginia Commonwealth University.[32] None of the six patients on dose level 1 (SIB1) and two of the six patients initially enrolled on dose level 2 (SIB2) developed dose-limiting toxicity. Both patients treated on dose level 3 (SIB3) required a 3-day treatment break and a dose reduction after grade 3 toxicity. Six additional confirmatory patients subsequently enrolled on SIB2 completed treatment without dose-limiting toxicity. With a median follow-up of 20 months from the date of enrolment, 28 months for surviving patients, the actuarial 2-year local control was 76.3%, which compared favorably with other accelerated regimens. Therefore, SIB2 at the dose level of 70.8 Gy was defined as the maximum tolerable dose to the gross tumor using this form of accelerated SIB-IMRT.

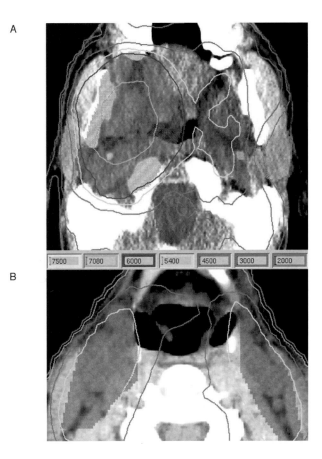

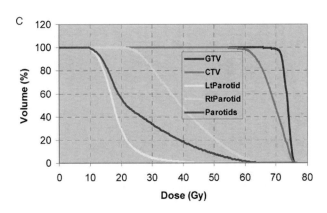

FIGURE 18.7-1. Dose distributions for one patient at the 70.8 Gy level. The gross tumor volume (GTV) is located on the right side; therefore, the left parotid gland is spared more than the right parotid gland. (*A*) Isodose distributions on one transverse computed tomographic slice at the GTV level with parotid glands. (*B*) Isodose lines on another slice that is 6 cm inferior; clinical target volume (CTV)1 and spinal cord are shown. (*C*) Corresponding dose-volume histograms for GTV, CTV, and parotid glands. Structures shown include the GTV (*red*), brainstem (*blue*), spinal cord (*green*), parotid glands (*light blue*), and uninvolved lymph nodes (*dark red*). (To view a color version of this image, please refer to the CD-ROM.) Reproduced with permission from Wu Q et al.[7]

A

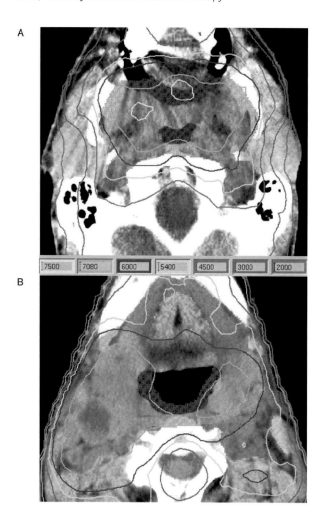

| 7500 | 7080 | 6000 | 5400 | 4500 | 3000 | 2000 |

B

C

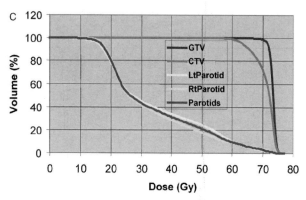

FIGURE 18.7-2. Dose distributions for another patient at the 70.8 Gy level. The tumor is located at the midline; therefore, doses to both parotid glands are minimized. (*A*) Isodose distributions on one transverse computed tomographic (CT) slice with gross tumor. (*B*) Isodose distributions on another CT slice, which is 3.6 cm inferior, showing two involved nodes, also prescribed at 70.8 Gy. (*C*) Corresponding dose-volume histograms for gross tumor volume (GTV), clinical target volume (CTV), and parotid glands. The structures are shown in the same colors as in Figure 18.7-1. (To view a color version of this image, please refer to the CD-ROM.) Reproduced with permission from Wu Q et al.[7]

Discussion

The hot spots inside the tumor volume may not be critical for tumors at other sites; however, they are generally not desirable for head and neck cancers. Realizing that the IMRT treatment is delivered in the form of SIB, the dose per fraction to PTV3 can be much higher than the conventional fixed 1.8 to 2.0 Gy; therefore, a constraint on the maximum dose or homogeneity to the PTV3 is necessary.[33] For example, if the prescription dose to PTV3 is 70 Gy in 30 fractions and the homogeneity index is 10%, then the maximum dose is 77 Gy, which translates into a maximum dose per fraction of 2.56 Gy. There is little clinical experience available currently at this dose level. As another example, normal tissues embedded inside the GTV can also receive very high doses (see Table 18.7-2). Note that the NTD corresponding to an ND of 77 Gy in 30 fractions is 90 Gy for tumors and 93 Gy for bone.

Because of the unique mode of delivery, the SIB-IMRT strategy can not only produce dose distributions superior to those of optimized conventional treatment plans but is, in principle, also an easier, more efficient, and safer way of planning and delivering IMRT because it uses a single plan for the entire treatment course. Furthermore, there is no need for the electron beams, and the field-matching problems are removed.

In this chapter, it has been assumed that the tumor shape remains the same throughout the treatment course, so the single plan can be used for the entire course of treatment. This may not be true because head and neck tumors usually respond well to the radiation treatment. For cases in which significant changes occur in the tumor sizes or shapes, additional treatment planning, including CT and modifications of immobilization devices, may be necessary. This applies to both conventional 3DCRT and SIB-IMRT.

Analyses performed on the patterns of local-regional recurrence of head and neck cancer patients after RT imply the need to escalate the doses to high-risk regions to improve local control.[34,35] However, the tumor dose cannot be escalated infinitely owing to the fact that as the tumor dose escalates, the doses to the normal tissues, either embedded or nearby, are also increased. The ability of IMRT to deliver nonuniform doses to the target volume and anywhere else inside patients offers a unique opportunity to escalate the biologically equivalent doses to the tumors without escalating the physical dose significantly by modifying the fractionation schemes to optimize the therapeutic ratio.

SIB can be applied to other tumor sites as well. For example, whole-pelvis treatment of prostate cancer has been shown to be more effective than prostate-only treatment for some intermediate-risk patients with prostate cancer.[36] In these cases, the lymph nodes will receive different dose levels than the prostate gland. By treating the lymph nodes and the prostate in the SIB arrangement, critical structures, such as the small bowel and rectum, can be spared to a greater degree compared with the conventional sequential boost technique.[37] Even for prostate-only treatment, the SIB arrangement has been shown to reduce the doses to the rectal wall.[38] It is relevant to mention that several recent studies have suggested that the α/β ratio for prostate cancer is lower than was previously thought,[39–43] leading to potential benefits of hypofractionated RT in which the dose per fraction is much higher than the usual 1.8 Gy. With the advancements made recently in the area of magnetic resonance spectroscopy, it is possible to identify the higher-risk regions inside the prostate gland to which a higher prescription dose may be of benefit. Such higher doses can be delivered simultaneously with a somewhat lower dose to the rest of the prostate gland.

Conclusions

In contrast to conventional RT for head and neck cancer, which requires highly complex, protracted treatment schemes with multiple portals and sequential field reductions, the SIB-IMRT approach provides two simultaneous opportunities for biologic dose escalation: (1) increased daily tumor doses achieved by dose or fraction escalation from the standard 2 Gy/fraction and (2) acceleration of the RT course through the shortening of the overall treatment time.

SIB-IMRT of head and neck cancers is feasible and yields highly conformal dose distributions. SIB-IMRT is more efficient, less error prone, and more accurate than traditional 3DCRT planning and delivery. However, tissues embedded in the target volume may be at higher risk, and caution should be observed when applying higher than conventional fraction sizes.

The combination of IMRT and SIB offers opportunities to improve radiation treatments. However, the potential benefits and drawbacks of the SIB-IMRT should be carefully evaluated before the clinical implementation for each site. Special attention should be paid to the total dose and dose per fractions for each target volume. Biologic constructs such as the LQ model are helpful in guiding the designing of the clinical protocols; however, it should be realized that the parameters in these models have some uncertainties, and their predictions can vary significantly with these parameters. Therefore, clinical implementation of SIB-IMRT remains a work in progress.

References

1. Boyer AL, Butler EB, DiPetrillo TA, et al. Intensity-modulated radiotherapy: current status and issues of interest. Int J Radiat Oncol Biol Phys 2001;51:880–914.

2. Ezzell GA, Galvin JM, Low D, et al. Guidance document on delivery, treatment planning, and clinical implementation of IMRT: report of the IMRT Subcommittee of the AAPM Radiation Therapy Committee. Med Phys 2003;30:2089–115.

3. Mohan R, Wu Q, Wang X, et al. Intensity modulation optimization, lateral transport of radiation, and margins. Med Phys 1996;23:2011–21.

4. Chen Z, Wang X, Bortfeld T, et al. The influence of scatter on the design of optimized intensity modulations. Med Phys 1995;22:1727–33.

5. Vicini FA, Sharpe M, Kestin L, et al. Optimizing breast cancer treatment efficacy with intensity-modulated radiotherapy. Int J Radiat Oncol Biol Phys 2002;54:1336–44.

6. Zelefsky MJ, Fuks Z, Hunt M, et al. High-dose intensity modulated radiation therapy for prostate cancer: early toxicity and biochemical outcome in 772 patients. Int J Radiat Oncol Biol Phys 2002;53:1111–6.

7. Wu Q, Mohan R, Morris M, et al. Simultaneous integrated boost intensity-modulated radiotherapy for locally advanced head-and-neck squamous cell carcinomas. I: dosimetric results. Int J Radiat Oncol Biol Phys 2003;56:573–85.

8. Hong L, Alektiar K, Chui C, et al. IMRT of large fields: whole-abdomen irradiation. Int J Radiat Oncol Biol Phys 2002;54:278–89.

9. Lebesque JV, Keus RB The simultaneous boost technique: the concept of relative normalized total dose. Radiother Oncol 1991;22:45–55.

10. Morris MM, Schmidt-Ullrich RK, DiNardo L, et al. Accelerated superfractionated radiotherapy with concomitant boost for locally advanced head-and-neck squamous cell carcinomas. Int J Radiat Oncol Biol Phys 2002;52:918–28.

11. Kavanagh BD, Segreti EM, Koo D, et al. Long-term local control and survival after concomitant boost accelerated radiotherapy for locally advanced cervix cancer. Am J Clin Oncol 2001;24:113–9.

12. Eisbruch A, Marsh LH, Martel MK, et al. Comprehensive irradiation of head and neck cancer using conformal multisegmental fields: assessment of target coverage and noninvolved tissue sparing. Int J Radiat Oncol Biol Phys 1998;41:559–68.

13. Withers HR, Taylor JM, Maciejewski B The hazard of accelerated tumor clonogen repopulation during radiotherapy. Acta Oncol 1988;27:131–46.

14. Withers HR, Peters LJ, Taylor JM, et al. Local control of carcinoma of the tonsil by radiation therapy: an analysis of patterns of fractionation in nine institutions. Int J Radiat Oncol Biol Phys 1995;33:549–62.

15. Hansen O, Overgaard J, Hansen HS, et al. Importance of overall treatment time for the outcome of radiotherapy of advanced head and neck carcinoma: dependency on tumor differentiation. Radiother Oncol 1997;43:47–51.

16. Wang CC. Local control of oropharyngeal carcinoma after two accelerated hyperfractionation radiation therapy schemes. Int J Radiat Oncol Biol Phys 1988;14:1143–6.

17. Johnson CR, Khandelwal SR, Schmidt-Ullrich RK, et al. The influence of quantitative tumor volume measurements on local control in advanced head and neck cancer using concomitant boost accelerated superfractionated irradiation. Int J Radiat Oncol Biol Phys 1995;32:635–41.

18. Ang KK. Altered fractionation trials in head and neck cancer. Semin Radiat Oncol 1998;8:230–6.

19. Ang KK. Altered fractionation in the management of head and neck cancer. Int J Radiat Biol 1998;73:395–9.

20. Fu KK, Pajak TF, Trotti A, et al. A Radiation Therapy Oncology Group (RTOG) phase III randomized study to compare

hyperfractionation and two variants of accelerated fractionation to standard fractionation radiotherapy for head and neck squamous cell carcinomas: first report of RTOG 9003. Int J Radiat Oncol Biol Phys 2000;48:7–16.

21. International Commission on Radiation Units and Measurements. ICRU-50: prescribing, recording and reporting photon beam therapy. Bethesda (MD): International Commission on Radiation Units and Measurements; 1993.

22. International Commission on Radiation Units and Measurements. ICRU-62: prescribing, recording and reporting photon beam therapy (supplement to ICRU report 50). Bethesda (MD): International Commission on Radiation Units and Measurements; 1999.

23. Martinez-Monge R, Fernandes PS, Gupta N, et al. Cross-sectional nodal atlas: a tool for the definition of clinical target volumes in three-dimensional radiation therapy planning. Radiology 1999;211:815–28.

24. Nowak PJ, Wijers OB, Lagerwaard FJ, et al. A three-dimensional CT-based target definition for elective irradiation of the neck. Int J Radiat Oncol Biol Phys 1999;45:33–9.

25. Som PM, Curtin HD, Mancuso AA. An imaging-based classification for the cervical nodes designed as an adjunct to recent clinically based nodal classifications. Arch Otolaryngol Head Neck Surg 1999;125:388–96.

26. Wu Q, Manning M, Schmidt-Ullrich R, et al. The potential for sparing of parotids and escalation of biologically effective dose with intensity-modulated radiation treatments of head and neck cancers: a treatment design study. Int J Radiat Oncol Biol Phys 2000;46:195–205.

27. Withers HR, Peters LJ, Taylor JM, et al. Late normal tissue sequelae from radiation therapy for carcinoma of the tonsil: patterns of fractionation study of radiobiology. Int J Radiat Oncol Biol Phys 1995;33:563–8.

28. Maciejewski B, Withers HR, Taylor JM, et al. Dose fractionation and regeneration in radiotherapy for cancer of the oral cavity and oropharynx: tumor dose-response and repopulation. Int J Radiat Oncol Biol Phys 1989;16:831–43.

29. Mohan R, Wu Q, Manning M, et al. Radiobiological considerations in the design of fractionation strategies for intensity-modulated radiation therapy of head and neck cancers. Int J Radiat Oncol Biol Phys 2000;46:619–30.

30. Eisbruch A, Chao KS, Garden AS. RTOG H-0022: phase I/II study of conformal and intensity modulated irradiation for oropharyngeal cancer. Available at: http://rtog.org/members/protocols/h0022/h0022.pdf.

31. Wu Q, Mohan R. Algorithms and functionality of an intensity modulated radiotherapy optimization system. Med Phys 2000;27:701–11.

32. Lauve A, Morris M, Schmidt-Ullrich R, et al. A phase I trial using a parotid-sparing, accelerated intensity-modulated radiotherapy (IMRT) regimen to treat locally advanced head and neck squamous cell carcinoma. Int J Radiat Oncol Biol Phys 2003;57:S302–3.

33. Zhou J, Fei D, Wu Q. Potential of intensity-modulated radiotherapy to escalate doses to head-and-neck cancers: what is the maximal dose? Int J Radiat Oncol Biol Phys 2003;57:673–82.

34. Dawson LA, Anzai Y, Marsh L, et al. Patterns of local-regional recurrence following parotid-sparing conformal and segmental intensity-modulated radiotherapy for head and neck cancer. Int J Radiat Oncol Biol Phys 2000;46:1117–26.

35. Chao KS, Ozyigit G, Tran BN, et al. Patterns of failure in patients receiving definitive and postoperative IMRT for head-and-neck cancer. Int J Radiat Oncol Biol Phys 2003;55:312–21.

36. Roach M, Lu JD, Lawton C, et al. A phase III trial comparing whole-pelvic (WP) to prostate only (PO) radiotherapy and neoadjuvant to adjuvant total androgen suppression (TAS): preliminary analysis of RTOG-9413. Int J Radiat Oncol Biol Phys 2001;51:3.

37. Wu Q, Arthur D, Benedict S, et al. Intensity-modulated radiotherapy for prostate cancer treatment with nodal coverage. Int J Radiat Oncol Biol Phys 2002;54:321.

38. Bos LJ, Damen EM, de Boer RW, et al. Reduction of rectal dose by integration of the boost in the large-field treatment plan for prostate irradiation. Int J Radiat Oncol Biol Phys 2002;52:254–65.

39. Brenner DJ, Martinez AA, Edmundson GK, et al. Direct evidence that prostate tumors show high sensitivity to fractionation (low alpha/beta ratio), similar to late-responding normal tissue. Int J Radiat Oncol Biol Phys 2002;52:6–13.

40. Fowler JF, Ritter MA, Chappell RJ, et al. What hypofractionated protocols should be tested for prostate cancer? Int J Radiat Oncol Biol Phys 2003;56:1093–104.

41. Wang JZ, Guerrero M, Li XA. How low is the alpha/beta ratio for prostate cancer? Int J Radiat Oncol Biol Phys 2003;55:194–203.

42. Wang JZ, Li XA, Yu CX, et al. The low alpha/beta ratio for prostate cancer: what does the clinical outcome of HDR brachytherapy tell us? Int J Radiat Oncol Biol Phys 2003;57:1101–8.

43. D'Souza WD, Thames HD. Is the alpha/beta ratio for prostate cancer low? Int J Radiat Oncol Biol Phys 2001;51:1–3.

Modulated Electron Radiation Therapy

Emerging Technology

Yulin Song, PhD, Arthur L. Boyer, PhD, Todd Pawlicki, PhD, Steve Jiang, PhD, Yulong Yan, PhD, C.-M. Charlie Ma, PhD, Lei Xing, PhD

Radiation therapy (RT) is commonly used in the treatment of parotid gland tumors, primarily combined with surgery.[1-4] As in other head and neck sites,[5-8] intensity-modulated radiation therapy (IMRT) is receiving increasing attention in parotid gland tumors.[9,10] This is not surprising because these tumors are located in close proximity to multiple critical structures, including the oral cavity, brainstem, auditory apparatus, spinal cord, optic nerves, and lenses. Highly conformal IMRT plans may reduce the risk of untoward treatment sequelae and provide a potential means of escalating the dose, improving local control.

A concern, however, with the application of IMRT in these patients is that most tumors arise in the superficial lobe of the parotid gland. Thus, unlike other head and neck tumors, the target tissues are located near the skin. Although photon beams are well suited for more deep-seated tumors, they are not ideal for superficial targets. Unsurprisingly, conventional RT approaches in these patients are often delivered with a combination of electrons and photons or exclusively with electrons.

Several investigators have used scanned beam systems (MM50 racetrack microtron, Scanditronix Medical AB, Uppsala, Sweden) to improve dose distributions for superficial targets using intensity- and energy-modulated high-energy electron beams.[11,12] Others have considered proton beams for targets close or distal to critical structures.[13] Clinical proton beams have several desirable physical characteristics, including uniform high dose (the spread out Bragg peak) in the target, a sharp falloff dose, and a small lateral penumbra. However, because of the high capital cost of these facilities, proton beam therapy is available at only a few large centers in the world.

We present here a novel approach known as modulated electron radiation therapy (MERT) in the treatment of parotid gland tumors. MERT is capable of delivering high-ly conformal dose distributions to superficial targets with increased sparing of underlying critical tissues, offering distinct advantages over photon IMRT. Moreover, MERT may be delivered on a standard linear accelerator using a customized multileaf collimator (MLC) that attaches to an electron cone.

Electron MLC

We previously described a prototype manually driven electron multileaf collimator (EMLC) for the delivery of MERT.[14-16] The EMLC had 30 steel leaf pairs, with each leaf being 0.476 cm wide, 20.0 cm long, and 2.54 cm thick, and was inserted into a 25 × 25 cm^2 electron applicator (Varian Medical Systems, Palo Alto, CA). Both sides and ends of the leaves were made parallel with the central beam axis. The maximum opening was 14.2 × 15.5 cm^2 when all leaves were completely retracted, giving the largest radiation field of 15.0 × 16.3 cm^2 projected at a 100 cm source-to-surface distance (SSD). The EMLC leaves could be pushed in and pulled out easily. For each of the beam segments, the corresponding field shape was obtained by manually positioning the leaves according to their coordinates, which were computed from the electron beam leaf-sequencing program. To set the field shapes more efficiently, we first drew the field shapes on a piece of hard cardboard at a ratio of 1:1 and cut them out. The field shapes were then set using these precut cardboard templates. In the near future, we will develop a faster and more accurate technique of setting field shapes.

Our initial configuration resulted in a 10 cm air gap between the bottom of the EMLC leaves and the patient skin for a nominal 100 cm SSD (Figure 18.8-1A). To further lower the EMLC leaves and, thus, reduce in-air electron scattering and the penumbra, we have now removed

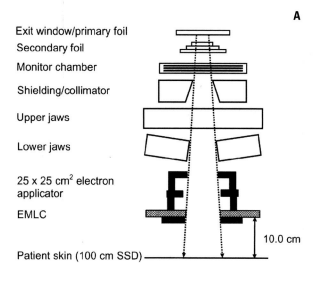

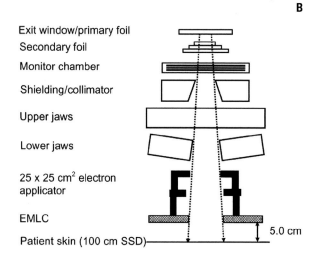

FIGURE 18.8-1. Schematic of the electron multileaf collimator (EMLC) and a Varian Clinac 2100C treatment head. (*A*) The manually driven EMLC was originally placed at the last scraper of a standard Varian 25 × 25 cm² electron applicator. (*B*) The entire last scraper of the electron applicator and its electronic circuitry have now been removed. The EMLC was placed immediately at the bottom of the modified electron applicator and stabilized with eight screws. SSD = source-to-surface distance.

the entire last scraper of the electron applicator and its electronic accessories. The EMLC frame was placed at the bottom of the modified electron applicator and stabilized with eight screws. This modification reduced the air gap to 5.0 cm between the bottom of the EMLC leaves and the patient skin (Figure 18.8-1B). Given that the electronic circuitry for detecting the electron cutout was completely removed, we were able to avoid activating interlocks associated with electron beam accessory malfunction while inserting the EMLC assembly into the linear accelerator treatment head. Thus, even if the linear accelerator was in the electron mode,

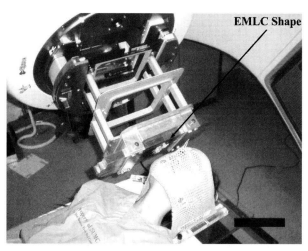

FIGURE 18.8-2. The electron multileaf collimator (EMLC) assembly mounted on a Varian Clinac 2100C linear accelerator. The air gap between the bottom of the EMLC leaves and the patient's skin is 5.0 cm. The gantry angle is 235°.

the gantry could still be rotated, making the delivery of MERT plans with multiple beam angles possible. Figure 18.8-2 shows a photograph of the newly modified EMLC assembly inserted on the treatment head of a Varian Clinac 2100C linear accelerator.

MERT Planning Study

Based on the manufacturer's specifications of the beam production system and the electron applicator design, electron beams produced by a Varian Clinac 2100C linear accelerator and collimated by the EMLC were simulated using the EGS4/BEAM code. Monte Carlo simulations were carried out using a group of 22 Pentium Pro central processing units (cpu) (200 MHz) (Intel Corporation, Santa Clara, CA) and 10 Pentium III cpu (450 MHz), all running *EGS4/BEAM, MCDOSE,* and their utilities under the Linux (Red Hat, Inc., Raleigh, NC) operating system.[17,18] All simulation parameters, such as the electron and photon energy cutoffs (ECUT and PCUT), the maximum fractional energy loss per electron step (ESTEPE), and the number of initial electron histories, were specified in the *EGS4/BEAM* input file. In this study, we used ECUT = 700 keV and PCUT = 10 keV, below which all remaining energy was assumed to deposit on the spot. ESTEPE was set to 0.04. The EMLC was included in the *EGS4/BEAM* simulations as an MLC component module. The number of initial electron histories ranged from 2 to 30 million, depending on the electron energy. Phase space data were scored at a plane of 100 cm SSD after the particles had transported through the linear accelerator treatment head, the EMLC, and the air gap beneath it. The 1σ statistical uncertainty in the dose was, in general, less than 2% of the $D_{maximum}$ value. Based on this simulated electron beam, the MERT plans were then created using our modified *EGS4/MCDOSE* code.

In this treatment planning study, a computed tomography (CT) scan was acquired with the patient in the supine position. A thermoplastic facial mask with three fiducials was used for the purpose of patient immobilization and target localization for the subsequent treatments. Approximately 90 images with a slice thickness of 3.0 mm were acquired over the entire treatment area. Each CT image had an in-plane resolution of 512 × 512 pixels, with each voxel being 0.94 × 0.94 × 3.0 mm^3 in size. The CT images were transferred to the AcQSim workstation (Philips Medical Systems, Andover, MA) for further processing.

The gross tumor volume (GTV) and critical structures were contoured on the axial CT images by a radiation oncologist using the AcQSim workstation. The GTV was defined based on diagnostic imaging and clinical findings and consisted of gross primary and nodal tumors. The clinical tumor volume (CTV) was constructed by expanding the GTV by 1.0 cm in all directions to cover microscopic extension of the tumor. The planning tumor volume was obtained by adding a 0.5 cm margin uniformly to CTV to account for patient setup uncertainty and organ shift. The critical structures to be protected included the spinal cord, brainstem, optic chiasm, optical nerve, and orbits. Like photon beam IMRT, only those structures that were contoured were considered in the plan and included in the final statistics.

The CT images, along with the outlined structures, were transferred to a workstation using the DICOM (Digital Imaging and Communication in Medicine) 3.0 protocol and then converted into a format that was compatible with the *EGS4/MCDOSE* code so that they could be sent to our designated Monte Carlo treatment planning machines. The final CT images used in MERT planning had an in-plane resolution of 128 × 128 pixels with a voxel size of 0.35 × 0.35 × 0.30 cm^3. This voxel size balanced resolution and Monte Carlo dose calculation time. Additionally, the CT numbers were converted into mass densities and material types for these simulations. Based on the CT numbers, each voxel was designated as being one of the three materials: air, tissue, or bone. This provided the approximate effective atomic numbers, cross-sections, and stopping powers for each voxel.

Figure 18.8-3 shows the simplified MERT planning flowchart. To facilitate the description of the flowchart, we use the term *field* to specify each beam angle and electron energy combination and reserve the term *port* to indicate a single beam orientation (gantry angle). Thus, a plan in which five electron energies are delivered at a single gantry angle may be said to have one port and five fields. In this study, the MERT plans consisted of three ports and 15 fields, as summarized in Tables 18.8-1 and 18.8-2.

The first step in creating a MERT plan was to select a set of suitable beam orientations to fully cover the target volume while sparing the adjacent critical structures as much

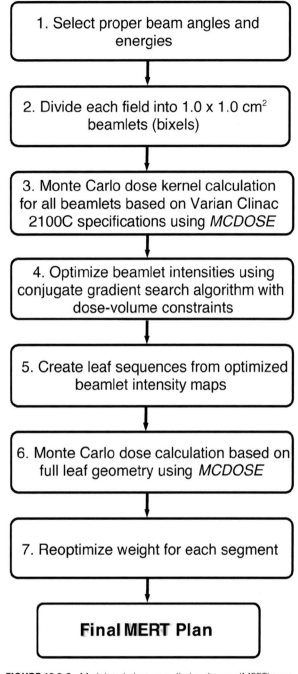

FIGURE 18.8-3. Modulated electron radiation therapy (MERT) treatment planning flowchart.

TABLE 18.8-1. List of Ports Used in the Modulated Electron Radiation Therapy Plans

Port No.	Gantry Angle, degrees
1	205
2	235
3	270

TABLE 18.8-2. List of Fields Used in the Modulated Electron Radiation Therapy Plans

Field No.	Gantry Angle, degrees	Beam Energy, MeV
1	205	6
2	205	9
3	205	12
4	205	16
5	205	20
6	235	6
7	235	9
8	235	12
9	235	16
10	235	20
11	270	6
12	270	9
13	270	12
14	270	16
15	270	20

as possible. Each port was then divided into 1.0×1.0 cm^2 beamlets. All beamlets smaller than 1×1 cm^2 at the edges of the field were rounded to 1×1 cm^2. The beamlet size was defined at the isocenter plane. The goal of this step was to determine how many beamlets were required to simulate each port. The user specified the isocenter, gantry, collimator, and couch angles; the desired beamlet size; and the dimension of the search space. A program calculated which beamlets intersected the target and created a text file containing these beamlets and their coordinates. This file was used by *MCDOSE* to precalculate the beamlet dose kernels. The total number of beamlets was the sum of the beamlets over all ports. A beamlet could be turned off (ie, assigned a weight of zero) but continue to remain active throughout optimization.

Next, we needed to determine which electron energies to use for each beam angle. To do so, we computed a tumor depth map for each beam angle whose pixel size was the same as that of a beamlet, that is, 1.0×1.0 cm^2. Based on the tumor depth distribution and assuming that the electrons lose energy at ~ 2 MeV/cm in tissue, we were able to determine a suitable set of electron energies for each beam angle. Given that, in most of the cases, the target was not spherical in shape, different beam angles could have different sets of electron energies. The advantage of this approach was the removal of those electron energies that contributed less to the target dose, thus reducing the number of fields and the delivery time.

The next step was to calculate beamlet dose kernels using *MCDOSE*. The beamlet dose kernel was the Monte Carlo calculated dose array for all structures owing to a single beamlet. Each element of the dose kernel represented the dose delivered to a dose calculation point or voxel, assuming a unit beamlet weight. These values were also referred to as dose deposition coefficients. To optimize beamlet weights or intensity maps, a quadratic objective function

augmented with dose-volume constraints was constructed. This was based on the assumption that a quadratic relationship existed between the delivered dose and the biologic effect. The overall objective function contained a linear component for each structure. Within each structure, each of the individual constraints contributed linearly to the objective function.

The core of the optimization procedure was the well-known conjugate gradient search algorithm. The major advantage of the gradient search technique was its fast convergence speed, compared with stochastic optimization techniques, such as simulated annealing. During the optimization, care was exercised to avoid negative weights. These nonphysical results were eliminated by scaling step sizes to avoid stepping over the boundary of the acceptable solution space and by projecting gradients onto the boundaries.

Following the beamlet weight optimization, the resulting 15 optimized continuous intensity maps were stratified into 5 discrete intensity levels in preparation for leaf sequencing. These discrete intensity maps were then converted to 15 step-and-shoot leaf sequences[19] based on the technique proposed by Bortfeld and colleagues.[20] Given that the dose distribution delivered by the ideal beamlets could be different from that delivered by the leaf sequences, a Monte Carlo dose calculation was performed again based on the discrete intensity maps reconstructed from the corresponding leaf sequences. With these new dose kernels, the leaf sequence segment weights were reoptimized. This second optimization differed from the first in two aspects. The first optimization was entirely based on idealized beamlets, without considering the EMLC geometry or the leaf scatter effect, whereas the second optimization took into account not only the EMLC geometry but also leaf end transmission and bremsstrahlung leakage. Thus, the first optimization produced the best dose distribution possible, whereas the second one gave the actual delivered dose.

The MERT plans with three coplanar beams (gantry angles: 205°, 235°, and 255°) were created using our modified *EGS4/MCDOSE* treatment planning system. Each gantry angle was treated with five nominal electron energies (6, 9, 12, 16, and 20 MeV), separately. The intensities of each energy for each particular gantry angle were determined by the optimizer. The goal dose to the target was 50.0 Gy, with a conventional fractionation scheme of 2.0 Gy per fraction, 5 fractions per week, and 25 fractions in total. The minimum and maximum target doses were 49.0 Gy and 54.0 Gy, respectively. The dose limit for critical structures ranged from 37.0 to 42.0 Gy, with the volume allowed above the limit dose being 5%. Isodose lines were normalized to 55.0 Gy for all plans.

Photon IMRT Planning

For comparison purposes, a photon beam IMRT plan was computed using a commercial treatment planning system

(*CORVUS*, North American Scientific, NOMOS Radiation Oncology Division, Cranberry Township, PA). Similar to MERT planning, the goal dose to the target was 50.0 Gy, with the minimum and maximum doses being 49.0 Gy and 54.0 Gy, respectively. For both MERT and IMRT treatment planning, the objective was to cover the entire target with isodose lines between 95% and 107% of the target dose as recommended by International Commission on Radiation Units and Measurements (ICRU) report 50.[21] The *CORVUS* system also allows the user to specify a percent target volume allowed below the goal dose. In this study, we used 4% for this value. For the critical structures, the limit dose also ranged from 37.0 to 42.0 Gy, with the volume allowed above the limit dose being 5%. The maximum allowable dose to the critical structures was set to be 40.0 Gy. IMRT plans using other combinations of the dose-volume constraints were also tried. It was found that the above-described constraints optimized target dose coverage and conformity against critical structure sparing.

Tissue heterogeneity corrections were performed during the beamlet intensity optimization and final dose calculation. Like the MERT planning system, the *CORVUS* system also uses an integral dose-volume histogram (DVH)-based cost function. The current version of the *CORVUS* IMRT software supports only one optimization technique, simulated annealing.[22] To obtain the best possible beamlet intensities and, thus, the optimal dose distribution, the optimizer mode was set to continuous. This mode determines the internal representation of the beamlet intensities and is, in general, the best choice for most treatment plans.

The final IMRT plan consisted of five coplanar gantry angles, each being treated with a 4 MV photon beam. The gantry angles were selected in such a way as to minimize unnecessary normal tissue and critical structure irradiation. However, in this study, beam orientations were not optimized. IMRT plans of different beam number and angle combinations were generated. Plan evaluation indicated that the plan with coplanar beams at angles of 0°, 205°, 235°, 270°, and 320° gave the best results. Therefore, this beam arrangement was used in this study. Isodose lines were also normalized to 55.0 Gy for all IMRT plans. The plan used in this study was created based on a Varian Clinac 2100C linear accelerator and delivered in the step-and-shoot mode. The machine was equipped with a 26-leaf pair photon MLC capable of producing 1.0×1.0 cm^2 beamlets.

Intensity Maps

Figure 18.8-4A shows a three-dimensional beam's eye view of a representative parotid gland tumor viewed at the beam angle of 235°. Figure 18.8-4B shows the corresponding tumor depth map at the same beam angle. Different pixel grayscale levels represent different depths of the target. Darker pixels indicate the area where the tumor extended deeper into the tissue at this particular beam angle. As clear-

ly demonstrated in the tumor depth map, this particular case was a good candidate for a MERT treatment because the target was superficial and had an irregular boundary. Based on the tumor depth map, a histogram was created, showing the tumor depth distribution (Figure 18.8-5).

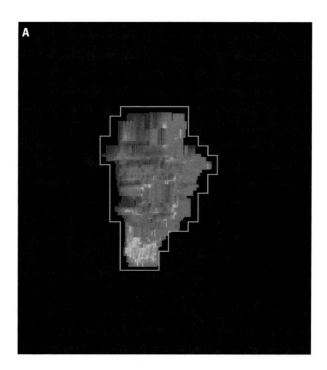

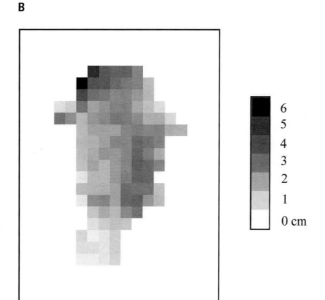

FIGURE 18.8-4. A representative parotid gland tumor and corresponding tumor depth map. (*A*) A three-dimensional beam's eye view of a parotid gland tumor at a beam angle of 235°. (*B*) Corresponding tumor depth map, with darker pixels indicating the deeper parts of the tumor at this viewing angle. (To view a color version of this image, please refer to the CD-ROM.)

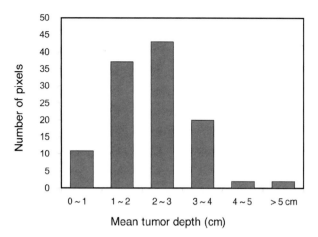

FIGURE 18.8-5. A representative tumor depth histogram. This histogram was created based on Figure 18.8-4B, showing the number of pixels as a function of the mean tumor depth. Based on this distribution, a suitable set of electron energies was selected for this particular beam angle.

From the histogram, we determined that the electron beams of 12, 16, and 20 MeV would be the best choices for this case in terms of depth dose conformity at this beam angle. However, we chose to use all available electron energies.

Figure 18.8-6A to Figure 18.8-6E show representative beam intensity maps for a MERT plan for the 6, 9, 12, 16, and 20 MeV fields at the beam angle of 235°. In all parts of the figure, each pixel represents a 1×1 cm^2 beamlet projected at the isocenter. Darker pixels indicate higher beam intensity levels, which correspond to a longer beam-on time. A white background indicates zero beam intensity. These are areas in which beams were blocked all the time by the EMLC leaves. In reality, however, there was about 1% radiation leakage through the EMLC leaves. As can be seen in the intensity maps, the optimizer gave significant weights to the 12, 16, and 20 MeV fields, whereas small weights were assigned to the 6 and 9 MeV fields. These different electron energy weights brought about the energy modulation. By carefully examining the intensity maps and the tumor depth map, we noticed that the MERT intensity maps largely reflected the tumor depth distribution. The superposition of these intensity maps yielded not only the optimal lateral dose conformity but, more importantly, the optimal depth dose conformity.

The number of segments needed to produce these intensity maps were 18 (for 6 MeV), 18 (for 9 MeV), 12 (for 12 MeV), 18 (for 16 MeV), and 14 (for 20 MeV), giving a total of 80 segments for this port. This number was comparable to the number of segments for a photon field in a typical *CORVUS* head and neck plan that has a similar target volume. For comparison, the corresponding optimized photon beam IMRT intensity map for the 4 MV field at the same beam angle is shown in Figure 18.8-6F. This intensity map, actually consisting of two separate maps, was

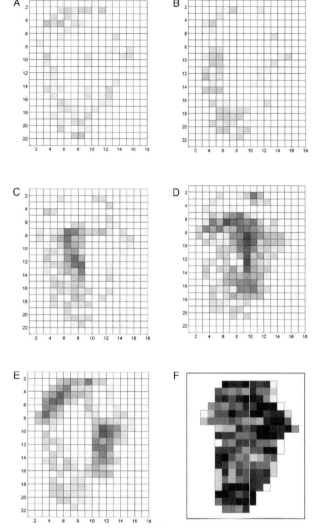

FIGURE 18.8-6. Representative beam intensity maps. Intensity maps for the modulated electron radiation therapy plan for the 6 (*A*), 9 (*B*), 12 (*C*), 16 (*D*), and 20 (*E*) MeV fields at a beam angle of 235°. (*F*) Corresponding photon beam intensity-modulated radiation therapy intensity map for the 4 MV field at the same beam angle. This intensity map consists of two separate intensity maps that were combined manually.

combined manually. This was because the size of the target in the anterior-posterior direction was fairly large; the MLC leaves could not cover the entire target with one field only. Thus, this 235° port was split into two subfields. Like the MERT intensity maps, each pixel in the photon beam IMRT map represents a 1×1 cm^2 beamlet projected at the isocenter. Compared with its MERT counterparts, the photon beam IMRT intensity map shows a relatively uniform intensity distribution, indicating a lack of depth dose modulation. The combined photon beam IMRT intensity map required 120 segments to deliver, divided into 62 and 58 segments for each subfield, respectively.

For both the MERT and the IMRT plans, we counted both "step" and "shoot" that were listed in the step-and-shoot leaf sequence files as a segment. However, some IMRT treatment planning systems count only "shoot" as a segment. Thus, in the case of the combined photon beam IMRT intensity map, it required 60 steps and 60 shoots to produce. Given that the delivery time is approximately linearly proportional to the number of "shoot" segments in a leaf sequence file, we can say that the MERT plan required relatively less time to deliver.

It is worth pointing out that in this study, we used all five available electron energies, which, in most cases, is not necessary. Let us take the 6 and 9 MeV electron beams as examples. As shown in Figure 18.8-6A and Figure 18.8-6B, the optimizer gave them very low weights. Their contributions to the dose distribution in the final MERT plan were not significant. Therefore, they could have been deleted from the plan, leaving only three electron beams in the plan. The final three leaf sequence files would have had

fewer segments, and the total delivery time would have been even less. At this point, for a typical MERT treatment, the total treatment time was about 40 minutes.

Dose Distributions

Figure 18.8-7A and Figure 18.8-7D show the comparison of the MERT and IMRT isodose distributions for the central axial slices from a representative case of parotid gland cancer. Figure 18.8-7B and Figure 18.8-7E show the comparison of the isodose distributions for the central coronal slices from the same example. Figure 18.8-7C and Figure 18.8-7F show the comparison of the isodose distributions for the central sagittal slices also from the same example. The isodose distributions are shown in color lines. In both plans, the isodose curves were normalized to 55.0 Gy, representing 10, 20, 30, 40, 50, 60, 70, 80, 90, and 100%, respectively. Only selected isodose lines are labeled in the figures.

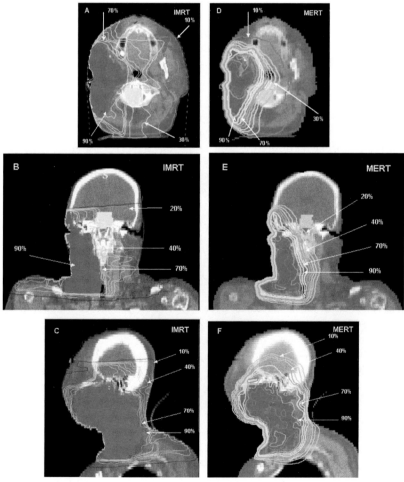

FIGURE 18.8-7. Comparison of the modulated electron radiation therapy (MERT) and photon intensity-modulated radiation therapy (IMRT) plan isodose distributions. (*A*) and (*D*) Isodose distributions for the central axial slices for a representative case of parotid gland cancer. (*B*) and (*E*) Isodose distributions for the central coronal slices from the same case. (*C*) and (*F*) Isodose distributions for the central sagittal slices from the same case. The isodose curves, normalized to 55.0 Gy, represent 10, 20, 30, 40, 50, 60, 70, 80, 90, and 100%, respectively. Only selected isodose lines are shown. (To view a color version of this image, please refer to the CD-ROM.)

It is evident from the isodose distributions that higher isodose lines covered the target well in terms of conformity in both plans, with the MERT plan showing an overall better conformity for all isodose lines in all three anatomic planes. As to the lower isodose lines, the photon beam IMRT plan exhibited a relatively poor conformity. As anticipated, the exit doses of the photon beams penetrated much more deeply than the doses delivered by the electron beams. This resulted in significant but unnecessary doses to deeper tissues, including some of the critical structures. This is demonstrated in the axial and coronal slices of the IMRT plan, in which the 30% isodose line covered the spinal cord fully and the 40% isodose line partly covered the brainstem and the orbits. In contrast, the corresponding MERT plan showed an excellent critical structure sparing because of the rapid falloff of the electron beams. The 30% isodose line covered only small portions of the spinal cord, brainstem, and right orbit. The left orbit was almost completely spared, as shown in Figure 18.8-7D and Figure 18.8-7E. Thus, it is clear that the MERT plan provided a better target dose coverage and normal tissue sparing than the photon beam IMRT plan.

Dose-Volume Histograms

To evaluate the plans objectively, we analyzed the cumulative DVHs of the plans. The DVHs for the target and the critical structures for this representative patient are shown in Figure 18.8-8. Based on the DVHs, it is evident that the MERT plan provided a more homogeneous dose coverage to the target than the corresponding photon beam IMRT plan because the former's DVH is more vertical than is the latter's. In the MERT plan, the maximum, minimum, and mean doses delivered to the CTV were 55.82, 40.50, and 50.32 Gy, respectively, whereas the corresponding doses delivered to the CTV in the IMRT plan were 60.38, 17.30, and 50.24 Gy, respectively, resulting in some undesirable hot and cold spots. The photon beam IMRT plan exhibited some degree of dose inhomogeneity. In addition, in the photon beam IMRT plan, about 3% of the CTV received a dose of ≥ 55 Gy and 5% of the CTV received a dose of ≤ 45 Gy. In contrast, the MERT plan gave much better statistics. Less than 0.5% of the CTV received a dose of ≥ 55 Gy and approximately 1.5% of the CTV received a dose of ≤ 45 Gy. All of these suggest that the MERT plan provides a better dose homogeneity.

It is well known that conventional treatment modalities using electron beams exhibit a higher degree of dose inhomogeneity in comparison with photon beam techniques. In part, this is caused by tissue heterogeneity and skin surface irregularity. Here we see that with electron energy and intensity modulations, it is possible to reduce the degree of dose heterogeneity and achieve a satisfactory dose distribution and uniformity.

The differences between the two DVHs for the critical structures indicate that the MERT plan also delivered much fewer doses to the critical structures than the photon beam IMRT plan. It is clear from Figure 18.8-8 that the MERT plan showed superior normal tissue sparing. The maximum and mean doses to the spinal cord in the MERT plan were 16.62 and 5.24 Gy, respectively, whereas the corresponding doses in the photon beam IMRT plan were 36.22 and 17.50 Gy. Only 16% of the spinal cord volume in the MERT plan received a dose of greater than or equal to 10 Gy compared with 97% in the IMRT plan. Similar sparing for other structures was also observed in the MERT plan. The maximum and mean doses given to the brainstem in the MERT plan were 13.65 and 2.66 Gy, respectively. In contrast, the corresponding doses given in the photon beam IMRT plan were 29.88 and 16.66 Gy, much higher than the doses delivered in the MERT plan. As for the orbits, both

A

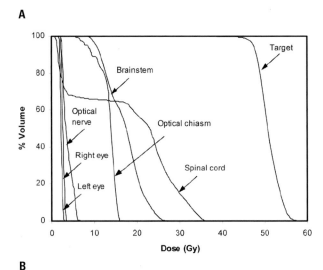

B

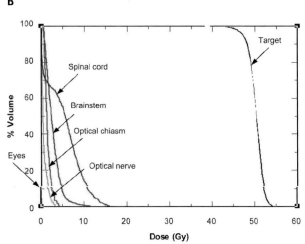

FIGURE 18.8-8. Comparison of dose-volume histograms for the photon beam intensity-modulated radiation therapy (*A*) and modulated electron radiation therapy (MERT) (*B*) plans. The MERT plan shows a superior normal tissue sparing and a better dose distribution.

the MERT and the photon beam IMRT plans gave very low doses. In particular, the MERT plan delivered an extremely low dose to the contralateral orbit, with the maximum and mean doses being 0.15 and 0.05 Gy, respectively. This is clinically relevant because the tolerance dose for the lenses is only 10 to 15 Gy.

In this case, the contralateral parotid gland was not contoured as an independent critical structure. However, based on the isodose distributions shown in Figure 18.8-7, it is clear that the dose delivered to the contralateral parotid gland for the MERT plan was well under the established tolerance dose of 20 to 30 Gy.[23] Even if we increased the prescribed dose to 60 Gy, the dose delivered to the contralateral parotid gland for the MERT plan would be within tolerance. It is important to point out that the mean dose to the nontarget tissue in the photon beam IMRT plan was 7.54 Gy compared with 3.95 Gy in the MERT plan. This is also of clinical significance because the MERT plan could greatly reduce low radiation doses to large normal tissue volume.

For many years, parotid gland cancers have been largely treated using one of these three techniques: an ipsilateral wedged pair of photon beams oriented at oblique angles, an ipsilateral field treated with high energy electrons, and a combination of high-energy photon and electron beams with carefully chosen weights. Unfortunately, because of the intrinsic limitation of the underlying physics, all of these techniques are not able to produce treatment plans that provide both a high degree of target dose conformity and good normal tissue sparing. Recently, photon IMRT has shown some success in treating certain head and neck cancers, but it is still not suitable to treat shallow tumors owing to an extremely low surface dose and an excessively high exit dose. The low surface dose is not effective in killing tumor cells in superficial tissues. The high exit dose constitutes a significant risk to the normal function of the distant critical structures, such as the spinal cord and the contralateral orbit and parotid gland. Therefore, it would be desirable to develop a technique that can eliminate these drawbacks. As the results presented here indicate, through both electron intensity and energy modulations, MERT was able to deliver highly conformal doses to targets with complex shapes. In the meantime, it provided sufficient protection of the critical structures and substantial normal tissue sparing. Considering the radiation side effects and the quality of life limiting organs at risk such as the contralateral parotid gland and orbit, it is necessary to keep the dose to the normal tissues to a minimum and preserve the organ function as much as possible. In this respect, MERT had a clear advantage.

However, the current MERT technique has two major disadvantages compared with photon IMRT. First, the poor clearance of the EMLC compared with the existing electron applicator makes it more apt to come into contact with the patient at some configurations of gantry and collimator angles. This could become one of the limitations of MERT for wide clinical applications. Therefore, further research and development are needed to improve EMLC design. Second, relatively long treatment times are needed for beamlet-based MERT, especially for cases in which multiple electron energies and gantry angles are used. Recently, aperture-based approaches have been proposed in an effort to overcome this problem.[24–26] In addition, because the current EMLC is manually driven, the MERT treatment is still a labor-intensive process in terms of planning, quality assurance, and delivery. This could cause potential problems associated with logistics and human resources. Before MERT becomes a practical and standard treatment modality, all of these problems have to be solved.

Acknowledgments

This study was supported in part by grants DAMD17-00-1-0443 (Yulin Song and Steve Jiang), DAMD17-00-1-0444 (Todd Pawlicki), and DAMD17-01-1-0635 (Lei Xing) from the US Department of Defense. We would like to express our sincere thanks to Varian Medical Systems for providing the electron applicators for this study.

References

1. Garden AS, El-Naggar AK, Morrison WH, et al. Postoperative radiotherapy for malignant tumors of the parotid gland. Int J Radiat Oncol Biol Phys 1997;37:79–85.

2. Spino IJ, Wang CC, Montogmery WW. Carcinoma of the parotid gland. Analysis of treatment results and patterns of failure after combined surgery and radiation therapy. Cancer 1993;71:2699–705.

3. Lenhard RE Jr, Osteen RT, Gansler T. Clinical oncology. American Cancer Society; Atlanta, GA, 2001.

4. North CA, Lee D-J, Piantedosi S, et al. Carcinoma of the major salivary glands treated by surgery plus postoperative radiotherapy. Int J Radiat Oncol Biol Phy 1990;18:1319–26.

5. Wu Q, Manning M, Schmidt-Ullrich R, et al. The potential for sparing of parotids and escalation of biologically effective dose with intensity-modulated radiation treatments of head and neck cancers: a treatment design study. Int J Radiat Oncol Biol Phys 2000;46:195–205.

6. Vineberg KA, Eisbruch A, Coselmon MM, et al. Is uniform target dose possible in IMRT plans in the head and neck? Int J Radiat Oncol Biol Phys 2002;52:1159–72.

7. Chao KS, Ozyigit G, Tran BN, et al. Patterns of failure in patients receiving definitive and postoperative IMRT for head-and-neck cancer. Int J Radiat Oncol Biol Phys 2003;55:312–21.

8. Lin A, Kim HM, Terrell JE, et al. Quality of life after parotid-sparing IMRT for head-and-neck cancer: a prospective longitudinal study. Int J Radiat Oncol Biol Phys 2003;57:61–70.

9. Nutting CM, Rowbottom CG, Cosgrove VP, et al. Optimization of radiotherapy for carcinoma of the parotid gland: a comparison of conventional, three-dimensional conformal, and intensity-modulated techniques. Radiother Oncol 2001;60:163–72.

10. Bragg CM, Conway J, Robinson MH. The role of intensity-modulated radiotherapy in the treatment of parotid tumors. Int J Radiat Oncol Biol Phys 2002;52:729–38.

11. Karlsson MK, Karlsson MG, Zackrisson B. Intensity modulation with electrons: calculations, measurements and clinical applications. Phys Med Biol 1998;43:1159–69.

12. Korevaar EW, Huizenga H, Lof J, et al. Investigation of the added value of high-energy electrons in intensity-modulated radiotherapy: four clinical cases. Int J Radiat Oncol Biol Phys 2002;52:236–53.

13. Suit HD. Protons to replace photons in external beam radiation therapy? Clin Oncol 2003;15:S29–31.

14. Lee MC, Deng J, Li J, et al. Monte Carlo based treatment planning for modulated electron radiation therapy. Phys Med Biol 2001;46:2177–99.

15. Ma C-M, Pawlicki T, Lee MC, et al. Energy-and intensity-modulated electron beams for radiotherapy. Phys Med Biol 2000;45:2293–311.

16. Song Y, Jiang SB, Lee MC, et al. A multileaf collimator for modulated electron radiation therapy (MERT) for breast cancer. In: The Department of Defense Breast Cancer Research Program meeting proceedings. The Department of Defense Vol I. Orlando, FL. 2002. p. 15–17.

17. Nelson WR, Hirayama H, Rogers DWO. The EGS4 code system. SLAC-report-265. Stanford Linear Accelerator Center; Stanford, CA,1985.

18. Rogers DWO, Faddegon BA, Ding GX, et al. BEAM: a Monte Carlo code to simulated radiotherapy treatment units. Med Phys 1995;22:503–24.

19. Boyer AL, Yu CX. Intensity modulated radiation therapy with dynamic multileaf collimators. Semin Radiat Oncol 1999;9:48–59.

20. Bortfeld T, Kahler DL, Waldron TJ, et al. X-ray field compensation with multileaf collimators. Int J Radiat Oncol Biol Phys 1994;28:723–30.

21. International Commission on Radiation Units and Measurements. Prescribing, recording, and reporting photon beam therapy. Report 50. Washington (DC): International Commission on Radiation Units and Measurements; 1993.

22. Webb S. Optimization of conformal radiotherapy dose distribution by simulated annealing. Phys Med Biol 1989;34:1349–70.

23. Chao KSC, Low DA, Perez CA, et al. Intensity modulated radiation therapy in head and neck cancers: the Mallinckrodt experience. Int J Cancer 2000;90:92–103.

24. Bednarz GD, Michalski D, Houser C, et al. The use of mixed-integer programming for inverse treatment planning with pre-defined field segments. Phys Med Biol 2002;47:2235–45.

25. Shepard DM, Earl MA, Naqvi S, et al. Direct aperture optimization: a turnkey solution for step-and-shoot IMRT. Med Phys 2002;29:1007–18.

26. Cotrutz C, Xing L. Segment-based dose optimization using a simple genetic algorithm. Phys Med Biol. 2003;48:2987-98.

Impact of Prolonged Treatment Times

Emerging Technology

Steven J. Chmura, MD, PhD, Karl Farrey, MS, Steve Wang, PhD,
Michael C. Garofalo, MD, John C. Roeske, PhD

Intensity-modulated radiation therapy (IMRT) is receiving increasing attention in the treatment of head and neck cancer.[1,2] Multiple investigators have demonstrated the superiority of IMRT planning over conventional approaches in terms of normal sparing, particularly sparing of the parotid glands in oropharyngeal and nasopharyngeal tumors.[3–5] Others have shown that highly conformal IMRT plans may also provide a means of safely escalating radiation dose.[6,7] To date, clinical outcome studies in head and neck patients undergoing IMRT have been promising.[8–10] However, longer follow-up is needed to truly evaluate tumor control and late toxicity in these patients.

Despite these promising results, several concerns exist regarding the routine use of IMRT in head and neck cancer. To date, most attention has been focused on the issue of target delineation.[11,12] However, an additional concern is prolongation of treatment delivery. At most centers, IMRT is delivered using a linear accelerator equipped with a multileaf collimator (MLC), which varies the radiation fluence across the treatment field. Unlike conventional radiation therapy (RT), the complicated fluence patterns used in IMRT typically require longer treatment times (15–40 minutes). Radiobiologically, increased treatment times may reduce the therapeutic efficacy of IMRT compared with conventional radiation therapy by allowing for the repair of sublethal damage.[13] Consequently, the potential benefits of IMRT in terms of reduced treatment toxicity may be offset by compromised tumor control.

The purpose of this chapter is to examine the issue of treatment delivery time and its implications for IMRT in head and neck cancers. The use of biologic modeling and new experimental designs are presented to test the hypothesis that prolonged delivery times may adversely impact the therapeutic efficacy of IMRT. Interested readers are encouraged to refer to Chapter 3, "Radiobiology of IMRT," for an in-depth review of radiobiologic issues in IMRT.

Factors Affecting Daily Treatment Times

The overall treatment time for a single fraction of IMRT is due to the complex interplay between the planning goals and available IMRT technologies. To illustrate this, consider a head and neck cancer patient who was treated using IMRT (Figure 18.9-1). The complexity of treatment (related to treatment time) depends on the target size and shape and its positional relationship to the surrounding normal tissues (eg, parotid glands, spinal cord, salivary glands, oral cavity). Moreover, the planning goals and desired degree of conformity affect the overall treatment time. Highly conformal IMRT plans, in general, require more monitor units (MUs) and hence longer delivery times.

From a planning perspective, a number of variables are used to generate an optimal IMRT plan, including beam number and orientation of the gantry angles. IMRT plans in head and neck patients typically use 5 to 11 equally spaced beams, which is significantly more than the 2 to 3 beams commonly used in conventional RT. Moreover, if noncoplanar beams are used, the therapist must enter the treatment room each time the couch needs to be rotated, further increasing treatment time. The planning system and variables chosen within this system also impact the overall treatment time, including the number of intensity levels, optimization algorithm used (eg, simulated annealing, iterative algorithms), and relative weightings of the planning goals.[14,15]

Once an acceptable plan has been generated, the fluence patterns must be converted to a leaf sequence.[16] The

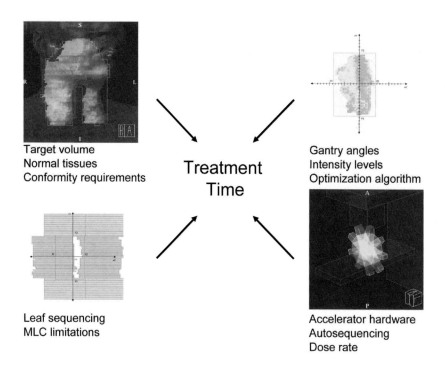

Target volume
Normal tissues
Conformity requirements

Treatment Time

Gantry angles
Intensity levels
Optimization algorithm

Leaf sequencing
MLC limitations

Accelerator hardware
Autosequencing
Dose rate

FIGURE 18.9-1. Schematic diagram illustrating the complex interplay between the various aspects of treatment planning and delivery and how these relate to the overall treatment time. MLC = multileaf collimator. (To view a color version of this image, please refer to the CD-ROM.)

efficiency of the dynamic MLC delivery depends on the MLC characteristics (eg, leaf speed, leaf overtravel, carriage limitations) and the algorithm used to generate these sequences.[17] Lastly, treatment time is also determined by the linear accelerator design. Factors associated with the linear accelerator include the dose rate (MU/minute), delivery methods (static vs dynamic), availability of automatic beam sequencing software, and physical limits imposed by the MLC.[18] Given the complexity of the planning process, it is not possible to identify a single factor that is most responsible for the prolonged delivery times associated with IMRT.

In the example shown in Figure 18.9-1, the IMRT plan was generated using the *CORVUS* system (North American Scientific, NOMOS Radiation Oncology Division, Cranberry Township, PA), which uses a simulated annealing algorithm. The planner selected nine equally spaced coplanar fields. This plan was subsequently delivered (step and shoot) using a Varian 2100EX linear accelerator (Varian Medical Systems, Palo Alto, CA) equipped with a Millennium 120-leaf MLC. Because of the limitations of carriage movement, the fields were split by the leaf sequencer to form 14 individual fields. The overall daily treatment time was 17 minutes (first beam "on" to last beam "off"). On a different linear accelerator, the daily treatment time for a plan with comparable complexity is estimated to be > 40 minutes.[19] A conventional head and neck plan (opposed laterals + anterior field) may require only 5 to 10 minutes.

Radiobiologic Studies

Tumor cell killing following ionizing radiation results from the induction of apoptosis, necrosis, or other mechanisms.[20] Dysregulation of the apoptotic response to ionizing radiation or alterations in cell-cycle checkpoints and deoxyribonucleic acid (DNA) repair play critical roles in determining tumor radiocurability.[21] Recent data demonstrate that chromatin, in combination with DNA, represents a target of DNA damage and is altered within minutes of DNA double-strand breaks.[22] For example, the histone H2AX, a minor histone H2A variant, is rapidly phosphorylated within minutes of exposure to ionizing radiation,

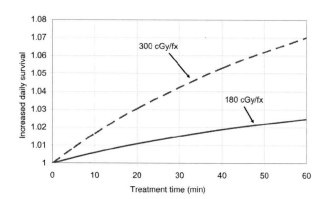

FIGURE 18.9-2. Increase in cell survival as a function of treatment time for SQ-20B cells. Parameters used in the calculation (equation 3) are $\alpha = 0.13$ Gy^{-1} and $\beta = 0.017$ Gy^{-2}.

thereby affecting regulation of gene expression and DNA repair.[23] Owing to the speed of phosphorylation and repair of initial strand breaks, H2AX phosphorylation, the initiation of DNA repair, and subsequent nonhomologous DNA end joining may be different with different IMRT techniques.

Data from our laboratory at the University of Chicago demonstrate that radioresistant lines clear γH2AX foci more rapidly than radiosensitive cells lines, suggesting that DNA repair efficiency within a given cell line may be monitored using H2AX foci as a surrogate.[24] Further experiments are under way to examine the effect of prolonged dose delivery on DNA damage and repair by assaying for γH2AX. By correlating clonogenic assay results (see below) with γH2AX assay results, it may be possible to further characterize the biologic impact of prolonged dose delivery on a molecular level.

Classic radiobiologic experiments support the hypothesis that extended treatment times adversely impact tumor cell killing. In vitro studies conducted by Emery and colleagues compared tumor cell killing using "two-hit" radiation treatments.[25] In these experiments, cells were exposed to a single fraction of 5 Gy or two fractions of 2.5 Gy separated by 45 minutes. The data demonstrated that a single 5 Gy fraction was significantly more effective than when the same dose was delivered in two fractions over the course of 45 minutes. In an analogy closer to the extended IMRT treatment times, dose rate has been found also to impact tumor cell killing.[26] Cells derived from a squamous cell carcinoma of the uterine cervix (HTB-35) were irradiated at dose rates ranging from 0.38 to 22.6 Gy/h. At the extremes for the dose rates evaluated, the dose required to produce a surviving fraction of 0.01 varied by a factor of two. Similar results have been demonstrated across numerous cell lines.[26–28] It is likely that this difference in tumor cell kill would decrease local tumor control in a subset of patients.

The impact of overall treatment time on cell survival was evaluated by Benedict and colleagues.[29] Human glioma tumor (U-87 MG) cells were irradiated with 6 MV x-rays using doses of 6 to 18 Gy and irradiation times of 0.25 to 3 hours. These doses and irradiation times were selected to simulate the treatment time and intermittent nature of stereotactic radiosurgery. Tumor cell killing decreased with increasing delivery time and with the delivery of the same total dose with repeated interruptions. For example, at 12 Gy, cell survival increased by a factor of 4.7 as the treatment time was increased from 16 to 112 minutes. These results suggest that delivery protraction with a discontinuous dose, similar to that used with some forms of IMRT, may result in a significant decrease in the efficacy of a given radiation dose. In addition, these results also suggest that in the fractionated RT setting, even larger effects on cell survival may be observed.

Recently, IMRT delivery was simulated in vitro by protracting treatment with various delivery schedules.[30] Tumor cells grown in monolayers were irradiated with a simulated conventional treatment regimen (2 Gy delivered at 1 Gy/min), and a schedule was made to simulate an IMRT delivery system (7 fractions, 0.29 Gy/fraction, dose rate 1 Gy/min, each fraction separated by a 3-minute time interval, for a total delivery time of 20 minutes). The simulated IMRT regimen appeared to enhance clonogenic survival significantly. However, although this study simulated the time course and lower dose rate of a typical IMRT treatment, it did not use actual IMRT beams, in which both temporal and spatial distributions are varied.

Mathematical Modeling

The generalized linear-quadratic (LQ) model for cell survival has been used in most dose protraction modeling studies.[31–33] The surviving fraction (S) for a total dose (D) is given by

$$S(D) = \exp[-n(\alpha d + \beta G(t)d^2) + \gamma T]$$ (1)

where n is the total number of fractions, d is the dose per fraction, α and β characterize the intrinsic radiosensitivity, G is the dose protraction factor, γ represents the effective tumor cell repopulation rate, and T is the overall time of a treatment course. The dose protraction factor, G, accounts for the repair of sublethal damage. A functional form of G used in many of these studies is given by

$$G = \frac{2}{\mu T}\left(1 - \frac{1 - e^{-\mu T}}{\mu T}\right)$$ (2)

where T is the daily treatment time and μ is a repair constant that is inversely proportional to the repair half-life (T_{repair}). Note that this functional form of G assumes that the dose is delivered continuously over a given treatment fraction. However, Fowler and colleagues point out that the repair of sublethal damage is likely to have multiple repair constants and that use of a single constant (μ) is an oversimplification.[34]

Wang and colleagues modeled the response of prostate tumors as the treatment time was protracted from 15 to 45 minutes using clinical IMRT plans.[13] Typical prostate cancer parameters ($\alpha/\beta = 3.1$ Gy) were used to derive the equivalent uniform dose and tumor control probability (see Chapter 3). Based on a prescription dose of 81 Gy in 1.8 Gy daily fractions, the equivalent uniform dose was observed to decrease by 12% (compared with conventional RT) when IMRT plans were delivered over 30 minutes. Fowler and colleagues recently reached similar conclusions by modeling repair rates for a wide range of fractionation dose schedules.[34] Using published in vivo half-times of repair, a model was constructed based on two components of repair. Similar to the study by Wang and colleagues,[13] it was concluded that IMRT plans that protract dose delivery beyond 30 minutes in a fractionated setting may result in a significant decrease in tumor cell killing.

Recently, Roeske and Chmura simulated the effects of prolonged treatment times in IMRT delivery.[35] Using the LQ model, an expression was derived for the fractional increase in cell survival owing to the prolongation in treatment time. This was obtained by dividing equation 1 with the prolongation factor G by the same equation, where G = 1 (instantaneous dose delivery). The resulting equation is given by

$$\frac{S}{S_o} = \exp[\ \beta\,(1 - G\,)d^{\,2}\,]$$

(3)

where S is the surviving fraction for a given treatment delivery, S_0 is the expected survival for instantaneous dose delivery, and the other factors are those discussed previously. A plot of the fractional increase in survival (S/S_0) is shown in Figure 18.9-2 for SQ-20B cells derived from a human epithelial tumor of the larynx.[36] The parameters used are $\alpha = 0.13$ Gy^{-1} and $\beta = 0.017$ Gy^{-2}.[37] In this example, T$_{repair}$ = 20 minutes.[13] The model predicts that for a daily dose/fraction of 1.8 Gy, treatment times of 20 to 40 minutes will increase cell survival by 1 to 2%. For higher than conventional doses (3 Gy/fraction), the increase in cell survival is 3 to 5% on a daily basis. Thus, prolonged treatment times may have a greater impact on hypofractionated regimens and techniques that use the simultaneous integrated boost technique.

The effects of prolonged treatment during the course of treatment are shown in Table 18.9-1 for the SQ-20B cell line. Table 18.9-2 shows the effects for the SCC25 cell line ($\alpha = 0.57$ Gy^{-1} and $\beta = 0.031$ Gy^{-2}),[37] which was derived from a human epithelial tumor of the tongue.[36] Note that in the case of the SCC25 cell line, the β value is nearly a factor of two higher than the SQ-20B cell line. In both cell lines, the model predicts a significant increase in the surviving fraction (relative to instantaneous dose delivery) over 30 fractions and when treatment protraction extends beyond 20 minutes.

Given the projected increase in cell survival, the next logical question is how much the daily dose per fraction should be increased to overcome the effects of prolonged treatment times. Roeske and Chmura applied the LQ model (equation 1) to derive an expression to determine the required daily fractional increase in prescription dose (f)[35]:

$$f = \frac{-\left(\alpha\!\big/\!\beta\right) + \sqrt{\left(\alpha\!\big/\!\beta\right)^2 + 4dG\left[\left(\alpha\!\big/\!\beta\right) + d\right]}}{2dG}$$

(4)

A plot of the f versus the treatment time is shown in Figure 18.9-3 for the SQ-20B cell line using the previously defined values. For a fraction size of 180 cGy, the dose needs to be increased by 3 to 6% for delivery times of 20 to 40 minutes. Given that IMRT plans often result in increased dose heterogeneity within the target volume, these doses are often achieved without significant effort from the planner. However, as the dose/fraction is increased to 300 cGy/fraction, the required fractional increase ranges from 5 to 10% to achieve the same level of cell kill as nearly instantaneous delivery.

In Vitro Experiments Using Linear Accelerator–Based IMRT Delivery

To date, no basic radiobiologic study has attempted to assess differences in the efficacy of actual IMRT delivery techniques compared with conventional RT regimens. To address this issue, we have developed an in vitro system that will permit delivery of both conventional and IMRT fractionated plans to cells in a manner that closely resembles those techniques employed during patient treatment, with the end point being clonogenic survival. The significance of using realistic IMRT plans is that surrounding critical structures will result in a fraction of the tumor cell population

TABLE 18.9-1. Fractional Increase in Cell Survival vs Treatment Time (SQ-20B Cells)

Time (min)	1 Fraction	5 Fractions	30 Fractions
0	1.000	1.000	1.000
5	1.003	1.014	1.090
10	1.006	1.028	1.180
20	1.010	1.052	1.358
40	1.018	1.092	1.694

TABLE 18.9-2. Fractional Increase in Cell Survival vs Treatment Time (SCC25 Cells)

Time (min)	1 Fraction	5 Fractions	30 Fractions
0	1.000	1.000	1.000
5	1.006	1.028	1.181
10	1.011	1.055	1.377
20	1.020	1.103	1.804
40	1.035	1.184	2.767

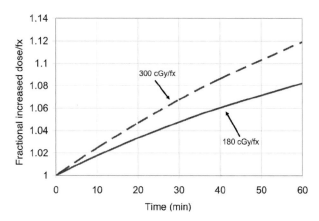

FIGURE 18.9-3. Required increase in daily dose/fraction to compensate for prolonged treatment times for SQ-20B cells. Parameters used in the calculation (equation 4) are $\alpha = 0.13$ Gy^{-1} and $\beta = 0.017$ Gy^{-2}.

being "shielded" from the beam at a variety of gantry angles. Thus, in a protracted scenario, these cells may be "shielded" for up to half of the total treatment time. The result is that the dose rate delivered to these cells is not only time but also spatially dependent. These experiments, therefore, present a unique opportunity to explore the interplay of these two variables that has not been previously studied.

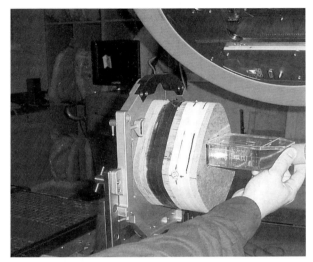

FIGURE 18.9-4. A head and neck phantom designed to permit delivery of actual intensity-modulated radiation therapy plans to cultured cells grown in suspension or monolayers. A stereotactic head frame holds the phantom in place and is mounted at the end of the treatment table. The stereotactic positioning system ensures daily reproducibility of 1 to 2 mm. (To view a color version of this image, please refer to the CD-ROM.)

A human head and neck cell line (SQ-20B) was selected for the initial studies owing to its relatively short cell cycle and large proliferation fraction in vitro and in vivo.[36] An IMRT phantom was designed to mimic a patient with head and neck cancer and was engineered to accommodate a 150 mm tissue culture flask (T-150) (Figure 18.9-4). Cells were grown in the bottom of the flask and were used to represent the gross tumor volume (GTV). The phantom is mounted stereotactically; thus, the daily positioning accuracy is ~ 1 to 2 mm. A computed tomography (CT) scan of the phantom was obtained, and the CT scan of a previous patient with head and neck cancer was fused to the study to provide a realistic planning target volume (Figure 18.9-5).

A seven-field IMRT plan and a conventional (opposed lateral) plan were generated. Both plans were normalized such that 99% of the cells received the daily prescription dose (180 cGy) and that the mean dose was the same (104% of the prescription dose). Individual thermoluminescent dosimeters were used to verify the dose delivered using the two techniques.

Two IMRT regimens were used. The "fast" IMRT treatment was delivered over 10 minutes and was based on the minimum treatment time using our available hardware and software. A second treatment regimen denoted as "slow" IMRT was delivered over 40 minutes. This time was based on documented treatment times for some commercial linear accelerators. Additionally, such extended treatment times may occur if one were using compensators, if the accelerator were not equipped with an autosequencing program, or if a malfunction occurred (eg, MLC motor failed during

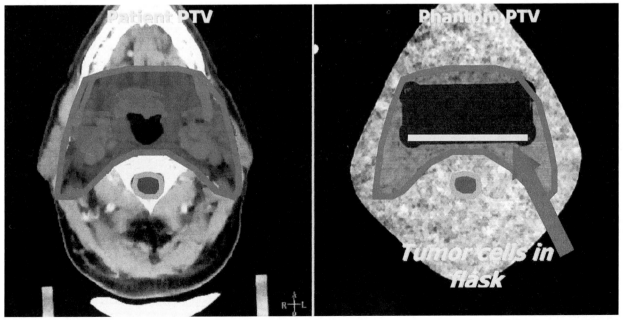

FIGURE 18.9-5. Planning target volume (PTV) and avoidance structures from an actual patient intensity-modulated radiation therapy plan (A) and the one represented by the phantom (B). The phantom and patient images were fused together to allow realistic structures to be used in generating the phantom plan. The tumor cell monolayer is denoted in the figure. (To view a color version of this image, please refer to the CD-ROM.)

treatment). The 40-minute delivery was achieved by allowing a 4- to 5-minute break between each gantry angle. All plans were delivered over 5 days on a Varian 2100 CD linear accelerator (Varian Medical Systems). Seven days after the last fractionated treatment, a clonogenic assay was performed.

In our preliminary experiments, only the opposed lateral and "slow" IMRT techniques were evaluated.[38] As shown in Figure 18.9-6, cell survival following 5 consecutive days of irradiation using the opposed lateral technique resulted in a surviving fraction of 33%. However, when the same dose was delivered using a seven-field IMRT plan that was protracted over 40 minutes (delivered over 5 days), the surviving fraction was 41%. Thus, in this case, dose protraction of 40 minutes resulted in a 24% increase in cell survival ($p < .02$ Mann-Whitney rank sum test). These preliminary data thus provide experimental evidence that increased treatment times adversely impact the biologic efficacy of fractionated IMRT. Further experiments are planned evaluating the effects of prolonged treatment times for a variety of disease sites and cell lines.

The data from these experiments may be used to refine models and develop future strategies for overcoming the effects of prolonged treatment times. For example, in Table 18.9-1, modeling studies for the same cell line predicted a 9.2% increase in cell survival as treatment is protracted to

40 minutes over 5 fractions. However, the preliminary experiments showed a larger increase in cell survival. These differences in theory and experiment suggest that the repair half-life for this cell line may be significantly shorter than the 20 minutes used in these calculations. Furthermore, the modeling studies did not take into account the "shielding" that portions of the flask receive at different gantry angles owing to the IMRT planning constraints. Refinements to the model, based on experimental data, may be used to determine the additional dose that is required to compensate for prolonged treatment (equation 4). Additionally, these models may be used to determine the maximum acceptable treatment time, from a biologic viewpoint, and therefore guide manufacturers in developing the next generation of IMRT planning and delivery systems.

Summary and Future Directions

IMRT represents a broad range of hardware and software technologies that usually result in protracted dose delivery. Despite widespread adoption of IMRT clinically, little attention has been drawn to the potential decrease in tumor cell killing that some IMRT delivery techniques and plans may produce. IMRT plans that protract treatment times beyond 20 minutes may significantly decrease tumor cell killing, especially in the fractionated therapy setting. Further experimental data are essential to (1) determine the length of time an IMRT plan may be delivered to maximize tumor cell killing, (2) optimize beam arrangement both spatially and temporally to minimize the "beam-off" time, and (3) determine whether the different IMRT treatment regimens and their effects can be monitored by examining DNA repair induction. Although IMRT has demonstrated initial promise in many malignancies through decreased normal tissue toxicity, long-term follow-up of these patients is essential given the radiobiologic concerns outlined here. Clinical studies should clearly report the type of hardware, software, and treatment time so that failure analysis can be done with respect to these factors.

Acknowledgment

This work was partially supported by a grant from Varian Medical Systems.

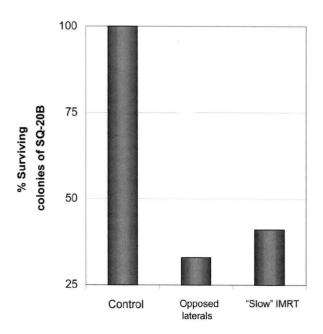

FIGURE 18.9-6. Clonogenic assay employing the intensity-modulated radiation therapy (IMRT) phantom with SQ-20B head and neck cells to simulate opposed lateral treatment and protracted IMRT ("slow") treatment. The IMRT plan (seven fields) was protracted to a delivery time of 40 minutes. Five fractions of 180 cGy were delivered over 5 consecutive days. Over 2,000 colonies were scored for each point. The results are presented as a percentage of colonies counted after 7 days of incubation at 37°C normalized to the plating efficiency of 45%.

References

1. Ozyigit G, Yang T, Chao KS. Intensity modulated radiation therapy for head and neck cancer. Curr Treat Options Oncol 2004;5:3–9.
2. Penagaricano JA, Papanikolaou N. Intensity modulated radiotherapy for carcinoma of the head and neck. Curr Oncol Rep 2003;5:131–9.
3. Hunt MA, Zelefsky MJ, Wolden S, et al. Treatment planning and delivery of intensity-modulated radiation therapy for primary nasopharynx cancer. Int J Radiat Oncol Biol Phys 2001;49:623–32.

4. Claus F, De Gershem W, De Wagter C, et al. An implementation strategy for IMRT of ethmoid sinus cancer with bilateral sparing of the optic pathways. Int J Radiat Oncol Biol Phys 2001;51:318–31.

5. Xia P, Fu KK, Wong GW. Comparison of treatment plans involving intensity-modulated radiotherapy for nasopharyngeal carcinoma. Int J Radiat Oncol Biol Phys 2000;48:329–37.

6. Butler EB, Teh BS, Grant WH, et al. SMART (simultaneous modulated accelerated radiation therapy) boost: a new accelerated fractionation schedule for the treatment of head and neck cancer with intensity modulated radiotherapy. Int J Radiat Oncol Biol Phys 1999;45:21–32.

7. Mohan R, Wu Q, Manning M, et al. Radiobiological considerations in the design of fractionation strategies for intensity-modulated radiation therapy of head and neck cancers. Int J Radiat Oncol Biol Phys 2000;46:619–30.

8. Chao KS, Deasy JO, Markman J, et al. A prospective study of salivary function sparing in patients with head-and-neck cancers receiving intensity-modulated or three-dimensional radiation therapy: initial results. Int J Radiat Oncol Biol Phys 2001;49:907–16.

9. Dawson LA, Anzai Y, Marshi L, et al. Patterns of local-regional recurrence following parotid-sparing conformal and segmental intensity-modulated radiotherapy for head and neck cancer. Int J Radiat Oncol Biol Phys 2000;46:1117–26.

10. Lee N, Xia P, Quivey JM, et al. Intensity-modulated radiotherapy in the treatment of nasopharyngeal carcinoma: an update of the UCSF experience. Int J Radiat Oncol Biol Phys 2002;53:12–22.

11. Gregoire V, Levendag P, Ang KK, et al. CT-based delineation of lymph node levels and related CTVs in the node-negative neck: DAHANCA, EORTC, GORTEC, NCIC, RTOG consensus guidelines. Radiother Oncol 2003;69:227–36.

12. Chao KS, Wippold FJ, Ozyigit G, et al. Determination and delineation of nodal target volumes for head-and-neck cancer based on patterns of failure in patients receiving definitive and postoperative IMRT. Int J Radiat Oncol Biol Phys 2002;53:1174–84.

13. Wang JZ, Li XA, D'Souza WD, et al. Impact of prolonged fraction delivery times on tumor control: a note of caution for intensity-modulated radiation therapy (IMRT). Int J Radiat Oncol Biol Phys 2003;57:543–52.

14. Xing L, Chen GTY. Iterative algorithms for inverse treatment planning. Phys Med Biol 1996;41:2107–23.

15. Webb S. Optimization by simulated annealing algorithms for three-dimensional conformal treatment planning for radiation fields defined with a multileaf collimator. Phys Med Biol 1991;36:1201–26.

16. Ping X, Verhey LJ. Multileaf collimator leaf sequencing algorithm for intensity modulated beams with multiple static segments. Med Phys 1998;25:1424–34.

17. Spirou SV, Chui CS. Generation of arbitrary modulated fields by dynamic collimation. Phys Med Biol 2001;46:2457–65.

18. Ping X, Verhey LJ. Delivery systems of intensity-modulated radiotherapy using conventional multileaf collimators. Med Dosim 2001;26:169–77.

19. Price RA, Murphy S, McNeeley SW, et al. A method for increased dose conformity and segment reduction for SMLC delivered IMRT treatments of the prostate. Int J Radiat Oncol Biol Phys 2003;57:843–52.

20. Chmura S J, Gupta N, Advani S J, et al. Prospects for viral-based strategies enhancing the anti-tumor effects of ionizing radiation. Semin Radiat Oncol 2001;11:338–45.

21. Meyn RE, Stephens LC, Milas L. Programmed cell death and radioresistance. Cancer Metastasis Rev 1996;15:119–31.

22. Rogakou EP, Pilch DR, Orr AH, et al. DNA double-stranded breaks induce histone H2AX phosphorylation on serine 139. J Biol Chem 1998;273:5858–68.

23. Smerdon MJ, Conconi A. Modulation of DNA damage and DNA repair in chromatin. Prog Nucleic Acid Res Mol Biol 1999;62:227–55.

24. Taneja N, Davis M, Choy JS, et al. Histone H2AX phosphorylation as a predictor of radiosensitivity and target for radiotherapy. J Biol Chem 2004;279:2273–80.

25. Emery E, Denekamp J, Ball M. Survival of mouse skin epithelial cells following single and divided doses of x-rays. Radiat Res 1970;41:450–66.

26. Amdur RJ, Bedford JS. Dose-rate effects between 0.3 and 30 Gy/h in a normal and malignant human cell line. Int J Radiat Oncol Biol Phys 1994;30:83–90.

27. Mothersill C, Cusak A, MacDonnell M, et al. Differential response of normal and tumour oesophageal explant cultures to radiation. Acta Oncol 1988;27:275–80.

28. Bedford J, Mitchell J. Dose rate effects in synchronous mammalian cells in culture. Radiat Res 1973;54:316–27.

29. Benedict SH, Lin PS, Zwicker RD, et al. The biological effectiveness of intermittent irradiation as a function of overall treatment time: development of correction factors for linac-based stereotactic radiosurgery. Int J Radiat Oncol Biol Phys 1997;37:765–9.

30. Morgan WF, Naqvi SA, Yu C, et al. Does the time required to deliver IMRT reduce its biological effectiveness [abstract]? Int J Radiat Oncol Biol Phys 2002;54:222.

31. Thames HD. An incomplete-repair model for survival after fractionated and continuous irradiations. Int J Radiat Oncol Biol Phys 1985;47:319–39.

32. Dale RG. The application of the linear-quadratic dose-effect equation to fractionated and protracted radiotherapy. Br J Radiol 1985;58:515–28.

33. Dale RG. Radiobiological assessment of permanent implants using tumor repopulation factors in the linear-quadratic model. Br J Radiol 1989;62:241–4.

34. Fowler JF, Welsh JS, Howard SP. Loss of biological effect in prolonged fraction delivery. Int J Radiat Oncol Biol Phys 2004;9:242–9.

35. Roeske JC, Chmura SJ. Biological impact of prolonged treatment times during intensity modulated radiation therapy (IMRT). Presented at the 51st Annual Meeting of the Radiation Research Society; April 24-27, 2004, St. Louis, MO.

36. Weichselbaum RR, Rotmensch J, Ahmed-Swan S, et al. Radiobiological characterization of 53 human tumor cells. Int J Radiat Oncol Biol Phys 1988;15:575–9.

37. Belli M. Bettega D, Calzolari P, et al. Inactivation of human normal and tumour cells irradiated with low energy protons. Int J Radiat Biol 2000;76:831–9.

38. Chmura SJ, Salama J, Roeske JC. Does the dose protraction inherent to IMRT decrease tumor cell killing in vitro [abstract]? Presented at the 46th Annual Meeting of the Society for Therapeutic Radiology and Oncology; October 3-7, 2004, Atlanta, GA.

Chapter 19

LUNG CANCER OVERVIEW

CRAIG W. STEVENS, MD, PhD, THOMAS GUERRERO, MD, PhD, KENNETH M. FORSTER, PhD, GEORGE STARKSCHALL, PhD, REGINALD MUNDEN, MD

More than 60% of patients with lung cancer will receive radiation therapy (RT) at some point during the course of their disease, 45% for initial treatment and 17% for palliation.[1] About 170,000 patients will develop lung cancer this year in the United States alone,[2] resulting in over 100,000 patients undergoing RT. It is therefore critical that the best of new technologies are aggressively implemented because, with such large numbers, even small advances can improve the lives of many patients.

RT approaches in lung cancer are rapidly evolving. The ability to define target volumes and avoid normal structures has been aided by advancements in computed tomography (CT) technology and in ^{18}F-labeled fluorodeoxyglucose ([18]FDG) positron emission tomography (PET) ([18]FDG-PET) scanning. It is also now possible to measure and account for individual variations in respiratory tumor motion and to replan periodically during treatment accounting for changes in tumor motion. Treatment planning algorithms can also now account for tissue inhomogeneity, which can improve dose distributions to target volumes, the choice of beam energies, and beam weighting. Lung cancer treatment has changed to using the International Commission on Radiation Units and Measurements (ICRU) Report 62 definitions of volumes and doses so that true three-dimensional conformal radiation therapy (3DCRT) is routinely achieved.

Increasing interest has been focused recently on the application of intensity-modulated radiation therapy (IMRT) techniques in the treatment of lung cancer. This is not surprising because IMRT has been shown to increase dose conformity and reduce normal tissue sparing in a number of disease sites. In fact, preliminary dosimetric studies evaluating IMRT in lung cancer have been promising. However, serious concerns remain regarding the application of IMRT in these patients, precluding its routine use at the present time.

The purpose of this chapter is to provide a review of the important concepts and issues in the radiotherapeutic management of patients with lung cancer, including anatomy, imaging, target design, and organ motion. An understanding of such concepts and issues is critical not only for the optimal delivery of 3DCRT but for the eventual incorporation of IMRT. In addition, concerns regarding the application of IMRT in patients with lung cancer and the available published IMRT literature in this setting are reviewed. Finally, the use of IMRT in patients with mesothelioma is discussed.

Technical Considerations
Normal Thoracic Anatomy

Correctly delineating the tumor in a patient with lung cancer requires an understanding of normal anatomy. Several excellent CT atlases are available for more detailed study,[3] and at least one should be available for review while contouring. Representative noncontrast CT slices are shown in Figure 19-1, displayed from superior to inferior. Note that the superior mediastinum has only five structures: the right and left brachiocephalic veins, right brachiocephalic artery, left common carotid artery, and left subclavian artery. Superior mediastinal images with more than five structures are suggestive of enlarged lymph nodes, although these may or may not be involved with malignancy. Suspicious structures should be evaluated for fluid content to exclude pericardial fluid in a recess[4] and also traced from slice to slice to determine if the structure is a vascular variant. Those failing to join identifiable vessels should be considered enlarged lymph nodes.

Normally, there should be no structures between the superior vena cava (see panels C, D, and E in Figure 19-1) and the trachea, but several small lymph nodes can be seen in this case. Note that lymphadenopathy would be extremely difficult to discern among the hilar structures (see panels G, H, and I in Figure 19-1).

Treatment Planning CT

After obtaining informed consent, patients with lung cancer are set up at our institution in the supine position using a Vac-Lok hemibody cast (MED-TEC, Orange City, IA),

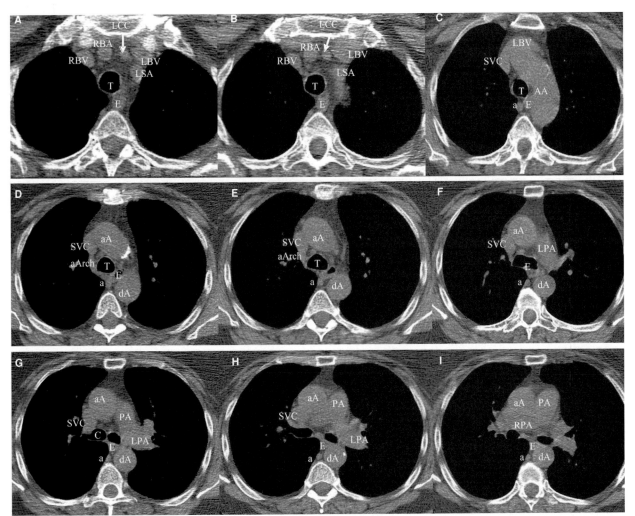

FIGURE 19-1. Normal patient anatomy illustrated on a computed tomography (CT) scan. Multiple CT slices from one patient are shown from superior (*A*) to inferior (*I*). a = azygos vein; aA = ascending aorta; AA = aortic arch; aArch = azygos arch; C = carina; dA = descending aorta; E = esophagus; LBV = left brachiocephalic vein; LCC = left common carotid artery; LPA = left pulmonary artery; LSA = left subclavian artery; PA = main pulmonary artery; RBA = right brachiocephalic artery; RBV = right brachiocephalic vein; RPA = right pulmonary artery; SVC = superior vena cava; T = trachea.

wing board, and T-bar. This technique was chosen because it reduced setup uncertainty (see below). Treatment planning CT scans typically are obtained with a 3 mm slice thickness from the low neck to the bottom of the liver. This slice thickness results in high-quality digitally reconstructed radiographs, which simplifies portal image verification. Scanning over this large volume ensures that the entire lung and heart are included within the treatment planning scan, so that dose-volume histogram (DVH) analysis will be meaningful.

Intravenous contrast has been used in our department only in selected patients with lung cancer (Figure 19-2). In our experience, contrast aids in the delineation of hilar and, occasionally, mediastinal lymph nodes. Both hilar and mediastinal lymph node metastases can be easily visualized with PET/CT, and this has supplanted our use of contrast. However, if PET/CT scanning is not available, then intravenous contrast-enhanced planning CTs can be useful. The

procedure for the use of contrast initially involved the training of therapists, nurses, and physicians regarding the management of contrast reactions. Although the risk of reaction is low for nonionic contrast, it is not zero. Clinical parameters for safe contrast administration should be cleared with one's radiology department, as should the procedure for management of contrast reactions.

A noncontrast study should be obtained first. Contrast is then infused according to a schema used by our diagnostic radiology group, and the contrast-enhanced CT scan is obtained. Contours are then drawn on the contrast study and transferred to the noncontrast study for treatment planning. This is important because planning should be done with heterogeneity corrections. The presence of intravenous contrast can result in dosimetric errors of 2 to 5% in regions (such as the aortopulmonary window) that are surrounded by vessels containing contrast. The use of intravenous contrast is becoming less common with the integration of PET scanning in our practice; however, it can be very useful for identifying hilar adenopathy (see the arrows in Figure 19-2). Intravenous contrast is most useful when hilar tumor volumes are small or the PET scan is negative (as is often the case for bronchoalveolar cancers).

We have actively involved our diagnostic imaging physicians in the calibration of our CT simulators and treatment planning workstations to ensure that the lung and mediastinal settings are similar in our departments and across all platforms. This makes it somewhat easier to compare diagnostic and treatment planning studies. We perform monthly calibrations of every monitor with access to our CT simulator data sets to comply with a Society of Motion Picture and Television Engineers (SMPTE) test pattern. This ensures that the programmed window or level will be displayed in an identical way on each monitor.

18FDG-PET

PET is another imaging modality that is a very important guide for RT treatment planning.[5,6] This is true both for staging and target delineation. First, because PET scans

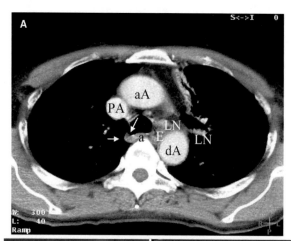

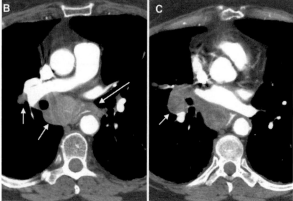

FIGURE 19-2. Effect of intravenous contrast on anatomic definition. In A, the lymph nodes (LN) are easily seen in the aortopulmonary (AP) window and also lateral to the azygos vein (a) (*arrows*). In B and C, the LNs (*arrows*) can be easily identified in the hila and mediastinum. aA = ascending aorta; dA = descending aorta; E = esophagus.

detect distant metastases in about 30% of patients with non-small lung cancer (NSCLC) (particularly those with an otherwise advanced disease), it can significantly help with patient triage.[7] Because of this, PET staging has a measurable impact on survival. [8] One caveat is that PET will make it difficult to compare the results of PET-staged patients with those of earlier studies because of significant stage migration. Investigators at the Peter MacCallum Cancer Institute compared the survival of patients treated on two similar protocols, one of which required PET scanning, whereas the other was performed before PET scanning was available.[9] The median survival of PET-staged patients was 31 months compared with 16 months for patients undergoing conventional staging.

However, the true value of PET/CT may lie in radiotherapy target delineation. In one study, the use of PET scans altered the target volumes in 11 of 11 cases, with 7 volumes increased and 4 decreased.[8] It can reduce interobserver differences in gross tumor volume (GTV) contouring.[10] It can also help categorize suspicious mediastinal and hilar lymph node adenopathy as either benign or malignant, with higher standard uptake values being predictive of metastatic disease. Moreover, it can aid in the identification of tumor within an atelectatic lobe and thereby decrease the amount of normal lung irradiated. It is not clear, however, what impact PET will have on patterns of failure.

Techniques for integrating PET scans into RT treatment planning are currently being developed. Several important technical points should be made. First, it is desirable to minimize the time between PET and the planning CT scan, lessening potential changes in tumor size or lung collapse that may render image registration difficult. Second, whenever possible, PET scans should be performed on flat tables with patients immobilized in the treatment position, minimizing systematic errors in soft tissue location (eg, the carina can move > 2 cm by changing the arm position). Moreover, it is important to note that the internal diameter of PET gantries (~ 50 cm) is usually smaller than that of the gantries of most CT simulators (~ 70 cm). It may thus be necessary to confirm the physical size of all patient immobilization devices prior to simulation, ensuring clearance through the PET gantry. Third, PET and CT images should be registered using both surface fiducial markers and the spine. This practice reduces registration error. Fortunately, most of these technical issues will be resolved when dedicated PET-CT units become more widely available.

An example case is illustrated in Figure 19-3. In this patient, a PET scan was obtained as part of the initial staging workup (see Figure 19-3A) and then registered with the treatment planning CT scan. It was assumed that the differences in tumor shape were due to motion artifacts between the PET (which is acquired over several minutes) and the CT (in which a slice is acquired over ~ 1 second). For unrelated medical reasons, the patient could not start treatment as scheduled. When the patient was ready to begin, a repeat simulation

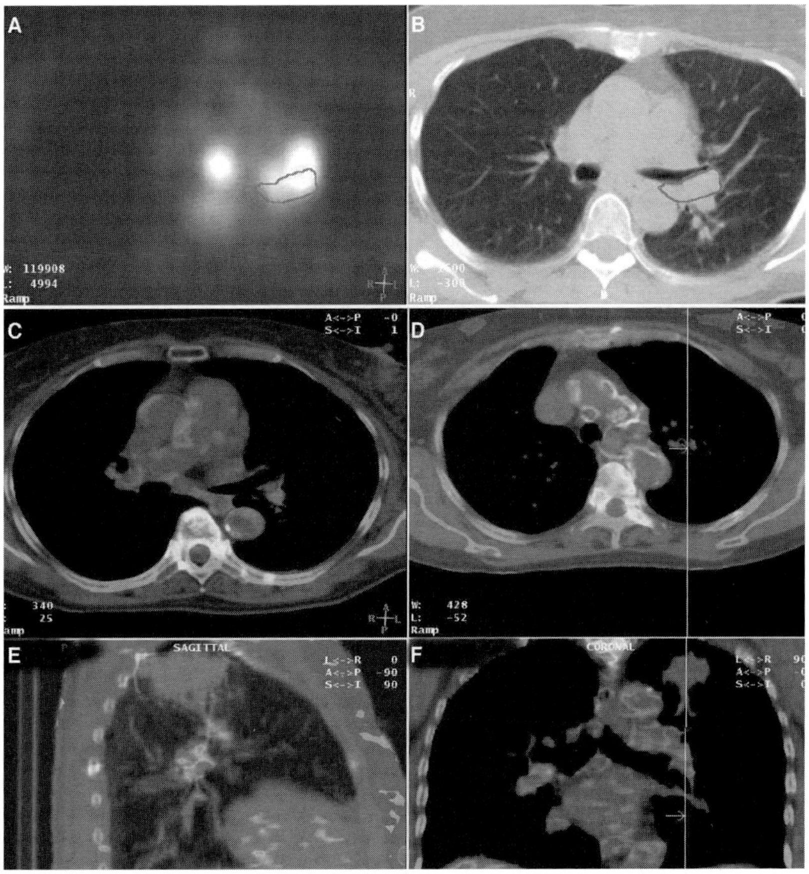

FIGURE 19-3. The importance of image registration in multimodality imaging. A fluorodeoxyglucose (FDG)–positron emission tomography (PET) scan was obtained for staging (*A*), followed by a treatment planning computed tomography (CT) (*B*). It was assumed that the difference between the red contours between modalities was due to tumor motion. The patient's treatment was delayed, and a repeat PET-CT (on a dedicated unit) was performed for staging and planning (*C–F*), with the PET image in overlapping color on the CT. The FDG-avid regions (*red*) overlap perfectly with the CT image, suggesting that soft tissue registration of the initial studies was flawed. Note that the spiculations are not particularly FDG-avid, although they may contain tumor cells (*E*). (To view a color version of this image, please refer to the CD-ROM.)

was performed on a dedicated PET-CT unit. Panels C to F in Figure 19-3 demonstrate excellent concordance between the CT and PET findings. In retrospect, our sequence of PET followed by CT probably represents misregistration caused by changes in arm position (because the patient was not immobilized for the PET scan). Note also that the spiculations seen easily on CT are not very ^{18}FDG-avid. Given that spiculations contain relatively few tumor cells per cubic centimeter, it is likely that the PET scan is falsely negative in this region. Contouring on the registered image sets can also be challenging. PET scanning is very poor at delineating tumor edges, particularly in areas of spiculation, because the number of tumor cells per voxel may be rather low. Also, the time course of the PET scan (~ 5 minutes per couch position) is long relative to CT scanning (1 second or less per slice). This causes a poorly characterized blurring of the edges along the axis of motion. Because of these edge effects, it is best to contour suspected mediastinal and hilar lymph nodes using CT (with reference to the contrast-enhanced scans) and use the PET image data to confirm or reject nodal involvement. PET scanning is rarely useful for contouring of the primary tumor but can sometimes identify hilar tumors in the setting of lobar and lung atelectasis (Figure 19-4). In this setting, the GTV should

be generously estimated because the edge cannot be identified unequivocally. As shown in Figure 19-4, the lung spared by this approach is most likely to be within the uninvolved adjacent lobe (denoted by arrows in the figure), not the involved lobe.

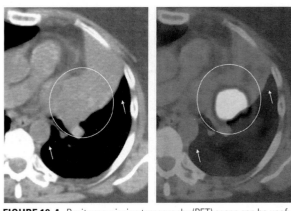

FIGURE 19-4. Positron emission tomography (PET) scans can be useful in identifying tumor within an atelectatic lung. The tumor has obstructed the upper lobe. PET helps identify the tumor so that additional normal lung can be spared (*arrow*). (To view a color version of this image, please refer to the CD-ROM.)

Defining Target Volumes
Treatment Volumes for Lung Cancer

Several target volumes are delineated in the modern treatment of lung cancer. The GTV represents all tumor that is visible on imaging studies. The clinical target volume (CTV) is the volume likely to contain microscopic disease. The planning target volume (PTV) includes the CTV with a margin accounting for daily setup error and target motion. An additional volume, the internal target volume (ITV), was defined in ICRU Report 62 and is an expansion of the CTV in which target motion is explicitly measured and taken into account. The final PTV is then formed by adding a setup margin (accounting for daily setup variations) to the ITV.

Gross Tumor Volume

Delineation of the GTV in patients with lung cancer is controversial. Radiologists and radiation oncologists define

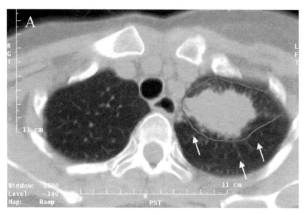

Lung Window
(W1000/L-300)

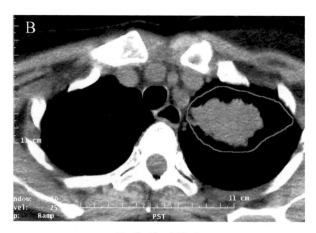

Mediastinal Window
(W340/L25)

FIGURE 19-5. Proper window and level settings help to identify tumor edges. Window and level settings were developed with assistance from our diagnostic imaging group. Using these presets, pulmonary windows (*A*) show tumor spiculations that are not seen on mediastinal windows (*B*). Spiculations do not branch, unlike blood vessels (*arrows*).

GTVs somewhat differently, suggesting that radiation oncologists must be well trained in imaging.[11] The pulmonary extent of lung tumors must be delineated on pulmonary windows, and their mediastinal extent must be delineated using mediastinal windows. Improper windowing or leveling may result in GTVs that vary by several centimeters (Figure 19-5). All treatment planning CT scans should be reviewed using both pulmonary (to determine the extent of the tumor within the lung) and mediastinal windows or levels (to determine any soft tissue invasion). Figure 19-6 demonstrates the need for this approach. The extension of tumor into the chest wall was not apparent on the pulmonary windows (see panels A and C in Figure 19-6), and the spiculations were not apparent on the mediastinal windows (see panels B and D in Figure 19-6).

Another important issue involves the contouring of spiculations. Figure 19-7 illustrates three tumors with different levels of spiculations but similar core sizes. Failure to contour spiculations would have little impact on the contours in Figure 19-7A but a significant impact on the others. Data from the 1970s suggest that spiculations contain tumor cells more often with adenocarcinomas than with squamous carcinomas. Our policy is to assume that all spiculations contain tumor. By

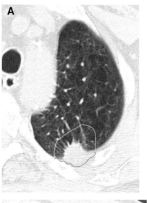
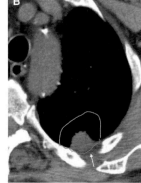
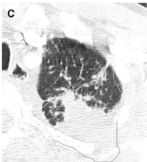
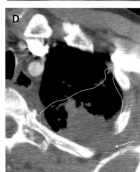

FIGURE 19-6. Window and level settings are important to determine chest wall invasion. The pulmonary extent of tumor (*yellow contours*) was drawn using pulmonary settings, and the chest wall invasion was delineated using mediastinal settings (*blue contours*). Note that both were needed to accurately define tumor edges. In the second case (*C* and *D*), there is significant tumor infiltration of the lobe (however, it does not cross the interlobar fissure). Again, the chest wall extent is appreciated only on the mediastinal windows (*arrow*).

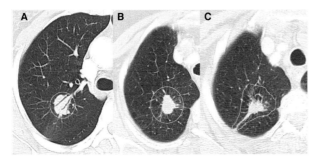

FIGURE 19-7. Tumors with similar solid components can have very different gross tumor volumes. Each of these tumors has a solid component that measures about 2 cm. However, the size and density of the spiculations can vary dramatically. Note that the contoured spiculations do not branch.

definition, these are considered GTV and are treated to the full dose. It is important to differentiate spiculations (which do not branch) from branching vessels (see Figure 19-5A, arrows), and this can sometimes be easier with a contrast-enhanced scan.

Clinical Target Volume

It has historically been difficult to determine the extent of microscopic disease in patients with lung cancer, both adjacent to the primary GTV and in the mediastinum. A radiographic-histopathologic comparison of lung tumor size was recently reported.[12] This study demonstrated that including the tumor within the CTV with 95% accuracy required GTV-to-CTV expansions of 6 mm for squamous cancers and 8 mm for adenocarcinomas. Expansions for other histologies have not been determined, but our approach has been to use 8 mm. Generally, CTVs should not extend beyond anatomic boundaries unless there is evidence of invasion. For example, CTVs should not extend across interlobar fissures, into the chest wall, or into the mediastinum without documented evidence of invasion.

Appropriate CTVs for mediastinal lymph nodes have not been rigorously determined. At our center, we empirically use 8 to 10 mm expansions around involved mediastinal and hilar lymph nodes (either gross involvement or PET positive). Obviously, these expansions should not necessarily be uniformly applied along all axes. CTV expansions of lymph node disease should not extend into the major airways, vessels, or lung. When using ITVs (see below), CTV editing should be done for each CTV on each CT scan.

Internal Target Volume

Fluoroscopy has traditionally been used to assess tumor motion and adjust target volumes. However, two-dimensional measurement of tumor motion, such as might be done by fluoroscopy, is inadequate. Fluoroscopic detection of anterior-posterior tumor motion is often quite poor owing to the superposition of the mediastinal structures.

We had also hoped that two-dimensional tumor motion might be predictable but found that it is not.[13]

To better understand lung tumor motion in three dimensions, we recently studied respiratory-driven lung tumor motion in 25 patients. All had pathologically proven lung cancer, were able to be trained to use the spirometer, and had a planned treatment course of at least 6 weeks. Patients with more than segmental atelectasis were excluded. A SensorMedics Vmax22 computer-controlled occlusion spirometer (SensorMedics, Yorba Linda, CA) and a Marconi PQ 5000 CT scanner (Philips Medical Systems, Andover, MA) were employed. Pulmonary function tests were performed primarily to assess the vital capacity of the patients. Patients held their breath for 15 to 20 seconds. CT images over the entire lung volume were acquired at 100% tidal volume (normal inspiration) and at 0% tidal volume (end expiration). For each CT data set, the GTV was contoured and reviewed by two physicians. All CT image sets were registered, using the vertebral bodies, to the treatment planning CT for the assessment of tumor motion.

Figure 19-8 demonstrates that lung motion is not uniform. For this example, the diaphragm moved anteriorly and inferiorly with inspiration, whereas the anterior chest wall moved slightly anteriorly. The carina can also move, in this case, anteriorly and slightly inferiorly. The mediastinum generally narrows with inspiration, and the heart rotates. In this example, the upper lobe lung tumor moved about 6 mm anteriorly as well.

The geometric tumor center was determined on the inspiration and expiration CT, and the displacement was measured. Figure 19-8B shows that under normal respiration, only 8 of the 25 patients had tumors that moved 3 to 5 mm, and no lesions moved less than 3 mm. The mean tumor displacement was 9.3 mm, and the standard deviation was 4.3 mm. Most of the observed motion was in the superior-inferior and anterior-posterior directions, whereas medial-lateral motion was smaller in magnitude. The mean magnitudes of motion for lower lobe and upper lobe lesions were 12.5 and 7.8 mm, respectively. However, the standard deviation was quite large (30–50%). GTV, T stage, and tumor location (upper vs lower, free vs fixed) were not correlated with motion direction or magnitude. Tumors adjacent to the mediastinum tended to move medially with inspiration (consistent with the motion of the mediastinum), but, again, the standard deviations were large. These results suggest that the direction and magnitude of lung tumor motion cannot be predicted with sufficient reliability.

Using these data, we evaluated whether "standard" margins could be constructed to account for tumor motion. Tumors were contoured on the free-breathing treatment planning CT scans. The GTV-to-CTV expansion was 8 mm, and a 7 mm margin was added for setup uncertainty. If this volume was then expanded uniformly by 5 mm, both the inspiration and the expiration target volumes were within the free-breathing PTV in only 10 of 25 cases (40%). If this volume was expanded by 10 mm, only 20 cases (80%) were adequately covered. Thus, the total expansion around the GTV would be 25 mm (8 mm CTV + 7 mm setup uncertainty + 10 mm tumor motion). Based on this analysis, we concluded that tumor motion should be measured in each patient and the margins individualized.

A motion study was also repeated at the end of treatment in 10 patients with lung cancer. Tumor motion changed significantly over the course of treatment, with both the direction and the magnitude of tumor motion changing in all

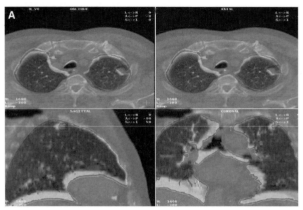

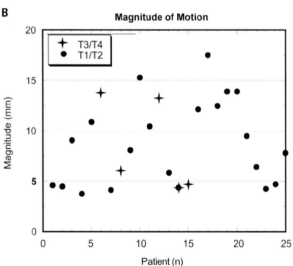

FIGURE 19-8. Lung tumor motion is complex and unpredictable. In *A*, inspiration and expiration computed tomography (CT) scans were obtained using spirometry-assisted breath-holds. The inspiration CT is in color, whereas the expiration CT is in black and white. (To view the color version of this image, please refer to the CD-ROM.) This tumor fixed to the chest wall in the upper lobe moved more than 1 cm anterior-posterior. The mediastinum moved medially, the carina moved inferiorly, the hila rotated, and the diaphragm moved inferiorly and posteriorly with inspiration. Using this technique, we measured tumor motion in 25 patients with unresectable lung cancer. No patients had significant atelectasis. Tumor motion (*B*) ranged from 3 to 17 mm and was not predictable by tumor size, stage, or location or pulmonary function. Also, two-dimensional superior-inferior motion (eg, fluoroscopically visible motion) did not predict motion along the other axes.

cases. Some tumors moved more, some moved less, and some changed direction! In two cases, the final ITV was outside the initial ITV by more than 1 cm, although the others were adequately covered. It was noted by spirometry that the amplitude and frequency of respiration changed with treatment, which was not surprising considering that the vital capacity could change by as much as 35%. The magnitude of motion change was surprising because no patient had large amounts of lung collapse at presentation. These data suggest that three-dimensional tumor motion should be assessed in each patient and probably several times during treatment.

Based on these studies, the application of a uniform margin to account for motion seems inappropriate because the tumor motion for our patients appears to be mainly in two directions. Following the guidelines of ICRU Report 62, we attempted to explicitly account for the tumor motion. The ITV represents the volume occupied by the CTV during normal quiet respiration. To determine this volume, CT image data sets at normal expiration (0% tidal volume) and at normal inspiration (100% tidal volume), as well as quiet-breathing image sets, need to be acquired. The GTV is delineated on each CT image and expanded to form the CTV. Finally, the two breath-hold data sets are registered to the quiet respiration data set, and the envelope of the three CTVs represents the ITV.

As can be seen in Figure 19-9 (and as previously discussed), lung tumors can move significantly, and often the motion is along the anterior-posterior direction and along the superior-inferior axis. CT images were obtained in the treatment position during inspiration and expiration, and the images were registered. Figure 19-9A demonstrates the expansion that would be used to take motion into account if only the anterior-posterior view had been used (as would be typical with fluoroscopy). Had this been done, the tumor would have been outside the target volume for part of the treatment, which would have resulted in significant underdosing. If tumor motion were measured in three dimensions, as shown in Figure 19-9B, the tumor would be properly irradiated. This technique also aids in the selection of beam angles because beam angles parallel to the axis of motion will usually irradiate less normal tissue. In this example, lateral fields or very oblique fields should be avoided.

Our experience with three-dimensional measurement of lung tumor motion suggests that about one-third of lung tumors move less than 0.5 cm with respiration. For this third of patients, simple expansion along the axis motion is adequate. For the remaining patients, the treatment machine can be gated with respiration, the patient can use an assisted breath-hold technique, or an ITV-based approach can be used.

A commercially available system can be used to gate the linear accelerator.[14] This technique uses an externally placed fiducial marker, which is tracked as the patient breathes.

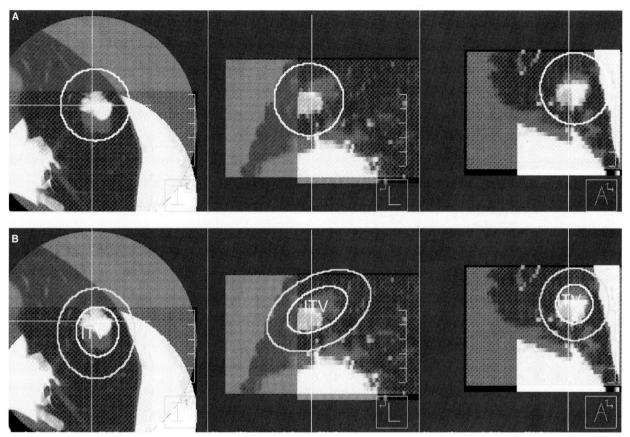

FIGURE 19-9. Constructing internal target volumes (ITVs). Computed tomography scans were obtained at inspiration (*yellow*) and expiration (*black and white*). The scans were subsequently registered. If margins had been decided based on the superior-inferior motion (*A*), the tumor would have been very close to the posterior-superior edge of the field. However, if an ITV had been constructed based on the measured tumor motion, the target volume would have expanded along the axis of motion. (To view a color version of this image, please refer to the CD-ROM.)

The beam can be triggered at a chosen point in the respiratory cycle, typically end-expiration because this is the longest, most reproducible portion of the cycle. Use of this gating system requires that patients be able to breathe slowly in a regular pattern.

Active breathing control[15] and deep inspiration breathhold[16] are two techniques that have been developed to help patients hold their breath at reproducible points in the respiratory cycle. These two techniques limit patient respiratory excursion to fixed volumes. The radiation beam is then initiated. Diaphragmatic excursion is limited to about 5 mm instead of 10 to 15 mm.[17] These techniques require very cooperative patients who are able to hold their breath for at least 15 seconds. Unfortunately, patients with poor pulmonary function (who would most benefit from reduction in irradiated lung volumes) are the very patients least able to comply with breath-holding techniques. Thus, the optimal method to temporally immobilize lung tumors remains unclear. Our feeling is that, until gating techniques are improved, an ITV-based approach offers the most reliable method of explicitly accounting for respiratory-dependent lung tumor motion.

Planning Target Volume

The PTV is designed to account for setup uncertainty (and motion if the ITV approach is not used). Because several respiratory cycles and associated motion typically occur during the treatment of a single fraction, the margin for motion and setup uncertainty should be combined linearly. Preliminary data at our institution have shown that when immobilizing patients with a Vac-Lok bag and T-bar, an expansion along all axes of 7 mm will account for 95% of the day-to-day setup uncertainty. Setup uncertainty is likely both technique dependent and institution dependent and should be measured individually for each technique and in each department.

Treatment Planning

Traditionally, RT treatment planning for thoracic tumors has assumed a homogeneous patient. In fact, the clinical trials using RT for lung cancer have almost all been based on dose planned in a homogeneous body.[18] Radiation Therapy Oncology Group (RTOG) protocols for thoracic tumors continue to require homogeneous treatment planning owing to fears of underdosing the primary tumor when correcting for heterogeneity and to allow comparisons with previous results. Nevertheless, the need for lung heterogeneity correction has been debated for some time,[19–21] and dose calculations taking into account the presence of heterogeneity have become commercially available.[21] Even though some studies have indicated that heterogeneity correction may result in isocenter doses 6 to 18% greater than those calculated without correction,[22] the use of heterogeneity corrections in treatment planning systems warrants serious consideration. However, it is important to note that any method incorporating heterogeneity correction factors make use of the clinical knowledge already gained from traditional homogeneous treatment planning.

To address this issue, we recently developed a heterogeneity-corrected dose-volume prescription method that allows prescription to an isodose that circumscribes and ensures coverage of at least 95% of the PTV. This prescription accounted for heterogeneity using a commercially available convolution-superposition algorithm. With the change in prescription technique using ICRU-defined parameters, there was concern that our technique might significantly affect the isocenter dose. Therefore, we studied the effect of this change on dose distributions and target volume coverage.[22]

Thirty patients with stage I and II NSCLC tumors were treated from 1998 to 2001 at our institution using heterogeneity-corrected plans. Treatment planning was performed using 6 MV beams in the clinically used geometries. Three treatment plans were generated for each case. The first treatment plan was generated using the traditional homogeneous point-dose method in which each prescription delivered a dose of 60 to 66 Gy to the isocenter. The dose distribution for this plan was recalculated using heterogeneity corrections while maintaining the same number of monitor units (MUs) per beam and wedges to more accurately reflect the actual clinical dose received. This second treatment plan incorporated heterogeneity corrections into the dose calculations while ensuring 95% coverage of the PTV. For the third technique (which is what is currently used in our clinic), beam weighting and MUs were allowed to vary so as to produce an acceptable plan.

Maximum CTV and PTV doses were not statistically different for these planning techniques, nor were the doses to the isocenter and the normal structures (lung, heart, esophagus, spinal cord) that are normally included in the evaluation of treatment plans. Total MUs delivered were indistinguishable between prescription techniques. However, accounting for heterogeneity significantly improved the PTV coverage compared with traditional homogeneous methods ($p = .05$). Most importantly, the dose prescribed by traditional treatment planning for 14 of 30 tumors covered less than 90% of the PTV when heterogeneity was taken

into account. Analysis of these 14 cases revealed no trends in tumor location, beam geometry, or target volume.

Figure 19-10 demonstrates a representative case. Figure 19-10A represents our initial plan using an isocenter-base prescription technique without heterogeneity corrections. When the MUs from this calculation are used to generate a dose distribution using heterogeneity corrections, there is actually slightly better target volume coverage (see Figure 19-10B). However, this distribution can be improved to cover 95% of the PTV by slightly adjusting the beam weighting (see Figure 19-10C). Of note, the MUs required are very similar. Review of the DVH demonstrates that the lung DVH is identical with all three techniques in the region from ~ 8 to 60 Gy. However, the dose to the PTV is much improved when the PTV dose is included as a planning constraint than when the dose is prescribed to the isocenter.

These data demonstrate that changing prescription techniques from the isocenter of a homogeneous target to 95% of the PTV does not significantly change the dose delivered to the isocenter but usually improves coverage of the PTV. It also reduced the use of higher-energy beams (especially for tumors surrounded by lung) because underdosing at the lung-tumor interface can result from the buildup of high-energy photons and electronic disequilibrium at the tumor surface. This results in a tumor-sparing effect similar to the skin-sparing effect produced by high-energy photons at the air-skin interface.[23] The prescription change has also slightly increased the distance from the PTV to the block edge (previously ~ 5 mm to now ~ 8–10 mm, particularly near the PTV edges that are surrounded by lung), but this can be individualized based on the calculated effect of tissue heterogeneity.

It is not yet known if this change in prescription technique will improve local control. However, we recently reviewed the outcome of 83 patients with stage I NSCLC treated at our institution and found that the only predictor of outcome was the margin from the GTV to the block edge. Tumor size, stage (Ia vs Ib), location, and dose were not predictive of local control (unpublished data). Although these patients were not planned using heterogeneity corrections, it is likely that larger margins resulted in better PTV coverage.

Intensity-Modulated Radiation Therapy

Technical Concerns

Compared with conventional techniques, IMRT improves conformity to the PTV and better avoids normal structures. Because the intensity distribution within each beam can be optimized according to the desired dose distribution, IMRT is more capable of delivering a higher dose to the target volume while sparing surrounding normal tissues. In principle, IMRT is clearly an appealing approach for

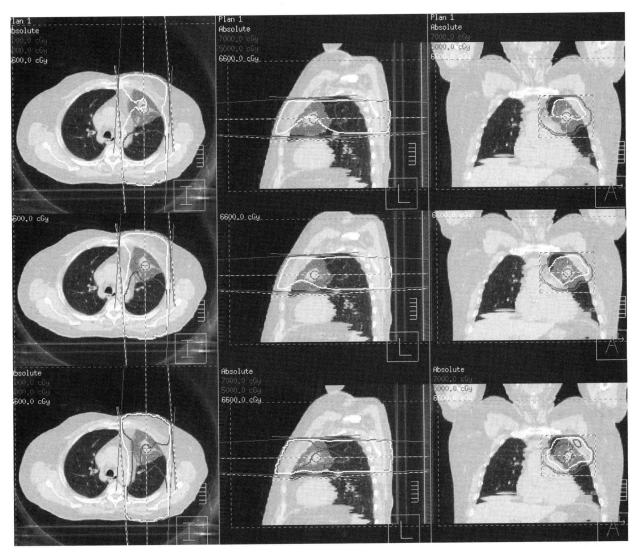

FIGURE 19-10. Heterogeneity corrections are important for accurately calculating the dose. In this example, the dose (66 Gy) was prescribed at the isocenter and the dose was calculated without accounting for tissue density heterogeneity (*A*). When the monitor units calculated for each beam from this plan are used to recalculate the dose using heterogeneity corrections (*B*), the dose is found to be slightly higher than originally calculated. Using the same beam geometry, it is possible to obtain a more homogeneous dose (with the high-dose region within the tumor) by setting an objective for 95% of the planning target volume to achieve the goal dose (*C*). (To view a color version of this image, please refer to the CD-ROM.)

patients with NSCLC, particularly those with locally advanced disease, who may benefit from dose escalation.

However, there are several technical reasons to delay the widespread use of IMRT for lung cancer at the present time. First is the issue of tumor motion. IMRT is not appropriate for mobile targets. Our recent data suggest that about two-thirds of lung tumors move more than 0.5 cm. Given that this motion cannot be predicted, it must be measured for each patient. Certainly, these motion issues will be averaged over many days; however, the day-to-day variation can be as much as 30% voxel by voxel. For very mobile tumors, even 3DCRT will tend to spread the dose into adjacent normal lung as it moves into and out of the radiation beam with respiration. Thus, IMRT may result in significant underdosing of tumor while irradiating additional volumes of lung. IMRT

plans are designed so that nonuniform dose distributions from various beam geometries add up appropriately to achieve a very conformal dose distribution. Because of the nature of the dynamic delivery of IMRT, it is not clear how the doses will add when the target is also moving.

Second, there is still some uncertainty about the algorithms used to calculate beamlet doses in very inhomogeneous structures,[24] although these problems can be minimized by the eventual use of Monte Carlo–based planning algorithms. The dose calculation algorithms used in most treatment planning systems are quite good at predicting the dose in heterogeneous structures (such as the lung) if the fields are large. However, as the field size decreases, there can be significant dose calculation errors. This is particularly problematic at tumor edges.

Third, IMRT achieves conformal high-dose regions by increasing volumes that receive relatively low doses. This may be a significant problem because the lung is so sensitive to radiation. Our experience suggests that when concurrent chemotherapy is used, the dose volume most predictive of lung injury is not the volume receiving 20 Gy (V_{20}) but the volume receiving 14 Gy. Thus, for lung IMRT to be safe, the dose-volume constraints of the lung must be better defined and validated. Dose-volume constraints may also need to be defined more as surfaces than as points (such as V_{20}). This is because 3DCRT uses a small number of beam geometries or weightings to achieve conformity. This means that the V_{20} is not independent (or the volume receiving 10 [V_{10}] or 30 Gy [V_{30}] or mean lung dose, all of which have been suggested as predictors of lung toxicity). With IMRT, the relationship between one part of the DVH and another is not so clear-cut because of the huge number of beamlets used to create a dose distribution.

Because of the above concerns, we have not yet implemented IMRT into widespread use in the clinic. We are particularly concerned about the lack of long-term clinical outcome data with IMRT. Careful, long-term follow-up of many patients treated with concurrent chemotherapy and IMRT will be needed to accurately determine toxicity profiles. Ideally, this will be done in prospective randomized trials.

Dosimetric (Planning) Studies

To explore the feasibility of IMRT in patients with lung cancer, we recently presented two dosimetric (planning) studies performed at M. D. Anderson Cancer Center. In our initial study, 3DCRT and IMRT planning were compared in a cohort of 10 previously treated patients with stage I to IIIb lung cancer.[25] Patients with a variety of tumor sizes and locations, nodal involvement, and number of primaries were selected. All had lesions with potentially a minimal degree of tumor motion caused by respiration based on an earlier in-house tumor motion study.[26] Compared with 3DCRT, IMRT was noted to have a higher degree of dose conformity. Moreover, IMRT was associated with significant reductions in the V_{20}, V_{30}, and mean lung dose. The integral thorax dose and the heterogeneity indices, however, were similar between the two approaches. Significant sparing of the heart and esophagus was achieved with IMRT planning. Of note, the degree of lung sparing was more pronounced with more advanced tumors, and the use of fewer beams in IMRT was associated with further reductions of the lung volume exposed to low radiation doses.

Based on these promising results, we extended our analysis to a larger cohort of 41 patients with locally advanced lung cancer.[27] We elected to focus on patients with locally advanced stage cancer because these represent the most typical patient population undergoing RT for NSCLC. Moreover, they remain a challenge for conventional 3DCRT. Consistent with our earlier results, IMRT significantly improved target coverage and reduced the volume of normal lung irradiated above low doses. Overall, the mean absolute reductions in the percentage of the V_{10} and V_{20} were 7% and 10%, respectively. These differences translated into a 10% reduction in the risk of pneumonitis.

At William Beaumont Hospital, Grills and colleagues recently compared different RT techniques to irradiate the primary tumor ± hilar and mediastinal lymph nodes in 18 patients with stage I to IIIb NSCLC.[28] Four approaches were evaluated: IMRT, 3DCRT (multiple beams), 3DCRT (two to three beams), and traditional RT using elective nodal irradiation. IMRT planning was associated with a higher mean PTV dose, and tumor control probabilities were 7 to 8% greater than 3DCRT and 14 to 16% greater than traditional RT. Of note, although IMRT had limited benefit in node-negative patients, it was beneficial in node-positive patients. Meeting all normal tissue constraints in node-positive patients, IMRT was able to deliver doses 25 to 30% greater than 3DCRT and 130 to 140% greater than traditional RT.

Other investigators in the United States,[29–32] Europe,[33–38] and Canada[39] have also reported promising dosimetric results evaluating IMRT in patients with lung cancer. To date, however, no series of patients with lung cancer treated with IMRT have yet been published. Clearly, the efficacy and long-term clinical outcome of IMRT in these patients should be rigorously investigated before any firm conclusions are drawn.

Mesothelioma

Although IMRT remains problematic for lung cancer, it has been successfully applied to the treatment of mesothelioma. We recently updated our technique and results.[40–42] Essential to this approach is the accurate definition of the target volume. Based on previous experience, the ipsilateral mediastinum should be delineated and included in the target volume.[41,43,44] The superior border is at the thoracic inlet. The medial border should include the ipsilateral nodal regions, trachea, and subcarinal regions[40] or the vertebral body[45] depending on whether three-dimensional or two-dimensional target definitions are used. The posterior mediastinal structures behind the heart have not been included in our trial, and, to date, there have been no retrocardiac failures (unpublished data).

Three other regions should be delineated carefully: the anterior-medial pleural reflection, the insertion of the diaphragm (which can range from L1 to L4), and the medial extent of the crus of the diaphragm, especially at its most inferior extent. All chest tube or biopsy sites are also included because of the risk of tumor tracking along the instrumentation track. These should be contoured to the skin, as should any regions of subcutaneous tissue disruption. Typically, the skin incision does not directly overlie the regions where the ribs are entered. Given that there is tunneling under the subcutaneous fat, the entire disturbed region should be irradiated. Disrupted tissue planes can often be identified at postoperative CT simulation and should be included in the CTV.

When the entire region is extensively clipped intraoperatively, regions of potential pitfall can be highlighted. Ideally, the surgeon, radiation oncologist, treatment planner, and physicist should discuss the target volumes at the planning workstation. This allows for unambiguous target volume identification and helps the radiation oncologist better understand the anatomy and extent of disease. Likewise, the surgeon gains an appreciation of the limits of target volume identification or clipping. Furthermore, the treatment planner gains insight into which regions of this very large CTV are critical, and the physicist appreciates the planning constraints for each case.

Unlike in lung cancer, there was little motion of the involved hemithorax compared with the contralateral hemithorax. This was important because respiratory motion can be significant in the chest, and such motion would be a contraindication to IMRT. With the lung removed, there also was little density heterogeneity from air-equivalent volumes. Finally, concurrent chemotherapy was not used in this trial, so this potential toxicity source is eliminated. However, unlike lung cancer RT, most of the remaining lung receives a mean dose ~ 7 to 8 Gy.

The target doses and the dose-volume limits for the critical structures are listed in Table 19-1. Treatment is delivered with 12 to 27 intensity-modulated fields using 7 to 11 gantry angles, typically with 100 segments per field. Because patients have only one lung after surgery, the volumes of contralateral lung irradiated should be limited such that the mean lung dose is less than 9.5 Gy, and the V_{20} should be less than 20%. This is consistent with the results of whole-lung irradiation.[46] It is often difficult to spare the ipsilateral kidney because of its proximity to the posterior diaphragmatic recess. Therefore, all patients must demonstrate adequate renal function prior to treatment (> 40% of contralateral kidney function by renal scan).

Treatment planning and quality assurance techniques in our patients with mesothelioma undergoing IMRT have been described in detail.[40] On the first day of treatment, anterior-posterior and lateral isocenter verification films

are acquired. During the first week of treatment, two sets of isocenter verification films are acquired on consecutive days. Subsequently, additional portal images are acquired twice weekly.

Clearly, IMRT is more complicated to deliver than conventional techniques in these patients; however, excellent target coverage can be achieved. Review of the DVH for a representative case (Figure 19-11) demonstrated that the target volume is well covered and that the normal tissue constraints are met. The liver and contralateral lung are spared with this technique. In this patient, it was possible to spare the ipsilateral kidney because the organ was particularly low. In most patients, the ipsilateral kidney receives a high dose because the CTV typically abuts its posterior edge. For left-sided lesions, the spleen is also likely to receive a high dose. Therefore, pneumococcal prophylaxis is recommended.

Outcomes in our first 50 patients have been promising. To date, we have had only one in-field failure and two failures at the field edge (one at the anterior-medial pleural reflection and one at the crus of the diaphragm). One patient died secondary to radiation pneumonitis, and five patients died from infectious pneumonias. However, 20 patients died from distant metastases (18 in the lung, 2 in the abdomen, and 3 in both). All five abdominal failures were the result of diffuse peritoneal mesothelioma, not localized failure. The 3-year actuarial survival rate for patients with uninvolved lymph nodes is 55%. It is not yet clear if these results can be attributed to target volume delineation or to

TABLE 19-1. Target Doses and Dose-Volume Constraints of the Organs at Risk

Target or Organ	Goal or Constraint Dose
CTV	50 Gy in 25 fractions
bCTV	60 Gy in 25 fractions
Lung	< 20% to receive > 20 Gy and mean < 9.5 Gy
Liver	< 30% to receive > 30 Gy
Contralateral kidney	< 20% to receive > 15 Gy
Heart	< 50% to receive > 45 Gy
Spinal cord	< 10% to receive > 45 Gy; no portion to receive > 50 Gy
Esophagus	< 30% to receive > 55 Gy

CTV = clinical target volume.

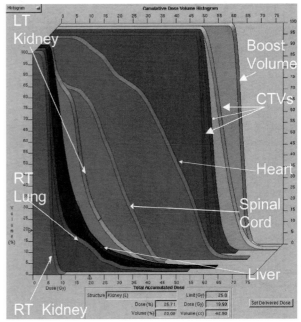

FIGURE 19-11. Dose-volume histograms from an intensity-modulated radiation therapy mesothelioma plan. The goal dose of 50 Gy to the clinical target volume (CTV) and 60 Gy to the gross tumor volume (positive surgical margin) was achieved. The liver, kidneys, spinal cord, heart, and esophagus were all within tolerance. (To view a color version of this image, please refer to the CD-ROM.)

superior target volume coverage by IMRT compared with three-dimensional plans.[42]

Others have reported promising dosimetric and clinical results in patients with mesothelioma. Tobler and colleagues at the University of Utah presented an IMRT technique using photon arcs, which significantly improved the dose distribution to the pleural surface with a concomitant decrease in dose to the lung parenchyma compared with traditional techniques.[47] In a preliminary feasibility study, Munter and colleagues at the German Cancer Research Center reported the results of IMRT treatment in seven patients with locally advanced unresectable mesothelioma.[48] All patients were treated after failure of chemotherapy. Overall, treatment was well tolerated. Both the 1-year actuarial overall survival rate from the start of RT and the 2-year overall survival rate since diagnosis were 28%.

Summary

Local control is dismal in most patients with NSCLC. Mathematical models suggest that radiation doses > 100 Gy are required to sterilize most lung tumors.[49] Although this can be achieved for small tumors using radiosurgery, it is impossible to achieve for most patients (who have locally advanced disease at presentation). One important hope for radiation dose escalation will be the use of IMRT and possibly proton therapy, allowing the delivery of highly conformal dose treatments. Until such aggressive therapy has been developed and evaluated, significant benefit can be achieved with 3DCRT by correctly identifying the GTV, CTV, and PTV for each patient. ITVs can also be individualized. Dose calculations should be performed while accounting for tissue heterogeneity. These techniques must be clinically applied before IMRT is routinely clinically implemented.

Acknowledgments

We would like to thank Drs. Lei Dong, H. Helen Liu, George Starkschall, and Steven Frank for their input on this chapter and Ms. Cora Bartholomew for her excellent administrative assistance in the preparation of the manuscript.

References

1. Tyldesley S, Boyd C, Schulze K, et al. Estimating the need for radiotherapy for lung cancer: an evidence-based, epidemiologic approach. Int J Radiat Oncol Biol Phys 2001;49:973–85.
2. Ahmedin J, Ram CT, Taylor M, et al. Cancer statistics 2004. CA Cancer J Clin 2004;54:8–29.
3. Bo WJ. Thorax. In: Bo WJ, Wolfman NT, Krueger WA, editors. Basic atlas of cross sectional anatomy. Philadelphia: WB Saunders; 1998. p. 87–158.
4. Truong MT, Erasmus JJ, Gladish GW, et al. Anatomy of pericardial recesses on multidetector CT: implications for oncologic imaging. AJR Am J Roentgenol 2003;181:1109–13.
5. Vanuytsel LJ, Vansteenkiste JF, Stroobants SG, et al. The impact of (18)F-fluoro-2-deoxy-D-glucose positron emission tomography (FDG-PET) lymph node staging on the radiation treatment volumes in patients with non-small cell lung cancer. Radiother Oncol 2000;55:317–24.
6. Seltzer MA, Yap CS, Silverman DH, et al. The impact of PET on the management of lung cancer: the referring physician's perspective. J Nucl Med 2002;43:752–6.
7. MacManus MP, Hicks RJ, Matthews JP, et al. High rate of detection of unsuspected distant metastases by PET in apparent stage III non-small-cell lung cancer: implications for radical radiation therapy. Int J Radiat Oncol Biol Phys 2001;50:287–93.
8. Erdi YE, Rosenzweig K, Erdi AK, et al. Radiotherapy treatment planning for patients with non-small cell lung cancer using positron emission tomography (PET). Radiother Oncol 2002;62:51–60.
9. MacManus MP, Wong K, Hicks RJ, et al. Early mortality after radical radiotherapy for non-small-cell lung cancer: comparison of PET-staged and conventionally staged cohorts treated at a large tertiary referral center. Int J Radiat Oncol Biol Phys 2002;52:351–61.
10. Caldwell CB, Mah K, Ung YC, et al. Observer variation in contouring gross tumor volume in patients with poorly defined non-small-cell lung tumors on CT: the impact of 18FDG-hybrid PET fusion. Int J Radiat Oncol Biol Phys 2001;51:923–31.
11. Giraud P, Grahek D, Montravers F, et al. CT and (18)F-deoxyglucose (FDG) image fusion for optimization of conformal radiotherapy of lung cancers. Int J Radiat Oncol Biol Phys 2001;49:1249–57.
12. Giraud P, Antoine M, Larrouy A, et al. Evaluation of microscopic tumor extension in non-small-cell lung cancer for three-dimensional conformal radiotherapy planning. Int J Radiat Oncol Biol Phys 2000;48:1015–24.
13. Stevens CW, Munden RF, Forster KM, et al. Respiratory-driven lung tumor motion is independent of tumor size, tumor location, and pulmonary function. Int J Radiat Oncol Biol Phys 2001;51:62–8.
14. Ramsey CR, Scaperoth D, Arwood D, et al. Clinical efficacy of respiratory gated conformal radiation therapy. Med Dosim 1999;24:115–9.
15. Sixel KE, Aznar MC, Ung YC. Deep inspiration breath hold to reduce irradiated heart volume in breast cancer patients. Int J Radiat Oncol Biol Phys 2001;49:199–204.
16. Rosenzweig KE, Hanley J, Mah D, et al. The deep inspiration breath-hold technique in the treatment of inoperable non-small-cell lung cancer. Int J Radiat Oncol Biol Phys 2000;48:81–7.
17. Ford EC, Mageras GS, Yorke E, et al. Evaluation of respiratory movement during gated radiotherapy using film and electronic portal imaging. Int J Radiat Oncol Biol Phys 2002;52:522–31.
18. Orton CG, Chungbin S, Klein EE, et al. Study of lung density corrections in a clinical trial (RTOG 88-08). Int J Radiat Oncol Biol Phys 1998;41:787–94.
19. Orton CG, Mondalek PM, Spicka JT, et al. Lung corrections in photon beam treatment planning: are we ready? Int J Radiat Oncol Biol Phys 1984;10:2191–8.
20. Klein EE, Morrison A, Purdy JA, et al. A volumetric study of measurements and calculations of lung density corrections for 6 and 18 MV photons. Int J Radiat Oncol Biol Phys 1997;37:1163–70.

21. Papanikolaou N, Klein EE. Point/counterpoint: heterogeneity corrections should be used in treatment planning for lung cancer. Med Phys 2000;27:1702–4.

22. Frank SJ, Forster KM, Stevens CW, et al. Treatment planning for lung cancer: traditional homogeneous point-dose prescription compared with heterogeneity-corrected dose-volume prescription. Int J Radiat Oncol Biol Phys 2003;56:1308–18.

23. Klein EE, Chin LM, Rice RK, Mijnheer BJ. The influence of air cavities on interface doses for photon beams. Int J Radiat Oncol Biol Phys 1993;27:419–27.

24. Wang L, Yorke E, Desobry G, et al. Dosimetric advantage of using 6 MV over 15 MV photons in conformal therapy of lung cancer: Monte Carlo studies in patient geometries. J Appl Clin Med Phys 2002;3:51–9.

25. Liu HH, Wang X, Dong L, et al. Feasibility of sparing lung and other thoracic structures with intensity-modulated radiotherapy for non-small cell lung cancer. Int J Radiat Oncol Biol Phys 2004;58:1268–79.

26. Seppenwoolde Y, Shirato H, Kitamura K, et al. Precise and real-time measurement of 3D tumor motion in lung due to breathing and heartbeat, measured during radiotherapy. Int J Radiat Oncol Biol Phys 2002;53:822–34.

27. Murshed H, Liu HH, Lioa X, et al. Dose and volume reduction for normal lung using intensity modulated radiotherapy for advanced stage non-small cell lung cancer. Int J Radiat Oncol Biol Phys 2004;58:1258–67.

28. Grills IG, Yan D, Martinez AA, et al. Potential for reduced toxicity and dose escalation in the treatment of inoperable non-small-cell lung cancer: a comparison of intensity-modulated radiation therapy (IMRT), 3D conformal radiation, and elective nodal irradiation. Int J Radiat Oncol Biol Phys 2003;57:875–90.

29. Dogan N, King S, Emami B, et al. Assessment of different IMRT boost delivery methods on target coverage and normal-tissue sparing. Int J Radiat Oncol Biol Phys 2003;57:1480–91.

30. Xiao Y, Werner-Wasik M, Michalski D, et al. Comparison of three IMRT inverse planning techniques that allow partial esophagus sparing in patients receiving thoracic radiation therapy for lung cancer [abstract]. Int J Radiat Oncol Biol Phys 2002;54:153.

31. Manon RR, Patel R, Zhang T, et al. CT-based analysis of free-breathing vs. maximum inspiratory breath hold techniques for 3-D conformal radiation therapy and intensity modulated radiation therapy in lung cancer: a potential basis for dose-escalation. Int J Radiat Oncol Biol Phys 2003;57:S417.

32. Jiang SB, Pope C, Al Jarrah KM, et al. An experimental investigation on intra-fractional organ motion effects in lung IMRT treatments. Phys Med Biol 2003;48:1773–84.

33. Dirkx MLP, Essers M, van Sornsen de Koste JR, et al. Beam intensity modulation for penumbra enhancement in the treatment of lung cancer. Int J Radiat Oncol Biol Phys 1999;44:449–54.

34. Derycke S, de Gersem WRT, van Duyse BB, et al. Conformal radiotherapy of stage III non-small cell lung cancer: a class solution involving non-coplanar intensity modulated beams. Int J Radiat Oncol Biol Phys 1998;41:771–7.

35. van Sornsen de Koste J, Dirkx M, van Meerbeeck J, et al. An evaluation of two techniques for beam intensity modulation in patients irradiated for stage III non-small cell lung cancer. Lung Cancer 2001;32:145–53.

36. Marnitz S, Stuschke M, Bohsung J, et al. Intraindividual comparison of conventional three dimensional radiotherapy and intensity modulated radiotherapy in the therapy of locally advanced non-small cell lung cancer: a planning study. Strahlenther Onkol 2002;178:651–8.

37. Brugmans MJ, van der Horst A, Lebesque JV, et al. Beam intensity modulation to reduce the field size for conformal irradiation of lung tumors: a dosimetric study. Int J Radiat Oncol Biol Phys 1999;43:893–904.

38. Nioutsikou E, Redford JL, Christian JA, et al. Segmentation of IMRT plans for radical lung radiotherapy delivery with step-and-shoot technique. Med Phys 2004;31:892–901.

39. Underwood LJ, Murray BR, Robinson DM, et al. An evaluation of forward and inverse radiotherapy planning using Helax-TMS (version 6.0) for lung cancer patients treated with RTOG 93-11 dose-escalation protocol. Med Dosim 2003;28:167–70.

40. Forster KM, Smythe WR, Starkschall G, et al. Intensity modulated radiation therapy following extrapleural pneumonectomy for the treatment of malignant mesothelioma: clinical implementation. Int J Radiat Oncol Biol Phys 2003;55:606–16.

41. Ahamed A, Stevens CW, Smythe WR, et al. Intensity-modulated radiation therapy: a novel approach to the management of malignant pleural mesothelioma. Int J Radiat Oncol Biol Phys 2003;55:768–75.

42. Ahamad A, Stevens CW, Smythe WR, et al. Promising early local control of malignant pleural mesothelioma following postoperative intensity modulated radiotherapy (IMRT) to the chest. Cancer J 2003;9:476–84.

43. Sugarbaker DJ, Flores RM, Jaklitsch MT, et al. Resection margins, extrapleural nodal status and cell type determine postoperative long-term survival in trimodality therapy of malignant pleural mesothelioma: results in 183 patients. J Thorac Cardiovasc Surg 1999;117:54–65.

44. Rusch VW, Rosenzweig K, Venkatraman E, et al. A phase II trial of surgical resection and adjuvant high-dose hemothoracic radiation for malignant pleural mesothelioma. J Thorac Cardiovasc Surg 2001;122:788–95.

45. Yajnik S, Rosenzweig KE, Mychalczak B, et al. Hemithoracic radiation after extrapleural pneumonectomy for malignant pleural meothelioma. Int J Radiat Oncol Biol Phys 2003;56:1319–26.

46. Della Volpe A, Ferreri AJ, Annaloro C, et al. Lethal pulmonary complications significantly correlate with individually assessed mean lung dose in patients with hematologic malignancies treated with total body irradiation. Int J Radiat Oncol Biol Phys 2002;52:483–8.

47. Tobler M, Watson G, Leavitt DD. Intensity-modulated photon arc therapy for treatment of pleural mesothelioma. Med Dosim 2002;27:255–9.

48. Munter MW, Nill S, Thilmann C, et al. Stereotactic intensity-modulated radiation therapy (IMRT) and inverse treatment planning for advanced pleural mesothelioma. Feasibility and initial results. Strahlenther Onkol 2003;179:535–41.

49. Martel MK, Ten Haken RK, Hazuka MB, et al. Estimation of tumor control probability model parameters from 3-D dose distributions of non-small cell lung cancer patients. Lung Cancer 1999;24:31–7.

TARGET DEFINITION IN NON–SMALL CELL LUNG CANCER CASE STUDY

THOMAS GUERRERO, MD, PHD, YERKO BORGHERO, MD, CRAIG W. STEVENS, MD, PHD

Patient History

A 61-year-old male smoker developed a persistent respiratory infection 1 month prior to presentation. A chest radiograph was obtained and revealed a right middle lobe lung opacity suspicious for malignancy (Figure 19.1-1). A computed tomography (CT) scan demonstrated a 3.2 cm mass in the right lower lobe and a 1 cm nodule in the right hilum. A positron emission tomography (PET) study revealed hypermetabolic activity in the right middle lobe mass. No suspicious activity was seen in the hilum, in the mediastinum, or outside the thorax. A CT-guided fine-needle aspiration was performed, and the pathology was consistent with poorly differentiated non–small cell carcinoma.

Owing to his poor pulmonary function, the patient was felt to be ineligible for surgical resection and was referred for definitive radiation therapy (RT). The remainder of his metastatic workup was negative. He was thus staged with T2N0M0 (stage IB) disease.

Simulation

The patient was immobilized in the supine position. The breath-hold CT imaging technique for determination of the internal margin owing to respiratory motion was used and is described here.[1,2] The patient was immobilized using a Vac-Lok device (MED-TEC, Orange City, IA) with his arms above his head grasping a T-bar, designed to reduce setup uncertainty. The patient was aligned with the axis of the scanner based on a CT scout film, and three radiopaque markers were placed at the level of the carina for identification of the isocenter reference point. The treatment isocen-

ter was set at the time of the planning. All CT data sets were acquired on a commercial multislice helical CT scanner (MX8000 IDT, Philips Medical Systems, Andover, MA).

An external fiducial marker was placed on the patient's abdomen, and a video tracking system monitored the respiratory phase and relative respiratory effort of the patient during the simulation session (Real-time Position Management system, version 1.5.1, Varian Medical Systems, Palo Alto, CA). The patient was provided with video feedback of the respiratory cycle and was coached on normal breathing to provide a regular breathing pattern. The patient was also coached on breath-hold techniques to maintain a normal inspiration and expiration breath-hold for 10 to 15 seconds (required for a fast thoracic CT acquisition). The patient setup is illustrated in Figure 19.1-2A, and a sample of his regular breathing pattern is shown in Figure 19.1-2B.

Three CT scans, with 3 mm slices, were obtained for this portion of the treatment planning session to define

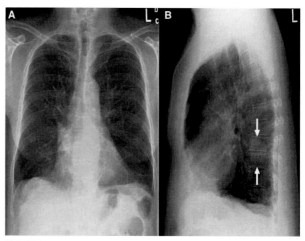

FIGURE 19.1-1. Posterior-anterior (*A*) and lateral (*B*) chest radiographs obtained prior to treatment. Arrows indicate the location of the 3.2 cm mass in the lateral radiograph.

Editor's note: This case was not treated with intensity-modulated radiation therapy. It is presented here to illustrate important issues surrounding target delineation in patients with non–small cell lung cancer undergoing radiation therapy.

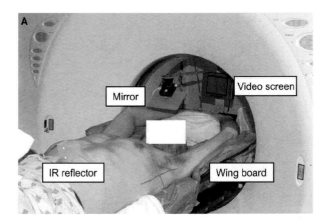

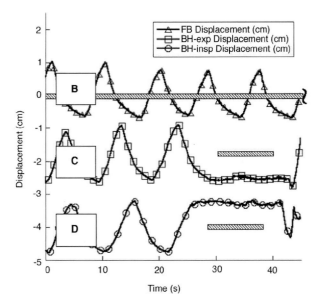

FIGURE 19.1-2. Respiratory feedback. The patient was positioned supine on a Vac-Lok bag and wing board with his arms above his head, where he grasps a T-bar (*A*). The video monitor used for feedback guidance and the three respiratory traces are shown. Free-breathing (FB) computed tomography (CT) has a prolonged expiratory phase indicative of this patient's chronic obstructive pulmonary disease (*B*). The inspiration breath-hold (BH-insp) CT (*C*) and the expiration breath-hold (BH-exp) CT (*D*) were obtained at the time indicated by the horizontal bar. (To view a color version of this image, please refer to the CD-ROM.)

TABLE 19.1-1. Comparison of CT Parameters Used for Free-Breathing Slow CT versus Breath-Hold Fast CT Scans Used in the Planning of Thoracic Radiation Therapy

CT Technique	Pitch	Detector Configuration	Rotational Speed	Table Speed	1 m Acquisition Time
Slow CT	0.33	8 × 3 mm	1.0 s/rotation	0.80 cm/s	125 s
Fast CT	1.5	8 × 3 mm	0.42 s/rotation	8.6 cm/s	11.6 s

CT = computed tomography.

inspiration BH-CT (iBH-CT) and expiration BH-CT (eBH-CT) images were obtained at normal breathing efforts (table pitch 1.5). The monitored respiratory traces obtained are shown in Figure 19.1-2.

The CT planning session was coordinated with the patient's staging PET-CT imaging session so that the immobilization devices would be available for data acquisition. The PET-CT imaging session was performed on a GE Discovery ST PET/CT scanner with a 74 cm bore (GE Healthcare, Milwaukee, WI), which accommodates the use of thoracic immobilization devices. The PET images were acquired with 3 minutes per couch position, for a total of five couch positions or 87.3 cm axial length, with the patient undergoing normal, quiet breathing. The CT component (PET/CT-CT) was obtained with the patient instructed to hold his breath at midinspiration, although no feedback guidance was used. The registration of the PET emission and the CT image sets was verified at the time of the aquisition because the CT image set was also used for the attenuation correction of the PET emission data prior to reconstruction.

The entire set of imaging studies was sent to the planning workstation running *Pinnacle³*, version 6.2b (Phillips Medical Systems, Andover, MA). A region of interest defining the spine and vertebrae was defined on the FB-CT, as shown in Figure 19.1-3A and Figure 19.1-3B. A CT-to-CT 6 degrees of freedom rigid body registration was performed between FB-CT and the eBH-CT, iBH-CT, and PET/CT-CT using a mutual information algorithm.[3] The FB-CT was the primary set in each case. A resulting registered image pair is shown in Figure 19.1-3C and 19.1-3D. The result of the registration of the iBH-CT and eBH-CT with the FB-CT is illustrated in Figure 19.1-4.

Target and Tissue Delineation

The breath-hold CT-based target delineation process used at our institution is described first.[1,2] The gross tumor volume (GTV) was defined as the volume of radiographically apparent disease, including both the primary tumor and involved nodes. The GTV was outlined on transaxial images on the FB-CT, eBH-CT, and iBH-CT image volumes. In cases such as this, in which the tumor is completely surrounded by normal lung, the initial contour set was drawn

the internal target volume (ITV). Two CT acquisition modes (fast and slow) were used, and their parameters are given in Table 19.1-1. The fast and slow acquisition modes scan 1 meter in 11.6 and 125 seconds, respectively. The first CT image acquisition was obtained with the patient breathing normally or freely breathing (FB-CT) using slow acquisition parameters (table pitch 0.33). The scan extended from the mandible to the tip of the liver to include the entire thoracic cavity and upper abdomen. The patient was next instructed on breath-holding at normal inspiration and at normal expiration for the subsequent breath-hold (BH-CT) CT acquisitions. The fast CT acquisition was used, and

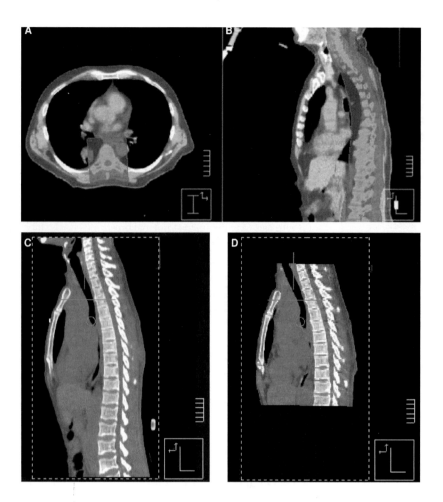

FIGURE 19.1-3. Image registration. This process assumes a stationary spine and uses mutual information to perform a 6 degrees of freedom registration. In (A) a simple square contour surrounds the vertebral body on this transaxial image from the free-breathing computed tomography (FB-CT) volume, and (B) shows a sagittal view through the entire image and contour set. The sagittal images from the FB-CT (C) and the expiration breath-hold computed tomography (eBH-CT) (D) are registered. The eBH-CT is resliced to correspond to the registration results with the FB-CT as a reference. (To view a color version of this image, please refer to the CD-ROM.)

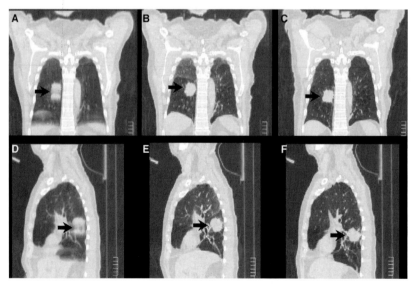

FIGURE 19.1-4. The registered free-breathing computed tomography (FB-CT), expiration breath-hold computed tomography (eBH-CT), and inspiration breath-hold computed tomography (iBH-CT) are shown in coronal (A–C) and sagittal (D–F) cross-sectional images. The FB-CT images (A and D) show the tumor (arrow) smeared over the motion range limits indicated by the dotted line. The tumor and normal structures demonstrate motion artifact, which appears as the nonuniform modulation. The eBH-CT images (B and E) show the tumor (arrow) adjacent to the upper dotted line. The iBH-CT images (C and F) show the tumor (arrow) at the lower dotted line.

using lung window and level values on the CT image display. In tumors contiguous with the hilum, mediastinum, or chest wall, two passes should be made in delineating the contours, the first with the lung-optimized display and the second with mediastinal soft tissue–optimized display. The green contour shown in sagittal section in Figure 19.1-5 represents the eBH-CT–determined contour (see Figure 19.1-5A), and the red contour represents the iBH-CT–determined contour (see Figure 19.1-5B). These two contours are shown to completely envelop the tumor present on the

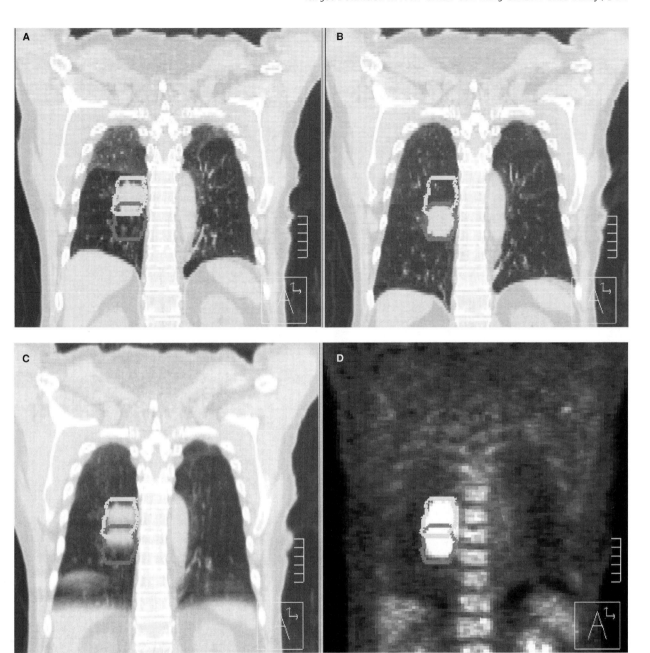

FIGURE 19.1-5. Computed tomography and positron emission tomography (PET) registration. The coronal sections illustrating the gross tumor volume (GTV) from the expiration breath-hold computed tomography (eBH-CT) (*green*) and inspiration breath-hold computed tomography (iBH-CT) (*red*) scans. (*A*) A coronal section through the eBH-CT (note that the green contour encloses the tumor). (*B*) A coronal section through the iBH-CT, with the red contour enclosing the tumor. (*C*) A coronal section through the free-breathing computed tomography; note that the tumor extends into both contours, although the extent of the combined breath-hold–derived GTV is greater. (*D*) A registered coronal section through the fluorodeoxyglucose (FDG)-PET scan, now that the FDG avid tumor is nearly completely enclosed by the breath-hold–derived GTV. (To view a color version of this image, please refer to the CD-ROM.)

slow CT (see Figure 19.1-5C) and on the fluorodeoxyglucose PET (see Figure 19.1-5D).

The clinical target volume (CTV) was defined as the GTV plus margin to account for subclinical or microscopic disease extension. Giraud and colleagues provide an excellent analysis of the microscopic extension observed in 70 non–small cell lung cancer (NSCLC) pathologic specimens.[4] The margin necessary to include 95% of the microscopic extension has been reported as 6 mm for squamous carcinoma and 8 mm for adenocarcinoma. Typically, we have used an 8 mm expansion as the default (as in this poorly differentiated NSCLC). The expansion of the GTV to the CTV should include knowledge of anatomic spread patterns.[5] For example, the microscopic spread will not occur freely across pleural or other anatomic boundaries unless there is invasion of adjacent structures. In this case (Figure 19.1-6), the tumor was positioned against the thoracic vertebral body and rib; the expansion should not cross the lung pleura. The uniform three-dimensional expansion of the GTV drawn on the iBH-CT and the eBH-CT (see Figure 19.1-6B) required editing to remove their extension across the pleural anatomic boundary (see Figure 19.1-6C). The resulting nonuniform expansion (see Figure 19.1-6D and Figure 19.1-6E) may then be combined to form the ITV (see Figure 19.1-6E).

The internal margin has been designed to account for variations in size, shape, and position of the CTV in relation to anatomic reference points. The variation of the CTV size, shape, and position owing to respiratory motion can then be included in the internal margin. Three methods have been reported to measure the resulting ITV: gated or breath-hold CT imaging,[1,2] slow CT imaging,[6] and PET imaging.[7] Using the BH-CT imaging approach, the ITV should be formed as the combination of the nonuniform expanded CTVs from the iBH-CT, eBH-CT, and FB-CT. The iBH-CT and eBH-CT account for the extremes of breathing, and the FB-CT accounts for lateral extent of motion in midcycle. Finally, the expansion to the planning target volume (PTV), which includes the effects of setup uncertainty and interfraction target positioning error, proceeds from the ITV. The positioning uncertainties were measured at our institution[8]; hence, the PTV is derived from the ITV plus 1.0 cm (see Figure 19.1-6F).

The second internal margin method can simply use expansions from the GTV drawn on the slow FB-CT study applied in two steps: first the expansion to the CTV and then the expansion to the PTV. As before, the expansion to the CTV should follow anatomic spread patterns. The overlap into the bony spine and ribs should be edited from a uniform expansion (Figure 19.1-8). However, because of motion within the FB-CT image set, any expansion into the mediastinum or anterior chest wall should remain.

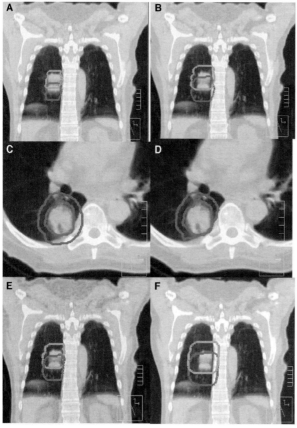

FIGURE 19.1-6. Clinical target volume (CTV) and planning volume (PTV) expansion using breath-hold computed tomography (CT). In (A) the gross tumor volume (GTV) contours derived from expiration breath-hold CT (eBH-CT) and inspiration breath-hold CT are shown superimposed on a coronal section through the free-breathing computed tomography (FB-CT). Uniform expansion of the contours of 8 mm results in the contours seen in panels (B) and (C) (note the overlap into the vertebral body and adjacent rib). In (D) the areas of the expanded GTV that extend across anatomic boundaries were edited. (E) is a coronal section through the two nonuniformly expanded CTVs obtained from the eBH-CT and iBH-CT. The resulting PTV is shown in (F). (To view a color version of this image, please refer to the CD-ROM.)

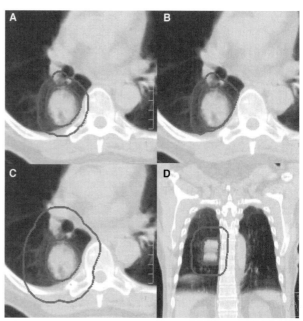

FIGURE 19.1-7. Clinical target volume (CTV) and planning volume (PTV) expansion using free-breathing computed tomography (FB-CT). (A) The gross tumor volume (GTV) contours are delineated based on the FB-CT. Uniform expansion of the contours by 8 mm results in the contours overlapping the vertebral body and adjacent rib. (B) Manual editing of the expanded GTV contours results in the nonuniform expanded CTV (outer contour). (C) A uniform expansion of 1.5 cm to account for internal margin and setup error results in the PTV. (D) The GTV and PTV are shown in coronal section. (To view a color version of this image, please refer to the CD-ROM.)

These structures may contain the lung lobe for a portion of the respiratory cycle. The posterior chest wall and spine do not move. An uncertainty of 0.5 cm can then be added to the CTV to account for residual tumor motion not seen on the FB-CT. The PTV would be constructed by adding 1.0 cm to the ITV (see Figure 19.1-8D).

The third internal margin method assumes that the range of motion would be captured in the prolonged PET acquisition, in which the emission acquisition may range from 3 to 5 minutes per couch position. The emission acquisition would be ungated and with the patient freely breathing. The GTV for this method would then be drawn on the FB-CT and coregistered PET image sets (Figure 19.1-9A). Object size depends on the choice of window and level for the PET emission images and results from low spatial resolution of the PET emission images. This effect on object size and activity quantification was described earlier.[9] The resulting contour set would then be assumed to include the internal margin, and no additional expansion is required

to explicitly include motion. The PTV would again be constructed using a 1.0 cm margin to account for setup uncertainty. The resulting three PTVs are compared in Figure 19.1-9. We are investigating the significance of the differences between these three methods to define the internal margin and subsequent PTV.

Treatment Planning and Treatment Delivery Issues

This case was planned and treated using three-dimensional conformal RT owing to the large amount of tumor motion observed during the treatment planning session and the issue of dose uncertainty owing to the interplay between tumor motion and IMRT delivery.[10–12] This patient was treated to 66 Gy in 33 fractions.

Clinical Outcome

At 4 months following completion of treatment, the patient is alive and well, with no evidence of disease progression, recurrence, or distant metastasis. A follow-up CT imaging study (Figure 19.1-10) revealed that the tumor had a partial response, with a greater than 50% reduction in tumor diameter.

References

1. Forster KM, Stevens CW, Liao Z, et al. Defining the internal target volume (ITV) using respiratory-gated CT image data sets. Int J Radiat Oncol Biol Phys. 2004. [In press]
2. Shih HA, Jiang SB, Aljarrah KM, et al. Planning target volume determined with fused CT images of fast, breath-hold, and four second simulation CT scans to account for respiratory movement in 3D-CRT in lung cancer. Int J Radiat Oncol Biol Phys. 2004;60:613–22.
3. Studholme C., Hawkes DJ, Hill DLG. A normalised entropy measure for multi-modality image alignment. Proc SPIE Med Imaging 1998;3338:132–42.
4. Giraud P, Antoine M, Larrouy A, et al. Evaluation of microscopic tumor extension in non-small-cell lung cancer for three-dimensional conformal radiotherapy planning. Int J Radiat Oncol Biol Phys 2000;48:1015–24.
5. Armstrong JG. Target volume definition for three-dimensional conformal radiation therapy of lung cancer. Br J Radiol 1998;71:587–94.
6. Lagerwaard FJ, Van Sornsen de Koste JR, Nijssen-Visser MR, et al. Multiple "slow" CT scans for incorporating lung tumor mobility in radiotherapy planning. Int J Radiat Oncol Biol Phys 2001;51:932–7.
7. Caldwell CB, Mah K, Skinner M, et al. Can PET provide the 3D extent of tumor motion for individualized internal target volumes? A phantom study of the limitations of CT and the promise of PET. Int J Radiat Oncol Biol Phys 2003;55:1381–93.
8. Forster KM, Stevens CW, Kitamura K, et al. Changes of tumor motion patterns during a course of radiation therapy for lung cancer. Int J Radiat Oncol Biol Phys 2003;57:1–7.

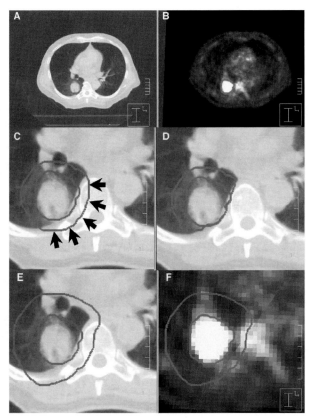

FIGURE 19.1-8. Clinical target volume (CTV) and planning target volume (PTV) expansion using positron emission tomography (PET)-derived gross tumor volume (GTV). (*A*) and (*B*) The GTV is delineated based on the fused PET data as shown. (*C*) Uniform expansion of the contours by 8 mm results in the contours overlapping the vertebral body and adjacent rib (*arrows*). (*D*) Manual editing of the expanded GTV contours results in the nonuniform expanded CTV (outer contour). (*E*) and (*F*) The resulting PTV created and original GTV are shown. (To view a color version of this image, please refer to the CD-ROM.)

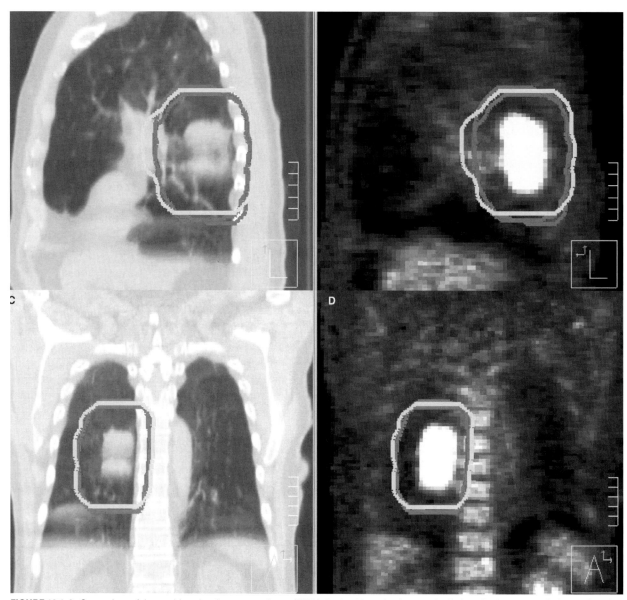

FIGURE 19.1-9. Comparison of the resulting planning target volumes (PTVs) obtained from the three methods described to account for internal motion: the breath-hold computed tomography (CT) (*red*), the slow CT (*green*), and the PET imaging (*blue*). In this example, the PTVs are quite similar, irrespective of the method used to generate the PTV. This is usually not the case. (To view a color version of this image, please refer to the CD-ROM.)

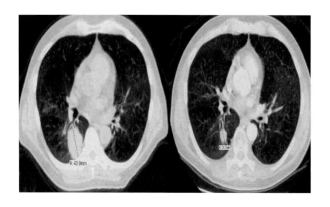

FIGURE 19.1-10. Pre- and post-treatment computed tomography (CT) images. Pre- and post-treatment transaxial CT images with the maximum tumor diameter (*A*) prior to treatment (43.9 mm) and (*B*) 1 month after treatment (21.2 mm). The tumor has responded modestly to treatment.

9. Hoffman EJ, Huang SC, Phelps ME. Quantitation in positron emission computed tomography: 1. Effect of object size. J Comput Assist Tomogr 1979;3:299–308.

10. Jiang SB, Pope C, Al Jarrah KM, et al. An experimental investigation on intra-fractional organ motion effects in lung IMRT treatments. Phys Med Biol 2003;48:1773–84.

11. Bortfeld T, Jiang SB, Rietzel E. Effects of motion on the total dose distribution. Semin Radiat Oncol 2004;14:41–51.

12. Bortfeld T, Jokivarsi K, Goitein M, et al. Effects of intra-fraction motion on IMRT dose delivery: statistical analysis and simulation. Phys Med Biol 2002;47:2203–20.

Chapter 19.2

Synchronous Bilateral Non–Small Cell Lung Cancer Case Study

Thomas Guerrero, MD, PhD, Stephen Bilton, CMD, Craig W. Stevens, MD, PhD

Patient History

A 64-year-old male nonsmoker developed bronchitis 1 month prior to presentation. A chest radiograph revealed a right lung opacity (Figure 19.2-1A) that did not resolve with antibiotics. A computed tomography (CT) scan demonstrated a 4.5 cm right lower lobe mass and a 2.5 cm mass in the left lower lobe. Enlarged left hilar lymph nodes and suspicious lymph nodes in the right mediastinum and subcarina region were noted. CT-guided fine-needle aspiration of the right lung mass was positive for high-grade spindle cell neoplasm mixed with high-grade adenocarcinoma, consistent with a sarcomatoid carcinoma. CT-guided fine-needle aspiration was performed of the left lower lobe

mass, and the pathology was positive for non–small cell lung cancer (NSCLC), favoring adenocarcinoma. No sarcomatoid elements were identified in the specimen.

Whole-body positron emission tomography (PET)-CT imaging was obtained revealing hypermetabolic activity in both the right and left lung lesions and in the bilateral hila, right paratracheal (level IVR), and subcarinal (level VII) nodal regions (Figure 19.2-2). Because of the planned

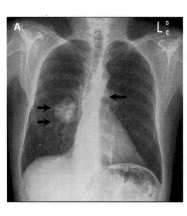
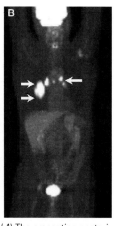

FIGURE 19.2-1. Presentation and staging. (*A*) The presenting posterior-anterior chest radiograph is shown. Two arrows delineate the primary tumor on the right, and one arrow delineates the primary tumor on the left. (*B*) An anterior projection of the fluorodeoxyglucose positron emission tomography (PET) imaging study obtained for staging is shown. The hypermetabolic primary tumors are delineated by two left-pointing arrows on the right and one right-pointing arrow on the left. The hilar and mediastinal lymph nodes are hypermetabolic, including the subcarinal nodal station seen on the patient's midline.

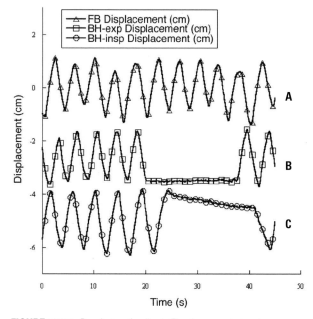

FIGURE 19.2-2. Respiratory feedback. The three respiratory traces were obtained using a commercial infrared video motion tracking device. (*A*) The free-breathing (FB) computed tomography (CT) has a regular breathing frequency of 15 breaths/s with the commonly observed variation in the baseline. The acquisition time was 1 minute 30 seconds, indicated by the striped bar. (*B*) The inspiration breath-hold (BH-insp) CT and (*C*) the expiration breath-hold (BH-exp) CT scans were obtained at the time indicated by the striped horizontal bar.

366

use of radiation therapy (RT), immobilization devices were constructed prior to PET-CT (see below). The imaging session was performed on a GE Discovery ST PET/CT scanner with a 70 cm bore (GE Medical Systems, Waukesha, WI), which accommodates the thoracic immobilization devices. The PET images were acquired with 3 minutes per couch position, for a total of five couch positions or 87.5 cm axial length, with the patient undergoing normal breathing. The CT component was obtained with the patient instructed to hold his breath at midinspiration. The registration of the two image sets was verified at the time of the aquisition because the CT scan was required for the attenuation correction of the PET data prior to reconstruction. A magnetic resonance image of the brain and a bone scan were negative for distant metastasis. Pulmonary function testing revealed excellent functional reserve.

The patient was staged as having T1N1 (stage IIA) NSCLC on the left and a synchronous T2N2M0 (stage IIIA) sarcomatoid carcinoma on the right. The patient elected to pursue concurrent chemo-RT with weekly carboplatin and paclitaxel. After comparing three-dimensional conformal radiation therapy (3DCRT) and intensity-modulated radiation therapy (IMRT) plans (see below), we elected to treat the patient with IMRT.

Simulation

A CT simulation was performed with the patient in the previously constructed immobilization devices, consisting of a Vac-Lok (MED-TEC, Orange City, IA), a T-bar, and a wing board with the patient's arm above his head (see Chapter 19.1, "Target Definition in Non–Small Cell Lung Cancer: Case Study"). The patient was aligned with the axis of the scanner based on a CT scout film, and three radioopaque markers were placed at the level of the carina for identification of this CT reference point. All CT data sets were acquired on a multislice helical CT scanner (MX8000 IDT, Philips Medical Systems, Andover, MA).

An external infrared reflective fiducial marker was placed on the patient's abdomen and tracked using a video tracking system, which monitored the patient's respiratory phase and relative respiratory effort during the simulation session (Real-time Position Management, version 1.5.1 system, Varian Medical Systems, Palo Alto, CA). The patient was provided with video feedback of the respiratory cycle and was coached on normal breathing to provide a regular breathing pattern. The patient was also coached on breath-hold techniques to maintain a normal inspiration and expiration breath-hold for the 10 to 15 seconds required for a fast CT acquisition. This patient's respiratory traces during the CT simulation are shown in Figure 19.2-2.

Three CT scans were obtained with 3 mm slice thickness to define the internal target volume (ITV).[1] The first CT scan was with the patient breathing normally (free-breathing computed tomography [FB-CT]), using slow CT

acquisition parameters. All scans extended from the mandible to the tip of the liver to ensure inclusion of the entire thoracic cavity and upper abdomen. The patient was then instructed to hold his breath at normal inspiration and at normal expiration during the subsequent breath-hold computed tomography (BH-CT). The BH-CT acquisitions used a fast acquisition mode. Inspiration breath-hold computed tomography (iBH-CT) and expiration breath-hold computed tomography (eBH-CT) scans were obtained at normal breathing efforts. The breathing cycle traces during the acquisition are shown in Figure 19.2-2 for the iBH-CT (see Figure 19.2-2C) and the eBH-CT (see Figure 19.2-2B) scans.

All imaging studies were then sent to the treatment planning computer running *Pinnacle[3]*, version 6.2b (Phillips Medical Systems). The registration process described in Chapter 18.1 was used to coregister the spine of each scan with the FB-CT imaging study. Target delineation occurred next and was performed with reference to the FB-CT as described below.

Target and Tissue Delineation

The gross tumor volume (GTV) was delineated on each of the treatment planning CT imaging studies (the FB-CT, iBH-CT, and eBH-CT scans), including the gross tumors and nodal disease. The PET study was used as a reference in the delineation process to identify regions and nodes suspicious for malignancy. There was no direct target delineation on the PET images owing to its intrinsically lower spatial resolution. The delineated GTV is shown in Figure 19.2-3. Note the change in GTV of both the primary tumor and the involved lymph nodes. The motion of the lymph nodes in this case was different from the motion of either primary tumor. The GTV was expanded to account for microscopic spread or subclinical involvement by 0.8 cm.[1,2] The CTVs from the iBH-CT, eBH-CT, and FB-CT were combined to form the ITV accounting for internal motion. The planning target volume (PTV) was formed from the ITV plus a 1.0 cm additional margin, accounting for daily setup error and interfraction target position uncertainty.

Treatment Planning

Both 3DCRT and IMRT treatment plans were generated for this patient using *Pinnacle[3]* treatment planning software, version 6.2b. The collapsed cone convolution dose calculation algorithm was used for all dose calculations,[3] which includes an accurate model to account for patient and target heterogeneity.

The normal tissue dose constraints used for both plans are given in Table 19.2-1. The esophagus and heart constraints were derived from Emami and colleagues,[4] the lung constraints from Graham and colleagues[5] and Lee and colleagues,[6] and the spinal cord constraints from Martel and

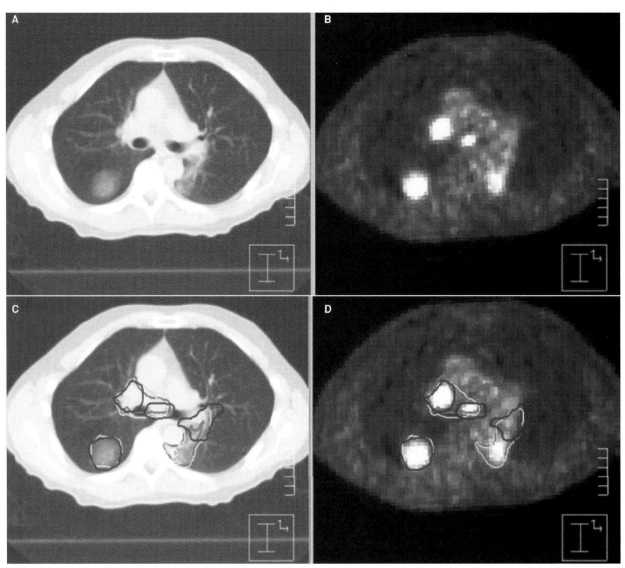

FIGURE 19.2-3. Tumor and target delineation. The gross tumor volume (GTV) was delineated on the free-breathing computed tomography (FB-CT) (*green*), the inspiration breath-hold computed tomography (BH-CT) (*red*), and the expiration BH-CT (*green*) scans. After applying an expansion for microscopic extension of disease and editing out expansions across anatomic boundaries, a set of clinical target volumes was obtained. These were combined to form the internal target volume, accounting for the internal motion. The positron emission tomography images were referenced during the contouring process. In (*A*) and (*B*) the involvement of the bilateral synchronous primaries, the presence of left hilar nodal involvment, and the presence of subcarinal nodal involvement are illustrated. In (*C*) and (*D*), the resulting contours are superimposed on an adjacent image. Note that the motion of the primary tumors and the motion of the lymph nodes are different. (To view a color version of this image, please refer to the CD-ROM.)

colleagues.[7] An initial 3DCRT plan was designed but required a large deviation from dose constraints (especially for the lung dose). Murshed and colleagues showed that a reduction in lung dose can be achieved using IMRT,[8] so an IMRT plan was devised with the goal of reducing the total lung dose to within the clinical constraints (see Table 19.2-1). Each plan is described below.

The 3DCRT plan was designed using four uniformly weighted beams: an anterior-posterior, a posterior-anterior, a left anterior oblique, and a right posterior oblique field, with a spinal cord block placed on the oblique fields. The

resulting isodose distribution is shown in Figure 19.2-4 through a plane designed to show the bilateral tumors. The cumulative dose-volume histogram is shown in Figure 19.2-5. The planning goal was to provide 95% coverage of the PTV; however, owing to the large volumes of normal tissues required in the treatment plan, the constraint was relaxed. The plan was normalized to provide 95% coverage of the ITV at the prescription dose (63 Gy). Complete coverage of the ITV occurred at 49 Gy (Table 19.2-2). The percentage of the total lung volume that received a dose ≥ 20 Gy (V_{20}) was 53.5%, far exceeding the planning constraint of 40%. The maximum spinal cord dose was 52.1 Gy owing to a direct trade-off between cord dose and ITV coverage.

TABLE 19.2-1. Normal Tissue Dose-Volume Constraints Used in Thoracic Radiation Therapy Treatment Planning

	RT Alone, Gy (%)	Chemo-RT, Gy (%)	Preoperative RT, Gy (%)
Spinal cord	50	45	45
Total lung	20 (< 40)	20 (< 35)	10 (< 40)
Heart	40 (< 100)	40 (< 100)	40 (< 100)
	50 (< 50)	50 (< 50)	50 (< 50)
Esophagus	60 (< 50)	55 (< 50)	55 (< 50)
Kidney	20 (< 50 both kidneys)	20 (< 50 both kidneys)	20 (< 50 both kidneys)
Liver	30 (< 40)	30 (< 40)	30 (< 40)

RT = radiation therapy.

A five-field IMRT plan was generated using equispaced 6 MV beams, every 72°. The two posterior beam angles were arranged obliquely to provide spinal cord avoidance (Figure 19.2-6). The initial planning goal to provide 95% coverage of the PTV to the prescribed dose was abandoned owing to the excessive volume of lung irradiated. The inverse planning goals were set to ensure 100% coverage of the ITV to the prescribed dose (63 Gy in 1.8 Gy/fraction) while reducing the V_{20} to < 40%.

The dose constraints for the normal structures are listed in Table 19.2-1, and the achieved dose-volume values are summarized in Table 19.2-2 (bottom row). For the heart, the goal was to keep the volume receiving ≥ 40 Gy (V_{40}) and the volume receiving ≥ 50 Gy (V_{50}) at < 100% and < 50%, respectively. For the spinal cord, the planning constraint was set at a maximum dose of < 45 Gy. The IMRT plan achieved a maximum spinal cord dose of 46.8 Gy, which was felt to be acceptable. The resulting isodose distribution is shown in Figure 19.2-4 through the

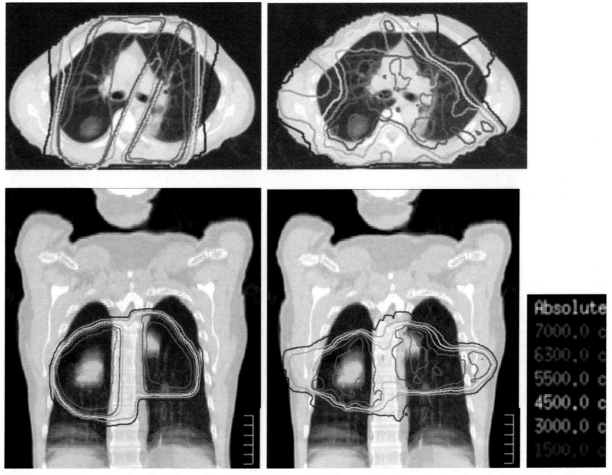

FIGURE 19.2-4. Plan comparison: intensity-modulated radiation therapy (IMRT) versus three-dimensional conformal radiation therapy (3DCRT). The isodose lines from the 3DCRT plan are shown in (*A*) and (*C*) The necessity to limit the spinal cord dose and provide uniform coverage over the target volumes, including the bilateral primary tumors, bilateral hila, and the mediastinum, complicated the treatment plan. Four beams were chosen for the 3DCRT plan. The IMRT isodose distribution is illllustrated in (*B*) and (*D*). (To view a color version of this image, please refer to the CD-ROM.)

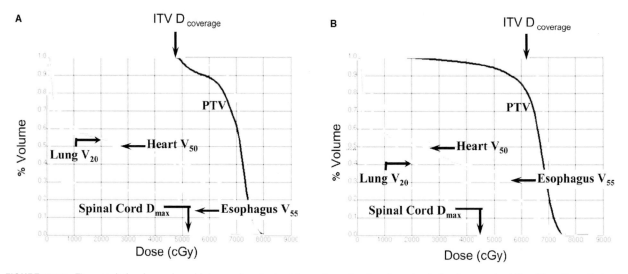

FIGURE 19.2-5. The cumulative dose-volume histogram from the best three-dimensional conformal radiation therapy plan (*A*) and from the optimized intensity-modulated radiation therapy plan (*B*). The treatment planning constraints shown on these distributions include the internal target volume (ITV) coverage dose, the total lung volume receiving 20 Gy (V_{20}), the spinal cord D_{max}, the heart volume receiving 50 Gy (V_{50}), and the esophagus volume receiving 55 Gy (V_{55}). PTV = planning target volume.

TABLE 19.2-2. Comparison of the Dose-Volume Histogram Results in the Three-Dimensional Conformal Radiation Therapy and Intensity-Modulated Radiation Therapy Plans

RT Plan	ITV 100% Coverage, Gy	PTV 95% Coverage, Gy	Lung V_{20}, %	Heart V_{55}, Gy	Spinal Cord D_{max}, Gy
3DCRT	47.9	50.4	53.5	31.5	52.10
IMRT	63.0	46.6	40.8	24.8	46.8

3DCRT = three-dimensional conformal radiation therapy; IMRT = intensity-modulated radiation therapy; ITV = internal target volume; PTV = planning target volume; RT = radiation therapy; V_{20} = volume receiving 20 Gy; V_{55} = volume receiving 55 Gy.

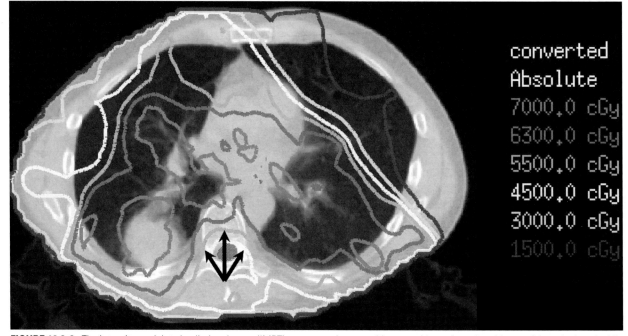

FIGURE 19.2-6. The intensity-modulated radiation therapy (IMRT) treatment plan was able to provide conformal avoidance of the spinal cord while simultaneously providing adequate coverage of the tumor targets in the lateral hila, mediastinum, and primary lung tumors. The arrows depict the avoidance of the spinal cord by the IMRT treatment plan's isodose distribution. (To view a color version of this image, please refer to the CD-ROM.)

same planes as for the 3DCRT plan. The IMRT plan was chosen for this patient's treatment as the best compromise between target coverage and normal tissue irradiation.

Treatment Delivery and Quality Assurance

Treatment was delivered in the "step-and-shoot" mode on a Varian 2100EX (Varian Medical Systems) equipped with the 120-Millennium multileaf collimator. The total treatment time was less than 20 minutes per fraction, including patient setup.

Prior to implementing IMRT for lung treatments, a series of commissioning measurements was performed to validate the planning system's inhomogeneity correction. Using a heterogeneous phantom, thermoluminescent dosimeter measurements were performed for both large and small fields. The standard deviation of these measurements was 2%, and no systematic difference between calculation and measurement was noted.

As part of the quality assurance process, the patient underwent weekly orthogonal portal film evaluation of the isocenter. Prior to treatment, dose calculations from the treatment planning system were verified using both ion chamber and film measurements in phantoms. Using a specially sealed water phantom, radiation intensity maps from the patient treatment plan were cast onto the CT scan of the phantom, and the dose to each of the ion chamber positions was then calculated. The phantom was then irradiated according to the patient treatment plan. The measured dose was compared with the calculated dose at the specific ion chamber location. A maximum discrepancy of 5% is allowed, although no deviations above 3% were observed in this patient. The relative dose distribution was verified using a plastic phantom (measuring $40 \times 40 \times 20$ cm^3) and radiographic films (EDR2, Eastman Kodak Corporation, Rochester, NY). Similar to the ionization chamber measurements, the patient geometry was replaced with that of the phantom in the treatment planning system. Isodose distributions were then calculated using the patient fluence maps. The film was then inserted in predetermined planes in the phantom, and the patient treatment was delivered. The resulting film images were analyzed using our in-house film dosimetry system (DoseLab). DoseLab reports the deviation from the calculated planer isodose in terms of relative dose agreement, distance to agreement, and normalized agreement test. Our acceptance criteria are a relative dose agreement of ≤ 3% and a distance to agreement of ≤ 3 mm. Both of these criteria were satisfied for this patient.

Given that the V$_{20}$ exceeded 40% in this patient, it was elected to administer daily amifostine (Ethyol, MedImmune Inc., Gaithersburg, PA) at a dose of 500 mg subcutaneously. In a randomized trial, amifostine has been shown to significantly reduce the risk of acute pneumonitis in patients with NSCLC receiving thoracic irradiation.[9] Moreover, amifostine reduced both the severity and the incidence of acute esophageal, pulmonary, and hematologic toxicity in patients receiving concurrent cisplatin-based chemotherapy and RT, without adversely impacting on tumor control. Amifostine has also been shown to reduce the reduction in DLCO resulting from lung irradiation.[10]

Clinical Outcome

The patient tolerated IMRT well and experienced only mild (grade 1) esophagitis. At 4 months following treatment, the patient was alive and well. His initial and follow-up chest radiographs are shown in Figure 19.2-7. Significant fibrosis is noted following the distribution of the isodose lines seen in the IMRT treatment plan (see Figure 19.2-4D). The similarity of the two distributions is also realized on a follow-up CT imaging study obtained at 4 months (Figure 19.2-8). There are similar features between the pattern of fibrosis and the 30 Gy isodose pattern. At his latest follow-up, the patient had no evidence of active disease or significant treatment sequelae.

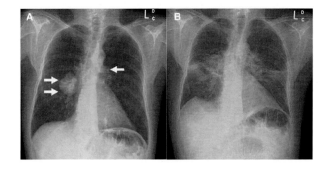

FIGURE 19.2-7. Tumor response. The presenting anterior-posterior chest radiograph is shown in (A) for comparison with the chest radiograph obtained 3 months after completion of therapy (B). The right-sided tumor is no longer evident owing to shrinkage and overlying fibrosis. There is radiation-induced fibrosis evident corresponding to the isodose distributions.

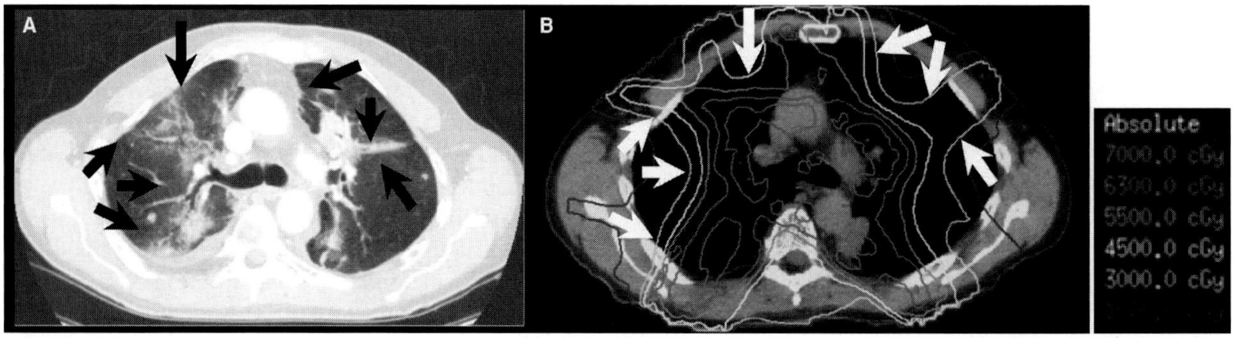

FIGURE 19.2-8. Pulmonary fibrosis corresponds to intermediate isodose distribution. (*A*) A computed tomography study was obtained 3 months after completion of intensity-modulated radiation therapy (IMRT). Using window and level values optimized to view the lung parenchyma, the developing lung fibrosis is readily apparent. (*B*) The IMRT dose distribution for a corresponding slice is shown. There are corresponding arrows indicating the similar pattern between the edge of the radiographically apparent fibrosis in (*A*) and the 30 Gy isodose line in (*B*). (To view a color version of this image, please refer to the CD-ROM.)

References

1. International Commission on Radiation Units and Measurements. Prescribing, recording, and reporting photon beam therapy (supplement to ICRU report 50). ICRU report 62. Washington (DC): International Commission on Radiation Units and Measurements; 1999.

2. Giraud P, Antoine M, Larrouy A, et al. Evaluation of microscopic tumor extension in non-small-cell lung cancer for three-dimensional conformal radiotherapy planning. Int J Radiat Oncol Biol Phys 2000;48:1015–24.

3. Mackie TR, Scrimger JW, Battista JJ. A convolution method of calculating dose for 15-MV x-rays. Med Phys 1985;12:188–96.

4. Emami B, Lyman J, Brown A, et al. Tolerance of normal tissue to therapeutic irradiation. Int J Radiat Oncol Biol Phys 1991;21:109–22.

5. Graham MV, Purdy JA, Emami B, et al. Clinical dose-volume histogram analysis for pneumonitis after 3D treatment for non-small cell lung cancer (NSCLC). Int J Radiat Oncol Biol Phys 1999;45:323–9.

6. Lee HK, Vaporciyan AA, Cox JD, et al. Postoperative pulmonary complications after preoperative chemoradiation for esophageal carcinoma: correlation with pulmonary dose-volume histogram parameters. Int J Radiat Oncol Biol Phys 2003;57:1317–22.

7. Martel MK, Eisbruch A, Lawrence TS, et al. Spinal cord dose from standard head and neck irradiation: implications for three-dimensional treatment planning. Radiother Oncol 1998;47:185–9.

8. Murshed H, Liu HH, Liao Z, et al. Dose and volume reduction for normal lung using intensity-modulated radiotherapy for advanced-stage non-small-cell lung cancer. Int J Radiat Oncol Biol Phys 2004;58:1258–67.

9. Komaki R, Lee JS, Milas L, et al. Effects of amifostine on acute toxicity from concurrent chemotherapy and radiotherapy for inoperable non–small cell lung cancer: report of a randomized comparative trial. Int J Radiat Oncol Biol Phys 2004;58:1369–77.

10. Werner-Wasik M., Scott C, Movsas B, et al. Amifostine as mucosal protectant in patients with locally advanced non-small cell lung cancer (NSCLC) receiving intensive chemotherapy and thoracic radiotherapy (RT): results of the Radiation Therapy Oncology Group (RTOG) 98-01 study. Int J Radiat Oncol Biol Phys 2003;57:S216.

HELICAL TOMOTHERAPY FOR LUNG CANCER EMERGING TECHNOLOGY

SCOTT P. TANNEHILL, MD, HAZIM A. JARADAT, PhD

Helical tomotherapy (TomoTherapy Inc., Middleton, WI) is a novel technique of delivering intensity-modulated radiation therapy (IMRT) using a linear accelerator mounted on a rotating ring gantry. The gantry rotates continuously through 360° while the patient is translocated through the gantry bore. The beam is modulated by a multileaf collimator array projecting a field up to 40 cm wide and 5 cm long at the isocenter. Highly conformal dose distributions can be achieved using this approach. The purpose of this chapter is to provide an overview of the application of IMRT delivered with tomotherapy in patients with lung cancer. Interested readers should also refer to Chapter 10, "Treatment Planning," and Chapter 12, "Delivery Systems," for general descriptions of tomotherapy IMRT planning and delivery.

Sample Case

A 60-year-old male presented with a T1N1 (stage IIA) non–small cell lung cancer of the right lower lobe. A positron emission tomography–computed tomography (PET-CT) scan and bronchoscopy confirmed the diagnosis, identifying a 2.5 cm mass in the medial right lower lobe and adenopathy in the distal bronchus intermedius. No mediastinal adenopathy or distant metastases were noted.

Owing to multiple comorbidities, the patient was felt to be medically inoperable and received three cycles of carboplatin and paclitaxel. A follow-up CT scan demonstrated a partial response. He subsequently received radiation therapy using a conventional three-dimensional treatment planning technique, consisting of opposed anterior-posterior and off-cord opposed oblique fields to 60 Gy, with appropriate beam weighting to maintain a spinal cord dose below 45 Gy. Treatment was planned and delivered with a maximum inspiration breath-hold technique using an in-house spirometer-based respiratory gating system.

With this system, monitor units are delivered only in maximum or near-maximum inspiration.

For this case, the gross tumor volume (GTV) was defined as all gross disease on the PET-CT scan; atelectatic lung on PET-CT was considered normal lung and not tumor. The clinical target volume (CTV) included the ipsilateral lower mediastinal, paratracheal, and subcarinal nodal regions (for elective irradiation). Also, the CTV included a 5 mm expansion of the GTV to account for subclinical disease extension. The GTV-to-CTV expansion did not include an adjacent vertebral body because spread to the bone was considered unlikely. The planning target volume (PTV) consisted of a 1.5 cm expansion of the CTV accounting for patient and organ motion. A 5 mm margin was applied between the PTV and the edge of each beam to account for penumbra. Normal tissues contoured included the lung, esophagus, and spinal cord.

Helical Tomotherapy Treatment Planning

For this comparison, the goal was to highlight the conformal avoidance feature of helical tomotherapy. Accordingly, the PTV and normal tissue contours were the same as for the three-dimensional plan. To obtain a meaningful comparison, the helical tomotherapy plan was optimized to minimize the dose to the lungs and esophagus while optimally treating the PTV to the same dose as the conventional plan: 60 Gy to 95% of the PTV. In actual practice, the image guidance capabilities of this unit (ie, the built in megavoltage CT) will permit smaller margins because of greater confidence in patient setup. The input parameters for the tomotherapy treatment planning are summarized in Table 19.3-1, including assigned importance and penalties.

TABLE 19.3-1. Intensity-Modulated Radiation Therapy Input Parameters

	Importance	Maximum Dose, Gy	Maximum Dose Penalty	DVH Volume, %	DVH Dose, Gy	DVH Pt Penalty	
Critical structure							
Spinal cord	1	25	5	15	15	5	
Esophagus	2	25	5	15	20	10	
Total lung	5	20	5	15	15	100	
	Importance	Maximum Dose, Gy	Maximum Dose Penalty	DVH Volume, %	DVH Dose, Gy	Minimum Dose, Gy	Minimum Dose Penalty
Target							
PTV	100	60	100	96	60	50	5

DVH = dose-volume histogram; PTV = planning target volume.
Field width = 2.46 cm; pitch = 0.21; dose calculation grid = normal (4 mm); modulation factor = 3.2.

Dose-Volume Histogram Comparison

Figure 19.3-1 illustrates the dose-volume histogram curves for helical tomotherapy and conventional three-dimensional treatment (*Pinnacle³*, Philips Medical Systems, Andover, MA). The radiation dose delivered to the lung and esophagus is substantially lower with helical tomotherapy. The lung volume receiving > 20 Gy (V_{20})—one parameter used to define the risk for pneumonitis—is 18% with tomother-apy versus 40% with three-dimensional planning. The esophageal dose is also significantly reduced. The spinal cord dose was also lower, but because the toxicity risk was insignificant in both plans, the curves are not displayed. However, for situations with vertebral body invasion, tomotherapy may offer distinct advantages in spinal cord sparing.

Figure 19.3-2 illustrates the isodose curves for conventional treatment and tomotherapy, respectively. Experts debate

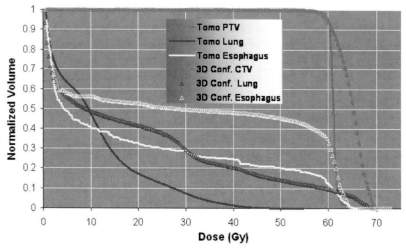

FIGURE 19.3-1. Comparison of dose-volume histogram curves for helical tomotherapy (TomoTherapy Inc.) and conventional three-dimensional (3D) conformal treatment planning (*Pinnacle³*) in the example patient. Note that the dose delivered to the lung and esophagus is substantially lower with helical tomotherapy. CTV = clinical target volume; PTV = planning target volume. (To view a color version of this image, please refer to the CD-ROM.)

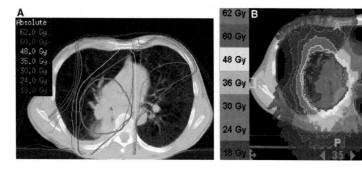

FIGURE 19.3-2. Axial computed tomography slice with isodose curves superimposed from the conventional three-dimensional (*A*) and helical tomotherapy (*B*) plans in the example patient. (To view a color version of this image, please refer to the CD-ROM.)

how to define appropriate target volumes for patients with lung cancer. However one defines the PTV for a patient, IMRT—illustrated with helical tomotherapy in this example—can substantially reduce the volume of lung and esophagus receiving high doses of radiation. IMRT will also probably improve dose homogeneity within the target volume compared with conventional techniques, illustrated by the steepness of the tomotherapy PTV line in Figure 19.3-1.

Discussion

Helical tomotherapy has distinct advantages over other IMRT delivery systems. First, helical tomotherapy offers image guidance capability using the built-in megavoltage CT scanner.[1] A megavoltage CT detector array is mounted 180° across from the beam source. This detector array uses the megavoltage treatment beam to create a CT image of the patient. Using very few monitor units, a megavoltage CT scan can be obtained immediately before treatment to verify patient setup. The patient position can then be adjusted using the software-driven couch to adapt to any changes in setup on a daily basis. By reducing the setup variability, CTV-to-PTV margins accounting for setup uncertainty can be reduced, further improving the sparing of normal tissues. Moreover, the unit can be integrated with a respiratory gating system. Clearly, this approach has considerable appeal in patients with lung cancer given the relationship between V_{20} and radiation pneumonitis.

Another important advantage of helical tomotherapy in these patients is fast delivery time. Increasing data suggest that IMRT is less efficacious when the daily treatment is protracted.[2] (See Chapter 18.9, "Impact of Prolonged Treatment Times: Emerging Technology.") With helical tomotherapy, patients are translocated through the machine while the treatment beam continuously rotates. This significantly reduces the delivery time of IMRT treatment, particularly when large fields are irradiated.

Although promising, clinical trials are needed to assess whether these benefits translate into better clinical outcomes. Several helical tomotherapy units are currently in operation, and clinical trials using helical tomotherapy for thoracic malignancies are ongoing at the University of Wisconsin-Madison and other centers.

References

1. Welsh JS, Patel RR, Ritter MA, et al. Helical tomotherapy: an innovative technology and approach to radiation therapy. Tech Cancer Res Treat 2002;1:55–63.
2. Fowler JF, Welsh JS, Howard SP. Loss of biological effect in prolonged fraction delivery. Int J Radiat Oncol Biol Phys 2004;59:242–9.

Intrafractional Organ Motion and Planning

Emerging Technology

Jong H. Kung, PhD, Piotr Zygmanski, PhD, George T. Y. Chen, PhD

As recommended by International Commission on Radiation Units and Measurements (ICRU) Report 50, a clinical target volume (CTV) to planning target volume (PTV) margin is necessary to account for geometric uncertainties, including patient setup error and organ motion. Organ motion is commonly categorized into interfractional and intrafractional motion. Interfractional motion pertains to organ shifts from one treatment session to another (on the time scale of days), whereas intrafractional motion describes motion during a treatment fraction. Intrafractional organ motion (IFOM) in the thorax is primarily due to respiration and cardiac motion, with time scales of 1 to 5 seconds.

Booth and Zavgorodni and Langen and Jones extensively reviewed and summarized the literature on organ motion.[1,2] More recently, the journal *Seminars in Radiation Oncology* devoted an issue to the high-precision treatment of moving targets.[3] This chapter reviews several facets of work in this area. The order of presentation here is imaging, beam delivery, and treatment planning because treatment planning approaches can be understood only after one appreciates the modes of beam delivery feasible with the current equipment. In reviewing the literature on these topics, emphasis will be placed on the characterization and management of IFOM for lung cancer; however, relevant studies for other sites (breast, abdomen) are also included.

Imaging

The magnitude of IFOM has been documented for various anatomic sites using an array of imaging devices. For example, the motion of the pancreas has been measured by ultrasonography.[4] The effects of intrafractional liver motion have been taken into account in gamma camera studies.[5] Kidney IFOM can be studied through magnetic resonance imaging (MRI).[6–9] Fluoroscopy has also been used to directly visualize radiopaque clips at the periphery of tumors.[10]

Each of these approaches has its strengths and weaknesses. Sonogram image quality can be limited, MRI near–real-time studies image only a single (arbitrary) plane, and fluoroscopy of radiopaque clips provides good spatial and temporal resolution but provides information only on the motion of the clips. Normal soft tissue organs, which are usually not clipped, would not be visible on videofluoroscopy. Ideally, a complete three-dimensional anatomic map as a function of time is needed in the treatment planning of moving targets.

In external beam treatment planning, the dominant imaging modality is computed tomography (CT).[11,12] Early CT scanners used in treatment planning were slow relative to physiologic processes such as respiration (early scanners required 30 minutes to scan 20 cm); therefore, CT studies in the presence of IFOM represented a time-averaged volume of the regions of interest. Today, a modern multislice helical CT scanner has a faster scanning speed (typical tube rotation < 0.5 seconds and couch travel velocity ~ 1 cm/s). Yet these scanners can still be subject to motion artifacts.[13,14] These artifacts are related to the organ size, scanning parameters, and amplitude of periodic motion. For example, Chen and colleagues showed that depending on the scanning time and respiratory period, a hypothetical lung tumor along the body axis can be imaged as either shortened or elongated and its centroid can be displaced (Figure 19.4-1).[15] Because of the presence of CT artifacts from IFOM, several investigators have proposed using breath-hold CT.[16,17]

Gated CT scanning is an alternative to scanning during voluntary breath-hold. In this acquisition mode, a patient breathes freely while an x-ray source is turned on and off (gated) at a predetermined respiratory phase. Gating techniques have been used for decades in imaging,

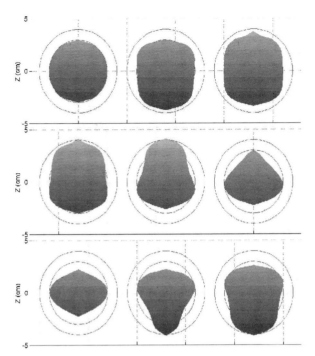

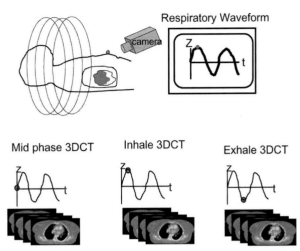

FIGURE 19.4-2. Four-dimensional computed tomography (CT) acquisition schematic. The patient is scanned during light breathing by a multislice CT scanner. The abdominal surface is monitored by tracking a fiducial marker with a video camera. Data are resorted based on respiratory phase to spatiotemporally coherent volumes at various instants of the respiratory cycle, indicated by the dots on the sinusoidal respiratory curve.

FIGURE 19.4-1. Numeric simulation of computed tomography artifacts from intrafractional organ motion. A hypothetical lung tumor (6 cm diameter) is oscillated along the craniocaudal axis with an amplitude of 1 cm and a period of 4 seconds. The circle in the upper left corner represents the true shape of the tumor, and the other objects estimate the shape and position for different phases of the periodic motion. The length of the tumor can be altered by twice the amplitude of the sinusoidal motion, or, in this case, a tumor that is 6 cm along the craniocaudal axis can be imaged as 4 cm along this axis. Reproduced with permission from Chen GT et al.[15]

and examples include electrocardiogram (ECG)-gated gamma camera studies,[18–20] ECG-gated positron emission tomography (PET),[21,22] ECG-gated MRI,[23–25] and ECG-gated CT of the heart.[26] Although fast helical scanners were introduced in the 1990s, CT has only recently been used for respiratory gating. There are two possible explanations for this delay. The first is a lack of a reliable surrogate signal needed to gate respiration. Unlike cardiac motion, respiration has both voluntary and involuntary components that can influence the reliability of a surrogate signal, such as abdominal height. The second reason is that with fast helical scanners, a simple breath-hold technique can, in principle, remove motion artifacts.

Ritchie and colleagues, Minohara and colleagues, and Kubo and colleagues described successful implementation of respiratory-gated CT.[27–29] In these systems, the chest wall or abdominal height is monitored. This signal (used for gating) is actually a surrogate for respiration. In one commercial implementation, known as Real-time Position Management (RPM) (Varian Medical Systems, Palo Alto, CA), a light plastic box with two reflective marker dots is placed on the patient's abdomen (between the umbilicus

and xyphoid). A camera and an infrared light source are mounted at the end of the treatment couch or on the wall of the treatment room. The reflected infrared light is captured by the camera, which is interfaced to a computer. The anterior-posterior block motion as a function of time is used as the respiratory waveform. The gating level is set by a user-specified threshold of the respiratory waveform.

An alternative approach uses four-dimensional imaging. Four-dimensional imaging of the beating heart obtained with ECG gating has been available with MRI,[30–32] CT,[33–35] and PET.[36] Direct four-dimensional CT of the heart and lungs has also been implemented with electron beam CT,[37] which is capable of scanning a 10 to 15 cm length of the body in a fraction of a second. Recently, a four-dimensional CT technique capable of imaging respiratory organ motion was reported by various groups.[38–42]

Figure 19.4-2 illustrates the schematic of a four-dimensional CT imaging method implemented using the RPM system. In this process, each part of the anatomy at a specific table index is imaged multiple times over a complete respiratory period (~ 4 seconds) to sample the full extent of organ motion. Furthermore, each axial image is indexed with a corresponding parameter of the surrogate respiratory signal (eg, abdominal motion amplitude or respiratory volume by spirometry) at the time of imaging. In the four-dimensional CT reconstruction process, three-dimensional images of the organ of interest at various phases can be generated by sorting and grouping all axial slices within the same respiratory phase window (Figure 19.4-3). The end result of this process is typically 500 to 1,500

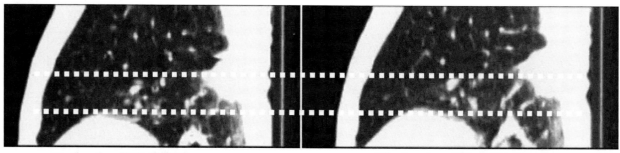

Inhale 3D(CT)
extracted from 4DCT

Exhale 3D(CT)
extracted from 4DCT

FIGURE 19.4-3. Examples of exhalation and inhalation three-dimensional computed tomography (3DCT) extracted from four-dimensional computed tomography (4DCT) illustrating respiratory organ motion. Courtesy of Eike Rietzel, MGH.

axial slices that are regrouped to create 10 or more spatiotemporally coherent volumes over the respiratory cycle. Details of the method can be found elsewhere.[41] Algorithms proposed to reduce motion artifacts during CT reconstruction have also been proposed.[43–45]

Beam Delivery

In gated radiation therapy (RT) treatment, the therapeutic beam is, in principle, turned on only when the target experiencing IFOM returns to the specified position (eg, treating lung tumors at the exhalation phase only). Approaches to gated RT treatment were devised early on for RT[28,46,47] because of the sensitivity of Bragg peak penetration to the depth changes that can occur during IFOM. The surrogate signals used by these investigators ranged from a strain gauge wrapped around a chest to measure expansion and contraction, to spirometry to measure exhaled and inhaled air volumes, to position-sensitive detectors to monitor the anterior-posterior movement of the abdominal surface.

IFOM management during beam delivery can be classified into three approaches: (1) gating the beam during normal respiration, (2) voluntary or forced breath-hold while the beam is continuously on, and (3) radiation aperture tracking of a moving tumor. Each of these is described briefly.

Gating the Beam during Normal Respiration

The goal in managing IFOM is to precisely target the tumor during its respiratory excursions. The difficulty with beam gating during respiratory motion is attributable to the lack of a verifiable surrogate signal that accurately describes tumor motion. The surrogate signals for tumor motion include the abdominal surface position as a function of time, the volume of lung-air exchange during respiration, the position of the diaphragm, and other surrogates that are, in principle, closely correlated with actual tumor motion

but may not have exact tumor correspondence at every instant. At the current time, these methods are under investigation.

Tada and colleagues described the feasibility of respiratory gating using a laser displacement sensor.[48] The sensor is placed over the patient's abdomen, and the variations in distance between the sensor and the surface of the abdomen are measured continuously. Their experience was limited to six patients with lung cancer. However, although the authors demonstrated a reliable method for synchronized treatment of lung tumors, they commented that further studies were needed for routine clinical use.

The Varian RPM gating system is currently used at many centers. Early work by Kubo and colleagues formed the basis of this product.[29] As noted by several investigators, patients tend to inhale more consistently (regular peak-to-peak abdominal amplitude and frequency) when audio coaching ("breathe in" and "breathe out") and visual feedback are provided.[49–51]

For fractionated RT, Ford and colleagues compared the diaphragmatic positions (not direct tumor position) of a gated port film with the digitally reconstructed radiograph of a gated CT to correct for daily patient setup error.[52] Vedam and colleagues studied the correlation between diaphragm motion (not tumor) and the respiratory waveform that was obtained simultaneously for each of 63 fluoroscopic sessions in five patients with lung cancer.[53] Vedam and colleagues concluded that there was a strong linear relationship over all sessions for all five patients, independent of audio coaching and/or visual feedback. The authors also found that gating parameters from the first treatment day can be used to predict diaphragm excursions of subsequent days to within 1 mm.

Wagman and colleagues described liver cancer treatment with gated beams.[54] The average superior-to-inferior diaphragmatic motion on initial fluoroscopy was reduced from 22.7 mm without gating to 5.1 mm with gating. Treatment was completed in less than 10 minutes with gating. The decrease in organ motion through gating enabled a 1 cm reduction in the gross tumor volume (GTV)-to-PTV expansion for patients with liver cancer. Theoretically, this margin reduction would allow the prescribed dose to be increased by 7 to 27%.

Mageras and colleagues obtained similar results for gated treatment of patients with lung cancer. Six patients receiving treatment for lung cancer participated in a study of system characteristics during treatment simulation with fluoroscopy.[55] From fluoroscopic observations, average patient diaphragm excursion was reduced from 1.4 cm (range 0.7–2.1 cm) without gating and without breathing instruction to 0.3 cm (range 0.2–0.5 cm) with instruction and with gating tolerances set for treatment at expiration for 25% of the breathing cycle.

These results should be weighed against critical observations made by Ozhasoglu and Murphy.[56] First, cardiac motion is not reflected in the respiratory waveform (abdominal motion), yet it can contribute up to 50% of the amplitude of tumor motion for targets near the heart. Additionally, comparing chest wall motion, abdominal motion, and tidal volume measured with a spirometer as functions of time, a typical patient may require up to 50 to 100 seconds to reach a steady breathing pattern. Lastly, in five patients with lung cancer, fiducial markers were implanted in the moving tumor, and fluoroscopic and respiratory waveforms were simultaneously recorded. In two of five patients, the correlation between internal and external surrogate signals either changed abruptly or could not be established even after 2 minutes of monitoring. These concerns suggest a more direct visualization of target position because a function of time is needed.

Another approach to mitigating the effects of IFOM during treatment is to directly determine the real-time position of the tumor through imaging or electronic sensing. This approach avoids inherent limitations of gating when a surrogate signal is used. Such limitations were noted in the early work of respiratory gating for charged particle beam RT. In work at the Heavy Ion Medical Accelerator in Chiba, Japan, Minohara and colleagues used orthogonal fluoroscopic imagers to monitor the respiratory motion of an implanted marker.[28] In parallel, Shimizu and colleagues used four diagnostic fluoroscopy systems for real-time tracking of 2.0 mm gold markers inserted into a tumor.[57] The imaging and decision system triggers the linear accelerator beam only when the target is within a specified region. In this report, four patients with lung cancer were treated, and gold marker movement that ranged from 5.5 to 15.9 mm in each of the three directions was reduced to within 5.3 mm with an image-based gating system. A technical issue of using diagnostic radiographs is the additional dose from the real-time imaging system. Shirato and colleagues estimated that the dose from fluoroscopy ranges from 0.01 to 1% of the target dose.[58] This dose should be significantly reduced when conventional fluoroscopy is replaced with amorphous silicon flat panel detectors, which have a higher quantum efficiency (and thus require less exposure).[59] Another issue is the placement of radiopaque (or other) fiducial markers. Placement of such markers in the lung, for example, may lead to complications, such as a pneumothorax.

In another approach to real-time localization of tumor motion, Seiler and colleagues at the Paul Scherrer Institute in Switzerland developed a prototype system capable of tracking tumor motion through an implanted sensor.[60] Positional information is determined by an external alternating magnetic field, thereby sparing the patient unnecessary radiation. In this technology, a 12 kHz alternating magnetic field penetrates the human body, inducing an electromagnetic field in the sensor (8.0×0.8 mm^2). The induced electromagnetic field is used to "decipher" the sensor's position in a room using established tracking applications. With the sensor 30 cm from the source, the sensor's location can be determined to within 2 mm. These systems are in the evaluation stage and are not widely available.

When respiratory-gated RT is implemented, it may alter the dosimetric characteristics of the therapeutic beam, depending on the details of the specific linear accelerator. It is therefore prudent to study the magnitude of such effects. Ramsey and colleagues evaluated the effect of gating on the central axis dose output, ionization ratios, beam flatness, and beam symmetry (for Varian linear accelerators, 6 and 18 MV photons).[61] The beam output, energy, flatness, and symmetry did not vary by more than 0.8% in most of the gating sequences. The maximum output deviations (0.8%), flatness deviations (1.9%), and symmetry deviations (0.8%) occurred when a low number of monitor units (MUs) (less than five) were delivered in the gating window. These results suggest that there are no significant perturbations of the beam characteristics when a typical linear accelerator is used in the gated mode.

Irradiation during Voluntary or Forced Breath-Hold

Voluntary or forced breath-hold typically uses spirometry or a surrogate to determine when to cease respiration at a given point. In the case of voluntary breath-hold, patients are asked to voluntarily hold their breath at some reproducible extrema. In the case of involuntary breath-holding, a spirometer may be used to measure air intake or outflow, and breathing is forcibly interrupted for several seconds while the beam is on. This requires good correlation between internal organs and the volume of air in the lungs. Several reports described gating treatment with a spirometer as the surrogate for tumor position.[46,56] Low and colleagues note that with spirometry, one can correlate instantaneous internal lung volume (instantaneous lung shape) with measured exhalation volume.[42] This was verified with four-dimensional CT studies of a patient with lung cancer obtained in conjunction with a spirometer. Therefore, spirometry can potentially provide a reliable surrogate signal for respiration.

Wong and colleagues developed a device known as active breathing control (ABC).[62] In ABC, the RT beam is turned on only when a specified point of respiration is reached and held by closing a valve to prevent normal respiration. The duration of forced breath-hold can be chosen to each patient's comfort level. The ABC method has also been used to gate CT scans. Stromberg and colleagues described how five patients with Hodgkin's disease underwent ABC-gated treatment.[63] A typical breath-hold achievable ranged from 34 to 45 seconds per segment.

In tangential field treatment of patients with left breast cancer, a scattered dose to the heart may result in long-term complications. At inhalation, the heart is displaced away from the chest wall; hence, the dose to the heart is reduced. Remouchamps and colleagues reported on using the ABC gating system for tangential field treatments of left-sided breast cancers.[64–66] For each of the medial and lateral tangential beams, RT can be delivered over two to three breath-holds ranging from 18 to 26 seconds. "Step-and-shoot" intensity modulation was employed to achieve a uniform dose distribution. ABC treatments achieved a mean absolute reduction of 3.6% in heart volume receiving > 30 Gy.

Balter and colleagues and Dawson and colleagues used an ABC-gated beam in the treatment of patients with liver cancer to reduce the PTV margin to enable dose escalation.[67,68] Breath-holds of up to 35 seconds were used for treatment, and typical treatment times were 25 to 30 minutes. With a reduced PTV margin, the prescribed dose was increased using this approach by an average of 5 Gy. During a fluoroscopic session, the authors observed no motion of the diaphragm or microcoil markers implanted in the liver during ABC breath-holds. Based on an analysis of 158 sets of positioning radiographs, the average intrafractional craniocaudal reproducibility of the diaphragm and hepatic microcoil position relative to bony anatomy using ABC were 2.5 mm (range 1.8–3.7 mm) and 2.3 mm (range 1.2–3.7 mm), respectively.

Beam Tracking

Approaches to tracking a moving target have been under investigation for over a decade. Investigators at Stanford University, in collaboration with Accuray (Accuray Inc., Sunnyvale, CA), have been involved in an image-guided robotic irradiation system initially known as the Neurotron-1000. This type of device has evolved and is now known as the Cyberknife. The initial design focused on building an x-ray source whose mechanical motion is not limited to a plane, as is that of a linear accelerator.[69,70] The six degrees of freedom were hypothesized to result in better dose conformity.

The Cyberknife combined a robotic linear accelerator with a treatment room fitted with video cameras to monitor the patient and/or a fluoroscopy system to image bony anatomy and implanted markers.[71–73] These imaging devices allow for frameless stereotactic procedures. The robotic linear accelerator compensates for daily patient setup error at the beginning of treatment and then adjusts for patient movement during a treatment by evaluating images acquired at a rate of one per second. The newest generation of the Cyberknife is equipped with an amorphous silicon imaging detector and can assess the position of a moving tumor based on real-time x-ray tumor imaging. The robotic arm can be used to follow the moving target.[74–76]

Linear accelerator–based image-guided RT has also been proposed. Keall and colleagues considered intensity-modulated radiation therapy (IMRT) of a moving tumor through a tracking approach known as motion-adaptive x-ray therapy (MAX-T).[77] In MAX-T, an IMRT plan and the corresponding dynamic mulileaf collimators (DMLCs) are generated based on static three-dimensional CT (eg, at the exhalation phase of respiration). During treatment, the real-time x-ray imaging system tracks tumor motion, and this motion is superimposed on each multileaf collimator (MLC) subfield; the center of each MLC subfield is, in principle, adjusted in real time to be in synchrony with tumor motion. There are two potential benefits to MAX-T. First, current IMRT treatment time with multiple ports takes longer to treat than conventional treatment. With gating, the treatment time can increase by a factor of 3. As a consequence of prolonged treatment times, a fraction of the sublethal damage may be repaired during treatment delivery, resulting in a decrease in efficacy. MAX-T has the potential of overcoming both of these problems.

However, MAX-T poses several technical hurdles. First, if the tumor and surrounding critical structures move as a rigid body, then MAX-T will deliver radiation to both the moving tumor and critical structures, as calculated by the treatment plan (ie, assumed static). However, as in lung tumors, if a tumor moves in relation to a stationary background that includes a critical structure (such as the spinal cord), then MAX-T could result in delivering more of the dose than calculated to the cord. Second, studies have shown that tumors can deform during respiration. Gierga and colleagues observed this during fluoroscopy,[10] and Aruga and colleagues, Giraud and colleagues, and Brock and colleagues showed this by comparison of inhalation and exhalation breath-hold CT scans.[78–80] If the tumor deforms, then simply shifting the center of the MLC subfields may not be sufficient for precise irradiation. Third, the spatial resolution of commercially available MLCs is ~ 0.5 cm. This means that the MAX-T technique typically must be discretized to steps of 0.5 cm (particularly if IFOM is perpendicular to a leaf motion direction), which may or may not be adequate.

Treatment Planning

Gating allows one to use a smaller CTV-to-PTV margin in treatment planning. Yu and colleagues noted that in MLC-based IMRT delivery, gating is necessary not only to reduce the CTV-to-PTV margin but also to ensure accurate dose delivery to the internal voxels of a moving organ.[81] In the extreme case, an interplay between the DMLC and periodic respiratory motion can result in as much as ± 100% fluence errors to portions of the tumor volume (Figure 19.4-4). Even in gated treatment, residual IFOM may be present owing to a finite gating window. Therefore, such an interplay can occur even with a gated treatment.

Kung and colleagues described a practical method to estimate such a dosimetric interplay effect.[82] A virtually identical approach was also independently proposed by Chui and colleagues to analyze the dose error in IFOM for patients with breast and lung cancer IMRT.[83] In the IMRT process, the treatment planning software generates a nonuniform x-ray intensity, $\Phi(x, y)$, for each portal, based on a desired input dose-volume histogram (DVH). $\Phi(x, y)$ is then decomposed into a DMLC sequence. The three-dimensional dose to a static organ would be based on this $\Phi(x, y)$. For an organ with IFOM, the dose can be calculated based on an effective incident fluence, $EIF(x, y)$. Simply stated, EIF is the x-ray fluence as seen moving from the perspective of the moving tumor. $EIF(x, y)$ can be calculated as follows: From the target's eye view (TEV), the target itself is stationary, and the MLC executes a trajectory, $-z(t)$, superimposed on the conventional DMLC leaf motion (Figure 19.4-5). Therefore, in the TEV, the function $-z(t)$ characterizes a beam delivery variation as a function of time. $EIF(x, y)$ can be analytically calculated from a given DMLC file by projecting each subfield aperture, weighted with its corresponding MUs, onto a calculational grid that incorporates the periodic motion $z(t)$. The $EIF(x, y)$ is then reintroduced into the dose calculation engine of the planning system to

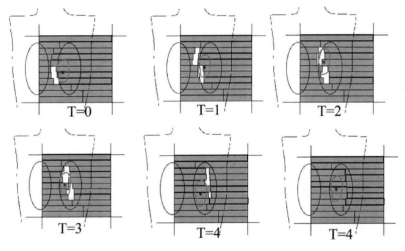

FIGURE 19.4-4. A schematic of possible dose error owing to interplay between the multileaf collimator (MLC) and intrafractional organ motion. The lung tumor (*red ellipse with specified tumor voxel, asterisk*) is visualized from an anterior direction. In the six panels, the tumor moves in the craniocaudal direction as the MLC sweeps across the field from left to right. Although the aperture length is sufficiently long to cover the target, the asterisked voxel in this illustration is found to be behind the MLC leaf during the collimator motion. (To view a color version of this image, please refer to the CD-ROM.) Reproduced with permission from Kung JH et al.[82]

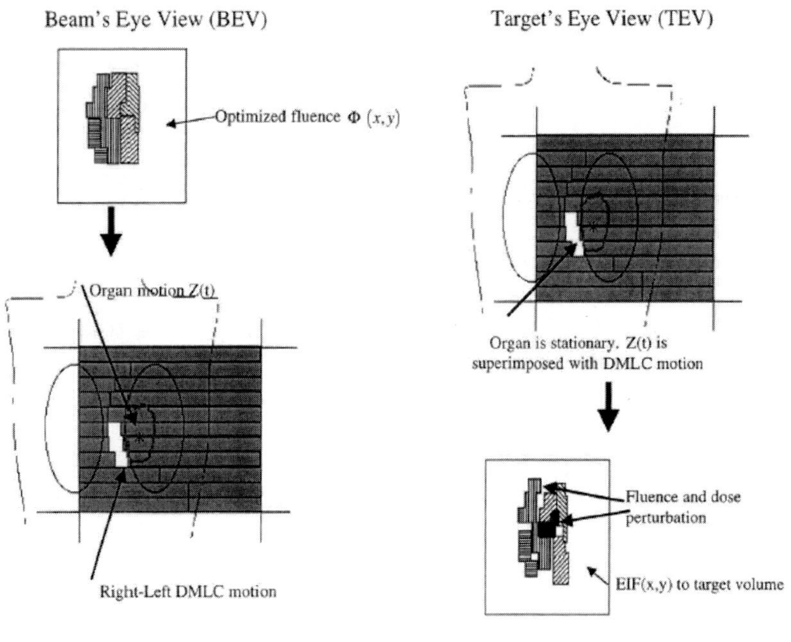

FIGURE 19.4-5. A schematic showing the principle behind the effective incident fluence (EIF) calculations. The left panel displays the beam's eye view perspective, whereas the right side shows the target's eye view (TEV). The fluence pattern is recalculated to the TEV, and the dose can then be appropriately summed. This assumes no target volume deformation. DMLC = dynamic multileaf collimator. Reproduced with permission from Kung JH et al.[82]

recalculate the three-dimensional dose to the gross tumor volume (GTV) (Figure 19.4-6). In the calculation of the $EIF(x, y)$ for gated treatment with an irradiation window (w), $z(t)$ is truncated for an amplitude greater than (w) as shown in Figure 19.4-7.

To evaluate the dosimetric effects of IFOM, the methodology of Kung and colleagues[82] was applied to the planning CT scan of a representative patient with lung cancer. Images were acquired on a helical CT scanner with a slice thickness of 3.75 mm. The CT scan was ungated, and in this study, it was assumed that the tumor volume as acquired represented the true mean position and shape. The GTV was contoured on axial CT slices, and a GTV-to-PTV margin of 1 cm was applied. An IMRT plan consisting of five coplanar fields was generated. Each beam had a nominal energy of 6 MV. Inhomogeneity corrections were used for the dose calculation. The IMRT plan output consisted of the MUs, DMLC, gantry angle, collimator angle, couch angle, and jaws for each IMRT port.

The $EIF(x, y)$ was calculated from each field using the previously described methodology. In the calculation of $EIF(x,,y)$ for each DMLC file, respiratory motion was modeled by a sinusoidal function with an amplitude of 10 mm in the superior-inferior direction, a period of 5 seconds, and a phase of zero. No additional motion was modeled in the other principal axes. A grid spacing of 2.5×2.5 mm^2 was used to match the resolution of the dose grid used by HELIOS (Varian Medical Systems). Subsequently, the $EIF(x, y)$ for each port was imported into the dose calculation engine to determine the three-dimensional dose to the GTV that would result if an IMRT plan were delivered without gating.

The resultant IMRT plans were computed for a dose rate of 300 MU/min (~ 5 MU/s). The Varian MLC hardware verifies leaf position every 50 milliseconds. With a DMLC tolerance setting of 2 mm, an effective dose rate for these IMRT plans was, on average, 4 MU/s. This latter value was used to convert from leaf positions as a function of MU to leaf positions as a function of time. Figure 19.4-8 shows an axial isodose distribution of a lung IMRT plan as generated by a *Helios/Cadplan* IMRT System (Varian Medical Systems).

Figure 19.4-9 shows the DVH(GTV) (not DVH[PTV]) calculated with and without organ motion. Note that when motion is included, the DVH has a "softer" shoulder over the 98 to 103% isodose levels. In this particular example, the dose error to the GTV from DMLC and organ motion interplay are small, and in comparison with the static field case, the GTV-to-PTV margin was adequate (data not shown). Thus, the need for a gated treatment can be based solely on the need to improve normal tissue sparing by decreasing the GTV-to-PTV margin. In other planning examples, the effect of IFOM has been more dramatic. Kung and colleagues showed the DVHs of a patient in whom the volume of the GTV receiving the prescription dose decreased by 18%.[82]

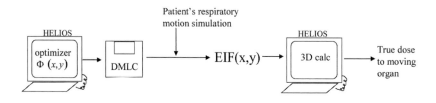

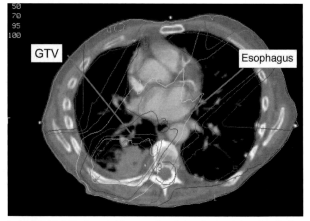

FIGURE 19.4-6. A block diagram indicating how organ motion is incorporated into the effective incident fluence (EIF) calculation, and the subsequent dose calculation with the HELIOS system (Varian Medical Systems). DMLC = dynamic multileaf collimator. Reproduced with permission from Kung JH et al.[82]

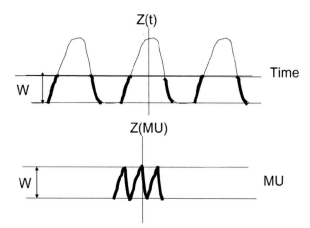

FIGURE 19.4-7. Amplitude of an organ motion as a function of beam-on time (monitor unit [MU]) for a gating window (W). Reproduced with permission from Kung JH et al.[82]

FIGURE 19.4-8. An axial image of an intensity-modulated radiation therapy plan in a patient with lung cancer used for organ motion calculation. GTV = gross tumor volume. (To view a color version of this image, please refer to the CD-ROM.) Reproduced with the permission from Kung JH et al.[82]

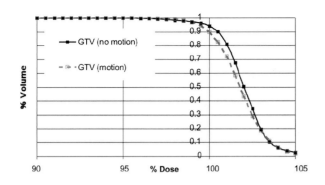

FIGURE 19.4-9. A comparison of gross tumor volume (GTV) dose-volume histograms with and without intrafractional organ motion from the patient in Figure 19.4-8. A = 1 cm; T = 5 seconds. Reproduced with permission from Kung JH et al.[82]

Thus, the dosimetric effects of IFOM will depend on the size, location, and three-dimensional dose distribution. Although the EIF method is a postprocessing technique, such an approach could be incorporated directly into the optimization process to determine fluence patterns that are the least sensitive to IFOM.

One can also estimate the dose delivered over many fractions when motion is present. Bortfeld and colleagues used numeric simulation to demonstrate that for treatment consisting of N fractions (N_f), a percent dose error (cumulative dose error/cumulative delivered dose) from the EIF calculation is reduced by a factor of

$$\frac{1}{\sqrt{N_f}}$$

in comparison with an unfractionated treatment.[84] This result is expected from the central limits theorem. Jiang and colleagues performed chamber and film studies.[85] The results of this study support the calculation by Bortfeld and colleagues.[84]

Summary and Conclusions

Currently, treatment planning is primarily based on static image data sets. This simplification can sometimes lead to rather large artifacts in imaging moving tumors and normal organs, with subsequent implications in dose calculations. Approaches to gating are actively being developed and may reduce the uncertainties in irradiating moving targets. Technology and issues to precisely deliver RT to a moving target are an area of active development and research. Recent capabilities to acquire four-dimensional CT scans provide an opportunity to examine the effects of IFOM on dynamic delivery systems. However, we are only in the initial phases of four-dimensional treatment planning, and many technical hurdles remain. As IMRT is applied to sites where IFOM is present, such as in lung cancer, new technologies and approaches toward accurate dose delivery and calculation will be required.

References

1. Booth JT, Zavgorodni SF. Set-up error and organ motion uncertainty: a review. Australas Phys Eng Sci Med 1999;22:29–47.
2. Langen KM, Jones DT. Organ motion and its management. Int J Radiat Oncol Biol Phys 2001;50:265–78.
3. Bortfeld T, Chen GT. Introduction: intrafractional organ motion and its management. Semin Radiat Oncol 2004;14:1.
4. Bryan PJ, Custar S, Haaga JR, et al. Respiratory movement of the pancreas: an ultrasonic study. J Ultrasound Med 1984;3:317–20.
5. Harauz G, Bronskill MJ. Comparison of the liver's respiratory motion in the supine and upright positions: concise communication. J Nucl Med 1979;20:733–5.
6. Korin HW, Ehman RL, Riederer SJ, et al. Respiratory kinematics of the upper abdominal organs: a quantitative study. Magn Reson Med 1992;23:172–8.
7. Moerland MA, van den Bergh AC, Bhagwandien R, et al. The influence of respiration induced motion of the kidneys on the accuracy of radiotherapy treatment planning, a magnetic resonance imaging study. Radiother Oncol 1994;30:150–4.
8. Schwartz LH, Richaud J, Buffat L, et al. Kidney mobility during respiration. Radiother Oncol 1994;32:84–6.
9. Shimizu S, Shirato H, Xo B, et al. Three-dimensional movement of a liver tumor detected by high-speed magnetic resonance imaging. Radiother Oncol 1999;50:367–70.
10. Gierga D, Sharp G, Brewer J, et al. Correlation between external and internal markers for abdominal tumors: implications for respiratory gating. Int J Radiat Oncol Biol Phys 2003;57:S186–7.
11. Hounsfield GN. Computerized transverse axial scanning (tomography). 1. Description of system. Br J Radiol 1973;46:1016–22.
12. Hounsfield GN. Historical notes on computerized axial tomography. J Can Assoc Radiol 1976;27:135–42.
13. Balter JM, Ten Haken RK, Lawrence TS, et al. Uncertainties in CT-based radiation therapy treatment planning associated with patient breathing. Int J Radiat Oncol Biol Phys 1996;36:167–74.
14. Shimizu S, Shirato H, Kagei K, et al. Impact of respiratory movement on the computed tomographic images of small lung tumors in three-dimensional (3D) radiotherapy. Int J Radiat Oncol Biol Phys 2000;46:1127–33.
15. Chen GT, Kung JH, Beaudette KP. Artifacts in computed tomography scanning of moving objects. Semin Radiat Oncol 2004;14:19–26.
16. Vock P, Soucek M, Daepp M, et al. Lung: spiral volumetric CT with single-breath-hold technique. Radiology 1990;176:864–7.
17. Kalender WA, Seissler W, Klotz E, et al. Spiral volumetric CT with single-breath-hold technique, continuous transport, and continuous scanner rotation. Radiology 1990;176:181–3.
18. Bulkley BH, Rouleau J, Strauss HW, et al. Proceedings: detection of hypertrophic cardiomyopathy by thallium 201 myocardial perfusion imaging and gated cardiac blood pool scans. Z Kardiol 1975;Suppl 2:5.
19. Green MV, Ostrow HG, Douglas MA, et al. High temporal resolution ECG-gated scintigraphic angiocardiography. J Nucl Med 1975;16:95–8.

20. Rigo P, Pitt B, Straus HW. The combined use of gated cardiac blood pool scanning and myocardial imaging with potassium-43 in the evaluation of patients with myocardial infarction. Radiology 1975;115:387–91.

21. Hoffman EJ, Phelps ME, Wisenberg G, et al. Electro-cardiographic gating in positron emission computed tomography. J Comput Assist Tomogr 1979;3:733–9.

22. Geltman EM, Roberts R, Sobel BE. Cardiac positron tomography: current status and future directions. Herz 1980;5:107–19.

23. Herfkens RJ, Higgins CB, Hricak H, et al. Nuclear magnetic resonance imaging of the cardiovascular system: normal and pathologic findings. Radiology 1983;147:749–59.

24. Lanzer P, Botvinick EH, Schiller NB, et al. Cardiac imaging using gated magnetic resonance. Radiology 1984;150:121–7.

25. Nishikawa J, Machida K, Iio M, et al. ECG-gated NMR-CT for cardiovascular disease. Radiat Med 1983;1:274–80.

26. Sagel SS, Stanley RJ, Levitt RG, et al. Gated computed tomography of the human heart. Invest Radiol 1977;12:563–6.

27. Ritchie CJ, Hsieh J, Gard MF, et al. Predictive respiratory gating: a new method to reduce motion artifacts on CT scans. Radiology 1994;190:847–52.

28. Minohara S, Kanai T, Endo M, et al. Respiratory gated irradiation system for heavy-ion radiotherapy. Int J Radiat Oncol Biol Phys 2000;47:1097–103.

29. Kubo HD, Len PM, Minohara S, et al. Breathing-synchronized radiotherapy program at the University of California Davis Cancer Center. Med Phys 2000;27:346–53.

30. Waterton JC, Jenkins JP, Zhu XP, et al. Magnetic resonance (MR) cine imaging of the human heart. Br J Radiol 1985;58:711–6.

31. Sechtem U, Pflugfelder P, Higgins CB. Quantification of cardiac function by conventional and cine magnetic resonance imaging. Cardiovasc Intervent Radiol 1987;10:365–73.

32. Utz JA, Herfkens RJ, Heinsimer JA, et al. Cine MR determination of left ventricular ejection fraction. AJR Am J Roentgenol 1987;148:839–43.

33. Johnson GA, Godwin JD, Fram EK. Gated multiplanar cardiac computed tomography. Radiology 1982;145:195–7.

34. Joseph PM, Whitley J. Experimental simulation evaluation of ECG-gated heart scans with a small number of views. Med Phys 1983;10:444–9.

35. Moore SC, Judy PF. Cardiac computed tomography using redundant-ray prospective gating. Med Phys 1987;14:193–6.

36. Klein GJ, Huesman RH. Four-dimensional processing of deformable cardiac PET data. Med Image Anal 2002;6:29–46.

37. Ross CS, Hussey DH, Pennington EC, et al. Analysis of movement of intrathoracic neoplasms using ultrafast computerized tomography. Int J Radiat Oncol Biol Phys 1990;18:671–7.

38. Ford EC, Mageras GS, Yorke E, et al. Respiration-correlated spiral CT: a method of measuring respiratory-induced anatomic motion for radiation treatment planning. Med Phys 2003;30:88–97.

39. Vedam SS, Keall PJ, Kini VR, et al. Acquiring a four-dimensional computed tomography dataset using an external respiratory signal. Phys Med Biol 2003;48:45–62.

40. Rietzel E, Chen GT, Doppke KP, et al. 4D computed tomography for treatment planning. Int J Radiat Oncol Biol Phys 2003;57:S232–3.

41. Pan T, Lee TY, Rietzel E, et al. 4D-CT imaging of a volume influenced by respiratory motion on multi-slice CT. Med Phys 2004;3:333–40.

42. Low DA, Nystrom M, Kalinin E, et al. A method for the reconstruction of four-dimensional synchronized CT scans acquired during free breathing. Med Phys 2003;30:1254–63.

43. Ritchie CJ, Crawford, C.R., Godwin, J.D., et al. Correction of computed tomography motion artifacts using pixel-specific back-projection. IEEE Trans Med Imaging 1996;15:333–42.

44. Dhanantwari AC, Stergiopoulos S, Zamboglou N, et al. Correcting organ motion artifacts in x-ray CT systems based on tracking of motion phase by the spatial overlap correlator. II. Experimental study. Med Phys 2001;28:1577–96.

45. Dhanantwari AC, Stergiopoulos S, Iakovidis I. Correcting organ motion artifacts in x-ray CT medical imaging systems by adaptive processing. I. Theory. Med Phys 2001;28:1562–76.

46. Ohara K, Okumura T, Akisada M, et al. Irradiation synchronized with respiration gate. Int J Radiat Oncol Biol Phys 1989;17:853–7.

47. Inada T, Tsuji H, Hayakawa Y, et al. [Proton irradiation synchronized with respiratory cycle]. Nippon Igaku Hoshasen Gakkai Zasshi 1992;52:1161–7.

48. Tada T, Minakuchi K, Fujioka T, et al. Lung cancer: intermittent irradiation synchronized with respiratory motion—results of a pilot study. Radiology 1998;207:779–83.

49. Kubo HD, Wang L. Introduction of audio gating to further reduce organ motion in breathing synchronized radiotherapy. Med Phys 2002;29:345–50.

50. Yokokawa T, Shintani H. [Development of picture and voice gated intermittent irradiation system connected without linear accelerator for voluntary breath-hold synchronized with respiration]. Nippon Igaku Hoshasen Gakkai Zasshi 2002;62:290–1.

51. Kini VR, Vedam SS, Keall PJ, et al. Patient training in respiratory-gated radiotherapy. Med Dosim 2003;28:7–11.

52. Ford EC, Mageras GS, Yorke E, et al. Evaluation of respiratory movement during gated radiotherapy using film and electronic portal imaging. Int J Radiat Oncol Biol Phys 2002;52:522–31.

53. Vedam SS, Kini VR, Keall PJ, et al. Quantifying the predictability of diaphragm motion during respiration with a noninvasive external marker. Med Phys 2003;30:505–13.

54. Wagman R, Yorke E, Ford E, et al. Respiratory gating for liver tumors: use in dose escalation. Int J Radiat Oncol Biol Phys 2003;55:659–68.

55. Mageras GS, Yorke E, Rosenzweig K, et al. Fluoroscopic evaluation of diaphragmatic motion reduction with a respiratory gated radiotherapy system. J Appl Clin Med Phys 2001;2:191–200.

56. Ozhasoglu C, Murphy MJ. Issues in respiratory motion compensation during external-beam radiotherapy. Int J Radiat Oncol Biol Phys 2002;52:1389–99.

57. Shimizu S, Shirato H, Ogura S, et al. Detection of lung tumor movement in real-time tumor-tracking radiotherapy. Int J Radiat Oncol Biol Phys 2001;51:304–10.

58. Shirato H, Shimizu S, Kunieda T, et al. Physical aspects of a real-time tumor-tracking system for gated radiotherapy. Int J Radiat Oncol Biol Phys 2000;48:1187–95.

59. Kubo HD, Shapiro EG, Seppi EJ. Potential and role of a prototype amorphous silicon array electronic portal imaging

device in breathing synchronized radiotherapy. Med Phys 1999;26:2410–4.

60. Seiler PG, Blattmann H, Kirsch S, et al. A novel tracking technique for the continuous precise measurement of tumour positions in conformal radiotherapy. Phys Med Biol 2000;45:N103–10.

61. Ramsey CR, Cordrey LL, Oliver AL. A comparison of beam characteristics for gated and nongated clinical x-ray beams. Med Phys 1999;26:2086–91.

62. Wong JW, Sharpe MB, Jaffray DA, et al. The use of active breathing control (ABC) to reduce margin for breathing motion. Int J Radiat Oncol Biol Phys 1999;44:911–9.

63. Stromberg JS, Sharpe MB, Kim LH, et al. Active breathing control (ABC) for Hodgkin's disease: reduction in normal tissue irradiation with deep inspiration and implications for treatment. Int J Radiat Oncol Biol Phys 2000;48:797–806.

64. Remouchamps VM, Letts N, Yan D, et al. Three-dimensional evaluation of intra- and interfraction immobilization of lung and chest wall using active breathing control: a reproducibility study with breast cancer patients. Int J Radiat Oncol Biol Phys 2003;57:968–78.

65. Remouchamps VM, Letts N, Vicini FA, et al. Initial clinical experience with moderate deep-inspiration breath hold using an active breathing control device in the treatment of patients with left-sided breast cancer using external beam radiation therapy. Int J Radiat Oncol Biol Phys 2003;56:704–15.

66. Remouchamps VM, Vicini FA, Sharpe MB, et al. Significant reductions in heart and lung doses using deep inspiration breath hold with active breathing control and intensity-modulated radiation therapy for patients treated with locoregional breast irradiation. Int J Radiat Oncol Biol Phys 2003;55:392–406.

67. Balter JM, Brock KK, Litzenberg DW, et al. Daily targeting of intrahepatic tumors for radiotherapy. Int J Radiat Oncol Biol Phys 2002;52:266–71.

68. Dawson LA, Brock KK, Kazanjian S, et al. The reproducibility of organ position using active breathing control (ABC) during liver radiotherapy. Int J Radiat Oncol Biol Phys 2001;51:1410–21.

69. Webb B. What does robotics offer animal behaviour? Anim Behav 2000;60:545–58.

70. Webb S. Conformal intensity-modulated radiotherapy (IMRT) delivered by robotic linac-conformality versus efficiency of dose delivery. Phys Med Biol 2000;45:1715–30.

71. Adler JR Jr, Chang SD, Murphy MJ Jr, et al. The Cyberknife: a frameless robotic system for radiosurgery. Stereotact Funct Neurosurg 1997;69:124–8.

72. Chang SD, Murphy M, Geis P, et al. Clinical experience with image-guided robotic radiosurgery (the Cyberknife) in the treatment of brain and spinal cord tumors. Neurol Med Chir (Tokyo) 1998;38:780–3.

73. Chang SD, Main W, Martin DP, et al. An analysis of the accuracy of the CyberKnife: a robotic frameless stereotactic radiosurgical system. Neurosurgery 2003;52:140–6.

74. Murphy MJ. Image-guided radiosurgery for the spine and pancreas. Comput Aided Surg 2000;5:278–88.

75. Schweikard A, Glosser G, Bodduluri M, et al. Robotic motion compensation for respiratory movement during radiosurgery. Comput Aided Surg 2000;5:263–77.

76. Murphy MJ. Tracking moving organs in real time. Semin Radiat Oncol 2004;14:91–100.

77. Keall PJ, Kini VR, Vedam SS, et al. Motion adaptive x-ray therapy: a feasibility study. Phys Med Biol 2001;46:1–10.

78. Aruga T, Itami J, Aruga M, et al. Target volume definition for upper abdominal irradiation using CT scans obtained during inhale and exhale phases. Int J Radiat Oncol Biol Phys 2000;48:465–9.

79. Giraud P, De Rycke Y, Dubray B, et al. Conformal radiotherapy (CRT) planning for lung cancer: analysis of intrathoracic organ motion during extreme phases of breathing. Int J Radiat Oncol Biol Phys 2001;51:1081–92.

80. Brock KK, Hollister SJ, Dawson LA, et al. Technical note: creating a four-dimensional model of the liver using finite element analysis. Med Phys 2002;29:1403–5.

81. Yu CX, Jaffray DA, Wong JW. The effects of intra-fraction organ motion on the delivery of dynamic intensity modulation. Phys Med Biol 1998;43:91–104.

82. Kung, JH, Zygmanski P, Choi N, et al. A method of calculating a lung clinical target volume DVH for IMRT with intrafractional motion. Med Phys 2003;30:1103–9.

83. Chui CS, Yorke E, Hong L. The effects of intra-fraction organ motion on the delivery of intensity-modulated field with a multileaf collimator. Med Phys 2003;30:1736–46.

84. Bortfeld T, Jiang SB, Rietzel E. Effects of motion on the total dose distribution. Semin Radiat Oncol 2004;14:41–51.

85. Jiang SB, Pope C, Al Jarrah KM, et al. An experimental investigation on intra-fractional organ motion effects in lung IMRT treatments. Phys Med Biol 2003;48:1773–84.

Chapter 20

BREAST CANCER OVERVIEW

FRANK A. VICINI, MD, DOUGLAS ARTHUR, MD, JOHN WONG, PHD, LARRY KESTIN, MD

In recent years, research in the investigation and clinical application of intensity-modulated radiation therapy (IMRT) for the treatment of all stages of breast cancer has increased throughout the radiation oncology community. The main goal of IMRT in this setting is the delivery of a much more homogeneous and/or conformal treatment plan to the patient. IMRT has the potential to improve target volume coverage compared with that obtained with conventional treatment plans and to reduce inhomogeneities. Perhaps more importantly, IMRT also has the potential to significantly reduce doses delivered to the heart and lung and therefore promises to minimize the risk of complications from treatment in patients receiving comprehensive regional nodal radiation therapy (RT).[1]

Rationale
Breast-Only Treatment

The necessity for IMRT in "breast-only" treatment has been questioned because standard tangential beams have resulted in excellent local control rates, low rates of cardiac and pulmonary complications, and excellent cosmetic results in the vast majority of patients.[2–5] However, it is important to remember that despite these excellent results, standard tangential fields have numerous limitations. First, dose homogeneity throughout the entire breast is difficult to produce because the breast is invariably a nonuniform structure. Typically, dose inhomogeneities are observed with tangents at the entrance and exit points of the beams, in the nipple, and in the superior and inferior portions of the breast. These areas of overdosage can and will produce unnecessary acute and chronic toxicities in many patients. The use of wedges and lung inhomogeneity correction further reduces these dose inhomogeneities; however, a homogeneous dose distribution across the entire breast is difficult to achieve in three dimensions with "unmodulated" tangential beams. In large-breasted women, these dose inhomogeneities can be further exaggerated and may be responsible for the suboptimal cosmetic results frequently observed in such patients.[6]

A second concern with standard tangential fields is that a small amount of the ipsilateral lung is invariably irradiated, and in left-sided patients, a portion of the heart can sometimes be irradiated to significant doses as well. Reducing unnecessary normal tissue radiation exposure is difficult to achieve with standard tangential fields because of the concave geometry of the breast and chest wall. Consequently, compromises in target volume coverage must frequently be made by the treating physician to avoid needless irradiation of normal tissues.

IMRT allows the possibility to reduce unnecessary heart and lung doses. One of the first clinical benefits for IMRT was in the treatment of concave structures, such as the chest wall, which wraps around the lung and the anterior portion of the heart.[7] With IMRT, it is possible to reduce the volume of the lung irradiated to full doses by tangential fields, and in left-sided cases, the heart can also be partially spared.[8]

Several approaches using either physical compensators or IMRT delivery of intensity-modulated beams have been applied to the treatment of the breast alone.[9] One of the first methods of IMRT delivery was the use of a segmental multileaf collimator (sMLC) technique to improve dose inhomogeneity.[10,11] This technique uses several discrete fields of radiation to modulate the composite intensity of the beam across the entire treatment volume. Three-dimensional treatment planning tools and calculations are employed to optimize the multileaf collimator (MLC) segments, producing the desired result. Additional techniques available to calculate areas of dose inhomogeneity throughout the breast include the use of equivalent path-length maps or transit dosimetry information from electronic portal imaging devices.[12,13] Through this iterative process, the addition of MLC segments facilitates the reduction or elimination of either under- or overdosed areas.

Recently, the William Beaumont Hospital (WBH) group reported a method of IMRT for whole-breast treatment.[8,14]

Using this technique, the dose distribution is described by a prescribed dose that is to be delivered to all points within the defined breast volume. Limitations are placed on the volume of tissue that can exceed the prescription. In terms of treatment parameters, the field number, gantry angles, and field size are constrained to match the existing clinical technique. A set of rules is then used to derive a sequence of field apertures, and the weights of these apertures are the free parameters in the optimization. This approach is referred to as "limited parameter set" optimization because the number of free parameters is small compared with so-called pixel-based or fluence map optimizations. Others have referred to this as aperture-based inverse planning or segmental IMRT. These tools are used (along with modern dose calculation algorithms and computed tomography [CT] simulation) to improve on conventional clinical treatment techniques. In addition, this technique employs all of the typical methodologies involved with IMRT, including the application of inverse planning with systematic target dose-volume constraints, consideration of the dose to the adjacent heart and lung tissue, and the use of an objective function.

Using the WBH technique, multileaf segments are designed based on isodose surfaces that result from an open set of tangent fields, with each segment weight optimized using a computerized algorithm. This approach (through an optimized combination of open fields and customized field apertures) allows one to compensate precisely for the changing breast contour, which, in turn, minimizes areas of inhomogeneity, thereby potentially reducing both acute and chronic breast toxicity. Although not primarily designed for this purpose, there is some ability to incorporate dose-volume constraints for other normal tissues, such as the lung and heart, in the optimization process (as needed).

Although several other comprehensive IMRT dosimetric studies for breast-only treatment have been reported in which objective functions of normal tissue complication constraints can direct the optimization process, these systems are quite time-consuming (both in treatment planning and delivery) and are as yet impractical. Groups that have explored IMRT in this setting (breast-only treatment) have included Memorial Sloan-Kettering Cancer Center,[15] the University of North Carolina,[16] and Stanford University.[17] Others have also shown improved dose distributions to the breast using IMRT compared with standard planning.[18] These studies are summarized in Table 20-1.

Clinical Data (Breast-Only Treatment)

The largest clinical experience with breast-only IMRT was recently published by the WBH group.[14] Two hundred eighty-one patients with breast cancer with stage 0, I, and II disease undergoing breast-conserving therapy received whole-breast RT after lumpectomy using the sMLC IMRT technique. The technical and practical aspects of implementing this technique on a large scale in the clinic were analyzed. The clinical outcome of patients treated with this technique was also reviewed.

The median times required for three-dimensional alignment of the tangential fields and dosimetric IMRT planning were 40 and 45 minutes, respectively. The median

TABLE 20-1. Breast-Only Intensity-Modulated Radiation Therapy Techniques

Institution	IMRT Technique Employed	Primary IMRT Planning Method	Significant Dosimetric Findings	Current Clinical Implementation	Clinical Findings
William Beaumont Hospital[14]	Static	MLC fields modulate high-dose areas Inverse planning	↓ Inhomogeneity Improved dose coverage	Yes (281 patients)	↓ Skin reactions
University of Massachusetts[30]	Static	Reduced MLC fields Iterative process	↓ Inhomogeneity	Yes (20 patients)	↓ Skin reactions
Netherlands Cancer Institute[31]	Static	Intensity of pencil beams based on treatment volume	Reduction in cardiac NTCP by > 50%	Anticipated	—
Royal Marsden Hospital[10,12]	Static	EPID used to construct MLC fields	↓ Inhomogeneity	Anticipated	—
Umea University[11]	Static	MLC fields exclude high-dose regions	Improved dose distribution	—	—
Stanford University[17]	Static	Electron beam combined with 4 static IMRT beams	Better dose conformity ↓ Normal tissue dose	—	—
Memorial Sloan-Kettering Cancer Center[32]	Static	Intensity of pencil beams based on treatment volume	Improved homogeneity, reduced dose to heart, lung, and contralateral breast	Yes	—
Memorial Sloan-Kettering Cancer Center[15]	Dynamic	Inverse planning algorithm used	↓ Inhomogeneity Improved dose coverage	—	—

EPID = electronic portal imaging device; IMRT = intensity-modulated radiation therapy; MLC = multileaf collimator; NTCP = normal tissue complication probability.

number of sMLC segments required per patient to meet predefined dose-volume constraints was 6 (range 3–12). The median percentage of the treatment given with open fields (no sMLC segments) was 83% (range 38–96%), and the median treatment time was < 10 minutes. The median volume of breast receiving 105%, 110%, and 115% of the prescribed dose was 11% (range 0–67.6%), 0% (range 0–39%), and 0%, respectively.

Overall, treatment was well tolerated, with 157 patients (56%) experiencing Radiation Therapy Oncology Group (RTOG) grade 0 or 1 acute skin toxicity. One hundred two patients (43%) developed grade 2 acute skin toxicity, and only three patients (1%) experienced grade 3 toxicity. Cosmetic results at 12 months (in 95 evaluable patients) were rated as excellent or good in 94 patients (99%). No skin telangiectasias, significant fibrosis, or persistent breast pain was noted.

Factors predicting an increased risk of acute skin toxicity were analyzed on univariate analysis in a subset of 95 patients (Table 20-2). These factors included race, age, the number of nodes excised, the development of a breast infection, menopausal status, the volume of the breast receiving 105% (V_{105}) and 110% of the prescribed dose (V_{110}), and the administration of chemotherapy. Only V_{105} ($p = .06$) and V_{110} ($p = .05$) were associated with increased skin toxicity on univariate analysis. Of note, both remained significant in the multivariate model. In patients with V_{110} < 200 cc ($n = 59$), the risk of developing grade 2 or 3 acute skin toxicity was 31% versus 61% in patients ($n = 36$) with $V_{110} \geq 200$ cc ($p = .005$).

The authors concluded that the use of intensity modulation using the sMLC technique for tangential breast-only RT was an efficient method for achieving a uniform and standardized dose throughout the whole breast. Strict dose-volume constraints could be readily achieved with the technique, resulting in both uniform coverage of breast tissue and a potential reduction in acute and chronic toxicities. Because the median number of sMLC segments required per patient was only six, treatment time was equivalent to their conventional wedged tangent treatment techniques. As a result, widespread implementation of this technology can be achieved with minimal imposition on clinic resources and time constraints.

At the present time, numerous other groups are also exploring modified versions of this breast-only IMRT technology.[11,12,17] In addition, randomized studies comparing conventional tangential techniques with IMRT for breast-only treatment have been initiated in both Europe and Canada. Data from these trials will be useful in quantifying the need for and benefits of IMRT in this setting.

Regional Nodal IMRT

All of the IMRT studies presented in Table 20-1 have primarily investigated dose distributions in the breast or chest wall only rather than in the breast or chest wall and regional lymphatics. Although improved dose distributions in the breast alone can result in clinical improvements (as discussed above), the need for improved dose distribution with comprehensive locoregional RT is more compelling and challenging.[1,19]

Comprehensive RT often involves treatment to the breast or chest wall and supraclavicular, infraclavicular, and internal mammary nodes, which increases the complexity of treatment planning owing to the convoluted target volume and the proximity of the heart and mediastinum.[19,20] Although three-dimensional treatment planning can improve the dosimetric coverage of this complex target volume and reduce normal tissue irradiation, conventional techniques have not yet been shown to reproducibly achieve target coverage goals in all patients. Recent randomized studies have demonstrated an improvement in overall survival secondary to locoregional RT.[21–23] However, long-term survival using this more comprehensive RT can clearly be compromised by irradiation of the heart.[24] Thus, to maximize survival, comprehensive RT must be fully optimized. To this end, research into the application of IMRT for comprehensive treatment of the breast or chest wall and regional nodes is ongoing. At the present time, this research has been limited to dosimetric studies only.

Cho and colleagues compared IMRT and non-IMRT techniques in the treatment of the left breast and internal mammary nodes and demonstrated superior breast and internal mammary node target coverage.[25] Using a nine-field coplanar IMRT plan, Krueger and colleagues reported improved uniform chest wall coverage using IMRT compared with that achieved with standard tangents while minimizing normal tissue complication probability (NTCP) for cardiac ischemia.[1]

In a subsequent analysis, Krueger and colleagues attempted to develop an IMRT technique for postmastectomy RT that improved target coverage while sparing all appropriate normal tissues using an in-house optimization system.[26] Priority was given to matching the heart doses achieved with partially wide tangent fields (PWTFs) while maintaining 50 Gy ± 5% to the chest wall, internal mammary, and supraclavicular nodes. Other normal tissue doses were

TABLE 20-2. Predictive Factors for Acute Skin Toxicity with Breast-Only Intensity-Modulated Radiation Therapy

Variable	p *Value*
V_{105}	.06
V_{110}	.05
Infection	.14
Race	.44
Chemotherapy	.18
Age (continuous)	.32
Number of nodes excised (continuous)	.16

V_{105} = volume of breast receiving 105% of prescribed dose; V_{110} = volume of breast receiving 110% of prescribed dose.

then minimized. Their results showed that IMRT resulted in more uniform chest wall coverage than PWTFs. The average chest wall minimal dose was 43.7 ± 1.1 Gy for IMRT and 31.2 ± 16.5 Gy for PWTFs ($p = .04$). The average internal mammary node minimal dose was 42.8 ± 2.1 Gy for IMRT and 21.8 ± 13.2 Gy for PWTFs ($p = .001$). IMRT matched the < 1% heart NTCP achieved using PWTFs. The average contralateral breast mean dose was 2.8 ± 1.7 Gy for IMRT, but a greater breast volume was exposed compared with PWTFs. The mean ipsilateral lung NTCP was lower for IMRT (0.0) than for PWTFs (0.07 ± 0.07; $p = .02$). The mean contralateral lung dose was greater for IMRT (5.8 ± 1.8 Gy) than for PWTFs (1.6 ± 0.1 Gy; $p \leq .0001$). Overall, this novel IMRT technique achieved excellent target coverage while maintaining doses to the heart and ipsilateral lung similar to those of conventional techniques. However, contralateral lung and breast volumes were exposed to low doses with IMRT.[26]

Finally, an IMRT planning study performed on only one patient at the University of Wisconsin-Madison demonstrated benefits in breast, internal mammary nodes, left lung, and heart doses compared with a technique using standard tangents matched to a separate mixed-beam field for internal mammary nodal coverage.[1]

At the present time, clinical use of IMRT for comprehensive regional-nodal irradiation remains investigational. The impact of breathing motion and treatment setup uncertainties on the delivery of these more complex treatment fields has not yet been fully evaluated (see below). In addition, the impact of exposing larger volumes of normal tissue (not generally irradiated with conventional techniques) to low radiation doses remains uncertain.

Recently, the WBH group demonstrated how incorporating short breath-holds timed to treatment delivery (using an active breathing control [ABC] device) can also further reduce normal tissue exposure with comprehensive regional nodal RT while improving target volume coverage.[27] Moderate deep inspiration breath-holds were found to displace the heart from the chest wall while aligning the internal mammary nodes with the treatment field.

In their published dosimetric analysis, 15 patients with stage 0–III breast cancer (9 left-sided and 6 right-sided lesions) underwent standard free breathing and ABC CT scans in the treatment position. A dosimetric study was then performed to evaluate the heart- and lung-sparing effects of moderate deep inspiration breath-holds achieved using the ABC device compared with free breathing during treatment. For locoregional RT, the treatment fields used for this study were deep tangent fields designed to cover the breast and chest wall and the internal mammary nodes. The study also compared the deep tangent moderate deep inspiration breath-hold technique with other standard techniques and evaluated the dosimetric effect of IMRT.

First, focusing on the free breathing scans, the nine patients with left-sided lesions were planned with a five-field technique with a standard supraclavicular field matched to a combination of electron fields treating the internal mammary node region and shallow tangents using wedges covering the breast and chest wall (Southwest Oncology Group [SWOG] protocol S9927 technique A). This method was compared with a three-field deep tangent technique with deep tangents covering the breast and the internal mammary nodes matched to a standard supraclavicular field (SWOG S9927 technique B). Compensation with IMRT was then compared with wedges for each technique. In 15 patients studied, dosimetric planning using deep tangents with IMRT was then reoptimized on the moderate deep inspiration breath-hold CT data set for comparison. Dose-volume histograms (DVHs) for the clinical target volume (CTV) (including the internal mammary nodes), planning target volume (PTV), ipsilateral and contralateral breast, and organs at risk were analyzed. In addition, NTCPs for the lung and heart, mean lung doses, and the number of monitor units (MUs) for a 1.8 Gy fraction were compared.

For the nine cases with left-sided lesions, the mean percentage of heart receiving > 30 Gy (heart V_{30}) was lower with the five-field wedged technique than with the deep tangent wedged technique (6.8% and 19.1%, respectively; $p < .004$). For the deep tangent technique, the replacement of wedges with IMRT slightly diminished the mean heart V_{30} to 16.3% ($p < .51$). The introduction of moderate deep inspiration breath-holds to the deep tangent IMRT technique reduced the heart V_{30} by 81% to a mean of 3.1% ($p < .0004$). Compared with five-field IMRT, deep tangent IMRT with moderate deep inspiration breath-holds reduced the heart V_{30} for six of the nine patients, entirely avoiding heart irradiation in two of six patients. For deep tangent IMRT, moderate deep inspiration breath-holds reduced the mean lung dose and NTCP to levels obtained with the five-field IMRT technique. For the 15 patients planned with deep tangent IMRT in free breathing, the use of moderate deep inspiration breath-holds reduced the mean percentage of both lungs receiving more than 20 Gy from 20.4 to 15.2% ($p < .00007$). With deep tangent IMRT, more than 5% of the contralateral breast received more than 10 Gy for six of the nine patients with left-sided lesions in free breathing, three of nine patients in moderate deep inspiration breath-holds, and only one of nine patients planned with five-fields. The mean percentage of the PTV receiving > 55 Gy (110% of the prescribed dose) was 36.4% for five-field wedges, 33.4% for five-field IMRT, 28.7% for deep tangent wedges, 12.5% for deep tangent IMRT, and 18.4% for deep tangent IMRT moderate deep inspiration breath-holds. The CTV remained covered by the 95% isodose in all of the deep tangent plans but one (99.1% of the volume covered). Deep tangent wedges required more MUs than deep tangent IMRT (mean of 645 and 416 MU, respectively; $p < .00004$).

The authors concluded that moderate deep inspiration breath-holds significantly reduced heart and lung doses when deep tangents were used for locoregional breast irradiation including the internal mammary nodes. Compared with shallow tangents matched to an electron field, deep tangents with moderate deep inspiration breath-holds reduced the heart dose (in most patients), resulting in comparable lung toxicity parameters, but potentially increased the dose to the contralateral breast. IMRT also improved dose homogeneity, slightly reduced the dose to the heart, and diminished the number of MUs required.

The same group also recently published their preliminary clinical experience treating patients (to the breast only) with left-sided breast cancer and demonstrated the practical application of this technology.[28] From February through August 2002, five patients with stage I–II left-sided breast cancer received RT to the whole breast using an ABC device. After standard virtual simulation, patients with > 2% of the heart receiving > 30 Gy in free breathing were selected. Patients underwent a training session with the ABC apparatus to determine their ability to comfortably maintain moderate deep inspiration breath-holds at 75% of the maximum inspiration capacity. Three patients received 45 Gy to the whole breast in 25 fractions, and two patients received 50.4 Gy in 28 fractions. For each of the medial and lateral tangential beams, radiation was delivered during two or three breath-hold durations that ranged from 18 to 26 seconds. "Step-and-shoot" intensity modulation was employed to achieve uniform dose distribution.

Comparing treatment plans performed on breath-hold and free-breathing CT scans, ABC treatments achieved a mean absolute reduction of 3.6% in heart V_{30} and 1.5% in the heart NTCP. One hundred thirty-four ABC sessions were performed in the five patients. The average number of breath-holds required per beam direction was 2.5 (four to six per treatment), with a median duration of 22 seconds per breath-hold (range 10–26). Patients tolerated moderate deep inspiration breath-holds well. The median treatment time was 18.2 minutes (range 13–32 minutes), which was progressively shortened with increasing experience.

The authors concluded that a reduction in heart V_{30} can be achieved in patients with left-sided breast cancer using moderate deep inspiration breath-holds assisted with an ABC device. With increasing experience, ABC treatments were streamlined and could be performed within a 15-minute treatment slot. These results suggest that moderate deep inspiration breath-holds using an ABC device may provide one of the most promising methods of improving the efficacy of RT in patients with left-sided breast cancer, particularly when wide tangential beams are employed. The use of moderate deep inspiration breath-holds in combination with IMRT provides the tools needed to optimize homogeneity and normal tissue avoidance when treating the breast and internal mammary nodes. The challenge that

remains is to practically, safely, and reproducibly integrate these technologic improvements of dose delivery into a busy clinic.

Issues and Challenges
Target and Tissue Delineation

Inverse planning IMRT for locoregional treatment requires accurate target and normal tissue delineation. This creates significant problems in a tumor site that traditionally uses clinically defined field borders. Target and normal tissue delineation are critical because the optimization algorithm uses these volumes to generate optimal intensity patterns. For example, an irregular edge in a contour may produce a high-intensity beamlet that increases the dose to a nearby critical structure. As a result, contours must be drawn with meticulous care and increased precision compared with traditional three-dimensional treatment planning.

Adding additional concern is the fact that defining the chest wall or breast is not straightforward, particularly when using CT scans. A reasonable approach in defining the tissues at risk for IMRT planning (for breast-only treatment) is to outline the tissues that would have been irradiated when the clinical borders of tangent fields are applied. This ensures, at a minimum, coverage of the traditional target volume.

In the case of locoregional treatment, accurate target and normal tissue delineation is even more critical. As stated above, target structures have traditionally been clinically defined. However, for IMRT treatment, the supraclavicular fossa, infraclavicular nodes, and internal mammary nodes must now be contoured. Published guidelines for these anatomic boundaries should be used for CT-based contouring.[1] In addition, all adjacent normal tissues traversed by a beam must be contoured for IMRT planning. Contouring the cardiac silhouette is relatively straightforward, although the lungs can be autocontoured in most planning systems. If all normal tissues are not defined and assigned a cost function (see below), excessively high doses may be delivered to these structures in an attempt to attain a clinical goal, such as a minimum target dose. Thus, all normal tissues (eg, great vessels, contralateral breast, bilateral lungs, spinal cord, brachial plexus) need to be outlined very carefully.

Cost Function Specification

Inverse planning requires clinical goals to be expressed in a mathematical term known as the "cost function." (See Chapter 2, "Physics of IMRT," and Chapter 11, "Plan Evaluation") Assuming that this cost function has been defined accurately, the inverse planning algorithm will then iterate to generate the beam parameters that minimize this cost function and produce the specified dose distribution. It cannot be overemphasized that the desired outcome must be accurately expressed for all clinical targets and normal tissues in the irradiated fields. In addition, these objectives must be reasonable so that trade-offs between normal tissue avoidance and target volume coverage can be allowed. Otherwise, the potential advantages of IMRT will not be realized because an impossible set of criteria will be requested and a plan will be aborted (ie, impossible to produce).

A reasonable approach to specify cost functions is to use normal tissue dose tolerances derived from data observed in other organ sites or to use clinically acceptable dose or volume data generated from standard plans or techniques that have resulted in acceptable rates of local control and complications. For example, standard tangents typically deliver between 0.5 and 2.5 Gy to the contralateral breast. Rather than establishing a cost function that specifies zero dose to the opposite breast (a goal that may be impossible to meet if target volume coverage criteria are prioritized), allowing a limited dose to the opposite breast (that has been shown to be safe in clinical practice) may make more sense.

This concept also holds true for doses to the heart and lung. Again, reasonable and achievable dose goals (rather than stipulating zero dose to these structures) should be set using NTCP data or DVHs. In effect, normal tissue complication data or DVH cost functions are used to set the upper limits on the acceptable safe doses that these structures can receive. It is also important to remember that these cost functions will not necessarily specify where the dose is to be deposited within designated critical structures. This is exemplified in the realization that even though a DVH of the heart may look acceptable, the highest dose could be delivered to the most critical part of that structure, creating a dangerous, unacceptable plan. Extreme care must be exercised in the comprehensive evaluation of each plan.

Finally, it must also be remembered that when IMRT is used, radiation may be delivered to normal tissues outside the breast that would typically not have been irradiated. This is particularly true if multiple new beam angles are used.[4] The long-term effect of irradiating these normal tissues remains unknown. Because patients with breast cancer generally experience long survival times, they may be at risk of developing secondary malignancies or other late complications.[29] As a result, the determination of an optimal plan for an individual patient must not be based exclusively on cost function specifications but rather on clinical judgment that balances the potential risks of irradiating soft tissues (some of which may not have been previously irradiated) against the potential benefits of a more homogeneous dose with reduced exposure to normal vital structures.

Future Directions

Owing to the benefits of dose homogeneity and normal tissue avoidance, IMRT may someday become the "gold standard" of RT in patients with breast cancer. Nevertheless, issues regarding treatment delivery accuracy and long-term outcome need to be resolved before IMRT can be applied routinely in the clinic.

The most obvious issue that requires additional evaluation is the adjustments needed to counteract the adverse effects that breathing motion and daily setup variations have on the accuracy of IMRT treatment delivery. This problem is further accentuated when taking into account the rapid dose falloff owing to sharp dose gradients inherent in IMRT planning. For successful widespread adoption of this treatment technique, quality assurance standards need to be in place at each institution to monitor the accuracy and safety of these complex, computer-controlled treatment delivery systems.

Additionally, many questions regarding the risks and benefits of IMRT are yet unanswered. The improvements in dose homogeneity throughout the target volume and restriction of high dose to normal tissue may come at the expense of increased exposure of other normal tissues to lower doses of RT (not previously irradiated), the consequences of which remain uncertain at the present time.[29] Finally, it remains unclear if the dosimetric improvements that can be obtained with IMRT will translate into improvements in clinical outcome. These are some of the many challenges that need to be addressed in future clinical studies.

TABLE 20-3. Reductions in Heart Doses Using the Breath-Hold Technique

Patient No.	Prescribed Dose, Gy	Heart V30, %		% V30 Reduction	Heart NTCP, %		% NTCP Reduction
		FB	BH		FB	BH	
1	50.4	3.6	0.0	100	1.0	0.0	100
2	45.0	3.3	0.6	82	0.8	0.4	50
3	50.4	2.3	0.1	96	0.9	0.0	100
4	45.0	5.9	0.1	98	1.5	0.2	87
5	50.4	9.7	0.1	99	3.9	0.0	100

BH = breath-hold; FB = free breathing; NTCP = normal tissue complication probability; V_{30} = volume of heart receiving 30% of prescribed dose.

References

1. Krueger EA, Fraass BA, Pierce LJ. Clinical aspects of intensity-modulated radiotherapy in the treatment of breast cancer. Semin Radiat Oncol 2002;12:250–9.

2. Potters L, Steinberg M, Wallner P, et al. How one defines intensity-modulated radiation therapy. Int J Radiat Oncol Biol Phys 2003;56:609–10.

3. Glatstein E. The return of the snake oil salesmen. Int J Radiat Oncol Biol Phys 2003;55:561–2.

4. Glatstein E. Intensity-modulated radiation therapy: the inverse, the converse, and the perverse. Semin Radiat Oncol 2002;12:272–81.

5. Clarke DH, Le MG, Sarrazin D, et al. Analysis of local-regional relapses in patients with early breast cancers treated by excision and radiotherapy: experience of the Institut Gustave-Roussy. Int J Radiat Oncol Biol Phys 1985;11:137–45.

6. Gray JR, McCormick B, Cox L, et al. Primary breast irradiation in large-breasted or heavy women: analysis of cosmetic outcome. Int J Radiat Oncol Biol Phys 1991;21:347–54.

7. Bortfeld T. Optimized planning using physical objectives and constraints. Semin Radiat Oncol 1999;9:20–34.

8. Kestin LL, Sharpe MB, Frazier RC, et al. Intensity modulation to improve dose uniformity with tangential breast radiotherapy: initial clinical experience. Int J Radiat Oncol Biol Phys 2000;48:1559–68.

9. Aref A, Thornton D, Youssef E, et al. Dosimetric improvements following 3D planning of tangential breast irradiation. Int J Radiat Oncol Biol Phys 2000;48:1569–74.

10. Evans PM, Donovan EM, Partridge M, et al. The delivery of intensity modulated radiotherapy to the breast using multiple static fields. Radiother Oncol 2000;57:79–89.

11. Zackrisson B, Arevarn M, Karlsson M. Optimized MLC-beam arrangements for tangential breast irradiation. Radiother Oncol 2000;54:209–12.

12. Donovan EM, Johnson U, Shentall G, et al. Evaluation of compensation in breast radiotherapy: a planning study using multiple static fields. Int J Radiat Oncol Biol Phys 2000;46:671–9.

13. van Asselen B, Raaijmakers CP, Hofman P, et al. An improved breast irradiation technique using three-dimensional geometrical information and intensity modulation. Radiother Oncol 2001;58:341–7.

14. Vicini FA, Sharpe M, Kestin L, et al. Optimizing breast cancer treatment efficacy with intensity-modulated radiotherapy. Int J Radiat Oncol Biol Phys 2002;54:1336–44.

15. Hong L, Hunt M, Chui C, et al. Intensity-modulated tangential beam irradiation of the intact breast. Int J Radiat Oncol Biol Phys 1999;44:1155–64.

16. Chang SX, Deschesne KM, Cullip TJ, et al. A comparison of different intensity modulation treatment techniques for tangential breast irradiation. Int J Radiat Oncol Biol Phys 1999;45:1305–14.

17. Li JG, Williams SS, Goffinet DR, et al. Breast-conserving radiation therapy using combined electron and intensity-modulated radiotherapy technique. Radiother Oncol 2000;56:65–71.

18. Landau D, Adams EJ, Webb S, et al. Cardiac avoidance in breast radiotherapy: a comparison of simple shielding techniques with intensity-modulated radiotherapy. Radiother Oncol 2001;60:247–55.

19. Pierce LJ, Butler JB, Martel MK, et al. Postmastectomy radiotherapy of the chest wall: dosimetric comparison of common techniques. Int J Radiat Oncol Biol Phys 2002;52:1220–30.

20. Arthur DW, Arnfield MR, Warwicke LA, et al. Internal mammary node coverage: an investigation of presently accepted techniques. Int J Radiat Oncol Biol Phys 2000;48:139–46.

21. Overgaard M, Hansen PS, Overgaard J, et al. Postoperative radiotherapy in high-risk premenopausal women with breast cancer who receive adjuvant chemotherapy. Danish Breast Cancer Cooperative Group 82b Trial. N Engl J Med 1997;337:949–55.

22. Overgaard M, Jensen MB, Overgaard J, et al. Postoperative radiotherapy in high-risk postmenopausal breast-cancer patients given adjuvant tamoxifen: Danish Breast Cancer Cooperative Group DBCG 82c randomised trial. Lancet 1999;353:1641–8.

23. Ragaz J, Jackson SM, Le N, et al. Adjuvant radiotherapy and chemotherapy in node-positive premenopausal women with breast cancer. N Engl J Med 1997;337:956–62.

24. Favourable and unfavourable effects on long-term survival of radiotherapy for early breast cancer: an overview of the randomised trials. Early Breast Cancer Trialists' Collaborative Group. Lancet 2000;355:1757–70.

25. Cho BC, Hurkmans CW, Damen EM, et al. Intensity modulated versus non-intensity modulated radiotherapy in the treatment of the left breast and upper internal mammary lymph node chain: a comparative planning study. Radiother Oncol 2002;62:127–36.

26. Krueger EA, Fraass BA, McShan DL, et al. Potential gains for irradiation of chest wall and regional nodes with intensity modulated radiotherapy. Int J Radiat Oncol Biol Phys 2003;56:1023–37.

27. Remouchamps VM, Vicini FA, Sharpe MB, et al. Significant reductions in heart and lung doses using deep inspiration breath hold with active breathing control and intensity-modulated radiation therapy for patients treated with locoregional breast irradiation. Int J Radiat Oncol Biol Phys 2003;55:392–406.

28. Remouchamps VM, Letts N, Vicini FA, et al. Initial clinical experience with moderate deep-inspiration breath hold using an active breathing control device in the treatment of patients with left-sided breast cancer using external beam radiation therapy. Int J Radiat Oncol Biol Phys 2003;56:704–15.

29. Hall EJ, Wuu CS. Radiation-induced second cancers: the impact of 3D-CRT and IMRT. Int J Radiat Oncol Biol Phys 2003;56:83–8.

30. Lo YC, Yasuda G, Fitzgerald TJ, et al. Intensity modulation for breast treatment using static multi-leaf collimators. Int J Radiat Oncol Biol Phys 2000;46:187–94.

31. Hurkmans CW, Saarnak AE, Pieters BR, et al. An improved technique for breast cancer irradiation including the locoregional lymph nodes. Int J Radiat Oncol Biol Phys 2000;47:1421–9.

32. Chui CS, Hong L, Hunt M, et al. A simplified intensity modulated radiation therapy technique for the breast. Med Phys 2002;29:522–9.

INTACT BREAST CANCER

CASE STUDY

FRANK A. VICINI, MD, DOUGLAS ARTHUR, MD, JOHN WONG, PhD, LARRY KESTIN, MD

Patient History

A 52-year-old postmenopausal female with no family history of breast cancer underwent a routine screening mammogram and was found to have a suspicious lesion in the upper outer quadrant of her right breast. No breast masses or adenopathy was palpated on physical examination. A needle localization biopsy was performed, which revealed a 2.2 cm infiltrating ductal carcinoma (moderately differentiated) with a minor component of ductal carcinoma in situ. Estrogen and progesterone receptors were negative. No angiolymphatic invasion was seen. The margins of excision were focally involved, both medially and posteriorly. The patient desired breast conservation therapy and underwent a lumpectomy and axillary lymph node dissection, which revealed no residual carcinoma in the breast and 12 negative lymph nodes. A metastatic workup was performed and was negative. The patient's cancer was thus staged as T2N0M0 (stage IIa).

Adjuvant systemic chemotherapy was recommended consisting of four cycles of doxorubicin-based chemotherapy. After the fourth cycle, the patient was referred for postlumpectomy radiation therapy. Owing to the proximity of the lumpectomy cavity to the chest wall, it was elected to use intensity-modulated radiation therapy (IMRT) to (1) provide an efficient method for achieving a uniform and standardized dose throughout the whole breast and (2) help avoid normal tissue irradiation (reducing acute and chronic toxicities).

Simulation

An immobilization device (Alpha Cradle, Smithers Medical Products, Hudson, OH) was fabricated with the patient supine and both of her arms extended above her head. After a planning computed tomography (CT) scan (Tomoscan, Philips Medical Systems, Andover, MA) was acquired, the entrance and exit points of coplanar tangential fields were aligned three-dimensionally on a treatment planning workstation. Field borders were designed to encompass the whole breast using transverse, sagittal, and coronal CT images. The tangent beams were initially aligned so that their deep edges passed through radiopaque markers placed clinically by the physician to define the medial and lateral extent of breast tissue at the time of CT scanning. Beam depth, gantry angle, and collimator angle were adjusted at the computer workstation as needed to (1) avoid unnecessary normal tissue irradiation (eg, heart, lung, humeral head, contralateral breast) and (2) to ensure full coverage of the breast and lumpectomy cavity with a "sufficient" margin (Figure 20.1-1).

Target and Tissue Delineation

Normal tissue volumes used for dose evaluation were generated for the lungs and skin. No attempt was made to delineate the breast tissue per se to avoid the inherent uncertainties in its definition on CT scan slices. Instead, an irradiated volume was identified with the superior and inferior

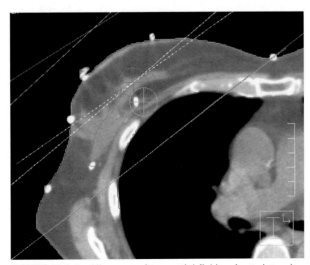

FIGURE 20.1-1. Alignment of tangential fields prior to intensity-modulated radiation therapy planning. (To view a color version of this image, please refer to the CD-ROM).

borders defined by the placement of the superior and inferior edges of the tangent beams. The skin on each axial CT slice was delineated as the superficial boundary, whereas the deep edge of the chest wall and tangential borders of the medial and lateral beams formed the posterior boundary of the irradiated volume, excluding the lung.

Treatment Planning

A dose of 45 Gy was prescribed to the whole breast in 1.8 Gy fractions to be followed by a supplemental boost to the tumor bed of 16 Gy (in 2.0 Gy fractions) using electron beam teletherapy. In terms of treatment parameters, the number of fields, gantry angles, and field size were constrained to match the definition used in a typical clinical technique. A set of rules (see below) was then used to derive a sequence of field apertures, and the weights of these apertures were the free parameters in the optimization. This approach is referred to as "limited parameter set" optimization because the number of free parameters is small compared with so-called pixel-based or fluence map optimizations. Others have referred to this as aperture-based inverse planning or segmental IMRT. These tools were used (along with modern dose calculation algorithms and CT simulation technologies) to improve the conventional clinical treatment technique.

The sequence of static multileaf collimator (sMLC) segments used in the optimization process was generated as follows. Maintaining the same beam orientation above, the dose distribution was initially calculated for equally weighted, open tangential fields (ie, no blocks, no wedges) (Figure 20.1-2). The normalization point was defined at approximately mid-depth and 1 cm superficial to the deep edge of the chest wall in the plane of the central axis of the beams. Regions of

nonuniform dose were delineated by contouring isodose surfaces in 5% increments. These surfaces were modestly smoothed, and the resulting volumes were displayed in the beam's eye view (Figure 20.1-3). From this perspective, the autoblocking utility of the treatment planning software was then used to create discrete multileaf collimator (MLC) segments that conformed to each of the isodose surfaces. In combination with the open field shape, these segments formed a sequence of blocks focusing on thicker portions of the breast sorted in order of decreasing area. The autoblocking utility was used to create an open aperture conforming to the maximal beam's eye view projection of a particular isodose surface. Additional medial and lateral segments were also constructed to conformally avoid lung exposed within the open field, limiting unnecessary dose to lung tissue. Including the open field and lung-block segments, seven sMLC segments were constructed for each tangent beam and made available for dose optimization (Figure 20.3-4). The number of segments could later be reduced to three or four per beam following the optimization step described below. For patients with large breasts (separations > 22 cm), additional 18 MV beams can be used, increasing the total sMLC segments available for each tangent field.

A special "script" (program) was created within the treatment planning system (*Pinnacle*[3], Version 6.2b, Philips Medical Systems) to automate the generation of the MLC segments and the optimization of their relative weights to achieve a uniform dose distribution. Originally, when the sMLC technique was developed, the dose was optimized for 100 reference points distributed randomly throughout

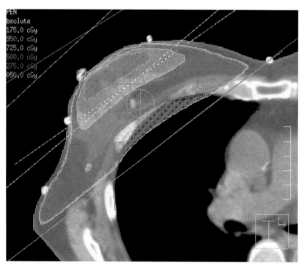

FIGURE 20.1-2. Dose distribution for equally weighted, open tangential fields (ie, no blocks, no wedges). (To view a color version of this image, please refer to the CD-ROM).

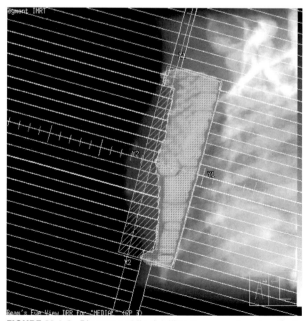

FIGURE 20.1-3. Discrete multileaf collimator segment conforming to the isodose surface. DRR = digitally reconstructed radiograph; IMRT = intensity-modulated radiation therapy. (To view a color version of this image, please refer to the CD-ROM).

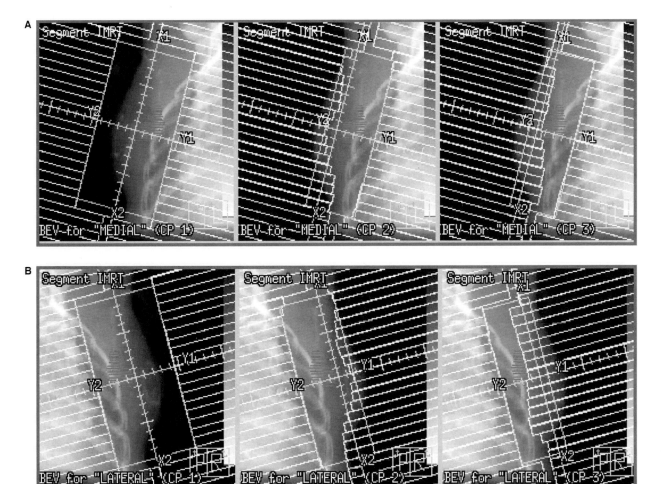

FIGURE 20.1-4. (*A*) Medial multileaf collimator (MLC) segments conforming to the isodose surface in 5% increments. (*B*) Lateral MLC segments conforming to the isodose surface in 5% increments. BEV = beam's eye view; IMRT = intensity-modulated radiation therapy. (To view a color version of this image, please refer to the CD-ROM).

the breast (ie irradiated volume defined above). Using the beam-weight optimization utility of the treatment planning system, the necessary segment weights were derived to deliver the most uniform dose to all of the reference points included in the irradiated volume.[1]

The treatment planning system has been enhanced to permit dose optimization over the entire breast using dose-volume objectives and constraints, obviating the need for the randomly distributed points. The dose-volume histogram (DVH) constraints used with this new system and for this patient were as follows[2]:

- Deliver the prescribed dose (PD) (45 Gy) uniformly and minimize the dose variation
- < 15% of the irradiated volume should receive > 105% of the PD
- < 10% of the irradiated volume should receive > 110% of the PD
- < 5% of the irradiated volume should receive > 115% of the PD

To minimize the number of segments required and to avoid transient start-up fluctuations, sMLC segments

delivering < 4 monitor units (MUs) were initially excluded. With recent enhancements to the IMRT delivery technology, segments with as few as 2 MU are now used routinely (including in this patient).

For the purpose of assessing the quality of the IMRT plan objectively (and to standardize dose delivery), the DVH of the irradiated volume was analyzed prior to finalizing the treatment plan (Figure 20.1-5). If the prescribed dose-volume prescription and objectives could not be met with the initial optimization, higher-energy beams (ie, 18 MV) could be used as needed to help achieve the whole-breast dose-volume constraint recommendations listed above (Figure 20.1-6). After calculating, evaluating, and accepting an IMRT treatment plan, the patient returned for a simulation to verify beam placement.

The times required for three-dimensional alignment of the tangential fields and dosimetric IMRT planning in this patient were 40 and 45 minutes, respectively. The median number of sMLC segments required per patient to meet pre-defined dose-volume constraints with this technique depends on breast size and the use of higher-energy beams. The expe-

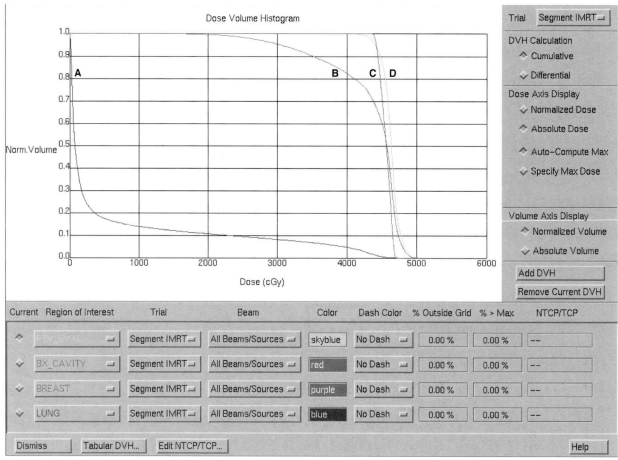

FIGURE 20.1-5. Dose-volume histogram (DVH) analysis of irradiated volume (breast) as analyzed prior to finalizing the treatment plan. IMRT = intensity-modulated radiation therapy; NTCP = normal tissue complication probability; TCP = tissue complication probability; A = lung; B = breast; C = biopsy cavity; D = planning target volume.

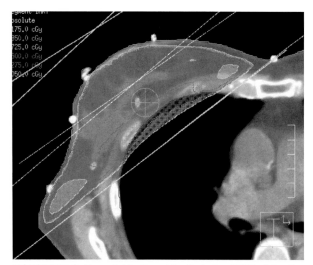

FIGURE 20.1-6. Dose distribution of the final plan. IMRT = intensity-modulated radiation therapy. (To view a color version of this image, please refer to the CD-ROM).

rience from William Beaumont Hospital using this approach can be found in Tables 20.1-1 and 20.1-2. The percentage of the treatment that is generally given with open fields (no sMLC segments) is quite high (60–80%) and also depends

TABLE 20.1-1. Intensity-Modulated Radiation Therapy Parameters versus Breast Volume (William Beaumont Hospital Experience)

Breast Volume,* cc	sMLC Segments, Median	Median Percentage of Treatment with Open Fields	Use of Dual-Energy Photon Beams, Median %
≤ 975 (n = 27)	5	88	11
975–1,600 (n = 34)	6	84	12
≥ 1,600 (n = 34)	8	78	74
All patients (n = 95)	6	83	34

sMLC = static multileaf collimator.
*Breast volume = irradiated volume.

TABLE 20.1-2. Breast Volume Irradiated versus Acute Skin Toxicity %/Cosmesis (William Beaumont Hospital Experience)

Breast Volume, cc	RTOG Acute Skin Toxicity, %			Cosmetic Results, %
	Grade ≤ 1	Grade 2	Grade 3	Good/Excellent
≤ 975 (n = 27)	73	27	0	100
975–1,600 (n = 34)	79	21	0	100
≥ 1,600 (n = 34)	38	59	3	94
All patients (n = 281)	56	43	1	99

RTOG = Radiation Therapy Oncology Group.

heavily on breast size and beam energy. Treatment time to deliver IMRT in this fashion should not be significantly greater than with conventional wedged techniques (< 10 minutes).

Treatment Delivery and Quality Assurance

Treatment was delivered on an SL20 linear accelerator (Elekta Oncology, Crawley, UK) equipped with a 40–leaf-pair MLC. During treatment, placement of the beams was documented and verified daily using an electronic portal imaging device. Previous work with film dosimetry measurements on an anthropomorphic phantom irradiated with the sMLC IMRT technique revealed that dose measurements were within ± 3% of the treatment plan calculations. In addition, 12 patients underwent an active breathing control study to evaluate the impact of respiratory motion on dose delivery. No significant effects of breathing motion were identified using this sMLC technique.

Clinical Outcome

The patient tolerated treatment without significant sequelae. She experienced only minor, diffuse breast erythema after the fourth week of IMRT delivery. She underwent her supplemental boost (16 Gy) to the tumor bed using 12 MeV electrons, bringing the total dose to the tumor bed to 61 Gy. On completion of treatment, only moderate erythema was noted over the lumpectomy site (no dry or moist desquamation developed). At her 6-month follow-up visit, only mild hyperpigmentation was noted.

References

1. Kestin LL, Sharpe MB, Frazier RC, et al. Intensity modulation to improve dose uniformity with tangential breast radiotherapy: initial clinical experience. Int J Radiat Oncol Biol Phys 2000;48:1559–68.
2. Vicini FA, Sharpe M, Kestin L, et al. Optimizing breast cancer treatment efficacy with intensity-modulated radiotherapy. Int J Radiat Oncol Biol Phys 2002;54:1336–44.

Accelerated Concomitant Boost Emerging Technology

Eugene P. Lief, PhD, J. Keith DeWyngaert, PhD,
Stella C. Lymberis, MD, Silvia C. Formenti, MD

Despite level I evidence of efficacy comparable to that of mastectomy,[1–5] breast-conserving therapy (BCT) remains underused in the United States.[6–10] The demands of the standard radiation therapy (RT) schedule most likely play an important role in its underuse.[11] Practically speaking, women who choose BCT must commit to approximately 6 weeks of daily treatments. Not surprisingly, distance from an RT facility plays an important role in women's decision to undergo a mastectomy instead of BCT.[12–16] Overall, 15 to 30% of patients who select BCT, particularly older patients, do not receive postoperative RT.[12,13,17–20]

The major reason underlying the long duration of treatment in these patients is that adjuvant RT is typically delivered in 1.8 to 2.0 Gy daily fractions. Consequently, a total dose of 45 to 50.4 Gy to the whole breast requires 23 to 25 daily office visits. Treatment duration could be significantly reduced by administering larger than conventional fraction sizes using an accelerated (hypofractionated) approach. Such schedules were common in the 1940s and 1950s. Although effective in terms of tumor control, hypofractionated schedules were associated with inferior cosmetic results owing to increased fibrosis and telangiectasias.[21,22] Although more recent data have revived interest in this approach,[23–25] significant concerns remain about potential toxicities.

An additional reason for the protracted duration of adjuvant RT in breast cancer is the delivery of a tumor bed boost following whole-breast treatment. Although only 10 to 16 Gy is prescribed, this adds 5 to 8 fractions to the overall treatment. Two modern randomized trials, however, have shown that the tumor boost is an important component of BCT.[26,27]

Intensity-modulated radiation therapy (IMRT) may provide a means of shortening the overall duration of adjuvant RT in patients with breast cancer. Compared with conventional approaches, IMRT improves dose homogeneity and normal tissue sparing in patients with breast cancer,[28–33] thus allowing the issue of accelerated fractionation to be revisited. Moreover, IMRT provides the ability to deliver a tumor bed boost during whole-breast treatment via a simultaneous integrated boost (SIB).[34] Combining an accelerated fractionation schedule together with an SIB, an approach known as accelerated concomitant boost IMRT, significantly shortens overall treatment time without potentially adversely impacting on local control or cosmesis. Such an approach could markedly reduce the demands of BCT and increase the use of adjuvant RT in patients with breast cancer.

The purpose of this chapter is to provide an overview of the accelerated concomitant boost approach as developed at New York University (NYU) Hospital. Technical issues and early clinical results are presented.

Accelerated Concomitant Boost IMRT

Several investigators are exploring the accelerated concomitant boost approach in early-stage breast cancer. Krueger and colleagues at the University of Michigan described a technique using cone intensity-modulated radiation therapy.[35] Beamlet IMRT plans (cone IMRT) were generated using five anterior oblique beams arranged in a cone shape. Optimization goals included delivery of 46 Gy to the breast, with 60 Gy to the lumpectomy bed, resulting in 23 daily fractions over 4.5 weeks.[35–37]

A technique proposed by investigators at Stanford University consisted of multiple-segment RT for concurrent breast boost treatment using a manual forward planning and step-and-shoot delivery.[36] A dose of 50.4 Gy is prescribed to the entire target volume with a concurrent boost dose of 18 Gy to the tumor bed. After setting up standard opposed wedged tangential fields, an additional multileaf collimator (MLC) segment is added to one or both beams boosting the surgical region. In some cases, more segments are added to improve homogeneity. Additional segments are added if necessary to reduce the dose to the ipsilateral lung and heart. The static MLC files are exported and concatenated to form a step-and-shoot delivery file.

Song and colleagues showed better uniformity in the target with a significant dose reduction in the ipsilateral lung and heart, as well as reduced target volume receiving high doses.[36]

Teh and colleagues at Baylor College of Medicine reported their experience of IMRT with a simultaneous modulated accelerated radiation therapy (SMART) boost in patients with pectus excavatum.[37] Forty-five Gy was prescribed to the whole breast, whereas 50 Gy was given to the tumor bed using a SMART boost in 25 fractions over 5 weeks. Treatment was delivered with multiple small fields in a 270° arc around the patient. With IMRT, a smaller volume of the ipsilateral lung received doses above the tolerance threshold of 15 Gy compared with that of a conventional plan. However, with IMRT, a larger volume of surrounding normal tissues (heart, spinal cord, and contralateral breast and lung) received low doses. The authors demonstrated that the SMART boost was feasible, allowing a mean dose of 57 Gy to be delivered to the tumor bed, simultaneously, during treatment of the whole breast.

NYU Hospital Approach

In contrast to the above techniques, the accelerated concomitant boost technique developed at NYU Hospital delivers treatment in a significantly shorter interval.[38] Patients treated with this approach at our institution are enrolled in an in-house clinical trial with appropriate informed consent. A dose of 40.5 Gy in 2.7 Gy fractions is delivered to the whole breast combined with an SIB (total dose 48 Gy in 3.2 Gy daily fractions). The entire treatment is thus completed in 15 fractions over 3 weeks. This dose is chosen to achieve a dose that is biologically equivalent to that of standard fractionation.[39]

Patient Selection

Eligibility criteria include patients with stage I–II cancer in whom postlumpectomy breast RT is recommended. Patients must have biopsy-proven invasive breast cancer, excised with negative margins of at least 1 mm, and have undergone either sentinel node biopsy or axillary node dissection. Excluded from the trial are women with more than three involved axillary nodes requiring axillary RT and patients with connective tissue disorders, such as lupus or scleroderma. Study end points are safety, feasibility, and local recurrence.

Simulation and Treatment Planning

Patients treated in this study are placed in the prone position on a dedicated treatment table for computed tomography (CT) planning and treatment (Figure 20.2-1). Experience derived from our previous work in partial breast RT has justified the merging of IMRT with prone positioning, with the aim of optimally sparing heart and lung tissue. Additionally, our study of three-dimensional conformal external beam RT for accelerated partial breast irradiation has provided us with experience in prone breast RT.[40,41] Several advantages are associated with this approach. For instance, prone positioning considerably reduces breathing motion, limiting the excursion of the chest wall to less than 5 mm.[18,19] Using our triangulation positioning technique, the breast tissue remains a predictably fixed target. In addition, prone positioning allows for a reduction of lung and heart tissue within the treatment fields. The sparing of heart and lung is particularly relevant in view of the growing evidence of the late morbidities that these organs derive from breast irradiation in the supine position.[42–45] Moreover, in women with pendulous and/or large-size

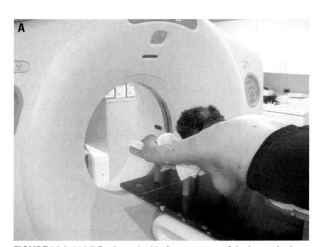
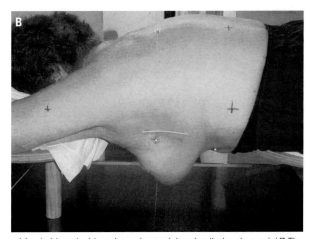

FIGURE 20.2-1. (*A*) Dedicated table for treatment of the breast in the prone position (with and without intensity-modulated radiation therapy). (*B*) The table design provides clearance for two or three beams coming from different directions. (To view a color version of this image, please refer to the CD-ROM.)

breasts, treatment in the prone position allows the breast tissue to fall away from the chest wall, preventing skin desquamation along the inframammary fold, a common occurrence when the patient is treated supine.

Our dedicated table has an aperture opened to the side, allowing the breast to fall away from the chest wall.[18] Patient positioning on the table is established by two lateral lasers and an overhead laser. Noncontrast CT images are acquired at 3.75 mm–thick intervals from the level of the mandible to below the diaphragm using a GE Light Speed helical CT scanner (GE Medical Systems, Waukasha, WI). CT images are transferred to a Varian *Eclipse/Cadplan* treatment planning system (Varian Medical Systems, Palo Alto, CA). The surgical cavity, identified as the area of architectural distortion in the breast tissue, defines the clinical target volume (CTV_{cav}) (Figure 20.2-2). When necessary, information is obtained from the surgical report, mammography, and other imaging. Although not intentionally included within the CTV_{cav}, the surgical incision is outlined with the aid of a wire placed over the incision.

A 1 cm margin is added to the CTV_{cav} to generate the planning target volume (PTV_{cav}). Following uniform expansion, PTV_{cav} is limited anteriorly by the 5 mm buildup region under the skin and posteriorly by the chest wall. The ipsilateral lung and heart are also outlined. The ipsilateral breast tissue volume is defined by applying radiopaque wires to the patient in the supine position, at the site of the medial, lateral inferior, and superior borders of classic opposed tangent breast fields, defining the volume that would have been treated by classic whole-breast tangents in the supine position (Figure 20.2-3). These wires are placed at midline, 2 cm below the breast fold inferiorly,

below the head of the clavicle, superiorly, and 2 cm lateral to the breast tissue to define the ipsilateral breast. The ipsilateral breast tissue volume is outlined on CT based on these markers, encompassing breast tissue to the skin anteriorly and the anterior chest wall posteriorly.

Spatial Beam Arrangements and Optimization

Prone accelerated concomitant boost IMRT was performed using either two coplanar or three to four noncoplanar fields. Often the physical constraints of the setup, coupled with the dosimetric constraints of limiting "dose dumping" to normal tissue, lead to the use of the more familiar two-field arrangement. An anterior oblique field is always coupled with either one or two posterior oblique fields. The isocenter is located approximately 4 cm lateral of midline, close to the chest wall. This location provides enough clearance for unobstructed rotation of the linear accelerator.

General constraints for beam geometry include the physical limitations imposed by the couch rotation in relation to the gantry and the dosimetric constraints imposed by increased path length and avoidance of structures. When using two posterior oblique fields (the three-field technique), a couch rotation of 20° to 30° is employed for each field to reduce the high-dose region (PTV_{cav}) overlap. This results in a 40° to 50° hinge angle between these two posterior fields. Further increasing the hinge angle between the posterior oblique fields increases the volume of normal tissue within the irradiation fields. The largest hinge angle is selected, which prevents the interception of the superior oblique with the ipsilateral arm and inferior oblique with the mandible in those cases in which the mandible extends below the plane of the treatment table.

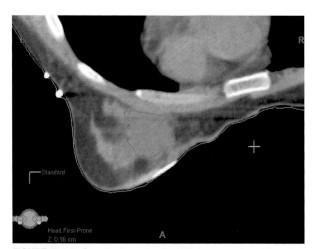

FIGURE 20.2-2. Computed tomography (CT) demonstration of the tumor bed cavity. The clinical target volume (CTV_{cav}) location is defined by the surgical cavity encompassed by the red contour in the left breast. The lateral fiducial marker of the isocenter is imaged as a larger (more anterior) round white spot, whereas the smaller white spot is a wire indicating the lateral border. A wire placed over the scar may also be seen on the medial side of the breast. (To view a color version of this image, please refer to the CD-ROM.)

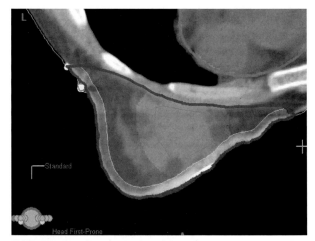

FIGURE 20.2-3. Characterization of the volumes used in optimization. Planning target volume (PTV_{cav} (equal to clinical target volume (CTV_{cav} + 1 cm margin in the residual breast region) is shown in orange, the heart and arteries are shown in pink, the lateral isocenter fiducial is shown in magenta, and the residual breast volume is shown in light blue. The shaded yellow area represents the buildup region, which is subtracted from the ipsilateral breast volume. (To view a color version of this image, please refer to the CD-ROM.)

An "opposed" pair of tangents can also be used to produce adequate dose coverage of the breast and boost volume. Because the breast hangs freely below the table, the separation of the breast along the beam path is reduced compared with the supine position. If the tumor bed is situated far enough from the chest wall, it will be located in this narrow, hanging region of the breast. Consequently, the amount of non-PTV$_{cav}$ breast tissue included in the shadow of the PTV$_{cav}$ for each beam is reduced. In these instances, the three-field noncoplanar geometry loses much of its dosimetric advantage over a more standard two-field arrangement.

Planning is performed using *Helios* inverse planning software (Varian Medical Systems). First, the ipsilateral breast volume is outlined by a physician as described previously (see the blue contour shown in Figure 20.2-3). To determine the volume of breast outside the PTV$_{cav}$, which can be used for optimization purposes, the ipsilateral breast volume has to be manipulated in two steps. The first step accounts for the dose buildup region, and the second step is used to subtract the PTV$_{cav}$.

Initally, we subtract a 5 mm layer of skin and subcutaneous tissue (the subtracted volume is shown in yellow in Figure 20.2-3) from the ipsilateral breast volume. This is done to exclude the buildup region from the volume in which the dose distribution is being optimized. Because intensity-modulated x-rays, like conventional open beams, deposit inherently lower doses in the buildup region, it is impossible to achieve the desired dose distribution in this region. Although some treatment planning systems, to eliminate potential instability of the optimization results, ignore the buildup effects, we have followed this approach[32] to exclude the problematic region from the optimized volume.

Next, we subtract PTV$_{cav}$ (shown as the orange area in Figure 20.2-3) from the volume obtained after the first step to obtain the final volume required for optimization. The remaining domain is defined as the residual breast tissue volume (shown as the light blue shaded area in Figure 20.2-3). This subtraction simply reflects the fact that in the process of optimization, we need to satisfy two different objectives: the PTV$_{cav}$ receives 48 Gy, whereas the residual breast receives 40.5 Gy. Certainly, these two objectives could not be completely achieved simultaneously using a restricted number of beams.

For the optimization procedure, we define two pairs of constraints signifying the upper and lower dose limits for the residual breast and PTV$_{cav}$, respectively. In addition to the previous dose objectives, we require two additional constraints. First, < 30% of the residual breast volume receives 105% of the prescription dose (40.5 Gy), and, second, the maximum dose within the PTV$_{cav}$ volume (as well as within the residual breast) should be kept below 52 Gy. We have learned that our ability to satisfy the first constraint was dependent on the volume and location of the PTV$_{cav}$. The prone treatment technique is, by design, favorable for sparing lung and heart tissues. A dose constraint

limiting the volume receiving 18 Gy and more to 5% of the total organ volume is applied to the heart and lung. After optimization, we arrive at a dose distribution similar to the one shown in Figure 20.2-4.

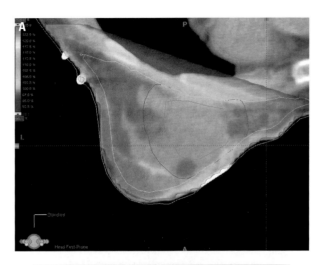

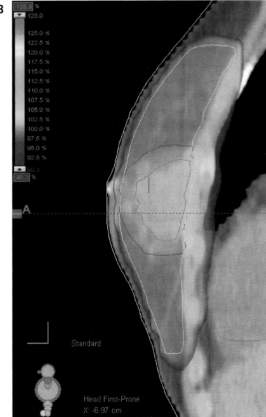

FIGURE 20.2-4. (*A*) Dose distribution in a transverse section. Owing to the limited number of beams, the dose in this plane to the residual breast at the level of planning target volume (PTV)$_{cav}$ is comparable to the boost dose. (*B*) Dose distribution in the sagittal section. Because the sagittal plane is almost perpendicular to the beam direction, the dose in the residual breast is much more homogeneous than in the transverse section shown in (*A*). (To view a color version of this image, please refer to the CD-ROM.)

The fluence patterns are subsequently converted to a leaf sequence using a sliding window technique (dynamic multileaf collimation). Despite the dose constraints provided during optimization, small regions of high dose are detected after this procedure. The field fluence pattern most responsible for the high-dose region is manually edited to reduce the dose to that volume. Similarly, additional editing of the fluence pattern is required to extend dose coverage to the first 5 mm of the breast volume that was purposely excluded from the optimization and to generate skin flash to account for setup variations. A skin flash tool included within the treatment planning software is used to extend the fluence 2.5 cm beyond the skin.

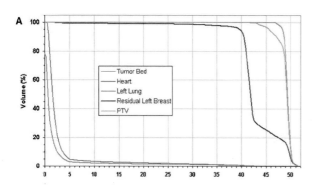

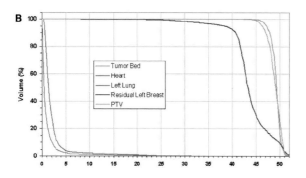

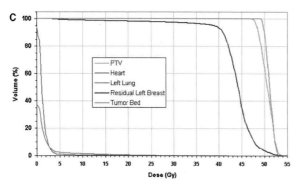

FIGURE 20.2-5. Dose-volume histograms for patients planned using (*A*), two fields; (*B*) three fields; and (*C*), four fields.

Dosimetric Considerations

From a physics prospective, the problem of placing a high-dose target within a low-dose target cannot be perfectly solved using a finite number of beams. Under these conditions, if the coverage of the tumor bed is not compromised, there will be regions of the residual breast, surrounding the boost area, that receive a higher dose than desired (Figure 20.2-5). Naturally, with an increased number of beams coming from different directions, one can spread and "dilute" high-dose regions in parts of intact breast, adjacent to the tumor bed. At the same time, there is virtually no dose to the contralateral breast, lung, and other normal tissues.

For our patients, IMRT with three to four beams compared with two beams achieved better coverage of the tumor bed (Figure 20.2-6A) at the expense of the residual breast tissue receiving a higher dose (Figure 20.2-6B). As shown in Figure 20.2-6C, for all field arrangements, ~ 50% of the residual breast volume received an average dose about 10% higher than prescribed. At the same time, 10 to 20% of the breast volume received a dose comparable to the boost area (see Figure 20.2-6C). Generally, it is easier to achieve better tumor bed coverage if the residual breast volume is overdosed, and, vice versa, it is easier to restrict the dose to the residual breast at the expense of dose homogeneity in the boost area.

To evaluate the relationship between optimal tumor bed coverage and residual breast high-dose regions, we studied the correlation between the dose delivered to 95% of the volume (D_{95}) of the boost compared to the volume receiving 120% of the dose (V_{120}) of the residual breast (Figure 20.2-7A). As mentioned earlier, the ideal coverage, indicated by the red triangle, cannot be achieved using a restricted number of either conventional or IMRT beams. Therefore, the distance between the point, corresponding to the dose distribution for a particular patient, and the red triangle provides a measure of the plan quality. Although preliminary, the data suggest that there is improved homogeneity using a larger number of beams. We also examined the correlation between the volume of the high-dose region (V_{120}) in the residual breast and the total volume of the breast. As shown in Figure 20.2-7B, the two values appear to be approximately directly proportional.

The use of the prone position for IMRT reduces the dose delivered to 5% of the volume (D_5) to the heart by half compared with supine IMRT techniques[27] and about four times compared with conventional supine treatments. With the proposed method, the dose to the heart is about two times larger for treatments of the left breast than for the right breast; however, overall, the D_5 of the heart was consistently below 6 Gy. Precautions taken in the beam arrangements for left-sided breast treatment to minimize the heart dose also lead to reduced ipsilateral lung dose.

Dose Delivery and Quality Assurance

A

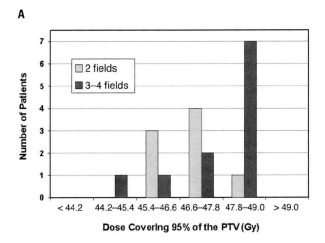

B

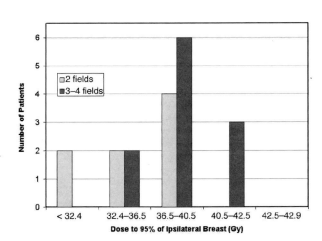

C

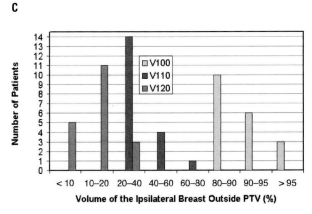

Intensity-modulated beams are produced using a Millennium-120 dynamic MLC (Varian Medical Systems). The leaf width is 0.5 cm in the center of the field (± 10 cm from the central axis) and 1 cm at the periphery. The maximum field length of 40 cm is sufficient for most patients. A limitation of this MLC is that 15 cm is the maximum width of the intensity-modulated fields that can be achieved without breaking the field in two or more subfields. This

A

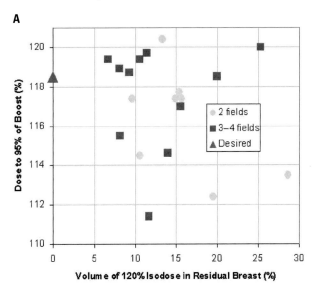

B

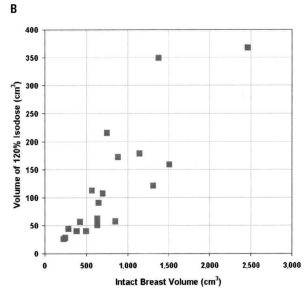

FIGURE 20.2-6. (*A*) Dose to the boost area with IMRT using two-field and multifield setups. The dose prescribed to the planning volume (PTV)$_{cav}$ is 48 Gy, or 118.5% of the prescription dose for the ipsilateral breast outside the PTV$_{cav}$. (*B*) Dose to the ipsilateral breast tissue outside the PTV$_{cav}$. (*C*) Prescription-dose and high-dose regions in the ipsilateral breast tissue outside the PTV$_{cav}$. V$_{100}$ represents the volume covered by 100% of the isodose (40.5 Gy), and, similarly, V$_{110}$ and V$_{120}$ represent volumes covered by 110% and 120% of the isodoses, respectively.

FIGURE 20.2-7. (*A*) Correlation between coverage of the boost area and high-dose regions in the ipsilateral breast. Each point corresponds to a set of parameters for a particular patient. The ideal coverage shown by the red triangle is 48Gy/40.5Gy × 100% = 118.5% dose to the boost area with minimal volume of the high dose in the residual breast. Higher doses in the boost area can be more easily achieved if hot spots in the ipsilateral breast tissue outside the planning target volume (PTV)$_{cav}$ are accepted. (*B*) Correlation between the volume of high-dose regions and the volume of the whole breast. This figure suggests a proportional relationship between the volume of the high-dose region within the breast and the total volume of the breast.

limitation exists because carriages on each side of the MLC allow the difference of the leaf positions only up to 15 cm. If the field has to be wider than 15 cm, the treatment planning system automatically breaks it into two subfields and calculates leaf motion and monitor units accordingly.

For quality assurance, two independent measurements are used. First, the output at the central axis is measured with an ion chamber in a flat solid water phantom. A cylindrical Farmer chamber (Capintec, Inc., Ramsey, NJ) with the volume of 0.6 cc at a depth of 5 cm is used. The treatment field fluence patterns are applied and calculated using the solid water phantom. The mean dose-volume histogram value for the actual size of the chamber is determined and then is compared with the measured reading. These values are expected to be within 2% agreement.

For the second measurement, a planar chamber array is used (MapCHECK, Sun Nuclear Corporation, Melbourne, FL) (Figure 20.2-8). This tool contains 445 diodes in a flat phantom. After the measurements, the software generates an isodose distribution at the depth of measurement (usually 5 cm). This distribution can be compared on a point-by-point basis with the distribution generated by the planning system. All points of measurement are compared with calculation points using typical criteria of 3% agreement of corresponding points or 3 mm distance between the corresponding isodoses. We expect 90% of the points to satisfy these criteria.

Preliminary Data

Since September 2003, 23 patients with stage I ($n = 16$) and stage IIa ($n = 7$) breast cancer entered the study. Nineteen of them have completed treatment on the accelerated concomitant boost IMRT protocol with two to four IMRT fields. Three- and four-beam arrangements used noncoplanar IMRT beams. The average volume of breast treated was 817 cm^3, with a standard deviation of 551 cm^3. For PTV$_{cav}$, the average volume was 138 cm^3, with a standard deviation of 134.2 cm^3. A more detailed dosimetric analysis for these 19 patients is summarized in Table 20.2-1. Current preliminary results support feasibility and suggest reduced acute skin reaction when compared with standard fractionation in the prone position.[45] However, it is too early to assess the efficacy or long-term morbidity of this approach.

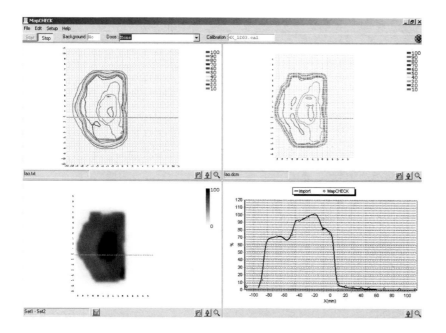

FIGURE 20.2-8. Quality assurance of an intensity-modulated radiation therapy beam with a concomitant boost, using the MapCHECK detector array from Sun Nuclear Corporation. The measured isodose distribution (*top left*) is compared with the one calculated by the treatment planning system (Varian Eclipse) (*top right*). The grayscale view is shown on the bottom left, whereas the bottom right compares the calculated profile (*line*) with measurements (*color circles*). A blue circle shows the dose discrepancy more than 3%. If 90% of the points are within the 3% tolerance, the measured beam passes the quality assurance test. (To view a color version of this image, please refer to the CD-ROM.)

Table 20.2-1. Dosimetric Summary for the First 19 Patients Treated with Accelerated Concomitant Boost IMRT

	Residual Breast Volume Receiving, % Dose					
	100	110	120	125	D$_{95}$ of PTV	D$_{90}$ of PTV
Average, %	89.2	38.6	14.1	4.8	117.1	118.3
Standard deviation, %	5.9	11.5	6.1	3.5	5.4	2.5

D$_{90}$ = dose covering 90% of the volume; D$_{95}$ = dose covering 95% of the volume; PTV = planning target volume.

Acknowledgments

This study was supported by the Department of Defense grant DAMD17-01-1-0345. 2001-2004.

References

1. Veronesi U, Luini A, Galimberti V, et al. Conservation approaches for the management of stage I/II carcinoma of the breast. Milan Cancer Institute Trials. World J Surg 1994;18:70–5.

2. Arriagada R, Le MG, Rochard F, et al. Conservative treatment versus mastectomy in early breast cancer: patterns of failure with 15 years of follow-up data. Institut Gustave-Roussy Breast Cancer Group. J Clin Oncol 1996;14:1558–64.

3. Fisher B, Anderson S, Redmond CK, et al. Reanalysis and results after 12 years of follow-up in a randomized clinical trial comparing total mastectomy with lumpectomy with or without irradiation in the treatment of breast cancer. N Engl J Med 1995;333:1456–61.

4. Jacobson JA, Danforth DN, Cowan KH, et al. Ten-year results of a comparison of conservation with mastectomy in the treatment of stage I and II breast cancer. N Engl J Med 1995;332:907–11.

5. Blichert-Toft M, Rose C, Andersen JA, et al. Danish randomized trial comparing breast conservation therapy with mastectomy: six years of life-table analysis. Danish Breast Cancer Cooperative Group. J Natl Cancer Inst Monogr 1992;19–25.

6. Hokanson P, Seshadri R, Miller KD. Underutilization of breast-conserving therapy in a predominantly rural population: need for improved surgeon and public education. Clin Breast Cancer 2000;1:72–6.

7. Madan AK, Aliabadi-Wahle S, Beech DJ. Age bias: a cause of underutilization of breast conservation treatment. J Cancer Educ 2001;16:29–32.

8. Du X, Freeman JL, Goodwin JS. Information on radiation treatment in patients with breast cancer: the advantages of the linked Medicare and SEER data. Surveillance, Epidemiology and End Results. J Clin Epidemiol 1999;52:463–70.

9. Morrow M, Bucci C, Rademaker A. Medical contraindications are not a major factor in the underutilization of breast conserving therapy. J Am Coll Surg 1998;186:269–74.

10. Fisher B, Ore L. On the underutilization of breast-conserving surgery for the treatment of breast cancer. Ann Oncol 1991;4:96–8.

11. Truong M, Hirsch A, Formenti S. Novel approaches to post-operative radiation therapy as part of breast conserving therapy for early stage breast cancer. Clin Breast Cancer 2003;4:253–63.

12. Ballard-Barbash R, Potosky AL, Harlan LC, et al. Factors associated with surgical and radiation therapy for early stage breast cancer in older women. J Natl Cancer Inst 1996;88:716–26.

13. Farrow DC, Hunt WC, Samet JM. Geographic variation in the treatment of localized breast cancer. N Engl J Med 1992;326:1097–101.

14. Joslyn SA. Racial differences in treatment and survival from early-stage breast carcinoma. Cancer 2002;95:1759–66.

15. Joslyn SA. Geographic differences in treatment of early stage breast cancer. Breast J 1999;5:29–35.

16. Joslyn SA. Radiation therapy and patient age in the survival from early-stage breast cancer. Int J Radiat Oncol Biol Phys 1999;44:821–6.

17. Hebert-Croteau N, Brisson J, Latreille J, et al. Time trends in systemic adjuvant treatment for node-negative breast cancer. J Clin Oncol 1999;17:1458–64.

18. Jozsef G, Luxton G, Formenti SC. Application of radiosurgery principles to a target in the breast: a dosimetric study. Med Phys 2000;27:1005–10.

19. Formenti SC, Rosenstein B, Skinner KA, et al. T1 stage breast cancer: adjuvant hypofractionated conformal radiation therapy to tumor bed in selected postmenopausal breast cancer patients—pilot feasibility study. Radiology 2002;222:171–8.

20. Cuzick J, Stewart H, Rutqvist L, et al. Cause-specific mortality in long-term survivors of breast cancer who participated in trials of radiotherapy. J Clin Oncol 1994;12:447–53.

21. Clark RM, Whelan T, Levine M, et al. Randomized clinical trial of breast irradiation following lumpectomy and axillary dissection for node-negative breast cancer: an update. Ontario Clinical Oncology Group. J Natl Cancer Inst 1996;88:1659–64.

22. Liljegren G, Holmberg L, Bergh J, et al. 10-year results after sector resection with or without postoperative radiotherapy for stage I breast cancer: a randomized trial. J Clin Oncol 1999;17:2326–33.

23. Shelley W, Brundage M, Hayter C, et al. A shorter fractionation schedule for post-lumpectomy breast cancer patients. Int J Radiat Oncol Biol Phys 2000;47:1219–28.

24. Baillet F, Housset M, Maylin C, et al. The use of a specific hypofractionated radiation therapy regimen versus classical fractionation in the treatment of breast cancer: a randomized study of 230 patients. Int J Radiat Oncol Biol Phys 1990;19:1131–3.

25. Whelan T, MacKenzie R, Julian J, et al. Randomized trial of breast irradiation schedules after lumpectomy for women with lymph node-negative breast cancer. J Natl Cancer Inst 2002;94:1143–50.

26. Romestaing P, Lehingue Y, Carrie C, et al. Role of a 10-Gy boost in the conservative treatment of early breast cancer: results of a randomized clinical trial in Lyon, France. J Clin Oncol 1997;15:963–8.

27. Bartelink H, Horiot JC, Poortmans P, et al. Recurrence rates after treatment of breast cancer with standard radiotherapy with or without additional radiation. N Engl J Med 2001;345:1378–87.

28. Lo YC, Yasuda G, Fitzgerald TJ, et al. Intensity modulation for breast treatment using static multi-leaf collimators. Int J Radiat Oncol Biol Phys 2000;46:187–94.

29. Evans PM, Donovan EM, Partridge M, et al. The delivery of intensity modulated radiotherapy to the breast using multiple static fields. Radiother Oncol 2000;57:79–89.

30. Zackrisson B, Arevarn M, Karlsson M. Optimized MLC-beam arrangements for tangential breast irradiation. Radiother Oncol 2000;54:209–12.

31. Li JG, Williams SS, Goffinet DR, et al. Breast-conserving radiation therapy using combined electron and intensity-modulated radiotherapy technique. Radiother Oncol 2000;56:65–71.

32. Hong L, Hunt M, Chui C, et al. Intensity-modulated tangential beam irradiation of the intact breast. Int J Radiat Oncol Biol Phys 1999;44:1155–64.

33. Vicini FA, Sharpe M, Kestin L, et al. Optimizing breast cancer treatment efficacy with intensity-modulated radiotherapy. Int J Radiat Oncol Biol Phys 2002;54:1336–44.

34. Galvin JM, Ezzell G, Eisbruch A, et al. Implementing IMRT in clinical practice: a joint document of the American Society for Therapeutic Radiology and Oncology and the American Association of Physicists in Medicine. Int J Radiat Oncol Biol Phys 2004;58:1616–34.

35. Krueger EA, Coselmon M, Pierce L, et al. Accelerated whole breast radiotherapy with a concomitant boost using a cone IMRT (cIMRT) technique. Int J Radiat Oncol Biol Phys 2003;57:S364.

36. Song Y, Peng P, Boyer AL, et al. Concurrent boost using forward multiple-segment planning and step-and-shoot delivery: a novel technique of breast-conserving radiation therapy. Int J Radiat Oncol Biol Phys 2003;57:S368.

37. Teh BS, Lu HH, Sobremonte S, et al. The potential use of intensity modulated radiotherapy (IMRT) in women with pectus excavatum desiring breast-conserving therapy. Breast J 2001;7:233–9.

38. Lief EP, DeWyngaert J, Formenti SC. IMRT for concomitant boost to the tumor bed for breast cancer radiation therapy. Int J Radiat Oncol Biol Phys 2003;57:S366.

39. Rosenstein BS, Lymberis SC, Formenti SC. Biological comparison of partial breast irradiation protocols. [Submitted]

40. Formenti S, Truong MT, Goldberg JD, et al. Prone accelerated partial breast radiation (P-APBI) after breast conserving surgery: preliminary clinical results and dose volume histogram (DVH) analysis. Int J Radiat Oncol Biol Phys 2004;60:493–504

41. DeWyngaert J, Lymberis SC, MacDonald S, et al. Accelerated IMRT with concomitant boost after breast-conserving therapy (BCT): preliminary clinical results and dose volume histogram (DVH) analysis. Int J Radiat Oncol Biol Phys 2004;60:493–504

42. Paszat LF, Mackillop WJ, Groome PA, et al. Mortality from myocardial infarction after adjuvant radiotherapy for breast cancer in the Surveillance, Epidemiology, and End-Results cancer registries. J Clin Oncol 1998;16:2625–31.

43. Paszat LF, Mackillop WJ, Groome PA, et al. Mortality from myocardial infarction following postlumpectomy radiotherapy for breast cancer: a population-based study in Ontario, Canada. Int J Radiat Oncol Biol Phys 1999;43:755–62.

44. Deutsch MLS, Begovic M, Wieand HS, et al. The incidence of lung carcinoma after surgery for breast carcinoma with and without postoperative radiotherapy. Results of National Surgical Adjuvant Breast and Bowel Project (NSABP) clinical trials B-04 and B-06. Cancer 2003;98:1362–8.

45. Marks LB YX, Zhou S, Prosnitz RG, et al. The impact of irradiated left ventricular volume on the incidence of radiation-induced cardiac perfusion changes. Int J Radiat Oncol Biol Phys 2003;57(2 Suppl):S129.

Real-Time-3D-Video-Guided IMRT Emerging Technology

Shidong Li, PhD, Jason Geng, PhD

Increasing interest is focused on the use of intensity-modulated radiation therapy (IMRT) for the treatment of breast cancer. Numerous investigators have reported the dosimetric benefits of IMRT planning compared with conventional approaches.[1–9] Moreover, preliminary clinical results have been promising and suggest less acute toxicity.[10] However, more patients and longer follow-up are needed to assess its impact on chronic toxicity and patient outcome.

Given the complex fluence patterns produced by IMRT planning software, accurate and reproducible patient positioning is essential for the success of this approach. Currently, patient positioning and verification are based on weekly portal imaging. This approach may be acceptable for conventional radiation therapy (RT) but may not satisfy the patient positioning requirements of IMRT.[11–14] In particular, although portal imaging provides information on internal anatomy, it does not provide information on the position and shape of the breast itself.

Recent developments, including on-line computed tomography (CT) and ultrasound-guided RT techniques, may assist in daily positioning. However, these techniques have not been applied to breast cancer treatment owing to the inefficiency in the large target volume acquisition. Remote video-based patient-positioning systems may potentially be used for breast cancer IMRT.[15,16] Baroni and colleagues described a system based on optoelectronics and close-range photogrammetry that captures in real time the position of a set of passive markers on the patient.[17–20] These marks have been used to monitor and adjust the patient's position by comparing the current positions of the marks with an initial reference position acquired at the time of simulation. However, this technique does not provide three-dimensional (3D) surface information of the breast itself.

In this chapter, a real-time 3D video image–guided IMRT approach is described that addresses the weaknesses of current imaging systems. This system allows the user to capture a 3D surface of the patient with a single video snapshot. Using real-time surface images of the treatment area, one can semiautomatically determine the external beam setup parameters and modify IMRT leaf segments while the patient is on the treatment table. Thus, it is possible to compensate for changes in the surface topology by modifying individual beamlets rather than by adjusting the patient position (as is done in current practice). The real-time-3D-video imaging technique and automatic beam reconfiguration are described below. The results of feasibility tests and the potential for real-time-3D-video-guided IMRT are also discussed.

System Overview

A schematic diagram of the 3D video image–guided approach is shown in Figure 20.3-1. In this system, a CT scan is initially acquired to provide the necessary information for treatment planning. A specific beam configuration is then defined according to the selected treatment technique, and a treatment plan is generated. In addition to the 3D dose distribution, this plan also provides a geometric relationship between the skin marks (beam setup marks and breast outline) and the internal structures (the ipsilateral lung and heart) that can be used for image-guided therapy.

When the patient is placed in the treatment position, a 3D surface image of the breast is acquired using a 3D optic camera that is rigidly mounted on the ceiling of the treatment room and controlled by a computer located outside the treatment vault. The 3D surface image shows the breast and skin marks used for conventional planning (Figure 20.3-2). Hence, one can semiautomatically determine the beam setup parameters by digitizing the beam setup marks and subsequently modify the leaf sequence

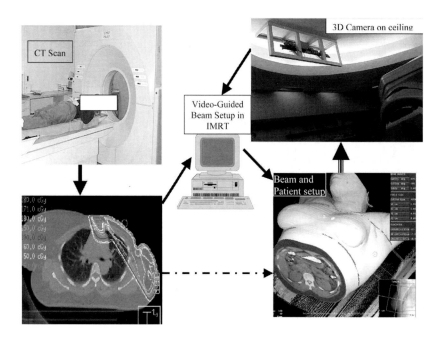

FIGURE 20.3-1. Illustration of the 3D-video-image-guided approach for breast cancer intensity-modulated radiation therapy (IMRT). CT = computed tomography. (To view a color version of this image, please refer to the CD-ROM.)

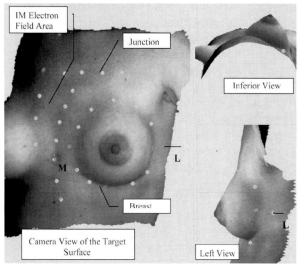

FIGURE 20.3-2. A 3D video image of a left breast showing skin marks used for setting daily (conventional) treatment fields. IM = intensity modulated.

accounting for daily positioning. An additional dose calculation may be performed if the new beams are significantly different from the original beams. However, a complete monitor unit (MU) and dose calculation may not be necessary if the modified beams are not very different (eg, < 5%) from the original beams. The newly defined beam parameters and leaf segments are then transferred to the multileaf collimator and linear accelerator computers via a local area network. An independent computer-aided verification is then performed prior to dose delivery. The entire process, including acquisition of a 3D surface image, subsequent calculation, data transfer, and computerized

dosimetry verification, typically requires 1 to 2 minutes. Therefore, it is possible to use real-time-3D-video image-guided IMRT in a clinical setting.

Video Components

A Rainbow 3D Camera (Genex Technologies, Inc., Kensington, MD) is capable of acquiring full-frame 3D surface images of an object through a single video snapshot.[21–23] The full-frame 3D surface image means that the coordinates (x, y, z) for all visible points on the object surface are provided by a single 3D image. The operating principle of the 3D camera is illustrated in Figure 20.3-3. Point O is the origin of the light source, and P is the pixel position in the image plane within a charged-coupled device (CCD) camera that receives the light reflected by point Q on the object surface. The light projection angle, α, the angle of the reflected light relative to the CCD camera, β, and the length between points O and P uniquely define the triangle, OPQ. The 3D coordinate (x, y, z) of the object surface point Q can be analytically determined through geometric methods. By setting the camera coordinate system origin at the light source, O, and known location of P in the camera coordinate system, one can determine Q (x, y, z) from the following equations:

$$Q = \sqrt{x^2 + y^2 + z^2} = P\,\frac{\sin(\beta)}{\sin(\alpha + \beta)} \tag{1}$$

The difficulty in determining all α angles corresponding to all the visible points on an object's surface was solved by the Rainbow light projection technique shown in Figure 20.3-4. The light projector first generates a fan beam of light with a broad spectrum (white light) that passes through a linear variable wavelength filter (LVWF) to illuminate a

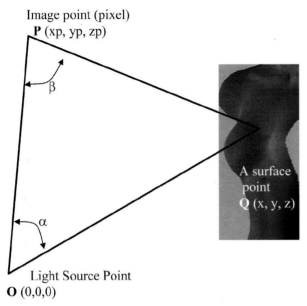

Image point (pixel)
P (xp, yp, zp)

β

α

Light Source Point
O (0,0,0)

A surface
point
Q (x, y, z)

FIGURE 20.3-3. Schematic diagram illustrating the geometry used in the 3D video imaging technique.

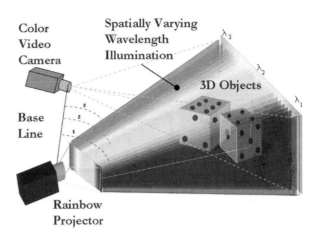

Color Video Camera

Spatially Varying Wavelength Illumination

λ_3

λ_2

3D Objects

λ_1

Base Line

Rainbow Projector

FIGURE 20.3-4. Illustration of the rainbow light projection and reconstruction used by the 3D video camera. (To view a color version of this image, please refer to the CD-ROM.)

3D object with a bundle of light rays with a rainbow-like spectrum distribution. The darker and lighter shadow sheets of light depict light stripes with different wavelengths. Owing to the fixed geometry between the light source, lens, and the LVWF, there exists a one-to-one correspondence between the projection angle α of the plane of light and the wavelength λ of the light ray. The color video camera is used to determine the wavelength (thus the projection angle of α) of the plane of light according to the proportion of its primary color (red, green, and blue components). The geometric arrangement of the CCD camera and coordinates of each pixel on the camera's imaging plane determine the other angle, β. Thus, the 3D surface of a given object can be analytically determined.

Image Registration in the Machine Coordinate System

The 3D surface images captured by the Rainbow camera are defined in the camera's coordinate system, which must then be transformed to the machine coordinate system. A custom-developed template-based calibration is used for the coordinate transformation. This template is a planar surface with two axes and four marks with a known distance, d, from the origin marker. The template is set with its origin at the machine isocenter, and the two axes are aligned with the x and y axes of the machine coordinate system, respectively. This setup ensures that the four marked points are located at $R_1 = (d, 0, 0)N$, $R_2 = (0, -d, 0)N$, $R_3 = (-d, 0, 0)N$, and $R_4 = (0, d, 0)N$ in the machine coordinate system. The camera then captures the 3D image of the template. Three points, $r_1 = (x_1, y_1, z_1)N$, $r_2 = (x_2, y_2, z_2)N$,

and $r_3 = (x_3, y_3, z_3)N$, in the camera coordinate system are identified and digitized. All of the points can then be transformed into the machine coordinate system as

$$\begin{bmatrix} a_{11} & a_{12} & a_{13} & t_x \\ a_{21} & a_{22} & a_{23} & t_y \\ a_{31} & a_{32} & a_{33} & t_z \\ 0 & 0 & 0 & 1 \end{bmatrix} \begin{bmatrix} x_i \\ y_i \\ z_i \\ 1 \end{bmatrix} = \begin{bmatrix} X_i \\ Y_i \\ Z_i \\ 1 \end{bmatrix}$$

(2)

The upper left 3 by 3 submatrix is the 3D rotation matrix and $T = (t_x, t_y, t_z)N$ is the translation vector. By setting the rotation pivot at the origin of the machine coordinate system, one can determine $T = (r_1 + r_3)/2$. The rotation matrix with nine unknown variables can then be uniquely determined from the nine linear equations for the three specific points.

The determined transformation matrix is stored as the camera calibration transformation file for the patient setup with no table rotation. Application of this calibration transformation to the treatment image (without table rotation) will transform the image to the room coordinate system automatically. However, in certain clinical situations, for example, left breast cancer treatment, it is desirable to rotate the treatment table by 90° to capture the anterior and lateral surfaces of the breast and chest wall. In this case, the same template setup is used, and the table is rotated by 90°. A second template image is then captured, and the three points are digitized to generate the coordinate transformation matrix with a table rotation of 90°. The resultant coordinate transformations have an accuracy of ~ 0.5 mm.

Automatic Field Setup According to the 3D Surface Image

In conventional tangential field techniques, the chest wall plane is usually defined by the medial sternum slope, measured by the average sternum angle from the horizontal plane, and the entry slope, given by the two beam-edge entrances.[24–31] Using the 3D surface images, the chest wall plane is defined through the midpoint between the medial entrance, M, lateral entrance, L, and multiple points that outline the medial edge of the irradiated area, E_i. Then the normal vector to the chest wall plane is defined as follows:

$$\mathbf{n}_c = \eta \cdot \mathrm{midial}\left\{ \begin{array}{l} \dfrac{(\mathbf{M}-\mathbf{L})\times(\mathbf{E}_i-\mathbf{L})}{|(\mathbf{M}-\mathbf{L})\times(\mathbf{E}_i-\mathbf{L})|} \,\Big|\, \forall \mathbf{E}_i \in \text{med - upper edge} \\ \dfrac{(\mathbf{M}-\mathbf{L})\times(\mathbf{E}_i-\mathbf{L})}{|(\mathbf{M}-\mathbf{L})\times(\mathbf{E}_i-\mathbf{L})|} \,\Big|\, \forall \mathbf{E}_i \in \text{med - lower edge} \end{array} \right\} \qquad (3)$$

where the η is equal to +1 or −1 for the right or left breast, respectively. The normal vector n_c of the chest wall plane is always pointing to the anterior-lateral direction. The distance from each 3D data point r_i to the chest wall plane can then be calculated. The maximum distance over all data points gives us the height of the breast relative to the chest wall plane as follows:

$$\mathbf{H} = \max\{(\mathbf{r}_i - \mathbf{M})\cdot\mathbf{n} \;|\; \forall\, \mathbf{r}_i \in \text{target}\} \qquad (4)$$

The treatment isocenter is placed in the plane bisecting the line segment of M to L and at a distance H/2 normal to the chest wall plane as

$$\mathbf{ISO} = \frac{1}{2}(\mathbf{M}+\mathbf{L}) + \frac{1}{2}\mathbf{H}\cdot\mathbf{n} \qquad (5)$$

Isocenter setup is performed by initially positioning the patient on the treatment table and acquiring a video image. At this time, the patient is positioned such that the isocenter is located at the medial entrance point, M. Using the video image and equations 3 to 5, the treatment table is then moved according to the 3D vector (ISO – M). Note that this isocenter setup is different from the current field setup that is restricted to the transverse plane.

Image-Guided IMRT

Consider an IMRT breast treatment plan based on opposed tangential beams. Each field is divided into beamlets with different intensity levels. Figure 20.3-5A illustrates an intensity map (with 10 levels) for a tangential IMRT field with the beamlet size of 0.5 × 0.5 cm^2. This plan was designed to provide a uniform dose to the breast. Thus, each intensity level is proportional to the breast separation along a given beamlet. The goal of our approach is to use the real-time video images to adjust the intensity levels based on the position and shape of the breast at the time of treatment.

The algorithm for adjusting the intensity levels is as follows. Using the previously described approach, in conjunction with the real-time surface image of the breast, the isocenter and beam parameters for a given treatment day are determined. Next, the pathlength for each beamlet is

A

9	9	9	8	8	7	7	7	6	5	4	0	0	0	0	0	0	0
9	9	9	8	8	7	7	6	6	5	4	3	0	0	0	0	0	0
9	9	9	8	8	7	7	6	6	5	4	3	2	0	0	0	0	0
9	9	9	8	8	7	7	7	6	6	5	4	2	0	0	0	0	0
9	9	9	8	8	8	7	7	7	6	5	5	4	0	0	0	0	0
9	9	9	8	8	8	7	7	7	6	5	5	4	2	0	0	0	0
8	9	9	8	8	8	7	7	7	6	5	5	4	3	0	0	0	0
8	9	9	8	8	8	7	7	7	6	5	5	4	3	0	0	0	0
8	9	9	8	8	8	7	7	7	6	5	5	4	3	1	0	0	0
8	8	9	8	8	8	7	7	7	6	5	5	4	3	2	0	0	0
8	8	9	8	8	8	7	7	7	6	5	5	4	3	3	0	0	0
8	8	9	8	8	8	7	7	7	6	5	5	4	3	3	0	0	0
8	9	9	8	8	8	7	7	6	6	5	5	4	3	3	0	0	0
8	9	9	8	8	8	7	7	6	6	5	5	4	3	3	3	0	0
8	9	9	8	8	8	7	7	6	6	5	5	4	3	3	3	0	0
8	9	9	8	8	8	7	7	6	6	5	5	4	3	3	3	0	0
8	9	9	8	8	8	7	7	6	6	5	5	4	3	3	0	0	0
8	9	9	8	8	8	7	7	6	6	5	5	4	3	3	0	0	0
9	9	9	8	8	8	7	7	6	6	5	5	4	3	0	0	0	0
9	9	9	8	8	8	7	7	6	6	5	5	3	0	0	0	0	0
9	9	9	8	8	8	7	7	6	6	5	4	2	0	0	0	0	0
9	9	9	8	8	8	7	7	6	6	4	3	0	0	0	0	0	0
9	9	9	8	8	8	7	7	6	6	3	0	0	0	0	0	0	0
9	9	9	8	8	8	7	7	6	3	0	0	0	0	0	0	0	0
9	9	9	8	8	8	7	7	6	3	0	0	0	0	0	0	0	0
9	9	9	8	8	8	7	7	6	0	0	0	0	0	0	0	0	0
9	9	9	8	8	8	7	7	3	0	0	0	0	0	0	0	0	0
9	9	8	8	8	8	7	4		0	0	0	0	0	0	0	0	0

B

0	0	0	0	0	0	0	0	0	0	-2	0	0	0	0	0	0	0
0	0	0	0	0	0	0	0	0	0	-1	0	0	0	0	0	0	0
0	0	0	0	0	0	0	0	0	0	-1	0	0	0	0	0	0	0
0	0	0	0	0	0	0	0	0	0	0	-1	0	0	0	0	0	0
0	0	0	0	0	0	0	0	0	0	0	-2	0	0	0	0	0	0
0	0	0	0	0	0	0	0	0	0	0	0	-1	-1	0	0	0	0
0	0	0	0	0	0	0	0	0	0	0	0	0	-1	0	0	0	0
0	0	0	0	0	0	0	0	0	0	0	0	0	-1	0	0	0	0
0	0	0	0	0	0	0	0	0	0	0	0	0	-1	0	0	0	0
0	0	0	0	0	0	0	0	0	0	0	0	0	-2	-1	0	0	0
0	0	0	0	0	0	0	0	0	0	0	0	0	-1	-1	0	0	0
0	0	0	0	0	0	0	0	0	0	0	0	0	0	-1	0	0	0
0	0	0	0	0	0	0	0	0	0	0	0	0	0	-1	0	0	0
0	0	0	0	0	0	0	0	0	0	0	0	0	0	-1	0	0	0
0	0	0	0	0	0	0	0	0	0	0	0	0	0	1	1	0	0
0	0	0	0	0	0	0	0	0	0	0	0	0	0	1	0	0	0
0	0	0	0	0	0	0	0	0	0	0	0	0	0	1	0	0	0
0	0	0	0	0	0	0	0	0	0	0	0	0	1	0	0	0	0
0	0	0	0	0	0	0	0	0	0	0	0	0	1	0	0	0	0
0	0	0	0	0	0	0	0	0	0	0	0	2	0	0	0	0	0
0	0	0	0	0	0	0	0	0	0	1	2	2	0	0	0	0	0
0	0	0	0	0	0	0	0	1	1	1	2	0	0	0	0	0	0
0	0	0	0	0	0	0	0	1	2	0	0	0	0	0	0	0	0
0	0	0	0	0	0	0	0	1	2	0	0	0	0	0	0	0	0
0	0	0	0	0	0	0	0	2	1	0	0	0	0	0	0	0	0
0	0	0	0	0	0	0	0	2	0	0	0	0	0	0	0	0	0
0	0	0	0	0	0	0	1	0	0	0	0	0	0	0	0	0	0
0	0	0	0	0	0	1	2		0	0	0	0	0	0	0	0	0

C

9	9	9	8	8	7	7	7	6	5	2	0	0	0	0	0	0	0
9	9	9	8	8	7	7	6	6	5	3	3	0	0	0	0	0	0
9	9	9	8	8	7	7	6	6	5	3	3	2	0	0	0	0	0
9	9	9	8	8	7	7	7	6	6	5	5	2	0	0	0	0	0
9	9	9	8	8	8	7	7	7	6	5	5	4	0	0	0	0	0
9	9	9	8	8	8	7	7	7	6	5	5	3	1	0	0	0	0
8	9	9	8	8	8	7	7	7	6	5	5	4	2	0	0	0	0
8	9	9	8	8	8	7	7	7	6	5	5	4	2	0	0	0	0
8	9	9	8	8	8	7	7	7	6	5	5	4	2	1	0	0	0
8	8	9	8	8	8	7	7	7	6	5	5	4	1	1	0	0	0
8	8	9	8	8	8	7	7	7	6	5	5	4	2	2	0	0	0
8	8	9	8	8	8	7	7	7	6	5	5	4	3	2	0	0	0
8	9	9	8	8	8	7	7	6	6	5	5	4	3	2	0	0	0
8	9	9	8	8	8	7	7	6	6	5	5	4	3	2	3	0	0
8	9	9	8	8	8	7	7	6	6	5	5	4	3	4	4	0	0
8	9	9	8	8	8	7	7	6	6	5	5	4	3	4	3	0	0
8	9	9	8	8	8	7	7	6	6	5	5	4	3	4	0	0	0
8	9	9	8	8	8	7	7	6	6	5	5	4	4	3	0	0	0
9	9	9	8	8	8	7	7	6	6	5	5	4	4	0	0	0	0
9	9	9	8	8	8	7	7	6	6	5	5	5	0	0	0	0	0
9	9	9	8	8	8	7	7	6	6	6	6	4	0	0	0	0	0
9	9	9	8	8	8	7	7	6	6	5	5	0	0	0	0	0	0
9	9	9	8	8	8	7	7	7	8	3	0	0	0	0	0	0	0
9	9	9	8	8	8	7	7	7	5	0	0	0	0	0	0	0	0
9	9	9	8	8	8	7	7	8	4	0	0	0	0	0	0	0	0
9	9	9	8	8	8	7	7	8	0	0	0	0	0	0	0	0	0
9	9	9	8	8	8	7	8	3	0	0	0	0	0	0	0	0	0
9	9	8	8	8	8	8	6	0	0	0	0	0	0	0	0	0	0

FIGURE 20.3-5 (*A*) Planned intensity map for a medial tangential intensity-modulated radiation therapy field. (*B*) Equivalent pathlength changes in the medial tangential field based on the 3D patient surface obtained at the time of treatment. (*C*) Image-guided intensity map for the tangential field as a result of a planned intensity map (*A*) plus the equivalent pathlength changes (*B*) for the medial tangential field.

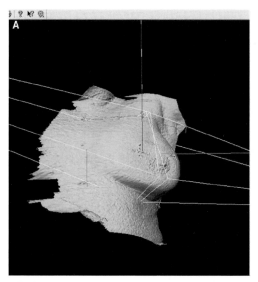
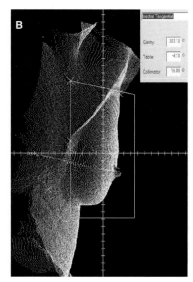
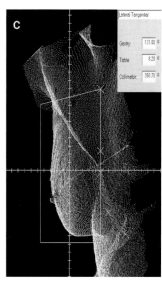

FIGURE 20.3-6. An automatic three-field setup according to the real-time surface image (*A*) and setup marks for the chest wall and junction plan matched on the medial tangential (*B*) and lateral tangential fields (*C*). (To view a color version of this image, please refer to the CD-ROM.)

calculated according to the intersection of the beamlet central ray with the 3D surface image. Subtraction of the real-time pathlength map from the planned beam pathlength map generates the relative increase (positive values) or decrease (negative values) in the depth of each beamlet. The pathlength changes as shown in Figure 20.3-5B can be presented in units of intensity. The planned intensity map (see Figure 20.3-5A) and the pathlength changes (see Figure 20.3-5B) across the field yield the desired intensity distribution, as shown in Figure 20.3-5C. The planned dose distribution would be preserved if the new intensity distribution was delivered. For easy comparison, the same leaf segmentation algorithm as that of the planning system should be used.[32–35] In general, the total segments and MUs should not be significantly different from those of the original planned field after the proper beam angle and isocenter adjustment. For a quick and accurate MU calculation, a modified Clarkson segmental integration can be used.[36,37]

The 3D video imaging–guided IMRT technique has been tested through a series of phantom experiments. The results for simulation of possible movements demonstrated that the accuracy of the surface is within 1 mm in shift and 1° in rotation. The precision of the 3D surface images is within 0.5 mm. The proposed real-time image-based beam adjustment and leaf sequence modification have also been experimentally verified. Figure 20.3-6 illustrates the automatic beam setup and beam's eye view of the medial and lateral tangential fields for the three-field technique according to the real-time video images. All of the setup marks located on the junction line and on the posterior field edges indicated the perfect matching on the junction plane and the chest wall plane. The leaf sequence change is usually small after the modification of the isocenter and beam setup.

The feasibility of this approach has also been evaluated on patients in an institutionally approved clinical trial. The patient 3D surface images shown in Figure 20.3-7 demonstrated that the required 3D information for the target and setup marks is achievable with a single 3D video image. The intensity of the light source can be computer controlled, and the relative intensity from 100 to 220% is used to capture clear surface images for patients with a range of skin tones.

Future Directions

The real-time 3D video-based system can be used to take into account daily setup variation. A very useful extension of this technology is to include real-time monitoring capability for taking into account respiratory motion. Improvements will need to be made to eliminate limitations on the time for image registration, beam calculation,

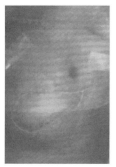
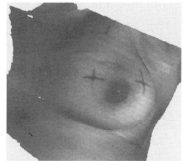

FIGURE 20.3-7. 3D images of two patients that clearly show the surgical (*left*) and beam setup (*right*) marks.

data transfer, and record and verification procedures. The 3D camera technique also needs to improve its calculation time in reconstructing the 3D surfaces to meet the real-time requirements. More importantly, we need to understand the mechanics of breathing and the anatomic relationship between the surface landmarks and internal structures.[38]

A deformable breast model may be useful for the image-guided respiration-gated breast IMRT. Based on careful clinical observations of breast patients at simulation and treatment setup, there appears to be a significant difference between the upper and lower ribs during inspiration and expiration. In general, the breast is located superiorly-inferiorly between the second and seventh ribs and laterally from the border of the sternum to beyond the anterior axillary fold. During respiration, the lung contacts the inner surface of the chest cage. Because of this regular pattern of internal motion, we may be able to use the lower rib motion to predict the entire lung motion. The lower chest wall motion could be monitored through surface images. Subtracting the lung anterior surface from the breast surface could provide the planning target volume and organs at risk during the respiration. The deformable breast model and this respiration model require further investigation.

Acknowledgments

This research is partially supported by a SPORE grant of NIH CA 88843.

References

1. Smitt MC, Li SD, Shostak CA, et al. Breast-conserving radiation therapy: potential of inverse planning with intensity modulation. Radiology 1997;203:871–6.
2. Krueger E, Coselmon M, Pierce L, et al. Accelerated whole breast radiotherapy with a concomitant boost using a cone IMRT (cIMRT) technique. Int J Radiat Oncol Biol Phys 2003;57:S364.
3. Lief EP, DeWyngaert J, Formenti SC. IMRT for concomitant boost to the tumor bed for breast cancer radiation therapy. Int J Radiat Oncol Biol Phys 2003;57:S366.
4. Teh BS, Lu HH, Sobremonte S, et al. The potential use of intensity modulated radiotherapy (IMRT) in women with pectus excavatum desiring breast-conserving therapy. Breast J 2001;7:233–9.
5. Cho BC, Hurkmans CW, Damen EM, et al. Intensity modulated versus non-intensity modulated radiotherapy in the treatment of the left breast and upper internal mammary lymph node chain: a comparative planning study. Radiother Oncol 2002;62:127–36.
6. Hong L, Hunt M, Chui C, et al. Intensity-modulated tangential beam irradiation of the intact breast. Int J Radiat Oncol Biol Phys 1999;44:1155–64.
7. Kestin LL, Sharpe MB, Frazier RC, et al. Intensity modulation to improve dose uniformity with tangential breast radiotherapy: initial clinical experience. Int J Radiat Oncol Biol Phys 2000;48:1559–68.
8. Remouchamps VM, Vicini FA, Sharpe MB, et al. Significant reductions in heart and lung doses using deep inspiration breath hold with active breathing control and intensity-modulated radiation therapy for patients treated with locoregional breast irradiation. Int J Radiat Oncol Biol Phys 2003;55:392–406.
9. Thilmann C, Sroka-Perez G, Krempien R, et al. Inversely planned intensity modulated radiotherapy of the breast including the internal mammary chain: a plan comparison study. Technol Cancer Res Treat 2004;3:69–75.
10. Vicini FA, Sharpe M, Kestin L, et al. Optimizing breast cancer treatment efficacy with intensity-modulated radiotherapy. Int J Radiat Oncol Biol Phys 2002;54:1336–44.
11. Carter DL, Marks LB, Bentel GC. Impact of setup variability on incidental lung irradiation during tangential breast treatment. Int J Radiat Oncol Biol Phys 1997;38:109–15.
12. McGee KP, Fein DA, Hanlon AL, et al. The value of setup portal films as an estimate of a patient's position throughout fractionated tangential breast irradiation: an on-line study. Int J Radiat Oncol Biol Phys 1997;37:223–8.
13. Pouliot J, Lirette A. Verification and correction of setup deviations in tangential breast irradiation using EPID: gain versus workload. Med Phys 1996;23:1393–8.
14. VanAken ML, Breneman JC, Elson HR, et al. Incorporation of patient immobilization, tissue compensation and matchline junction technique for three-field breast treatment. Med Dosim 1988;13:131–5.
15. Johnson LS, Milliken BD, Hadley SW, et al. Initial clinical experience with a video-based patient positioning system. Int J Radiat Oncol Biol Phys 1999;45:205–13.
16. Wilks RJ. An optical system for measuring surface shapes for radiotherapy planning. Br J Radiol 1993;66:351–9.
17. Baroni G, Ferrigno G, Orecchia R, et al. Real-time opto-electronic verification of patient position in breast cancer radiotherapy. Comput Aided Surg 2000;5:296–306.
18. Baroni G, Troia A, Riboldi M, et al. Evaluation of methods for opto-electronic body surface sensing applied to patient position control in breast radiation therapy. Med Biol Eng Comput 2003;41:679–88.
19. Baroni G, Troia A, Troia A, et al. [Opto-electronic techniques and 3D body surface reconstruction for the control of patient positioning in the radiotherapy of breast cancer]. Radiol Med (Torino) 2001;102:168–77.
20. Riboldi M, Baroni G, Orecchia R, et al. Enhanced surface registration techniques for patient positioning control in breast cancer radiotherapy. Technol Cancer Res Treat 2004;3:51–8.
21. Li S, Frassica D, DeWeese T, et al. A real-time image-guided intraoperative high-dose-rate brachytherapy system. Brachytherapy 2003;2:5–16.
22. Geng Z. Rainbow 3D Camera - A New Concept for High Speed and Low-Cost 3D Vision SPIR Journal Optical Engineering 1996;35:376.
23. Galdino GM, Manson PN, Nahabedian M, et al. Three dimensional photography in plastic surgery: clinical applications for breast surgery. Plast Reconstr Surg 2002;110:1–13.

24. Siddon RL, Buck BA, Harris JR, et al. Three-field technique for breast irradiation using tangential field corner blocks. Int J Radiat Oncol Biol Phys 1983;9:583–8.

25. Siddon RL, Tonnesen GL, Svensson GK. Three-field technique for breast treatment using a rotatable half-beam block. Int J Radiat Oncol Biol Phys 1981;7:1473–7.

26. Svensson GK, Bjarngard BE, Larsen RD, et al. A modified three-field technique for breast treatment. Int J Radiat Oncol Biol Phys 1980;6:689–94.

27. Chu JC, Solin LJ, Hwang CC, et al. A nondivergent three field matching technique for breast irradiation. Int J Radiat Oncol Biol Phys 1990;19:1037–40.

28. Butker EK, Helton DJ, Keller JW, et al. A totally integrated simulation technique for three-field breast treatment using a CT simulator. Med Phys 1996;23:1809–14.

29. Jansson T, Lindman H, Nygard K, et al. Radiotherapy of breast cancer after breast-conserving surgery: an improved technique using mixed electron-photon beams with a multileaf collimator. Radiother Oncol 1998;46:83–9.

30. Rosenow UF, Valentine ES, Davis LW. A technique for treating local breast cancer using a single set-up point and asymmetric collimation. Int J Radiat Oncol Biol Phys 1990;19:183–8.

31. Lu XQ, Sullivan S, Eggleston T, et al. A three-field breast treatment technique with precise geometric matching using multileaf collimator-equipped linear accelerators. Int J Radiat Oncol Biol Phys 2003;55:1420–31.

32. Geis P, Boyer AL, Wells NH. Use of a multileaf collimator as a dynamic missing-tissue compensator. Med Phys 1996;23:1199–205.

33. Bortfeld TR, Kahler DL, Waldron TJ, et al. X-ray field compensation with multileaf collimators. Int J Radiat Oncol Biol Phys 1994;28:723–30.

34. Yu CX. Intensity-modulated arc therapy with dynamic multileaf collimation: an alternative to tomotherapy. Phys Med Biol 1995;40:1435–49.

35. Xia P, Hwang AB, Verhey LJ. A leaf sequencing algorithm to enlarge treatment field length in IMRT. Med Phys 2002;29:991–8.

36. Kung JH, Chen GT, Kuchnir FK. A monitor unit verification calculation in intensity modulated radiotherapy as a dosimetry quality assurance. Med Phys 2000;27:2226–30.

37. Xing L, Chen Y, Luxton G, et al. Monitor unit calculation for an intensity modulated photon field by a simple scatter-summation algorithm. Phys Med Biol 2000;45:N1–N7.

38. Cherniack RM, Cherniack L, Naimark A. Respiration in health and disease. 2nd ed. Philadelphia: Saunders; 1972.

Chapter 21

GASTROINTESTINAL TUMORS

OVERVIEW

MICHAEL C. GAROFALO, MD, STEVEN J. CHMURA, MD, PhD

Intensity-modulated radiation therapy (IMRT) is increasingly employed in the treatment of gastrointestinal (GI) malignancies. A recent survey found that approximately one-third of practicing radiation oncologists in the United States use IMRT in their clinical practice.[1] Of these, 15% of physicians have treated a patient with a GI malignancy.

At present, reports on the use of IMRT in GI tumors are limited. Existing studies have largely focused on pancreatic cancer, a disease in which outcomes remain poor and improvements may lie in dose-escalated chemoradiation therapy (chemo-RT).[2–8] As modern treatments for GI cancers have evolved toward more dose-intensive, combined-modality regimens, the potential for toxicity has increased. IMRT represents a fundamental improvement in the planning and delivery of radiation therapy (RT). It may improve modern treatment of GI malignancies through more conformal dose delivery, reducing the risk of toxicity and allowing safe escalation of chemotherapy and/or radiation dose.

The purpose of this chapter is to provide an overview of the rationale, current literature, and challenges associated with the IMRT planning and delivery in patients with GI malignancies.

Rationale

GI malignancies are a heterogeneous group of tumors spanning the alimentary tract from the cervical esophagus to the anal canal. Several solid organ tumors (pancreatic and hepatobiliary) are also included. Although randomized trials have established the therapeutic benefit of chemo-RT in the treatment of both operable and inoperable GI tumors, toxicity has also been substantially increased over RT alone. Further dose escalation of either chemotherapy or RT has been limited by concerns over normal tissue toxicity. IMRT promises reductions in treatment-related toxicity and safer dose escalation of modern multimodality regimens in GI malignancies. All existing IMRT outcome studies include chemotherapy.[9–19]

It has been well established that IMRT facilitates delivery of RT in a more conformal manner than conventional approaches, thereby minimizing the dose to surrounding normal tissues.[20] The dose to critical tissues (eg, spinal cord, lungs, kidneys) can be further minimized through inverse planning. By imposing predefined dose constraints for both normal tissues and target volumes, one can tailor the dose delivered to these tissues without compromising target coverage, thereby improving the therapeutic index.

The potential for improved outcomes with IMRT in the various GI tumors is dependent on several site-specific factors: the tolerance of surrounding normal tissues (which are often dose-limiting), the expected motion of the target tissues and normal tissues, the three-dimensional shape of the target, and the expected toxicity and efficacy of the best modern treatment (ie, is there room for improvement).

Organized in craniocaudal order, a site-specific rationale for the potential role and benefit of IMRT is presented for the GI sites that have garnered the most attention in the IMRT literature: esophageal, gastric, pancreatic, and anal cancers.

Esophageal Cancer

Irradiation of patients with carcinoma of the esophagus represents a challenging clinical problem. Conventional RT doses have been limited primarily by the proximity of the spinal cord and lungs. Consequently, improvements in therapy have been sought through the addition of chemotherapy. Several randomized trials have established the benefit of chemo-RT in both operable and inoperable cases of esophageal cancer.[14–18] The long-term survival benefit of concomitant chemo-RT over RT alone was established by Radiation Therapy Oncology Group (RTOG) study 85-01. Patients receiving combined-modality treatment had an improved 5-year overall survival (26 vs 0%) than did those treated with RT alone. Although locoregional failure was reduced, it remained the most prevalent type of failure, occurring in 47% of patients. Unsurprisingly, toxicity was increased compared with RT alone.[14,16,18] Local control and survival remain particularly poor in patients with locally advanced, unresectable disease.

IMRT may permit a reduction of dose to surrounding normal tissues without compromising target coverage, allowing for safer dose escalation strategies. However, a recently reported phase III trial calls into question the potential benefit of dose-escalated chemo-RT in the treatment of locally advanced disease.[21] It remains to be established if dose escalation in the adjuvant setting of resectable cases will meet a similar fate. Irrespective of the questionable efficacy of dose escalation, reductions in dose to surrounding normal tissues will likely translate into reduced acute and chronic toxicity in these patients.

Gastric Cancer

The standard of care for operable gastric cancer is resection followed by chemo-RT. A multi-institutional Intergroup trial demonstrated a reduced locoregional relapse (19 vs 29%) and an improved survival in resected stage Ib–IV patients receiving adjuvant chemo-RT compared with no further therapy.[19] However, toxicity was significant with the combined approach.

Radiation treatment volumes in the postoperative setting are large, accounting for the patterns of failure established in earlier surgical series.[22,23] Target volumes include the stomach bed (to include surgical clips), a portion of the left hemidiaphragm, and regional lymphatic glands. The standard dose of 45 Gy well exceeds the tolerance of surrounding critical normal tissues (notably the kidneys and liver). As a result, volumes are often "tailored" to reduce potential renal and liver damage, compromising target coverage. This practice, however, may lead to poorer local control and survival rates. Conformal IMRT plans may provide a means of improving target coverage in these patients, increasing locoregional control while reducing treatment-related toxicity.

Pancreatic Cancer

Pancreatic cancer represents a biologically aggressive disease with poor treatment outcomes. Despite advances in treatment and a relatively low incidence, pancreatic cancer represents the fourth leading cause of cancer-related death in the United States.[24] Randomized studies performed by the Gastrointestinal Tumor Study Group have established a survival advantage through the use of 5-fluorouracil (5-FU) in combination with RT in both operable and inoperable disease.[9,12,25] Recently, treatment has evolved toward more intensive chemo-RT regimens. Split-course RT has been replaced by dose-escalated, continuous-course treatment, and gemcitabine has moved to front-line therapy. However, gemcitabine-based chemo-RT approaches result in increased toxicity.[26] Poor outcomes and increased toxicity of modern multimodality treatments provide a strong rationale for the use of treatment technologies that reduce

toxicity and allow for safer dose escalation. IMRT may provide a means to safely deliver increasing amounts of radiation to the tumor by reducing the damage to the surrounding normal tissues whose tolerances have traditionally limited dose escalation.

Anal Carcinoma

RT occupies an important role in the treatment of anal carcinoma. In the past, radical surgery was commonly used consisting of an abdominoperineal resection. Based on the work of Nigro,[27] however, radical surgery has been replaced by chemo-RT approaches, allowing avoidance of a colostomy.[28] Abdominoperineal resection is now reserved for patients with persistent or recurrent disease.[29] Unsurprisingly, combined chemo-RT approaches are quite toxic owing to the inclusion of multiple normal tissues, including the small bowel, rectum, bladder, and pelvic bone marrow. Moreover, the inclusion of the genitalia in the conventional treatment fields is associated with considerable acute toxicity and may compromise long-term sexual function. IMRT may provide a means to deliver curative doses of RT in these patients, with improved sparing of surrounding normal tissues, thereby reducing the risk of normal tissue toxicity.

Planning Studies

A number of investigators have performed preclinical planning studies evaluating the potential role of IMRT in GI malignancies. As shown in Table 21-1, these studies focus on a variety of tumor sites and use different study end points. However, a common finding is that all suggest a benefit in terms of normal tissue sparing to IMRT planning compared with conventional techniques.

Esophageal Cancer

As shown in Table 21-1, four IMRT planning studies have been performed in esophageal cancer.[30–33] Nutting and colleagues at the Royal Marsden Hospital compared three-dimensional conformal radiation therapy (3DCRT) and IMRT planning in five patients with esophageal carcinoma.[30] The 3DCRT plans consisted of four fields (anterior-posterior and two posterior oblique), whereas the IMRT plans used either the same four fields (4F-IMRT) or nine equally spaced fields (9F-IMRT). Treatment was optimized to deliver a total dose of 55 Gy to the planning target volume (PTV) while minimizing the dose to the spinal cord ($\leq$ 45 Gy) and lungs. Dose-volume histograms (DVHs) and normal tissue complication probabilities (NTCPs) were calculated for both approaches.

Although no differences were seen in PTV coverage or homogeneity among the three approaches, a trend toward increased PTV dose inhomogeneity was noted in the 9F-IMRT plan. Moreover, no significant difference in maximum dose to the spinal cord was seen. Interestingly, the

TABLE 21-1. Gastrointestinal Intensity-Modulated Radiation Therapy Planning Studies

Study	Insitution	Site	No. of Patients	Study Design	End Points
Nutting et al[30]	Royal Marsden Hospital	Esophagus	5	4F/9F IMRT vs 3DCRT	DVH, NTCP
Nutting et al[31]	Royal Marsden Hospital	Esophagus	5	5F IMRT vs 3DCRT	DVH, NTCP
Chandra et al[32]	M. D. Anderson Cancer Center	Distal esophagus, GE junction	10	4F/7F/9F IMRT vs 3DCRT	DVH
Fu et al[33]	Beijing	Upper esophagus	2	3F/5F/7F/9F SIB-IMRT	DVH
Lohr et al[34]	Heidelberg	Stomach	1	IMRT vs 3DCRT (± KS)	DVH
Ringash et al[35]	Princess Margaret Hospital	Stomach GE junction	20	IMRT vs 3DCRT Blinded evaluation	Physician evaluation
Cheng et al[36]	Sun Yat-Sen Cancer Center (Taipei)	Liver	12	5F IMRT vs 3DCRT	DVH, NTCP
Aoki et al[2]	Kyoto	Pancreas	5	IMRT vs IORT	DVH
Landry et al[3]	Emory University	Pancreas	10	IMRT vs 3DCRT	DVH, NTCP
Chmura and Heimann[4]	University of Chicago	Pancreas, bile duct	7	IMRT vs 3DCRT	DVH, NTCP

3DCRT = three-dimensional conformal radiation therapy; DVH = dose-volume histogram; F = field; GE = gastroesophageal; IMRT = intensity-modulated radiation therapy; IORT = intraoperative radiation therapy; KS = kidney sparing; NTCP = normal tissue complication probability; SIB = simultaneous integrated boost.

4F-IMRT plan was associated with reductions of normal lung irradiation and a lower calculated NTCP for the lung. For example, the percent volume of lung receiving $\geq$ 18 Gy (V_{18}) was 22.2, 18.8, and 14.1% for the 9F-IMRT, 3DCRT, and 4F-IMRT, respectively. Corresponding means doses of the normal lung were 11.7, 11.0, and 9.5 Gy, respectively. NTCPs for the lung were 1.0, 1.0, and 0.6% for the 9F-IMRT, conformal RT, and 4F-IMRT plans, respectively. A statistically significant benefit to the use of 4F-IMRT compared with 3DCRT was seen on all surrogate measures of lung toxicity while maintaining similar PTV coverage and homogeneity. The data demonstrate that 4F-IMRT planning using conventional beam angles reduces normal lung irradiation without compromising PTV coverage when compared with 3DCRT or 9F-IMRT.

In a subsequent study, Nutting and colleagues compared five-field IMRT with 3DCRT planning in five patients with esophageal cancer using the same field arrangement.[31] As in the prior study, treatment was planned in two phases, delivering a total of 55 Gy while minimizing the dose to the spinal cord ($\leq$ 45 Gy) and lung parenchyma. The first phase used opposed anterior-posterior fields, and the second phase used an anterior and two posterior oblique fields. The clinical target volume (CTV) included the primary tumor with circumferential and craniocaudal margins of 2 and 5 cm, respectively. A 1.5 cm CTV-PTV expansion was used to account for setup uncertainty and organ motion.

Inhomogeneity was significantly increased in the 3DCRT plans compared with the IMRT plans ($p = .03$). Whereas the maximum spinal cord dose was similar, the mean lung dose (9.5 vs 11.0 Gy; $p = .001$) and V_{18} (9.5 vs 11.0 Gy; $p = .001$) were significantly lower using IMRT planning. NTCP calculations revealed a lower risk of $\geq$ grade 2 pneumonitis with IMRT versus 3DCRT (0.6 vs 1.0%; $p = .008$). These data again suggested a dosimetric benefit to IMRT when compared with 3DCRT.

Researchers at the M. D. Anderson Cancer Center recently suggested a benefit to IMRT in distal esophageal tumors.[32] To investigate whether IMRT planning could reduce the dose to uninvolved lung in these patients, 10 patients were planned with both IMRT (using four, seven, and nine fields) and conventional (four field) 3DCRT techniques. The 4F-IMRT plans were generated using the same beam orientation as the clinically treated 3DCRT plans. 9F-IMRT plans were equally spaced, and 7F-IMRT plans used the same angles as the nine-field plans minus the lateral beams. Treatment plans were optimized to deliver 50.4 Gy to the PTV while minimizing total lung volumes receiving $\geq$ 10 Gy and 20 Gy (V_{10} and V_{20}). IMRT plans resulted in significant decreases in lung dose, as represented by every dosimetric end point calculated (V_{10}, V_{20}, mean lung dose, and mean integral lung dose) compared with 3DCRT plans. Conformity indices were slightly better for the 7F-IMRT and 9F-IMRT plans. Additionally, no clinically meaningful differences were observed in terms of the heart, liver, spinal cord, and total body integral doses between the various plans.

In a small feasibility study, Fu and colleagues evaluated the simultaneous integrated boost technique in two patients with intact upper esophageal cancers.[33] The total dose to the primary tumor was 67.2 Gy, and the dose to the electively treated region (including lymph nodes) was 50.4 Gy. Using identical dose-volume constraints, IMRT plans were generated using three, five, seven, or nine equally spaced coplanar beams. Significant improvements were seen in dose conformity and normal tissue sparing with increasing beam number; however, little difference was noted between the seven- and nine-field plans.

Gastric Cancer

Two IMRT planning studies have been performed in patients with gastric cancer (see Table 21-1).[34,35] Lohr and colleagues compared IMRT and conventional planning in a patient with node-positive gastric cancer receiving adjuvant RT.[34] In this study, four plans (or plan combinations) were generated: (1) a conventional four-field plan, (2) a combination of a four-field plan with a kidney-sparing boost, (3) a conventional plan with noncoplanar fields for improved kidney sparing, and (4) an IMRT plan. IMRT provided better sparing of the left kidney and liver than all of the conventional plans. However, a small increase in the dose to the right kidney and the spinal cord was seen. Of note, both the spinal cord (median dose 37.6 Gy with IMRT) and right kidney (median dose 7.8 Gy with IMRT) remained well below tolerance. By contrast, the left kidney was above tolerance with conventional four-field plans (median dose 26.9 Gy), and IMRT was more effective in reducing the dose (median dose 10.5 Gy) than either of the conventional plans with kidney-sparing strategies (median doses of 14.8 and 19.8 Gy).

Investigators at the Princess Margaret Hospital assessed the feasibility and potential advantage of IMRT in patients with resected gastric cancer.[35] Twenty patients previously treated to 45 Gy with 3DCRT were replanned with IMRT using seven to nine fields. For each case, DVH data for the two plans (IMRT and 3DCRT) were provided to two independent radiation oncologists blinded to the plan type. The oncologists were asked to indicate which of the two plans provided better PTV coverage and better sparing of critical organs (spinal cord, kidneys, liver, and heart) and which they would choose to treat the patient.

Agreement between the evaluating oncologists was high. In 18 of 20 cases (90%), both chose the same plan. Overall, a "preferred plan" could be determined in 19 of the 20 cases. Of these, 17 (89%) were the IMRT plan. IMRT was felt to provide better PTV coverage in 86% of plans reviewed. Moreover, IMRT was felt to result in better sparing of the spinal cord (74%), kidneys (69%), liver (71%), and heart (69%).

Hepatoma

Cheng and colleagues at the Sun Yat-Sen Cancer Center in Taiwan recently reported the results of a dosimetric study of IMRT in patients with hepatoma.[36] Of 68 patients previously irradiated with conventional RT, 12 who had developed documented radiation-induced liver disease were selected for this study. These patients were replanned with five-field IMRT plans, and dosimetric differences between the targets and normal tissues were compared between conventional and IMRT plans. Comparable target coverage was achieved with both approaches. Moreover, no significant differences were seen in terms of kidney and stomach sparing. Of note, IMRT planning significantly reduced the volume of spinal cord irradiated. IMRT planning was associated with a significantly lower NTCP for the liver (23.7 vs 36.6%; $p = .009$) compared with conventional RT. However, the mean dose to the liver was higher in the IMRT plan (29.2 vs 25.0 Gy; $p = .009$).

Pancreatic Cancer

As shown in Table 21-1, three IMRT planning studies have been presented in pancreatic cancer.[2–4] Aoki and colleagues investigated whether IMRT could substitute for intraoperative radiation therapy (IORT) in patients with unresectable disease.[2] The treatment plan called for an initial

12 Gy fraction to the CTV, with a cone-down field receiving an additional 18 Gy in a single fraction. The volume of CTV receiving 24 Gy or more was significantly greater with IMRT planning compared with IORT (92.2 vs 32.9%; $p = .04$). However, improvements in target coverage and conformity came at the cost of increased dose to the small bowel. The volume of small bowel receiving ≥ 14 Gy was higher using IMRT planning (4.2 vs 0.1%; $p = .04$) compared with IORT. Despite a biologically and clinically insignificant trend toward increased maximum spinal cord dose (4.4 Gy for IMRT vs 0.8 Gy for IORT), these data demonstrate that IMRT may represent a potential replacement for IORT in this setting.

In a comprehensive planning study, Landry and colleagues at Emory University evaluated IMRT planning in 10 patients with locally advanced adenocarcinoma of the pancreatic head.[3] The goal of treatment planning was to deliver 61.2 Gy to the gross tumor volume (GTV) and 45 Gy to the CTV while maintaining critical normal tissues below specified tolerances. IMRT plans were significantly more conformal and effectively reduced the dose to surrounding normal tissues. The average dose delivered to one-third of the small bowel volume was 30.2 Gy for IMRT (vs 38.5 Gy for 3DCRT; $p = .006$).

Given that the risk of small bowel injury increases significantly with doses above 50 Gy, the investigators compared DVH results at 50 and 60 Gy as well. The median volume of small bowel receiving > 50 Gy was 19.2% for IMRT (vs 31.4% for 3DCRT; $p = .048$). The median volume of small bowel receiving > 60 Gy was 12.5% for IMRT (vs 19.8% for 3DCRT; $p = .034$). Using the Lyman-Kutcher model, the probability of small bowel injury was calculated to be 9.3% for IMRT (vs 24.4% for 3DCRT; $p = .021$). With these reductions in small bowel dose and injury probability, the authors concluded that IMRT has the potential to significantly improve treatment of pancreatic cancers by reducing normal tissue toxicity and allowing safer escalation of dose (see Chapter 21.1, "Pancreatic Cancer: Case Study").

In a similar study, Chmura and Heimann analyzed seven patients with either locally advanced pancreatic cancer or cholangiocarcinoma.[4] IMRT and conventional treatment plans were compared. All plans were normalized to deliver 59.4 Gy to the PTV while minimizing the dose to surrounding normal tissues. IMRT resulted in significant reductions in the volume of small bowel, liver, and kidney irradiated compared with conventional planning. Further, IMRT resulted in a > 50% relative decrease in the volume of small bowel receiving > 35 Gy and a 30 to 60% reduction in the volume of liver receiving > 30 Gy. Of note, IMRT reduced the liver NTCP threefold. For tumors in the head of the pancreas, a 30% decrease in the right kidney volume receiving > 22 Gy was achieved with IMRT. An IMRT plan in a patient with pancreatic cancer is shown in Figure 21-1.

Although no dosimetric studies exclusively focusing on IMRT in the postoperative setting for pancreatic cancer have been published, researchers at the University of Chicago included a comparison as part of their recently reported experience treating pancreatic malignancies with IMRT.[8] Of the 25 patients treated, 8 underwent adjuvant chemo-RT and 5 were planned with conventional four-field treatment for dosimetric comparison with IMRT. Compared with conventional planning, IMRT reduced the median dose to the liver, kidneys, stomach, and small bowel and resulted in more conformal treatment.

Anal Carcinoma

Chmura and colleagues at the University of Chicago evaluated the role of IMRT planning in five patients with anal carcinoma.[37] Opposed anterior-posterior fields (based on RTOG study 98-11) were compared with seven- to nine-field IMRT planning. All plans were used to deliver a total dose to the primary tumor of 50.4 Gy. IMRT significantly reduced the volume of small bowel, bladder, and genitalia irradiated. On average, the volume of small bowel receiving > 40 Gy in the IMRT and conventional plans was 3% and 55%, respectively. Corresponding volumes of bladder irradiated to > 40 Gy in the two plans were 15% and 100%, respectively. Of particular note, IMRT planning reduced the volume of genitalia receiving > 40 Gy from 70 to 0%. An IMRT plan in a representative patient with anal cancer is shown in Figure 21-2 (see Chapter 21.3, "Anal Cancer: Case Study").

Outcome Studies

Despite promising preclinical IMRT studies in patients with GI malignancies, outcome studies in patients treated with IMRT remain limited (Table 21-2). Most studies have focused on patients with pancreatic carcinoma. Moreover, although most of the studies suggested a potential benefit to IMRT, follow-up is short, and the number of patients treated in most reports is small.

Pancreatic Cancer

Landry and colleagues treated nine patients with locally advanced pancreatic cancer with IMRT, seven of whom were considered unresectable.[5] Total doses ranged from 49.5 to 60 Gy delivered in 1.8 Gy daily fractions, except in three patients who received 1.5 Gy twice daily to a total of 49.5 Gy in a phase I study. All patients received concomitant continuous-infusion 5-FU. At a median follow-up of 5 months, the most common acute GI symptoms were nausea and vomiting (one grade 3, three grade 2, and one grade 1). Diarrhea was the second most common side effect noted in two patients, both grade 1. No acute genitourinary sequelae were seen.

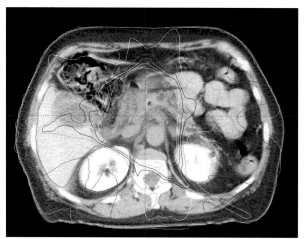

FIGURE 21-1. An isodose distribution overlaid on the treatment planning computed tomography scan of a patient with pancreatic cancer. (To view a color version of this image, please refer to the CD-ROM.)

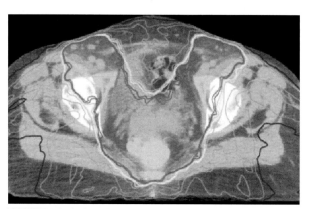

FIGURE 21-2. An intensity-modulated radiation therapy plan of a patient with anal cancer. (To view a color version of this image, please refer to the CD-ROM.)

TABLE 21-2. Gastrointestinal Intensity-Modulated Radiation Therapy Outcome Studies

Study	Institution	Site	No. of Patients	Study Design	End Points
Landry et al[5]	Emory University	Pancreas	9	IMRT, 5-FU	Toxicity
Bai et al[7]	Xinhua Hospital of Shanghai	Pancreas	16	IMRT, GEM and 5-FU	Toxicity, outcome, CA 19-9, KPS, pain control
Crane et al[6]	M. D. Anderson Cancer Center	Pancreas	5	IMRT, GEM, dose escalation	Toxicity
Milano et al[8]	University of Chicago	Pancreas, bile duct	25	IMRT, 5-FU	Toxicity, outcome
Chmura et al[37]	University of Chicago	Anus	11	IMRT, 5-FU, mitomycin	Toxicity, outcome

CA = cancer antigen; 5-FU = 5-fluorouracil; GEM = gemcitibine; IMRT = intensity-modulated radiation therapy; KPS = Karnofsky Performance Scale.

Bai and colleagues reported their experience of IMRT and chemotherapy (5-FU or gemcitabine) in 16 patients with locally advanced pancreatic carcinoma.[7] Most cases were unresectable, without evidence of distant metastases. One of four escalating total doses was planned: 51, 54, 57, or 60 Gy. Treatment was delivered in two phases: the first phase consisted of conventional RT (30 Gy in 2 Gy daily fractions), and IMRT was given during the second phase (21–30 Gy in 3 Gy fractions). A 5 mm GTV-PTV expansion was used.

With dose-limiting toxicity defined as grade 4 hematologic sequelae, patients were successfully dose-escalated to 60 Gy. Following treatment, improvements were noted in cancer antigen (CA) 19-9 levels, oral analgesic requirements, and performance status. Prior to treatment, CA 19-9 levels were elevated in 13 of 16 patients (median value 716 U/mL). At the end of treatment, the levels had decreased to a median value of 255 U/mL ($p < .001$). Of note, 14 patients had a reduction in oral analgesic consumption, of whom 10 had reductions of > 50%. GI toxicity was mild, with no patients developing grade 2 or higher sequelae. With an unstated follow-up period and local control rate, a 1-year survival rate of 35% was reported. These outcome data demonstrate the safety of dose escalation using IMRT and resulted in a definite palliative benefit when combined with chemotherapy (see Chapter 21.1).

In contrast, researchers at M. D. Anderson recently reported a negative dose escalation trial using IMRT in pancreatic cancer.[6] The study was designed to evaluate the escalating doses of gemcitabine in patients treated with concomitant hypofractionated IMRT (30–33 Gy in 3 Gy daily fractions). All three patients in the starting cohort suffered dose-limiting toxicity when receiving 350 mg/m[2] of gemcitabine. A second cohort of two patients received a lower gemcitabine dose (250 mg/m[2]); however, both patients again suffered dose-limiting toxicity, resulting in the closure of the trial.

Milano and colleagues at the University of Chicago reported the outcome of 25 patients treated with IMRT for pancreatic or bile duct malignancies.[8] The study included 17 adenocarcinomas and 1 peripheral neuroectodermal tumor (PNET). All patients received concomitant 5-FU, except the patient with PNET, who received ifosfamide and etoposide therapy, and one patient refused chemotherapy. Four patients were treated postoperatively. Seven- or nine-field coplanar IMRT plans were used in all patients. Uninvolved regional lymphatic glands received 45 Gy, whereas gross disease received 59.4 Gy in the unresectable cases (or 45–50.4 Gy to the tumor bed in the postoperative cases).

Overall, two patients developed grade 4 toxicity (an ileus requiring hospitalization and a duodenal fistula that was successfully repaired). Of note, no excessive hot spots could be identified in the treatment plans of these patients to account for these toxicities. Twenty patients experienced ≤ grade 2 toxicity. At a median follow-up of 12.3 months, the median and metastasis-free survival rates were 13.4 and

7.3 months, respectively. The 1- and 2-year actuarial survival rates for the entire group were 55 and 22%, respectively. Resected patients had significant improvements in 1- and 2-year survival when compared with unresectable patients (83 and 50% vs 40 and 8%; $p = .04$).

Anal Cancer

Investigators at the University of Chicago reported the results of a small feasibility study of IMRT in anal carcinoma.[38] Eight patients with squamous cell carcinoma of the anal canal (T2–3,N0–3) were treated to an initial dose of 30.6 Gy using a nine-field IMRT plan. A subsequent boost field was treated with IMRT for an additional 14.4 to 18.8 Gy. Concurrent 5-FU and mitomycin C were also given. Overall, treatment was well tolerated, with no unplanned interruptions. Grade 4 hematologic toxicity occurred in three patients, with two patients requiring transfusions after the completion of RT. No patient developed grade 3 or higher skin toxicity. At a median follow-up of 15 months, the 2-year actuarial colostomy-free and disease-free survival rates were 80% and 55%, respectively. The 2-year ultimate local control rate was 88%.

Issues and Challenges

The challenges associated with the implementation of IMRT in the treatment of GI tumors are similar across many of the GI sites. Pancreatic cancer has been the focus of the majority of GI IMRT studies published to date. For the purposes of discussion, the issues and challenges associated with the implementation of IMRT are discussed in this context. One can extrapolate the principles of the analysis in pancreatic cancer to less studied GI sites.

The potential clinical advantages of IMRT are contingent on increased target conformity and consequent reductions in dose to surrounding normal tissues. In the postoperative setting, the treatment target for pancreatic cancer has been historically defined by bony landmarks for conventional treatment. For purposes of IMRT treatment planning, a three-dimensional target must be defined. PTV design must account for gross and microscopic disease, setup uncertainty, and organ motion. For patients with inoperable pancreatic cancers, PTV design is relatively intuitive as the primary tumor and draining lymphatic glands at risk are typically well visualized on computed tomography (CT) scans or magnetic resonance images (MRIs). One of the challenges associated with IMRT treatment is the need to delineate both the target volume(s) and normal structures prior to IMRT planning. It is crucial that clinicians continue to familiarize themselves with modern imaging technologies to ensure a high level of accuracy and consistency when entering these structures.

In contrast to patients with inoperable disease, three-dimensional PTV design in postoperative cases is less intuitive. Should the design be based on the preoperative location of the tumor and at-risk lymphatic glands? Should it be influenced by the postoperative anatomy and surgical clips? How much margin should be added to account for setup uncertainty and organ motion? Does the target need to be "tailored" after expansion to keep adjacent normal tissues under tolerance? These are some of the questions that a clinician confronts when designing a three-dimensional target for adjuvant treatment of pancreatic carcinoma. Without appropriate target coverage and expansion, local control could be compromised as a result of attempts to selectively contour the radiation dose around critical structures.

Upper abdominal organ motion represents perhaps the greatest challenge to the use of IMRT for pancreatic cancer. Recent studies suggest that, in the absence of respiratory gating, a target expansion of 2.5 cm may be appropriate to account for respiratory-induced organ motion. In a sophisticated, modern analysis of upper abdominal organ motion, Bussels and colleagues assessed respiration-induced movement of the upper abdominal organs in 12 subjects using dynamic MRI. The largest movements were noticed in the craniocaudal direction for the pancreas and liver (23.7 and 24.4 mm, respectively).[39] In a similar volumetric analysis of abdominal organ motion using clip coordinates and CT scans during various phases of the respiratory cycle, researchers from Massachusetts General Hospital reported maximal craniocaudal pancreatic motion of 16 mm.[40] With the increased treatment time associated with IMRT, intrafraction organ motion is an even greater concern.[20]

When reported, there has been significant heterogeneity in three-dimensional target design among the published clinical studies in pancreatic cancer. For instance, the expansion margins reported in the literature have ranged from 1 to 3 cm for initial treatment volumes and from 0.5 to 2 cm for boost volmes.[5–8] After appropriate target expansion, it is probable that nearby normal tissues will never be completely excluded from the PTV. Given the likelihood that a portion of the small bowel will always be included in the initial treatment PTV, there is an obvious limitation to RT dose escalation. Small bowel complications are known to increase with doses in excess of 50 Gy. Historical reports in the literature suggest that radiation doses of 45 to 50 Gy to the small bowel will result in a 5% incidence of injury at 5 years when one-third of the volume is irradiated. Doses above 60 Gy are associated with a 50% risk of small bowel ulcer or stricture at 5 years.[41–43] Therefore, dose escalation may be limited to "boost" strategies with IMRT to smaller volumes.

Inherent in the nature of inverse-planned IMRT, increased conformity is achieved at the cost of increases in

both inhomogeneity and integral dose. Given the increased integral dose with IMRT, the overall risk of secondary tumors may be increased.[44] This is an issue to be considered when treating pediatric malignancies or younger adults with favorable cancers. However, treatment outcomes for GI tumors such as pancreatic and biliary cancers suggest that the majority of treated patients would be unlikely to live long enough to experience this complication. With regard to increased inhomogeneity, the clinical significance of relatively small hot spots or cold spots is unknown. In pancreatic cancer, in which organ motion is significant, many argue that these areas of inhomogeneity would autofeather over time. However, in sites in which organ motion is minimal and immobilization is effective, one could hypothesize that cold spots in the target (of adequate size) may result in compromised tumor control. Likewise, hot spots in surrounding normal tissues may result in increased toxicity, particularly in serial organs such as the spinal cord. The clinical significance of increased inhomogeneity (both in the target and in normal tissues) has yet to be established and merits further investigation.

Future Directions

Although preliminary data suggest a role for IMRT in the treatment of GI malignancies, caution must be used when interpreting these early reports. Conclusions from the existing literature are difficult to make because they are small studies with inconsistent target design and limited follow-up. Further, there is considerable variation in radiation planning parameters and treatment dose from study to study. Well-designed phase III studies are needed to provide definitive evidence that clinically relevant improvements in treatment can be achieved through the use of IMRT. Although two randomized studies in prostate cancer suggest that reduced treatment toxicity can be achieved with more conformal treatment techniques, there are currently no published randomized clinical studies investigating the potential for reduced toxicity with inverse-planned IMRT.[45,46]

Before inverse-planned IMRT can be evaluated in phase III trials, a cooperative group mechanism is needed to facilitate standardization of target design and planning parameters. Without consensus standardization, accrual to such a trial would likely be poor. Toward a similar end, IMRT working groups have been established for several sites. As of yet, no such working group has been established for GI malignancies. Organ motion presents perhaps the greatest limitation to conformal target design in GI tumors; therefore, respiratory-gated treatment approaches warrant further investigation. Given the continued evolution toward dose-intensive multimodality therapies for GI malignancies, future research will likely continue to center around the use of IMRT toward reduced toxicity and safer escalation of chemotherapy or radiation dose.

Editor's Note: As this text was going to press, the first article evaluating IMRT planning in rectal cancer was published. Interested readers should refer to Duthoy W et al. Int J Radiat Oncol Biol Phys 2004;50:794–806.

References

1. Mell LK, Roeske JC, Mundt AJ. A survey of intensity-modulated radiation therapy use in the United States. Cancer 2003;98:204–11.

2. Aoki T, Mizowaki T, Nagata Y, et al. Can intensity modulated radiation therapy replace intraoperative radiation therapy in patients with unresectable pancreatic cancer. Int J Radiat Oncol Biol Phys 2001;51 Suppl 1:397–8.

3. Landry JC, Yang GY, Ting JY, et al. Treatment of pancreatic cancer tumors with intensity-modulated radiation therapy (IMRT) using the volume at risk approach (VARA): employing dose-volume histogram (DVH) and normal tissue complication probability (NTCP) to evaluate small bowel toxicity. Med Dosim 2002;27:121–9.

4. Chmura SJ, Heimann R. Normal tissue toxicity using intensity modulated radiation therapy (IMRT) in pancreatic cancer and cholangiocarcinoma [abstract]. Proc Am Soc Clin Oncol 2001.

5. Landry J, Esiashvili N, Ting J, et al. Intensity modulated radiation therapy employing the volume at risk approach to minimize small bowel and renal toxicity when treating patients with locally advanced pancreatic carcinomas. Int J Radiat Oncol Biol Phys 2001;51 Suppl 1:270.

6. Crane CH, Antolak JA, Rosen II, et al. Phase I study of concomitant gemcitabine and IMRT for patients with unresectable adenocarcinoma of the pancreatic head. Int J Gastrointest Cancer 2001;30:123–32.

7. Bai YR, Wu GH, Guo WJ, et al. Intensity modulated radiation therapy and chemotherapy for locally advanced pancreatic cancer: results of a feasibility study. World J Gastroenterol 2003;9:2561–4.

8. Milano MT, Chmura SJ, Garofalo MC, et al. Intensity modulated radiation therapy (IMRT) in the treatment of pancreatic and bile duct malignancies: toxicity and clinical outcome. Int J Radiat Oncol Biol Phys. 2004;59(2):445-53.

9. Moertel CG, Frytak S, Hahn RG, et al. Therapy of locally unresectable pancreatic carcinoma: a randomized comparison of high dose (6000 rads) radiation alone, moderate dose radiation (4000 rads + 5-fluorouracil), and high dose radiation + 5-fluorouracil: the Gastrointestinal Tumor Study Group. Cancer 1981;48:1705–10.

10. Kalser MH, Ellenberg SS. Pancreatic cancer. Adjuvant combined radiation and chemotherapy following curative resection. Arch Surg 1985;120:899–903.

11. Gastrointestinal Tumor Study Group. Further evidence of effective adjuvant combined radiation and chemotherapy following curative resection of pancreatic cancer. Cancer 1987;59:2006–10.

12. Gastrointestinal Tumor Study Group. Treatment of locally unresectable carcinoma of the pancreas: comparison of combined-modality therapy (chemotherapy plus radiotherapy) to chemotherapy alone. J Natl Cancer Inst 1988;80:751–5.

13. Krook JE, Moertel CG, Gunderson LL, et al. Effective surgical adjuvant therapy for high-risk rectal carcinoma. N Engl J Med 1991;324:709–15.

14. Herskovic A, Martz K, al-Sarraf M, et al. Combined chemotherapy and radiotherapy compared with radiotherapy alone in patients with cancer of the esophagus. N Engl J Med 1992;326:1593–8.

15. Walsh TN, Noonan N, Hollywood D, et al. A comparison of multimodal therapy and surgery for esophageal adenocarcinoma. N Engl J Med 1996;335:462–7.

16. Bartelink H, Roelofsen F, Eschwege F, et al. Concomitant radiotherapy and chemotherapy is superior to radiotherapy alone in the treatment of locally advanced anal cancer: results of a phase III randomized trial of the European Organization for Research and Treatment of Cancer Radiotherapy and Gastrointestinal Cooperative Groups. J Clin Oncol 1997;15:2040–9.

17. Bosset JF, Gignoux M, Triboulet JP, et al. Chemoradiotherapy followed by surgery compared with surgery alone in squamous-cell cancer of the esophagus. N Engl J Med 1997;337:161–7.

18. Cooper JS, Guo MD, Herskovic A, et al. Chemoradiotherapy of locally advanced esophageal cancer: long-term follow-up of a prospective randomized trial (RTOG 85-01). JAMA 1999;281:1623–7.

19. Macdonald JS, Smalley SR, Benedetti J, et al. Chemoradiotherapy after surgery compared with surgery alone for adenocarcinoma of the stomach or gastroesophageal junction. N Engl J Med 2001;345:725–30.

20. Intensity Modulated Radiation Therapy Collaborative Working Group. Intensity- modulated radiotherapy: current status and issues of interest. Int J Radiat Oncol Biol Phys 2001;51:880–914.

21. Minsky BD, Pajak TF, Ginsberg RJ, et al. INT 0123 (Radiation Therapy Oncology Group 94-05) phase III trial of combined-modality therapy for esophageal cancer: high-dose versus standard-dose radiation therapy. J Clin Oncol 2002;20:1167–74.

22. Gunderson LL, Sosin H. Adenocarcinoma of the stomach: areas of failure in a re-operation series (second or symptomatic look) clinicopathologic correlation and implications for adjuvant therapy. Int J Radiat Oncol Biol Phys 1982;8:1–11.

23. Landry J, Tepper JE, Wood WC, et al. Patterns of failure following curative resection of gastric carcinoma. Int J Radiat Oncol Biol Phys 1990;19:1357–62.

24. Jemal A, Murray T, Samuels A, et al. Cancer statistics 2003. CA Cancer J Clin 2003;53:5–26.

25. Gastrointestinal Tumor Study Group. Radiation therapy combined with Adriamycin or 5-fluorouracil for the treatment of locally unresectable pancreatic carcinoma. Cancer 1985;56:2563–8.

26. Talamonti MS, Catalano PJ, Vaughn DJ, et al. Eastern Cooperative Oncology Group phase I trial of protracted venous infusion fluorouracil plus weekly gemcitabine with concurrent radiation therapy in patients with locally advanced pancreas cancer: a regimen with unexpected early toxicity. J Clin Oncol 2000;18:3384–9.

27. Nigro ND. An evaluation of combined therapy for squamous cell cancer of the anal canal. Dis Colon Rectum 1984;27:763–6.

28. Bendell JC, Ryan DP. Current perspectives on anal cancer. Oncology (Huntingt) 2003;17:492–7.

29. Nilsson PJ, Svensson C, Goldman S, et al. Salvage abdominoperineal resection in anal epidermoid cancer. Br J Surg 2002;89:1425–9.

30. Nutting CM, Bedford JL, Cosgrove VP, et al. A comparison of conformal and intensity-modulated techniques for oesophageal radiotherapy. Radiother Oncol 2001;61:157–63.

31. Nutting CM, Bedford JL, Cosgrove VP, et al. Intensity-modulated radiotherapy reduces lung irradiation in patients with carcinoma of the oesophagus. Front Radiat Ther Oncol 2002;37:128–31.

32. Chandra A, Liu H, Tucker SL, et al. IMRT reduces lung irradiation in distal esophageal cancer over 3DCRT. Int J Radiat Oncol Biol Phys 2003;57(2 Suppl):S384–5.

33. Fu WH, Wang LH, Zhou ZM, et al. Comparison of SIB-IMRT treatment plans for upper esophageal carcinoma. Zhongguo Yi Xue Ke Xue Yuan Xue Bao 2003;25:337–42.

34. Lohr F, Dobler B, Mai S, et al. Optimization of dose distributions for adjuvant locoregional radiotherapy of gastric cancer by IMRT. Strahlenther Onkol 2003;179:557–63.

35. Ringash J, Perkins G, Lockwood G, et al. IMRT for adjuvant radiation in gastric cancer: a preferred plan? Int J Radiat Oncol Biol Phys 2003;57(2 Suppl):S381–2.

36. Cheng JC, Wu JK, Huang CM, et al. Dosimetric analysis and comparison of 3-dimensional conformal radiotherapy and intensity modulated radiation therapy for patients with hepatocellular carcinoma and radiation-induced liver disease. Int J Radiat Oncol Biol Phys 2003;56:229–34.

37. Chmura SJ, Kim S, Johnson S, et al. Intensity modulated radiation therapy (IMRT) in anal cancer [abstract]. Proc Am Soc Clin Oncol 2002.

38. Chmura SJ, Milano M, Garofalo M, et al. Initial outcome with intensity-modulated radiation (IMRT) and chemotherapy (CTX) in anal cancer [abstract]. Proc Am Soc Clin Oncol 2003;22:368.

39. Bussels B, Goethals L, Feron M, et al. Respiration-induced movement of the upper abdominal organs: a pitfall for the three-dimensional conformal radiation treatment of pancreatic cancer. Radiother Oncol 2003;68:69–74.

40. Chen GT, Jiang SB, Kung J, et al. Abdominal organ motion and deformation: implications for IMRT. Int J Radiat Oncol Biol Phys 2001;51 Suppl 1:210.

41. Emami B, Lyman J, Brown A, et al. Tolerance of normal tissue to therapeutic irradiation. Int J Radiat Oncol Biol Phys 1991;21:109–22.

42. Letschert JG, Lebesque JV, Aleman BM, et al. The volume effect in radiation-related late small bowel complications: results of a clinical study of the EORTC radiotherapy cooperative group in patients treated for rectal carcinoma. Radiother Oncol 1994;32:116–23.

43. Coia LR, Myerson RJ, Tepper JE. Late effects of radiation therapy on the gastrointestinal tract. Int J Radiat Oncol Biol Phys 1995;31:1213–36.

44. Hall EJ, Wuu CS. Radiation-induced second cancers: the impact of 3D-CRT and IMRT. Int J Radiat Oncol Biol Phys 2003;56:83–8.

45. Koper PC, Stroom JC, van Putten WL, et al. Acute morbidity reduction using 3DCRT for prostate carcinoma: a randomized study. Int J Radiat Oncol Biol Phys 1999;43:727–34.

46. Dearnaley DP, Khoo VS, Norman AR, et al. Comparison of radiation side-effects of conformal and conventional radiotherapy in prostate cancer: a randomized trial. Lancet 1999;353:267–72.

PANCREATIC CANCER

CASE STUDY

JEROME LANDRY, MD, NATIA ESIASHVILI, MD, MARY KOSHY, MD

Patient History

A 57-year-old male presented with persistent and worsening epigastric pain radiating to his back for 3 to 4 months. He also noticed yellowing of his skin and conjunctiva. Initially, his primary care physician evaluated the patient and noted an elevated bilirubin consistent with obstructive jaundice. An abdominal computed tomography (CT) scan revealed dilated intra- and extrahepatic bile ducts and an irregular mass in the head of the pancreas. The pancreatic mass extended to the celiac axis with encasement of the superior mesenteric artery and the hepatic and left gastric arteries. The portal, splenic, and superior mesenteric veins were patent. There was no evidence of extrapancreatic disease.

A CT-guided biopsy was performed, and the pathology was consistent with adenocarcinoma of the pancreas. The patient was staged according to the American Joint Committee on Cancer (AJCC) TNM system as T4N0M0 (stage IVa). An oncologic surgeon concluded that resection could not be performed owing to vessel encasement. Endoscopic retrograde cholangiopancreatography with biliary stenting was performed to alleviate his symptoms of biliary obstruction.

The patient was then referred to radiation and medical oncology for consideration of preoperative treatment. The multidisciplinary gastrointestinal cancer team recommended induction chemotherapy followed by concurrent radiation therapy (RT) and chemotherapy according to a phase II in-house protocol. Induction chemotherapy consisted of cisplatin, 5-fluorouracil (5-FU), and gemcitabine for two cycles followed by concurrent continuous venous infusion 5-FU during twice-daily RT. Intensity-modulated radiation therapy (IMRT) was used in this patient to reduce the volume of normal tissues irradiated.

Simulation

The patient was placed in the supine position in a Vac-Lok device (MED-TEC Inc., Orange City, IA) for immobilization. His arms were extended overhead in order not to limit the gantry angles used for treatment (Figure 21.1-1). A planning CT scan was performed with 3.0 mm spacing on a GE Light Speed scanner (GE Healthcare, Waukesha, WI). The planning scan extended from above the diaphragm and down to the bottom of the ischial tuberosities and was performed during normal respiration. To ensure accurate visualization of the small bowel, oral contrast was administered 30 minutes prior to CT simulation.

Target and Tissue Delineation

All of the volumes of interest were then contoured on the planning CT scan (Figure 21.1-2). The gross tumor volume (GTV) consisted of all gross disease seen on the planning CT scan. Diagnostic and planning CT scans were carefully compared to ensure proper target delineation.

The clinical target volume (CTV) in this patient consisted of the GTV plus regional lymph nodes. In patients with pancreatic head tumors, the regional lymph node sites include the porta hepatic and celiac axis.[1–6] Accurate delineation of these nodal regions is crucial. The celiac axis is typically located at T11–12 (often the celiac truck can be visualized) (see Figure 21.1-2). During contouring, the celiac axis should be delineated on approximately three to five CT slices. The porta hepatis is located at the level of the hepatic duct bifurcation.

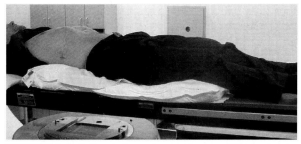

FIGURE 21.1-1. Patient in the supine position immobilized using the Vac-Lok system. (To view a color version of this image, please refer to the CD-ROM.)

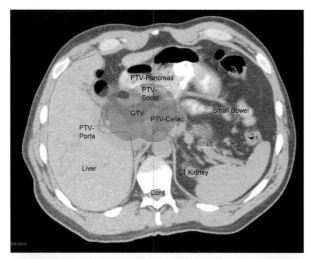

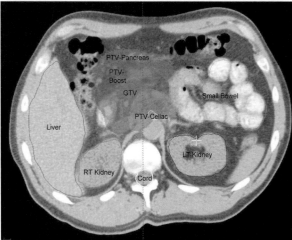

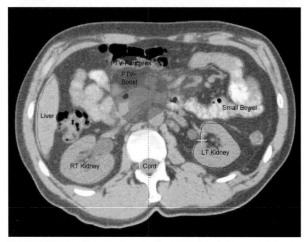

FIGURE 21.1-2. Planning target volume (PTV) and organs at risk contoured on axial computed tomography images. GTV = gross tumor volume. (To view a color version of this image, please refer to the CD-ROM.)

Two planning target volumes (PTVs) were designated in this patient. The initial planning target volume (PTV₁) consisted of the CTV with a 2.5 cm uniform expansion, accounting for setup uncertainties and organ motion.[7–10] PTV₁ was modified at the vertebral column, the borders of the organs at risk (OAR), and the skin. A boost PTV (PTV₂) was created with reduced margins of 1.75 cm around the GTV.

The OAR contoured in this patient included the right and left kidneys, liver, small bowel, and spinal cord. Each of these tissues was contoured separately, as shown in Figure 21.1-2.

Treatment Planning

The IMRT plan in this patient was generated using the *Eclipse* treatment planning system (Varian Medical Systems, Palo Alto, CA). The treatment plan was composed of seven coplanar beams with gantry angles consisting of 204, 225, 306, 0, 51, 102, and 153 degrees. Our treatment planning goals in patients with pancreatic cancer include homogeneous coverage of the PTV by the prescription dose with a maximum dose of 110% within the PTV. Dose constraints for the OAR are based on normal organ tolerance data.[11–14] The input parameters for inverse planning in this patient are shown in Table 21.1-1.

According to our in-house protocol, 45 Gy in 1.5 Gy twice-daily fractions (6-hour minimum interfraction interval) was prescribed to the PTV₁ followed by 14.5 Gy (also delivered twice daily), for a total dose of 59.5 Gy. Isodose distributions overlaid on an axial CT slices are shown in Figure 21.1-3. Composite dose-volume histograms for the OAR for both the initial and boost portions of treatment are shown on Figure 21.1-4.

TABLE 21.1-1. Intensity-Modulated Radiation Therapy Inverse Treatment Planning Algorithm Constraint Template

Structure	Volume (%)	Constraint Criteria
Planning treatment volume	100	Prescription dose: 50.4 Gy Minimum dose: 45 Gy Priority: 90%
Gross tumor volume	100	Prescription dose: 61.2 Gy Minimum dose: 59.4 Gy Priority: 90%
Small bowel	100	Maximum dose: 45 Gy Maximum dose: 48 Gy Maximum dose: 50 Gy Maximum dose: 55 Gy Priority: 80%

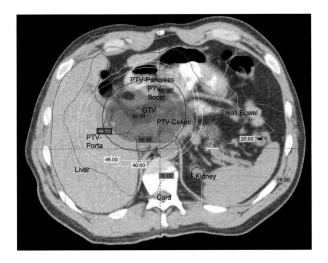

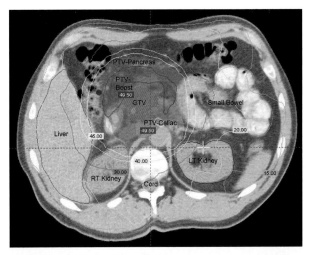

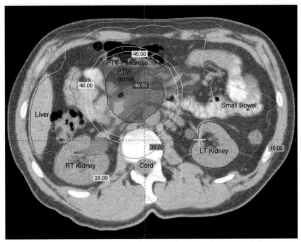

FIGURE 21.1-3. Axial computed tomomgraphy images with corresponding isodose lines. GTV = gross tumor volume; PTV = planning target volume. (To view a color version of this image, please refer to the CD-ROM.)

Treatment Delivery and Quality Assurance

IMRT was delivered using 18 MV photons on a Varian CL 2300 linear accelerator (Varian Medical Systems) equipped with a 120 dynamic multileaf collimator. Treatment was delivered using a sliding window approach.

Careful quality assurance is crucial for all patients undergoing IMRT. In our patients, port film verification is performed prior to the initiation of treatment and is continued on a weekly basis. Orthogonal films, including both anterior-posterior and lateral views, are used to confirm the isocenter position. The isocenter position is compared to the digitally reconstructed radiograph from the treatment planning computer.

Clinical Outcome

Following completion of induction chemotherapy, a repeat abdominal CT scan was performed, which failed to reveal any significant change in the tumor. The patient was still felt to be unresectable and was thus treated with definitive chemoradiotherapy. He tolerated treatment well without

significant acute toxicity. Following completion of IMRT, the patient was enrolled in a protocol evaluating pancreatic vaccine therapy. He subsequently expired 10 months later secondary to progressive disease.

We recently reported the outcome of patients with pancreatic cancer treated at our institution with IMRT.[15] Between March 2000 and March 2001, nine patients with locally advanced pancreatic cancer were treated. Seven underwent neoadjuvant chemoradiotherapy owing to unresectable T4 disease; two received chemoradiotherapy following surgery. The total radiation dose ranged from 49.5 to 60 Gy. Three patients received 1.5 Gy twice daily to a total dose of 49.5 Gy on a phase I clinical trial (the remainder received 1.8 Gy daily fractions). All patients received continuous infusion 5-FU.

Overall, treatment was well tolerated. The most common gastrointestinal complaints were nausea and emesis. One patient developed grade 3, three patients grade 2, and one patient grade 1 nausea. Diarrhea was observed in only two patients (both grade 1). Only one patient required a treatment break for external biliary stent revision. At a median follow-up of 5 months, no late toxicities were reported. Although preliminary, these results suggest that IMRT may allow dose escalation strategies to be safely employed in these patients.

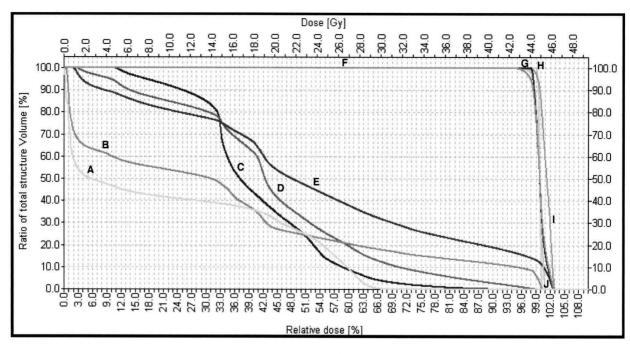

Dose Constrained Organs

Liver   Kidney-LT   Kidney-RT   Small Bowel   Spinal Cord

FIGURE 21.1-4. Composite dose-volume histograms for the organs at risk. LT = left; RT = right. (To view a color version of this image, please refer to the CD-ROM.)

References

1. Tepper J, Nardi G, Suit H. Carcinoma of the pancreas: review of MGH experience from 1963 to 1973. Analysis of surgical failure and implications for radiation therapy. Cancer 1976;37:1519–24.

2. Cubilla AL, Fortner J, Fitzgerald PJ. Lymph node involvement in carcinoma of the head of the pancreas area. Cancer 1978;41:880–7.

3. Griffin JF, Smalley SR, Jewell W, et al. Patterns of failure after curative resection of pancreatic carcinoma. Cancer 1990;66:56–61.

4. Johnstone PA, Sindelar WF. Lymph node involvement and pancreatic resection: correlation with prognosis and local disease control in a clinical trial. Pancreas 1993;8:535–9.

5. Gunderson LL, Martenson JA, Smalley SR, et al. Upper gastrointestinal cancers: rationale, results, and techniques of treatment. Front Radiat Ther Oncol 1994;28:121–39.

6. Dobelbower RR, Borgelt BB, Strubler KA, et al. Precision radiotherapy for cancer of the pancreas: technique and results. Int J Radiat Oncol Biol Phys 1980;6:1127–33.

7. Gierga DP, Chen GTY, Kung JH, et al. Quantification of respiration-induced abdominal tumor motion and its impact on IMRT dose distributions. Int J Radiat Oncol Biol Phys 2004;58:1584–1595.

8. Bussels B, Goetals L, Feron M, et al. Respiration-induced movement of the upper abdominal organs: a pitfall of the three-dimensional conformal radiation treatment of pancreatic cancer. Radiother Oncol 2003;68:69–74.

9. Balter JM, Lam KL, McGinn CJ, et al. Improvement of CT-based treatment planning models of abdominal targets using static exhale imaging. Int J Radiat Oncol Biol Phys 1998;41:939–43.

10. Horst E, Micke O, Moustakis C, et al. Conformal therapy for pancreatic cancer: variation of organ position due to gastrointestinal distention—implications for treatment planning. Radiology 2002;222:681–6.

11. Coia LR, Myerson RJ, Tepper JE. Late effects of radiation therapy on the gastrointestinal tract. Int J Radiat Oncol Biol Phys 1995;31:1213–36.

12. Emami B, Lyman J, Brown A, et al. Tolerance of normal tissue to therapeutic irradiation. Int J Radiat Oncol Biol Phys 1991;21:109–15.

13. Lyman JT. Complication probabilities as assessed from dose-volume histograms. Radiat Res 1985;104:S13–9.

14. Letschert JG, Lebesque JV, Aleman BM, et al. The volume effect in radiation-related late small bowel complications: results of a clinical study of the EORTC radiotherapy cooperative group in patients treated for rectal carcinoma. Radiother Oncol 1994;32:116–23.

15. Landry JC, Yang GY, Ting JY, et al. Treatment of pancreatic cancer tumors with intensity-modulated radiation therapy (IMRT) using the volume at risk approach (VARA): employing dose-volume histogram (DVH) and normal tissue complication probability (NTCP) to evaluate small bowel toxicity. Med Dosim 2002;27:121–9.

RECTAL CANCER CASE STUDY

JAVIER ARISTU, MD, PhD, JUAN D. AZCONA, MSc, MARTA MORENO, MD, RAFAEL MARTÍNEZ-MONGE, MD, PhD

Patient History

A 64-year-old male presented with a 3-month history of rectal bleeding and a 2 kg weight loss. Physical examination and a digital rectal examination were unremarkable. Colonoscopy and endorectal ultrasonography identified an ulcerated mass arising from the lateral wall of the distal rectum 4 cm above the external anal sphincter. The mass involved 40% of the rectal circumference and extended to the subserosa. Several suspicious perirectal lymph nodes were identified. The biopsy was positive for well-differentiated adenocarcinoma.

Computed tomography (CT) of the pelvis was performed and demonstrated thickening of the distal rectum with involvement of the perirectal fat. No enlarged pelvic lymph nodes were seen. The remainder of his workup, including chest and abdominal CT scans, revealed no evidence of metastatic disease. Liver function tests and carcinoembryonic antigen levels were within normal limits. According to the TNM staging system, the tumor was staged as T3N1M0.

The patient was enrolled in a prospective phase I–II study of escalating doses of intensity-modulated radiation therapy (IMRT) chemoradiation for locally advanced rectal cancer. He was assigned to receive the upper dose level of preoperative IMRT (47.5 Gy in 19 fractions) with concomitant capecitabine 825 mg/m^2 (twice daily) and oxaliplatin 60 mg/m^2 (on days 1, 8, and 15).

Simulation

The patient was immobilized in the prone position using a combination of a foam cushion and a prone head cushion. Three lasers were used to align the patient, and marks were drawn on the patient's skin and the bag to assist in daily setup reproducibility. Three radiopaque adhesive setup markers (one midline anteroposterior and two lateral) were placed on the skin. A planning CT scan was performed using a diagnostic CT scanner (Somatron Plus 4, Siemens Oncology Care Systems, Heidelberg, Germany)

with a flat table insert. The scan extended from the L2 vertebral body to below the perineum with a slice thickness of 5 mm. The patient was asked to empty his bladder and rectum prior to the CT scan. No contrast was administered during the CT scan.

Target and Tissue Delineation

The tumor target and organs at risk (OAR) were contoured on axial CT slices in the Helax-TMS treatment planning system (Nucletron Scandinavia, Uppsala, Sweden) (Figure 21.2-1). The gross tumor volume (GTV) was defined as the primary tumor and suspicious lymph nodes visualized on the CT scan. The clinical target volume (CTV) included the GTV, the presacral region, and the common and internal iliac lymph nodes. A planning target volume (PTV) was generated by adding a margin of 1 cm uniformly around the CTV. In areas in which the tumor was in close proximity to the small bowel and bladder, a 0.5 cm expansion was used.

The OAR outlined in this case were the bladder and the small bowel. The small bowel was outlined 1 cm above and below the PTV. Only the small bowel outside the PTV was contoured.

Treatment Planning

IMRT treatment planning was performed using the *KonRad* inverse planning system, version 2.0 (Siemens Oncology Care Systems). Seven coplanar equally spaced fields (gantry angles 0, 51, 103, 154, 206, 257, and 308 degrees) were used with 53 segments. The isocenter was placed at the geometric center of the PTV. The beam energy of all seven beams was 15 MV.

In the *KonRad* system, the treatment planner specifies both maximum and minimum dose constraints for the PTV. For the OAR, only a maximum dose constraint is required, but the user can also manipulate the dose-volume histogram (DVH) shape with a set of five dose-volume constraints. The final solution obtained depends on the

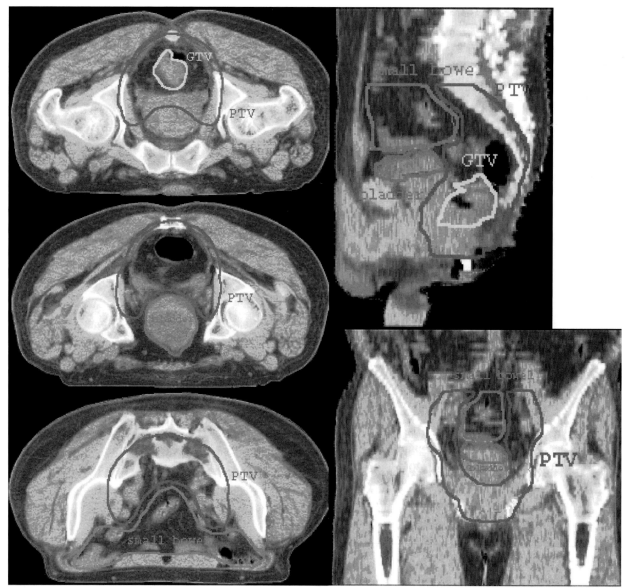

FIGURE 21.2-1. The gross tumor volume (GTV), planning target volume (PTV), and organs at risk contoured on the axial, sagittal, and coronal computed tomography (CT) slices. (To view a color version of this image, please refer to the CD-ROM).

steps followed during the optimization process. In our experience, the input parameters are modified from one solution to another until the DVHs and the dose statistics are found to satisfy all clinical requirements.

The initial and final sets of input parameters for this patient are listed in Table 21.2-1. The minimum doses for the GTV and the PTV were 47.5 Gy and 40 Gy, respectively, and the median dose was 50 Gy for both volumes. The desired dose delivered to 5% of the volume and median target doses for the bladder and small bowel were 45 Gy and 35 Gy and 40 Gy and 25 Gy, respectively. Figure 21.2-2 and Table 21.2-2 illustrate the DVH and final dose statistics respectively, in this patient. The isodose curves of the optimized IMRT plan are shown in Figure 21.2-3.

Treatment Delivery and Quality Assurance

IMRT treatment was delivered on a Mevatron Primus linear accelerator (Siemens Oncology Care Systems, Concord, CA). The Primus multileaf collimator consists of 29 pairs of leaves (double-focused) 1 cm wide at the isocenter and two peripheral pairs of leaves 6.5 cm wide at the isocenter. Treatment was delivered in the step-and-shoot mode. The average delivery time for each fraction was approximately 20 minutes. The mean total treatment time, including patient positioning, was 30 minutes.

Before treatment delivery, the accuracy of the calculations performed by the inverse planning software was

TABLE 21.2-1. Intensity-Modulated Radiation Therapy Input Parameters

Name	Organ Type	Overlap Priority	Maximum Dose, Gy	Maximum Penalty	Minimum Dose, Gy	Minimum Penalty
Initial input parameters						
GTV	Target	—	51	10	51	10
PTV	Target	1	51	10	51	10
Small bowel	OAR	2	30	2	—	—
Bladder	OAR	3	40	1	—	—
Final input parameters						
GTV	Target	—	51	500	1,000	10
PTV	Target	1	51	800	1,000	10
Small bowel	OAR	2	30	40	—	—
Bladder	OAR	3	40	25	—	—

GTV = gross tumor volume: OAR = organ at risk; PTV = planning target volume.

verified. Using the patient plan parameters, dose was calculated to a white polystyrene phantom (PTW Freiburg, Freiburg, Germany), which was previously scanned and introduced into into the *KonRad* software. The phantom was composed of 30 × 30 cm² slices of 1 cm thickness. Dose distribution verification was performed with Kodak EDR2 (Eastman Kodak, Rochester, NY) radiographic films inserted between the phantom slices. The phantom was irradiated with the films in the axial position, and the calculated dose matrices were compared with the corresponding measured dose matrices. *VeriSoft* (PTW Freiburg) software was used for the comparison. The acceptance criterion is agreement within 5% of the dose for all points or 3 mm difference in the distance for points in a high-gradient area. The calculation of the gamma index takes these two criteria into account.[1] Figure 21.2-4 shows the gamma index map and the superposition of calculated and measured isodose lines.

For single points, verification with a 0.125 cm³ volume ionization chamber (PTW Freiburg, model 31002) was performed in a high-dose, low-gradient area. Three different points were irradiated. The agreement between the calculated dose and the measured absolute dose was 1.5%, −1.4%, and 1.7% (mean 0.6%).

Patient positioning and isocenter verification were initially checked using x-ray films for each gantry position by visual comparison of digitally reconstructed radiograms (DRRs). Weekly verifications were made before treatment delivery with orthogonal x-ray films fused with created DRRs in the Helax planning system. The patient was repositioned or the isocenter was readjusted if a discrepancy of more than 3 mm was observed.

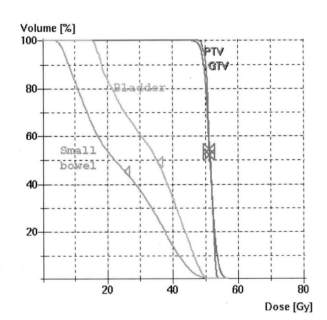

FIGURE 21.2-2. Dose-volume histogram showing the gross tumor volume (GTV), planning target volume (PTV), and organs at risk. (To view a color version of this image, please refer to the CD-ROM).

TABLE 21.2-2. Final Dose Statistics for the Volumes of Interest

Name	Volume, cm³	Minimum, Gy	Maximum, Gy	Mean Value, Gy	SD, Gy	5% Volume, Gy	50% Volume, Gy	95% Volume, Gy
GTV	69.9	50.65	55.11	52.10	0.50	53.14	52.12	51.56
PTV	1,439.0	40.46	56.53	51.04	1.51	53.48	51.22	48.62
Small bowel	588.3	4.08	52.89	23.65	12.41	44.43	21.82	6.78
Bladder	72.4	12.19	49.11	28.49	9.71	43.87	28.61	14.36

GTV = gross tumor volume; PTV = planning target volume.

Patient Outcome

The patient received the prescribed treatment dose (19 fractions of 2.67 Gy to a total GTV minimum dose of 50.65 Gy) without unplanned treatment interruptions. Overall, treatment was well tolerated, with only grade 2 rectal and grade 1 bladder acute sequelae noted. An abdominal-perineal resection with total mesorectal resection was performed 5 weeks following completion of treatment without any significant postoperative complications. The pathology revealed isolated tumor cells located in the submucosa,

and the lymph nodes were negative. The patient is currently receiving the first cycle of adjuvant chemotherapy with oxaliplatin and capecitabine.

From March 2003 to March 2004, 16 patients have been enrolled in this phase I–II study. The first three patients received 37.5 Gy, the next three patients received 42.5 Gy, and the remaining patients were treated with 47.5 Gy. All patients received 19 fractions. The tolerance was good, with acute grade 2 gastrointestinal toxicity in 50% of the patients. None developed grade 3 or higher toxicity. The pathologic response has been excellent, with an 85% downstaging rate.

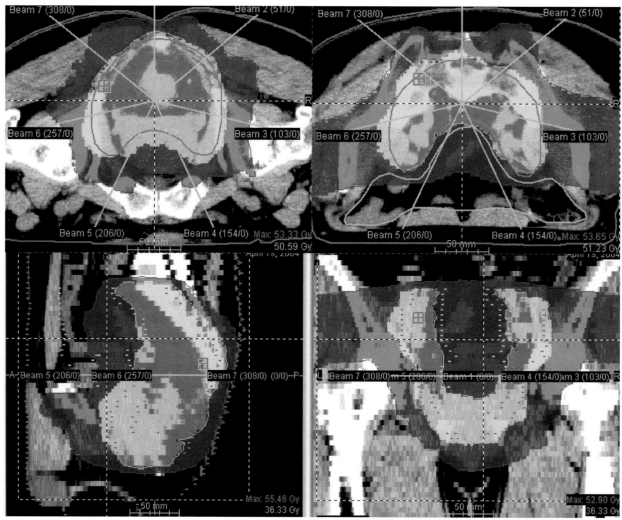

FIGURE 21.2-3. Axial, sagittal, and coronal computed tomography (CT) slices with superimposed dose distributions. The 47.5 Gy isodose surface (*green*) encompasses the gross tumor volume (GTV) and planning target volume (PTV), with the blue region representing the 25 Gy isodose. (To view a color version of this image, please refer to the CD-ROM).

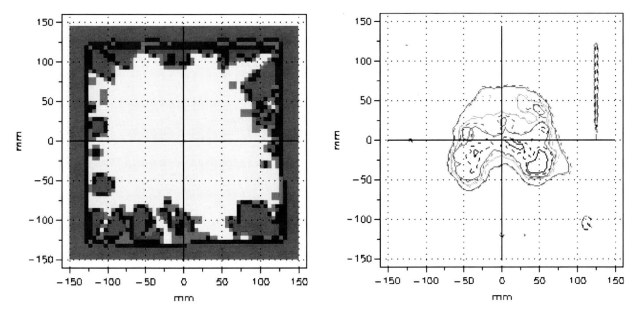

FIGURE 21.2-4. Gamma index map (*left*) and isodose comparison (*right*). The green color in the gamma map means that the acceptance criterion has been passed ($\gamma \leq 1$). The red color means that the test failed ($\gamma > 1$). The red color appears in the very low-dose area, where the measurement accuracy is lower. Below, the continuous lines represent the calculated isodoses and the dashed lines are the measured isodoses. The blue, orange, and red colors represent the 80%, 90%, and 95% isodose lines, respectively. (To view a color version of this image, please refer to the CD-ROM).

Reference

1. Low DA, Harms WB, Mutic S, Purdy JA. A technique for the quantitative evaluation of dose distributions. Med Phys 1998; 25:656–61.

ANAL CANCER

CASE STUDY

ANTHONY M. BERSON, MD, GREGORY M. RICHARDS, MD, RICHARD EMERY, MS, DABR

Patient History

A 57-year-old human immunodeficiency virus (HIV)-positive male presented with a 4-month history of hematochezia. Anoscopy revealed a 1 cm ulcerated lesion in the anal canal. On physical examination, there were no palpable inguinal lymph nodes. Biopsy of the lesion was consistent with an invasive moderately differentiated squamous cell carcinoma. Metastatic workup, including a computed tomography (CT) scan of the abdomen and pelvis, was negative for metastatic disease. The tumor was thus staged as a stage I (T1N0M0) anal carcinoma.

Previous experience treating HIV-positive patients with anal cancer revealed an increased incidence of acute toxicity from chemoradiation compared with HIV-negative patients. Based on this observation, we decided to treat the patient with intensity-modulated radiation therapy (IMRT) to reduce the dose to the surrounding normal tissues while delivering the prescribed dose to the target volumes.

Simulation

To minimize setup variability, the patient was positioned supine and immobilized with a custom vacuum-locking immobilization device. Oral and intravenous contrast were administered, and a radiopaque marker was placed at the anal verge, just inferior to the tumor. The patient was then scanned (NXi PRO, GE Healthcare, Waukesha, WI) from the L3 level down to 5 cm inferior of the anus, in 3 mm increments. An isocenter was chosen at midline, 6 cm posterior to the anterior-superior edge of the pubic symphysis. The completed CT scan was imported into our treatment planning system (*Eclipse*, Varian Medical Systems, Palo Alto, CA), where target delineation was performed.

Target and Tissue Delineation

Two clinical target volumes (CTVs) were delineated: an anal canal CTV and a nodal CTV. The inferior border of the anal canal CTV was delineated by the opaque marker

at the anal verge, and the CTV was continued superiorly for 12 slices to ensure coverage of the anal canal. This CTV includes the soft tissues surrounding the anal canal and the lymphatic plexus of the rectal mucosa. The nodal CTV included the inguinal nodes; common, internal, and external iliac nodes; obturator nodes; and presacral nodes. The contrast-enhanced vessels were used to define the nodal CTVs, which were contoured inferiorly to the level of the anal verge and superiorly to the L4–L5 interspace. In addition, critical avoidance structures consisted of bony anatomy, bladder, bowel, rectum, and genitals and were contoured on each CT slice.

To minimize underdosing of the target tissues, owing to organ motion and setup variation, margins were uniformly added to each CTV to create a planning target volume (PTV). The PTV of the anal canal was created by adding a uniform 1 cm margin in three dimensions to the anal canal CTV. To define the nodal PTV, a uniform 2 cm margin in three dimensions was added to the nodal CTV. Subsequently, this PTV was reduced in areas where it overlapped the bone, bladder, and bowel while carefully maintaining a minimum 1 cm margin from the nodal CTV. Any portion of the nodal PTV that extended outside the body was subtracted from each CT slice. Figure 21.3-1 illustrates the contouring of the target and avoidance structures. Not pictured in this figure is the contouring of the small bowel. To prevent the high-density oral contrast from affecting the dose calculation owing to heterogeneity corrections, the contoured small bowel's density was forced to 1.0, as illustrated in Figure 21.3-2.

Treatment Planning

A five-field coplanar IMRT plan was designed to deliver 54 Gy in three phases using gantry angles spaced at 72° intervals (36, 108, 180, 252, and 324 degrees; Varian IEC scale, Varian Medical Systems). Six-megavolt photons were used to treat the anterior-oblique fields, whereas the posterior and posterior-oblique fields were delivered with

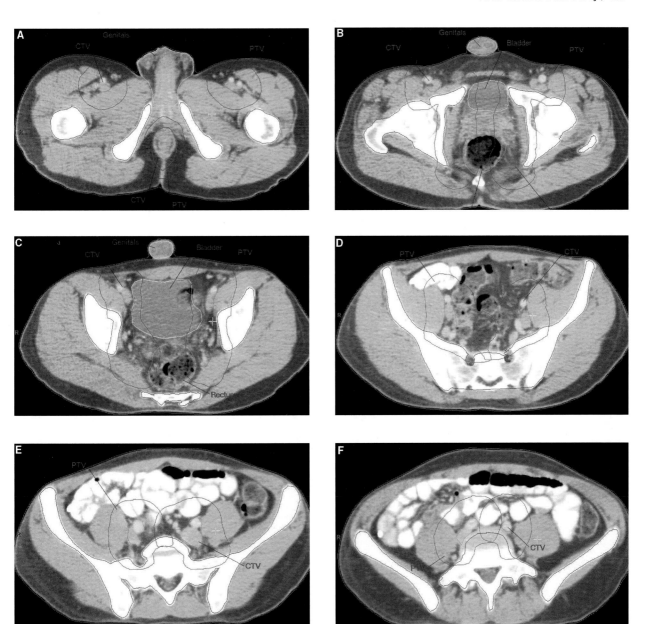

FIGURE 21.3-1. Axial computed tomography slices demonstrating the clinical target volume (CTV), planning target volume (PTV), and critical structures from the lower pelvis (*A*) superiorly to L5 (*F*).

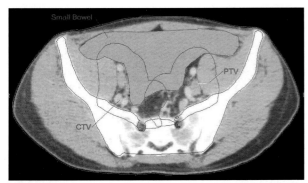

FIGURE 21.3-2. Contour of the small bowel with the density forced to 1.0 to allow for the use of heterogeneity corrections. CTV = clinical target volume; PTV = planning target volume.

15 MV photons. Six-megavolt photons were chosen for the anterior-oblique fields because the smaller skin-sparing effect improves target coverage to the shallow portion of the inguinal nodes compared with 15 MV photons. Phase I delivered 30.6 Gy to all PTVs. For phase II, the superior border was lowered to the bottom of the sacroiliac joints to deliver an additional 14.4 Gy. After 45 Gy, a final boost of 9 Gy was delivered to the anal canal PTV alone (phase III). The dose-volume constraints for all three phases are summarized in Table 21.3-1. Isodose curves are shown in Figure 21.3-3. A dose-volume histogram for the anal canal PTV, bladder, bone, bowel, genitalia, and rectum is shown in Figure 21.3-4.

TABLE 21.3-1. Input Parameters

	Phase I			Phase II			Phase III		
	Volume, %	Dose, Gy	Priority	Volume, %	Dose, Gy	Priority	Volume, %	Dose, Gy	Priority
PTV anal canal									
Upper	0	31.3	100	0	15.2	100	0	9.2	100
Lower	100	30.6	105	100	14.5	100	100	9.0	100
PTV nodes									
Upper	0	31.8	100	0	15.2	100			
Lower	100	30.6	100	100	14.5	100			
Bladder									
Upper	0	31.5	90	0	15.0	65			
Upper	63	26.1	65	66	13.3	65			
Upper	78	22.3	65	85	11.4	65			
Upper	91	17.8	65	97	9.3	65			
Small bowel									
Upper	0	31.3	65	0	15.0	65			
Upper	40	22.5	60	14	11.3	65			
Bone									
Upper	0	31.4	65	0	15.0	70	3	3.4	70
Upper	40	24.5	60	30	11.7	60	0	6.7	70
Rectum									
Upper	0	31.5	90	0	15.0	65			
Upper	68	26.8	65	62	13.7	65			
Upper	84	23.6	65	81	12.0	65			
Upper	95	19.1	65	94	9.3	65			
Genitalia									
Upper	0	25.0	95	0	11.5	80	0	3.0	90
Upper	30	20.5	65						

PTV = planning target volume.
Note: the optimization was performed using "upper" and "lower" points. Lower points refer to the minimum dose and percent volume that a specified structure should receive. Upper points refer to the maximum dose and percent volume that a structure should receive. When used together, upper and lower optimization points specify the bounds for the optimization. Multiple upper bounds are designated for critical structures to better define the shape of the desired dose-volume histogram. There is no lower bound for normal structures.

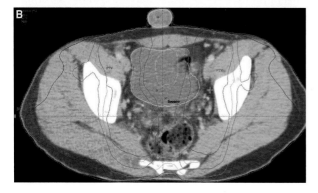

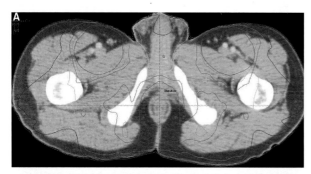

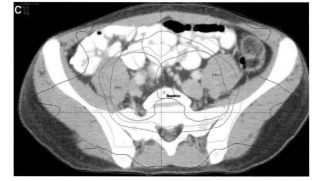

FIGURE 21.3-3. Axial computed tomography scans with isodose distribution of the intensity-modulated radiation therapy plan. The distribution lines represent the following isodose levels: 50% (*blue*), 70% (*green*), 90% (*magenta*), and 100% (*pink*). The planning target volumes (PTV) are outlined with the red lines. (To view a color version of this image, please refer to the CD-ROM.)

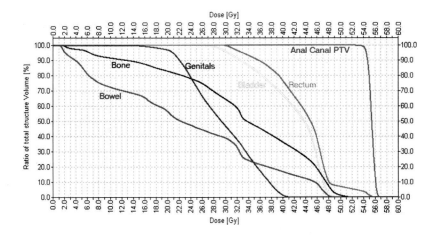

FIGURE 21.3-4. Dose-volume histogram of the sum of all three intensity-modulated radiation therapy phases totaling 54 Gy. Included are the anal canal planning target volume (PTV) (*red*), rectum (*pink*), bladder (*yellow*), genitals (*brown*), bone (*blue*), and bowel (*green*). (To view a color version of this image, please refer to the CD-ROM.)

Treatment Delivery and Quality Assurance

The patient was treated with sliding-window IMRT using a Varian 21EX linear accelerator (Varian Medical Systems) with a 120-leaf multileaf collimator. Setup accuracy was confirmed daily with anterior-posterior and lateral electronic portal images to verify the location of the isocenter and the patient setup. Because the penis lies adjacent to and can potentially fall into the radiation fields targeting the inguinal nodes and anal canal, it is important to position it identically for daily treatment as it was during the initial simulation. Typically, the optimal position when using a five-field coplanar IMRT as described above is taped in the midsagittal plane, preferably pointing toward the patient's feet. However, optimal positioning may vary on an individual basis. Daily setup time and treatment time were approximately 3 to 5 minutes and 12 to 15 minutes, respectively.

Patient-specific quality assurance was performed by comparing the expected and measured dose distributions in the phantom using the patient's specific IMRT treatment fields. The relative dose distribution was measured using film placed in the phantom's coronal plane. The resultant distribution was compared with the predicted distribution in the same plane. Agreement was within 3 mm or 3%. Additionally, an absolute dose measurement was performed using a MOSFET detector (Thompson and Nielson Electronics Ltd., Ontario, Canada). The absolute dose agreed with the predicted dose within 3%.

Clinical Outcome

This patient tolerated treatment extremely well and was able to complete the full course of radiation with concomitant 5-fluorouracil (two cycles) and mitomycin C (one cycle). He exhibited a complete clinical response in 43 days. He developed mild acute skin and lower gastrointestinal toxicities at approximately 21.6 Gy. The skin reaction, mild erythema and dry desquamation, was treated topically and completely resolved within 12 weeks of beginning treatment. His main complaint was uncomfortable bowel movements that resolved within 2 weeks with topical hydrocortisone. He developed a severe, although asymptomatic, leukopenia (700/μL) and thrombocytopenia (36,000/μL) during the third week of treatment that resolved quickly without the use of colony-stimulating factors. After 12 months of follow-up, the patient remained clinically free of disease, without any chronic toxicities.

Intact Prostate Cancer

Overview

Alan Pollack, MD, PhD, Robert Price, PhD, Lei Dong, PhD, Steven J. Feigenberg, MD, Eric M. Horwitz, MD

Rationale for IMRT

The goal for the radiation oncologist treating prostate cancer is to maximize tumor control while minimizing toxicity. Improved disease control through dose escalation should not be at the expense of unacceptable toxicity. Any advance in the treatment of prostate cancer must satisfy this condition. The preliminary results using intensity-modulated radiation therapy (IMRT) indicate that the gains in disease control and toxicity reduction may be substantial when appropriate treatment parameters are used. The development of criteria for the application of IMRT to the treatment of any site is of the utmost importance. For prostate cancer, there is an even greater need because of the slow-growing natural history and the fact that many patients die from other causes. The rule of *do no harm* is especially apropos in the treatment of this disease.

Prostate Cancer Dose Response

Improved disease control through dose escalation using three-dimensional conformal radiation therapy (3DCRT) or IMRT has been the subject of several prostate-specific antigen (PSA)-era studies.[1–7] In nearly every retrospective or prospective sequential analysis, increased radiation dose has been associated with a reduction in disease failure, using the rising PSA profile as a surrogate end point. The subdivision of patients into risk groups (favorable, intermediate, and high) has led to the recognition that patients at intermediate risk benefit the most when doses are escalated above 70 Gy.

Table 22A-1 shows two common risk stratification schemes,[8] and Table 22A-2 summarizes the results of some of the dose escalation studies that subdivide patients by risk. In contrast to intermediate-risk patients, only modest gains in freedom from biochemical failure (FFBF) have been realized in high-risk patients, based solely on increasing the radiation dose from 70 to ≥ 75.6 Gy.[1,5,9] The dose response of favorable-risk patients has been limited mainly to doses ≤ 70 Gy. When going from < 70 to 70 Gy, a clear

dose response is evident.[1,4,9,10] In all of these existing reports, when a dose response in favorable-risk patients has been observed and doses ≥ 75.6 Gy were used, the comparison group contained patients treated to < 70 Gy. Recently, Zelefsky and colleagues presented data from the Memorial Sloan-Kettering Cancer Center (MSKCC) sequential dose escalation series indicating that with longer follow-up, even favorable-risk patients benefited from an increase in dose from 70 to > 75.6 Gy.[11] Perhaps with longer follow-up and, more importantly, randomized trials, others will confirm the importance of doses above 70 Gy in favorable-risk patients with prostate cancer.

The main end point used in prostate cancer external beam dose escalation trials is FFBF. The American Society for Therapeutic Radiology and Oncology (ASTRO) consensus definition served to standardize the classification of the rising PSA profile.[12] Although many discount the

TABLE 22A-1. Single- and Double-Factor High-Risk Models

Risk	Single Factor	Double Factor
Low	PSA ≤ 10 ng/mL GS 2–6 T1–T2c*	PSA < 10 ng/mL GS 2–6 T1–T2c
Intermediate	Presence of 1 or more PSA 10–20 ng/mL GS 7	Presence of 1 PSA > 10 ng/mL GS 7 T3
High	Presence of 1 or more PSA > 20 ng/mL GS 8–10 T3	Presence of 2 or 3 PSA > 10 ng/mL GS 7 T3

Adapted from Chism DB et al.[8] The single- and double-factor high risk models are patterned after those described by D'Amico et al and Zelefsky et al.[39,117] GS = Gleason score; PSA = prostate-specific antigen.
*T2b has sometimes been considered intermediate risk and T2c has sometimes been considered intermediate or high risk (see Lyons et al[4] and D'Amico and colleagues[117]). In the Fox Chase Cancer Center database, these patients have about the same prognosis as patients with T2a disease in univariate and multivariate analysis and so have been grouped in a favorable-risk category here.

TABLE 22A-2. Sequential Retrospective or Prospective Dose Escalation Results

Study (Institution)	Year	N	Risk	5-Year Results		p
				%bNED (Dose 1, Gy)	%bNED (Dose 2, Gy)	
Lyons (Cleveland Clinic)	2000	738	Low	81 (< 72)	98 (≥ 72)	.02
			High	41 (< 72)	75 (≥ 72)	.0001
Hanks (FCCC)	2000	618	Low*	86 (< 70)	80 (> 70)	NS
			Intermediate	29 (< 71.5)	66 (≥ 71.5)	< .05
			High	8 (< 71.5)	29 (≥ 71.5)	< .05
Pollack (MDACC)	2000	1,213	Low	84 (< 67)	91 (> 67–70)	NS
			Low	91 (> 67–77)	100 (> 77)	NS
			Intermediate	55 (≤ 67)	100 (> 77)	.0001
			Intermediate	79 (> 67–77)	89 (> 77)	NS
			High	27 (≤ 67)	47 (> 67–77)	.0001
			High	47 (> 67–77)	67 (> 77)	.016
Zelefsky (MSKCC)	2001	1,100	Low	77 (≤ 70)	90 (≥ 75.6)	.05
			Intermediate	50 (≤ 70)	70 (≥ 75.6)	.001
			High	21 (≤ 70)	47 (≥ 75.6)	.002

Adapted from Pollack A.[118]

%bNED = % biochemical no evidence of disease; FCCC = Fox Chase Cancer Center; MDACC = M. D. Anderson Cancer Center; MSKCC = Memorial Sloan-Kettering Cancer Center; NS = not significant.
*Based on pretreatment prostate-specific antigen level.

use of FFBF as a surrogate for clinical failure and death, reports are emerging that link biochemical failure to other disease end points, such as distant metastasis, cause-specific death, and overall death.[13–20] Long follow-up is required to measure the power of these associations, and, eventually, there will be greater confidence in using FFBF as a surrogate end point.

Although the application of the ASTRO definition on a broad basis has resulted in much needed standardization of PSA as an end point so that data between research groups may be compared, there are clearly pitfalls to the current definition that should be recognized. The ASTRO definition is based on three consecutive rises at follow-up of 3 to 6 months, with backdating of the failure to the midpoint between the nadir and the first rise in PSA. Under these conditions, 20 to 30% of patients who receive neoadjuvant or adjuvant androgen deprivation therapy are misclassified because of a transient rise in PSA and then a subsequent leveling off or fall in PSA.[21] Backdating distorts the shape of Kaplan-Meier curves, causing a flattening at the end of the later time points, resulting in falsely high estimates of FFBF, which is exacerbated by short follow-up.[22,23] Other definitions are being entertained as possible alternatives.[23–29] The "Houston definition" of a PSA rise of 2 ng/mL above the PSA nadir eliminates the effects of backdating and appears to be a better correlate of clinical outcome compared with the ASTRO definition.[25,27,28] Dose escalation data from retrospective and prospective sequential dose escalation studies are compelling, yet they all suffer from time-dependent confounding factors, which cannot be adequately controlled for in multivariate analysis. Because of the implementation of PSA in screening, transrectal

ultrasound-directed prostate biopsies, and more complete prostate biopsies (sextant or more), there has been a shift to earlier diagnosis and stage migration.[30–34] Perhaps more disturbing is that upgrading in Gleason scoring by pathologists has been observed over the last 10 years.[8,35,36] For example, a diagnostic sample graded as a Gleason score of 5 or 6 might now be upgraded to 6 or 7. Additionally, in sequential dose escalation analyses, follow-up is always shorter in the patients who received the higher radiation doses. As mentioned above, the ASTRO consensus definition of biochemical failure overestimates FFBF in Kaplan-Meier curves. These factors mar the interpretation of sequential dose escalation studies. The true impact of radiation dose requires a randomized comparison.

A number of randomized prostate cancer dose escalation trials are in progress around the world. The M. D. Anderson Cancer Center (MDACC) trial is the most mature.[6] Three hundred one assessable men were randomized between 70 and 78 Gy (isocenter doses). All were initially treated with a four-field box to 46 Gy, prescribed to the isocenter. The men in the 70 Gy arm received the remaining dose through a reduced four-field arrangement, whereas those in the 78 Gy arm were then treated with a six-field conformal boost. The margins (clinical target volume [CTV] to block edge) on the conformal boost were 0.75 to 1.0 cm posteriorly and superiorly and 1.25 to 1.5 cm anteriorly and inferiorly. The CTV consisted of the prostate and seminal vesicles. The freedom from failure results, based mainly on biochemical criteria, supported the conclusions of the sequential dose escalation trials. With 60 months median follow-up, the intermediate- to high-risk patients (initial pretreatment PSA > 10 ng/mL) experienced the

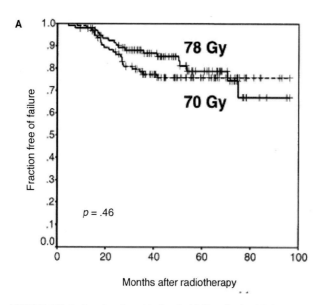
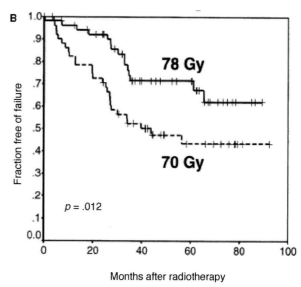

FIGURE 22A-1. Freedom from biochemical failure Kaplan-Meier results of the M. D. Anderson Cancer Center randomized trial. Figures display the patients with a pretreatment prostate-specific antigen (PSA) ≤ 10 and > 10 ng/mL, *A* and *B*, respectively. Reproduced with permission from Pollack A et al.[6]

greatest benefit (Figure 22A-1), whereas the 8 Gy radiation dose increase had no effect on the more favorable-risk patients (initial pretreatment PSA ≤ 10 ng/mL).

One limitation of the MDACC trial is that different boost field arrangements were used in the two randomization arms, conventional versus conformal. However, computed tomography (CT) was performed in all cases to ensure that the CTV was adequately covered by the boost treatment fields. The other limitation that was raised earlier is the use of FFBF as the main end point. The MDACC trial showed a trend toward a reduction in distant metastasis (*p* = .056, log rank) in the subset of patients with an initial pretreatment PSA level > 10 ng/mL, but there were only eight patients with distant metastasis at the time of the analysis. Certainly, larger clinical trials powered to detect differences in clinical disease and survival end points, such as distant metastasis and cause-specific death, are needed.

Radiation Dose and Morbidity

The effects of dose and volume on late rectal toxicity are well recognized.[6,37–47] The establishment of well-defined bladder dose-volume relationships for morbidity has been elusive, probably owing to the inconsistent volume of the bladder at simulation and the day-to-day (interfraction) variation during treatment, combined with the requirement for long follow-up owing to the late onset of symptoms.[48]

The associations of radiation dose and rectal volume to toxicity are summarized in Tables 22A-3 and 22A-4. Table 22A-3 shows that the relationship of radiation dose to grade 2 or higher rectal reactions has been observed by a number of groups with remarkably similar conclusions. In nearly every study, an association between higher doses and increased

rectal complications has been identified. Only the recently described randomized trial results from the Netherlands have yet to show an effect of dose; however, the follow-up in that study is relatively short.[47] In the MDACC randomized trial, it was not until the median follow-up was 5 years that a significant increase in the rectal complication risk was found in the patients who received the higher dose (Figure 22A-2).

The effect of rectal volume that receives higher radiation doses is displayed in Table 22A-4. These findings demonstrate that the volume of the rectum exposed to a specific radiation dose level is as important as the dose prescribed. The implication is that high radiation doses (≥ 75.6 Gy) may be used as long as the amount of rectum

TABLE 22A-3. Relationship of Radiation Dose to Grade 2 or Higher Rectal Morbidity

Study	Year	Dose, Gy	GI Toxicity, %
Smith	1990	≤ 70	22 (2 yr actuarial)
		> 70–75	20
		> 75	60
Shipley	1995	67.2	12 (10 yr actuarial)
		75.6 CGE	32
Lee	1996	< 72	7 (18-mo actuarial)
		72–76	16
		> 76	23
Zelefsky	1998	≤ 70.2	6 (5 yr actuarial)
		> 75.6	17
Pollack	2002	70	12 (5 yr actuarial)
		78	24
Lebesque	2003	68	18 (2.5 yr crude)
		78	24

GI = gastrointestinal.

TABLE 22A-4. Relationship of Rectal Volume Exposed to Radiation Marker Doses and Grade 2 or Higher Rectal Morbidity

Study	Year	Dose	Rectum	GI Toxicity, %
Benk	1993	67–76 CGE	V76$_{CGE}$ < 40% ARW	19 (40 mo actuarial)*
			V76$_{CGE}$ ≥ 40% ARW	71
Lee	1996	74–76 Gy	Rectal block	10 (18 mo actuarial)
			No block	19
Dearnaley	1999	64 Gy	3DCRT	8 (5 yr actuarial)
			Conventional RT	18
Boersma	1998	70 Gy	≤ 30	0 (crude)†
			> 30	9
Pollack	2002	70–78 Gy	V70$_{Gy}$ ≤ 25%	16 (6 yr actuarial)
			V70$_{Gy}$ > 25%	46
Kupelian	2002	78 Gy	≤ 15 cc	5 (24 mo actuarial)
			> 15 cc	22
Fiorino	2003	70–78 Gy	V50$_{Gy}$ ≤ 66%	8
			V50$_{Gy}$ > 66	32
			V70$_{Gy}$ ≤ 30%	8
			V70$_{Gy}$> 30%	24

ARW = anterior rectal wall; CGE = cobalt - Gy - equivalent ; 3DCRT = three-dimensional conformal radiation therapy; GI = gastrointestinal; RT = radiation therapy.
*Any rectal bleeding.
†Severe rectal bleeding.

exposed to specific marker doses remains lower than the thresholds defined. These thresholds vary from group to group, which complicates the adoption of criteria that should be used in IMRT planning. In implementing planning constraints that have been promulgated by a particular investigative team, one must carefully attempt to mimic all aspects of the features used in the planning process. These features include, for example, how the normal structures were identified (eg, whole rectum vs rectal wall, entire rectal length vs a smaller segment).

Kupelian and colleagues from the Cleveland Clinic reported that the absolute volume of the rectum that received the prescription radiation dose or higher was a more significant predictor of grade 2 or higher toxicity than the percentage of the rectum.[45] When > 15 cc of the rectum received greater than the prescription dose (78 Gy in 2 Gy fractions or 70 Gy in 2.5 Gy fractions), the risk of rectal bleeding was 22%, whereas the risk was 5% when ≤ 15 cc received greater than the prescription dose. They outlined only a segment of the rectum (not the entire length), extending from just above and below the prostate. Pollack and colleagues[6] and Huang and colleagues,[49] using data from MDACC, observed a stronger association of complication risk with the percentage of the rectum treated to certain marker doses as opposed to the absolute volume of the rectum. In these reports, the rectum was outlined from the ischial tuberosities, superiorly for an 11 cm segment. The 11 cm length was done because the initial fields extended 11 cm in the superior-inferior dimensions. Pollack and colleagues found that when ≤ 25% of the rectal volume received ≥ 70 Gy, grade 2 or higher rectal morbidity was 16% at 5 years versus 46% when > 25% of the rectal volume received ≥ 70 Gy (Figure 22A-3).[6] Huang and colleagues extended these observations by testing multiple rectal dose-volume (absolute and percentage) relationships.[49] The percentage of rectal volume correlated significantly with the incidence of rectal complications at multiple radiation therapy (RT) dose levels, whereas the absolute rectal volume criteria were significant only at the higher RT doses (70, 75.6, and 78 Gy). Fiorino and colleagues also found that the percentage of the rectum treated to specified dose levels was a robust determinant of rectal complication risk; they outlined from the anal verge to the sigmoid flexure superiorly.[44,46] This

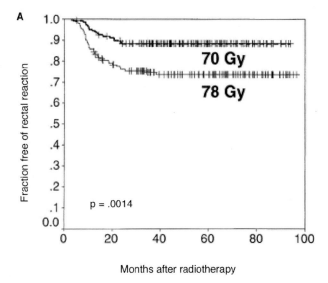

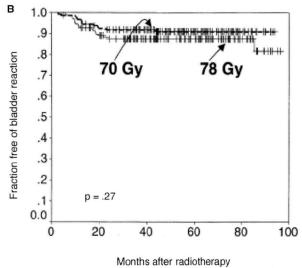

FIGURE 22A-2. Kaplan-Meier plots of the risk of grade 2 or higher rectal (*A*) or bladder (*B*) toxicity. Reproduced with permission from Pollack A et al.[6]

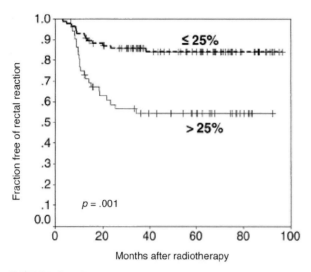

FIGURE 22A-3. Relationship of the percentage of rectum (≤ 25% vs > 25%) treated to ≥ 70 Gy to grade 2 or higher rectal morbidity. Reproduced with permission from Pollack A et al.[6]

is the volume of rectum that has been used in Radiation Therapy Oncology Group (RTOG) protocols and is the volume most commonly used.

The results of Skwarchuck and colleagues[50] and Jackson[43] from MSKCC were mixed in terms of whether absolute or percentage rectal wall volume should be used. The rectal wall was defined from just above the anal verge to just below the sigmoid flexure. They found that the maximum rectal dose and the rectal wall volume (a shorter volume implies a higher percentage exposed to a significant dose) were both correlates of ≥ grade 2 rectal bleeding. Enclosure of the rectum by the 50% line at the isocenter, age, and diabetes were also predictive of rectal morbidity. The significance of age and diabetes was small in comparison with the dose-volume histogram (DVH) factors.[43] Diabetes has been described by others to be a risk factor previously. Recently, Feigenberg and colleagues found that a history of diabetes was primarily a correlate of grade 3, not grade 2, complications.[51] Diabetes was not a factor in the MDACC study reported by Huang and colleagues.[49] The analysis by Jackson and colleagues found that the greatest significance of the relationship between rectal toxicity and dose was with the percentage of the rectal wall exposed to intermediate doses of 40 to 50 Gy.[43] They recommended DVH constraints of ≤ 60% rectal wall volume treated to ≥ 40 Gy and ≤ 30% rectal wall volume treated to ≥ 75.6 Gy. The DVH data in aggregate, therefore, indicate that a single dose-volume constraint is not optimal for minimizing rectal reactions. Our DVH constraints now include a second cutpoint in the 40 Gy range (see below).

Motion and Margin Considerations

The prostate is a moving target; its position is affected pri-marily by bladder and rectal volume changes. The majority of studies have estimated that day to day, or interfraction, prostate positional changes are considerable and, in general, are more influenced by rectal volume than by bladder volume.[52–57] Intrafraction prostate motion, which occurs during treatment delivery, could potentially result in inadequate coverage of the CTV and must also be considered. The extent of intrafraction motion is dependent on multiple factors, especially patient positioning (eg, prone vs supine, use of a thermoplastic shell).

Antolak and colleagues estimated that the planning target volume (PTV) margin required to contain the CTV 95% of the time was 1.1 cm in the anterior-posterior, 0.7 cm in the superior-inferior, and 0.7 cm in the left-right planes.[56] These calculations were based on considering uncertainties from interfraction motion and setup error. The extent of the uncertainties was in line with the reports of others. The major limitation of adhering to the 1.1 cm PTV anterior-posterior margin has been rectal toxicity, mainly in the form of increased rectal bleeding. Lee and colleagues showed in patients treated with conformal RT that when the fields extended 1.5 cm from the prostate to the block edge (ie, PTV = 1.0 cm, 0.5 cm additional margin for penumbra), rectal bleeding was substantial.[38] The results were improved by reducing the rectal volume irradiated through the use of a rectal block placed when the prostate dose was 60 to 70 Gy. A somewhat analogous approach has been in use at MSKCC, where a dose gradient in the overlap region of the PTV with the rectum, and hence the posterior aspect of the prostate as well, has been used to maintain maximum doses to the rectum in the 72 Gy range.[2,58,59] Although the FFBF results from MSKCC[2] and Fox Chase Cancer Center (FCCC)[9] have held up over time in patients who had such blocking, the margin is insufficient to adequately ensure coverage of the posterior aspect of the prostate—typically the region of greatest tumor involvement.

A better solution is to reduce or correct for interfraction motion such that rectal planning constraints may be met by using tighter margins throughout treatment. There are a number of methods for correcting for prostate motion. One approach is to immobilize the prostate against the pubic symphysis by placing a balloon in the rectum.[60,61] The use of a rectal balloon without imaging results in some variability in the position of the prostate from day to day.[62–64] The more common methods for localizing the prostate on a daily basis involve imaging. Ultrasonography has become a popular tool for the determination of prostate position.

The B-mode acquisition and targeting (BAT) system (North American Scientific, NOMOS Radiation Oncology Division, Cranberry Township, PA) was the first commercial ultrasound imaging device designed specifically to adjust for interfraction motion. The initial reports described a close correlation of the corrections from transabdominal ultrasonography with pelvic CT scan measurements.[65,66] Although suboptimal images occur in patients who cannot maintain fluid in the bladder or are obese, the quality of the images and the accuracy of the shifts by the therapists are usually acceptable.[67] The success of ultrasonography for the correction of interfraction prostate motion hinges on diligent quality assurance by the team of treating physicians, medical physicists, and radiation therapists. The group must periodically review and agree on policies regarding the shifts. The physicians must also check each daily ultrasonography-based shift and must constantly give feedback to the therapists. Without such practices, the value of the ultrasonography method has been questioned.[68] Recently, Patel and colleagues described using both a rectal balloon and ultrasonography to target the prostate more precisely.[69] The advantages of this technique are that the prostate position is defined by the sonogram and the prostate is immobilized to prevent intrafraction motion.

The other popular prostate localization strategy is to implant radiopaque metallic (usually gold) seed markers in the prostate that may be visualized via electronic portal imaging.[54,70–73] Software is available to triangulate the position of the seeds in three-dimensional space from orthogonal images with considerable accuracy. Concern over seed migration has been largely unfounded,[74] but how representative the limited number of seeds are to the three-dimensional shape of the prostate is still unknown.

The prostate may also be imaged just prior to treatment using CT. Lattanzi and colleagues accomplished daily prostate CT by moving patients on a stretcher between the CT simulator and the treatment room.[75] More recently, CT scanners have been placed within linear accelerator rooms, allowing for prostate position measurements and adjustments with the patients on a table that shuttles between the CT scanner and linear accelerator.[76–78] Hua and colleagues reported that using standard weekly port film alignments on bony anatomy, a portion of the prostate falls outside the 6 mm posterior PTV (prostate-rectum dimension) about 35% of the time.[77] These conclusions are remarkably similar to those obtained with daily BAT ultrasonography.[67,79] In the near future, it will be possible to acquire cone beam megavoltage (using the megavoltage beam) or kilovoltage (using a gantry-mounted device) CT images by rotating the gantry with the patient in the treatment position.[80,81]

Advances in imaging have substantially improved the ability to correct for interfraction prostate positional changes. Further advances along these lines are anticipated in the near future. One example is the development of nonionizing electromagnetic transponders (1.85 × 8 mm; Calypso Medical Technologies, Seattle, WA) that can be permanently positioned in the prostate, like gold seeds, and the resultant magnetic field-monitored with a high degree of positional accuracy.[82] The transponders may be tracked in real time, not only to correct for interfraction uncertainty in prostate location but also to track intrafraction motion. One must consider that the chance for intrafraction motion during an IMRT treatment (~ 15–20 minutes) is much greater than

that for conformal RT (~ 10 minutes). There may be changes in bladder and rectal volume during this time, as well as in patient compliance with remaining in the same position. In most cases, intrafraction motion is inconsequential when the patient is positioned supine without a thermoplastic shell over the pelvis and lower abdomen.[73,83,84] Effects from respiration are minimized in this position.[72,85,86]

IMRT versus 3DCRT
Dosimetric Studies

The prostate is a nearly ellipsoid structure, and, as such, the gains from using IMRT over 3DCRT might be negligible. Dong and colleagues systematically investigated this question in patients with favorable-risk prostate cancer who did not have much of the seminal vesicles outlined.[87] They rationalized that the inclusion of the seminal vesicles in this test might give IMRT an advantage. Therefore, the conditions used were heavily weighted in favor of 3DCRT. The same CTV-to-PTV expansion margins were used in all plans. Two different IMRT delivery methods (a Peacock MIMiC system [North American Scientific] and a 10-field static multileaf collimator system [Varian Medical Systems, Palo Alto, CA]) were compared with four 3D-conformal plans. The conformal plans were based on a 4-field technique, two 7-field techniques with different weightings from the laterals (40% and 50%), and the 10-field conformal boost technique used in the MDACC randomized dose escalation trial (four-field conventional followed by a 6-field conformal boost). All plans were prescribed to the PTV to 75.6 Gy, with the exception of the MDACC protocol method, which was prescribed to 78 Gy to the isocenter, as was done in the original trial. The 78 Gy isocenter plan actually had a lower CTV mean dose (Figure 22A-4). Figure 22A-4 shows that the highest mean CTV doses were achieved in the two IMRT plans. Figure 22A-5 demonstrates that the IMRT plans resulted in the lowest percentage of the rectum treated to over ≥ 70 Gy. The IMRT plans were also associated with lower volumes of the bladder and femoral heads treated to ≥ 70 Gy and ≥ 50 Gy, respectively. The two IMRT plans were nearly identical in terms of the DVH parameters. The benefits of IMRT over 3DCRT were both in the achievement of higher doses to the CTV and the limitation of exposure of the nearby normal tissues to the higher radiation doses. The FCCC IMRT approach in early stage prostate cancer patients is presented in Chapter 22.1, "Intact Prostate Cancer: Case Study." Others have come to similar conclusions.[59,88–90]

Several investigators have evaluated the use of IMRT to irradiate the pelvic lymph nodes in prostate cancer patients.[91–95] Investigators at Stanford compared intensity-modulated nodal RT with 3DCRT planning in 20 prostate cancer patients.[94] IMRT reduced the mean volumes of rectum, bladder, and bowel receiving > 40 Gy by 50.2%, 69.8%,

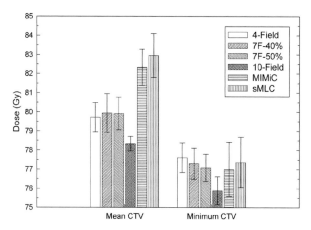

FIGURE 22A-4. Comparison of mean and minimum clinical target volume (CTV) doses in six different plans (four three-dimensional conformal radiation therapy and two intensity-modulated radiation therapy). The CTV included the prostate and proximal seminal vesicles and was identical for all of the different plans. The prescription for five of the plans was for the planning target volume to receive 75.6 Gy; the 10-field plan was prescribed to 78 Gy to the isocenter, as was done in the M. D. Anderson Cancer Center randomized trial. MIMiC = multileaf intensity-modulating collimator; sMLC = static multileaf collimator.

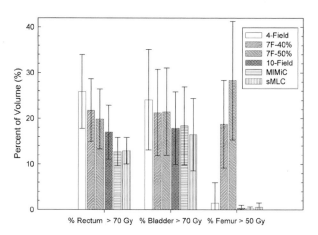

FIGURE 22A-5. Comparison of the percentages of the rectum treated to ≥ 70 Gy, bladder treated to ≥ 70 Gy, and femoral heads treated to ≥ 50 Gy. The prescription for five of the plans was for the planning target volume to receive 75.6 Gy; the 10-field plan was prescribed to 78 Gy to the isocenter, as was done in the M. D. Anderson Cancer Center randomized trial. Reproduced with permission from Pollack A.[9]

and 60.8%, respectively (see Chapter 22.3, "Targeted Lymph Node Irradiation: Case Study").

Another potential role for IMRT in prostate cancer is the delivery of an intraprostatic boost. Investigators at University of California San Francisco (UCSF) have demonstrated the feasibility of treating the entire prostate to a total dose of > 70 Gy while concurrently treating a dominant intraprostatic lesion identified by endorectal MR and MR spectroscopy (MRS) to 90 Gy.[96,97] The Royal Marsden Hospital intraprostatic IMRT boost approach is described in detail in Chapter 22.5, "Intra-Prostatic Boost: Emerging Technology."

Other novel uses of IMRT in prostate cancer patients are to reduce dose to the penile bulb and other penile structures without compromising target coverage[98–100] and to potentially "repair" an acceptable interstitial prostate implant (see Chapter 22.6, "Repair of Unacceptable Implants: Emerging Technology").[101]

Clinical Studies

Several centers have reported promising clinical results in prostate cancer patients treated with IMRT, substantiating the dosimetric conclusions of the superiority of IMRT over 3DCRT.[1,2,59,60,102] The most mature data are from MSKCC. In a series of reports[1,2,59] Zelefsky and coworkers have reported high rates of biochemical control with low rectal toxicity in patients treated to ≥ 81 Gy (Figure 22A-6). In their initial report,[59] the outcomes of 171 IMRT and 61 3DCRT patients treated to 81 Gy were compared. The 2-year actuarial risk of grade 2–3 rectal injury in the 3DCRT and IMRT patients were 24% and 2%, respectively (p < .001). No dif-

ference was seen in late urinary toxicity. In a follow-up report of 772 patients,[2] the 3-year actuarial risk grade ≥ 2 late rectal toxicity was 4%. Three-year actuarial PSA control for favorable-, intermediate-, and high-risk patients was 92%, 86%, and 81%, respectively (Figure 22A-7).

Investigators at the Cleveland Clinic have explored the use of hypofractionated IMRT (70 Gy in 2.5 Gy fractions) (see Chapter 22.2, "Hypofractionated IMRT: Case Study").[103–106] In a comparison of 166 IMRT and 116 3DCRT patients, IMRT patients had a better 30 month actuarial PSA control (94 vs 88%); however, the difference failed to reach statistical significance (p = .08). On multivariate analysis, the most significant factors correlated with PSA control were pretreatment PSA level and Gleason score. Grade 2–3 rectal injury rates at 30 months for the 3DCRT and IMRT groups were 12% and 5%, respectively (p = .24). In their most recent report,[106] Djemil and colleagues reported a 4-year late rectal toxicity rate of 3.6%. Others have reported promising preliminary results using hypofractionated approaches.[107,108]

More limited outcome data are available in prostate cancer patients treated with an IMRT intraprostatic boost[109] or intensity-modulated pelvic RT.[110] As noted above, the Stanford targeted nodal IMRT approach is described in detail in Chapter 22.3.

IMRT Planning Considerations

Inverse planning is a powerful method for escalating dose and reducing toxicity. Central to obtaining this goal is the adoption of strict normal tissue constraints. The latest

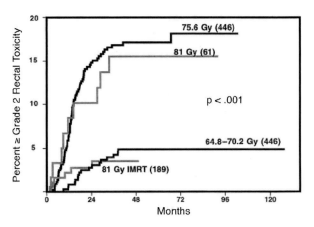

FIGURE 22A-6. Effect of intensity-modulated radiation therapy (IMRT) on grade 2 or higher rectal complications. These data are from the Memorial Sloan-Kettering Cancer Center group sequential prospective dose escalation study. The ≥ grade 2 rectal reactions are shown for patients treated with three-dimensional conformal radiation therapy to 64.8 to 70.2 Gy, 75.6 Gy, and 81 Gy and with IMRT to 81 Gy. Reproduced with permission from Zelefsky MJ et al.[1]

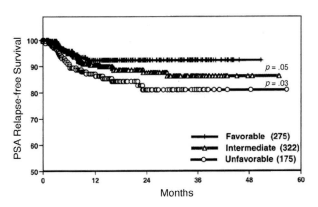

FIGURE 22A-7. Kaplan-Meier freedom from biochemical failure for men with prostate cancer treated at Memorial Sloan-Kettering Cancer Center with intensity-modulated radiation therapy. Six hundred ninety-eight patients were treated to 81 Gy and 74 patients were treated to 86.4 Gy. Four hundred twenty-six patients received 3 months of neoadjuvant androgen deprivation. The double-factor risk stratification scheme (see Table 22A-1) was used. PSA = prostate-specific antigen. Reproduced with permission from Zelefsky MJ et al.[2]

inverse planning software allows for exceptional dose conformity, but the attainment of an optimal plan requires an understanding of such constraints on several levels and the intricacies of the planning system. The latter is almost as important as the constraints because there are methods for forcing dose into the PTV and reducing dose to the surrounding normal tissue such that constraints are met with fewer segments and shorter treatment times.[112] As described above, objective DVH criteria have clearly been associated with rectal toxicity. Rectal side effects are manifest by 2 to 4 years,[6] whereas bladder side effects mature over a much longer time course.[48] The rectal constraints that have been implemented are based on sound data. Bladder constraints are less well defined. As a consequence of this and the considerable variability in interfraction bladder volume, bladder planning restrictions have, in general, been less strict.

Of key importance in adopting planning parameters from published studies is an understanding of how the patient has been simulated (supine vs prone) and how anatomy has been defined. Investigators at MSKCC use rectal and bladder wall volumes, whereas those at MDACC, FCCC, and the Cleveland Clinic include the entire rectal contents. If the rectum is simulated empty (after an enema), it is difficult to discern the rectal wall in many cases. Simulating with the rectum empty also serves to plan under the worst conditions if a percentage parameter is used; the lower the rectal volume, the more sensitive the DVH is to overlap with higher RT doses. We simulate with the rectum empty and the bladder about half-full. If patients are told to have a completely full bladder, they end up having more fluid in the bladder than they are able to achieve during treatment.

Target Volumes

The prostate cancer gross tumor volume (GTV) is ill-defined on three-dimensional imaging studies, such as CT and magnetic resonance imaging (MRI). The prostate (± seminal vesicles) represents the CTV. The prostate, particularly at the bladder–prostate base superiorly and the prostate apex–urogenital diaphragm inferiorly, is better defined on MRI than on CT. Also, the boundaries of the surrounding normal structures (bladder, rectum, penile bulb) are more easily defined on MRI.

Adequate coverage of the apex of the prostate is of particular concern. In over 30% of cases, there is tumor involvement at the apex of the prostate at prostatectomy.[113,114] Because the prostatic capsule is absent from this region, microscopic extension inferiorly is frequent. Moreover, distinct identification of the prostate apex, even on MRI, is not unqualified. For these reasons, the CTV should extend about two imaging slices (each slice is 3 mm) below where the prostate apex is believed to end. Another consideration for extended margins in the superior-inferior dimensions is that localization of the prostate by ultrasonography or CT in these planes is more subject to error, although this type of misalignment may be accounted for by adding to the PTV.

Absolute (Hard) PTV Constraints

The absolute conditions for plan acceptance should include the criterion that 95 to 100% of the PTV receives the prescription dose. At FCCC, the dose encompassing 95% of the volume (D_{95}) for the PTV is used. The CTV should receive 100% of the prescription dose. The maximum dose to the PTV should not exceed 17% of the prescribed dose, and < 1% (usually it is < 0.5%) of the PTV should receive < 65 Gy. These constraints have been easier to maintain with the newer planning software versions.

The FCCC absolute PTV margins are 8 mm in all dimensions, except posteriorly at the prostate-rectum interface, where a 5 mm margin is planned. Because the computer will consider the three-dimensional shape of the PTV, this margin, when examined on a slice-by-slice basis, may be larger or smaller than what is desired.

Effective (Soft) PTV Constraints

The effective or soft PTV constraints are those that are not put into the planning system but are still viewed as important for plan acceptance. The prescription line (the effective PTV) does not encompass the desired PTV on every slice. The physician should evaluate every transverse slice to determine the relationship between the prescription line and the PTV. If the prescription line deviates into the PTV on several slices or deviates into the CTV on any slice, the physician may opt to have the plan redone.

Absolute (Hard) Normal Tissue Constraints

The FCCC hard normal tissue constraints are derived in part from the MDACC randomized trial.[6] In that study, there was a very dramatic increase in ≥ grade 2 rectal complications when ≥ 25% of the rectal volume received ≥ 70 Gy. The rectum was outlined from the ischial tuberosities to 11 cm superiorly. The prescription was 78 Gy in 2 Gy fractions to the isocenter. Since that time, a number of changes have been made that make the constraints now used much stricter. First, a shorter segment is outlined, extending superiorly from the ischial tuberosities to the sigmoid flexure (about 10 cm on average). Second, the prescription has changed to deliver 74 to 78 Gy to the PTV at 2 Gy per fraction; thus, the cutpoint was reduced from 70 to 65 Gy. Third, the percentage of rectum that receives the cutpoint dose was lowered from 25 to 17% because the risk of complications is a continuous function, and we found that we could consistently meet this stricter constraint. Fourth, a second cutpoint at 40 Gy was added. Thus, the hard constraints for the rectum are ≤ 17%, and ≤ 35% of the rectal volume receives ≥ 65 Gy and ≥ 40 Gy, respectively.

No well-defined bladder constraints have been identified. As a consequence, we have initiated constraints that seem reasonable. These constraints serve as a guide. Many plans do not meet the constraints because the bladder was not sufficiently full during simulation. The hard constraints for the bladder are that ≤ 25% and ≤ 50% of the bladder volume receives ≥ 65 Gy and ≥ 40 Gy, respectively.

There is infrequently a problem limiting the dose to the femoral heads, such that ≤ 10% receives over 50 Gy. The femoral heads are outlined down to the level of the bottom of the greater trochanters and the top of the lesser trochanters.

Effective (Soft) Normal Tissue Constraints

The transverse 3 mm CT images should be examined on a slice-by-slice basis. If the 90% line encompasses more than the half-width of the rectum or the 50% line encompasses the full width of the rectum on any slice, the plan is usually adjusted. There may be some slices in which the rectum is very small and these soft constraints are violated. However, the goal is to have a relatively sharp dose falloff. These constraints are a surrogate measure of dose falloff.

Beam Energy, Number, and Arrangement

Reasonable IMRT plans are obtained with 6, 10, or 18 MV photons. With 18 MV, there is greater neutron production through photonuclear interactions, and at FCCC, a precautionary age limit of ≥ 65 has been set for the use of this energy. The optimal energy in our hands has been 10 MV.

At FCCC, the beam number and arrangement have not been standardized, whereas at other institutions, standard five- to six-field arrangements have been used. We usually start with six beams and then add beams as needed to meet the above-described constraints. The use of nine beams is not uncommon. Our typical six-beam configuration consists of the following directions and associated beam angles: left posterior oblique (gantry 135° and gantry 105°), left anterior oblique (gantry 75°), anterior-posterior (gantry 0°), right lateral (gantry 270°), and right posterior oblique (gantry 225°). Additional beam directions are added in an iterative manner while attempting to meet our acceptance criteria for normal structures and maximize dose conformity to the target. The use of parallel opposed beams is avoided. The collimator angle is evaluated through each beam's eye view to achieve geometric separation between target and normal structures where possible. Five intensity levels are used in all plans, resulting in approximately 45 to 110 total segments given over 10 to 25 minutes for 6 MV and 7 to 18 minutes for 10 and 18 MV. The inclusion of the pelvic lymph nodes greatly enhances the number of segments and overall treatment time. When confronted with difficulty in meeting the planning criteria, noncoplanar beam arrangements are explored.[115] We now use, on a routine basis, a planning technique that has resulted in a significant reduction in the number of segments used.[116] Tissue regions outside the outlined target and normal tissues have been defined by concentric rings, each with dose constraints added. This maneuver results in an increased control over the dose gradient outside the target boundaries. We have built standardized templates for input parameters for each specific dose scheme for the treatment of prostate cancer at the FCCC. These parameters, including dose constraints, gantry angles, number of beam directions, and collimator angles, are varied in an iterative manner on a case-by-case basis in an attempt to arrive at the best plan for each individual. Target conformity, normal tissue sparing, and efficient delivery time are the primary end points for plan acceptance.

References

1. Zelefsky MJ, Fuks Z, Hunt M, et al. High dose radiation delivered by intensity modulated conformal radiotherapy improves the outcome of localized prostate cancer. J Urol 2001;166:876–81.

2. Zelefsky MJ, Fuks Z, Hunt M, et al. High-dose intensity modulated radiation therapy for prostate cancer: early toxicity and biochemical outcome in 772 patients. Int J Radiat Oncol Biol Phys 2002;53:1111–6.

3. Pollack A, Smith L, von Eschenbach A. External beam radiotherapy dose-response characteristics of 1127 men with prostate cancer treated in the PSA era. Int J Radiat Oncol Biol Phys 2000;48:507–12.

4. Lyons J, Kupelian P, Mohan D, et al. Importance of high radiation doses (72 Gy or greater) in the treatment of stage T1-T3 adenocarcinoma of the prostate. Urology 2000;55:85–90.

5. Hanks GE, Hanlon AL, Epstein B, et al. Dose response in prostate cancer with 8-12 years' follow-up. Int J Radiat Oncol Biol Phys 2002;54:427–35.

6. Pollack A, Zagars GK, Starkschall G, et al. Prostate cancer radiation dose response: results of the M. D. Anderson phase III randomized trial. Int J Radiat Oncol Biol Phys 2002;53:1097–105.

7. Bey P, Carrie C, Ginestet C, et al. French study of dose escalation from 66 to 80 Gy with 3D-CRT in prostate cancer: results at 5 years. Int J Radiat Oncol Biol Phys 2003;57:S272.

8. Chism DB, Hanlon AL, Troncoso P, et al. The Gleason score shift: score four and seven years ago. Int J Radiat Oncol Biol Phys 2003;56:1241–7.

9. Pollack A, Hanlon AL, Horwitz EM, et al. Prostate cancer radiotherapy dose response: an update of the Fox Chase Cancer Center experience. J Urol 2004;171:1132–6.

10. Pinover W, Hanlon A, Hanks G, et al. Defining the appropriate radiation dose for pretreatment PSA </=10 ng/ml prostate cancer. Int J Radiat Oncol Biol Phys 2000;47:649–54.

11. Zelefsky M, Fuks Z, Chan H, et al. Ten-year results of dose escalation with 3-dimensional conformal radiotherapy for patients with clinically localized prostate cancer. Int J Radiat Oncol Biol Phys 2003;57:S149–50.

12. Cox J, Grignon D, Kaplan R, et al. Consensus statement: guidelines for PSA following radiation therapy. Int J Radiat Oncol Biol Phys 1997;37:1035–41.

13. Zagars GK, Pollack A. The fall and rise of prostate-specific antigen. Kinetics of serum prostate-specific antigen levels after radiation therapy for prostate cancer. Cancer 1993;72:832–42.

14. Pollack A, Zagars GK, Kavadi VS. Prostate specific antigen doubling time and disease relapse after radiotherapy for prostate cancer. Cancer 1994;74:670–8.

15. Zagars GK, Pollack A. Kinetics of serum prostate-specific antigen after external beam radiation for clinically localized prostate cancer. Radiother Oncol 1997;44:213–21.

16. Hanks G, Hanlon A, Pinover W, et al. Survival advantage for prostate cancer patients treated with high dose 3D conformal radiation. Cancer J Sci Am 1999;5:152–8.

17. Sandler HM, Dunn RL, McLaughlin PW, et al. Overall survival after prostate-specific-antigen-detected recurrence following conformal radiation therapy. Int J Radiat Oncol Biol Phys 2000;48:629–33.

18. Valicenti R, Lu J, Pilepich M, et al. Survival advantage from higher-dose radiation therapy for clinically localized prostate cancer treated on the Radiation Therapy Oncology Group trials. J Clin Oncol 2000;18:2740–6.

19. Kupelian PA, Buchsbaum JC, Patel C, et al. Impact of biochemical failure on overall survival after radiation therapy for localized prostate cancer in the PSA era. Int J Radiat Oncol Biol Phys 2002;52:704–11.

20. Pollack A, Hanlon AL, Movsas B, et al. Biochemical failure as a determinant of distant metastasis and death in prostate cancer treated with radiotherapy. Int J Radiat Oncol Biol Phys 2003;57:19–23.

21. Buyyounouski MK, Hanlon AL, Pollack A. The temporal kinetics of PSA after 3D-conformal radiotherapy with androgen deprivation. Int J Radiat Oncol Biol Phys 2003;57 Suppl:S147–8.

22. Vicini F, Kestin L, Martinez A. The importance of adequate follow-up in defining treatment success after external beam irradiation for prostate cancer. Int J Radiat Oncol Biol Phys 1999;45:553–61.

23. Horwitz EM, Thames HD, Kuban DA, et al. Definitions of biochemical failure that best predict clinical failure in prostate cancer patients treated with external beam radiation alone—a multi-institutional pooled analysis. Int J Radiat Oncol Biol Phys 2003;57:S147.

24. Kestin LL, Vicini FA, Ziaja EL, et al. Defining biochemical cure for prostate carcinoma patients treated with external beam radiation therapy. Cancer 1999;86:1557–66.

25. Kestin LL, Vicini FA, Martinez AA. Practical application of biochemical failure definitions: what to do and when to do it. Int J Radiat Oncol Biol Phys 2002;53:304–15.

26. Kuban DA, Thames HD, Levy LB, et al. Failure definition-dependent differences in outcome following radiation for localized prostate cancer. Can one size fit all? Int J Radiat Oncol Biol Phys 2003;57:S146–7.

27. Thames H, Kuban D, Levy L, et al. Comparison of alternative biochemical failure definitions based on clinical outcome in 4839 prostate cancer patients treated by external beam radiotherapy between 1986 and 1995. Int J Radiat Oncol Biol Phys 2003;57:929–43.

28. Pickles T, Kim-Sing C, Morris WJ, et al. Evaluation of the Houston biochemical relapse definition in men treated with prolonged neoadjuvant and adjuvant androgen ablation and assessment of follow-up lead-time bias. Int J Radiat Oncol Biol Phys 2003;57:11–8.

29. Horwitz EM, Uzzo RG, Hanlon AL, et al. Modifying the ASTRO definition of biochemical failure to minimize the influence of backdating in patients with prostate cancer treated with 3D conformal radiation therapy alone. J Urol 2003;169:2153–9.

30. Amling CL, Blute ML, Lerner SE, et al. Influence of prostate-specific antigen testing on the spectrum of patients with prostate cancer undergoing radical prostatectomy at a large referral practice. Mayo Clin Proc 1998;73:401–6.

31. Hankey BF, Feuer EJ, Clegg LX, et al. Cancer surveillance series: interpreting trends in prostate cancer—part I: evidence of the effects of screening in recent prostate cancer incidence, mortality, and survival rates. J Natl Cancer Inst 1999;91:1017–24.

32. Jhaveri FM, Klein EA, Kupelian PA, et al. Declining rates of extracapsular extension after radical prostatectomy: evidence for continued stage migration. J Clin Oncol 1999;17:3167–72.

33. Ung JO, Richie JP, Chen MH, et al. Evolution of the presentation and pathologic and biochemical outcomes after radical prostatectomy for patients with clinically localized prostate cancer diagnosed during the PSA era. Urology 2002;60:458–63.

34. Berger AP, Spranger R, Kofler K, et al. Early detection of prostate cancer with low PSA cut-off values leads to significant stage migration in radical prostatectomy specimens. Prostate 2003;57:93–8.

35. Schellhammer PF, Moriarty R, Bostwick D, et al. Fifteen-year minimum follow-up of a prostate brachytherapy series: comparing the past with the present. Urology 2000;56:436–9.

36. Smith EB, Frierson HF Jr, Mills SE, et al. Gleason scores of prostate biopsy and radical prostatectomy specimens over the past 10 years: is there evidence for systematic upgrading? Cancer 2002;94:2282–7.

37. Shipley WU, Verhey LJ, Munzenrider JE, et al. Advanced prostate cancer: the results of a randomized comparative trial of high dose irradiation boosting with conformal protons compared with conventional dose irradiation using photons alone. Int J Radiat Oncol Biol Phys 1995;32:3–12.

38. Lee WR, Hanks GE, Hanlon A, et al. Lateral rectal shielding reduces late rectal morbidity following high dose three-dimensional conformal radiation therapy for clinically localized prostate cancer: further evidence for a significant dose effect. Int J Radiat Oncol Biol Phys 1996;35:251–7.

39. Zelefsky M, Leibel S, Gaudin P, et al. Dose escalation with three-dimensional conformal radiation therapy affects the outcome in prostate cancer. Int J Radiat Oncol Biol Phys 1998;41:491–500.

40. Benk VA, Adams JA, Shipley WU, et al. Late rectal bleeding following combined x-ray and proton high dose irradiation for patients with stages T3-T4 prostate carcinoma. Int J Radiat Oncol Biol Phys 1993;26:551–7.

41. Boersma LJ, van den Brink M, Bruce AM, et al. Estimation of the incidence of late bladder and rectum complications after high-dose (70-78 Gy) conformal radiotherapy for prostate cancer, using dose-volume histograms. Int J Radiat Oncol Biol Phys 1998;41:83–92.

42. Wachter S, Gerstner N, Goldner G, et al. Rectal sequelae after conformal radiotherapy of prostate cancer: dose-volume histograms as predictive factors. Radiother Oncol 2001; 59:65–70.

43. Jackson A, Skwarchuk MW, Zelefsky MJ, et al. Late rectal bleeding after conformal radiotherapy of prostate cancer. II. Volume effects and dose-volume histograms. Int J Radiat Oncol Biol Phys 2001;49:685–98.

44. Fiorino C, Cozzarini C, Vavassori V, et al. Relationships between DVHs and late rectal bleeding after radiotherapy for prostate cancer: analysis of a large group of patients pooled from three institutions. Radiother Oncol 2002;64:1–12.

45. Kupelian PA, Reddy CA, Carlson TP, et al. Dose/volume relationship of late rectal bleeding after external beam radiotherapy for localized prostate cancer: absolute or relative rectal volume? Cancer J 2002;8:62–6.

46. Fiorino C, Sanguineti G, Cozzarini C, et al. Rectal dose-volume constraints in high-dose radiotherapy of localized prostate cancer. Int J Radiat Oncol Biol Phys 2003;57:953–62.

47. Lebesque J, Koper P, Slot A, et al. Acute and late GI and GU toxicity after prostate irradiation to doses of 68 Gy and 78 Gy; results of a randomized trial. Int J Radiat Oncol Biol Phys 2003;57:S152.

48. Gardner BG, Zietman AL, Shipley WU, et al. Late normal tissue sequelae in the second decade after high dose radiation therapy with combined photons and conformal protons for locally advanced prostate cancer. J Urol 2002;167:123–6.

49. Huang EH, Pollack A, Levy L, et al. Late rectal toxicity: dose-volume effects of conformal radiotherapy for prostate cancer. Int J Radiat Oncol Biol Phys 2002;54:1314–21.

50. Skwarchuk MW, Jackson A, Zelefsky MJ, et al. Late rectal toxicity after conformal radiotherapy of prostate cancer (I): multivariate analysis and dose-response. Int J Radiat Oncol Biol Phys 2000;47:103–13.

51. Feigenberg SJ, Hanlon AL, Horwitz EM, et al. Androgen deprivation increases late morbidity in prostate cancer patients treated with 3D conformal radiation therapy. Int J Radiat Oncol Biol Phys 2003;57:S176.

52. Schild SE, Casale HE, Bellefontaine LP. Movements of the prostate due to rectal and bladder distension: implications for radiotherapy. Med Dosim 1993;18:13–5.

53. van Herk M, Bruce A, Kroes AP, et al. Quantification of organ motion during conformal radiotherapy of the prostate by three dimensional image registration. Int J Radiat Oncol Biol Phys 1995;33:1311–20.

54. Crook JM, Raymond Y, Salhani D, et al. Prostate motion during standard radiotherapy as assessed by fiducial markers. Radiother Oncol 1995;37:35–42.

55. Beard CJ, Kijewski P, Bussiere M, et al. Analysis of prostate and seminal vesicle motion: implications for treatment planning. Int J Radiat Oncol Biol Phys 1996;34:451–8.

56. Antolak J, Rosen I, Childress C, et al. Prostate target volume variations during a course of radiotherapy. Int J Radiat Oncol Biol Phys 1998;42:661–72.

57. Zelefsky MJ, Crean D, Mageras GS, et al. Quantification and predictors of prostate position variability in 50 patients evaluated with multiple CT scans during conformal radiotherapy. Radiother Oncol 1999;50:225–34.

58. Burman C, Chui CS, Kutcher G, et al. Planning, delivery, and quality assurance of intensity-modulated radiotherapy using dynamic multileaf collimator: a strategy for large-scale implementation for the treatment of carcinoma of the prostate. Int J Radiat Oncol Biol Phys 1997;39:863–73.

59. Zelefsky MJ, Fuks Z, Happersett L, et al. Clinical experience with intensity modulated radiation therapy (IMRT) in prostate cancer. Radiother Oncol 2000;55:241–9.

60. Teh BS, Mai WY, Uhl BM, et al. Intensity-modulated radiation therapy (IMRT) for prostate cancer with the use of a rectal balloon for prostate immobilization: acute toxicity and dose-volume analysis. Int J Radiat Oncol Biol Phys 2001;49:705–12.

61. Teh BS, McGary JE, Dong L, et al. The use of rectal balloon during the delivery of intensity modulated radiotherapy (IMRT) for prostate cancer: more than just a prostate gland immobilization device? Cancer J 2002;8:476–83.

62. Ciernik IF, Baumert BG, Egli P, et al. On-line correction of beam portals in the treatment of prostate cancer using an endorectal balloon device. Radiother Oncol 2002;65:39–45.

63. McGary JE, Teh BS, Butler EB, et al. Prostate immobilization using a rectal balloon. J Appl Clin Med Phys 2002;3:6–11.

64. Wachter S, Gerstner N, Dorner D, et al. The influence of a rectal balloon tube as internal immobilization device on variations

of volumes and dose-volume histograms during treatment course of conformal radiotherapy for prostate cancer. Int J Radiat Oncol Biol Phys 2002;52:91–100.

65. Lattanzi J, McNeeley S, Hanlon A, et al. Ultrasound-based stereotactic guidance of precision conformal external beam radiation therapy in clinically localized prostate cancer. Urology 2000;55:73–8.

66. Lattanzi J, McNeely S, Pinover W, et al. A comparison of daily CT localization to a daily ultrasound-based system in prostate cancer. Int J Radiat Oncol Biol Phys 1999;43:719–25.

67. Chandra A, Dong L, Huang E, et al. Experience of ultrasound-based daily prostate localization. Int J Radiat Oncol Biol Phys 2003;56:436–47.

68. Langen KM, Pouliot J, Anezinos C, et al. Evaluation of ultrasound-based prostate localization for image-guided radiotherapy. Int J Radiat Oncol Biol Phys 2003;57:635–44.

69. Patel RR, Orton N, Tome WA, et al. Rectal dose sparing with a balloon catheter and ultrasound localization in conformal radiation therapy for prostate cancer. Radiother Oncol 2003;67:285–94.

70. Wu J, Haycocks T, Alasti H, et al. Positioning errors and prostate motion during conformal prostate radiotherapy using on-line isocentre set-up verification and implanted prostate markers. Radiother Oncol 2001;61:127–33.

71. Nederveen AJ, Lagendijk JJ, Hofman P. Feasibility of automatic marker detection with an a-si flat-panel imager. Phys Med Biol 2001;46:1219–30.

72. Kitamura K, Shirato H, Seppenwoolde Y, et al. Three-dimensional intrafractional movement of prostate measured during real-time tumor-tracking radiotherapy in supine and prone treatment positions. Int J Radiat Oncol Biol Phys 2002;53:1117–23.

73. Kitamura K, Shirato H, Shimizu S, et al. Registration accuracy and possible migration of internal fiducial gold marker implanted in prostate and liver treated with real-time tumor-tracking radiation therapy . Radiother Oncol 2002;62:275–81.

74. Pouliot J, Aubin M, Langen KM, et al. (Non)-migration of radiopaque markers used for on-line localization of the prostate with an electronic portal imaging device. Int J Radiat Oncol Biol Phys 2003;56:862–6.

75. Lattanzi J, McNeely S, Barnes S, et al. Initial results of using daily CT localization to correct portal error in prostate cancer. Int J Radiat Oncol Biol Phys 1997;39:193.

76. Uematsu M, Shioda A, Suda A, et al. Computed tomography-guided frameless stereotactic radiotherapy for stage I non-small cell lung cancer: a 5-year experience. Int J Radiat Oncol Biol Phys 2001;51:666–70.

77. Hua C, Lovelock M, Mageras GS, et al. Development of a semi-automatic alignment tool for accelerated localization of the prostate. Int J Radiat Oncol Biol Phys 2003;55:811–24.

78. Court LE, Dong L. Automatic registration of the prostate for computed-tomography-guided radiotherapy. Med Phys 2003;30:2750–7.

79. Little DJ, Dong L, Levy LB, et al. Use of portal images and BAT ultrasonography to measure setup error and organ motion for prostate IMRT: implications for treatment margins. Int J Radiat Oncol Biol Phys 2003;56:1218–24.

80. Jaffray DA, Siewerdsen JH, Wong JW, et al. Flat-panel cone-beam computed tomography for image-guided radiation therapy. Int J Radiat Oncol Biol Phys 2002;53:1337–49.

81. Sidhu K, Ford EC, Spirou S, et al. Optimization of conformal thoracic radiotherapy using cone-beam CT imaging for treatment verification. Int J Radiat Oncol Biol Phys 2003;55:757–67.

82. Russell K, Skrumeda L, Gisselberg M, et al. Biocompatibility of a wireless electromagnetic transponder permanent implant for accurate localization and continuous tracking of tumor targets. Int J Radiat Oncol Biol Phys 2003;57:S396–7.

83. Mah D, Freedman G, Milestone B, et al. Measurement of intrafractional prostate motion using magnetic resonance imaging. Int J Radiat Oncol Biol Phys 2002;54:568–75.

84. Padhani AR, Khoo VS, Suckling J, et al. Evaluating the effect of rectal distension and rectal movement on prostate gland position using cine MRI. Int J Radiat Oncol Biol Phys 1999;44:525–33.

85. Malone S, Crook JM, Kendal WS, et al. Respiratory-induced prostate motion: quantification and characterization. Int J Radiat Oncol Biol Phys 2000;48:105–9.

86. Dawson LA, Litzenberg DW, Brock KK, et al. A comparison of ventilatory prostate movement in four treatment positions. Int J Radiat Oncol Biol Phys 2000;48:319–23.

87. Dong L, O'Daniel JC, Smith LG, et al. Comparison of 3D conformal and intensity-modulated radiation therapy for early-stage prostate cancer. Int J Radiat Oncol Biol Phys 2001;51:320–20.

88. Oh CE, Antes K, Darby M, et al. Comparison of 2D conventional, 3D conformal, and intensity-modulated treatment planning techniques for patients with prostate cancer with regard to target-dose homogeneity and dose to critical, uninvolved structures. Med Dosim 1999;24:255–63.

89. Fiorino C, Broggi S, Corletto D, et al. Conformal irradiation of concave-shaped PTVS in the treatment of prostate cancer by simple 1D intensity-modulated beams. Radiother Oncol 2000;55:49–58.

90. Corletto D, Iori M, Paiusco M, et al. Inverse and forward optimization of one- and two-dimensional intensity-modulated radiation therapy-based treatment of concave-shaped planning target volumes: the case of prostate cancer. Radiother Oncol 2003;66:185–95.

91. Wu Q, Arthur D, Benedict S, et al. Intensity-modulated radiotherapy for prostate cancer treatment with nodal coverage [abstract]. Int J Radiat Oncol Biol Phys 2002;54:321.

92. Nutting CM, Convery DJ, Cosgrove VP, et al. Reduction of small and large bowel irradiation using an optimized intensity-modulated pelvic radiotherapy technique in patients with prostate cancer. Int J Radiat Oncol Biol Phys 2000;48:649-56.

93. Clark CH, Mubata CD, Meehan CA, et al. IMRT clinical implementation: prostate and pelvic node irradiation using Helios and a 120-leaf multileaf collimator. J Appl Clin Med Phys 2002;3:273-84.

94. Luxton G, Hancock SL, Chen Y, et al. Reduction of bowel dose in lymph node irradiation with IMRT treatment of prostate cancer [abstract]. Int J Radiat Oncol Biol Phys 2000;48:352.

95. Adams EJ, Convery DJ, Cosgrove VP, et al. Clinical implementation of dynamic and step-and-shoot IMRT to treat prostate cancer with high risk of pelvic lymph node invovlement. Radiother Oncol 2004;70:1-10.

96. Nutting CM, Corbishley CM, Sanchez-Nieto B, et al. Potential improvements in the therapeutic ratio for prostate cancer irradiation: dose escalation of pathologically identified tumour nodules using intensity modulated radiotherapy. Br J Radiol 2002;75:151–161.

97. Xia P, Pickett B, Vigneault E, et al. Forward or inversely planned segmental multileaf collimator IMRT and sequential tomotherapy to treat multiple dominant intraprostatic lesions of prostate cancer to 90 Gy. Int J Radiat Oncol Biol Phys 2001;51:244–54.

98. Pickett B, Vigneault E, Kurhanewicz J, et al. Static field intensity modulation to treat a dominant intra-prostatic lesion to 90 Gy compared to 3-dimensional radiotherapy. Int J Radiat Oncol Biol Phys 1999;44:921 9.

99. Sethi A, Mohideen N, Leybovich L, et al. Role of IMRT in reducing penile doses in dose escalation for prostate cancer. Int J Radiat Oncol Biol Phys 2003;55:970–8.

100. Kao J, Turian J, Meyers A, et al. Sparing of the penile bulb and proximal penile structures with intensity-modulated radiation therapy for prostate cancer. Br J Radiol 2004;77:129–36.

101. Boyyounouski MK, Horwitz EM, Price RA, et al. Intensity-modulated radiotherapy with MRI simulation to reduce doses received by erectile tissue during prostate cancer treatment. Int J Radiat Oncol Biol Phys 2004;58:743 9.

102. Li X, Wang LZ, Amin PP, et al. Using IMRT to repair unacceptable dose distributions of prostate implants [abstract]. Int J Radiat Oncol Biol Phys 2003;57:434.

103. Vora SA, Ezzell G, Wong W, et al. High-dose radiation therapy for prostate cancer delivered by intensity modulated radiation therapy (IMRT): report of acute toxicity. Proc Am Soc Clin Oncol 2002; Abstract 2453.

104. Kupelian PA, Reddy CA, Klein EA, et al. Short-course intensity modulated radiotherapy (70 Gy at 2.5 Gy per fraction) for localized prostate cancer: preliminary results on late toxicity and quality of life. Int J Radiat Oncol Biol Phys 2001;51:988–93.

105. Kupelian PA, Willoughby TR. Short-course, intensity modulated radiotherapy for localized prostate cancer. Cancer J 2001;7:421–6.

106. Kupelian PA, Reddy CA, Carlson TP, et al. Preliminary observations on biochemical relapse free survival rates after short-course intensity-modulated radiotherapy (70 Gy at 2.5 Gy/fractions) for localized prostate cancer. Int J Radiat Oncol Biol Phys 2002;53:904–12.

107. Djemil T, Reddy CA, Willoughby TR, et al. Hypofractionated intensity-modulated radiotherapy (70 Gy at 2.5 Gy per fraction) for localized prostate cancer. Int J Radiat Oncol Biol Phys 2003;57:S275.

108. Cheung P, Morton G, Loblaw A, et al. Hypofractionated IMRT boost for prostate carcinoma with on-line targeting of the prostate gland: patient-specific PTV margins and acute toxicity results. Int J Radiat Oncol Biol Phys 2003;57:S276.

109. Catton CN, Chung P, Haycocks T, et al. Hypofractionated intensity modulated radiation therapy for prostate cancer. Int J Radiat Oncol Biol Phys 2002;54:188.

110. Shu HK, Lee TT, Vigneault E, et al. Toxicity following high-dose three-dimensional conformal and intensity-modulated radiation therapy for clinically localized prostate cancer. Urology 2001;57:102-7.

111. Hancock SL, Luxton G, Chen Y, et al. Intensity modulated radiotherapy for localized or regional treatment of prostate cancer: clinical implementation and improvement in acute tolerance [abstract]. Int J Radiat Oncol Biol Phys 2000;48:251.

112. Price R, Murphy S, McNeeley SW. A method for increased dose conformity and segment reduction for sMLC delivered IMRT treatment of the prostate. Int J Radiat Oncol Biol Phys 2003. [Submitted]

113. Stamey TA, Villers AA, McNeal JE, et al. Positive surgical margins at radical prostatectomy: importance of the apical dissection. J Urol 1990;143:1166–73.

114. Ohori M, Abbas F, Wheeler TM, et al. Pathological features and prognostic significance of prostate cancer in the apical section determined by whole mount histology. J Urol 1999;161:500–4.

115. Price R, Hanks GE, McNeeley SW. Advantages of using non-coplanar vs axial beam arrangements when treating prostate cancer with intensity modulated radiation therapy and the step-and-shoot delivery method. Int J Radiat Oncol Biol Phys 2002;53:236–43.

116. Price RA, Murphy S, McNeeley SW, et al. Department of Radiation Oncology, Fox Chase Cancer Center, Philadelphia, PA 19111, USA. r.price@fccc.edu

117. D'Amico A, Whittington R, Malkowicz S, et al. Biochemical outcome after radical prostatectomy, external beam radiation therapy, or interstitial radiation therapy for clinically localized prostate cancer. JAMA 1998;280:969–74.

118. Pollack A. The prostate. In: Cox J, Ang K, editors. Moss' radiation oncology: rationale, technique, results. 8th ed. St. Louis (MO): Mosby; 2002. p. 629–80.

POSTOPERATIVE PROSTATE CANCER OVERVIEW

BIN S. TEH, MD, THOMAS M. SCHROEDER, MD, WEI-YUAN MAI, MD, E. BRIAN BUTLER, MD

Although radiation therapy (RT) is commonly used in the definitive treatment of prostate cancer, it also occupies an important role following prostatectomy. Postoperative RT may be delivered either as adjuvant RT (in high-risk patients despite an undetectable prostate-specific antigen [PSA] level postoperatively) or as salvage RT (in patients with a rising or persistently elevated postoperative PSA or a clinical local recurrence). In properly selected patients, both approaches have been shown to be beneficial, particularly in terms of local and biochemical control.[1–10]

A common concern, however, with the routine use of postoperative RT in prostate cancer is the risk of potential increased treatment-related toxicity in patients who have undergone radical surgery. This is particularly the case because high doses have been shown to be required to achieve local control in both the adjuvant and the salvage RT setting.[11,12]

Intensity-modulated radiation therapy (IMRT) is receiving increasing attention in prostate cancer. To date, most of the attention has focused on its use in the treatment of patients with an intact prostate.[13–17] Nonetheless, an equally strong rationale exists for IMRT in the postoperative setting. The purpose of this chapter is to provide an overview of IMRT in patients with prostate cancer following surgery. Various issues and challenges, including target delineation and imaging, patient and organ motion, immobilization, and treatment planning, are discussed. In addition, a review of published data on postprostatectomy IMRT and future research directions are presented.

Background and Rationale

Prostatectomy

Prostatectomy has been used as a treatment for prostate cancer since Hugh Hampton Young performed the first radical perineal prostatectomy in 1904.[18] The technique evolved with the introduction of the radical retropubic prostatectomy in 1945[19] and the nerve-sparing radical prostatectomy in 1983.[20] The first sural nerve graft to restore erectile function was performed in 1997,[21] and the first series of laparoscopic prostatectomies were presented in 1998.[22] Today, prostatectomy remains the most used form of definitive treatment of prostate cancer. In recent years, surgical and anesthesia techniques have advanced, resulting in less risk of adverse outcome from both anesthesia and surgery,[23,24] leading to an even greater use of surgery in patients previously felt to be poor surgical candidates.

Despite the preoperative prognostic information available today, up to 35 to 60% of patients with clinical stage T1–2 cancers will develop a PSA recurrence within 10 years, with rates increasing with pathologically staged T3 and T4 disease.[1–3,25–28] Certain pathologic features have been correlated with increased recurrence, including positive surgical margins, seminal vesicle invasion, extraprostatic extension, and high Gleason scores.[4,5,28–30]

In a retrospective review of 1,000 patients undergoing prostatectomy alone, Scardino and colleagues reported a 10-year progression-free survival of 86.7 to 89.4% in patients with low-risk, organ-confined (≤ pT2) disease. However, less favorable results are seen in patients with extracapsular extension (ECE). The progression-free survival rates in patients with seminal vesicle involvement and positive margins were 37.4% and 36.4%, respectively.[31] The adverse impact of extracapsular disease is also evident in the CaPSURE database, a longitudinal disease registry of 1,383 men who underwent radical prostatectomy as definitive local treatment. Overall, positive margins were seen in one-third of the patients. Surgical margin status was shown to be an independent predictor of PSA recurrence and adjuvant or salvage treatment (p = .06 and .0011, respectively).[32] Although prostatectomy is a good therapy for clinical localized disease, a clear need for adjuvant therapy exists.

Radiation Therapy

The first report of a patient with prostate cancer undergoing RT was by Minet in 1909.[33] George and colleagues began treating patients with unresectable disease with external beam RT (cobalt 60) in the late 1950s,[34] and the first series of patients with residual or recurrent disease treated with megavoltage RT appeared in 1975.[35] In 1991, Soffen and colleagues published their technique on three-dimensional (3D) computed tomography (CT)-guided conformal therapy,[36] and on March 21, 1994, the first cancer patient was treated with IMRT at Baylor College of Medicine.

The use of postoperative RT remains controversial. Some advocate adjuvant RT in high-risk patients despite an undetectable PSA postoperatively.[6] The premise underlying adjuvant RT is that local recurrence precedes systemic, metastatic spread in many patients failing radical prostatectomy. Others are proponents of salvage RT in patients with a rising postoperative PSA level or a persistently elevated or clinical local recurrence.[6] Biochemical no evidence of disease rates for patients undergoing salvage RT were more than 70% (when the pre-RT PSA value was < 1–2 ng/mL) and less than 50% (when the pre-RT PSA was higher).[7,8] Thus, both adjuvant RT and salvage RT have been shown to be effective.

Patient Selection for Postoperative RT

In an effort to identify the patients who may benefit from postprostatectomy RT, numerous retrospective studies addressing predictors of outcome for both prostatectomy and postprostatectomy RT have been performed. These studies have shown predictable results, with pathologic stage, preoperative PSA level, postoperative PSA level, PSA velocity or doubling time, Gleason grade, ECE, and positive margins playing prominent roles. At the time of diagnosis, PSA level is a potent independent predictor of PSA failure after prostatectomy, but it cannot discriminate between local and distant recurrence. Furthermore, there are currently no good objective means of identifying the patients who have microscopic local recurrence versus those who have microscopic distant metastasis. Thus, the indications for prostatic bed RT are unclear.

The preoperative and postoperative factors that indicate a local recurrence predominantly reflect factors that indicate nonaggressive disease, whereas the factors indicative of a distant recurrence reflect more aggressive disease. Partin and colleagues demonstrated that patients with a PSA velocity > 0.75 ng/mL and patients with detectable PSA before reaching 1 year postoperatively were more likely to have distant metastasis.[37] In another publication, Han and colleagues demonstrated that Gleason scores ≥ 7 were more likely to have distant metastatic disease with PSA recurrence.[28] Numerous other studies have found that seminal vesicle invasion (SVI) and positive lymph nodes were associated with distant metastasis. Patel and colleagues demonstrated that a PSA doubling time of greater than 6 months was more likely to be associated with local recurrence.[38] Leventis and colleagues found similar results with a greater likelihood of a positive prostatic fossa biopsy and a greater likelihood of biochemical-free survival with a PSA doubling time of greater than 1 year.[39]

Although these indicators may be helpful in describing the prognosis and likelihood of a response to RT, the absence of an objective means of identifying either local or distant microscopic disease precludes clinical decisions based on these factors. Patients with adverse features but without an objective distant metastasis may benefit from salvage or adjuvant RT. Furthermore, with the advent of ultrasensitive PSA, the time of biochemical failure is significantly decreasing, making the decision to treat in the adjuvant setting moot. The likelihood of identifying bony metastasis in the postprostatectomy setting is less than 5% until the PSA reaches levels of 40 to 45 ng/mL.[40] As a result, the postprostatectomy patient with a rising PSA level and without preoperative metastatic disease may be salvaged with local RT.

A positive margin is considered a sign of local recurrence and indicates a need for adjuvant therapy or re-excision for nearly every type of cancer and tumor in the body. Apparently, this is not the case in prostate cancer. The poorly defined prostate "capsule" and the skip lesion nature of prostate cancer make margins difficult to evaluate and complete surgical excision difficult to obtain. As a result, the rate of positive margins with prostatectomy can vary from approximately 15% to as high as one-third of cases.[31,32] Kupelian and colleagues demonstrated that margin status was an independent predictor of local failure ($p = .015$) in a retrospective analysis of clinical patients with T1 or T2 cancer treated initially with prostatectomy.[41] However, Connolly and colleagues found that the rate of positive margins in proven local recurrence was nearly equivalent to the rate of positive margins in cases of no proven local recurrence.[42] The National Comprehensive Cancer Network guidelines for prostate cancer claim that the significance of positive surgical margins in determining local recurrence is controversial.[43] Transrectal ultrasound-guided prostatic fossa biopsy is the gold standard in establishing local recurrence. Unfortunately, this modality is subject to considerable sampling error. Furthermore, times to prostatic fossa biopsy vary from study to study, as have the definition of biochemical failure, the methods of pathologic evaluation of margins, and the definition of a positive margin.

These factors, combined with irregular use of adjuvant therapy and irregular time use of these therapies (both androgen ablation and radiation), result in data sets with considerable variation. Regardless, a positive margin is a proven independent risk factor of biochemical failure and likely results from local recurrence. In a nonrandomized comparison, we have shown that adjuvant RT provided a longer freedom from biochemical failure in patients with positive surgical margins and undetectable PSA. The 5- and 10-year cumulative freedom from biochemical recurrence rates were 90.9% and 90.9% for the adjuvant RT group ($n = 44$) and 66.4% and 54.5% for the observation group ($n = 189$).[44] We are eagerly awaiting the results of two prospective randomized trials (from the Southwest Oncology Group [SWOG] and the European Organization for the Research and Treatment of Cancer [EORTC]) to further address the role of adjuvant RT for patients with poor pathologic features on prostatectomy specimens. Although this does not yet represent the standard of care, a positive margin is probably an indication for local adjuvant therapy.

Potential Benefits of IMRT

A major concern with the use of postoperative RT in prostate cancer is the potential for increased toxicity. A radical prostatectomy may already have adverse effects on urinary and erectile function by disrupting nerves and blood vessels. Moreover, more normal tissues (including the rectum and bladder) may be present in the prostatic fossa (and thus target volume) owing to the absence of the prostate. The target tissues in the postprostatectomy setting are also highly irregularly shaped. In some patients, the seminal vesicle beds wrap around the rectum, rendering it necessary to include a considerable volume of rectum within the treatment field. Concerns also exist regarding the small bowel in patients treated with regional lymphatic RT.

Interestingly enough, published reports reveal that morbidity after radical prostatectomy and postoperative RT is comparable to that observed following surgery alone when conventional doses are delivered.[9,45] Treatment-related toxicity is a concern when higher than conventional doses are prescribed. Increasing data support the need for higher doses in the postprostatectomy setting. Valicenti and colleagues showed improved biochemical-free survival rates with increased dose.[10,11] Patients with an undetectable pre-RT PSA were found to have a biochemical-free survival of 91% versus 57% ($p = .01$) when treated above versus below 61.5 Gy. In patients with a detectable pretreatment PSA (> 0.2 and < 2.0 ng/mL), doses > 64.8 Gy were associated with a biochemical-free survival of 79% versus 33% ($p = .02$). In a review of 87 patients at Duke University treated for a rising PSA level after surgery, Anscher and colleagues noted a strong correlation between tumor control and dose. On multivariate analysis, doses > 65 Gy were associated with an improved disease-free survival rate.[12] The American Society for Therapeutic Radiology and Oncology (ASTRO) Consensus Panel advocated doses ≥ 64 Gy in the postoperative setting.[46]

IMRT may represent a means of safely delivering higher than conventional doses in patients with prostate cancer following surgery. Unlike conventional approaches, IMRT conforms the prescription dose to the shape of the target tissues in three dimensions, thereby sparing the surrounding normal tissues. By allowing conformal treatment of targets and avoidance of normal tissues, IMRT may overcome the limitations of conventional RT. In fact, with the irregularly shaped target in the postprostatectomy setting, IMRT appears to be ideal.

Issues and Challenges
Immobilization

Owing to the rapid dose gradients inherent in IMRT planning, optimal patient immobilization is critical in all patients undergoing IMRT, and postprostatectomy patients are no exception. At our institution, postprostatectomy patients are simulated in the prone position and immobilized in a customized Vac-Lok (MED-TEC, Orange City, IA) bag that conforms to both the patient's body contour and the treatment box. A representative patient immobilized in a Vac-Lok bag-box system is shown in Figure 22B-1.

In addition, owing to internal organ motion (see below), consideration should be given to immobilization of the target tissues as well. At the Baylor College of Medicine, immobilization of the prostate gland in patients treated with definitive IMRT has been accomplished with placement of a rectal balloon (Figure 22B-2). With the balloon in place, we have noted less prostate gland motion, especially in the anterior-posterior direction.[47,48] A similar approach can be applied in the postprostatectomy setting, decreasing the motion of prostatic fossa tissues. Furthermore, the distention of rectum, especially the lateral and posterior walls away from areas of higher dose, as well as the buildup effects owing to the air-filled balloon, increases rectal sparing.[49] Others have confirmed these results and used rectal balloons with 3D conformal RT.[50]

Target Delineation

Definition of the target volume is a difficult task in the postprostatectomy patient for one simple reason: there is no gross tumor volume (GTV) (ie, the prostate gland has been removed) on imaging studies. Traditional magnetic resonance imaging (MRI), computed tomography (CT), and

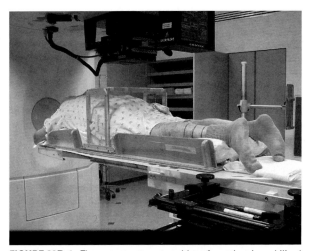

FIGURE 22B-1. The prone treatment position of a patient immobilized in a Vac-Lok bag-box system. Note the fiducial box (with laser beams) and the marks on the legs for setup purposes. (To view a color version of this image, please refer to the CD-ROM.)

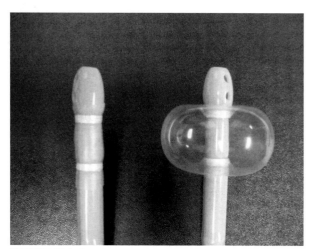

FIGURE 22B-2. Rectal balloon deflated and inflated with 100 cc air. (To view a color version of this image, please refer to the CD-ROM.)

ultrasonography can identify possible areas of involvement, but these modalities have previously been demonstrated to have relatively poor sensitivity or specificity. As a result, target volumes must be based in retrospective local recurrence and surgical studies.

Numerous retrospective studies of patients with positive prostatic fossa biopsies have been performed. Unfortunately, few of these include data on the location of positive biopsies. Connolly and colleagues found that local recurrences were most common at the site of urethral anastomosis (66%), with 16% at the bladder neck and 13% in the retrovesicle area.[42] Leventis and colleagues reported similar results in a study of transrectal ultrasonography compared with a digital rectal examination. In cases of positive ultrasonographic findings, positive biopsies were found at the site of anastomosis (55%), bladder neck (23%), and retrovesicle area (7%) and in multiple areas (16%).[51]

Studies on patients with an intact prostate also may be helpful in delineating the postprostatectomy target volume. Two studies have demonstrated a tendency of CT-guided planning to provide larger fields than may be necessary. Our institution performed CT-based IMRT planning on 10 patients who were not treated with RT but subsequently went on to prostatectomy. Comparison with the anatomic volume of the prostate gland demonstrated that planning volumes were significantly larger. The average GTV was 2 times larger than the pathologic prostate volume (PPV), and the average planning target volume (PTV) was 4.1 times larger than the PPV.[52] Roach and colleagues compared CT-based and MRI-based GTVs and found the CT-based GTVs to be 32% larger.[53] One other study of importance, given the propensity of recurrence at the site of urethral anastomosis, is a urethrogram study performed by Roach and colleagues. They studied 15 patients with cancer with retrograde urethograms and urethroscopy to identify the apex of the prostate and found that the location of the prostate

apex varied significantly. In particular, they observed that the inferior border of the ischial tuberosities did not provide sufficient coverage in 13% of the cases and provided excessive coverage in 40% of the patients. They went on to recommend placement of the prostatic apex 13 mm superior to the tip of the contrast column on a retrograde urethrogram.[54] In a postprostatectomy setting, the inferior border may be even lower.

Although there are no specific anatomic landmarks identifying areas of local recurrence in the postprostatectomy setting, the literature provides clues as to appropriate areas to cover. The locations of the bladder and rectum, as well as a cystourethrogram, will help delineate the prostatic bed or target volume. The operative note and pathology report will describe the areas of positive margin, ECE, seminal vesicle involvement, and greatest tumor involvement. As a result, those documents are invaluable in identifying areas that clearly require coverage. Furthermore, surgical clips identifying areas of tissue disruption by the surgeon, including the prostatic and seminal vesicle bed, should be included in the surgical bed. Surgical clips in the areas of lymphadenectomy should not be covered unless lymph node involvement was identified (discussed below). The gross pathologic description usually indicates dimensions, including volume or mass estimates. These are also helpful in determining the target volume. In addition, the preprostatectomy CT scan, if performed, is also very useful.

A bone scan, CT, MRI, biopsy of the prostatic bed, and/or a ^{111}In capromab pendetide immunoscintigraphy (ProstaScint, Cytogen Corp., Princeton, NJ) may be done in the postprostatectomy setting. Biopsy of the surgical bed and anastomotic site is not routinely performed because the yield is very low and may not change the outcome.[55]

ProstaScint scans use a whole murine antibody that is reactive with prostate-specific membrane antigen (PSMA), a glycoprotein on the surface of normal and abnormal prostate epithelium.[56] PSMA expression increases with the degree of dedifferentiation of tumors. PSA expression is down-regulated by hormone treatment, whereas PSMA is not. Many studies have emphasized the complementary diagnostic value of ProstaScint scans to the PSA level and Gleason score as independent indicators of prostate cancer recurrence and metastases and in identifying extrapelvic soft tissue metastases in both newly diagnosed and recurrent prostate cancer.[57,58]

Data are emerging on the usefulness of immunoscintigraphy with ProstaScint to locate the anatomic site of disease recurrence in patients with biochemical failure after prostatectomy,[59,60] particularly when registered with anatomic CT images. Interestingly, ProstaScint immunoscintigraphy can detect the site of relapse in patients with PSA levels < 4 ng/mL, even in patients with normal conventional imaging (bone and CT scans).[58] Immunoscintigraphy revealed disease in 108 of 181 patients (60%) with interpretable scans. The antibody was localized most frequently to the prostatic fossa

(34% of the cases), abdominal lymph nodes (23%), and pelvic lymph nodes (22%). The use of ProstaScint imaging in the planning of postoperative IMRT is shown in Chapter 22.4, "ProstaScint-Guided IMRT: Case Study."

However, the use of ProstaScint is not universal because of moderate accuracy (sensitivity 51%, specificity 71%).[60] Hopefully, with further refinement and improvement, ProstaScint scanning may be used to assist in the target delineation in the postprostatectomy setting. ^{18}F-labelled fluorodeoxyglucose–positron emission tomography ([18]FDG-PET) scanning has not been shown to be useful for the detection of local tumor recurrence following prostatectomy,[61] but there does appear to be a role for the detection of nodal involvement.[62] Recently, it has been suggested that ^{11}C-choline PET may be more useful than [18]FDG-PET for detecting local tumor relapse after prostatectomy.[63]

Following prostatectomy, scar tissue, surgical clips, and postoperative changes can impair image interpretation because of considerable soft tissue distortion of the surgical bed. Part of the seminal vesicles is usually left behind, and the presence of residual tissue at their location should be recognized. Turbo spin-echo T_2-weighted MRI minimizes susceptibility artifacts, and surgical scar tissue can be recognized at the bladder-urethra anastomosis. Contrast medium enhancement is mandatory for evaluation of the surgical bed. Any focal enhancement in the prostatectomy bed to the same degree or greater than that of rectal or urethral mucosa should be considered abnormal and should warrant biopsy confirmation. Recently, dynamic contrast-enhanced MRI has been shown to be able to detect cancer recurrence following a radical prostatectomy even before it can be detected by biopsy.[64]

It is important to remember, however, that contrast enhancement can be markedly reduced if the patient is receiving intercurrent androgen deprivation treatment, and this can lead to false-negative results. Blunting of contrast medium enhancement is due to fibrotic changes occurring histologically and to reduced vascularity of residual prostate cancer caused by androgen deprivation.[70] In the future, improved dynamic contrast-enhanced MRI may be helpful in assisting target delineation in the postprostatectomy setting.

Whether to irradiate the pelvic lymph nodes in the postprostatectomy patient remains controversial. The majority of patients undergoing adjuvant or salvage RT in the postprostatectomy setting already have a negative lymph node sampling. This means that they have already had a negative gold standard test for lymph node involvement. It also means that they have altered nodal draining. This not only confuses the issue as to whether nodes should or should not be treated but also what nodes to treat. Many radiation oncologists recommend treatment of the nodes when they are at increased risk of involvement in the postprostatectomy setting. However, others see no need unless there are positive nodes. At this time, there is a paucity of data on the issue of whole-pelvis irradiation in the postprostatectomy setting. In the future, technologies may evolve to allow for treatment of nodal areas by means other than the whole pelvis. A patient treated with postprostatectomy intensity-modulated pelvic RT is described in Chapter 22.3, "Targeted Lymph Node Irradiation: Case Study."

Organ Motion

Many studies have been performed regarding prostate motion. Exploring these results gives clues to the possible motions of prostatic fossa tissue. A review by Langen and Jones summarizes studies on several organs with relation to organ motion. Their summary describes prostate motion as being greatest in the anterior-posterior direction, followed closely by the superior-inferior direction. On average, anterior-posterior motion was on the order of 5 mm, with results similar to those of superior-inferior motion.[66] The largest anterior-posterior motion detected was 20 mm. This review also addressed seminal vesicle motion and found that seminal vesicle motion was larger than prostate motion and had greater variation from patient to patient.

Although numerous studies have examined prostate motion, few have evaluated prostatic fossa motion in the postoperative setting. Chinnaiyan and colleagues performed the only current published study on postprostatectomy motion.[67] Sixteen postprostatectomy patients were evaluated with ultrasonography and port films. Ultrasonography was used for bladder neck localization, and a comparison was made with port films to determine tissue motion. Motion on the order of 3 to 5 ± 3 to 4 mm was noted, greatest in the anterior-posterior dimension, and was similar to patients with an intact prostate. Of note, this daily internal motion was noted in patients treated with a daily rectal balloon, which, in the intact prostate setting at least, has been shown to effectively immobilize the prostate.[47–50,68] Thus, daily internal movement in the postprostatectomy setting might have been greater without it. Further studies on this issue are likely forthcoming. With tight isodose curves, 5 mm may make a difference, resulting in sparing of prostatic fossa tissue or treating excessive rectum. Treating in multiple fractions helps to average out these motions, but this limits the benefit of IMRT.

Treatment Planning

As noted earlier, postprostatectomy patients treated with IMRT at the Baylor College of Medicine are simulated in the prone position, immobilized in a Vac-Lok bag. Simulation involves performing a cystourethrogram and placement of a rectal catheter with 100 cc of air in an inflatable balloon. A planning CT scan (3 mm slices) is performed with the patient in the treatment position.

The essence of IMRT is the optimization of dose delivered to the targets and surrounding critical structures. Avoidance structures include the rectum, bladder, and femoral heads. At our institution, assigned radiation dose limits to partial volumes of these structures are 62 Gy for the rectum, 60 Gy for the bladder, and 41 Gy for the femoral heads. These normal tissue limits are considered by the optimization process, but target coverage is not sacrificed unless priority is placed on a particular critical structure.

A 5 mm margin is placed around the prostate fossa in a 3D fashion using the expansion function of the system, creating a PTV. The prescribed dose to the PTV is 60 to 66 Gy in a 2 Gy fraction for 30 to 33 fractions. Generally, this dose is prescribed to the 84 to 89% isodose line for full coverage of the PTV. The dose distributions are examined carefully on every axial slice. The mean target dose is 64 to 72 Gy.

Our first six patients were prescribed a dose of 60 Gy. All patients thereafter were prescribed 64 Gy, with the exception of those with palpable recurrent nodule or positive biopsy who received a prescribed dose of 66 Gy. In essence, this represents moderate dose escalation when compared with the conventional 45 to 60 Gy, as well as a higher fraction size (2.13–2.18 Gy) compared with the conventional 1.8 to 2.0 Gy.

The dose-response relationship in prostate cancer has been well demonstrated. More recently, it has been suggested that prostate cancer has a low α/β ratio of 1.5.[69,70] Current evidence suggests that prostate cancer may behave more like late-reacting tissues radiobiologically.[71,72] A higher fraction size may have added benefits in tumor control in view of this low α/β ratio. In fact, if one uses an α/β ratio of 1.5, a mean dose of 70 Gy, and a fraction size of 2.16 Gy (compared with a standard fraction size of 1.8 Gy), the biologic equivalent dose is approximately 77 Gy. This is a true dose-escalation trial. It is hoped that IMRT allows the feasibility and safety of both dose escalation and a higher fraction size. Such an approach could lead to an increase in local control while minimizing the treatment-related side effects.

The treatment planning parameters are evaluated, including the PTV mean dose, maximum dose, and volume of PTV below the prescribed dose, along with dose-volume histograms. Adequate coverage of the target without overdosage of normal tissues is used as a criterion for acceptability of the treatment plan. Generally, not more than 2% of the PTV is allowed to receive below the prescribed dose. The rectal wall is outlined, whereas the bladder is contoured as a whole structure. An effort is made to keep no more than 15% of rectal or bladder volumes above their respective thresholds. More recently, we also evaluated the doses delivered to the penile bulb and femoral heads.

Figures 22B-3 to 22B-5 show two axial (superior and inferior slice) and one sagittal CT image (with the patient in the prone position). As shown on the images, in addition to acting as an immobilization device, the rectal balloon contributes to the reduction in the rectal volume (especially lateral and posterior walls), receiving a high dose by distending the rectal wall. Also, note especially in the superior axial image that the "butterfly"-shaped target covering the surgical clips with the surrounding concave isodose lines demonstrates the benefits of IMRT.

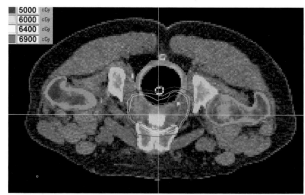

FIGURE 22B-3. Intensity-modulated radiation therapy dose distribution in the axial plane (inferior level). Note that the patient was treated in the prone position with an air-filled rectal balloon in place. Prostatic fossa (*brown*), rectum (*green*), pubic bone (*light blue*), femoral head (*dark blue*). (To view a color version of this image, please refer to the CD-ROM.)

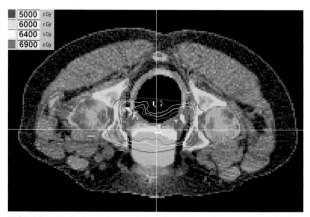

FIGURE 22B-4. Intensity-modulated radiation therapy dose distribution in the axial plane (superior level). Note that the patient was treated in the prone position with an air-filled rectal balloon in place. Also note the "butterfly"-shaped target volume covering the surgical clips. Prostatic fossa (*brown*), rectum (*green*), pubic bone (*light blue*), femoral head (*dark blue*), bladder (*purple*). (To view a color version of this image, please refer to the CD-ROM.)

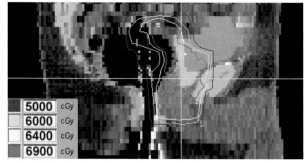

FIGURE 22B-5. Intensity-modulated radiation therapy dose distribution in the sagittal plane. Note rectal balloon posteriorly. Prostatic fossa (*brown*), rectum (*green*), pubic bone (*light blue*), femoral head (*dark blue*), bladder (*purple*). (To view a color version of this image, please refer to the CD-ROM.)

Published Data

To date, published data on postprostatectomy IMRT remain limited. More data are needed in both planning and clinical outcome studies.

Planning Studies

Postprostatectomy IMRT was first implemented at the Baylor College of Medicine in 1998. Initially, we were concerned about target (prostatic fossa with or without the seminal vesicle bed) delineation, especially in a surgically violated bed. There is no prostatic capsule to contain the disease. There were many issues, including the presence of ECE, SVI, high-grade tumor, multiple positive surgical margins, and residual or recurrent disease, especially in the context of no imaging avid tumor (cf, in patients with an intact prostate, the target delineation is more straightforward). We were also very concerned that we might underestimate the target volume.

We proceeded to examine 712 radical prostatectomy specimens evaluating the level of prostatic capsular invasion and the radial extent of ECE.[52] ECE (both focal and established level 3 prostatic capsular invasion) was noted in 299 of 712 patients (42%). Measurable disease extending radially outside the prostatic capsule was noted in 185 of 712 patients (26%). The median radial extension was 2 mm outside the capsule. Twenty of 712 patients (2.8%) had an ECE > 5 mm. We further reported that there were no predictors for the radial distance of ECE.[73]

Two other studies examining the issue of ECE were also published.[74,75] In addition, Kestin and colleagues evaluated SVI in 344 radical prostatectomy specimens.[76] Fifty-one patients (15%) demonstrated SVI in 81 seminal vesicles (21 unilateral and 30 bilateral). The median seminal vesicle length was 3.5 cm (0.7–8.5 cm). The median length of SVI was 1 cm (90th percentile: 2 cm, range 0.2–3.8 cm).

We next examined IMRT target volumes in 10 patients based on their preoperative CT scan and compared them with their PPV on radical prostatectomy specimens.[52] We found that the average GTV was 2 times larger than the PPV, and the average PTV was 4.1 times larger than the PPV. We then performed a treatment planning comparative study between the primary IMRT group ($n = 40$) (with an intact prostate) and the postprostatectomy IMRT group ($n = 125$) (prostatic fossa).[77] Table 22B-1 shows that the target volume

(prostatic fossa) is significantly larger in the postprostatectomy IMRT group when compared with the primary IMRT group (the prostate with or without the seminal vesicles). The larger postprostatectomy target volume may be related to the difficulty in delineating prostatic fossa. More importantly, from these volumetric comparison studies, we concluded that we are not underestimating the postprostatectomy volume when compared with the primary IMRT volume.

Outcome Studies

Only three clinical outcome articles have been published on postprostatectomy IMRT.[77–79] We addressed the treatment-related toxicity in these articles, but the treatment outcome, including biochemical control, local control, and freedom from PSA recurrence, is forthcoming. Despite the escalated dose with postprostatectomy IMRT, the acute toxicity profile was very acceptable, without any grade 3 or higher toxicity. In addition, postprostatectomy IMRT produced a more favorable acute genitourinary toxicity when compared with primary IMRT, in spite of a larger target volume and a higher mean dose to the bladder. This may be related to a combination of lower mean and maximum doses to the target and smaller bladder volumes receiving > 65 Gy in the postprostatectomy group. All of these factors, as well as RT-induced edema and inflammation of the prostate and the prostatic urethra rather than the bladder, may have contributed to the difference in the acute genitourinary toxicity.[77,78]

We have also published on the effects of post–nerve-sparing prostatectomy dose-escalated IMRT on erectile function.[79] Of 51 patients, 18 (35.3%) maintained their potency and 33 (64.7%) became impotent after nerve-sparing prostatectomy. Patients who underwent bilateral nerve-sparing prostatectomy had higher rates of postprostatectomy potency than did those who underwent unilateral nerve-sparing surgery (72.2% vs 27.8%; $p = .025$). All 18 patients (100%) who were potent postoperatively remained potent after IMRT despite the high dose (mean dose 69.6 Gy) to the prostatic bed and nerves. More results on the effects of postprostatectomy IMRT on sural nerve grafts and salvage versus adjuvant radiotherapy are also forthcoming.

Future Directions
Hypofractionation

The conventional postprostatectomy RT dose to the prostatic fossa ranges from 45 to 60 Gy. Two separate single-institution retrospective nonrandomized studies have demonstrated the improvement in biochemical disease-free survival when the radiation dose is above 60 Gy.[10–12] Our currently prescribed IMRT dose is 64 to 66 Gy, delivering a mean dose of 68 to 72 Gy in a higher fraction size. We have observed a favorable toxicity profile thus far.

In the future, further dose escalation with a higher than conventional fraction size (ie, hypofractionation approach)

TABLE 22B-1. Comparison of Target Volumes

	PI (n = 125)	PPI (n = 40)	p Value
Target volume (cc)	Prostate 81.6 (28.7–241.5)	Prostatic fossa 123.6 (28.7–241.5)	< .001
Target volume (cc)	Prostate + seminal vesicles 99.5 (44.2–241.5)	Prostatic fossa 123.6 (64.7–181.3)	< .001

PI = primary intensity-modulated radiation therapy; PPI = postprostatectomy intensity-modulated radiation therapy.

may be used in conjunction with IMRT. This post-prostatectomy IMRT dose-escalation approach, as in the setting of an intact prostate, may have a positive impact on the disease or biochemical control, especially in patients with palpable disease or biopsy-positive local recurrence (both suggesting higher tumor burden). Similar to the randomized dose-escalation trial with intact prostate,[80] a randomized dose-escalation trial in the postprostatectomy setting using IMRT is planned.

Penile Bulb Sparing

Erectile function is an important consideration after radical prostatectomy, especially with a nerve-sparing procedure or sural nerve graft for the cavernosal nerve sacrifice. The mechanisms of radiation-induced erectile dysfunction are complex: a decrease in vascular integrity, an adverse effect on the nerve, and dose to the bulb of the penis. When the patients receive both treatments (radical prostatectomy and postprostatectomy RT), it is unclear which plays a greater role in the development of erectile dysfunction. Some preliminary data appear to show that conformal RT as primary treatment for prostate cancer decreases the incidence of erectile dysfunction compared with nonconformal techniques.[81,82] We published the only article on postprostatectomy IMRT showing no negative effects on erectile function for patients who remained potent after nerve-sparing prostatectomy.[79] In the future, we plan to evaluate and limit the dose to the penile bulb to further refine the delivery of IMRT in this setting. One caution is that the urogenital diaphragm can descend after prostatectomy and the apical margin is often positive for significant apical tumors. Hence, the target volume is more inferior when compared with that of the intact prostate, and sparing the penile bulb may be difficult.

Advanced Imaging

Target delineation will significantly improve with the use of a more advanced imaging technique, for example, ProstaScint scanning, dynamic contrast-enhanced MRI, and ^{11}C-choline PET. With the capability of IMRT, different targets can be outlined, for example, image-positive local recurrence (target 1) and the subclinical disease (target 2), and treated to different total doses with different fraction sizes. The SMART (simultaneous modulated accelerated radiation therapy) approach,[83] initially implemented at the Baylor College of Medicine/The Methodist Hospital to overcome the rapid repopulation in head and neck cancer and to provide patients with the convenience of once-daily treatment, should be explored here.

Acknowledgment

We would like to acknowledge Dr. Anwar Padhani for his contribution to imaging of the prostatic bed.

References

1. Andriole GL. Adjuvant therapy for prostate cancer patients at high risk of recurrence following radical prostatectomy. Eur Urol 1997;32 Suppl 3:65–9.

2. Cheng WS, Frydenberg M, Bergstralh EJ, et al. Radical prostatectomy for pathologic stage C prostate cancer: influence of pathologic variables and adjuvant treatment on disease outcome. Urology 1993;42:283–91.

3. Schild SE, Wong WW, Grado GL, et al. The result of radical retropubic prostatectomy and adjuvant therapy for pathologic stage C prostate cancer. Int J Radiat Oncol Biol Phys 1996;34:535–41.

4. Shevlin BE, Mittal BB, Brand WN, et al. The role of adjuvant irradiation following primary prostatectomy, based on histopathologic extent of tumor. Int J Radiat Oncol Biol Phys 1989;16:1425–30.

5. Anscher MS, Prosnitz LR. Multivariate analysis of factors predicting local relapse after radical prostatectomy—possible indications for postoperative radiotherapy. Int J Radiat Oncol Biol Phys 1991;21:941–7.

6. Taylor N, Kelly JF, Kuban DA, et al. Adjuvant and salvage radiotherapy after radical prostatectomy for prostate cancer. Int J Radiat Oncol Biol Phys 2003;56:755–63.

7. Schild SE. Radiation therapy (RT) after prostatectomy: the case for salvage therapy as opposed to adjuvant therapy. Int J Cancer 2001;96:94–8.

8. Forman JD, Velasco J. Therapeutic radiation in patients with a rising post-prostatectomy PSA level. Oncology (Huntingt) 1998;12:33–9.

9. Valicenti RK, Gomella LG, Perez CA. Radiation therapy after radical prostatectomy: a review of the issues and options. Semin Radiat Oncol 2003;13:130–40.

10. Valicenti RK, Gomella LG, Ismail M, et al The efficacy of early adjuvant radiation therapy for pT3N0 prostate cancer: a matched-pair analysis. Int J Radiat Oncol Biol Phys 1999;45:53–8.

11. Valicenti RK, Gomella LG, Ismail M, et al. Durable efficacy of early postoperative radiation therapy for high-risk pT3N0 prostate cancer: the importance of radiation dose. Urology 1998;52:1034–40.

12. Anscher MS, Clough R, Dodge R. Radiotherapy for a rising prostate-specific antigen after radical prostatectomy: the first 10 years. Int J Radiat Oncol Biol Phys 2000;48:369–75.

13. Zelefsky MJ, Fuks Z, Hunt M, et al. High-dose intensity modulated radiation therapy for prostate cancer: early toxicity and biochemical outcome in 772 patients. Int J Radiat Oncol Biol Phys 2002;53:1111–6.

14. Pickett B, Vigneault E, Kurhanewicz J, et al. Static field intensity modulation to treat a dominant intra-prostatic lesion to 90 Gy compared to seven field 3-dimensional radiotherapy. Int J Radiat Oncol Biol Phys 1999;44:921–9.

15. Zelefsky MJ, Fuks Z, Hunt M, et al. High dose radiation delivered by intensity modulated conformal radiotherapy improves the outcome of localized prostate cancer. J Urol 2001;166:876–81.

16. Kupelian PA, Reddy CA, Carlson TP, et al. Preliminary observations on biochemical relapse-free survival rates after short-course intensity-modulated radiotherapy (70 Gy at

2.5 Gy/fraction) for localized prostate cancer. Int J Radiat Oncol Biol Phys 2002;53:904–12.

17. Nutting CM, Corbishley CM, Sancjez-Nieto B, et al. Potential improvements in the therapeutic ration of prostate cancer irradiation: dose escalation of pathologically identified tumour nodules using intensity modulated radiotherapy. Br J Radiol 2002;75:151–61.

18. Young HH. Four cases of radical prostatectomy. Johns Hopkins Bull 1905;16:315.

19. Millin T. Retropubic prostatectomy, a new extravesical technique. Lancet 1945;ii:693–6.

20. Walsh PC, Lepor H, Eggleston JC. Radical prostatectomy with preservation of sexual function: anatomical and pathological considerations. Prostate 1983;4:473–85.

21. Kim ED, Scardino PT, Hampel O, et al. Interposition of sural nerve restores function of cavernous nerves resected during radical prostatectomy. J Urol 1999;161:188–92.

22. Guillonneau B, Cathelineau X, Barret E, et al. [Laparoscopic radical prostatectomy. preliminary evaluation after 28 interventions]. Presse Med 1998;27:1570–4.

23. Pierce EC Jr. The 34th Rovenstine Lecture. 40 years behind the mask: safety revisited. Anesthesiology 1996;84:965–75.

24. Lepor H, Kaci L. Contemporary evaluation of operative parameters and complications related to open radical retropubic prostatectomy. Urology 2003;62:702–6.

25. Garnick MB, Fair WR. Prostate cancer: emerging concepts. Part I. Ann Intern Med 1996;125:118–25.

26. Lu-Yao GL, Potosky AL, Albertsen PC, et al. Follow-up prostate cancer treatments after radical prostatectomy: a population-based study. J Natl Cancer Inst 1996;88:166–73.

27. Epstein JI, Partin AW, Sauvageot J, et al. Prediction of progression following radical prostatectomy. A multivariate analysis of 721 men with long-term follow-up. Am J Surg Pathol 1996;20:286–92.

28. Han M, Partin AW, Pound CR, et al. Long-term biochemical disease-free and cancer-specific survival following anatomic radical retropubic prostatectomy. The 15-year Johns Hopkins experience. Urol Clin North Am 2001;28:555–65.

29. Pound CR, Partin AW, Epstein JI, et al. Prostate-specific antigen after anatomic radical retropubic prostatectomy. Patterns of recurrence and cancer control. Urol Clin North Am 1997;24:395–406.

30. Quinn DI, Henshall SM, Haynes AM, et al. Prognostic significance of pathologic features in localized prostate cancer treated with radical prostatectomy: implications for staging systems and predictive models. J Clin Oncol 2001;19:3692–705.

31. Hull GW, Rabbani F, Abbas F, et al. Cancer control with radical prostatectomy alone in 1,000 consecutive patients. J Urol 2002;167:528–34.

32. Grossfeld GD, Chang JJ, Broering JM, et al. Impact of positive surgical margins on prostate cancer recurrence and the use of secondary cancer treatment: data from the CaPSURE database. J Urol 2000;163:1171–7.

33. Minet H. Application du radium aux tumeurs vesicales, a l'hypertophie et au cancer de la prostate. Assoc Franc Urol 1909;13:629.

34. George FW, Carlton CE Jr, Dykhuizen RF, et al. Cobalt-60 telecurietherapy in the definitive treatment of carcinoma of the prostate: a preliminary report. J Urol 1965;93:102–9.

35. Ray GR, Cassady JR, Bagshaw MA. External-bean megavoltage radiation therapy in the treatment of post-radical prostatectomy residual or recurrent tumor preliminary results. J Urol 1975;114: 98–101.

36. Soffen EM, Hanks GE, Hwang CC, et al. Conformal static field therapy for low volume low grade prostate cancer with rigid immobilization. Int J Radiat Oncol Biol Phys 1991;20:141–6.

37. Partin AW, Pearson JD, Landis PK, et al. Evaluation of serum prostate-specific antigen velocity after radical prostatectomy to distinguish local recurrence from distant metastases. Urology 1994;43:649–59.

38. Patel A, Dorey F, Franklin J, et al. Recurrence patterns after radical retropubic prostatectomy: clinical usefulness of prostate specific antigen doubling times and log slope prostate specific antigen. J Urol 1997;158:1441–5.

39. Leventis AK, Shariat SF, Kattan MW, et al. Prediction of response to salvage radiation therapy in patients with prostate cancer recurrence after radical prostatectomy. J Clin Oncol 2001;19:1030–9.

40. Cher ML, Bianco FJ Jr, Lam JS, et al. Limited role of radionuclide bone scintigraphy in patients with prostate specific antigen elevations after radical prostatectomy. J Urol 1998;160:1387–91.

41. Kupelian PA, Katcher J, Levin HS, et al. Stage T1-2 prostate cancer: a multivariate analysis of factors affecting biochemical and clinical failures after radical prostatectomy. Int J Radiat Oncol Biol Phys 1997;37:1043–52.

42. Connolly JA, Shinohara K, Presti JC Jr, et al. Local recurrence after radical prostatectomy: characteristics in size, location, and relationship to prostate-specific antigen and surgical margins. Urology 1996;47:225–31.

43. Scherr D, Swindle PW, Scardino PT. National Comprehensive Cancer Network guidelines for the management of prostate cancer. Urology 2003;61:14–24.

44. Bastasch MD, Butler EB, Augspurger ME, et al. Adjuvant radiotherapy after prostatectomy for patients with high risk factors but an undetectable PSA. RSNA 2001. Radiology 2001;221:225.

45. Van Cangh PJ, Richard F, Lorge F, et al. Adjuvant radiation therapy does not cause urinary incontinence after radical prostatectomy: results of a prospective randomized study. J Urol 1998;159:164–6.

46. Cox JD, Gallagher MJ, Hammond EH, et al. Consensus statements on radiation therapy of prostate cancer: guidelines for prostate re-biopsy after radiation and for radiation therapy with rising prostate-specific antigen levels after radical prostatectomy. American Society for Therapeutic Radiology and Oncology Consensus Panel. J Clin Oncol 1999;17:1155.

47. McGary JE, Teh BS, Butler EB, et al. Prostate immobilization using a rectal balloon. J Appl Clin Med Phys 2002;3:6–11.

48. Teh BS, Mai WY, Uhl BM, et al. Intensity-modulated radiation therapy (IMRT) for prostate cancer with the use of a rectal balloon for prostate immobilization: acute toxicity and dose-volume analysis. Int J Radiat Oncol Biol Phys 2001;49:705–12.

49. Teh BS, McGary JE, Dong L, et al. The use of rectal balloon during the delivery of intensity modulated radiotherapy (IMRT) for prostate cancer: more than just a prostate gland immobilization device? Cancer J 2002;8:476–83.

50. Patel RR, Orton N, Tome WA, et al. Rectal dose sparing with a balloon catheter and ultrasound localization in conformal radiation therapy for prostate cancer. Radiother Oncol 2003;67:285–94.

51. Leventis AK, Shariat SF, Slawin KM. Local recurrence after radical prostatectomy: correlation of US features with prostatic fossa biopsy findings. Radiology 2001;219:432–52.

52. Teh BS, Bastasch MD, Wheeler TM, et al. IMRT for prostate cancer: defining target volume based on correlated pathologic volume of disease. Int J Radiat Oncol Biol Phys 2003;56:184–91.

53. Roach M III, Faillace-Akazawa P, Malfatti C, et al. Prostate volumes defined by magnetic resonance imaging and computerized tomographic scans for three-dimensional conformal radiotherapy. Int J Radiat Oncol Biol Phys 1996;35:1011–8.

54. Wilder RB, Fone PD, Rademacher DE, et al. Localization of the prostatic apex for radiotherapy treatment planning using urethroscopy. Int J Radiat Oncol Biol Phys 1997;38:737–41.

55. Koppie TM, Grossfeld GD, Nudell DM, et al. Is anastomotic biopsy necessary before radiotherapy after radical prostatectomy? J Urol 2001;166:111–5.

56. Yao D, Trabulsi EJ, Kostakoglu L, et al. The utility of monoclonal antibodies in the imaging of prostate cancer: Semin Urol Oncol 2002:20:211–8.

57. Freeman LM, Krynyckyi BR, Li Y, et al. The role of (111) in capromab pendetide (Prosta-ScintR) immunoscintigraphy in the management of prostate cancer. Q J Nucl Med 2002;46:131–7.

58. Sodee DB, Malguria N, Faulhaber P, et al. Multicenter ProstaScint imaging findings in 2154 patients with prostate cancer. The ProstaScint Imaging Centers. Urology 2000;56:988–93.

59. Raj GV, Partin AW, Polascik TJ. Clinical utility of indium 111-capromab pendetide immunoscintigraphy in the detection of early, recurrent prostate carcinoma after radical prostatectomy. Cancer 2002;94:987–96.

60. Kahn D, Williams RD, Manyak MJ, et al. [111]Indium-capromab pendetide in the evaluation of patients with residual or recurrent prostate cancer after radical prostatectomy. The ProstaScint Study Group. J Urol 1998;159:2041–6.

61. Hofer C, Laubenbacher C, Block T, et al. Fluorine-18-fluorodeoxyglucose positron emission tomography is useless for the detection of local recurrence after radical prostatectomy. Eur Urol 1999;36:31–5.

62. Chang CH, Wu HC, Tsai JJ, et al. Detecting metastatic pelvic lymph nodes by (18)F-2-deoxyglucose positron emission tomography in patients with prostate-specific antigen relapse after treatment for localized prostate cancer. Urol Int 2003;70:311–5.

63. Picchio M, Messa C, Landoni C, et al. Value of [11C]choline-positron emission tomography for re-staging prostate cancer: a comparison with [18F]fluorodeoxyglucose-positron emission tomography: J Urol 2003;169:1337–40.

64. Hricak H, Schoder H, Pucar D, et al. Advances in imaging in the postoperative patient with a rising prostate-specific antigen level. Semin Oncol 2003;30:616–34.

65. Bostwick DG, Grignon DJ, Hammond ME, et al. Prognostic factors in prostate cancer. College of American Pathologists Consensus Statement 1999. Arch Pathol Lab Med 2000;124:995–1000.

66. Langen KM, Jones DT. Organ motion and its management. Int J Radiat Oncol Biol Phys 2001;50:265–78.

67. Chinnaiyan P, Tomee W, Patel R, et al. 3D-ultrasound guided radiation therapy in the post-prostatectomy setting. Technol Cancer Res Treat 2003;2:455–8.

68. Teh BS, Woo SY, Butler EB. Intensity modulated radiation therapy (IMRT): a new promising technology in radiation oncology. Oncologist 1999;4:433–42.

69. Brenner DJ, Hall EJ. Fractionation and protraction for radiotherapy of prostate carcinoma. Int J Radiat Oncol Biol Phys 1999;43:1095–101.

70. King CR, Fowler JF. A simple analytic derivation suggests that prostate cancer alpha/beta ratio is low. Int J Radiat Oncol Biol Phys 2001;51:213–4.

71. Duchesne GM, Peters LJ. What is the alpha/beta ratio for prostate cancer? Rationale for hypofractionated high-dose-rate brachytherapy. Int J Radiat Oncol Biol Phys 1999;44:747–8.

72. D'Souza WD, Thames HD. Is the alpha/beta ratio for prostate cancer low? Int J Radiat Oncol Biol Phys 2001;51:1–3.

73. Teh BS, Bastasch MD, Mai WY, et al. Predictors of extracapsular extension and its radial distance in prostate cancer: implications for prostate IMRT, brachytherapy, and surgery. Cancer J 2003;9:454–60.

74. Davis BJ, Pisansky TM, Wilson TM, et al. The radial distance of extraprostatic extension of prostate carcinoma: implications for prostate brachytherapy. Cancer 1999;85:2630–7.

75. Sohayda C, Kupelian PA, Levin HS, et al. Extent of extracapsular extension in localized prostate cancer. Urology 2000;55:382–6.

76. Kestin L, Goldstein N, Vicini F, et al. Treatment of prostate cancer with radiotherapy: should the entire seminal vesicles be included in the clinical target volume? Int J Radiat Oncol Biol Phys 2002;54:686–97.

77. Teh BS, Mai WY, Augspurger ME, et al. Intensity modulated radiation therapy (IMRT) following prostatectomy: more favorable acute genitourinary toxicity profile compared to primary IMRT for prostate cancer. Int J Radiat Oncol Biol Phys 2001;49:465–72.

78. Teh BS, Woo SY, Mai WY, et al. Clinical experience with intensity-modulated radiation therapy (IMRT) for prostate cancer with the use of rectal balloon for prostate immobilization. Med Dosim 2002;27:105–13.

79. Bastasch MD, Teh BS, Mai WY, et al. Post-nerve-sparing prostatectomy, dose-escalated intensity-modulated radiotherapy: effect on erectile function. Int J Radiat Oncol Biol Phys 2002;54:101–6.

80. Pollack A, Zagars GK, Starkschall G, et al. Prostate cancer radiation dose response: results of the M. D. Anderson phase III randomized trial. Int J Radiat Oncol Biol Phys 2002;53:1097–105.

81. al-Abany M, Steineck G, Agren Cronqvist AK, et al. Improving the preservation of erectile function after external beam radiation therapy for prostate cancer. Radiother Oncol 2000;57:201–6.

82. Wilder RB, Chou RH, Ryu JK, et al. Potency preservation after three-dimensional conformal radiotherapy for prostate cancer: preliminary results. Am J Clin Oncol 2000;23:330–3.

83. Butler EB, Teh BS, Grant WH III, et al. Smart (simultaneous modulated accelerated radiation therapy) boost: a new accelerated fractionation schedule for the treatment of head and neck cancer with intensity modulated radiotherapy. Int J Radiat Oncol Biol Phys 1999;45:21–32.

Chapter 22.1

INTACT PROSTATE CANCER

CASE STUDY

ROBERT A. PRICE JR, PHD, ERIC M. HORWITZ, MD, STEVEN J. FEIGENBERG, MD, ALAN POLLACK, MD, PHD

Patient History

A 67-year-old male was found on routine screening to have an elevated prostate-specific antigen (PSA) of 5.4 ng/mL. He denied any urinary symptoms, except for nocturia once per night. His International Prostate Symptom Score (IPSS) was 7. A digital rectal examination revealed a 1.5 cm right-sided nodule between the apex and the midgland laterally. Prostate biopsies were obtained from the following regions: sextants, bilateral anterior horns (lateral aspects of the prostate), and the bilateral transition zone. These biopsies revealed a Gleason score of 3 + 3 carcinoma from the right apex (40% of one core), right anterior horn (10% of one core), right midgland (< 5% of one core), and left base (5% of one core). Metastatic workup, including a bone scan, and an abdominal/pelvic computed tomography (CT) scan were negative (note that these tests have a low yield in this patient and are not necessary).

The tumor was thus staged as a T2aN0M0 prostate carcinoma and was classified as intermediate risk owing to involvement of multiple prostate biopsy cores (4 of 10). To reduce the volume of bladder and rectum irradiated (and thus the risk of acute and chronic toxicity), intensity-modulated radiation therapy (IMRT) was used in this patient.

Simulation

At the Fox Chase Cancer Center, all patients with prostate cancer are simulated in the supine position. A customized alpha cradle (extending from the midback to the midthigh) is fabricated for immobilization. In addition, a custom Plexiglas foot-holder is used to position the patient's feet.

The patient was instructed to have a half-full bladder at simulation (because maintaining a full bladder during treatment is difficult). In addition, he was told to eat a low-residue diet the night prior to simulation to reduce intestinal gas. On the day of simulation, he was asked to empty his rectum using an enema. If, at simulation, the rectum is > 3 cm in width owing to gas or stool, patients are asked to try to expel any residual rectal contents. A retrograde urethrogram was not performed.

A planning CT scan was obtained in the treatment position using a flat table insert on a PQ5000 CT simulator (Philips Medical Systems, Andover, MA). Images were acquired from 2 cm above the iliac crests to the midfemur. This scanning extent facilitates the use of noncoplanar beams when necessary.[1] Slices in the region beginning 2 cm above the femoral heads to the bottom of the ischial tuberosities were acquired using a 3 mm slice thickness and 3 mm table increments. Outside this region, a 1 cm slice thickness was used.

At our center, patients with prostate cancer also undergo planning magnetic resonance imaging (MRI) using a 0.23 Tesla open scanner (Philips Medical Systems) located within the department. The scan is obtained within 30 minutes prior to or following the planning CT scan. The planning CT and MRI are obtained without contrast media. The resultant MRIs are processed using a gradient distortion correction (GDC) algorithm. After GDC, the CT scan and MRI are fused according to bony anatomy (using either chamfer matching or maximization of mutual information methods). Presently, we have the capability of performing MRI simulation without CT because the GDC software is approved by the US Food and Drug Administration (Philips Medical Systems).

Target and Tissue Delineation

Soft tissue structures were contoured based on the MRI information, whereas the external contour and bony structures were based on CT. A clinical target volume (CTV) was delineated consisting of the prostate and seminal vesicles. No gross tumor volume was delineated. The proximal seminal vesicles were outlined separately to facilitate B-mode acquisition and targeting (BAT) ultrasound localization (North American Scientific, NOMOS Radiation

Oncology Division, Cranberry Township, PA). We have found that outlining the proximal seminal vesicles separately from the prostate allows easier alignment with the BAT ultrasonography. The distal seminal vesicles are outlined as a separate structure as well; the ability to see the position of the distal seminal vesicles during the BAT ultrasound alignment process is useful.

MRI simulation greatly facilitates CTV delineation in patients with prostate cancer. In general, the borders of the prostate are often not well visualized on CT. The levator ani muscles are often difficult to distinguish from the lateral aspect of the prostate. Moreover, the base and apex of the prostate are also difficult to discern. As a consequence, our standard simulation procedure involves MRI.

If one uses CT-based planning, contrast in the bladder may help distinguish the prostate-bladder interface; intravenous contrast is preferred because catheter placement distorts the anatomy. If contrast is used, heterogeneity corrections should not be attempted. We do not routinely perform heterogeneity corrections even though we do not use contrast.

For delineation of the prostatic apex, a retrograde urethrogram may be used if CT simulation is performed. Of note, Malone and colleagues found that a retrograde urethrogram may alter the anatomy by displacing the prostate superiorly.[2] Although this has not been our experience, anytime a catheter is used, there is the potential for alteration of the anatomic relationships such that they are not representative of what occurs during treatment.

Another means of determining the prostatic apex is to identify the penile bulb and then go superiorly approximately 1 cm. This approach will overestimate the position of the apex inferiorly, which may be appropriate, given that there is no prostatic capsule inferiorly and tumor involvement is noted in this region in approximately one-third of cases. For these reasons, and the concern that the BAT ultrasound localization system is least accurate in the superior-inferior dimensions, we tend to overestimate the prostatic apex position even on MRI simulation.

The bilateral femoral heads, bladder, and rectum were also contoured for this patient. The femoral heads were contoured from the top of the femoral head to the level of the upper border of the lesser trochanters. The bladder was contoured in its entirety and was, as noted above, simulated half-full.

The rectum was defined according to the Radiation Therapy Oncology Group (RTOG) guidelines and was contoured from the bottom of the ischial tuberosities to the sigmoid flexure. As noted above, the rectum was simulated empty (facilitated by an enema), and the volume included the entire rectal contents. The goal was to limit the rectal diameter to 3 cm or less on any axial slice. By planning with an empty rectum, the acceptance dose-volume histogram (DVH) criteria represent the worst-case scenario; the smaller the rectal volume, the larger the volume of rectum receiv-

ing high doses owing to the overlap of the planning target volume (PTV). Using BAT localization on a daily basis allows for alignment of the prostate-rectum interface, such that if the rectum is larger on a given day, the absolute rectal wall volume exposed in the PTV-rectal overlap region (exposed to the higher radiation dose) is kept the same. The relationship between the posterior aspect of the prostate and anterior wall of the rectum changes by less than 1 mm daily as evaluated by in-house MRI. The target and normal tissue contours delineated in this case are summarized in Figure 22.1-1.

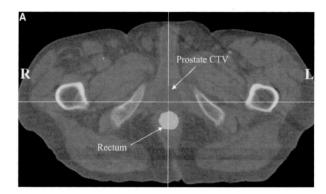

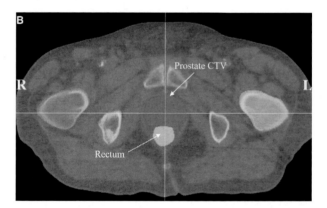

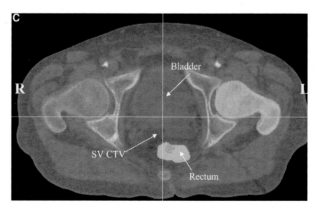

FIGURE 22.1-1. Illustration of contours used for planning. All soft tissues structures outlined were delineated on the associated magnetic resonance images and subsequently fused to the computed tomography study for planning. CTV = clinical target volume; SV = seminal vesicles. (To view a color version of this image, please refer to the CD-ROM.)

TABLE 22.1-1. Input Parameters

Target	Type	Goal, Gy	Volume below Goal, %	Minimum, Gy	Maximum, Gy	I
Prostate	Homogeneous	76.0	5	72.2	81.3	
Seminal vesicle	Homogeneous	56.0	5	53.2	76.0	

Sensitive Structure	Type	Limit, Gy	Volume above Limit, %	Minimum, Gy	Maximum, Gy	I
Tissue	Homogeneous	76.0	0	0.0	76.0	
Bladder	Basic	35.0	20	2.0	60.0	
Rt femoral head	Basic	40.0	30	10.0	45.0	
Lt femoral head	Basic	40.0	30	10.0	45.0	
Rectum	Critical	15.0	10	5.0	76.0	X
Region						
1	Basic	68.4	20	34.2	76.0	
2	Basic	60.8	20	30.4	68.4	
3	Basic	53.2	20	26.6	57.0	
4	Basic	38.0	1	19.0	41.8	
5	Basic	22.8	1	11.4	26.6	
6	Basic	15.2	1	7.6	19.0	

The prostate or target is assigned a dose goal, a percentage of the volume that may be underdosed, and minimum and maximum doses to be delivered. Each additional nontarget structure is assigned a dose limit, a percentage of the volume for each structure that may receive more than this limit, and minimum and maximum values. The "I" box is checked if the planner wants the system to improve on the input parameters.

Treatment Planning

The PTV is 8 mm larger than the CTV (prostate and proximal seminal vesicles) in all directions except posteriorly, where the margin is typically 5 mm. This margin is variable in that we evaluate the "effective margin." This margin is defined by the distance between the posterior aspect of the CTV and the prescription isodose line and typically falls between 3 and 8 mm.

Treatment planning was performed in this patient using the *CORVUS* inverse planning system, version 3.0 (North American Scientific). A dose of 76 Gy in 2 Gy daily fractions was planned for the prostate using the segmental multileaf collimation delivery technique. A dose of 56 Gy was planned for the proximal seminal vesicles (we now take the proximal seminal vesicles to 76 Gy) in 38 fractions, which is biologically equivalent to 45 to 50 Gy using standard fractionation. Input parameters for inverse planning are summarized in Table 22.1-1. The continuous annealing method was selected for optimization. A minimum beamlet size of 1 × 1 cm was used with five intensity levels throughout. Ellipsoid regions for dose constraints were used, and their associated input parameters are contained within Table 22.1-1.[3] Heterogeneity corrections were not used.

The treatment plan used in this patient consisted of seven coplanar beams using 18 MV photons.[4] The beam angles used in this patient are shown in Figure 22.1-2. The photon energy was used specifically for the dose rates available on this particular accelerator (6 MV: 300 monitor units/min; 18 MV: 500 monitor units/min) and was based on resultant treatment time only.

Our plan acceptance criteria in prostate cancer IMRT are as follows. A minimum of 95% of the prostate planning target volume (PTV_{95}) must receive 100% of the prescription dose (76 Gy). In addition, 95% of the proximal seminal vesicle PTV must receive 56 Gy. Rectal constraints must be met such that no more than 17% of the rectum may receive ≥ 65 Gy (R_{65}) and no more than 35% may receive ≥ 40 Gy (R_{40}). These criteria are based on the results of an M. D. Anderson Cancer Center phase III randomized trial.[5] In that study, significantly less grade 2 or higher rectal morbidity was noted when no more than 25% of the

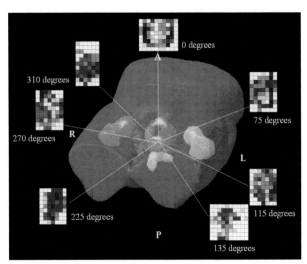

FIGURE 22.1-2. Illustration of the beam directions used in this case study and the resultant intensity patterns associated with each. (To view a color version of this image, please refer to the CD-ROM.)

rectum received 70 Gy or above. The cutpoint was reduced from ≥ 70 to ≥ 65 Gy or higher to account for the increase in daily fraction size to 2 Gy, and the percent rectal volume parameter was reduced from ≥ 25 to ≥ 17% owing to the ability to consistently meet or exceed this constraint. The relationship between rectal complication risk and the proportion of rectum exposed to high doses is likely a continuous function; the lower the percentage receiving ≥ 65 Gy, the lower the risk.

The second constraint parameter, R_{40}, was added to better define the shape of the DVH curve. Another constraint applied was that the 50% isosdose line must fall within the rectal contour (based on the Memorial Sloan Kettering Cancer Center Experience) on any individual CT slice, and the 90% isodose line should not exceed half the diameter of the rectal contour on any slice. These constraints are shown on the sagittal dose distribution in Figure 22.1-3.

From the M. D. Anderson study, no bladder DVH constraints were identified, although bladder complications occur later than rectal injuries.[6,7] At Fox Chase Cancer Center, we have, somewhat arbitrarily, adopted bladder constraints to minimize the dose to the bladder. The constraints are that no more than 25% of the bladder may receive ≥ 65 Gy (B_{65}) and no more than 50% may receive ≥ 40 Gy (B_{40}). It should be noted that in many cases, these bladder constraints are not possible because the bladder was not appropriately full at simulation. In such cases, the bladder volume is monitored during treatment via daily ultrasonography, and the patient is encouraged to have a full bladder during treatment. Figure 22.1-4 illustrates the resultant DVH for the target and normal tissues in this case. Figure 22.1-5 illustrates the resultant dose distributions of the treatment plan.

Treatment Delivery and Quality Assurance

This patient was treated on a Primus linear accelerator (Siemens Medical Systems, Concord, CA). The treatment plan consisted of 977 monitor units being delivered through 55 individual beam segments. The modified modulation scaling factor for this treatment was 3.57, and the treatment was delivered in ~ 9 minutes.

All prostate treatments at our center incorporate daily ultrasound localization using the BAT system. The treatment isocenter is chosen during the CT simulation such that it falls within the prostate volume. The planning isocenter is forced to be identical to that depicted during the CT simulation, ensuring that any isocenter shifts occurring on a daily basis are the result of localization. Treatment portal images are not routinely taken. Portal image evaluation is based on bony anatomy, whereas our localization method is based on soft tissue structures. Adjusting the isocenter based on portal images of our daily localized isocenter compared with the simulation digitally reconstructed radi-

ographs would result in treatment errors. We do, however, verify the original isocenter on a weekly basis through the use of a single set of orthogonal port films. This ensures that the starting point used in the localization process is the same throughout the course of treatment and allows us to minimize the required isocenter shifts.

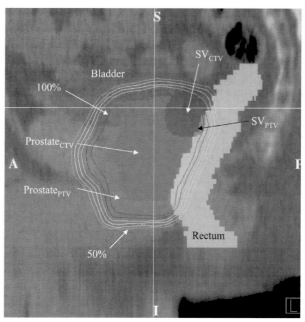

FIGURE 22.1-3. Sagittal dose distribution for this case study illustrating dose conformity and the positioning of the 90% and 50% isodose lines with respect to our rectal acceptance criteria. CTV = clinical target volume; PTV = planning target volume; SV = seminal vesicles. (To view a color version of this image, please refer to the CD-ROM.)

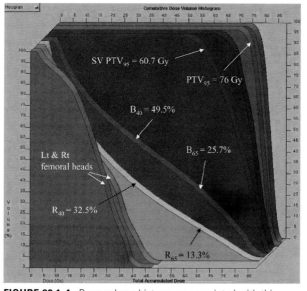

FIGURE 22.1-4. Dose-volume histograms associated with this case study. B_{40} = bladder receiving ≥ 40 Gy; B_{65} = bladder receiving ≥ 65 Gy; PTV_{95} = 95% of planning target volume; R_{40} = rectum receiving ≥ 40 Gy; SV PTV_{95} = 95% of the seminal vesicles planning target volume. (To view a color version of this image, please refer to the CD-ROM.)

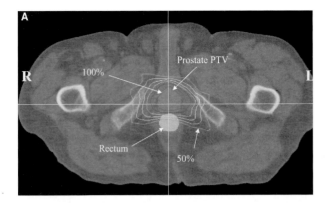

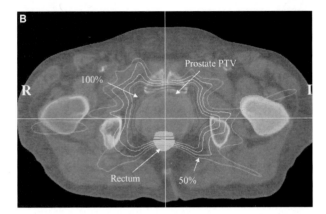

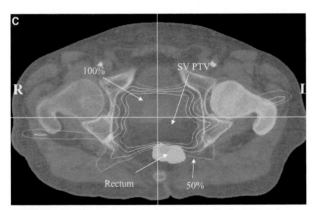

FIGURE 22.1-5. Illustration of resultant isodose distributions on images depicted in Figure 22.1-1 with planning target volume (PTV) applied. SV = seminal vesicles. (To view a color version of this image, please refer to the CD-ROM.)

Clinical Outcome

The patient tolerated the treatment well, with only mild irritative and obstructive urinary symptoms (which were relieved with the administration of an α-blocker). An increase in bowel movement frequency from one to two to three per day was also noted. At the 3-month follow-up visit, his PSA had dropped to 2 ng/mL, and most of his symptoms had resolved. His IPSS score was 8, with nocturia once per night. He noted that urgency of urination occurred occasionally and was a little more pronounced than prior to radiation therapy. He denied any gastrointestinal symptoms. At 9 months post-treatment, his PSA was 1.2 ng/mL, and at 1.25 years, it was 0.7 ng/mL. His symptoms had changed little, although he was no longer taking the α-blocker.

References

1. Price RA, Hanks GE, McNeeley SW, et al. Advantages of using noncoplanar vs. axial beam arrangements when treating prostate cancer with intensity-modulated radiation therapy and the step-and-shoot delivery method. Int J Radiat Oncol Biol Phys 2002;53:236–43.

2. Malone S, Donleer A, Broader M, et al. Effects of urethrography on prostate position: considerations for radiotherapy treatment planning of prostate carcinoma. Int J Radiat Oncol Biol Phys 2000;46:89–93.

3. Price RA, Murphy S, McNeeley SW, et al. A method for increased dose conformity and segment reduction for SMLC delivered IMRT treatment of the prostate. Int J Radiat Oncol Biol Phys 2003;57:843–52.

4. Price RA, Chibani O, Ma CM. Shielding evaluation for IMRT implementation in an existing accelerator vault. J Appl Clin Med Phys 2003;4:231–8.

5. Pollack A, Zagars GK, Starkshall G, et al. Prostate cancer radiation dose response: results of the M. D. Anderson phase III randomized trial. Int J Radiat Oncol Biol Phys 2002;53:1097–105.

6. Feigenberg SJ, Hanlon AL, Horwitz EM, Pollack A. Androgen deprivation increases late morbidity in prostate cancer patients treated with 3D conformal radiation therapy. Int J Radiat Oncol Biol Phys 2003;57(2 Suppl):S176.

7. Gardner BG, Seitman AL, Shipley W, et al. Late normal tissue sequelae in the second decade after high dose radiation therapy with combined photons and conformal protons for locally advanced prostate cancer. J Urol 2002;167:123–6.

Hypofractionated IMRT

Case Study

Patrick Kupelian, MD, Twyla Willoughby, MS

Patient History

A 63-year-old male presented with an elevated prostate-specific antigen (PSA) level of 8.7 ng/mL noted on a routine medical examination. He denied any symptoms, except for mild nocturia. His American Urological Association symptom index score was 8. A digital rectal examination failed to reveal any palpable abnormalities of the prostate. Transrectal ultrasound-guided biopsies of the prostate were performed. The pathology was consistent with adenocarcinoma, Gleason Score 3 + 3, from one of eight cores. The positive core was from the right apical area. No perineural invasion was noted. A bone scan was negative for metastatic disease. No additional workup was performed.

The patient's initial evaluation included an extensive discussion of various treatment options, including radical prostatectomy, brachytherapy, and different forms of external beam radiation therapy. He elected to proceed with definitive intensity-modulated radiation therapy (IMRT).

Simulation

To perform daily target localization, intraprostatic markers were placed on the day of the computed tomography (CT) planning scan. The patient was directed to take antibiotics on the day before and the day of the procedure, as well as an enema on the morning of the procedure. Using a transrectal ultrasound probe designed for prostate biopsies, three small gold markers were inserted through 18-gauge brachytherapy needles at the right base, right apex, and left midgland. The procedure took approximately 5 minutes and did not require any anesthesia.

After the seeds were placed, the patient underwent a planning CT simulation (PQ2000, Philips Medical Systems, Andover, MA) in the supine position with his feet taped and without any other external immobilization devices. Three-millimeter cuts were obtained throughout the lower pelvis, from the midsacrum to the bottom of the lesser trochanters. Contrast was not administered.

Target and Tissue Delineation

The clinical target volume (CTV) in this patient consisted of the prostate gland alone. The seminal vesicles were outlined but were not included in the CTV because the risk of seminal vesicle involvement in this patient was very low. The prostate was outlined on axial CT slices starting from the midgland and proceeding superiorly until the base and then inferiorly to the apex, excluding the venous plexus anterolaterally and the puborectalis muscle. Superiorly, the prostate gland was outlined, taking into consideration a certain thickness of the bladder wall. Inferiorly, it was outlined around the area of the urethra down to the level of the superior aspect of the crurae, thereby somewhat extending the CTV beyond the prostate per se.

The organs at risk outlined in this patient included the rectum, bladder, penile bulb, and femoral heads. The outer circumference of the rectum was outlined from 1 cm above to 1 cm below the prostate and seminal vesicles. The bladder was delineated using the outer bladder wall. The penile bulb and femoral heads were delineated in their entirety.

The planning target volume (PTV) in this patient was generated by expanding the CTV 4 mm posteriorly and anteriorly and 6 mm laterally, superiorly, and inferiorly. Figure 22.2-1 illustrates the PTV and organs at risk at the level of the mid–prostate gland.

Treatment Planning

The IMRT plan was generated using the *BrainSCAN* inverse planning software (BrainLAB AG, Heimstetten, Germany). A dose of 70 Gy was prescribed to the PTV in 2.5 daily fractions. Assuming an α/β ratio of 1.5 for prostate cancer tissues, this is the equivalent of approximately 83 Gy in 1.8 Gy daily fractions. Five treatment beams were selected: one anterior, two anterior oblique (45° off horizontal), and two shallow posterior oblique (10° off horizontal). All beams had a nominal energy of 6 MV.

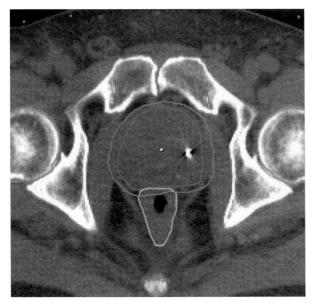

FIGURE 22.2-1. Simulation computed tomography scan at midgland with one of the markers visible in the left lobe. Highlighted are the clinical target volume (*red*), planning target volume (*magenta*), rectum (*green*), and femoral heads (*pink*). (To view a color version of this image, please refer to the CD-ROM.)

Our treatment planning goals are to deliver the prescription dose (70 Gy) to a minimum of 99% and 95% of the CTV and PTV, respectively. Over the years, different dose limits have been tried with the various normal structures. With the small margins used to design the PTV, the only important normal structure found to be crucial during plan optimization is the rectum. The femoral heads and bladder dose limits have all been consistently met. The dose limits for the normal tissues used at our center are summarized in Table 22.2-1. Although no limits are placed on the penile bulb in the optimization process, the doses are recorded. Typically, ≤ 50% of the penile bulb receives 40 Gy. In this patient, four limits were used for the rectum to optimize the rectal doses: (1) maximum dose < 74 Gy, (2) < 20% of the rectum receiving 50 Gy, (3) < 50% receiving 25 Gy, and (4) < 90% receiving 12 Gy.

The dose was prescribed to the 95% isodose line. Figure 22.2-2 shows the isodose lines at midgland; the 95% line corresponds to the 250 cGy line. After optimization, 100% of the CTV and 98.8% of the PTV were covered with the prescription dose. The volume of rectum receiving 70 Gy was 6.7 cc (9.4% of the rectal volume), and 20% received 56 Gy. In this patient, 11% of the penile bulb received 40 Gy. Figure 22.2-3 shows two separate three-dimensional

TABLE 22.2-1. Normal Tissue Dose Limits

Structure	Normal Tissue	Dose Limit, Gy
Bladder	≤ 25%	> 60
Rectum	≤ 25%	> 56
	< 10 cc	> 70
Femoral heads	≤ 10%	> 45
	Maximum dose	50 Gy

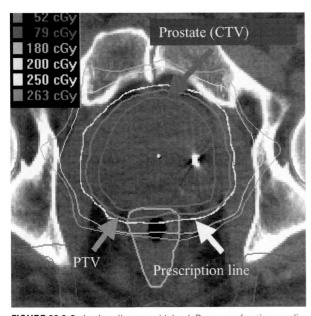

FIGURE 22.2-2. Isodose lines at midgland. Doses per fraction are displayed. The yellow line is the prescription line (250 cGy per fraction). CTV = clinical target volume; PTV = planning target volume. (To view a color version of this image, please refer to the CD-ROM.)

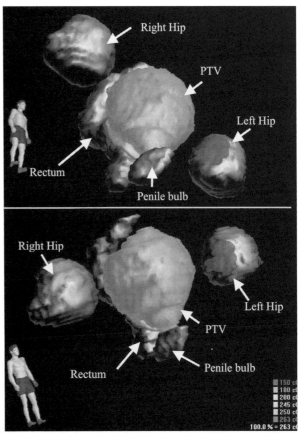

FIGURE 22.2-3. Three-dimensional renderings from two anterior viewpoints demonstrating the rapid dose falloff outside the planning target volume (PTV). (To view a color version of this image, please refer to the CD-ROM.)

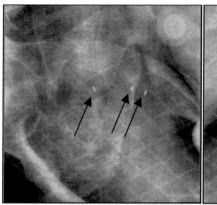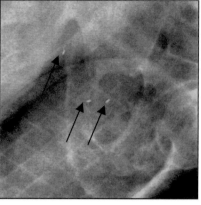

FIGURE 22.2-4. Markers identified on in-room kilovoltage radiographs prior to each treatment.

views of the delivered doses, demonstrating rapid dose falloff along the rectum and penile bulb, minimal dose to the hips, and excellent coverage of the PTV.

Treatment Delivery and Quality Assurance

Treatment was delivered to this patient on a Novalis linear accelerator (BrainLAB AG) equipped with a micromultileaf collimator (M3). The M3 consists of 52 leaves and has variable leaf thicknesses ranging from 3 mm near the isocenter to 5 mm at the periphery.

Prior to the initiation of treatment, careful quality assurance procedures were performed. Films were obtained of each fluence map and compared with those generated by the planning system. Additionally, an ion chamber measurement was performed at a point corresponding to the isocenter using a water-equivalent phantom.

For each treatment, the patient was instructed to keep his bladder somewhat full. He was set up everyday on skin marks. To visualize the intraprostatic markers, two separate kilovoltage radiographs were obtained from two different angles with the patient in the treatment position (Figure 22.2-4). The couch offsets were then generated after identifying the three markers on both radiographs. These offsets were subsequently applied automatically to the couch. The treatment was then delivered with the above-described five-field step-and-shoot IMRT technique. The total beam-on time was 5 minutes. The patient was on the treatment couch for 20 minutes every day.

Clinical Outcome

The patient tolerated treatment well, with only mild urinary frequency, dysuria, and decreased urinary stream occurring during week 3 of treatment, which responded well to oral medications. These symptoms subsided completely within 3 weeks of completing treatment. At 6 weeks following IMRT, his PSA level was 3.7 ng/mL. His follow-up PSA levels at 7 and 13 months were 0.9 ng/mL and 0.6 ng/mL, respectively. As of his last follow-up at 13 months after treatment, he had noted no urinary or rectal symptoms. He did notice a significant decrease in the volume of his ejaculate but no change in the quality of his erections or the quality of his orgasms. The plan is to continue his follow-ups and PSA levels with a 6-month frequency.

Dosimetric[1] and clinical[2–4] results of our hypofractionated IMRT approach have been published. In our most recent report, the outcomes of 100 consecutive patients were analyzed.[4] Sixty-two patients had high-risk disease (T3, PSA > 10, or Gleason Score > 6); the remainder had low-risk disease (T1–2, PSA ≤ 10, or Gleason Score ≤ 6). Fifty-one patients received androgen deprivation therapy (median duration 6 months). At a median follow-up of 43 months, the 4-year actuarial biochemical relapse-free survival of the entire group was 88% (low risk, 100%; high risk, 81%). Treatment was well tolerated, with only one patient developing a late grade 3 rectal toxicity (requiring a cauterization procedure). The 4-year actuarial risk of grade ≥ 2 rectal sequelae for the entire group was 6%.

References

1. Mohan DS, Kupelian PA, Willoughby TR. Short-course intensity-modulated radiotherapy for localized prostate cancer with daily transabdominal ultrasound localization of the prostate gland. Int J Radiat Oncol Biol Phys 2000;46:575–80.

2. Kupelian PA, Willoughby TR. Short-course intensity-modulated radiotherapy for localized prostate cancer. Cancer J Sci Am 2001;7:421–6.

3. Kupelian PA, Reddy CA, Carlson TP, et al. Preliminary observations on biochemical relapse-free survival rates after short-course intensity-modulated radiotherapy (70 Gy at 2.5 Gy per fraction) for localized prostate cancer. Int J Radiat Oncol Biol Phys 2002;53:904–12.

4. Djemil T, Reddy CA, Willoughby TR, et al. Hypofractionated intensity-modulated radiotherapy (70 Gy at 2.5 Gy per fraction) for localized prostate cancer. Int J Radiat Oncol Biol Phys 2003;57:S275.

TARGETED LYMPH NODE IRRADIATION Case Study

STEVEN L. HANCOCK, MD, TODD PAWLICKI, PhD, RAYMOND TAN, MD

Patient History

A 52-year-old male presented with a detectable and rising prostate-specific antigen (PSA) level of 0.11 ng/mL at 18 months following a radical retropubic prostatectomy performed for a stage T2b, Gleason grade 4 + 4 adenocarcinoma of the prostate. His maximum pretreatment PSA was 15.8 ng/mL. The pathology from the prostatectomy demonstrated extensive bilateral glandular involvement, with a cancer volume of 9.9 cc (60% Gleason grade 4 and 20% Gleason grade 5). Although the surgical margins were deemed uninvolved, there was a 2 cm zone of capsular penetration by tumor with focal penetration into the right seminal vesicle. Two right lymph nodes and one left pelvic lymph node were free of tumor.

On presentation, the patient was asymptomatic. Physical examination, including digital rectal examination, was within normal limits. Restaging radionuclide bone scan, magnetic resonance imaging (MRI) of the abdomen and pelvis, and computed tomography (CT) of the chest revealed no evidence of local or distant disease recurrence. Radiation to the prostatic fossa and regional pelvic lymph nodes was advised, combined with neoadjuvant and concurrent androgen blockade. Intensity-modulated radiation therapy (IMRT) was used to target the pelvic lymph nodes as an alternative to conventional whole-pelvis radiation therapy (RT).

Simulation

Because prone positioning has been shown to increase respiratory-induced movement of the prostate,[1] the patient was simulated and treated in the supine position. He was immobilized using a fixed Styrofoam pad extending from the thighs to his feet, with the foot position marked to improve reproducibility (Figure 22.3-1).

A CT reference plane was established through the pubic symphysis and was marked by anterior and lateral tattoo points. On a CT simulator (PQ 5000, Philips Medical Systems, Andover, MA), axial images were obtained at 3 mm intervals from 3 cm superior to the L4–L5 interspace to

3 cm below the ischial tuberosities. Intravenous contrast was not used. At our institution, urethral contrast is routinely used in these patients, unless MRI is available for image fusion, as was the case in this patient.

Target and Tissue Delineation

The clinical target volume (CTV) in this patient consisted of the prostatic fossa, proximal urethra, and pelvic lymph nodes. Because our planning approach involves the delivery of different doses per fraction to these structures, three separate CTVs were contoured: a prostatic fossa CTV (CTV_{fossa}), a pelvic lymph node CTV (CTV_{nodes}), and a proximal urethra CTV ($CTV_{urethra}$).

Fusing of the MRI and planning CT aided in identifying the proximal urethra and nodal regions and in differentiating the prostatic fossa from surgically displaced bladder and rectum. The nodal areas included within the CTV_{nodes} started inferiorly in the lateral perivesicular regions and generally followed the course of the obturator nerves. It included the pelvic sidewall regions between

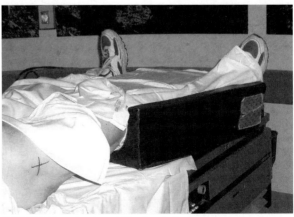

FIGURE 22.3-1. The immobilization device used in this patient consisted of a fixed Styrofoam pad extending from the midthigh to the ankles. This device reduces pelvic rotation. (To view a color version of this image, please refer to the CD-ROM.)

the external iliac vessels anteriorly and the internal iliac vessels posteriorly to their vascular juncture at the common iliac artery. Lymph node regions adjacent to the common iliac vessels and the distal aorta and inferior vena cava were included to the level of the L4–L5 interspace. Nodal regions at risk were identified by reference to a set of MRIs from another patient with disease recurrence after prostatectomy for Gleason grade 5 + 5 disease (Figure 22.3-2). These volumes were in accordance with published atlases of nodal drainage of the prostate.[2]

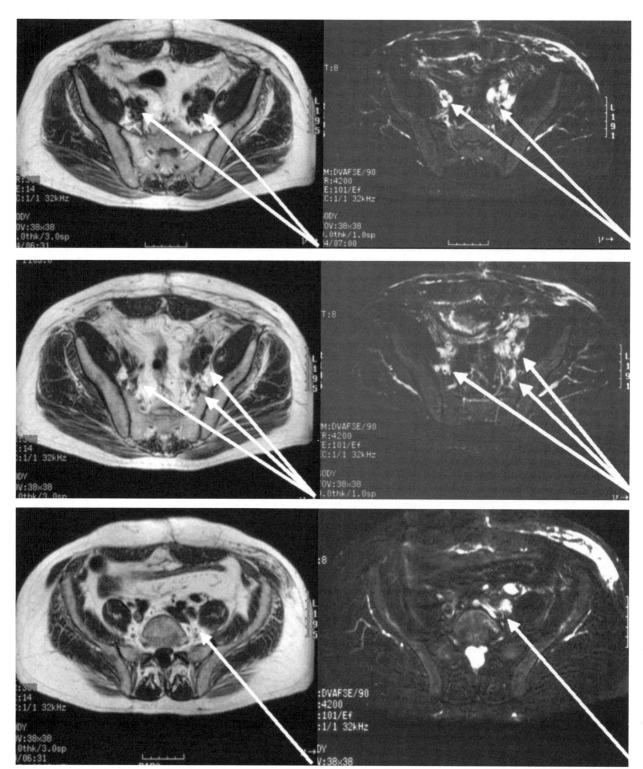

FIGURE 22.3-2. Axial pelvic magnetic resonance images illustrating disease recurrence in the common iliac (*A*), external iliac (*B*), and obturator (*C*) lymph nodes in a patient with prostate cancer following radical prostatectomy.

The CTV$_{urethra}$ included approximately 1.5 cm of proximal urethra distal to the urogenital diaphragm, as identified on MRI (or by the triangular "beak" of contrast on a urethrogram). Occasionally, remnants of the seminal vesicles are apparent on postoperative MRIs and/or CT scans. Unless such structures appear to be infiltrated with tumor, we do not routinely include them within the CTV$_{nodes}$ to limit the volumes of bladder and rectum irradiated to high doses. When treating patients with an intact prostate, the CTV$_{fossa}$ is replaced by the prostate CTV and a separate seminal vesicle CTV with separate dose specification is employed. The CTV$_{nodes}$ and CTV$_{urethra}$ are identical to those specified for postoperative treatment.

Organs at risk were segmented on axial CT slices as avoidance structures and for dose-volume histogram evaluation. The rectum was contoured at the serosa from the anus to the sigmoid flexure. It is often difficult to differentiate small bowel from large bowel on pelvic images obtained without gastrointestinal contrast, and the positions of these structures vary during therapy. Therefore, a single structure was designated as bowel that included the large bowel proximal to the rectum and the pelvic portions of the small bowel with associated portions of mesentery, mesocolon, and interposed pelvic fat. The bladder and femoral head regions were also segmented on the axial image set.

Treatment Planning

The CTV$_{fossa}$ and CTV$_{nodes}$ were expanded, creating planning target volumes (PTVs) (PTV$_{fossa}$ and PTV$_{nodes}$, respectively). The CTV-to-PTV margins for the prostatic fossa were 4 mm in the anterior direction, 2 mm in the posterior direction, and 4 mm in the left, right, superior, and inferior directions. The CTV-to-PTV margin for the pelvic lymph nodes was 3 mm in all dimensions. The PTV contours of the prostatic fossa were further expanded by 2 mm anteriorly and posteriorly and 4 mm in the lateral, inferior, and superior dimensions in the *CORVUS* system for inverse treatment planning (North American Scientific, NOMOS Radiation Oncology Division, Cranberry Township, PA). PTV$_{nodes}$ was similarly expanded by 3 mm in all dimensions to generate the best IMRT plan. The CTV$_{urethra}$ anterior to the urogenital diaphragm was considered a portion of the anterior-inferior margin on the prostatic apex region and intrapelvic, urethrovesicular anastomosis. For this reason, the CTV$_{urethra}$ was not expanded. Thus, the CTV$_{urethra}$ in this case was identical to the PTV$_{urethra}$. The target and normal tissue structures in this patient are shown in Figures 22.3-3 and 22.3-4.

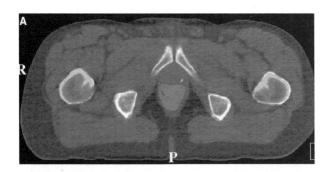

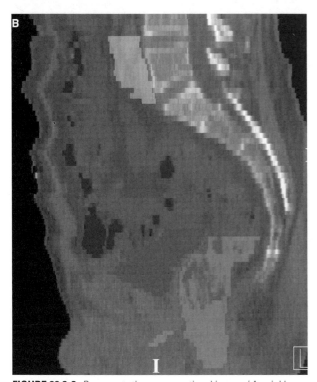

FIGURE 22.3-3. Representative cross-sectional images (*A*, axial lower pelvis; *B*, midsagittal) from the treatment planning computed tomography scan showing the planning target volume (PTV)$_{fossa}$ (*red*), PTV$_{nodes}$ (*yellow*), PTV$_{urethra}$ (*light blue*), rectum (*brown*), bladder (*blue*), bowel (*violet*), left femur (*purple*), and right femur (*pink*). (To view a color version of this image, please refer to the CD-ROM.)

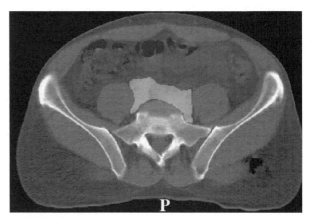

FIGURE 22.3-4. Representative cross-sectional image from the treatment planning computed tomography scan of the upper pelvis showing the planning target volume for the nodes (*yellow*) and bowel (*violet*). (To view a color version of this image, please refer to the CD-ROM.)

When planning IMRT treatment for patients with an intact prostate, similarly modest CTV-to-PTV expansions have been used (typically 4 mm posteriorly and 8 mm in other dimensions) despite concerns regarding organ movement. With more conventional margins of 10 to 15 mm, regions of higher dose frequently surround the CTV structures when using the *CORVUS* planning system. Doses appear to conform better to designated targets when more limited expansions are used. Whether this observation is unique to the *CORVUS* planning system or shared by other planning systems is unclear.

In this patient, the prescribed doses were 60 Gy in 30 fractions (2 Gy/fraction) to the PTV_{fossa}, 50 Gy in 30 fractions (1.67 Gy/fraction) to the PTV_{nodes}, and 42 Gy in 30 fractions (1.4 Gy/fraction) to the $PTV_{urethra}$. *CORVUS* inverse planning software, version 4.0, was used to generate the IMRT plan. Heterogeneity corrections were turned on during both beamlet optimization and final dose calculation. The input planning parameters specified for the targets and OAR in this case are summarized in Tables 22.3-1 and 22.3-2, respectively. The treatment plan in this patient consisted of seven coplanar beams. The beam angles were 0, 51, 103, 154, 206, 257, and 309 degrees. The energy of all seven beams was 15 MV.

Although the normal tissue structures designated above were used in the process of confining high-dose regions to the target structures, creating hypothetical tissue structures, called "tuning structures," has proven to be helpful in generating optimal conformal dose distributions in patients with prostate cancer planned using *CORVUS*. These tuning structures are added for the purpose of minimizing extraneous regions of excess dose outside the target volume(s) and improving dose conformity. Four tuning structures were used in the planning of this case. Two tuning structures were used as targets (similar to those described by Price and colleagues[3]), and the other two were used as normal tissue structures to help confine dose (Figures 22.3-5 and 22.3-6).

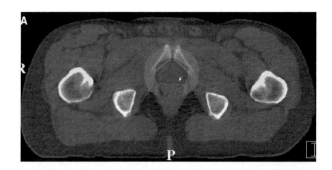

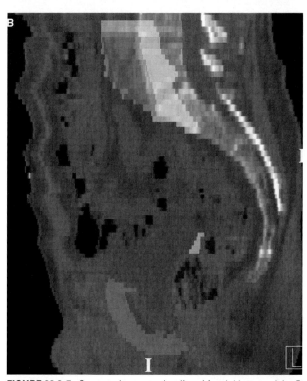

FIGURE 22.3-5. Computed tomography slices (*A*, axial lower pelvis; *B*, midsagittal) illustrating the tuning structure used to optimize the dose distribution conformity and homogeneity. The tuning structure specified as a target in the planning system is shown in blue (surrounding the planning target volume [PTV]$_{fossa}$) and light green (surrounding the PTV$_{nodes}$). The tuning structure specified as normal tissue in the planning system is shown in cyan (near the PTV$_{fossa}$) and yellow (near the PTV$_{nodes}$). (To view a color version of this image, please refer to the CD-ROM.)

TABLE 22.3-1. Input Parameters for the Targets

Structure	Goal Dose, Gy	Volume below Goal, %	Minimum, Gy	Maximum, Gy	Type
PTV$_{fossa}$	60	1	59	65	Homogeneous
PTV$_{nodes}$	50	2	49	55	Homogeneous
PTV$_{urethra}$	42	25	35	60	Basic
Tuning structure (prostatic fossa)	60	20	45	62	Basic
Tuning structure (lymph nodes)	50	20	40	52	Basic

PTV = planning target volume.

TABLE 22.3-2. Input Parameters for the Normal Tissues

Normal Tissue	Limit, Gy	Volume above Limit, %	Minimum, Gy	Maximum, Gy	Type
Bladder	48	5	40	56	Basic
Rectum	48	5	40	56	Basic
Right femoral head	40	3	0	40	Basic
Left femoral head	40	3	0	40	Basic
Bowel	42	2	40	47	Critical
Tuning structure (prostatic fossa)	45	1	42	50	Basic
Tuning structure (lymph nodes)	45	1	42	50	Basic

Note that the critical structure tissue type as specified in the *CORVUS* software adds an extra weighting factor to that structure.

The prescription for this patient's treatment plan specified a minimum peripheral or threshold dose for all target structures. Because IMRT frequently produces more heterogeneous dose distributions in tumor targets than were customary with conventional planning, regions within the designated target structures exceed the threshold dose. The goal in this patient was to achieve minimum doses of 60 and 50 Gy to the CTV_{fossa} and CTV_{nodes}, respectively. An isodose value of 89% was specified. This resulted in 0.13% of the CTV_{fossa} (0.02 cc) receiving < 60 Gy, an absolute minimum dose of 59.3 Gy, and mean and maximum doses of 63.3 Gy and 67.3 Gy, respectively. For the pelvic nodes, 0.92% (2.15 cc) of the CTV_{nodes} received less than the target dose of 50.0 Gy, with an absolute minimum of 47.5 Gy, a maximum dose of 63.7 Gy, and a mean dose of 54.2 Gy. Selected isodose distributions are shown in Figures 22.3-7 and 22.3-8.

The average and maximum target doses currently in use for postoperative RT of the prostatic fossa (generally 63–68 Gy in 30 fractions) are well within the expected tolerance of the rectum and bladder.[4] Therefore, the maximum dose to these structures is less of a concern in the postoperative setting than in patients with an intact prostate. In the present case, the treatment plan resulted in a mean rectal dose of 42.4 Gy and a maximum dose of 65.1 Gy. Because the structure designated as bowel includes portions of the small and large intestine, mesentery, mesocolon, and pelvic fat, it is important to review the isodose distributions on all of the axial images. In this case, the average dose to the bowel volume was 17.6 Gy, with a maximum dose of 57 Gy. A total of 14.5 cc of the bowel received > 50 Gy. Review of the isodose distributions confirmed that the regions exceed-

ing 50 Gy were small, dispersed, and often confined to pelvic fat. Plans in which a significant portion of the bowel receives higher doses are not acceptable.

The amount of dose heterogeneity in the targets and selected normal structures is summarized in Table 22.3-3, and the resultant dose-volume histograms are shown in Figure 22.3-9. The greater amount of dose heterogeneity within CTV_{nodes} is a reflection of the greater total volume of this target (234 cc vs 16 cc for the CTV_{fossa}), its irregular contour, and proximity to the bowel (a critical normal structure, which itself has a large volume and irregular shape). The dose heterogeneity in $CTV_{urethra}$ reflects

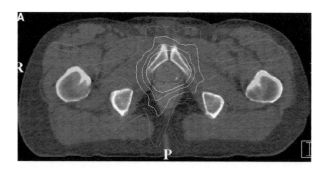

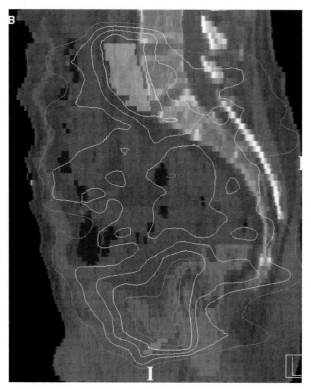

FIGURE 22.3-7. Isodose curves superimposed on an axial lower pelvis slice (*A*) and a midsagittal slice (*B*): 66 Gy (*dark blue*), 60 Gy (*magenta*), 50 Gy (*yellow*), 40 Gy (*green*), 30 Gy (*cyan*), and 20 Gy (*light blue*). The prescribed doses are 60 Gy at 2 Gy/fraction to the planning target volume $(PTV)_{fossa}$ and 50 Gy at 1.67 Gy/fraction to the PTV_{nodes}. Note that the $PTV_{urethra}$ is enclosed by the 40 Gy isodose line at 1.33 Gy/fraction. (To view a color version of this image, please refer to the CD-ROM.)

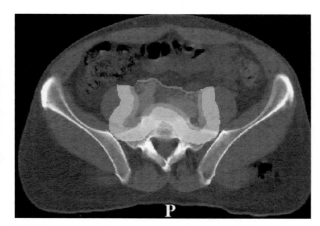

FIGURE 22.3-6. An axial computed tomography slice illustrating the tuning structure used to optimize the dose distribution conformity and homogeneity. The tuning structure specified as a target in the planning system is shown in light green (surrounding the lymph nodes), and the tuning structure specified as normal tissue in the planning system is shown in yellow (near the lymph nodes). (To view a color version of this image, please refer to the CD-ROM.)

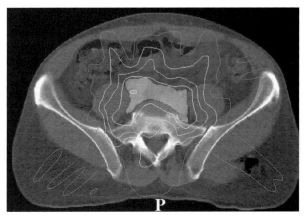

FIGURE 22.3-8. Isodose curves superimposed on an axial slice in the upper pelvis: 50 Gy (*yellow*), 40 Gy (*green*), 30 Gy (*cyan*), and 20 Gy (*light blue*). The prescribed dose to the lymph node planning target volume is 50 Gy at 1.67 Gy/fraction. (To view a color version of this image, please refer to the CD-ROM.)

the decreasing risk of microscopic tumor with increasing distance from the urethrovesicular anastomosis.

Multiple plans with differing numbers of incident beams and differing beam orientations were evaluated prior to selecting the final treatment plan used in this patient. Because of this patient's favorable anatomy, four plans appeared to be potentially acceptable based on similar coverage of the CTV_{fossa} and CTV_{nodes}, with normalization to high isodose levels keeping target dose heterogeneity within in a reasonable range (Table 22.3-4). A treatment plan using seven incident beams was selected owing to lower maximum doses to the bowel and the medial femoral heads.

TABLE 22.3-3. Dose Statistics for Targets and Normal Structures

Structure	Goal Dose, Gy	% of Structure > 105% of Goal	Volume Structure >105% of Goal, cc	% of Structure >110% of Goal	Volume Structure > 110% of Goal, cc	Maximum Dose/ Goal Dose
CTV_{fossa}	> 60	60	9.7	4	0.6	1.11
CTV_{nodes}	> 50	78	183.0	36	85.0	1.27
$CTV_{urethra}$	> 42	88	0.5	69	0.4	1.28
Bowel	< 42	65	85.0	68	57.0	1.36
Rectum	< 48	27	24.0	22	19.0	1.35

CTV = clinical target volume.

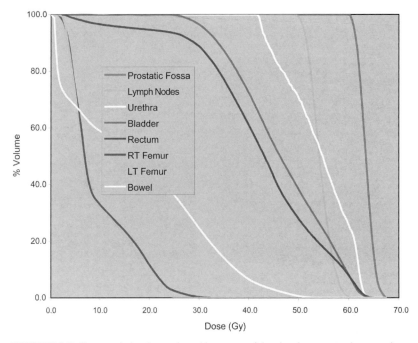

FIGURE 22.3-9. The cumulative dose-volume histograms of the planning target volumes and normal tissues. RT = right; LT = left. (To view a color version of this image, please refer to the CD-ROM.)

TABLE 22.3-4. Comparison of Clinical Target Volume Coverage and Maximum Normal Tissue Doses for the 4 Best Candidate Plans for This Patient's Postoperative Intensity-Modulated Radiation Therapy Treatment

Characteristics	Plan			
	1	2	3	4
No. of beams	7 (equally spaced from 0°)	6	5 (equally spaced from 0°)	5 (equally spaced from 180°)
Isodose normalization, %	89	90	88.7	88.7
CTV$_{fossa}$				
Minimum, Gy	59.33	59.33	59.86	59.53
Maximum, Gy	67.42	66.67	67.64	67.31
Mean, Gy	63.27	63.3	63.63	63.73
CTV$_{nodes}$				
Minimum, Gy	47.53	47.33	45.66	46.0
Maximum, Gy	63.71	64.0	63.92	64.95
Mean, Gy	54.16	55.12	55.63	55.4
Rectum	65.0	64.0	65.0	65.3
Bladder	65.0	65.7	64.6	66.0
Bowel	56.7	59.3	57.8	58.2
Femoral heads	33.4	33.0	41.6	41.3

CTV = clinical target volume.
Although the six-field plan offered slightly less dose heterogeneity in the CTV$_{fossa}$ and CTV$_{nodes}$, the seven-field plan resulted in less dose to the bowel. Likewise, the five equally spaced beams plan offered equivalent coverage and a shorter treatment time. However, doses exceeded 40 Gy to the medial portion of the femoral head and were considered less optimal.

Treatment Delivery and Quality Assurance

The patient was treated on a Varian 21EX dual-energy linear accelerator (Varian Medical Systems, Palo Alto, CA) equipped with a Millennium 120 multileaf collimator (MLC). On Varian accelerators, the maximum treatable field width for IMRT is limited to 14.5 cm owing to the finite length of the MLC leaves and the inability of collimator jaws to move during treatment. The *CORVUS* planning system automatically accounts for these limitations by splitting a field into two smaller fields if the target width exceeds 14.5 cm in the beam's eye view. Consequently, although the treatment plan was generated with seven coplanar beam angles, the actual number of treated fixed fields in this patient was 12.

Prior to treatment, multiple quality assurance (QA) checks are performed using software that was developed in-house. Initially, a monitor unit verification program is run to validate the dose to the isocenter.[5] The leaf sequences generated by *CORVUS* and the treatment depths for each field are used to independently calculate the dose to the isocenter. A separate program is then run to validate the fluence maps.[6] The software reads in the leaf sequences, simulates the motion of the MLC, and calculates the resultant fluence maps. These fluence maps are then quantitatively compared with those generated by the planning system. Our acceptance criteria are that the calculated dose discrepancy at the isocenter must be < 5% and the correlation coefficient for the fluence maps must be > 98%. In this particular case, both acceptance criteria were satisfied. However, in cases that are outside this range, the dose dis-

tribution is cast onto a phantom and is measured using an ion chamber. Once these QA checks are performed, the plan is transferred to our record and verify system (Varis, Varian Medical Systems). The beam parameters (leaf sequences) are then used to generate the individual intensity maps using *Shaper* software (Varian Medical Systems). These intensity maps are visually compared with those produced by *CORVUS* to ensure that no errors occurred during data transfer.

Before the initial treatment, the patient underwent a setup verification step, during which the immobilization system was checked, and orthogonal images of the isocenter were reproduced on simulation films for better visualization of bony landmarks. In addition, outlines of the modulated anatomic region for each beam angle were filmed at the beginning of treatment to ensure the accuracy of the isocenter location. During the active treatment period, portal images of the isocenter were taken weekly or more often if necessary.

Patient Outcome

While on treatment, the patient reported a mild increase in stool frequency and occasional loose stools. He characterized these symptoms as a "minor nuisance" and was managed with alterations in diet (decreased fiber). In addition, he reported occasional episodes of brief, spasmodic rectal discomfort and up to one episode of nocturia without urinary discomfort. Within 3 months after completing treatment, his bowel function normalized. He noted the development of a trace pedal edema that persisted after irradiation. At his most recent follow-up (2 years after therapy), he had no clinical or biochemical evidence of disease recurrence. A recent screening colonoscopy identified no inflammation or abnormalities in the colon or rectum.

Our initial experience using targeted lymph node IMRT in patients with prostate cancer was presented earlier.[7] Twenty-three patients with high-risk prostate cancer (T1c–3N0–1) underwent targeted pelvic lymph node IMRT. Initial treatment delivered 50 Gy over 5 weeks to the prostate, seminal vesicles, and pelvic lymph nodes using seven to nine fixed fields. Subsequently, the prostate and seminal vesicles were treated to a minimum dose of 70 Gy and 50 Gy, respectively, with six to nine fields. Treatment plans and acute toxicities were compared with a cohort of 38 patients treated with a split-course, conventional RT technique (four-field whole-pelvis treatment and a six-field prostate boost). Although the IMRT plans delivered a higher average and maximum dose to the prostate and pelvic nodes, the percent volume of pelvic bowel exposed to doses of > 25 Gy was significantly lower compared with that of conventional plans. Moreover, IMRT patients experienced less ≥ grade 2 acute gastrointestinal (13 vs 60.5%; $p = .001$) and genitourinary (17.4 vs 60.1%; $p = .003$) sequelae than the patients treated with conventional RT.

References

1. Dawson LA, Litzenbeg DW, Brock KK, et al. A comparison of ventilatory prostate movement in four treatment positions. Int J Radiat Oncol Biol Phys 2000;48:319–23.

2. Martinez-Monge R, Fernandes PS, Gupta N, et al. Cross sectional nodal atlas: a tool for the definition of clinical target volumes in three-dimensional radiation therapy planning. Radiology 1999;211:815–28.

3. Price RA, Murphy S, McNeeley SW, et al. A method for increased dose conformity and segment reduction for SMLC delivered IMRT treatment of the prostate. Int J Radiat Oncol Biol Phys 2003;57:843–52.

4. Jackson A, Skwarchuk MW, Zelefsky MJ, et al. Late rectal bleeding after conformal radiotherapy of prostate cancer. II. Volume effects and dose-volume histograms. Int J Radiat Oncol Biol Phys 2001;49:685–98.

5. Xing L, Chen Y, Luxton G, et al. Monitor unit calculation for an intensity modulated photon field by a simple scatter summation algorithm. Phys Med Biol 2000;45:N1–7.

6. Xing L, Li JG. Computer verification of fluence map for intensity modulated radiation therapy. Med Phys 2000;27:2084–92.

7. Hancock SL, Luxton G, Chen Y, et al. Intensity modulated radiotherapy for localized or regional treatment of prostatic cancer: clinical implementation and improvement in acute tolerance [abstract]. Int J Radiat Oncol Biol Phys 2000;48:252.

Chapter 22.4

PROSTASCINT-GUIDED IMRT

CASE STUDY

ASHESH B. JANI, MD, JOHN C. ROESKE, PHD

Patient History

A 68-year-old male presented with a prostate-specific antigen (PSA) level of 12 ng/mL. A digital rectal examination failed to reveal any palpable abnormalities of the prostate. An ultrasound-guided prostate biopsy was performed, and the pathology was consistent with adenocarcinoma, Gleason grade 4 + 3. Bone and computed tomography (CT) scans were negative for metastatic disease. The patient had no significant comorbid conditions and was thus considered to be an excellent candidate for surgery, brachytherapy, or external beam radiation therapy (RT). After weighing the trade-offs between RT and prostatectomy, he elected to undergo surgery.

He underwent a radical retropubic prostatectomy (RRP). During the initial part of this procedure, lymph nodes sampled on both sides of the pelvis and two nodes on the left and one node on the right were free of disease. The urologist then proceeded with a bilateral nerve-sparing RRP. On the pathologic specimen, there were tumor nodules on both sides of the apical portion of the prostate, each < 1 cm in size, and both were Gleason grade 4 + 3 adenocarcinoma. There was no seminal vesicle invasion, but there was extracapsular extension in the midportion of the prostate. The margins were focally positive at the apex on both sides but were negative elsewhere.

The patient recovered well post-RRP; he had no urinary incontinence, no rectal symptoms, and only mild erectile dysfunction. His PSA level was undetectable on the first draw 2 months post-RRP and remained undetectable on periodic follow-ups for approximately 2 years. His PSA then began to increase slowly over a period of a year to a maximum level of 0.43 ng/mL. At that time, he was referred for consideration of salvage RT.

Restaging with CT and bone scans was negative for metastatic disease. As an aid in the radiation decision-making process, a radioimmunoscintigraphy (RIS) scan (ProstaScint, Cytogen Corporation, Princeton, NJ) was performed.[1,2] The RIS scan showed no extrapelvic uptake or suspicious pelvic lymph nodes but did reveal uptake in the prostate fossa (Figure 22.4-1). Based on these results, the patient was offered a course of intensity-modulated radiation therapy (IMRT).

Simulation

Standard bowel preparation instructions were given to the patient, and on the morning of the CT planning scan, he was asked to perform an enema. At the University of Chicago, all patients with prostate cancer (post-RRP or intact prostate) are simulated and treated in the supine position. To immobilize the patient, customized upper and lower alpha cradles (Smithers Medical Products, Hudson, OH) were fabricated. A retrograde urethrogram was performed, and bladder contrast was used. Following the placement of a rectal tube, rectal contrast was injected. Intravenous contrast was used to assist in identifying the pelvic vasculature as part of the treatment planning process (see below).

A planning CT scan was performed in the treatment position using a flat table insert on an AcQSim CT simulator (Philips Medical Systems, Andover, MA). The table insert mimics the Varian Exact Couch (Varian Medical Systems, Palo Alto, CA). Notches located along its edges allow the immobilization devices to be positioned as they would on the treatment table. Using a 3 mm slice thickness, the patient was scanned from the top of the L4 vertebral body to 5 cm below the ischial tuberosities.

Target and Tissue Delineation

On this planning CT scan, the following structures were delineated:

1. *Prostate bed clinical target volume (CTV).* In the pre-CT era, there were standard guidelines for defining a post-RRP treatment volume.[3] In the CT era, these guidelines do not necessarily apply. In this patient, definition of the CTV was done first using all available information except the RIS scan. Specifically, information about the size or shape of the prostate and seminal vesicles from

the preoperative CT scan, digital rectal examination, operative and pathology reports, discussions with the urologist about areas of concern, and surgical clips visible on the planning CT scan were all used. Given that the RIS information was not used, this CTV was termed $CTV_{pre-RIS}$.

2. *Rectum.* This structure was defined according to the Radiation Therapy Oncology Group (RTOG) guidelines and was contoured from the bottom of the ischial tuberosities to the sigmoid flexure.

3. *Bladder.* As per RTOG guidelines, this structure was contoured in its entirety.

4. *Pelvic arteries.* The abdominal aorta, right and left common iliac arteries, and right and left internal and external iliac arteries were entered for later RIS and CT correlation (see below).

5. *Pelvic lymph nodes.* These are identified only in patients with uptake in the pelvic lymph nodes on RIS or who otherwise have high-risk features for nodal involvement; this structure was not outlined on our patient.

For the majority of patients treated at other institutions, treatment planning is initiated immediately after simulation. However, at the University of Chicago, we have developed and reported techniques to use the RIS scan to guide

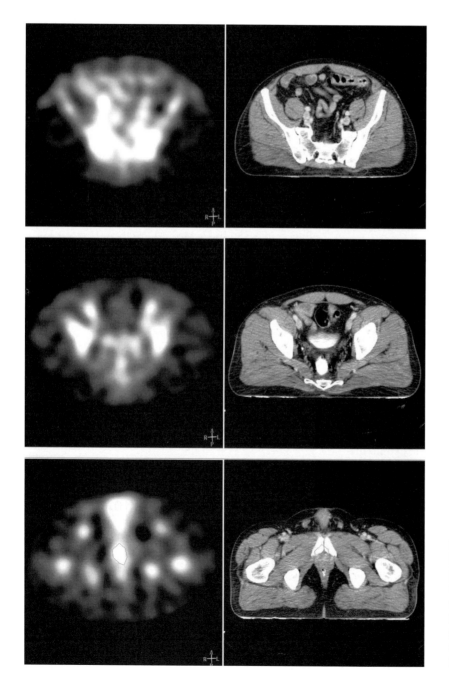

FIGURE 22.4-1. ^{111}In-labeled antibody scans (ProstaScint) and corresponding planning computed tomography images. The orange contour on the lower image set represents the clinical target volume from the radioimmunoscintigraphy scan. This contour was subsequently edited to exclude the uptake in the symphysis. (To view a color version of this image, please refer to the CD-ROM.)

the target definition.[4] This process involves image-correlating the RIS and CT scans, which allows the ability to project the region of interest on the RIS scan directly into the planning CT scan to assist in modifying the $CTV_{pre-RIS}$.

The RIS scan was obtained in the nuclear medicine department prior to the planning CT scan. The RIS scan has two components: a ^{99m}Tc-labeled red blood cell (RBC) single-photon emission computed tomography (SPECT) scan and a simultaneously acquired ^{111}In-capromab pendetide monoclonal antibody (7E11.C5) RIS-SPECT scan. After all image sets were obtained, the major arterial vessels (abdominal aorta, bifurcation into the common iliac arteries, subsequent bifurcation into the internal and external iliac arteries and the inferior extent to which these arteries could be visualized) were outlined on both the planning CT and RBC-SPECT scans. Using the AcQSim image fusion software (Philips Medical Systems), these two image sets were aligned by minimizing the distance between the outlines of the vessel surfaces. The resultant coordinate transformation was used to reslice the RIS-SPECT scans along the same planes as the planning CT images.

The nuclear medicine physician independently reads the RIS scan and outlines a CTV, termed CTV_{RIS}. The CTV_{RIS} is then projected onto the planning CT (by virtue of the fact that the RIS and RBC scans are simultaneously acquired and the vessel registration between the SPECT and planning CT has been done). The radiation oncologist then uses the CTV_{RIS} on the planning CT directly to modify the $CTV_{pre-RIS}$. Although the resulting modifications are case dependent, the general goal is to define a $CTV_{post-RIS}$ as the union of the $CTV_{pre-RIS}$ and CTV_{RIS}. However, in some cases, there can be significant artifact owing to uptake in the bladder or symphysis bone marrow (as occurred in the case of our patient), requiring "pruning" of the CTV_{RIS}. That is, inclusion of areas in the CTV_{RIS} that were not already included in $CTV_{pre-RIS}$ must be done while using the CT to avoid including uptake areas that are not consistent with potential sites of disease. In this patient, the $CTV_{post-RIS}$ was more generous in the region of the prostatic apex, consistent with the location of the positive margin.

Treatment Planning

A planning target volume (PTV) was then generated by expanding the $CTV_{post-RIS}$ uniformly by 1 cm. The planning process is subtly different in the post-RRP setting than for the intact prostate because the anatomy is different. Although the post-RRP PTV is smaller in absolute volume (compared with an intact prostate), it overlaps with the bladder and rectum to an extent similar to that in the intact prostate setting. Fortunately, the prescription dose is lower in the post-RRP setting. A consensus conference recommended the use of ≥ 64 Gy[5]; the prescription dose in this patient was 66 Gy in 2 Gy daily fractions. Figure 22.4-2 depicts the PTV, bladder, and rectal contours.

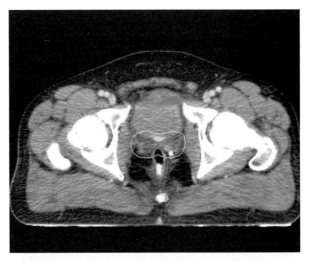

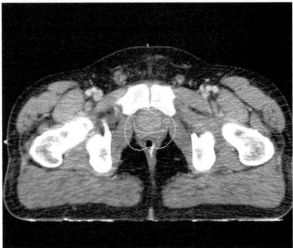

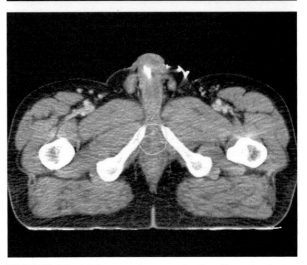

FIGURE 22.4-2. Axial computed tomography slices illustrating the target and normal tissues contoured in this patient. Highlighted are the bladder (*red*), rectum (*magenta*), planning target volume (*light blue*), clinical target volume (CTV) before the radioimmunoscintigraphy (RIS) scan (*yellow*), and CTV following the RIS scan (*orange*). The overlap of the CTV before and after the RIS scan is shown in blue. (To view a color version of this image, please refer to the CD-ROM.)

Treatment planning was performed using the *CORVUS* inverse planning system, version 5.0 (North American Scientific, NOMOS Radiation Oncology Division, Cranberry Township, PA). *CORVUS* uses a simulated annealing algorithm to determine the optimal fluence pattern based on a set of dose constraints entered by the treatment planner. The input parameters used in this patient are summarized in Table 22.4-1. Note that in this patient, we included an artificial organ called a "sparing" structure. This structure is contoured by the dosimetrists at the time of planning and is used to improve the dose conformity to the PTV.

The discrete annealer was selected for optimization. When the discrete annealer is combined with a homogeneous target type, the system attempts to minimize the dose heterogeneity within the PTV. A beamlet size of 0.5×0.5 cm was used with eight discrete intensity levels (30–100% in steps of 10%). Heterogeneity corrections were not used. The optimized IMRT plan consisted of seven coplanar beams using 6 MV photons. The following beam angles were selected: 240, 280, 320, 0, 40, 80, and 120 degrees (where 0° is an anterior beam). Note that none of these beams enter posteriorly to produce a sharper dose gradient through the rectum.

Because the *CORVUS* treatment planning system does not allow any voxel to be defined as more than one structure, the dose distribution was then exported to our three-dimensional treatment planning system (PlanUNC, University of North Carolina, Chapel Hill, NC). True dose-volume histograms were then generated for the bladder and rectum and were subsequently used in plan evaluation.

Our plan acceptance criteria in postprostatectomy IMRT patients are as follows. A minimum of 95% of the PTV (PTV$_{95}$) must receive 100% of the prescription dose (66 Gy). In general, we are able to encompass 95 to 98% of the PTV with the prescription dose. Our acceptance criteria for the rectum are the volume receiving 68 Gy or higher (V_{68}) should be < 15% and the volume receiving 40 Gy or higher (V_{40}) should be < 50%. The criteria for the bladder are the volume receiving 66 Gy or higher (V_{66}) should be < 20% and the V_{40} should be < 50%. These constraints were easily met in this patient. If, however, the rectal dose is prohibitively high, the PTV can be modified in stages. PTV$_1$ is the PTV described above but is prescribed to 50 Gy in 2 Gy daily fractions. A second PTV (PTV$_2$) consists of CTV$_{post-RIS}$ uniformly expanded by 1 cm, with the exception being a 0.6 cm expansion posteriorly. PTV$_2$ is prescribed to 16 Gy in 2 Gy daily fractions.

The normal tissue dose constraints used in this patient evolved from constraints used in the intact prostate setting and those reported in the post-RRP setting. Prior RTOG studies have suggested that the rectal volume receiving 70 Gy or higher (V_{70}) should be < 25%. Because the prescription dose is lower in the post-RRP setting, this constraint can almost always be met, so more stringent criteria have been adopted. One prior study (in the post-RRP IMRT era) lowered the rectum V_{70} constraint to the V_{68} and the 25% to 15%; also, the bladder constraints were lowered to the V_{65} < 15%.[6] These are what we strive for at our institution, with the exception that the bladder constraint is tailored to our prescription dose (ie, V_{66}) and is slightly more liberal (ie, V_{66} < 20%) because the expanded CTV$_{post-RIS}$ often overlaps with the bladder neck. The other constraints (ie, bladder and rectum V_{40} < 50%) serve to reduce the integral dose to these organs.

Figure 22.4-3 illustrates the optimized dose distributions for the IMRT treatment plan in this patient. Figure 22.4-4 illustrates the resultant dose-volume histograms for the PTV and normal structures.

Treatment Delivery and Quality Assurance

The IMRT treatment plan was delivered using a 2100EX Varian linear accelerator (Varian Medical Systems) equipped with a 120 multileaf collimator. The fields were treated sequentially in a clockwise direction starting at 240°. The treatment was delivered in approximately 5 minutes. Weekly portal images were routinely obtained and evaluated using bony anatomy. Transabdominal ultrasonography for patient positioning is not used routinely at our institution for post-RRP patients.

Careful quality assurance was performed prior to the first treatment. A monitor unit verification calculation (*RadCalc*, Version 4.3, Lifeline Software, Inc., Tyler, TX) was used to verify the dose delivered to the isocenter. Previous investigations from our institution have demonstrated that the average discrepancy for patients with prostate cancer between *RadCalc* and *CORVUS* is +1.6%, with a 1.1% SD.[7] Disparities outside this range are checked and resolved prior to treatment. In this particular patient, a +1.0% dose discrepancy between *RadCalc* and *CORVUS* was noted at the isocenter.

TABLE 22.4-1. Input Parameters

Target Name	Type	Goal, Gy	Volume below Goal, %	Minimum, Gy	Maximum, Gy
PTV	Homogenous	66.0	2	63.0	70.0

Sensitive Structure Name	Type	Limit, Gy	Volume above Limit, %	Minimum, Gy	Maximum, Gy
Tissue	Basic	34.0	26	0.0	63.0
Rectum	Basic	24.3	40	5.6	63.0
Bladder	Basic	7.4	44	3.0	63.0
Sparing structure	Basic	47.6	47	34.9	63.0

PTV = planning target volume.

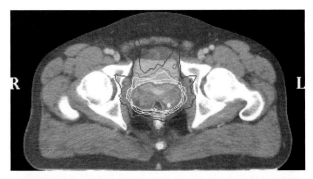

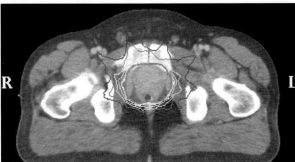

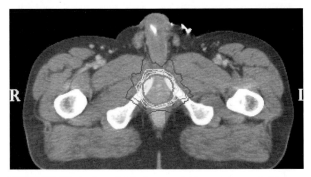

FIGURE 22.4-3. Isodose distributions overlaid on axial computed tomography images. Highlighted are the planning target volume (*dark green*), rectum (*light green*), and bladder (*light blue*). (To view a color version of this image, please refer to the CD-ROM.)

In addition, phantom plans are routinely generated using the fluence maps for individual patients. Our phantom consists of a 20 cm stack of solid water slabs. The isocenter is located at a depth of 10 cm from the anterior surface. The phantom was scanned and irradiated with a 0.1 cm³ ion chamber (PTW, Nuclear Associates, Hicksville, NY) at the isocenter. On average, the discrepancy between *CORVUS* and ion chamber measurements for patients with prostate cancer is −1.2%.

Clinical Outcome

During treatment, the patient developed mild diarrhea requiring the use of nonprescription Imodium (loperamide). Additionally, the patient had mild urinary symptoms not requiring pharmacologic intervention. He experienced no significant fatigue or skin toxicity. At his 1-month follow-up, all acute urinary and rectal side effects had resolved. Over the subsequent 9 months, his PSA level showed a slow trend downward and reached an undetectable level; it remained so when seen at the last follow-up.

Preliminary clinical results have been reported documenting a small biochemical survival advantage to the use of the RIS-CT correlation technique in the post-RRP setting when compared with a retrospective comparison group.[6] Of 107 post-RRP patients reviewed, 53 patients (49.5%) underwent an RIS study. Of these, 40 underwent the RIS-CT correlation described above. The 3-year biochemical failure-free survival rate was higher in patients who underwent an RIS study (80.7% vs 75.5%) owing to the higher biochemical failure-free survival rate in the patients who underwent an RIS-CT correlation (84.5%); the survival rate in patients in whom a RIS was obtained but no RIS-CT correlation was done was similar to that of patients who did not undergo a RIS scan (71.6% vs 75.5%). On multivariate

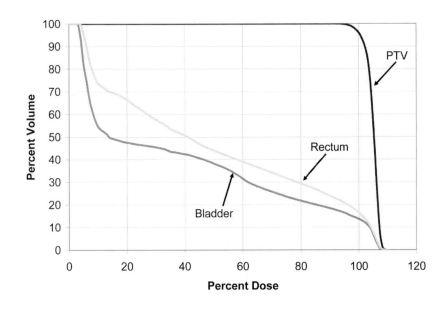

FIGURE 22.4-4. Dose-volume histograms of the planning target volume (PTV), bladder, and rectum; the prescription dose is 66 Gy.

analysis controlling for pretreatment factors, surgical staging factors, and treatment factors, only RIS-CT correlation reached statistical significance. Furthermore, although patients who had an RIS study had slightly higher acute rectal toxicity, no differences in acute urinary toxicity were observed. In addition, no differences in chronic toxicity were seen between the various groups, suggesting that IMRT to the larger CTV$_{post-RIS}$ is tolerable.

References

1. Sodee DB, Malguria N, Faulhaber P, et al. Multicenter ProstaScint imaging findings in 2154 patients with prostate cancer. The ProstaScint Imaging Centers. Urology 2000;56:988–93.

2. Jani AB, Blend MJ, Hamilton R, et al. The influence of radioimmunoscintigraphy on post-prostatectomy radiotherapy treatment decision-making. J Nucl Med 2004;45:571–8.

3. Pilepich MV, Prasad SC, Perez CA. Computed tomography in definitive radiotherapy of prostatic carcinoma, part 2: definition of target volume. Int J Radiat Oncol Biol Phys 1982;8:235–9.

4. Jani AB, Spelbring D, Hamilton R, et al. Impact of radioimmunoscintigraphy on definition of clinical target volume for radiotherapy after prostatectomy. J Nucl Med 2004;45:238–46.

5. Cox JD, Gallagher MJ, Hammond EH, et al. Consensus statements on radiation therapy of prostate cancer: guidelines for prostate re-biopsy after radiation and for radiation therapy with rising prostate-specific antigen levels after radical prostatectomy. J Clin Oncol 1999;17:1155–63.

6. Jani AB, Blend MJ, Hamilton R, et al. Radioimmunoscintigraphy for post-prostatectomy radiotherapy: analysis of toxicity and biochemical control. J Nucl Med 2004; 45: 1315-22.

7. Haslam JJ, Bonta DV, Lujan AE, et al. Comparison of dose calculated by an intensity modulated radiotherapy treatment planning system and an independent monitor unit verification program. J Appl Clin Med Phys 2003;4:224–30.

INTRAPROSTATIC BOOST

EMERGING TECHNOLOGY

MARIA T. GUERRERO URBANO, FRCR, MRCPI, CATHARINE CLARK, PhD, MIPEM, CHRIS M. NUTTING, MD, MRCP, FRCR, ECMO, DAVID P. DEARNALEY, MD, MRCP, FRCR

Patient History

A 56-year-old male presented with a 1-year history of erectile dysfunction and obstructive urinary symptoms. Clinical examination revealed an indurated prostate bilaterally. A prostate-specific antigen (PSA) level was obtained and was noted to be 6.2 ng/mL. The patient subsequently underwent transrectal ultrasound-guided prostatic biopsies. The pathology was consistent with adenocarcinoma, with a Gleason grade of 3 + 4, comprising approximately 80% of the biopsied tissue.

Pelvic magnetic resonance imaging (MRI) revealed a low signal intensity within the peripheral zone on the left extending through the prostatic capsule and no seminal vesicle involvement (Figure 22.5-1). Enlarged lymph nodes were noted in both obturator fossae and the left external and right common iliac regions. The remainder of the metastatic workup, including laboratory studies, bone scan, and computed tomography (CT) of the abdomen, was negative. The patient was thus staged as cT3N1M0.

Initially, the patient was treated with hormonal therapy and was subsequently enrolled in a phase I dose-escalation intensity-modulated radiation therapy (IMRT) protocol with treatment delivered to the prostate and pelvic nodes (see below). However, this patient is presented here to illustrate an intraprostatic boost technique developed at the Royal Marsden Hospital in patients with prostate cancer.[1] This approach involves the delivery of 85 Gy to an intraprostatic nodule with simultaneous treatment of the prostate and the base of the seminal vesicles to 74 Gy.

Simulation

At simulation, the patient was placed in the supine position with a foot and ankle rest and his arms on his chest. The pelvis was screened using a Varian Acuity simulator (Varian Medical Systems, Palo Alto, CA), and one anterior and two lateral tattoos were placed. The patient was then positioned on a Lightspeed CT scanner (GE Healthcare, Waukesha, WI). Using the previously marked tattoos, the patient was aligned to the CT lasers. A noncontrast planning CT scan was obtained extending from the diaphragm to the perineum with 5 mm slices.

Target and Tissue Delineation

All targets and normal tissues were delineated on axial slices of the planning CT scan (Figure 22.5-2). Two gross tumor volumes (GTVs) were contoured: GTV$_1$ consisted of the prostate gland, extraprostatic extension of disease, and the base of the seminal vesicles. GTV$_2$ consisted of the intraprostatic nodule identified on MRI.

The organs at risk (OAR) delineated in this case included the rectum, bladder, and femoral heads. The rectum was contoured from the anus to the rectosigmoid junction.

GTV$_1$ was expanded by 10 mm, creating a planning target volume (PTV$_1$), except posteriorly, where an 8 mm margin was used. No margin was added to GTV$_2$ to generate a PTV$_2$. A clinical target volume was not delineated in this patient.

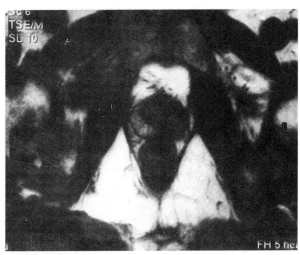

FIGURE 22.5-1. Diagnostic magnetic resonance (MR) image showing an intraprostatic tumor nodule.

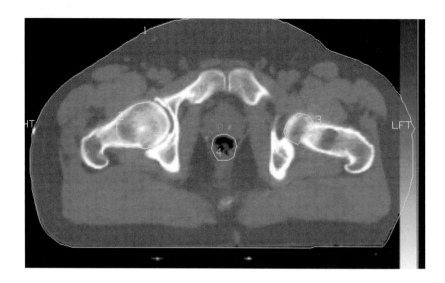

FIGURE 22.5-2. Axial computed tomography slice showing gross tumor volume (GTV)₁ (*red*), GTV₂ (*pink*), rectum (*blue*), and femoral heads (*blue*). (To view a color version of this image, please refer to the CD-ROM.)

Target and OAR volumes are summarized in Table 22.5-1. Of note, the GTV-to-PTV expansion resulted in the inclusion of considerable portions of the rectum and bladder within the PTV₁. A total of 9.1 and 28.7 cc of the rectum and bladder were included within PTV₁, respectively. These volumes represented 10% and 19.3% of the rectum and bladder, respectively.

TABLE 22.5-1. Target and Organ at Risk Volumes

Targets and OARs	Volume, cc
GTV₁	34.9
GTV₂ (IP boost)	1.3
PTV₁	148.8
PTV₂	1.3
Rectum	90.8
Bladder	148.8

GTV = gross tumor volume; IP = intraprostatic; PTV = planning target volume.

Treatment Planning

IMRT treatment plans were generated using *Cadplan* inverse planning software, version 6.3.5 (Varian Medical Systems). Five coplanar equispaced beams were selected (gantry angles: posterior, 180°; left anterior oblique, 36°; right anterior oblique, 324°; left posterior oblique, 108°; and right posterior oblique, 252°) (Figure 22.5-3). All beams had an energy of 6 MV.

The total prescribed doses in this case were 74 Gy in 37 daily fractions to PTV₁ and 85 Gy in 37 daily fractions to PTV₂. The plan was designed to cover 50% of each PTV with the respective prescription dose. Subsequently, 95% of each PTV was encompassed by the 95% isodose.

The PTV₁ and PTV₂ goals and achieved doses and OAR dose and volume goals are summarized in Table 22.5-2 and Table 22.5-3. The resultant dose-volume histograms for

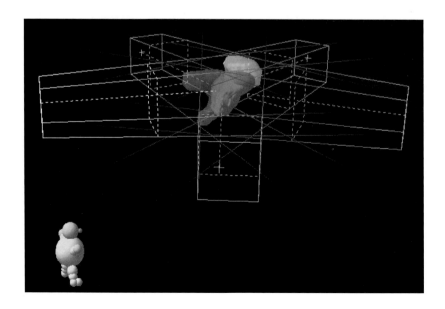

FIGURE 22.5-3. Three-dimensional reconstruction of planning target volume 1, bladder, and rectum with the beam arrangement. (To view a color version of this image, please refer to the CD-ROM.)

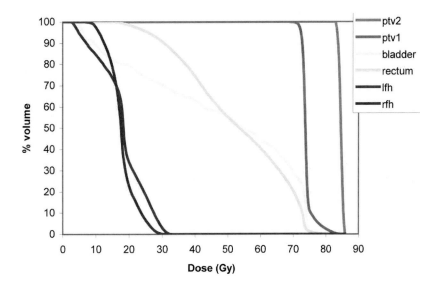

FIGURE 22.5-4. Dose-volume histograms of the individual planning target volumes (PTVs) and organs at risk. lfh = left femoral head; rfh = right femoral head.

the target volumes and OAR are shown in Figure 22.5-4. Isodose distributions on axial, coronal, and sagittal CT slices are illustrated in Figure 22.5-5.

In this patient, there was a large volume of rectum and bladder within PTV₁. This made achieving the target volumes and OAR goals more difficult. Nevertheless, the IMRT plan achieved excellent coverage of the targets while sparing the rectum and bladder.

Treatment Delivery and Quality Assurance

As noted above, this patient was not treated using the intraprostatic boost approach. However, the intraprostatic boost plan was designed to be delivered in the dynamic mode on a Varian 2100CD linear accelerator (Varian Medical Systems).

TABLE 22.5-2. Organs at Risk Dose Goals and Achieved Volumes

Rectum			Bladder			Femoral Heads		
Dose Constraint, Gy	Maximum Volume, %	Volume Achieved, %	Dose Constraint, Gy	Maximum Volume, %	Volume Achieved, %	Dose Constraint, Gy	Maximum Volume, %	Volume Achieved, %
50	60	55.0	50	50	55.3	50	50	0
60	50	40.5	60	25	44.3			
65	30	31.5	70	5	27.9			
70	15	20.0						
75	0	1.3						

TABLE 22.5-3. Planning Target Volume 1 and 2 Objective and Achieved Doses

PTV₁ (Prostate)			PTV₂ (Intraprostatic Boost)		
Volume Constraint, %	Dose Required, % (Gy)	Dose Achieved, Gy	Volume Constraint, %	Dose Required, % (Gy)	Dose Achieved, Gy
99	90 (66.6)	71.2	99	90 (76.5)	83.0
95	95 (70.3)	72.3	95	95 (80.8)	83.4
50	100 (74.0)	73.7	50	100 (85.0)	84.7
5	105 (77.7)	77.7	5	105 (89.3)	85.8

PTV = planning target volume.

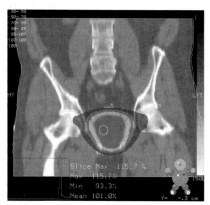
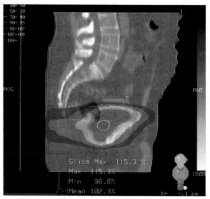
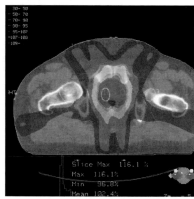

FIGURE 22.5-5. Coronal, sagittal, and axial computed tomography (CT) slices showing the 95% isodose (*red*) of planning target volume (PTV$_2$) (85 Gy) and the 95% isodose (*magenta*) of the PTV$_1$ (74 Gy). (To view a color version of this image, please refer to the CD-ROM.)

Our quality assurance (QA) protocol in prostate IMRT is as follows. Intensity maps for each field are produced and verified using Kodak verification film (Eastman Kodak, Rochester, NY). These films are irradiated at the isocenter in a solid water phantom at a depth of 10 cm. The dose through the plane of the film is calculated on *Cadplan*. The measured isodoses are then compared with the calculated isodoses. Intensity maps of the posterior and right posterior oblique fields in this hypothetical case are shown in Figure 22.5-6.

Next, the total dose delivered from the whole treatment plan and that from each field are verified. The patient plan is exported to a phantom, and suitable points are chosen for dose measurements with an ionization chamber. The percentage deviation in measured dose is then calculated for each individual field and for the whole plan. Tolerance is set at ±3%. This tolerance was achieved in the hypothetical prostate plan.

Isocenter verification is performed daily during the first week of treatment and once weekly thereafter provided that setup is within tolerance (5 mm). The method employed uses anterior (gantry 0°) and lateral (gantry 270°) electronic portal images, which are then compared with CT-derived digitally reconstructed radiographs.

Clinical Outcome

The patient was started on hormonal therapy (goserelin 3.6 mg monthly implants). After six months, his PSA was 0.8 ng/mL. In addition, a restaging pelvic MRI demonstrated a marked reduction in the lymphadenopathy and less extraprostatic extension.

In light of his good response, the patient was enrolled in a phase I dose-escalation IMRT protocol. Treatment was delivered to the prostate and pelvic lymph nodes (70 Gy to the prostate, 55 Gy to the pelvic nodes, and a nodal boost of the four involved nodes to 60 Gy all in 35 daily fractions). He tolerated treatment well, with grade 2 acute urologic and bowel toxicity. He fully recovered, and at 10 weeks postcompletion of IMRT, he had neither bowel nor urinary toxicity. At 9 months follow-up, the patient is alive and well. His most recent PSA was 0.22 ng/mL.

We and others explored the feasibility of simultaneously boosting intraprostatic nodules in patients with prostate cancer undergoing IMRT.[1–3] In our previous study, prostate maps were produced from six radical prostatectomy specimens from men with clinically staged T1c–2a prostate cancer.[1] After sectioning the specimens in the axial plane, large whole-mount sections were produced, and a histopathologist outlined areas of tumor. The largest tumor nodule

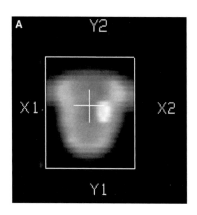
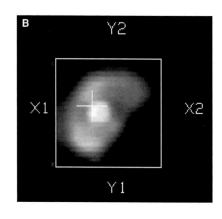

FIGURE 22.5-6. Measured intensity maps of the (*A*) posterior and (*B*) right posterior oblique fields.

was designated as the dominant intraprostatic tumor nodule (DIPTN) and smaller nodules as non-DIPTNs. The positions of the tumor nodules were transferred onto corresponding CT images. Each map was paired with a CT scan from a patient with a similar prostate size and stage. The nodules were delineated on the CT scan relative to the apex, base, urethra, and lateral gland borders.

The PTV was defined as the prostate gland with a margin of 10 mm in all directions. Normal tissues included the bladder, rectum, and prostatic urethra. Three IMRT plans were generated and compared. The first was designed to irradiate the PTV to 70 Gy in 2 Gy fractions. The second irradiated the PTV to 70 Gy but escalated the dose to all of the intraprostatic nodules to 90 Gy. A third plan was produced to escalate only the DIPTN to 90 Gy.

If all nodules were boosted, the mean dose to the nodules increased from 69.8 to 89.1 Gy ($p = .003$). Compared with the standard (nonboost) plan, the IMRT boost plan was associated with an increase in mean tumor control probability, ranging from 8.7 to 31.2% depending on the α/β ratio selected ($p < .001$). Of note, a 3% increase in the mean normal tissue complication probability (NTCP) for the rectum was noted ($p < .01$). If only the DIPTN were boosted, the tumor control probability was increased by 6.4 to 27.5% ($p < .003$) and the rectal NTCP was increased by 1.8% ($p < .01$). Unsurprisingly, the highest rectal NTCP was seen in patients with nodules in the posterior peripheral zone close to the anterior rectal wall.

These results suggest that it may be possible to deliver an intraprostatic boost in prostate cancer with IMRT, improving tumor control while sparing surrounding normal tissues. Clearly, although promising, many issues arise with the clinical implementation of such an approach. First, the prostate gland itself would require reproducible and accurate positioning. This could be achieved by immobilization with a rectal balloon catheter[4] or by image-guided patient setup using implanted gold seeds within the prostate[5] or a radiopaque urethral catheter.[6]

Moreover, advances in multimodality imaging are required to accurately define the position of the intraprostatic nodules. As shown in the above case study, MRI is an appealing approach. Contrast-enhanced dynamic MRI[7] and magnetic resonance spectroscopy[2,3] have the potential to produce the required definition. Nonetheless, a careful clinical trial design will be essential to confirm whether improvements in dose distributions can be translated into clinically relevant end points.

References

1. Nutting CM, Corbishley CM, Sanchez-Nieto B, et al. Potential improvements in the therapeutic ratio of prostate cancer irradiation: dose escalation of pathologically identified tumour nodules using intensity modulated radiotherapy. Br J Radiol 2002;75:151–61.

2. Pickett B, Vigneault E, Kurhanewicz J, et al. Static field intensity modulation to treat a dominant intra-prostatic lesion to 90 Gy compared to seven field 3-dimensional radiotherapy. Int J Radiat Oncol Biol Phys 1999;44:921–9.

3. Xia P, Pickett B, Vigneault E, et al. Forward or inversely planned segmental multileaf collimator IMRT and sequential tomotherapy to treat multiple dominant intraprostatic lesions of prostate cancer to 90 Gy. Int J Radiat Oncol Biol Phys 2001;51:244–54.

4. Gerstner N, Wachter S, Dorner D, et al. Significance of a rectal balloon as internal immobilization device in conformal radiotherapy of prostatic carcinoma. Strahlenther Onkol 1999;175:232–8.

5. Crook JM, Raymond Y, Salhani D, et al. Prostate motion during standard radiotherapy as assessed by fiducial markers. Radiother Oncol 1995;37:35–42.

6. Bergstrom P, Lofroth PO, Widmark A, et al. High precision conformal radiotherapy (HPCRT) of prostate cancer—a new technique for exact positioning of the prostate at the time of treatment. Int J Radiat Oncol Biol Phys 1998;42:305–11.

7. Padhani AR. Dynamic-contrast enhanced MRI studies in human tumours. Br J Radiol 1999;72:427–31.

REPAIR OF UNACCEPTABLE IMPLANTS EMERGING TECHNOLOGY

X. ALLEN LI, PHD, JIAN Z. WANG, PHD

For clinically localized prostate carcinomas, increasing data demonstrate that ultrasound-guided permanent brachytherapy, three-dimensional conformal radiation therapy (3DCRT), and intensity-modulated radiation therapy (IMRT) offer an equal likelihood of cure.[1–6] However, unacceptable dose distributions (eg, cold spots) in permanent implants are often observed owing to many anatomic and/or technical reasons, including pubic arch interference, prostate volume or shape change, image artifacts, seed placement errors, and seed migration. Clinical results and biologic modeling have shown that cold spots can significantly impact treatment outcome.[7–9] To repair unacceptable brachytherapy dose distributions, we investigated the use of IMRT.

Combining dose distributions from different modalities is challenging because each modality generates a unique spatial and temporal dose distribution. Compared with external beam radiation therapy (EBRT), brachytherapy possesses many different dosimetric and radiobiologic features. The most important one is the dose-rate effect. The low-dose rate (LDR) associated with prostate brachytherapy may alter the microradioenvironment of clonogenic tumor cells. These changes may lead to differences in radioresponse, oxygenation (ie, hypoxia effect), nutrient supply, and tumor kinetics. Such dose-rate differences have a significant impact on the repair of sublethal cell damage. Although brachytherapy provides a high degree of dose conformity, it also presents significant dose and dose-rate heterogeneity. This heterogeneity may also alter the response of tumor and normal tissues. Another distinct feature of brachytherapy versus EBRT is the overall treatment time. Owing to the intrinsic LDR, an ^{125}I implant takes more than 200 days to deliver the prescribed dose. This treatment duration is approximately four to five times longer than that of EBRT. Tumor cell repopulation may become an important issue and should be taken into account in any combined treatment.

Because of these differences, dosimetric treatment planning by simply adding the absolute doses from EBRT and brachytherapy, without considering the differences in biologic effects, is misleading. A biologic consideration of the above features is needed to determine the required IMRT dose distribution that compensates for an unacceptable implant dose distribution. Given that brachytherapy dose distributions are highly nonuniform, these biologic considerations need to be carried out on a voxel-by-voxel (small tissue region) basis, that is, in three-dimensional space. In this chapter, various radiobiologic models are used to calculate the required IMRT dose distributions in cases in which an implant has resulted in an unacceptable dose distribution. A commercial IMRT planning system is then used to generate the IMRT plans that deliver these required dose distributions.

Linear-Quadratic Survival Formula

Clonogenic cell death is an often used measure of the biologic effectiveness of a radiation treatment. The standard linear-quadratic (LQ) model has been widely used to describe cell killing and to model clinical data. The general LQ formalism, extended to include the effects of dose rate, repair of sublethal damage, and clonogen repopulation, is used to calculate cell-surviving fraction S, that is,[10–12]

$$S = e^{-(\alpha D + \beta G D^2 - \gamma T)} \tag{1}$$

where D is the total dose delivered within the effective treatment time T, α and β characterize intrinsic radiosensitivity, G is the protraction factor that accounts for sublethal damage repair, and γ is the repopulation rate ($\gamma = ln(2)/T_d$, where T_d is the effective clonogen doubling time). It has been reported that prostate cancer has a median potential doubling time of 42 days based on in situ measurements.[13,14] This median doubling time was used in this calculation.

For EBRT, the fraction delivery time is usually much shorter than the repair half-time T_r of the tumor cells. Thus, $G = 1/n$ and $D = nd$, where n is the number of dose fractions and d is the dose per fraction. However, for certain IMRT delivery techniques (eg, step-and-shoot IMRT), the fraction dose delivery time T_f may be comparable to or even longer than the repair half-time ($T_r = 16$ minutes for prostate tumor cells, as reported by Wang and colleagues[15]). In this situation, the dose protraction factor G should be given by[11]

$$G = \frac{2}{n\mu T_f}\left[1 - \frac{1}{\mu T_f}(1 - e^{-\mu T_f})\right] \quad (2)$$

where μ is the repair rate of tumor cells [$\mu = ln(2)/T_r$]. As described in a previous article,[16] the impact of the prolonged IMRT fraction delivery time on cell-surviving fraction S can be approximately calculated by considering the multisegment IMRT dose-time delivery pattern as a single segment with a constant dose rate over the entire delivery time. The overall treatment time or duration for EBRT can be simply calculated as the number of treatment fractions multiplied by 1.4 (7 days per week divided by 5 fractions per week).

For permanent brachytherapy, the dose delivered within the treatment time is given by

$$D = \frac{R_0}{\lambda}(1 - e^{-\lambda T}) \quad (3)$$

and the dose protraction factor G and the effective treatment time T are[10,11,15]

$$G = \frac{2R_0^2}{D^2(\mu-\lambda)}\left[\frac{1}{2\lambda}(1-e^{-2\lambda T}) - \frac{1}{\mu+\lambda}(1-e^{-(\mu+\lambda)T})\right], \quad (4)$$

$$T \approx -\frac{1}{\lambda}\ln\left(\frac{\gamma}{\alpha R_0}\right) \quad (5)$$

Here R_0 is the initial dose rate, D_0 is the prescribed dose ($R_0 = D_0 \cdot \lambda$), and λ is the decay constant for the implanted isotopes ($\lambda = ln(2)/T_s$, where T_s is the half-time of the isotope). T_s is equal to 60.2 days for the ^{125}I implant and 17 days for the ^{103}Pd implant.

Recently, the α/β ratio used in the LQ model for prostate cancer has become a highly debated topic.[15,17–21] By taking into account the effect of tumor cell repopulation, Wang and colleagues analyzed several reported clinical studies,[15,20] including those of the EBRT dose escalation data[22,23] and the high-dose rate (HDR) brachytherapy data.[19] A self-consistent set of LQ parameters ($\alpha = 0.14$–0.15 Gy^{-1}, $\alpha/\beta = 3.1$ Gy, and a repair time $T_r = 16$ minutes) was obtained in their analysis.[15,20] The number of clonogens was estimated to be 10^6 to 10^7 depending on the patient risk levels.[15] These results provide reasonable estimates for

radiosensitivity and the number of clonogens for human prostate cancer.[24,25] Radiobiologic modeling with these parameters offers a consistent interpretation for most clinical data currently available for prostate cancer, including data with different RT modalities: EBRT, permanent implant, HDR brachytherapy, and their combinations.[9,15,20] Except where explicitly noted otherwise, Wang and colleagues' LQ parameters[15,20] were used in this chapter to estimate prostate tumor cell survival as a function of dose and dose rate. To assess the dependence of the results on the parameters, calculations were also performed using several other sets of LQ parameters, including $\alpha/\beta = 1.5$ Gy as reported by Brenner and Hall,[17] Fowler and colleagues,[18] and Brenner and colleagues[19] and $\alpha/\beta = 10$ Gy as normally assumed for tumor.[26,27]

Equivalent Uniform Dose and Voxel Equivalent Dose

Because IMRT and brachytherapy generate very different spatial and temporal dose distributions, biologic effectiveness indicators are necessary to compare and combine these two modalities. The concept of equivalent uniform dose (EUD), which provides a useful means to assess the overall biologic effectiveness of a treatment plan, is selected as one of the indicators. The EUD concept was originally proposed for EBRT by Niemierko.[28] It is defined as the biologically equivalent dose that, if given uniformly, would lead to the same biologic effect as a given nonuniform dose distribution. The EUD can be applied to both tumor and normal tissue[29–31] and has recently been applied to LDR brachytherapy.[9] It has been shown that the EUD is a convenient quantity with which to compare the overall effectiveness of different EBRT and brachytherapy dosing schemes.[9]

However, the EUD is a spatially averaged quantity. The spatial (voxel by voxel based) information (eg, the hot and cold spots produced by the unacceptable implants in question) cannot be easily identified by using EUD. To address the effects of cold spots in a treatment plan, it is useful to have a voxel-by-voxel indicator of treatment effectiveness. For this purpose, we introduce a new concept, the voxel equivalent dose (VED), to characterize the biologic effectiveness of a treatment plan on a voxel-by-voxel basis. The VED is defined as the equivalent dose to a voxel, if delivered using a specified reference modality (such as the conventional EBRT in 2 Gy fractions), that will produce the same level of cell killing in that voxel as that of the time-dose delivery method of interest (such as brachytherapy or IMRT). In this formulation, the VED in the ith voxel can be given by

$$VED_i = \frac{-\log(S_i)}{\alpha + \beta d - 1.4\gamma/d} \quad (6)$$

where S_i is the surviving fraction of the ith voxel. The VED is conceptually similar to the biologically equivalent dose (BED), conventionally defined as $-ln(S)/\alpha$ (see Dale and colleagues[32]). Both quantities provide a quantitative method to investigate the potential impact of dose rate and fraction size on treatment outcome. However, the VED concept is a clinically more useful indicator of changes in treatment effectiveness than BED. This is because VED gives an absolute indication of the dose required to achieve a desired level of cell killing, whereas BED gives only an indication of relative treatment effectiveness. The numeric value of the VED is clinically relevant and relates to clinicians' experience. For a given voxel, the spatial and temporal pattern of radiation delivery should be very nearly the same throughout the entire voxel. A typical voxel size can be a cube of $0.5 \times 0.5 \times 0.5$ cm. Throughout this section, the numeric values of both the EUD and VED are expressed as an EBRT dose of 2 Gy per fraction.

Required Dose from IMRT

For an unsatisfactory implant, the surviving fraction in each voxel is calculated based on the dose distribution from postimplant computed tomography (CT) using equations 1 to 5. Equation 6 is used to calculate the VED value for each voxel. Then a three-dimensional VED distribution delivered by the unsatisfactory implant can be obtained. For a voxel within a cold spot, the required VED to compensate for the underdosing can be obtained by subtracting the VED value delivered by the implant from the desired EUD. Repeating this process for all voxels in all cold spots, the required three-dimensional VED distribution that would repair the unacceptable implant can be reconstructed. Because the VED values are expressed as the EBRT dose, the calculated three-dimensional VED distribution can be used directly as the prescription for IMRT planning.

It has been shown from clinical outcome data that a 145 Gy ^{125}I implant is biologically equivalent to 70 Gy of EBRT in 2 Gy fractions (ie, EUD = 70 Gy for these two treatments).[9,15,18] Based on this clinical finding, the required IMRT doses for various unacceptable implant dose levels are tabulated in Table 22.6-1. For practical purposes, all of the values in the table are converted back to the physical doses in Gray for both the implant and IMRT. The doses for IMRT are to be delivered in 2 Gy daily fractions. Data for two target EUD values of 70 and 80 Gy calculated using three sets of LQ parameters are included in the table. According to Table 22.6-1 (Wang and colleagues' para-

TABLE 22.6-1. Intensity-Modulated Radiation Therapy Doses Required to Compensate for Various Unacceptable Implant Dose Levels

Implant plus IMRT with EUD of 70 Gy				Implant plus IMRT with EUD of 80 Gy			
^{125}I + IMRT		^{103}Pd + IMRT		^{125}I + IMRT		^{103}Pd + IMRT	
^{125}I	IMRT	^{103}Pd	IMRT	^{125}I	IMRT	^{103}Pd	IMRT
Wang et al's parameters[15,20]*							
40	60	40	51	50	64	40	61
60	49	60	38	80	48	60	48
80	38	80	25	100	36	80	35
100	26	90	19	120	24	100	22
120	14	100	12	140	12	120	9
Brenner et al's parameters[17,19]†							
40	52	40	51	50	58	40	61
60	43	60	39	80	43	60	49
80	33	80	27	100	33	80	37
100	23	90	21	120	23	100	24
120	13	100	14	140	13	120	10
Generic parameters‡							
40	48	40	40	50	51	40	50
60	33	60	23	80	26	60	33
80	10	80	6	100	10	80	16
100	0§	90	0	120	0	100	0
120	0	100	0	140	0	120	0

EUD = equivalent uniform dose; IMRT = intensity-modulated radiation therapy.
*$\alpha = 0.14$ Gy^{-1}, $\alpha/\beta = 3.1$ Gy, $T_r = 16$ minutes, and $T_d = 42$ days.[14,15,20]
†$\alpha = 0.04$ Gy^{-1}, $\alpha/\beta = 1.5$ Gy, $T_r = 1.9$ hours, and with repopulation effect ignored.[17–19]
‡$\alpha = 0.3$Gy^{-1}, $\alpha/\beta = 10$ Gy, $T_r = 1$ hour as normally suggested for tumor, and $T_d = 42$ days.[14,26,27]
§No intensity-modulated radiation therapy dose is required.
All dose values are physical doses expressed in Gray. The doses for intensity-modulated radiation therapy are to be delivered in 2 Gy daily fractions. Data for two target equivalent uniform dose values of 70 and 80 Gy calculated using three sets of linear-quadratic parameters are included.

meters), for example, an underdosing of 45 Gy by an ^{125}I implant with a prescription of 145 Gy (EUD = 70 Gy) can be compensated by an IMRT dose of 26 (13 × 2.0) Gy.

Table 22.6-1 shows the calculational results with different LQ parameter sets. The LQ parameters obtained by Brenner and colleagues,[17,19] Fowler and colleagues,[18] and Wang and colleagues[15,20] were based on clinical data. The difference in the calculated IMRT doses between these two parameter sets is not significant, as illustrated in Table 22.6-1 (Wang and colleagues' and Brenner and colleagues' parameters). This demonstrates that, compared with tumor control probability, EUD or VED is less sensitive to LQ parameters and more reliable in evaluating and comparing different treatment plans. The differences between the IMRT doses in Table 22.6-1 (Wang and colleagues' and Brenner and colleagues' parameters) are mainly because the clonogenic cell repopulation was ignored in the data analysis by Brenner and colleagues[17,19] and Fowler and colleagues.[18] The results calculated with the generic LQ parameters (Table 22.6-1 [generic parameters]) are quite different from Wang and colleagues' and Brenner and colleagues' parameters, presented in Table 22.6-1, and are somewhat unrealistic. For example, no IMRT dose is required for a brachytherapy dose of 100 Gy based on the calculation with the generic parameters. This is inconsistent with clinical findings.

IMRT Planning

In principle, the IMRT plans that deliver the required three-dimensional dose distributions to compensate for an unacceptable implant can be designed using an inverse planning system. However, planning can be challenging, and several issues need to be considered. Generally speaking, the required IMRT dose distributions are highly nonuniform because of highly inhomogeneous dose distributions produced by brachytherapy. Another important issue is the sparing of critical structures (eg, urethra and rectum). High doses may already have been delivered to these organs from the implant. Different IMRT planning strategies may have to be employed to optimally achieve the desired dose distributions. For example, if underdosing is mainly in the

apex-anterior region (eg, owing to pubic arch interference), the fixed-gantry IMRT approach is preferred because of its low integral dose and simplicity. If underdosing is mainly in the anterior-lateral peripheral region (eg, owing to sonogram artifacts for a large prostate gland), rotational IMRT is advantageous because of its superior sparing of urethra and rectum. Because of the highly nonuniform dose distributions and/or small treatment volumes, the planned IMRT delivery needs to be guided by real-time imaging (eg, ultrasonography). The IMRT plans presented below were generated using a commercial planning system (ERGO^{++} Planning System, 3Dline USA, Inc., Reston, VA) with the application of a micromultileaf collimator (MLC).

Sample IMRT Plan

A sample IMRT plan was designed to repair an unacceptable permanent prostate implant. The implant was produced using ^{125}I seeds, and a prescribed dose of 145 Gy was intended to cover the entire prostate. Dosimetric evaluation on the postimplant CT indicated that only 70% of the prostate volume was covered by 90% of the prescribed dose. The IMRT plan was designed to add dose to the under-dosed regions using a series of rotational 6 MV photon beams with a micro-MLC. The required IMRT dose was delivered over 20 fractions (2 Gy/fraction) to the anterior-lateral regions of the prostate.

The dose distributions overlaid on an axial CT image of the implant alone, IMRT alone, and a combined approach are shown in Figure 22.6-1. The prostate, urethra, and rectum are shaded in red, blue, and yellow, respectively. The isodose lines displayed from inside to outside are 100% and 30% of 145 Gy of the ^{125}I implant (VED of 70 Gy); 100%, 90%, and 80% of the 2 Gy fraction dose for the IMRT; and 150%, 100%, and 70% of the 70 Gy VED for the combined modalities. As observed in Figure 22.6-1A, the prostate was encompassed by the 30% isodose line from the original implant. The IMRT compensates in the underdosed regions while sparing the urethra and the rectum, as seen from Figure 22.6-1B. It is clear from Figure 22.6-1C that the prostate is covered by 100% of the desired dose (VED of 70 Gy) by the combined dose distribution.

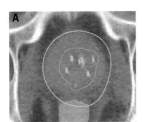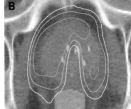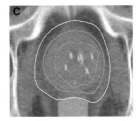

FIGURE 22.6-1. Dose distributions of (*A*) the original prostate permanent implant alone; (*B*) intensity-modulated radiation therapy (IMRT) alone; and (*C*) the combined brachytherapy and IMRT on an axial computed tomography (CT) image. The prostate, urethra, and rectum are shaded by red, blue, and yellow colors, respectively. The isodose lines displayed from inside to outside are (*A*) 100% and 30% of 145 Gy of the ^{125}I implant (voxel equivalent dose [VED] of 70 Gy); (*B*) 100%, 90%, and 80% of the 2 Gy fraction dose for the IMRT alone; and (*C*) 150%, 100%, and 70% of the 70 Gy VED for the combined brachytherapy and IMRT. (To view a color version of this image, please refer to the CD-ROM.)

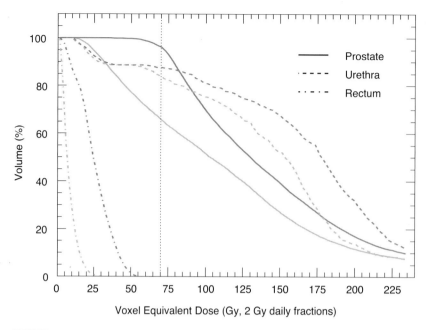

FIGURE 22.6-2. Voxel equivalent dose (VED)-based dose-volume histograms of the prostate, urethra, and rectum for brachytherapy alone (*blue curves*) and combined brachytherapy with intensity-modulated radiation therapy (*red curves*). The desired VED of 70 Gy, which is equivalent to 145 Gy of the ^{125}I implant, is indicated by a vertical dotted line. (To view a color version of this image, please refer to the CD-ROM.)

Figure 22.6-2 shows VED-based dose-volume histograms of the prostate, urethra, and rectum for the implant alone (blue curves) and the combined plans (red curves). Coverage of the prostate by the prescribed dose (70 Gy VED) is increased from 65% with the implant alone to 96% with the combined approach. The rectal dose, which is < 50 Gy VED, is acceptable.

Conclusions

The data presented here indicate that it is dosimetrically and biologically feasible to use IMRT to repair an unacceptable prostate permanent implant. Successful implementation of this technology requires careful consideration of the various biologic, dosimetric, and treatment delivery issues. The methodology for the use of VED or EUD to combine brachytherapy with IMRT can be applied to the combination of other radiation therapy modalities.

Acknowledgments

We would like to thank Pradip Amin, MD, Lijun Ma, PhD, Matt Earl, PhD, and David Shepard, PhD, of the University of Maryland for their valuable input in this work.

References

1. D'Amico AV, Whittington R, Malkowicz SB, et al. Biochemical outcome after radical prostatectomy, external beam radiation therapy, or interstitial radiation therapy for clinically localized prostate cancer. JAMA 1998;280:969–74.

2. Fuks Z, Leibel SA, Wallner KE, et al. The effect of local control on metastatic carcinoma of the prostate: long term results in patients treated with I-125. Int J Radiat Oncol Biol Phys 1991;21:537–47.

3. Kuban DA, El-Mahdi AM, Schellhammer PF. I-125 interstitial implantation for prostate cancer. What have we learned 10 years later? Cancer 1989;63:2415–20.

4. Koprowski CD, Berkenstock KG, Borofski AM, et al. External beam irradiation versus 125 iodine implant in the definitive treatment of prostate carcinoma. Int J Radiat Oncol Biol Phys 1991;21:955–60.

5. Blasko JC, Grimm PD, Ragde H. Brachytherapy and organ preservation in the management of carcinoma of the prostate. Semin Radiat Oncol 1993;3:240–9.

6. Blasko JC, Walker K, Grimm PD, et al. Prostate specific antigen based disease control following ultrasound guided [125]iodine implantation for stage T1/T2 prostatic carcinoma. J Urol 1995;154:1096–9.

7. Stock RG, Stone NN, Tabert A, et al. A dose-response study for I-125 prostate implants. Int J Radiat Oncol Biol Phys 1998;41:101–8.

8. Tome WA, Fowler JF. On cold spots in tumor subvolumes. Med Phys 2002;29:1590–8.

9. Wang JZ, Li XA. Evaluation of external beam radiotherapy and brachytherapy for localized prostate cancer using equivalent uniform dose. Med Phys 2003;30:34–40.

10. Thames HD. An incomplete-repair model for survival after fractionated and continuous irradiations. Int J Radiat Biol 1985;47:319–39.

11. Dale RG. The application of the linear-quadratic dose-effect equation to fractionated and protracted radiotherapy. Br J Radiol 1985;58:515–28.

12. Dale RG. Radiobiological assessment of permanent implants using tumor repopulation factors in linear-quadratic model. Br J Radiol 1989;62:241–4.

13. Haustermans KMG, Hofland I, Poppel HV, et al. Cell kinetic measurements in prostate cancer. Int J Radiat Oncol Biol Phys 1997;37:1067–70.

14. Haustermans K, Fowler JF. A comment on proliferation rates in human prostate cancer [letter]. Int J Radiat Oncol Biol Phys 2000;48:303.

15. Wang JZ, Guerrero M, Li XA. How low is the α/β ratio for prostate cancer? Int J Radiat Oncol Biol Phys 2003;55:194–203.

16. Wang JZ, Li XA, D'Souza WD, et al. Impact of prolonged dose-delivery time on tumor control: a note of caution for IMRT. Int J Radiat Oncol Biol Phys 2003;57:543–52.

17. Brenner DJ, Hall EJ. Fractionation and protraction for radiotherapy of prostate carcinoma. Int J Radiat Oncol Biol Phys 1999;43:1095–101.

18. Fowler J, Chappell R, Ritter M. Is α/β for prostate cancer really low? Int J Radiat Oncol Biol Phys 2001;50:1021–31.

19. Brenner DJ, Martinez AA, Edmundson GK, et al. Direct evidence that prostate tumors show high sensitivity to fractionation (low α/β ratio), similar to late-responding normal tissue. Int J Radiat Oncol Biol Phys 2002;52:6–13.

20. Wang JZ, Li XA, Yu CX, et al. The low α/β ratio for prostate cancer: what does the clinical outcome of HDR brachytherapy tell us? Int J Radiat Oncol Biol Phys 2003;57:1101–8.

21. Kal HB, Van Gellekom MPR. How low is the α/β ratio for prostate cancer? Int J Radiat Oncol Biol Phys 2003;57:1116–21.

22. Levegrün S, Jackson A, Zelefsky MJ, et al. Fitting tumor control probability models to biopsy outcome after three-dimensional conformal radiation therapy of prostate cancer: pitfalls in deducing radiobiologic parameters for tumors from clinical data. Int J Radiat Oncol Biol Phys 2001;51:1064–80.

23. Levegrün S, Jackson A, Zelefsky MJ, et al. Risk group dependence of dose-reponse for biopsy outcome after three-dimensional conformal radiation therapy of prostate cancer. Radiother Oncol 2002;63:11–26.

24. King CR, Mayo CS. Is the prostate α/β ratio of 1.5 from Brenner and Hall a modeling artifact [letter]? Int J Radiat Oncol Biol Phys 2000;47:536–8.

25. Wyatt RM, Beddoe AH, Dale RG. The effects of delays in radiotherapy treatment on tumor control. Phys Med Biol 2003;48:139–55.

26. Thames HD, Bentzen SM, Turesson I, et al. Time-dose factors in radiotherapy: a review of the human data. Radiother Oncol 1990;19:219–35.

27. Brenner DJ, Hall EJ. Conditions for the equivalence of continuous to pulsed low dose rate brachytherapy. Int J Radiat Oncol Biol Phys 1991;20:181–90.

28. Niemierko A. Reporting and analyzing dose distribution: a concept of equivalent uniform dose. Med Phys 1997;24:103–10.

29. Niemierko A. A generalized concept of equivalent uniform dose (EUD) [abstract]. Med Phys 1999;26:1100.

30. Wu Q, Mohan R, Niemierko A, et al. Optimization of intensity-modulated radiotherapy plans based on the equivalent uniform dose. Int J Radiat Oncol Biol Phys 2002;52:224–35.

31. Li AX, Wang JZ, Stewart RD, et al. Dose escalation in permanent brachytherapy for prostate cancer: dosimetric and biological considerations. Phys Med Biol 2003;48:2753–65.

32. Dale RG, Coles IP, Deehan C, et al. Calculation of integrated biological response in brachytherapy. Int J Radiat Oncol Biol Phys 1997;38:633–42.

Chapter 23

GYNECOLOGIC CANCER

OVERVIEW

LOREN K. MELL, MD, JOHN C. ROESKE, PHD, NEIL MEHTA, MD, ARNO J. MUNDT, MD

Radiation therapy (RT) has a long history in the treatment of gynecologic malignancies. In fact, the first gynecology patient received RT over a century ago.[1] In the following years, RT soon became commonplace in the treatment of a wide variety of gynecologic tumors, delivered with external beam and/or intracavitary brachytherapy approaches.[2–4]

Although effective, RT has a number of limitations in these patients. First, conventional techniques result in the treatment of large volumes of normal tissues, exposing patients to numerous treatment-related toxicities, primarily related to the gastrointestinal tract, including diarrhea and malabsorption of vitamins, lactose, and bile acids.[5,6] Genitourinary problems may also develop.[6,7] Given that much of the total-body bone marrow reserve is located within the pelvic bones, hematologic toxicity may also occur, particularly in women receiving chemotherapy during or following RT.[8,9] Unsurprisingly, treatment toxicities are even more prevalent when comprehensive fields are treated owing to the inclusion of even greater volumes of normal tissues.[10,11]

Concerns regarding treatment toxicities also limit the dose administered in gynecology patients. Although conventional doses result in high control rates in most patients, selected patients remain at increased risk of recurrence and may benefit from higher doses, for example, women with lymph node involvement.[12] Current techniques, however, allow the delivery of only modest dose increases.

Finally, the cornerstone of treatment for cervical cancer, brachytherapy, is not always feasible, particularly in elderly patients or in women with unfavorable vaginal geometry. In such cases, only modest additional doses are possible with external beam techniques.[13] Even when brachytherapy is possible, coverage of bulky tumors can be inadequate. Unsurprisingly, tumor control rates in these patients are often poor.

To overcome such limitations, attention is turning to intensity-modulated radiation therapy (IMRT).[14] Unlike conventional approaches, IMRT conforms the prescription dose to the shape of the target tissues in three dimensions, thereby sparing the normal surrounding tissues. Sparing of normal tissues may reduce the risk of toxicity in patients receiving conventional doses and provide a means to safely deliver higher doses in select patients. IMRT may even one day provide an alternative to (or replacement for) brachytherapy in gynecology patients.

This chapter examines the application of IMRT in gynecology patients, highlighting its benefits, risks, and challenges. Preclinical and clinical gynecologic IMRT studies are reviewed, and future directions are discussed.

IMRT Process: Issues and Challenges
Patient Selection

Debate exists over which gynecology patients should receive IMRT.[14] A simpler question is which patients should not receive it. IMRT often requires longer planning and treatment times. A patient in significant pain who is unable to tolerate prolonged treatment sessions is thus a poor candidate. Similarly, uncooperative patients should instead receive more conventional approaches. The additional time required also renders women requiring urgent treatment poor candidates, for example, cervical cancer patients with significant bleeding. One could initiate conventional therapy in these women, switching to IMRT once the plan is complete, provided that this transition is accomplished quickly. One of the few groups of patients unable to receive IMRT is the morbidly obese, owing to the inability to capture their entire external contour on the planning computed tomography (CT) scan.[15]

Of patients able to undergo IMRT, which ones should receive it? In theory, IMRT can be used in place of all external beam approaches performed in gynecology (pelvic, extended field, abdominopelvic, and pelvic-inguinal irradiation). In fact, as is reviewed later, favorable dosimetric results have been reported using IMRT planning in all of these settings.[16–24] However, outcome data remain limited almost exclusively to women receiving pelvic irradiation.[25–30] Some feel that not all patients undergoing pelvic irradiation should receive IMRT, restricting its use to the postoperative setting, citing concerns over organ motion.[14] Others have questioned the benefit of IMRT in obese patients.[18] Our clinical experience to date, however, has not supported these concerns, suggesting that IMRT is appropriate in most women undergoing pelvic irradiation. Future studies will determine its role in patients undergoing more comprehensive fields.

A more controversial role for IMRT is as an alternative to (or replacement for) brachytherapy.[31,32] As is discussed, several groups are examining its role in this setting.[29,30,33,34] However, no outcome data are available to date. Its use in place of brachytherapy should thus be considered experimental.

The same holds true for dose escalation using IMRT. Preclinical and preliminary outcome data have been promising, particularly using the simultaneous integrated boost (SIB) technique.[29,30,35,36] However, such approaches remain experimental and are best performed under the auspices of a controlled clinical trial.

An evolving role for IMRT is as a means of treatment of recurrent tumors within a prior irradiated field.[14] Although this is being done at a number of centers, no studies have been published to date evaluating its efficacy and toxicity. IMRT in the treatment of recurrent tumors is discussed further in Chapter 27, "Metastatic and Recurrent Tumors: Overview."

Simulation and Immobilization

Patients being treated with gynecologic IMRT must undergo a planning CT scan, preferably with thin slices (3–5 mm). Care is taken to encompass the entire volume of interest and the external patient contour. One should scan the entire volume of all normal tissues; otherwise, interpretation of dose-volume histograms (DVHs) may be difficult. The scan parameters selected in a particular patient depend on the volume of treatment. In patients undergoing pelvic irradiation, we scan from the L3 vertebral body to 5 cm below the ischial tuberosities.[15,16] A summary of scan parameters and other simulation details in selected gynecologic IMRT reports is shown in Table 23-1.

The optimal patient positioning in gynecologic IMRT remains unclear. As seen in Table 23-1, most favor the supine position, owing to ease of reproducibility and better patient tolerance.[16,19,21–23] However, recent data suggest that prone positioning may augment small bowel sparing in these patients.[17] Although prone positioning is often used with extended field irradiation, supine positioning is preferable in those treated with abdominopelvic[22,23] and pelvic-inguinal[24] irradiation, allowing the latter to be placed in the frog-leg position.

Considerable attention must be given to patient immobilization. In light of the rapid dose gradients inherent in

TABLE 23-1. Simulation Details: Gynecologic Intensity-Modulated Radiation Therapy Studies

Study	Positioning	Immobilization Approach	Planning CT Scan Parameters	Contrast	Vaginal Marker
Pelvic RT					
Adli et al [17]	Supine/prone*	NS	NS	Oral, IV, rectal	Yes
Ahamad et al [18]	NS	NS	NS	NS	NS
Chen et al [19]	Supine†	NS	NS	NS	NS
Heron et al [20]	Prone (belly board)	NS	NS	Oral	Yes
Roeske et al [16]	Supine	Upper and lower body alpha cradles	L3–5 cm below ischial tuberosities (3 mm slices)	Oral, rectal, IV, bladder	Yes
Schefter et al [30]	Prone	Customized body mold	T12 femoral lesser trochanters (3 mm slices)	Bladder‡	NS
Extended field RT					
Chen et al [19]	Supine†	NS	NS	NS	NS
Portelance et al [21]	Supine	NS	T2 ischial tuberosities (slice thickness NS)	NS	NS
Mutic et al [35]	Supine	Customized body mold	Diaphragm-peritoneum§ (3 mm slices)	NS	NA§
Abdominopelvic RT					
Duthoy et al [23]	Supine (arms overhead)	NS	10 cm cranial to the diaphragm-10 cm caudal to obturator foramen (5 mm slices)	None	NS
Hong et al [22]	Supine (arms overhead)	NS	Midthorax, 5 cm below below ischial tuberosities (5 mm slices)	NS	NS
Pelvic-inguinal RT					
Garofalo et al [24]	Supine (frog-leg)	Upper and lower body alpha cradles	L3–5 cm below the inferior extent of the vulva	Oral, rectal, IV, bladder	Yes

CT = computed tomography; IMRT = intensity-modulated radiation therapy; IV = intravenous; NA = not applicable; NS = not stated; RT = radiation therapy.
*A comparison study of prone versus supine positioning.
†Some patients simulated both supine and prone.
‡When disease is abutting or invading the bladder.
§Only the para-aortic lymph node region is treated with intensity-modulated radiation therapy; the pelvis is treated with conventional radiaton therapy.

IMRT, poor immobilization may increase the dose to normal tissues (and thus toxicity) and reduce the dose to the target tissues (and thus tumor control). At our institution, an upper and lower body alpha cradle is fabricated and indexed to the treatment table (Figure 23-1), reducing setup uncertainty to ≤ 5 mm.[37] Others use customized body molds.[30,35] The University of Colorado approach is described in detail in Chapter 23.1, "Cervical Cancer: Case Study."

Contrast is an important component of the simulation of gynecologic IMRT, aiding in the delineation of both the target and normal tissues. Oral, rectal, and intravenous contrast is typically sufficient. Bladder contrast is used in selected patients. Intravenous contrast is particularly useful in identifying lymph node regions, given the close association of lymphatic and vascular vessels. A vaginal marker should be placed in all patients at simulation.

Target and Tissue Delineation

Two targets are delineated in most patients: a gross tumor volume (GTV) and a clinical target volume (CTV). The GTV comprises all gross tumor sites. In patients with early-stage cancer, the GTV may include solely the primary tumor; in more advanced patients, it may also include enlarged lymph nodes and sites of residual disease. An unfortunate limitation is that gross disease is often poorly visualized on the planning CT, even with the aid of contrast. Attention is thus turning to more sophisticated imaging approaches, including positron emission tomography (PET)[35,38] and magnetic resonance imaging (MRI).[39]

The CTV consists of the GTV plus all sites of microscopic disease spread. In the postoperative patient, the CTV is the sole target delineated. CTV design is complex, requiring an understanding of the patterns of failure and sites of disease spread. Unfortunately, no consensus exists regarding which sites should be included within the CTV. Table 23-2 summarizes the CTV delineated in published gynecologic IMRT studies.

After selecting the components of the CTV, one must decide how to contour them. Currently, no guidelines exist regarding CTV delineation in patients receiving gynecologic IMRT. Fortunately, an increasing number of publications are focusing on this important issue.[40] Moreover, national cooperative groups, including the Gynecology Oncology Group (GOG), are developing guidelines for CTV design in these patients. Figure 23-2 illustrates the CTV in a patient with endometrial cancer treated at our center with adjuvant intensity-modulated pelvic irradiation. CTV design approaches at the University of Colorado and M. D. Anderson Cancer Center are described in Chapter 23.1 and Chapter 23.2, "Endometrial Cancer: Case Study," respectively

A controversial aspect of CTV design is the delineation of the lymph nodes. Most investigators use pelvic vessels as surrogates for lymphatic channels. The optimal margin around these vessels, however, remains unclear. Some include the vessels along with the "surrounding fat and connective tissues."[18] Others use "generous" margins.[20] We routinely use 0.5 to 1.0 cm margins. Only careful analyses of patterns of failure in treated patients will help determine the optimal approach. Sophisticated direct lymph node imaging may also help delineate lymph node regions in these women.[41]

Various normal tissues can be contoured in these patients. However, which should be contoured? The answer remains unclear. Table 23-2 summarizes the normal tissues included in representative IMRT series. In women treated with pelvic irradiation, most delineate the rectum, bladder, and small bowel.[17–20,25,30] Some include the femoral heads[19] and bone marrow.[26,28] The latter is particularly useful in patients undergoing chemo-RT to reduce hematologic toxicity.[28,42] When more comprehensive volumes are treated, additional organs are delineated, for example, the kidneys[19,21–23,35] and liver.[19,22,23,35] Examples of normal tissue contours in a patient undergoing intensity-modulated pelvic irradiation are shown in Figure 23-2.

Treatment Planning

Several commercial planning systems are currently available. Although inherent differences exist, there is no reason that one system should generate better IMRT plans than another. As seen in Table 23-3, most studies to date have used the *CORVUS* system (North American Scientific, NOMOS Radiation Oncology Division, Cranberry Township, PA). However, acceptable gynecologic IMRT plans have been produced on all of the major planning systems.

An important step in gynecologic IMRT planning is the expansion of the CTV to produce a planning target volume (PTV), accounting for setup uncertainty and organ motion. As seen in Table 23-3, many investigators expand

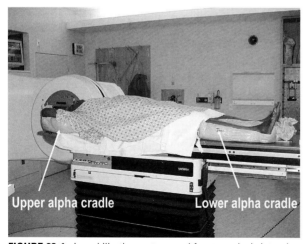

FIGURE 23-1. Immobilization system used for gynecologic intensity-modulated radiation therapy at the University of Chicago. (To view a color version of this image, please refer to the CD-ROM.) Adapted from Mundt AJ et al.[15]

TABLE 23-2. Target and Tissues: Gynecologic Intensity-Modulated Radiation Therapy Studies

Study	Tumor Site(s)	Target	Normal Tissues
Pelvic RT			
Adli et al[17]	Cervix, uterus	GTV: uterus, cervix, tumor/tumor extensions (intact uterus patients) and postoperative changes + vaginal cuff (postoperative patients) CTV: GTV + pelvic nodes, contrast-enhanced vessels (obturator to aortic bifurcation), upper 4 cm vagina, presacral region	Small bowel, large bowel, bladder
Ahamad et al[18]	Cervix, uterus*	CTV: vaginal vault, paravaginal tissues, pelvic nodes	Small bowel, rectum, bladder
Chen et al[19]	Uterus	CTV: uterus/cervix, parametria, upper half vagina and pelvic nodes (common, internal, external iliac)	Femoral heads, rectum, small bowel, bladder, cauda equina
Heron et al[20]	Cervix, uterus*	CTV: upper 4 cm vagina, pelvic lymph node regions (common, internal, and external iliac)	Small bowel, rectum, bladder
Mundt et al[25]	Cervix, uterus	CTV: upper half vagina, uterus/cervix, parametria, presacral region, pelvic node regions (common, external, and internal iliac)	Small bowel, bladder, rectum, pelvic bone marrow
Schefter et al[30]	Cervix†	GTV (CTV$_{cervix}$): tumor, enlarged nodes, uterus CTV$_{pelvis}$: PTV$_{cervix}$ + proximal uterosacral ligaments, parametria, proximal vagina, pelvic nodes (common, internal, external iliac)	Small bowel, bladder, rectum
Extended field RT			
Chen et al[19]	Uterine	CTV: uterus/cervix, parametria, upper half vagina, and pelvic node regions (common, internal, external iliac), para-aortic nodes (to the T11–12 interspace)	Femoral heads, rectum, small bowel, bladder, kidneys, liver, stomach, cord/cauda equina
Portelance et al[21]	Cervix	"Target": para-aortic, common iliac, external iliac, internal iliac lymph nodes and uterus	Small bowel, colon, rectum, kidney, bladder, vagina, spinal cord, femoral heads
Mutic et al[35]	Cervix	GTV: PET-enhancing para-aortic lymph nodes CTV: para-aortic lymph node region‡	Skin, kidneys, colon, liver, small bowel, stomach, cord
Abdominopelvic RT			
Duthoy et al[23]	Ovary*	CTV: total peritoneal cavity (including pelvic and para-aortic lymph node regions, 0.5 cm rim of liver (adjacent to peritoneum)	Liver (excluding 0.5 cm rim), kidneys
Hong et al[22]	Uterus*	"GTV" (CTV): entire peritoneal surface, pelvic and para-aortic lymph node regions, including aorta/inferior vena cava	Liver (except outer 1 cm), kidneys, spinal cord, thoracic and lumbar vertebral bodies, pelvic bones, femurs
Pelvic-inguinal RT			
Garofalo et al[24]	Vulva*	Vulva, inguinal and pelvic (common, internal, and external iliac) lymph nodes	Small bowel, bladder, rectum, femoral heads

CTV = clinical target volume; GTV = gross tumor volume; IMRT = intensity-modulated radiation therapy; RT = radiation therapy; PET = positron emission tomography; PTV = planning target volume; RT = radiation therapy.
*Postoperative patients only.
†Intact cervical cancer patients only.
‡Only the para-aortic lymph node region is treated with intensity-modulated radiation therapy; the pelvis is treated with conventional radiation therapy.

the CTV by 1 cm. A detailed analysis of the impact of various CTV-PTV expansions in patients who undergo gynecologic IMRT was recently presented by Ahamad and colleagues. The larger the CTV-PTV expansion, the less sparing of normal tissues was seen.[18] Some groups also expand the normal tissues, accounting for setup uncertainty and organ motion.[23,35]

Surprisingly little is known about organ motion in gynecology patients. Some studies noted significant organ motion, particularly in the region of the cervix, vagina, and rectum,[43–45] whereas others noted only small amounts of motion.[30] More detailed studies of gynecology patients are clearly needed. For now, we favor the use of a 1 cm margin. Investigators at M.D. Anderson Cancer Center have adopted an integrated target volume approach (see Chapter 23.2). Figure 23-3 illustrates a volume-rendered image of the PTV in a patient with endometrial cancer.

Although many aspects of IMRT planning are automated, the planner still specifies the number, angle, and energy of all beams. Details of planning parameters from selected IMRT reports are summarized in Table 23-3. Most centers use seven to nine equally spaced beams delivered with 6 MV photons. In contrast, Hong and colleagues used five equally spaced beams in patients undergoing intensity-modulated abdominopelvic irradiation delivered with 15 MV photons.[22] In patients receiving pelvic irradiation, we compared various beam numbers and configurations. Fewer than seven beams reduced the conformity of the treatment plan, whereas more than nine beams did not improve it. Conformity of the treatment plans was also superior using 6 MV rather than higher-energy photons.[16] Current work is focusing on beam angle optimization programs to improve IMRT planning.[46]

The dose prescribed in a gynecologic IMRT plan is a function of tumor site, stage, and treatment volume. As seen in Table 23-3, most investigators administer 45 Gy in 1.8 daily fractions.[16–20] More sophisticated dose prescriptions are currently being explored using the SIB technique.[29,30,35,36] The

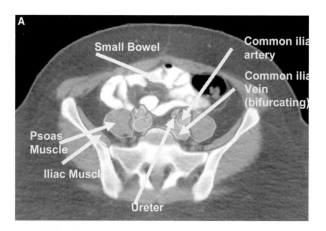

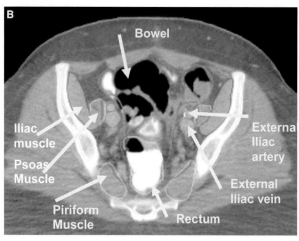

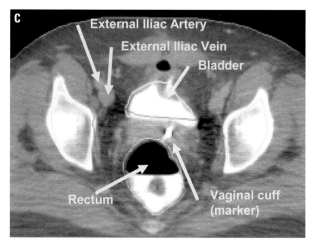

FIGURE 23-2. Axial computed tomography (CT) slices of a patient receiving gynecologic intensity-modulated radiation therapy illustrating the clinical target volume (CTV) and normal tissues. (*A*) Upper pelvis. The CTV (*red*) encompasses the bilateral common iliac lymph node regions. Note that the psoas muscles are lateral to the common iliac vessels. Critical normal tissues include the small bowel (*pink*) and pelvic (iliac crest) bone marrow (*light blue*). (*B*) Midpelvis. The CTV includes the bilateral internal and external iliac lymph node regions. At this level, the CTV is split into two structures. Note that the piriform muscles form the posterior border of the CTV. (*C*) Lower pelvis. The CTV includes the parametrial tissues and the external iliac vessels. Critical normal tissues include the bladder (*green*), rectum (*yellow*), and bone marrow. Note the vaginal marker identifying the vaginal cuff. (To view a color version of this image, please refer to the CD-ROM.)

TABLE 23-3. Planning Parameters: Gynecologic Intensity-Modulated Radiation Therapy Studies

Study Total/Fraction	Expansion CTV-PTV	Other*	Beams	No. of Coplanar	Angles (deg)	Beam Energy, MV	Beam System	Planning Dose (Gy)
Pelvic RT								
Adli et al[17]	1.5 cm	No	Arc technique	Yes	Limited arc (180), extended arc (340)	6	CORVUS	45/1.8
Ahamad et al[18]	Various†	No	4, 6, 8	NS	NS	6	CORVUS	45/1.8
Chen et al[19]	1 cm	No	9	Yes	Equally spaced	6	CORVUS	45/1.8
Heron et al[20]	0.5 cm	No	7	Yes	Equally spaced (0, 51, 102, 145, 215, 255, 306)	6	CORVUS	45/1.8
Roeske et al[16]	1 cm	No	7, 9	Yes	Equally spaced (40 or 51.4 intervals)	6	CORVUS	45/1.8
Schefter et al[15]	"Small"	No	5	Yes	Equally spaced (0, 72, 144, 216, 288)	15	FOCUS	PTV$_c$: 55/2.2 PYV$_p$: 45/1.8
Extended field RT								
Chen et al[19]	1 cm	No	9	Yes	Equally spaced	6	CORVUS	45/1.8
Portelance et al[21]	4 mm (nodes) 12.4 mm (cervix)	No	7, 9	Yes	Equally spaced 7 field (26, 77, 129, 180, 231, 283, 334) 9 field (20, 60, 100, 140, 180, 220, 260, 300, 340)	18	CORVUS	45/1.8
Mutic et al[35]	4 mm	Yes‡	7	Yes	Equally spaced (26, 77, 129, 180, 231, 283, 334)	18	CORVUS	GTV: 59.4/1.8 CTV: 50.4/1.53
Abdominopelvic RT								
Duthoy et al[23]	0.5 cm	Yes§	Arc technique	Yes	−128 to +128 arc 90° sliding window	18	Pinnacle	33/1.5
Hong et al[22]	0.5–1 cm‖	No	5	Yes	Equally spaced (255, 325, 180, 105, 35)	15	In-house	30/1.5
Pelvic-inguinal RT								
Garofalo et al[24]	1 cm	No	9	Yes	Equally spaced (51.4 intervals)	6	CORVUS	45/1.8

CTV = clinical target volume; IMRT = intensity-modulated radiation therapy; PTV = planning target volume; PTV$_c$ = planning target volume (cervix); PTV$_p$ = planning target volume (pelvis); RT = radiation therapy.

*Normal tissue expansion.

†This study focused on the impact of various clinical target volume–planning target volume expansions.

‡Expansions for the kidneys, colon, small intestine, liver, stomach, and spinal cord were 20, 10, 15, 20, 7, and 4 mm, respectively.

§Kidneys expanded by 5 mm.

‖0.5 cm axial; 1 cm superior and inferior.

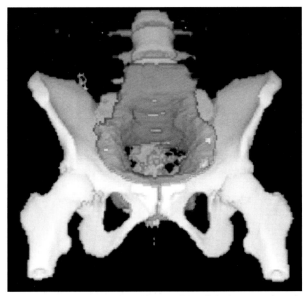

FIGURE 23-3. Volume-rendered image of the clinical target volume in a patient receiving gynecologic intensity-modulated radiation therapy. (To view a color version of this image, please refer to the CD-ROM.)

TABLE 23-4. Input Parameters: Gynecologic Intensity-Modulated Radiation Therapy Studies

	Goal, Gy	Volume below Goal, %	Minimum, Gy	Maximum, Gy
Pelvic irradiation (University of Chicago[25])				
PTV	45	3	42.8	47.3

Organ	Limit, Gy	Volume above Limit, %	Minimum, Gy	Maximum, Gy
Bladder	35.1	40	27.9	42.8
Rectum	35.8	54	27.5	42.8
Small bowel	38.1	0	8.2	42.8

	Goal, Gy	Volume below Goal, %	Minimum, Gy	Maximum, Gy
Pelvic irradiation (University of Iowa[17])				
PTV	45	5	43	45

Organ	Limit, Gy	Volume above Limit, %	Minimum, Gy	Maximum, Gy
Bladder	80	33	65	90
Large bowel	22	50	11	45
Small bowel	22	50	11	45

	Goal, Gy	Volume below Goal, %	Minimum, Gy	Maximum, Gy
Extended field irradiation (Washington University[21])				
Uterus	45	5	42.8	48.3
Nodes	45	5	42.8	48.3

Organ	Limit, Gy	Volume above Limit, %	Minimum, Gy	Maximum, Gy
Bladder	40	50	15	45
Rectum	30	50	15	40
Small bowel	30	50	20	40
Colon	30	50	10	45
Kidney	10	33	5	23
Spinal cord	45	5	10	45
Femoral head	40	10	15	50

IMRT = intensity-modulated radiation therapy.

SIB approach used at the University of Colorado is described in Chapter 23.1. Others are exploring the SIB approach in patients with involved para-aortic lymph nodes.[35]

Regardless of the system used, dose-volume constraints (for the PTV and normal tissues) must be specified. Such constraints serve as input parameters in the inverse planning process and are typically entered as DVHs. Some systems allow priority weights to be assigned to the PTV and normal tissues. Although priority is always given to PTV coverage, a small volume should be allowed to receive below the prescription dose. At our center, our goal is to cover ≥ 98% of the PTV with the prescription dose. Others recommend > 97%.[18] Input parameters for the normal tissues are less intuitive. Table 23-4 summarizes the input parameters used at our center[26] and other centers.[17,21]

An example IMRT plan in a patient with endometrial cancer treated with adjuvant pelvic irradiation is shown in Figure 23-4. Figure 23-5 illustrates an IMRT plan in another patient with the iliac crest bone marrow included as a planning constraint in the optimization process.

Plan Evaluation

By varying input constraints, several plans can be generated for each patient. Each should be evaluated jointly by the radiation oncologist and medical physicist, both qualitatively (dose conformity and hot and cold spots) and quantitatively (PTV and normal tissue DVHs). Unfortunately, no standards exist that aid one in the selection of the best plan. Each center must instead adopt its own criteria. At our center, a plan is acceptable only if the PTV receives ≥ 98% of the prescription dose.[16,25] Others have adopted less stringent criteria, particularly when large volumes are treated.[21–23] Care should be taken to ensure that all cold spots are on the periphery of the PTV, not within the CTV (and never within the GTV). It is unwise to insist on 100% of the PTV receiving the full prescription dose because sizable hot spots will result within the PTV and normal tissues.

Owing to the inhomogeneity of IMRT plans, hot spots will exist. Each center must adopt maximum allowable volumes for these hot spots. In the past, we accepted IMRT plans with up to 20% and 2% of the PTV receiving 110% and 115% respectively of the prescription dose.[15,16] With newer versions of planning software, however, the PTVs receiving 110% and 115% of the prescription dose have been ≤ 10% and ≤ 1%, respectively. Care should always be taken to avoid hot spots along the anterior rectal and posterior bladder walls in patients undergoing brachytherapy.

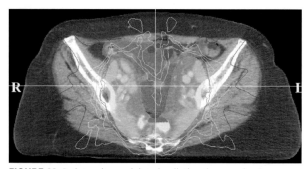

FIGURE 23-4. Intensity-modulated radiation therapy plan in a gynecology patient. Note that the high-dose lines conform to the shape of the lateral lymph nodes and the presacral region, sparing the small bowel. (To view a color version of this image, please refer to the CD-ROM.)

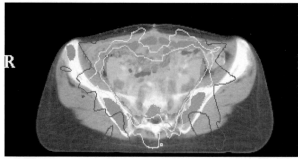

FIGURE 23-5. Bone marrow–sparing intensity-modulated radiation therapy plan in a gynecology patient. Note the sparing of the bone marrow (*red*) in the iliac crests. (To view a color version of this image, please refer to the CD-ROM.)

A challenging aspect of plan evaluation is the assessment of normal tissue DVHs. Just as no standards exist for assessing PTV DVHs, so do none exist for assessing normal tissue DVHs. In fact, little is known about what makes a normal tissue DVH acceptable (or not). At a minimum, one should specify a maximum allowable dose for each normal tissue. In their abdominopelvic IMRT study, Duthoy and colleagues specified that less than 5% and 20% of the kidneys (with a 5 mm expansion) could receive more than 30 Gy and 25 Gy, respectively, whereas the median dose had to be lower than 18 Gy. The median liver dose had to be ≤ 30 Gy.[23]

The ideal shape of the normal tissue DVHs in patients undergoing gynecologic IMRT remains unclear. What percentage of the prescription dose, for example, should 40% of the rectum receive? It is hoped that, over time, intermediate- and low-dose constraints can be developed for each normal tissue. At the present time, these constraints remain arbitrary. Only with follow-up of a large number of patients will these constraints become clear.

Treatment Delivery and Quality Assurance

IMRT plans can be delivered by a number of commercially available delivery systems. At our center, treatment is delivered with a Varian CL2100 CD accelerator (Varian Medical Systems, Palo Alto, CA) equipped with a 120-leaf multileaf collimator (MLC) and automatic beam sequencing software. Treatment is delivered in the step-and-shoot mode.[16] Gynecologic IMRT can also be delivered using intensity-modulated arc therapy.[23] Duthoy and colleagues used such an approach on a SLiPlus linear accelerator (Elekta, Stockholm, Sweden).[23] Another promising approach is helical tomotherapy. Important advantages of tomotherapy are fast delivery times and image guidance capability, allowing daily setup verification. Moreover, tomotherapy is ideal for treating large targets, for example, extended field RT fields (Figure 23-6). There is no evidence to date that one treatment planning or delivery system is superior to another in these patients.

Prior to (and throughout) the delivery of IMRT, rigorous quality assurance (QA) is essential to ensure proper delivery of the treatment plans. At our institution, the accuracy of setup is verified on the first treatment day and then weekly with orthogonal radiographs verifying the location of the isocenter. In addition, we perform a number of QA procedures. One such QA procedure uses an independent monitor unit verification calculation (MUVC). A recent study by Haslam and colleagues compared the doses calculated by our treatment planning system (*CORVUS*) with those estimated by the MUVC program (*RadCalc*, Lifeline Software Inc., Tyler, TX).[47] In 22 gynecology cases, they observed that the mean disparity between these two systems was 0.2%, with a standard deviation of 1.1%. Disparities outside this tight region require additional QA, including ion chamber and film measurements.

Duthoy and colleagues used gel dosimetry to determine the three-dimensional dose distribution for gynecology patients receiving whole abdominopelvic RT.[23] The gel was molded to conform to the shape of the Rando phantom (Alderson Research Laboratories, Stamford, CT). Patient treatment plans were subsequently delivered to the phantom. Using a magnetic resonance scanner, the amount of polymer formed, and hence the resultant dose distribution in the gel, was determined. A comparison of planned and delivered dose distributions showed good agreement within the PTV (~ 1%). However, disagreements of 16% and 13% were observed between the calculated and measured median doses for the liver and kidney, respectively. The authors attributed these differences to leaf transmission calculation errors and setup uncertainty. Both of these need to be considered before the widespread clinical implementation of this approach.

A problem that occurs for gynecologic IMRT treatment plans is that the field sizes may exceed the travel limits of the MLC. In these cases, the fields are split into two (or more) carriage movements. Hong and colleagues considered the dosimetric implications in patients receiving whole abdominal RT.[22] In cases in which the fields are split, adja-

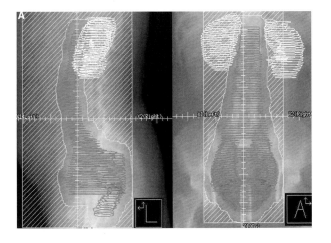

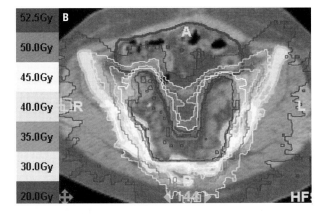

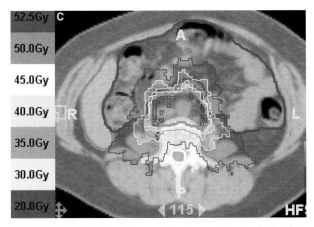

FIGURE 23-6. Helical tomotherapy intensity-modulated radiation therapy plan in a patient with cervical cancer undergoing extended field irradiation. (*A*) Sagittal and coronal views of the planning target volume (PTV) in this patient. (*B*) Axial computed tomography (CT) slice in the pelvis in this patient with superimposed isodose lines. Note the high degree of conformity of the 40 Gy (*green*) and 45 Gy (*yellow*) isodose lines to the PTV, resulting in sparing of the surrounding small bowel. (*C*) Axial CT slice in the para-aortic region in the same patient. Again note the high degree of conformity of the treatment plan and sparing of surrounding tissues. (To view a color version of this image, please refer to the CD-ROM.) Courtesy of Scott P. Tannehill, MD, University of Wisconsin-Madison.

cent subfields may contribute additional scatter and leakage dose that are not accurately calculated by the planning system. Using ion chamber and film, it was determined that this additional dose was dependent on the number of monitor units from these fields. On average, they determined that the additional dose was ~ 4% of the prescribed dose. Thus, in treatments involving large fields, this effect should be quantified, and, if necessary, the dose prescription should be altered to account for this additional dose.

Preclinical (Planning) Studies

Multiple investigators have evaluated IMRT planning in patients with gynecologic malignancies. The planning details of most of these studies have been discussed earlier and are summarized in Tables 23-1 to 23-4. This section focuses on the dosimetric results of these reports, particularly studies comparing IMRT and conventional planning.

Pelvic RT

Most planning studies focus on intensity-modulated pelvic irradiation. The first was presented by Roeske and colleagues and compared IMRT and conventional planning in five patients with cervical cancer and five patients with endometrial cancer.[16] Conventional plans consisted of a four-field "box" approach, and IMRT plans consisted of nine-field equally spaced beams. IMRT resulted in highly conformal dose distributions providing excellent coverage of the PTV while reducing the volume of small bowel irradiated to the prescription dose by a factor of 2 (17.4 vs 33.8%; $p < .001$). Significant reductions in the volume of bladder (76.6 vs 99.3%; $p < .001$) and rectum (57.7 vs 80.3%; $p < .001$) receiving 45 Gy or more were also seen. IMRT plans, however, were less homogeneous than conventional plans.

Heron and colleagues compared IMRT and four-field box plans in eight patients with endometrial cancer and two patients with cervical cancer.[20] Significant reductions in the volume of small bowel (14.8 vs 30.3%), bladder (59.7 vs 86.4%), and rectum (32.0 vs 92.8%) receiving ≥ 30 Gy were observed for IMRT plans. Volumes of normal tissue receiving > 45 Gy were significantly reduced: small bowel, 0.4 versus 10%; bladder, 4 versus 59%; and rectum, 1 versus 56%.

Chen and colleagues found significant reductions in small bowel irradiated to 45 Gy or more (5.2 vs 16.9%; $p = .02$) comparing IMRT with conventional plans in seven gynecology patients.[19] IMRT planning significantly reduced the volume of small bowel receiving more than 15 Gy (84.0 vs 67.2%; $p < .01$).

Adli and colleagues compared prone and supine positioning in 16 patients (13 with cervical cancer, 3 with endometrial cancer) undergoing intensity-modulated pelvic RT planning.[17] As seen in Table 23-3, IMRT planning in this study differed from other reports and consisted of limited (180°) and extended (340°) arc techniques. Significant reductions were observed in terms of the sparing of the small bowel, bladder, and rectum using IMRT planning. Reductions in the volume of small bowel receiving > 45 Gy were noted for prone compared with supine positioning (10.1 vs 13.6%; $p = .03$) in the extended arc plans. Greater reductions in small bowel irradiation were observed for prone positioning with limited arc plans. Significant reductions in large bowel and bladder irradiation were also observed for prone positioning when limited arc plans were used.

Chen and colleagues compared prone and supine positioning in two patients and similarly noted a benefit to prone positioning.[19] The volume of small bowel irradiated to more than 35 Gy was reduced by 60 to 70% for patients in the prone position.

Ahamad and colleagues at M. D. Anderson Cancer Center evaluated IMRT planning in 10 patients undergoing adjuvant pelvic RT.[18] A 40% reduction in the volume of small bowel receiving > 40 Gy was seen with IMRT planning, without sacrificing PTV coverage. Various CTV-PTV expansions were compared, and larger expansions reduced the sparing of normal tissues. Less small bowel sparing was observed with increasing body mass index and/or anterior-posterior diameter, whereas greater sparing was seen with increasing CTV length. The M. D. Anderson approach in patients with endometrial cancer treated with adjuvant intensity-modulated pelvic RT is highlighted in Chapter 23.2.

Huh and colleagues evaluated the impact of a small bowel displacement system (SBDS) on IMRT planning in patients with cervical cancer.[48] The SBDS consisted of a customized compression device, which displaces the small bowel out of the radiation fields, and an individualized immobilization abdominal board. In a cohort of 10 patients, the SBDS reduced the small bowel volume within the pelvic radiation field. The mean irradiated small bowel volume, with the SBDS, was 61.46 ± 4.97% smaller than with conventional IMRT. The SBDS-assisted IMRT plan was superior to the conventional one in terms of dose homogeneity in the PTV but not significantly different in the rectum and bladder. Of note, the mean monitor units and MLC segment numbers with the SBDS were 26.2% and 31.65% lower than without the SBDS, respectively (both $p < .0001$).

Lujan and colleagues investigated IMRT planning as a means to reduce the volume of pelvic bone marrow irradiated in gynecology patients.[42] The medullary canal of the iliac crests was entered as a constraint in the optimization process. Three plans were compared: a conventional four-field plan, an IMRT plan without bone marrow sparing, and an IMRT plan with bone marrow sparing. At all dose levels > 15 Gy, IMRT planning reduced the volume of bone marrow irradiated without compromising PTV coverage or sparing of other normal tissues. This approach is discussed in more detail in Chapter 23.4, "Bone Marrow–Sparing IMRT: Emerging Technology."

Extended Field RT

Portelance and colleagues at Washington University evaluated IMRT planning in 10 patients with advanced cervical cancer undergoing pelvic plus para-aortic lymph node irradiation.[21] Although equivalent target coverage was achieved, IMRT planning significantly reduced the volume of small bowel (13.6 vs 34.2%; $p < .05$), rectum (3.3 vs 46.4%; $p < .001$), and bladder (26.9 vs 60.5%; $p < .05$) receiving more than 45 Gy compared with a four-field approach. Comparable benefits were seen comparing IMRT and a two-field approach. In a smaller study, Chen and colleagues compared IMRT and conventional planning in four patients undergoing extended field irradiation and noted similar benefits.[19]

Abdominopelvic RT

Hong and colleagues used IMRT planning to simulate abdominopelvic irradiation in 10 patients with advanced endometrial cancer.[22] The target volume included the entire peritoneal surface and pelvic and para-aortic lymph nodes, with a 0.5 cm axial expansion and 1 cm superior and inferior expansion. The PTV also included the outer 1 cm border of the liver and the left renal hilum. IMRT plans were compared with opposed anterior-posterior plans. IMRT planning achieved superior target coverage, particularly near the kidneys. Reductions in the dose to the vertebral column and femoral heads were also seen. In fact, the volume of pelvic bones (and thus bone marrow) receiving ≥ 21 Gy was reduced by 60%. Mean doses to the kidney, liver, and spinal cord were comparable.

Duthoy and colleagues compared intensity-modulated arc therapy with conventional therapy in five patients with ovarian cancer.[23] The PTV was defined as the entire peritoneal cavity plus a 0.5 cm expansion. Conventional and IMRT plans were normalized to deliver a median dose of 33 Gy. IMRT was associated with less dose inhomogeneity compared with conventional planning ($p = .01$). Moreover, the median dose to the right kidney was lower (13.6 Gy vs 18.6 Gy; $p = .02$).

Pelvic-Inguinal RT

Garofalo and colleagues at the University of Chicago evaluated IMRT planning in four patients with vulvar carcinoma treated with pelvic-inguinal irradiation.[24] IMRT plans were compared with conventional two-field (opposed anterior-posterior) plans with standard blocking. Significant reductions in irradiated volumes of normal tissues (including the femoral heads) were observed at ≥ 75% and ≥ 100% of the prescription dose for the IMRT plans ($p < .01$).

In contrast, Gilroy and colleagues found that IMRT planning in a patient with vulvar cancer resulted in excess dose (57 Gy) to sensitive pelvic structures and increased setup complexity.[49] It is unclear, however, how the CTV and sensitive structures were contoured and whether these tissues were included in the optimization process.

Dose Escalation

Mutic and colleagues evaluated the SIB approach in four patients with cervical cancer with para-aortic lymph node metastases.[35] IMRT plans were generated to deliver 59.4 Gy in 1.8 Gy fractions to involved lymph nodes (identified on PET imaging) and 50.4 Gy in 1.53 fractions to the para-aortic lymph node region. On average, 97.6% of involved nodes and 89.0% of para-aortic region lymph nodes received 100% of the prescription dose. The median volume of normal tissue receiving the tolerance dose (in parentheses) was as follows: kidney, 23.1% (22 Gy); colon, 9.0% (25 Gy); small intestine, 42.0% (25 Gy); liver, 0.0% (30 Gy); stomach, 1.2% (30 Gy); and spinal cord, 0.0% (45 Gy). Recently, these investigators published treatment guidelines regarding this approach.[50]

Lujan and colleagues studied the SIB approach to escalate dose to involved nodes in patients undergoing pelvic irradiation.[36] Involved nodes were delineated as a separate target, with a larger target volume consisting of the upper vagina, uterus, parametria, and regional lymph nodes. The SIB approach allowed the simultaneous delivery of 54 Gy (in 2.14 Gy fractions) to the involved nodes and 45 Gy (in 1.8 Gy fractions) to the larger target, without compromising sparing of the normal pelvic tissues.

Investigators at the University of Colorado evaluated the SIB technique in patients with advanced cervical cancer undergoing external beam RT and brachytherapy.[29,30] Two separate CTVs were defined: CTV$_{cervix}$ and CTV$_{pelvis}$. CTV$_{cervix}$ consisted of the uterus, primary tumor, and contiguous involved lymph nodes, and a uniform 0.5 or 1.0 mm expansion was used generating the PTV$_{cervix}$. The CTV$_{pelvis}$ consisted of PTV$_{cervix}$ plus the presacral region (to at least S3) and the nodal regions of the internal and external iliac chains (to the lower common iliac nodes); PTV$_{pelvis}$ was defined by a 0.5 to 1 cm expansion of the CTV$_{pelvis}$. IMRT plans were generated to deliver 1.8 Gy fractions to the PTV$_{pelvis}$ and 2 to 2.2 Gy fractions to the PTV$_{cervix}$, prior to intracavitary brachytherapy. Compared with conventional techniques, this approach resulted in a reduced 60 Gy isodose volume with significant reductions in the mean bladder and rectal doses. A full discussion of this technique is provided in Chapter 23.1.

Alternative to Brachytherapy

Schefter and colleagues compared dose distributions achieved with high–dose rate (HDR) brachytherapy and IMRT in a patient with stage IIb cervical cancer.[30] HDR planning was simulated to deliver 6 Gy to point A. The resulting isodose curves were then contoured as target volumes, and an IMRT plan was generated. The investigators found that IMRT could closely replicate HDR dose distributions. The point A isodose volume was well covered for both plans; however, hot spots near the HDR source were avoided with IMRT. Moreover, the same volume of rectum received the prescription dose in both plans, whereas the volume of bladder receiving more than the point A dose was reduced with IMRT. A greater volume of rectum, however, received lower doses with the IMRT plan.

Low and colleagues at Washington University described a novel approach known as applicator-guided intensity-modulated radiation therapy (AG-IMRT) as a potential replacement for brachytherapy in patients with cervical cancer (see Chapter 23.5, "Applicator-Guided IMRT: Emerging Technology").[34] As envisioned, a CT-compatible applicator would be placed in the vagina and uterus to localize the target tissues and reproducibly position the bladder and rectum during treatment. MRI and/or PET would be used to delineate the target tissues, and treatment would be delivered using HDR schedules. In a recent treatment planning study, Wahab and colleagues compared dose distributions between HDR brachytherapy and AG-IMRT in 10 patients with cervical cancer. The average minimum tumor dose and mean percent volume receiving the prescription dose were greater with AG-IMRT (both $p = .0005$). Although the mean volume of rectum at the tolerance limit was higher with AG-IMRT (4.1 vs 2.2%) compared with HDR brachytherapy, the difference did not reach statistical significance.[51]

Roeske and Mundt evaluated IMRT planning in women unable to undergo intracavitary brachytherapy.[33] The CTV consisted of the residual tumor mass and was expanded by 1 cm to generate a PTV. Using dose constraints established for prostate cancer, these investigators demonstrated that total doses of 75 to 79 Gy to the primary tumor were feasible.[52] A patient with cervical cancer unsuitable for intracavitary brachytherapy who was treated with IMRT at Princess Margaret Hospital is discussed in Chapter 23.3, "Cervical Cancer Not Suitable for Brachytherapy: Case Study."

Clinical (Outcome) Studies

Mundt and colleagues at the University of Chicago described the first clinical experience with gynecologic IMRT in a series of reports.[25,26] In their most recent study, acute gastrointestinal and genitourinary sequelae in 40 gynecology patients treated with intensity-modulated pelvic irradiation were presented.[26] Toxicity was graded on a 4-point scale: 0, none; 1, mild (no medications required); 2, moderate (medications required); and 3, severe (treatment breaks or hospitalization required). The worst toxicity during treatment was compared with that experienced by 35 patients previously treated with conventional RT. The two groups were well matched with regard to clinicopathologic and treatment factors. IMRT treatment was associated with lower grade 2 (60 vs 91%; $p = .002$) and grade 1 (34 vs 75%; $p = .001$) gastrointestinal toxicity than conventional RT. Grade 2 genitourinary toxicity was also less common in the IMRT group (10 vs 20%); however, this difference did not reach statistical significance ($p = .22$).

To improve on the above results, Roeske and colleagues performed a detailed dosimetric analysis of acute gastrointestinal toxicity in 50 patients undergoing intensity-modulated pelvic irradiation.[53] Clinically significant gastrointestinal toxicity was defined as any grade ≥ 3 or grade 2 toxicity requiring frequent medications. Clinically significant toxicity was observed in 28% of patients. Normal tissue complication probability (NTCP) modeling demonstrated that the volume of small bowel receiving 100% of the prescription dose ($SB_{vol\ 100\%}$) was the most significant predictor of clinically significant acute toxicity. The NTCP model predicted a 77% risk of clinically significant toxicity with conventional pelvic irradiation compared with 27% with IMRT, consistent with clinical observations. These results demonstrate the importance of minimizing the $SB_{vol\ 100\%}$ in these patients.

Preliminary analysis of IMRT patients suggests that chronic gastrointestinal toxicity can also be reduced. Mundt and colleagues noted that chronic gastrointestinal toxicity was reduced from 50% in 30 women treated with conventional pelvic RT to 11.1% in 36 women treated with intensity-modulated pelvic irradiation ($p = .001$).[27] As in the previous study, chronic toxicity was scored on a 4-point scale, with the worst recorded toxicity serving as the primary outcome. Minimum follow-up in all patients was 8 months; median follow-up intervals were 19.6 and 30.2 months in IMRT and conventional therapy patients, respectively. The difference in chronic toxicity remained significant after adjusting for clinicopathologic characteristics, including length of follow-up, with logistic regression modeling (odds ratio = 0.16; 95% confidence interval 0.04–0.67; $p = .01$).

Other reductions in toxicity have been observed, somewhat fortuitously, in patients who received gynecologic IMRT. Brixey and colleagues noted marked reductions in hematologic toxicity in a group of 36 patients treated with intensity-modulated pelvic RT compared with 88 patients treated with conventional pelvic RT.[28] These reductions occurred despite the fact that the pelvic bone marrow was not included as a planning constraint. DVH analysis of 10 patients revealed that IMRT planning, even without intentional avoidance of the bone marrow, resulted in less bone marrow irradiated at ≥ 45 Gy (15.1 vs 32.1% for the IMRT and conventional plans, respectively; $p < .001$).

In this study, hemoglobin concentration and white blood cell, platelet, and absolute neutrophil counts were collected prior to RT and weekly during treatment. Among patients receiving RT and chemotherapy (cisplatin, 40 mg/m^2/wk), use of IMRT was associated with a higher white blood cell count (3.6 vs 2.8 µg/dL; $p = .05$) and absolute neutrophil count (2,669 vs 1,874; $p = .04$) nadir. Grade 2 hemoglobin toxicity (15.2 vs 35.2%; $p = .22$), blood transfusions (8.3 vs 37.5%; $p = .48$), and chemotherapy treatment breaks (3.7 vs 9.0%; $p = .16$) were also less frequent in IMRT patients, but these differences were not statistically significant. No

significant differences in hematologic toxicity were observed in patients receiving RT alone.

To improve on these results, Roeske and colleagues are exploring the incorporation of technetium 99m single-photon emission computed tomography (SPECT) bone marrow imaging in the IMRT planning process.[54] SPECT allows one to identify the areas of active bone marrow (red marrow), which then can be entered as an avoidance structure in the planning process (see Chapter 23.4). Clinical trials are under way at the University of Chicago to determine whether bone marrow–sparing approaches can reduce the risk of hematologic toxicity in gynecology patients treated with chemotherapy and IMRT.

Investigators at the University of Chicago recently reported high pelvic control rates in patients with endometrial cancer[55] and patients with cervical cancer[56] treated with IMRT. Knab and colleagues reviewed the outcome of 31 patients with endometrial cancer treated with adjuvant intensity-modulated pelvic RT.[55] Seventeen (54%) had unfavorable histologies (5 serous, 1 clear cell, 11 carcinosarcoma). Twenty patients (64%) had stage I–II and 11 patients had stage III–IV (pelvis only) disease. Twelve patients (38%) also received intracavitary vaginal vault brachytherapy, and five (all carcinosarcomas) received chemotherapy. The CTV consisted of the upper vagina, parametria, and regional lymph nodes (common iliac, internal iliac, and external iliac). In two patients with stage IIIc cancer, the para-aortic lymph nodes were included. The prescription dose was 45 Gy in 1.8 Gy fractions. At a median follow-up of 24 months (range 5.4–44.6 months), five patients (16.1%) had experienced a recurrence for a 3-year actuarial disease-free survival rate of 80.6%. The most significant factor correlated with relapse was histology. Patients with unfavorable histologies had a worse 3-year disease-free survival rate ($p = .04$) than those with adenocarcinomas. All five patients who experienced a recurrence failed in extrapelvic sites. No patient had a recurrence in the pelvis or vagina. Treatment was well tolerated, with no patient developing grade ≥ 2 chronic sequelae. Six patients (19%) developed grade 1 toxicity, predominantly mild diarrhea with select foods. One patient with a history of multiple abdominal surgeries developed an upper abdominal small bowel obstruction outside the irradiated field that required surgery.

Kochanski and colleagues reviewed the outcome of 34 patients with stage I–II cervical cancer treated with intensity-modulated pelvic RT.[56] Twenty-one patients had an intact uterus and underwent IMRT (20 received weekly cisplatin) followed by intracavitary brachytherapy, and six patients underwent simple hysterectomy. Thirteen (38%) patients with clinical stage I cancer underwent primary surgery and received adjuvant IMRT owing to adverse pathologic features (lymphovascular invasion, tumor > 4 cm, positive nodes). At a median follow-up of 26.4 months (range 4.2–42.4 months), five patients (15%) have had a recurrence, for a 3-year actuarial disease-free survival rate of 82%. All five patients had a recurrence in extrapelvic sites (lung, liver, bone). One (2.9%) patient also had a recurrence in the pelvis, for a 3-year actuarial pelvic control rate of 92%. This patient had stage IIB disease. None of the patients with stage IB-IIA cancer treated with an intact uterus or the 13 patients treated following surgery experienced a recurrence in the pelvis. No patient developed grade ≥ 2 gastrointestinal or genitourinary RT-related sequelae (two patients had grade 1 gastrointestinal toxicity and one patient had grade 1 genitourinary toxicity).

Published outcome studies involving larger treatment fields are limited. Kavanagh and colleagues reported on seven women with locally advanced, metastatic, or recurrent cervical cancer treated with concomitant boost IMRT and brachytherapy.[29] Three patients received RT to the para-aortic lymph nodes; the remainder received pelvic RT. All received four-field concomitant boost IMRT, followed in five patients by low-dose intracavitary brachytherapy and in one patient by intraperitoneal permanent seed implantation. Six of seven patients received weekly cisplatin (40 mg/m^2). In-field complete responses were observed in all patients. At 3 months follow-up, four patients were alive, with no evidence of disease, and two patients were alive with disease. Two patients with grade 3 toxicity experienced chemotherapy treatment delays. Of the remaining five patients, four developed grade 2 upper gastrointestinal toxicity and one had grade 2 lower gastrointestinal toxicity. One of seven patients had grade 2 genitourinary toxicity and two of seven patients had grade 1 genitourinary toxicity.

Future Directions

Current gynecologic IMRT data are limited by the fact that IMRT has been performed only for a short period of time. The available outcome studies include small numbers of patients, with limited follow-up, treated at only a few institutions. Moreover, outcomes have also been almost exclusively studied in women undergoing pelvic irradiation. More data are needed involving well-controlled, large, multicenter cohorts to fully investigate the potential IMRT in these patients. Fortunately, several national cooperative groups are currently developing gynecologic IMRT protocols. Hopefully, such protocols will contain more objective toxicity analyses and detailed quality-of-life measures as outcomes. Future studies regarding the economics of IMRT are also clearly needed to evaluate the cost-benefit ratio of this treatment modality. Theoretical concerns also exist regarding the risk of second malignancies in IMRT patients.[57] Such events may be associated with long time intervals between exposure and onset; thus, careful long-term follow-up of these patients is essential.

A second area of future research focuses on the incorporation of novel imaging approaches in the IMRT planning process. As noted earlier, several investigators are currently exploring the incorporation of PET, MRI, and SPECT into the planning process.[35,39,53] Other imaging approaches currently used in IMRT planning in other sites, including magnetic resonance spectroscopy[58] and Cu-ATSM (Cu(II)-diacetyl-bisN(4)-methylthiosemicarbazone) PET imaging,[59] may also prove useful.

Standards and guidelines for gynecologic IMRT are also clearly needed. At the present time, none exist regarding any aspect of IMRT planning and delivery in gynecology patients. Numerous questions remain unanswered. Which patients should be treated? Which tissues should be irradiated? Which ones should be avoided? How should the target be delineated? What are the best input parameters? What makes a plan acceptable or unacceptable? To this end, the Gynecologic IMRT Working Group was formed consisting of 45 institutions in the United States, Canada, Europe, and Asia. This group is in the process of developing a consensus statement on IMRT planning in patients undergoing adjuvant pelvic irradiation.[60] A joint RTOG-GOG collaboration is also under way to establish guidelines for CTV design in these patients. Such guidelines will not only help individual clinicians interested in adopting gynecologic IMRT but will also aid cooperative groups in the development of prospective trials.

References

1. Cleaves M. Radium: with a preliminary note on radium rays in the treatment of cancer. Med Rec 1903;64:1719–23.
2. Heyman J. The so-called Stockholm method and the results of treatment of uterine cancer at the Radiumhemmet. Acta Radiol 1935;16:129.
3. Laccasagne A. Results of the treatment of cancer of the cervix uteri. BMJ 1932;2:912–3.
4. Rutledge FN, Fletcher GH. Transperitoneal pelvic lymphadenectomy following supervoltage irradiation for squamous-cell carcinoma of the cervix. Am J Obstet Gynecol 1958;76:321–34.
5. Perez CA, Breaux S, Bedwinek JM, et al. Radiation therapy alone in the treatment of carcinoma of the uterine cervix. II. Analysis of complications. Cancer 1984;54:235–46.
6. Snijders-Keilholz A, Griffioen G, Davelaar J, et al. Vitamin B$_{12}$ malabsorption after irradiation for gynaecological tumours. Anticancer Res 1993;13:1877–81.
7. Creutzberg CL, van Putten WL, Koper PC, et al. Surgery and postoperative radiotherapy versus surgery alone for patients with stage-1 endometrial carcinoma. Multicentre randomized trial. Lancet 2000;355:1404–11.
8. Keys HM, Bundy BN, Stehman FB, et al. Cisplatin, radiation, and adjuvant hysterectomy compared with radiation and adjuvant hysterectomy for bulky stage IB cervical carcinoma. N Engl J Med 1999;340:1154–61.
9. Lhomme C, Fumoleau P, Fargeot P, et al. Results of the European Organization for Research and Treatment of Cancer/Early Clinical Studies Group phase II trial of first-line irinotecan in patients with advanced or recurrent squamous cell carcinoma of the cervix. J Clin Oncol 1999;17:3136–42.

10. Rose PG, Cha SD, Tak WK, et al. Radiation therapy for surgically proven para-aortic node metastases in endometrial carcinoma. Int J Radiat Oncol Biol Phys 1992;24:229–35.

11. Gibbons S, Martinez A, Schray M, et al. Adjuvant whole abdomino-pelvic irradiation for high risk endometrial carcinoma. Int J Radiat Oncol Biol Phys 1991;21:1019–24.

12. Stock RG, Chen AS, Flickinger JC, et al. Node-positive cervical cancer: impact of pelvic irradiation and patterns of failure. Int J Radiat Oncol Biol Phys 1995;31:31–6.

13. Ferreira PR, Braga-Filho A, Barletta A, et al. Radiation therapy alone in stage III-B cancer of the uterine cervix—a 17 year old experience in south Brazil. Int J Radiat Oncol Biol Phys 1999;45:441–6.

14. Implementation of intensity modulated radiation therapy for patients with carcinoma of the cervix. Panel 6. Presented at the 45th Annual Meeting of the American Society for Therapeutic Radiology and Oncology (ASTRO); 2003 Oct 20; Salt Lake City, UT.

15. Mundt AJ, Roeske JC, Lujan JC. IMRT in gynecologic malignancies. Med Dosim 2002;27:131–6.

16. Roeske JC, Lujan A, Rotmensch J, et al. Intensity-modulated whole pelvis radiation therapy in patients with gynecologic malignancies. Int J Radiat Oncol Biol Phys 2000;48:1613–21.

17. Adli M, Mayr NA, Kaiser HS, et al. Does prone positioning reduce bowel dose in pelvic radiation with intensity modulated radiation therapy (IMRT) for gynecologic cancer. Int J Radiat Oncol Biol Phys 2003;57:230–8.

18. Ahamad A, D'Souza W, Salehpour M, et al. Intensity modulated radiation therapy (IMRT) for post-hysterectomy pelvic radiation: selection of patients and planning target volume (PTV) [abstract]. Int J Radiat Oncol Biol Phys 2002;54:42.

19. Chen Q, Izadifar N, King S, et al. Comparison of IMRT with 3-D CRT for gynecologic malignancies [abstract]. Int J Radiat Oncol Biol Phys 2001;51:332.

20. Heron DE, Gerszten K, Selvaraj RN, et al. Conventional 3D conformal versus intensity-modulated radiotherapy for the adjuvant treatment of gynecologic malignancies: a comparative dosimetric study of dose-volume histograms. Gynecol Oncol 2003;91:39–45.

21. Portelance L, Chao KS, Grigsby PW, et al. Intensity-modulated radiation therapy (IMRT) reduces small bowel, rectum, and bladder doses in patients with cervical cancer receiving pelvic and para-aortic irradiation. Int J Radiat Oncol Biol Phys 2001;51:261–6.

22. Hong L, Alektiar K, Chui C, et al. IMRT of large fields: whole abdomen irradiation. Int J Radiat Oncol Biol Phys 2002;54:278–89.

23. Duthoy W, De Gersem W, Vergote K, et al. Whole abdomino-pelvic radiotherapy (WAPRT) using intensity-modulated arc therapy (IMAT): first clinical experience. Int J Radiat Oncol Biol Phys 2003;57:1019–32.

24. Garofalo M, Lujan AE, Roeske JC, et al. Intensity-modulated radiation therapy in the treatment of vulvar carcinoma. Presented at the 88th Annual Meeting of the Radiologic Society of North America; November 2002; Chicago, IL.

25. Mundt AJ, Roeske JC, Lujan AE, et al. Initial clinical experience with intensity modulated whole-pelvis radiation therapy in women with gynecologic malignancies. Gynecol Oncol 2001;82:456–63.

26. Mundt AJ, Lujan AE, Rotmensch J, et al. Intensity-modulated whole pelvic radiotherapy in women with gynecologic malignancies. Int J Radiat Oncol Biol Phys 2002;52:1330–7.

27. Mundt AJ, Mell LK, Roeske JC. Preliminary analysis of chronic gastrointestinal toxicity in gynecology patients treated with intensity-modulated whole pelvic radiation therapy. Int J Radiat Oncol Biol Phys 2003;56:1354–60.

28. Brixey CJ, Roeske JC, Lujan AE, et al. Impact of intensity modulated radiation therapy on acute hematologic toxicity in women with gynecologic malignancies. Int J Radiat Oncol Biol Phys 2002;54:1388–96.

29. Kavanagh B, Schefter TE, Wu Q, et al. Clinical application of intensity modulated radiotherapy for locally advanced cervical cancer. Semin Radiat Oncol 2002;12:260–71.

30. Schefter TE, Kavanagh BD, Wu Q, et al. Technical considerations in the application of intensity-modulated radiotherapy as a concomitant integrated boost for locally advanced cervix cancer. Med Dosim 2002;27:177–84.

31. Mundt AJ, Roeske JC. Could intensity modulated radiation therapy (IMRT) replace brachytherapy in the treatment of cervical cancer? Brachyther J 2002;1:195–6.

32. Alektiar K. Could intensity modulated radiation therapy (IMRT) replace brachytherapy in the treatment of cervical cancer? Brachyther J 2002;1:194–5.

33. Roeske JC, Mundt AJ. A feasibility study of IMRT for the treatment of cervical cancer patients unable to receive intracavitary brachytherapy. Med Phys 2000;27:1382.

34. Low DA, Grigsby PW, Dempsey JF, et al. Applicator-guided intensity-modulated radiation therapy. Int J Radiat Oncol Biol Phys 2002;52:1400–6.

35. Mutic S, Malyapa RS, Grigsby PW, et al. PET-guided IMRT for cervical carcinoma with positive para-aortic lymph nodes— a dose escalation treatment planning study. Int J Radiat Oncol Biol Phys 2003;55:28–35.

36. Lujan AE, Mundt AJ, Roeske JC. Sequential versus simultaneous boost in the female pelvis using intensity modulated radiation therapy. Presented at the 43rd Annual Meeting of the American Association of Physicists in Medicine; July 2001; Salt Lake City, UT.

37. Haslam JJ, Lujan AE, Mundt AJ, et al. Setup errors in patients treated with intensity modulated whole pelvic radiation therapy for gynecological malignancies. Med Dosim. In press.

38. Miller TR, Grigsby PW. Measurement of tumor volume by PET to evaluate prognosis in patients with advanced cervical cancer treated by radiation therapy. Int J Radiat Oncol Biol Phys 2002;53:353–9.

39. Wagenaar HC, Trimbos JB, Postema S, et al. Tumor diameter and volume assessed by magnetic resonance imaging in the prediction of outcome for invasive cervical cancer. Gynecol Oncol 2001;82:474–82.

40. Chao KS, Lin M. Lymphangiogram-assisted lymph node target delineation for patients with gynecologic malignancies. Int J Radiat Oncol Biol Phys 2002;54:1147–52.

41. Harisinghami MG, Barentsz J, Hahn PF, et al. Noninvasive detection of clinically occult lymph-node metastases in prostate cancer. N Engl J Med 2003;348:2491–9.

42. Lujan AE, Mundt AJ, Yamada D et al. Intensity-modulated radiotherapy as a means of reducing dose to bone marrow in gynecologic patients receiving whole pelvic radiotherapy. Int J Radiat Oncol Biol Phys 2003;57:516–21.

43. Malyapa RS, Chao KS, Williamson JF, et al. Pelvic organ motion and displacement during radiation therapy in patients with gynecological malignancies—a prospective study using serial CT imaging during external beam radiotherapy [abstract]. Int J Radiat Oncol Biol Phys 2001;51:218.

44. Buchali A, Koswig S, Dinges S, et al. Impact of the filling status of the bladder and rectum on their integral dose distribution and the movement of the uterus in the treatment planning of gynaecological cancer. Radiother Oncol 1999;52:29–34.

45. Huh SJ, Park W, Han Y. Interfractional variation in position of the uterus during radical radiotherapy for cervical cancer. Radiother Oncol 2004;71:73–9.

46. Pugachev A, Xing L. Computer-assisted selection of coplanar beam orientations in intensity modulated radiation therapy. Phys Med Biol 2001;46:2467–76.

47. Haslam JJ, Bonta DV, Lujan AE. et al. Comparison of dose calculated by an intensity modulated radiotherapy planning system and an independent monitor unit verification program. J Appl Clin Med Phys 2003;4:224–30.

48. Huh SJ, Kang MK, Han Y. Small bowel displacement system-assisted intensity-modulated radiotherapy for cervical cancer. Gynecol Oncol 2004;93:400–6.

49. Gilroy JS, Amdur RJ, Louis DA, et al. Irradiating the inguinal nodes without breaking a leg [abstract]. Int J Radiat Oncol Biol Phys 2002;54:68.

50. Esthappan J, Mutic S, Malyapa RS, et al. Treatment planning guidelines regarding the use of CT/PET-guided IMRT for cervical carcinoma with positive paraaortic lymph nodes. Int J Radiat Oncol Biol Phys 2004;58:1289–97.

51. Wahab SH, Malyapa RS, Mutic S, et al. A treatment planning study comparing HDR and AGIMRT for cervical cancer. Med Phys 2004;31:734–43.

52. Zelefsky MJ, Fuks Z, Hunt M, et al. High-dose intensity modulated radiation therapy for prostate cancer: early toxicity and biochemical outcome in 772 patients. Int J Radiat Oncol Biol Phys 2002;53:111–6.

53. Roeske JC, Bonta D, Lujan AE, et al. Dose volume histogram analysis of acute gastrointestinal toxicity in gynecologic patients undergoing intensity modulated whole pelvic radiation therapy. Radiother Oncol 2003;69:201–7.

54. Roeske JC, Lujan AE, Reba RC, et al. Incorporation of SPECT bone marrow imaging into intensity modulated whole-pelvic radiation therapy treatment planning for gynecologic malignancies. Radiother Oncol. In press.

55. Knab B, Mehta N, Roeske JC, et al. Outcome of endometrial cancer patients treated with adjuvant intensity modulated pelvic radiation therapy. Presented at the 46th Annual Meeting of the American Society for Therapeutic Radiology and Oncology; 2004 Oct 6–7; Atlanta, GA.

56. Kochanski JD, Roeske JC, Mell LK, et al. Outcome of FIGO stage I-II cervical cancer patients treated with intensity modulated pelvic radiation therapy. Presented at the 40th Annual Meeting of the American Society of Clinical Oncology; 2004 Jun 5–8; New Orleans, LA.

57. Hall E, Wuu CS. Radiation-induced second cancer: the impact of 3D-CRT and IMRT. Int J Radiat Oncol Biol Phys 2003;56:83–8.

58. Pickett B, Vigneault E, Kurhanewicz J, et al. Static field intensity modulation to treat a dominant intra-prostatic lesion to 90 Gy compared to seven field 3-dimensional radiotherapy. Int J Radiat Oncol Biol Phys 1999;44:921–9.

59. Chao KS, Bosch WR, Mutic S, et al. A novel approach to overcome hypoxic tumor resistance: Cu-ATSM-guided intensity-modulated radiation therapy. Int J Radiat Oncol Biol Phys 2001;49:1171–82.

60. Mell LK, Fyles AW, Small W, et al. Adjuvant intensity modulated pelvic radiation therapy in gynecologic malignancies: survey of the gynecologic IMRT Working Group. Presented at the 46th Annual Meeting of the American Society for Therapeutic Radiology and Oncology; 2004 Oct 3–7; Atlanta, GA.

CERVICAL CANCER

CASE STUDY

TRACEY E. SCHEFTER, MD, BRIAN D. KAVANAGH, MD

Patient History

A 44-year-old female presented with vaginal bleeding. Physical examination revealed a 6 cm cervical tumor with bilateral parametrial extension. Biopsy was consistent with squamous cell carcinoma. A computed tomography (CT) scan revealed pathologically enlarged pelvic and para-aortic lymph nodes. Her cancer was thus staged as clinical stage IVb.

Definitive treatment with a combination of radiation therapy (RT) and concurrent chemotherapy was recommended. In an effort to increase the daily fractional dose to gross nodal disease, conform the high-dose region to areas at risk of microscopic disease, and maintain conventional overall treatment times, intensity-modulated radiation therapy (IMRT), using a concomitant boost approach, was administered to this patient.

Simulation

The patient was simulated in the prone position. A customized body mold was fabricated to facilitate patient immobilization (Figure 23.1-1). The prone position (with

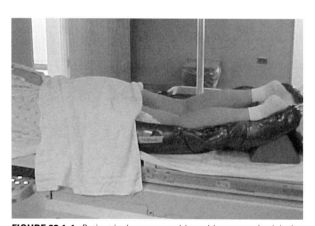

FIGURE 23.1-1. Patient in the prone position with a customized device to immobilize the lower extremities. (To view a color version of this image, please refer to the CD-ROM.)

or without a belly board) has been shown to reduce the dose to the small bowel regardless of whether IMRT or conventional RT treatment is used.[1] One caveat is that the prone position may be less comfortable and not as reproducible for obese patients. In addition, the longer daily treatment times with IMRT make intrafractional patient movement and resultant target motion an important factor.

Prior to simulation, the patient was instructed to have a modestly full bladder (drink two 8 ounce glasses of water within 1 hour of simulation and each daily treatment) and an empty rectum. Dilute (to minimize CT artifacts) bladder contrast was used to identify the bladder-tumor interface. A planning CT (FXi, General Electric Corporation, Waukesha, WI) scan was obtained using a 3 mm slice thickness extending from the T12 vertebral body to the femoral lesser trochanters. The data set was then transferred to the *FOCUS* (Computerized Medical Systems, Inc., St. Louis, MO) planning workstation.

Target and Tissue Delineation

Several target volumes required delineation and differential dose delivery. The largest were the planning target volumes (PTVs) for microscopic disease in the para-aortic lymph nodes and pelvis (PTV$_{PAN}$ + PTV$_{pelvis}$). These targets encompassed the para-aortic, common iliac, internal, and external iliac nodal regions, potential sites of microscopic local extension of primary tumor, plus a margin for positional uncertainty. Lymphangiogram-assisted target analysis for gynecologic malignancies has suggested the need for a 1 to 2 cm margin around corresponding vessels to define the clinical target volume (CTV) for nodal disease.[2] However, there are currently no widely accepted consensus guidelines for defining image-based CTVs and PTVs in this setting. Careful follow-up of treated patients, ideally within the context of formal clinical protocols, will help identify the frequency of marginal failures that might result from inaccurate estimations of the CTV and PTV.

In this patient, the gross nodal target volume (GTV$_{node}$) and gross primary cervical target volume (GTV$_{cervix}$) were contained within the PTV$_{PAN}$ + PTV$_{pelvis}$. The GTV$_{node}$ and GTV$_{cervix}$ were considered equivalent to the CTV$_{node}$ and CTV$_{cervix}$, respectively. These volumes were then expanded into a PTV$_{node}$ and PTV$_{cervix}$. The margin on the CTV$_{cervix}$ (GTV$_{cervix}$) used to define the PTV$_{cervix}$ accounts for variability in the position of the CTV$_{cervix}$ owing to set-up errors, variations in bladder and rectal filling, and shape deformations of the CTV$_{cervix}$ itself. In a small cohort of patients, margins as small as 5 mm appeared to be adequate to account for the net effect of all of these factors, but validation in a larger cohort of patients is required.[3] Representative axial, sagittal, and coronal sections illustrating these target volumes are shown in Figure 23.1-2.

Treatment Planning

The concomitant boost approach used in this patient is a form of accelerated fractionation. Gross disease is boosted during the course of conventionally fractionated daily treatment (to the entire region at risk of occult microscopic disease) by the use of a second daily fraction targeting only the gross disease. Conventional external beam RT techniques have been used to investigate concomitant boost RT in locally advanced cervical cancer, and a favorable effect on local control was observed at the expense of increased normal tissue toxicity.[4]

By permitting dose distributions in which electively treated volumes receive a standard dose per fraction while gross disease is simultaneously treated with a larger dose per fraction, IMRT can yield radiobiologic dose intensification by integrating the boost dose within a shorter overall treatment time. More conformal coverage of electively irradiated volumes using IMRT can also result in greater normal tissue sparing.[5] In an ongoing phase I-II study at the University of Colorado, IMRT using a concomitant boost approach is being evaluated in locally advanced cervix cancer. The hypothesis is based on two premises: intensifying the prebrachytherapy external beam component of treatment may yield improved tumor regression, thus allowing the residual gross primary cervical disease

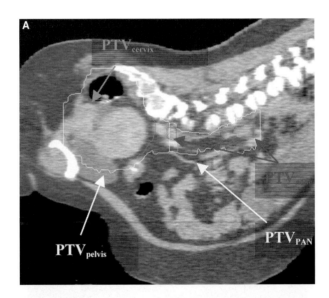

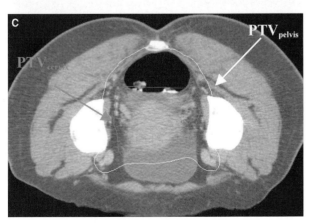

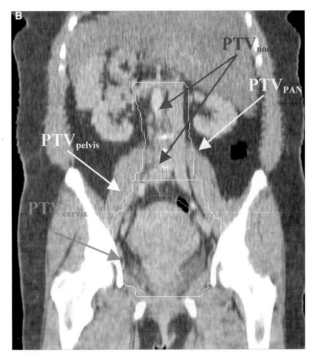

FIGURE 23.1-2. (*A*) Sagittal planning computed tomography (CT) reconstruction of the patient in the prone position (with a belly board). PTV$_{pelvis}$ is the microscopic planning target volume for the pelvis. PTV$_{PAN}$ is the microscopic planning target volume for the para-aortic lymph node region. PTV$_{cervix}$ is the planning target volume for the gross primary cervical tumor. PTV$_{node}$ is the planning target volume for the gross nodal disease in the para-aortic region and the pelvis. (*B*) Coronal CT reconstruction of the paraortic and pelvic regions. (*C*) Axial CT slice at the level of the primary tumor. (To view a color version of this image, please refer to the CD-ROM.). ***Continued on the next page.***

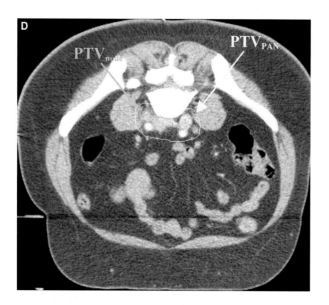

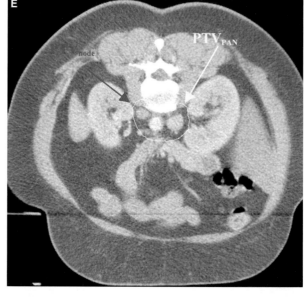

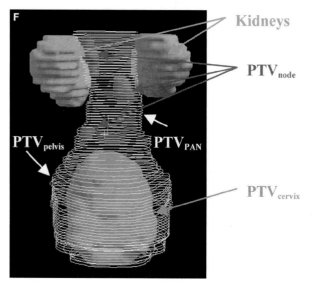

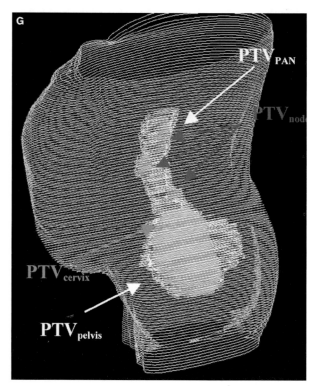

FIGURE 23.1-2. *Continued* (*D*) Axial CT slice in the upper pelvis. (*E*) Axial CT slice at the level of the kidney. (*F*) Three-dimensional rendering illustrating the proximity of the gross lymph nodes to the kidneys. (*G*) Three-dimensional rendering of target volumes and patient external surface. (To view a color version of this image, please refer to the CD-ROM.)

to be encompassed within a higher brachytherapy isodose volume, and increasing the daily fraction size to the primary disease, which might magnify the radiosensitization effects. It remains unclear whether concurrent cisplatin-based chemotherapy provides only additive cytotoxicity or exerts truly synergistic effects; if true radiosensitization is achieved, the magnitude of this effect is likely fraction size dependent.[3]

Commercial planning systems optimize beam intensity profiles but not the beam number, energy, or orienta-

tion. Consequently, either a class solution-type beam arrangement or an individually tailored beam orientation must be tried. The plans generated for this patient included five, seven, and nine coplanar and noncoplanar beams. Both 10 and 15 MV photon beams were considered for this case.

Inverse planning constraints that resulted in the most conformal IMRT plan in this patient are shown in Table 23.1-1. Represented is the final result after iterative changes to the number, energy, and orientation of fields, as well as

TABLE 23.1-1. Input Parameters

Overlap Structure	On/Off	Target, Yes/No	Minimum Dose, cGy	Maximum Dose, cGy	Goal Dose, cGy	Importance Weighting, 1–100	Priority
PTV$_{node}$	On	Yes	5,750	6,500	6,500	100	1
IMRT-node	On	Yes	4,500	5,750	4,600	100	4
PTV$_{cervix}$	On	Yes	5,000	5,750	5,300	100	2
Patient	On	No		0		5	19
Small bowel	On	No		0		5	12
IMRT-R kidney	On	No		0		20	5
IMRT-L kidney	On	No		0		5	7
Bladder	Off	No				100	12
Rectum	Off	No				100	13
PTV$_{pelvis}$	Off	Yes		5,500	4,500	100	10
PTV$_{PAN}$	Off	Yes		5,500	4,500	100	11
R kidney	Off	No				20	8
L kidney	Off	No				5	9
Bone marrow	Off	No				100	17
Spinal cord	Off	No				100	18
IMRT-PTV$_{cervix}$	Off	Yes		5,500		100	3

IMRT = intensity-modulated radiation therapy; L = left; PTV = planning target volume: R = right.

the optimization constraints. IMRT-PTV$_{cervix}$ and IMRT-PTV$_{node}$ are modified volumes derived by expanding the PTV$_{cervix}$ and PTV$_{node}$ by 5 mm in all directions. The extra few millimeters added to each true PTV are required by the planning system to ensure that when the final dose distribution is calculated, the true PTV is encompassed by the prescription dose.

The *FOCUS* planning system requires a priority rank for overlap regions in addition to the importance weighting. PTV$_{cervix}$ and PTV$_{node}$ are contained entirely within the PTV$_{pelvis}$ and PTV$_{PAN}$ (electively irradiated volumes); therefore, PTV$_{node}$ was given the highest overlap priority (1, highest goal dose of 5,750 cGy in 25 fractions, 2.3 Gy/fraction) and PTV$_{cervix}$ the second highest priority (2, goal dose of 5,000 cGy in 25 fractions, 2 Gy/fraction). These priority goals were used to deliver the different prescription doses to these volumes. The electively irradiated volumes, PTV$_{PAN}$ and PTV$_{pelvis}$, were given lower overlap priorities (10 and 11, respectively), and the goal dose was 4,500 cGy in 25 fractions (1.8 Gy/fraction).

Obtaining a deliverable plan from optimized intensity maps requires a process of clinical optimization in which a number of factors are selected by dosimetrists and physicians, each influencing both the conformity and the complexity of the plan.[6] With the treatment planning system used, the minimum distance between multileaf collimator (MLC) leaves can be varied between 0.5 and 3 cm (2 cm was selected for this case). MLC- and compensator-based modulation are the two options for static IMRT (MLC modulation was selected for this case). The number of intensity levels can vary between 5 and 25 (10 for this case). Selecting a high number of intensity levels and low minimum distance between MLC leaves improves the confor-

mity but also increases the complexity and number of segments. The net effect is an increase in total treatment time and resultant increased susceptibility to intrafractional movement and geographic miss. Therefore, any improvement in dose conformity and sharpness of dose gradients achieved with a larger number of segments must be weighed against the practical limitations associated with prolongation of daily treatment time.

Among the beam arrangements evaluated, the optimal deliverable "step-and-shoot" MLC-modulated plan resulted from five equally spaced coplanar 15 MV fields (0-, 72-, 144-, 216-, and 288-degree gantry angles) with an average of 14 segments per field. Representative axial, sagittal, and coronal isodose distributions are shown in Figure 23.1-3. Dose-volume histograms for all targets and organs at risk are shown in Figure 23.1-4.

Treatment Delivery and Quality Assurance

The optimized IMRT plan for this patient was delivered on an Elekta Precise linear accelerator (Elekta Inc., Norcross, GA) equipped with an 80-leaf MLC. The daily treatment time was approximately 15 to 20 minutes.

Prior to the initiation of treatment, extensive quality assurance checks were performed. Our process consists of calculating and measuring the dose to a phantom based on the individual beam profiles used for this patient (Figure 23.1-5). The ion chamber reading and dose profile were acquired simultaneously. The measured dose profile was compared with the calculated dose profile (both at the same depth) using the *RIT* software (Radiological Imaging Technology,

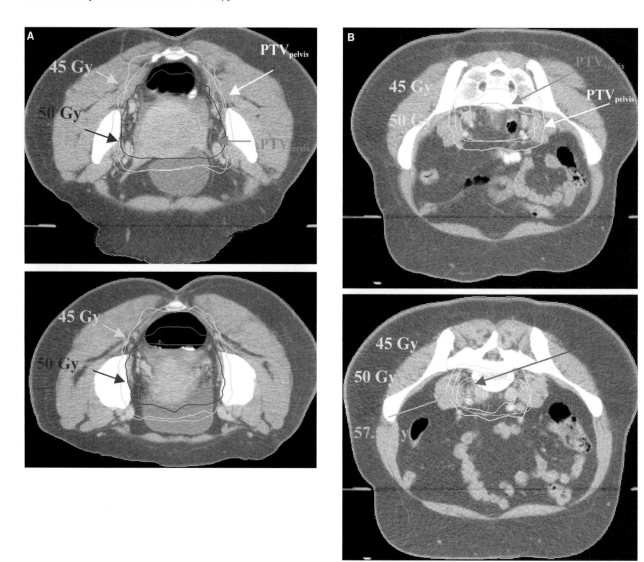

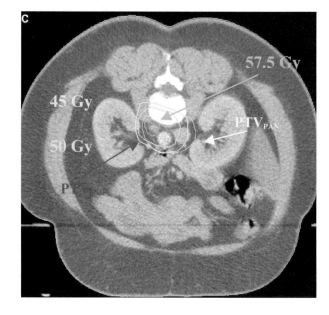

FIGURE 23.1-3. (*A*) Axial computed tomography (CT) slices at the lower and upper levels of the cervical tumor with superimposed isodose distribututions (color scheme same as that of Figure 23.1-2). (*B*) Axial CT slices at the level of the upper pelvis with superimposed isodose distributions. (*C*) Axial CT image at the level of the kidney with superimposed isodose distributions. PTV = planning target volume. (To view a color version of this image, please refer to the CD-ROM.) ***Continued on the next page.***

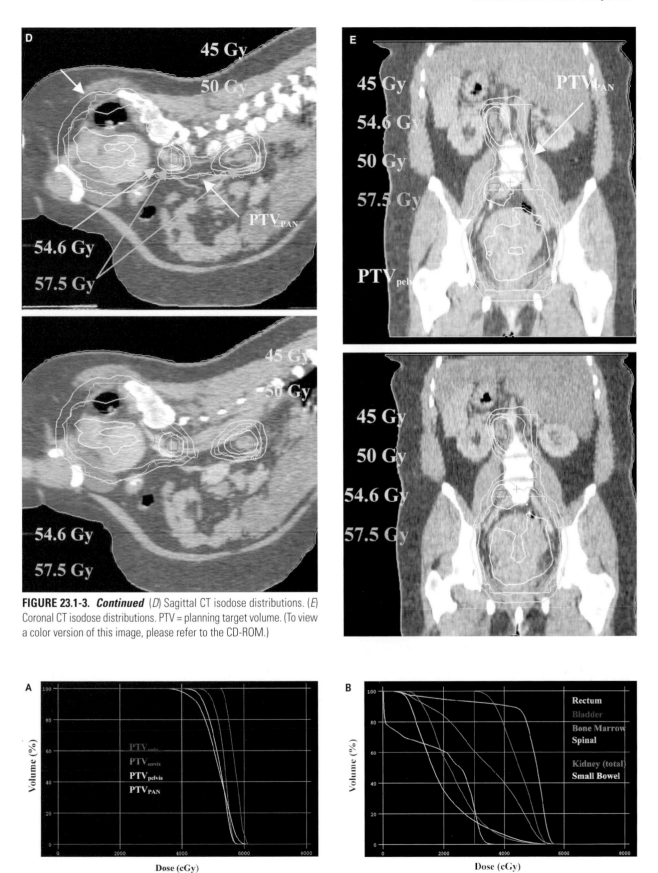

FIGURE 23.1-3. *Continued* (*D*) Sagittal CT isodose distributions. (*E*) Coronal CT isodose distributions. PTV = planning target volume. (To view a color version of this image, please refer to the CD-ROM.)

FIGURE 23.1-4. Dose-volume histograms of the planning target volume (PTV) and organs at risk in the treated patient. (*A*) Targets; (*B*) organs at risk. (To view a color version of this image, please refer to the CD-ROM.)

Inc., Colorado Springs, CO). Our acceptance criteria are that measured and calculated dose profiles must be within 2 to 5 mm and that ion chamber measurements and calculated point doses must agree within ± 5%. If the measured values exceed these tolerances, the process is repeated for the treatment fields that are out of acceptance. The IMRT segments for those treatment fields are analyzed, and a new location for the interest points in a low dose gradient region is determined. A region of low dose gradient is preferred owing to the size of the ion chamber (0.125 cc). In this particular case, all fields satisfied the established criteria.

Weekly orthogonal portal images were obtained throughout the course of treatment. Two planning CT scans were obtained during the 5-week course of IMRT to ensure no significant internal movement of the targets, which is especially relevant when escalating the daily dose to an intact primary cervical tumor.

Clinical Outcome

Treatment was well tolerated by the patient, without any unplanned treatment breaks. At a follow-up period of 12 months, her disease remained well controlled, with the enlarged lymph nodes exhibiting a complete response.

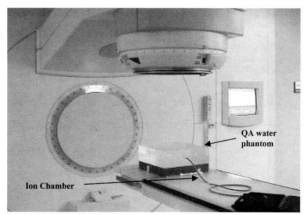

FIGURE 23.1-5. Quality assurance (QA) water phantom setup. (To view a color version of this image, please refer to the CD-ROM.)

Moreover, the patient has not developed any significant late genitourinary or late gastrointestinal toxicity.

Preliminary clinical results using a concomitant boost approach were presented earlier.[3,6] In a cohort of seven locally advanced, metastatic, or recurrent cervical cancer patients,[3] three received RT to the para-aortic lymph nodes; the remainder received pelvic RT. All received concomitant boost IMRT, followed in five patients by intracavitary brachytherapy, and in one patient by permanent seed implantation. Six patients received weekly cisplatin (40 mg/m[2]). In-field complete responses were observed in all patients. At three months, four were alive with no evidence of disease, and two were alive with disease. Two with grade 3 toxicity experienced chemotherapy treatment delays. Of the remaining five patients, four developed grade 2 upper gastrointestinal and one had grade 2 lower gastrointestinal toxicity. One patient had grade 2 and two of seven patients had grade 1 genitourinary toxicity.

References

1. Mustafa A, Mayr NA, Kaiser HS, et al. Does prone positioning reduce small bowel dose in pelvic radiation with intensity-modulated radiotherapy for gynecologic cancer? Int J Radiat Oncol Biol Phys 2003;57:230–8.
2. Chao CKS, Lin M. Lymphangiogram-assisted lymph node target delineation for patients with gynecologic malignancies. Int J Radiat Oncol Biol Phys 2002;54:1147–52.
3. Kavanagh BD, Schefter TE, Wu Q, et al. Clinical application of intensity-modulated radiotherapy for locally advanced cervical cancer. Semin Radiat Oncol 2002;12:260–71.
4. Kavanagh BD, Gieschen HL, Schmidt-Ullrich RK, et al. A pilot study of concomitant boost accelerated superfractionated radiotherapy for stage III cancer of the uterine cervix. Int J Radiat Oncol Biol Phys 1997;38:561–8.
5. Mundt AJ, Mell LK, Roeske JC. Preliminary analysis of chronic gastrointestinal toxicity in gynecology patients treated with intensity-modulated whole pelvic radiation therapy. Int J Radiat Oncol Biol Phys 2003;56:1354–60.
6. Schefter TE, Kavanagh BK, Wu Q, et al. Technical considerations in the application of intensity-modulated radiotherapy as a concomitant integrated boost for locally advanced cervix cancer. Med Dosim 2002;27:177–84.

ENDOMETRIAL CANCER

CASE STUDY

ANUJA JHINGRAN, MD, MOHAMMAD SALEHPOUR, PHD, BROOKE BROOKS, RT, CMD

Patient History

A 64-year-old female presented with a 1-year history of postmenopausal bleeding. Ultrasonography demonstrated a 2.8 cm thickened endometrial stripe. An endometrial biopsy was performed and was positive for well-differentiated endometrial adenocarcinoma. A computed tomography (CT) scan demonstrated an enlarged and irregular uterus with heterogeneous material in the uterine cavity and subcentimeter pelvic lymph nodes.

The patient subsequently underwent a total abdominal hysterectomy and bilateral salpingo-oophorectomy, assessment of peritoneal cytology, and lymph node sampling. The pathology was consistent with a grade 2 papillary adenocarcinoma of the endometrium. The depth of invasion was 22 mm of a total 40 mm myometrial thickness. Focal vascular invasion and endocervical stromal involvement were noted. Multiple pelvic lymph nodes were sampled, and all were negative. In addition, peritoneal cytology and the omentum were negative. The patient was thus staged as having International Federation of Gynecology and Obstetrics (FIGO) stage IIB cancer.

Adjuvant pelvic radiation therapy (RT) was recommended. Of note, the patient had a past medical history of irritable bowel syndrome, diabetes, and hypertension. In addition, she had had one prior abdominal surgery. Intensity-modulated radiation therapy (IMRT) was used in this patient to treat the vaginal cuff and pelvic lymph nodes to reduce the volume of normal tissues irradiated and thus the risk of treatment-related sequelae.

Simulation

The patient was simulated in the supine position with her arms overhead. Two separate Vac-Lok immobilization devices (MED-TEC, Orange City, IA) were fabricated: one for the legs as a cradle and one for the upper body (Figure 23.2-1). Planning CT scans were performed on a wide-bore CT simulator (AcQSim, Philips Medical Systems,

Andover, MA). A "mini"-scan was initially performed to place the isocenter (midline at the level of the top of the femoral heads). The patient was then scanned from the top of the L2 vertebral body to 1.0 cm below the vulva with a full bladder (the patient was instructed to drink four 8 oz glasses of water 15 to 30 minutes prior to simulation). She was then asked to empty her bladder and was rescanned. Contrast was not administered. For all scans, a slice thickness of 3 mm was used.

Target and Tissue Delineation

Target and normal tissues were delineated on each axial slice of the planning CT scan. Two separate clinical target volumes (CTVs) were delineated. The CTV consisted of the vagina and parametrial tissues; CTV$_{nodes}$ consisted of the pelvic lymph nodes, including the obturator, external iliac, internal iliac, and common iliac (up to the top of L5). In the case presented here, because the tumor involved the cervix, sacral nodes (to S2) were also included in the

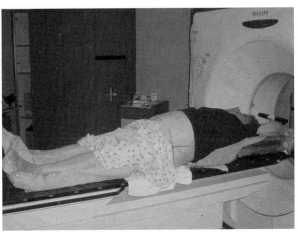

FIGURE 23.2-1. Patient immobilized in the treatment position with customized upper and lower Vac-Lok devices. (To view a color version of this image, please refer to the CD-ROM.)

CTV_{nodes}. If the cervix is not involved, we do not include the sacral nodes in patients with endometrial cancer undergoing IMRT. Since the patient was treated following surgery, no gross tumor volume was delineated.

An integrated tumor volume (ITV) of the vagina and parametrial tissues was also delineated. The ITV was derived by fusing the empty and full bladder planning CT scans. The ITV was drawn on the full bladder scan encompassing the vaginal and parametrial tissue volumes on both scans. However, CTV_{nodes} was delineated only on the full bladder scan because the position of the lymph node regions does not change with bladder and rectal filling. It was drawn based on the pelvic vessel and surgical clips. A 0.5 cm margin was placed anteriorly, superiorly, and inferiorly around the vessels and surgical clips. No margin was placed on the bone.

Normal tissues delineated included the bladder, small bowel, rectum, and femoral heads. The rectum was outlined up to the sigmoid flexure. The small bowel included the entire peritoneal cavity (not individual loops of bowel) up to L3. The normal tissues were outlined on the full bladder CT scan because the patient was treated with a full bladder (see below).

Planning target volumes (PTVs) were generated by expanding the ITV and the CTV_{nodes} in three dimensions by 5 mm to create PTV_{ITV} and PTV_{nodes}, respectively. In addition, margins were placed around the bladder, rectum, small bowel, and femoral heads. Table 23.2-1 summarizes the expansion margins used in this patient. Figure 23.2-2 illustrates the target and normal tissues delineated in this patient.

Treatment Planning

IMRT treatment planning was performed using *CORVUS* inverse planning software, version 5.0 (North American Scientific, NOMOS Radiation Oncology Division, Cranberry Township, PA.). The prescription dose to both the PTV_{ITV} and the PTV_{nodes} in this patient was 50 Gy in 27 fractions (185 cGy/d). The input parameters used in this patient are summarized in Table 23.2-2. The final plan delivered a minimum of 98% of the prescribed dose to the PTV.

TABLE 23.2-1. Expansion Margins for the Targets and Normal Tissues

Name	Expansion (mm)					
	Anterior	Posterior	Right	Left	Superior	Inferior
ITV	5.0	5.0	5.0	5.0	5.0	5.0
CTV_{nodes}	5.0	5.0	5.0	5.0	5.0	5.0
Bladder	30.0	32.0	5.0	5.0	30.0	10.0
Femoral heads	5.0	5.0	5.0	5.0	5.0	5.0
Rectum	8.0	8.0	2.0	2.0	10.0	10.0
Small bowel	20.0	30.0	20.0	20.0	20.0	20.0

CTV = clinical target volume; ITV = integrated tumor volume.

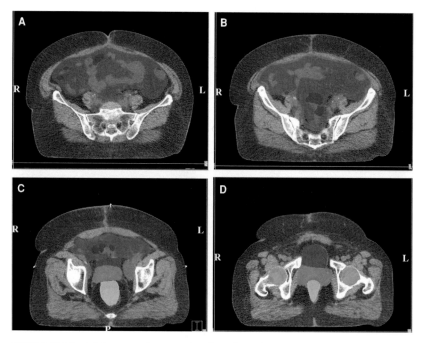

FIGURE 23.2-2. Axial computed tomography slices illustrating the planning treatment volume (PTV)_{nodes} (*brown*), integrated tumor volume (*red*), small bowel (*light blue*), bladder (*dark blue*), rectum (*green*), and femoral heads (*dark green*) in the upper (*A*), mid-upper (*B*), mid-lower (*C*), and lower (*D*) pelvis. (To view a color version of this image, please refer to the CD-ROM.)

TABLE 23.2-2. Intensity-Modulated Radiation Therapy Input Parameters

Target	Goal, Gy	Volume below Goal, %	Minimum Dose, Gy	Maximum Dose, Gy
PTV$_{ITV}$	50.0	2	48.0	52.0
PTV$_{nodes}$	50.0	2	48.0	51.0
Bladder	45.0	15	10.0	51.0
Femoral heads	40.0	40	5.0	45.0
Rectum	43.0	15	15.0	48.0
Small bowel	40.0	8	5.0	50.0

ITV = integrated tumor volume; PTV = planning target volume.

Eight coplanar, 6 MV treatment beams were used in this patient. The beam angles were 210, 240, 275, 340, 20, 85, 120, and 150 degrees. One thousand twenty beam segments were used. The source to surface distance varied from 76.3 to 84.5 cm depending on the beam angle. The resultant isodose distributions overlaid on axial CT slices are shown in Figure 23.2-3. Dose-volume histograms of the target and normal tissues are shown in Figure 23.2-4.

Treatment Delivery and Quality Assurance

Treatment was delivered in the "step-and-shoot" mode on a Varian 2100CD linear accelerator (Varian Medical Systems, Palo Alto, CA) equipped with the integrated Millennium 120-leaf multileaf collimator. On average, treatment took approximately 30 minutes per day. As noted above, the patient was treated everyday with a full bladder. She was given written instructions to drink four 8 oz glasses of fluid 20 to 30 minutes prior to their treatment. These instructions were reinforced at each doctor visit.

Prior to treatment, dose computations from the treatment planning system were verified using both ion chamber and film measurements in phantoms. A Wellhofer CC04 (Scanditronix/Wellhoffer Inc., Bartlett, TN) ion chamber with a sensitive volume of 0.04 cc was used to perform absolute dose measurements in a specially sealed water phantom. This water phantom allows for 10 different ion chamber positions. The radiation intensity maps from the patient treatment plan were applied to this water phantom in the treatment planning computer by substituting the phantom scan for that of the patient. The dose to each of

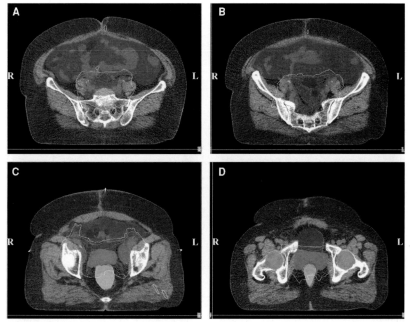

FIGURE 23.2-3. Isodose distributions overlaid on the axial computed tomography slices in the upper (*A*), mid-upper (*B*), mid-lower (*C*), and lower (*D*) pelvis: 40 Gy (*yellow*), 45 Gy (*orange*), 50 Gy (*magenta*), and 54 Gy (*red*). Targets and normal tissues shown include the planning target volume (PTV)$_{nodes}$ (*brown*), integrated tumor volume (*red*), small bowel (*light blue*), bladder (*dark blue*), rectum (*green*), and femoral heads (*dark green*). (To view a color version of this image, please refer to the CD-ROM.)

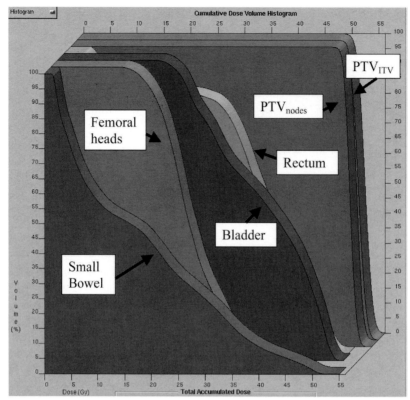

FIGURE 23.2-4. Dose-volume histograms of the PTV$_{ITV}$, PTV$_{nodes}$, and normal tissues (bladder, rectum, small bowel, and femoral heads). (To view a color version of this image, please refer to the CD-ROM.)

the ion chamber positions was then calculated. The phantom was irradiated according to the patient treatment plan. The measured dose was compared with the calculated dose at the specific ion chamber location. A maximum discrepancy of 5% is allowed, although no deviations above 3% were observed in this patient.

The relative dose distribution was verified using a plastic phantom (measuring 40 × 40 × 20 cm^3) and radiographic films (EDR2, Eastman Kodak Corporation, Rochester, NY). Similar to the ionization chamber measurements, the patient geometry was replaced with that of the phantom in the treatment planning system. Isodose distributions were then calculated using the patient fluence maps. The film was then inserted in predetermined planes in the phantom, and the patient's treatment was delivered. A calibration film was also exposed using eight unique and separated square segments of the multileaf collimator with different intensity levels. The calibration film and planer in-phantom films were scanned using a Vidar 16-bit film dosimetry scanner (Vidar Systems Corporation, Herndon, VA). The resulting film images were analyzed using our in-house film dosimetry system (DoseLab). DoseLab will report the deviation from the calculated planer isodose in terms of relative dose agreement, distance to agreement, and normalized agreement

test. Our acceptance criteria are a relative dose agreement of ≤ 3% and a distance to agreement of ≤ 3 mm. Both of these criteria were satisfied for this patient.

Orthogonal anterior-posterior and left lateral digital images of the treated region were taken on the first day of treatment and at least once weekly throughout the treatment course. These were compared with digitally reconstructed radiographs of the same projections made from the treatment planning CT scan. The field position was adjusted if there was a 2 mm or greater disparity in the anterior-posterior, superior-inferior, or medial-lateral direction between the digital portal images and the digitally reconstructed radiographs.

Clinical Outcome

The patient has a history of irritable bowel syndrome, and even before the initiation of treatment, the patient reported having 6 to 8 loose bowel movements a day. While on treatment, the patient was placed on Lomotil and Imodium to help with the fequent bowel movements. However, even with maximum doses of both medications, the patient reported having 6 to 8 bowel movements a day at the completion of therapy. However, the patient never lost any weight while on treatment. At the time of her 1-month follow-up, she had stopped taking the Lomitil but was still taking Imodium, with about three to four bowel movements a day. She described this as normal.

We recently presented an analysis of IMRT planning in patients with gynecologic cancer undergoing adjuvant pelvic RT.[1] The purpose of this study was to evaluate the impact of varying CTV-to-PTV margins on normal tissue sparing. Varying margins (0, 0.5, and 1 cm) were added to the CTV (vaginal vault, paravaginal tissues, and pelvic nodes) in 10 patients with cervical and endometrial cancer, generating a PTV. We found that the volume of small bowel irradiated to high doses treated with IMRT versus a conventional four-field technique increased markedly, even with increases in the PTV margin from 0 to 10 mm. Our results demonstrate the importance of accurate target delineation and the need for accurate patient positioning in gynecology patients undergoing IMRT.

Reference

1. Ahamad A, D'Souza W, Salehpour M, et al. Intensity modulated radiation therapy (IMRT) for post-hysterectomy pelvic radiation: selection of patients and planning target volume (PTV). Int J Radiat Oncol Biol Phys 2002;54:42.

Chapter 23.3

CERVICAL CANCER NOT SUITABLE FOR BRACHYTHERAPY

CASE STUDY

PHILIP CHAN, MBBS, MICHAEL MILOSEVIC, MD, JANET PATERSON, MRT(T), CMD,
INHWAN YEO, PhD, ANTHONY W. FYLES, MD

Patient History

A 46-year-old female presented to her gynecologist complaining of postcoital vaginal bleeding and discharge for 4 months. A pelvic examination revealed a firm, enlarged cervix measuring 4 to 5 cm with extension to the left parametrium but not the pelvic sidewall. The biopsy was consistent with a squamous cell carcinoma. Pelvic magnetic resonance imaging (MRI) demonstrated a 5 cm cervical mass with parametrial involvement and an 8 mm left external iliac lymph node of uncertain significance. The uterus was noted to be retroverted and retroflexed. A computed tomography (CT) scan of the abdomen revealed no evidence of hydronephrosis or extrapelvic metastasis. She was thus staged as having International Federation of Gynecology and Obstetrics (FIGO) stage IIb cervical cancer.

A definitive course of chemoradiotherapy was advised, with weekly cisplatin given during external whole-pelvis radiation therapy (RT) to a dose of 50 Gy, followed by intrauterine brachytherapy. Pelvic RT and chemotherapy were completed as planned; however, the initial brachytherapy insertion was complicated by a perforation, which was confirmed on MRI (Figure 23.3-1). A second attempt by a gynecologic oncologist was similarly unsuccessful, and the uterus was noted to be fixed in the sacral hollow. The patient was thus felt to be unsuitable for conventional brachytherapy, and it was elected to deliver a pelvic boost with intensity-modulated radiation therapy (IMRT).

Simulation

The patient was placed supine on an inflated Vac-Lok bag (MED-TEC, Orange City, IA) with her legs in a dual–foam leg immobilizer. Fiducial markers were placed on the patient's previous tattoos on the lateral and anterior pelvis.

The tattoos were then aligned using the lasers, and the Vac-Lok was shaped around the patient. Marks were drawn on the Vac-Lok at the level of the tattoos to ensure accurate placement of the bag during treatment.

The patient was instructed to empty her rectum prior to the planning session. On arrival in the department, she was asked to empty her bladder and, 1 hour prior to simulation, was given 500 mL of oral contrast. The patient was then scanned in the treatment position from the bottom of L5 to below the ischial tuberosities. Both MRI and CT were performed for treatment planning. T2-weighted axial MRIs were obtained (4 mm slice thickness, 1 mm

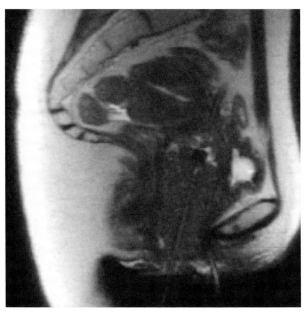

FIGURE 23.3-1. The patient had a retroverted and retroflexed fixed uterus with an intrauterine applicator perforated anteriorly.

spacing) using a 1.5 Tesla GE Excite MR scanner (GE Medical Systems, Waukesha, WI). She was then taken to a large-bore helical CT scanner (Philips Medical Systems, Andover, MA), repositioned in the Vac-Lok, and scanned over the same region (3 mm slice thickness).

Target and Tissue Delineation

Delineation of the target and organs at risk (OAR) was done with the aid of MRIs fused to the planning CT referenced to bony anatomy. Despite the MRI being completed approximately 15 minutes prior to CT, significant bladder filling was noted, affecting the tumor and OAR (Figure 23.3-2).

In this patient, the gross tumor volume (GTV) was defined as the imaged cervix and lower uterine segment and was contoured on axial CT slices with the aid of the corresponding MRIs (see Figure 23.3-2). No parametrial extension was evident on the planning MRI. OAR contours consisted of the outer outline of each organ (rectum, bladder, sigmoid colon, and femoral heads). The remaining bowel (including small bowel) was contoured by outlining the parietal peritoneum. The inner bladder wall was contoured, but not the inner rectal or sigmoid wall (Figure 23.3-3).

The clinical target volume (CTV) consisted of the GTV expanded by 10 mm in all directions except posteriorly, where a 7 mm expansion was used. The planning target volume (PTV) was generated by expanding the CTV uni-

formly by an additional 5 mm (except anteriorly). In light of the difference in bladder filling between the MRI and CT scan, the anterior CTV-to-PTV margin was 10 mm.

Planning organ at risk volumes (PRVs) were generated as follows: the outer rectal wall was expanded by 7 mm, the outer bladder wall by 10 mm, the sigmoid colon by 7 mm, and the femoral heads by 5 mm. The overlap regions between PTV and PRVs were subtracted from each PRV, and "pure" PRVs (ie, rectum: PRV-PTV, bladder: PRV-PTV, and sigmoid: PRV-PTV) were separately contoured, ensuring a minimum 3 mm distance from the PTV. By treating the overlap region as part of the PTV and providing this 3 mm separation between the PRV and PTV, plan optimization could be carried out while minimizing priority conflicts between these structures.

Treatment Planning

An IMRT plan was generated using *Cadplan/Helios* inverse planning software, version 6.2.7 (Varian Medical Systems, Palo Alto, CA). Beam arrangements and optimization constraints were based on our prior gynecologic IMRT planning study.[1] Our standard beam arrangement was slightly adjusted to accommodate the particular location of PTV relative to the critical organs (see Figure 23.3-2 and Figure 23.3-3). After a few iterative trials, the following six gantry angles were selected: 35, 80, 115, 245, 280, and 330 degrees. All beams had a nominal energy of 6 MV. We ensured that

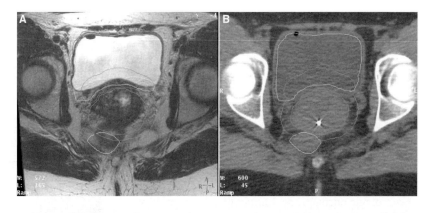

FIGURE 23.3-2. (*A*) Magnetic resonance imaging and (*B*) computed tomography fusion referenced to bony anatomy. Note that the cervix and rectum deviated significantly owing to increased bladder volume. The slice shown was at 2.4 cm superior to the inferior limit of the planning target volume (PTV). Highlighted are the bladder (*light blue*), bladder–planning organ at risk volume (*red*), rectum (*green*), gross tumor volume (blue), and PTV (*orange*). (To view a color version of this image, please refer to the CD-ROM.)

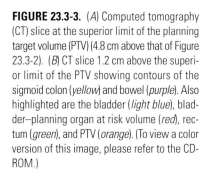

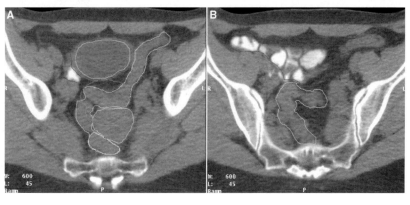

FIGURE 23.3-3. (*A*) Computed tomography (CT) slice at the superior limit of the planning target volume (PTV) (4.8 cm above that of Figure 23.3-2). (*B*) CT slice 1.2 cm above the superior limit of the PTV showing contours of the sigmoid colon (*yellow*) and bowel (*purple*). Also highlighted are the bladder (*light blue*), bladder–planning organ at risk volume (*red*), rectum (*green*), and PTV (*orange*). (To view a color version of this image, please refer to the CD-ROM.)

none of the beams passed through the couch directly because the patient was on the 10 cm–thick Styrofoam pad (Dow Chemical, Midland, MI). Two additional portal imaging fields, which delivered four monitor units with 18 MV x-rays, were placed at 0° and 270° and were included in the dose calculation.

Tables 23.3-1 to 23.3-3 summarize the input parameters used for IMRT planning in this patient. Figure 23.3-4 illustrates the isodose curves of the optimized treatment plan. The dose-volume histograms for the PTV and PRVs are shown in Figure 23.3-5.

TABLE 23.3-1. Constraints for the Planning Target Volume

Points	Dose, Gy	Volume, %	Priority
Minimum	95% of PD	100	100
Maximum	105% of PD	0	100
1	107% of PD	0.5	100
2	96% of PD	99	100

The highest priority was used to achieve an acceptable dose uniformity in the planning target volume (PTV). This was done by associating the values of the volume with the priority of 100% and providing two constraint points, respectively, at or near the maximum (95% and 96% of the prescribed dose [PD]) and minimum (105 and 107% of the PD) points of the targeted cumulative dose-volume histogram for the PTV.

TABLE 23.3-2. Constraints for Bladder:PRV-PTV, Rectum:PRV-PTV, and Sigmoid:PRV-PTV

Points	Dose, Gy	Volume, %	Priority
Minimum	0	100	0
Maximum	95% of PD	0	100
1	33% of PD	5	5
2	66% of PD	5	20

PD = prescribed dose; PRV = planning organ at risk volume; PTV = planning target volume.
The use of small volumes (points 1 and 2), coupled with relatively small priorities, speeds up the optimization process while achieving the same result as optimization to the combination of relatively large values of the volumes and priorities.

TABLE 23.3-3. Constraints for the Femoral Heads

Points	Dose, Gy	Volume, %	Priority
Minimum	0	100	0
Maximum	33% of PD	5	5

PD = prescribed dose.

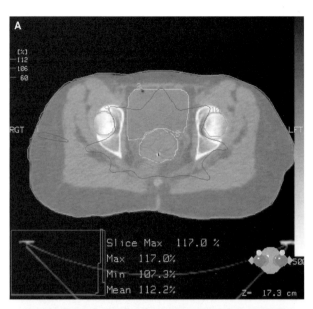

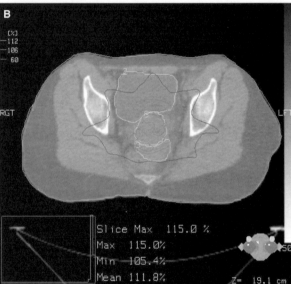

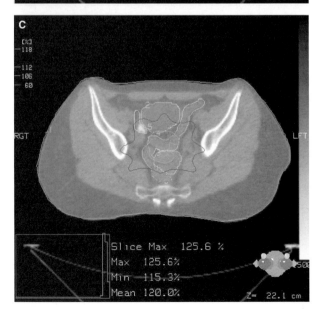

FIGURE 23.3-4. Dose distributions on representative computed tomography slices: (*A*) 2.4 cm superior to the inferior limit of the planning target volume (PTV); (*B*) 3 cm inferior to the superior limit of the PTV; (*C*) the superior limit of the PTV. The prescription isodose level was 112%. The maximum dose was 118% and was located at the superior limit of the PTV. (To view a color version of this image, please refer to the CD-ROM.)

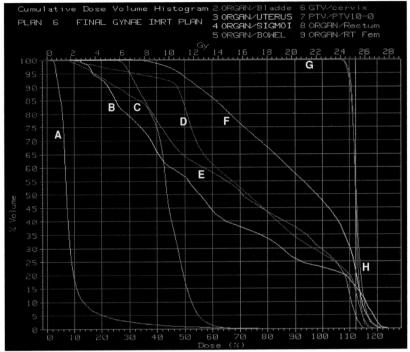

FIGURE 23.3-5. Dose-volume histograms. The dose distribution in the planning target volume (PTV) was maintained within 106 to 118% (clinical maximum) or ± 5% of the prescription dose. GTV = gross tumor volume; IMRT = intensity-modulated radiation therapy. (*A*) bowel; (*B*) rt fem; (*C*) sigmoid; (*D*) rectum; (*E*) bladder; (*F*) uterus; (*G*) cervix; (*H*) PTV10-0. (To view a color version of this image, please refer to the CD-ROM.)

A dose of 25.2 Gy in 1.8 Gy daily fractions was prescribed to the PTV in this patient. As seen in Figure 23.3-4 and Figure 23.3-5, an acceptable level of dose uniformity (within ± 5% of the prescription dose) was obtained. A minimum of 95% of the prescription dose was delivered to the PTV. The doses delivered to the OAR were found to be comparable to the predetermined set of criteria based on the past results with conformal therapy.[1] Specifically, the average doses delivered to 50% of the volume were 21, 13, and 5 Gy for the rectum, bladder, and small bowel, respectively. Given that part of the sigmoid volume was actually within the PTV, doses up to the prescription dose were accepted to avoid compromising tumor control. The doses to the femoral heads were minimal.

Treatment Delivery and Quality Assurance

The IMRT plan was delivered in this patient using a Varian 2100EX linear accelerator (Varian Medical Systems) equipped with a Millenium-120 multileaf collimator. Treatment was delivered using the sliding window technique. On average, treatment was delivered in 30 minutes, which included patient setup, delivery, and portal imaging.

Our quality assurance program included dose verification performed using an ion chamber measurement (0.6 cc) in the center of a cylindrical phantom (10 cm radius). The phantom was positioned on the treatment table such that the center was located at the isocenter. Next, the patient treatment was simulated by allowing each beam to be delivered at the corresponding gantry angle. Compared with the phantom plan, an underdose of 1.9% was measured. This fell well within our acceptance criterion of ± 3% dose disparity.

Patient Outcome

The patient tolerated treatment well, without any significant acute side effects. The patient has only recently completed treatment and will be followed closely for tumor response and chronic sequelae.

Our dosimetric study evaluating IMRT as an external beam boost in patients unsuitable for brachytherapy was presented earlier.[1] IMRT plans were generated in 10 gynecology patients (5 cervical cancer, 2 endometrial cancer, 3 vaginal cancer) previously treated with external beam pelvic RT and a conformal RT boost. The CTV consisted of the gross tumor, including the proximal vaginal and/or cervix. On average, the target coverage (PTV receiving 95% of the prescription dose) was significantly increased with IMRT. However, PTV dose inhomogeneity, as measured by the dose encompassing 5% of the volume, increased significantly. Significant benefits were seen in normal tissue sparing. The dose received by 50% of the rectum decreased from, on average, 80% of the prescription dose to 62% with IMRT ($p < .001$). IMRT also reduced the dose received by 50% of the bladder volume by 10% ($p = .04$). These results suggest that IMRT may be a valuable means of providing an external beam boost to gynecology patients unsuitable for brachytherapy. However, the clinical benefits of this approach need to be evaluated in clinical trials.

Reference

1. Chan P, Perkins G, Yeo I, et al. Intensity modulated radiation therapy as an external beam boost in gynaecologic cancer patients unsuitable for brachytherapy [abstract]. Proceedings of International Congress of Radiation Research (ICRR) 2003;PP14: 146, Brisbane, Australia.

BONE MARROW–SPARING IMRT

EMERGING TECHNOLOGY

JOHN C. ROESKE, PHD, ANTHONY E. LUJAN, PHD, ARNO J. MUNDT, MD

Increasing attention is being focused on the use of intensity-modulated radiation therapy (IMRT) in gynecologic malignancies. We and others have shown that IMRT planning significantly reduces the volume of small bowel and rectum irradiated to high doses compared with conventional techniques.[1–6] Moreover, clinical experience has suggested that such dosimetric benefits translate into less gastrointestinal toxicity in patients treated with IMRT.[7–10]

Although attention has focused primarily on the small bowel and rectum, an additional organ that should be considered in these patients is the pelvic bone marrow (BM). Most of the total-body BM reserve is located in the lower spine and pelvic bones, thus within standard radiation therapy (RT) fields.[11] Unsurprisingly, hematologic toxicity is common in patients receiving chemotherapy, often necessitating chemotherapy dose reductions and/or treatment interruptions.[12] Hematologic toxicity also adds to the cost of therapy by requiring the use of growth factors and transfusions.[13] Given the exquisite radiosensitivity of BM,[14] hematologic toxicity can occur without chemotherapy. Long-term BM suppression may even result, impairing the delivery of chemotherapy at the time of relapse.[15,16]

The purpose of this chapter is to provide an overview of BM-sparing approaches in patients with gynecologic cancer treated with intensity-modulated whole-pelvis radiation therapy (IM-WPRT). Many of the principles presented here are applicable to gynecology patients treated with more comprehensive fields and to nongynecology patients undergoing pelvic and/or abdominal irradiation.

Unintentional BM Sparing

Although developed to reduce the risk of gastrointestinal toxicity, we noted early on that patients treated with IM-WPRT developed less hematologic toxicity. As seen in Figure 23.4-1, the highly conformal plan designed to minimize the volume of small bowel and rectum irradiated also unintentionally reduced the dose to the pelvic BM compared with a standard four-field whole-pelvis radiation therapy (WPRT) plan.

To explore this finding further, an analysis of acute hematologic toxicity in our IM-WPRT patients was performed.[17] Hematologic sequelae were compared between 36 patients treated with IM-WPRT and a historical control group of 88 patients treated with conventional WPRT. Approximately one-third of patients received concomitant chemotherapy consisting of cisplatin (40 mg/m^2/wk).

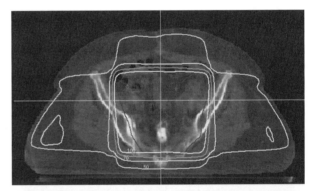

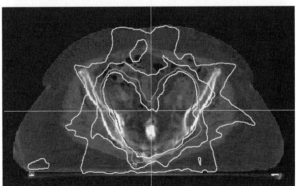

FIGURE 23.4-1. A comparison of conventional whole-pelvis radiation therapy and intensity-modulated whole-pelvis radiation therapy (IM-WPRT) treatment planning in a representative patient. Note that the highly conformal IM-WPRT plan reduces the dose to the bone marrow in the iliac crests, although the bone marrow was not included in the planning process. (To view a color version of this image, please refer to the CD-ROM.)

WPRT was delivered with a four-field "box" technique using standard blocking. In most WPRT patients, treatment planning was performed using three-dimensional techniques. Our IM-WPRT approach is described in Chapter 23, "Gynecologic Cancer: Overview," and in earlier publications.[1,2,7–9,18] In short, following fabrication of a customized immobilization device, patients underwent a contrast-enhanced planning computed tomography (CT) scan. The clinical target volume (CTV) consisted of the upper half of the vagina, parametria, uterus (if present), presacral region, and regional lymph node regions (common, internal, and external iliac crests). The CTV was then expanded by 1 cm to produce a planning target volume (PTV). IM-WPRT plans were generated using commercial inverse planning software (*CORVUS*, versions 3.0 and 4.0, North American Scientific, NOMOS Radiation Oncology Division, Cranberry Township, PA) consisting of equally spaced seven or nine coplanar fields using 6 MV photons. The planning goals were to encompass the PTV with the prescription dose while minimizing the dose to the small bowel, bladder, and rectum. Pelvic BM was not entered as a separate constraint.

Overall, 26 patients (20.9%) developed grade ≥ 2 acute white blood cell (WBC) toxicity. Grade ≥ 2 absolute neutrophil count (ANC) and hemoglobin (Hgb) toxicities were noted in 8.5% and 9.1% of patients, respectively. No patient developed grade ≥ 2 platelet toxicity. Acute hematologic toxicity was more common in chemotherapy patients. Grade ≥ 2 WBC, ANC, and Hgb toxicities occurred in 10.7%, 1.1%, and 6.8% of patients treated with RT alone, respectively. Corresponding values in the chemotherapy group were 47.2% ($p < .0001$), 16.6% ($p = .001$), and 19.4% ($p = .04$), respectively.

When subdivided by treatment, hematologic toxicity was noted to be low in patients receiving RT alone, regardless of technique. In contrast, IM-WPRT plus chemotherapy patients experienced less hematologic toxicity than those treated with WPRT plus chemotherapy. Grade ≥ 2 WBC toxicity was seen in 60% and 31.2% of WPRT and IM-WPRT patients combined with chemotherapy, respectively ($p = .08$). Corresponding ANC toxicities were 23.5% and 15.3%, respectively ($p = .58$).

Overall, WPRT plus chemotherapy patients developed lower WBC (2.8 vs 3.6 µg/dL; $p = .05$) and ANC (1,874 vs 2,669; $p = .04$) nadirs than those treated with IM-WPRT plus chemotherapy. As seen in Figure 23.4-2, IM-WPRT plus chemotherapy patients experienced a lower rate of decline of WBC counts during treatment versus WPRT plus chemotherapy patients. Consequently, the percentage of missed chemotherapy cycles was lower in the IM-WPRT group (12.5 vs 40%; $p = .06$).

Average dose-volume histograms (DVHs) of the BM within the iliac crests, lumbar spine, and sacrum in 10 women planned with WPRT and IM-WPRT were compared. The greatest difference was seen in the irradiation of the iliac crests (Figure 23.4-3). Although no reduction

was seen at the 10 and 30 Gy levels, significant reductions were seen in the IM-WPRT plans at 20 Gy ($p < .001$), 40 Gy ($p < .001$), and 45 Gy ($p < .001$). Significant differences in BM volume irradiated in the lumbar spine and sacrum were noted only at doses near the prescription dose.

Intentional BM Sparing

We next evaluated the inclusion of BM as a constraint in the inverse planning process of IM-WPRT.[19] BM-sparing IM-WPRT plans were generated in 10 gynecology patients by including BM as an additional normal tissue constraint

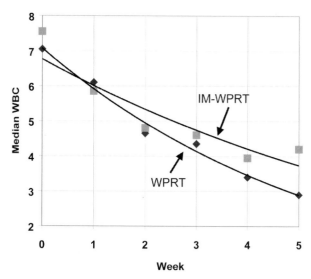

FIGURE 23.4-2. Plots of the median white blood cell (WBC) values versus time since the initiation of treatment. Patients treated with conventional whole-pelvis radiation therapy (WPRT) exhibited a higher rate of WBC decline compared with those treated with intensity-modulated whole-pelvis radiation therapy (IM-WPRT). Reproduced with permission from Brixey C et al.[17]

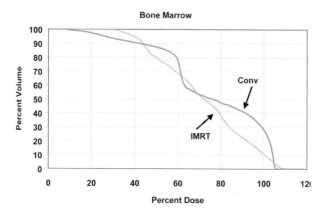

FIGURE 23.4-3. Average dose-volume histograms for 10 patients planned with conventional whole-pelvis radiation therapy and (WPRT) intensity-modulated radiation therapy (IM-WPRT). Conv = conventional RT. Adapted from Brixey C et al.[17]

(along with the small bowel, bladder, and rectum). Given that differences in the volume of BM irradiated in the lumbosacral spine were previously observed only at high doses, we limited our analysis to sparing of the iliac crest BM. IM-WPRT (without BM sparing) and conventional WPRT planning were also performed in the same patients as described above.

Visual inspection of the dose distribution in the 10 patients showed that BM-sparing IM-WPRT plans resulted in the higher isodose lines bending away from iliac crest BM compared with IM-WPRT and WPRT plans. As seen in a representative patient in Figure 23.4-4A, the isodose lines in a BM-sparing IM-WPRT plan conform more tightly to the PTV in the regions adjacent to iliac crest BM compared with the standard IM-WPRT (Figure 23.4-4B) and WPRT (Figure 23.4-4C) plans. Furthermore, the 40% isodose line does not fully encompass the BM in the BM-sparing plan, whereas it does in the other plans. In addition, the prescription and 95% isodose lines conform to the PTV in the standard and BM-sparing IM-WPRT plans, thus preserving small bowel sparing.

Figure 23.4-5 summarizes the average DVHs of the iliac crests in the 10 patients studied. As reported earlier,[17] IM-WPRT planning (without BM sparing) reduced the volume of BM receiving ≥ 20 Gy compared with the standard four-field WPRT plan. Here, on average, BM-sparing IM-WPRT planning resulted in a decrease in the volume of BM receiving doses ≥ 15 Gy compared with both WPRT and standard IM-WPRT planning. At all dose levels between 40% and 67% of the prescription dose, the BM-sparing IM-WPRT plan significantly reduced the volume of BM irradiated ($p < .001$). For doses above 70%, BM-sparing IM-WPRT plans all demonstrated a reduction in the volume of BM irradiated as well, but the differences were not statistically significant. However, compared with conventional WPRT plans, BM-sparing IM-WPRT plans showed a significant reduction in the volume of BM irradiated at all dose levels above 40%.

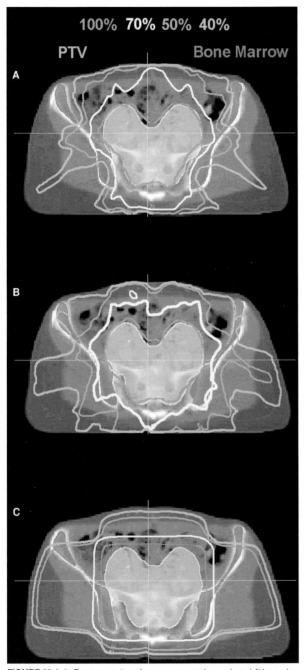

FIGURE 23.4-4. Treatment plans for a representative patient. (*A*) Intensity-modulated whole-pelvis radiation therapy (IM-WPRT) with bone marrow (BM) sparing; (*B*) IM-WPRT (without BM sparing); and (*C*) conventional whole-pelvis radiation therapy. PTV = planning target volume. (To view a color version of this image, please refer to the CD-ROM.) Reproduced with permission from Lujan AE et al.[19]

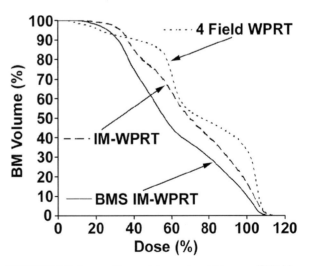

FIGURE 23.4-5. Average iliac crest dose-volume histograms (DVHs) for 10 patients planned using conventional whole-pelvis radiation therapy (WPRT), intensity-modulated radiation therapy (IM-WPRT) (without bone marrow sparing [BMS]), and IM-WPRT with BMS. Reproduced with permission from Lujan AE et al.[19]

In addition to reducing the dose to the BM, the BM-sparing IM-WPRT plans were designed to preserve PTV coverage. On average, the BM-sparing plans resulted in a slightly more inhomogeneous dose distribution than standard IM-WPRT planning. Specifically, the volume of the PTV receiving at least 110% of the dose in a BM-sparing plan was 15.9% compared with 12.9% ($p = .09$) with standard IM-WPRT planning. Similarly, the small bowel volume encompassed by the prescription dose was slightly greater in the BM-sparing plans (30.1 vs 28.6%; $p = .7$). Although not likely clinically significant, it is clear that BM-sparing cannot be achieved without some compromise in the dose distribution. The average DVHs for the bladder and rectum (data not shown) were similar for both BM-sparing and standard IM-WPRT treatment plans.

We are currently treating our gynecology patients with BM-sparing IM-WPRT to limit the dose to the iliac crests. To further evaluate the benefit of this approach, we initiated a two-part phase I trial. Part I was recently completed and consisted of patients treated with conventional WPRT, cisplatin (40 mg/m²/wk), and escalating doses of vinorelbine to determine the maximum tolerated dose (MTD) of vinorelbine in this setting. Twelve patients were enrolled, and the vinorelbine MTD was determined to be 15 mg/m²/wk, with predominantly hematologic dose-limiting toxicity.[20] In part II (which is ongoing), patients receive BM-sparing IM-WPRT, cisplatin, and escalating doses of vinorelbine. It is our hope that the BM-sparing IM-WPRT approach will allow a higher vinorelbine MTD owing to decreased hematologic dose-limiting toxicity.

Incorporation of Functional Imaging

To improve our BM-sparing approach, we recently sought to incorporate functional BM imaging into the planning process. The rationale for this is that much of the contents of the medullary canal within the iliac crests is composed of fatty inactive (yellow) BM.[21] Hematopoietically active (red) BM is poorly visualized on CT, necessitating the inclusion of the entire medullary canal as an avoidance structure. Inclusion of the entire canal thus overestimates the volume of active BM and unnecessarily constrains the IMRT planning process. It also ignores deposits of red BM elsewhere in the pelvis.

Active BM can be imaged using technetium 99m (^{99m}TC) sulfur colloids.[22,23] These colloids are sequestered by macrophages associated with red BM, providing a surrogate for its distribution. When imaged using single-photon computed emission tomography (SPECT), a three-dimensional map of the active BM regions can be produced.

To evaluate the potential of this technique, a patient with endometrial cancer undergoing IM-WPRT planning also underwent a functional BM imaging scan.[24] An hour prior to imaging, 12.2 mCi of ^{99m}Tc sulfur colloid was administered. The patient was positioned on the curved table of a PRISM 2000XP scanner (Philips Medical Systems, Andover, MA) and a SPECT scan of the pelvis was obtained from above the top of the iliac crest to below the ischial tuberosities using a low-energy, high-resolution collimator. Four SPECT scans were taken using 120 projection images, each 128×128 pixels and 8 seconds in duration (total scanning time 32 minutes). The four projection image sets were reviewed for motion and then added together. Axial scans were reconstructed with ramp-filtered backprojection, resulting in a 3.9 mm pixel size in the axial plane and a 4.7 mm slice thickness. The axial slice set was then smoothed using a three-dimensional Butterworth low-pass filter with an order of 4 and a cutoff frequency equal to 0.56 times the Nyquist frequency.

The SPECT BM images were subsequently fused with the planning CT scan using commercially available image fusion software (*AcQSim Multimodality Fusion*, Philips Medical Systems). The interactive mode of the fusion software was used, allowing manual translation and rotation of the SPECT scan to produce the best visual overlay of the two image sets. The CT and SPECT images (resliced along the planes of the CT scan) were then displayed side by side. The window and level of the SPECT images were adjusted such that only the regions of highest activity were visible, representing the sites of active BM. These sites were simultaneously displayed on the correlated CT image and contoured as active BM.

Three treatment plans were generated: a conventional WPRT plan, an IM-WPRT plan (without BM sparing), and a BM-sparing IM-WPRT plan. The prescribed dose in all three plans was 45 Gy in 1.8 Gy daily fractions. The WPRT and IM-WPRT plans were generated as described in the above sections. In the standard IM-WPRT plan, the active BM identified on the SPECT scan was included only as a reference structure, without dose constraints. In the BM-sparing IM-WPRT plan, the active BM sites were included as a constraint in the inverse planning process. The BM constraints were modified during the planning process so that target dose homogeneity and small bowel sparing would not be compromised.

BM-SPECT images through the pelvis are shown in Figure 23.4-6. Highlighted are individual slices through the upper, mid-, and lower pelvis. A high degree of activity is seen in the lumbar vertebrae, sacrum, and iliac crests. To a lesser degree, uptake is also shown in the symphysis and femoral heads.

Fusion of the planning CT and SPECT images was accomplished without difficulty in approximately 5 minutes. Alignment of the SPECT images with the planning CT showed good anatomic agreement (see Figure 23.4-6). The highest activity regions of the SPECT image are overlaid on the CT axial image using a colorwash technique. From the overlaid SPECT images, the most active BM sites were identified in the lumbar spine and the medial portion of the iliac crests. Slightly lower in the pelvis, a high concentration of active BM is seen in the anterior sacrum, medial iliac crests, and, to a lesser extent, lateral iliac crests.

Isodose curves of the conventional WPRT, IM-WPRT (without BM sparing), and BM-sparing IM-WPRT plans through the midpelvis are shown in Figure 23.4-7. The sites of active BM are shown as solid shaded areas superimposed on the pelvic bones. In the conventional WPRT plan, the majority of the active BM sites are included within the high-dose isodose (70–100%) lines. In contrast, the IM-WPRT plan (without BM sparing) reduces the volume of active BM included within the 90 to 100% isodoses. Further reduc-

tion in the BM volume irradiated is also seen at lower doses when the BM is entered as a constraint in the plan.

Figure 23.4-8 shows the DVH of active BM in the three treatment plans. The conventional WPRT plan results in 95% of the active BM receiving 60% of the prescription dose, whereas nearly 70% receives the entire prescription dose or greater. The IM-WPRT without BM-sparing plan reduces the active BM volume irradiated, particularly at the higher-dose levels. However, the BM-sparing IM-WPRT

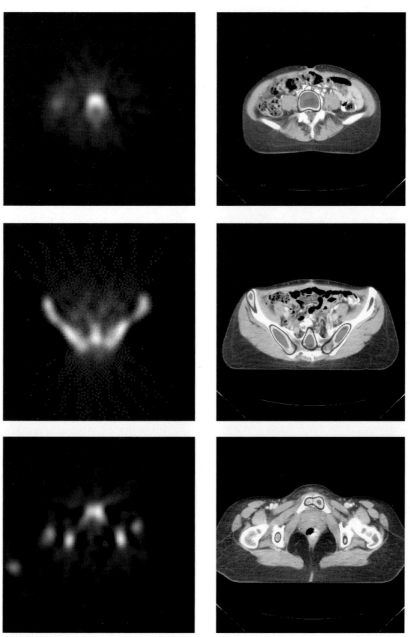

FIGURE 23.4-6. Representative technetium 99m sulfur colloid single-photon emission computed tomography (SPECT) images and the corresponding results of the SPECT–computed tomography (CT) image fusion. (To view a color version of this image, please refer to the CD-ROM.) Adapted from Roeske JC et al.[24]

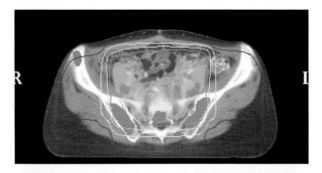

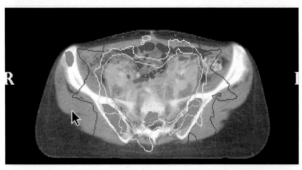

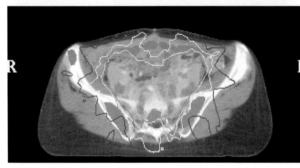

FIGURE 23.4-7. Isodose distributions overlaid on an axial computed tomography slice in the midpelvis. The red shaded regions represent the bone marrow identified from the technetium 99m sulfur colloid single-photon emission computed tomography (SPECT) images. Shown are plans produced using a conventional (four field) approach, as well as intensity-modulated whole-pelvis radiation therapy with and without bone marrow sparing. (To view a color version of this image, please refer to the CD-ROM.)

plan is associated with the largest reduction of BM irradiated relative to the other plans at all dose levels greater than 50%. The percentages of active BM receiving 20 Gy or higher in the conventional WPRT, IM-WPRT, and BM-sparing IM-WPRT plans are 96%, 95%, and 89%, respectively. At the 30 Gy and above level, corresponding percentages are 85%, 75%, and 40%, respectively. Finally, at the prescription dose (45 Gy), the corresponding percentages are 66%, 32%, and 16%, respectively.

The PTV DVHs of the three plans are nearly identical below the prescription dose. However, for doses above the prescription dose, the conventional WPRT plan provides the most uniform PTV with the maximum dose of 109%. The IM-WPRT without BM-sparing plan results in

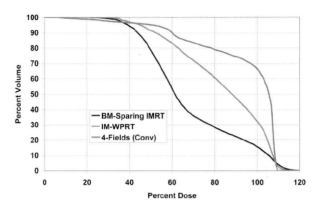

FIGURE 23.4-8. Dose-volume histograms for the single-photon emission computed tomography–defined bone marrow (BM) of the four-field conventional whole-pelvis radiation therapy plan and intensity-modulated whole-pelvis radiation therapy (IM-WPRT) plans (with and without BM sparing). IMRT = intensity-modulated radiation therapy.

slightly more dose heterogeneity, whereas the BM-sparing IM-WPRT plan is the most inhomogeneous. However, despite the slight increase in dose heterogeneity, the BM-sparing plan significantly reduces the volume of BM irradiated. The volume of PTV receiving 110% of the prescription dose in the IM-WPRT without BM sparing and BM-sparing IM-WPRT plans are 11% and 23%, respectively. In both plans, less than 4% of the PTV receives 115% of the prescription dose. Both IM-WPRT plans provide nearly identical sparing of the small bowel relative to the conventional WPRT plan. At the prescription dose, the percent volumes of small bowel irradiated in the conventional WPRT, IM-WPRT without BM sparing, and BM-sparing IM-WPRT plans are 65%, 26%, and 29%, respectively.

Future Directions

Numerous questions remain regarding the utility of our BM-sparing IMRT approach. First and foremost, it is unclear whether these dosimetric benefits will translate into improved clinical outcomes. Clearly, this question can be answered only in a prospective clinical trial. However, we are optimistic that the reductions in active BM volume irradiated will prove clinically significant. First, a clinical difference has already been seen with the more modest reductions achieved using our standard IM-WPRT approach.[17] Second, SPECT-guided IMRT improves BM sparing at low to moderate doses. Active BM is exquisitely radiosensitive, with histologic changes (reduction of precursor cells) evident at doses as low as 4 Gy.[14] Starting at doses of 10 Gy, progressively more significant damage is manifest, including dilated sinusoids and acute hemorrhage. Nonetheless, until doses of 50 Gy and above, regeneration can occur. Given this spectrum of damage, it is likely that increased BM sparing at low to moderate doses using the SPECT-guided IMRT approach will prove clinically significant.

Second, it is unclear whether functional BM imaging would need to be performed on every patient or if some generalizations can be made. The spatial distribution of active BM is highly individualized, varying with age and sex and whether the patient is a smoker or had previous RT or chemotherapy. For example, in women, the red BM proportion in the proximal femur decreases from age 25 through 70 years.[25] Variations such as these have been observed in other pelvic bones.[26] Because most of our patients fall into this age group, we believe that individualized, functional BM imaging studies will be required.

Finally, it remains unclear whether SPECT is the ideal BM imaging technique. An alternative BM imaging approach is T_1-weighted magnetic resonance imaging. On these images, active marrow exhibits a low-intensity signal (similar to that of muscle) and nonactive BM has a high-intensity signal similar to that of fat.[25] Preliminary studies have validated the feasibility of this approach.[27] Furthermore, as magnetic resonance simulators become more widely available, they may obviate the need for an additional imaging session.

References

1. Roeske JC, Lujan A, Rotmensch J, et al. Intensity-modulated whole pelvis radiation therapy in patients with gynecologic malignancies. Int J Radiat Oncol Biol Phys 2000;48:1613–21.
2. Mundt AJ, Roeske JC, Lujan JC. IMRT in gynecologic malignancies. Med Dosim 2002;27:131–6.
3. Heron DE, Gerszten K, Selvaraj RN, et al. Conventional 3D conformal versus intensity-modulated radiotherapy for the adjuvant treatment of gynecologic malignancies: a comparative dosimetric study of dose-volume histograms. Gynecol Oncol 2003;91:39–45.
4. Chen Q, Izadifar N, King S, et al. Comparison of IMRT with 3-D CRT for gynecologic malignancies [abstract]. Int J Radiat Oncol Biol Phys 2001;51:332.
5. Ahamad A, D'Souza W, Salehpour M, et al. Intensity modulated radiation therapy (IMRT) for post-hysterectomy pelvic radiation: selection of patients and planning target volume (PTV) [abstract]. Int J Radiat Oncol Biol Phys 2002;54:42.
6. Portelance L, Chao KS, Grigsby PW, et al. Intensity-modulated radiation therapy (IMRT) reduces small bowel, rectum, and bladder doses in patients with cervical cancer receiving pelvic and para-aortic irradiation. Int J Radiat Oncol Biol Phys 2001;51:261–6.
7. Mundt AJ, Roeske JC, Lujan AE, et al. Initial clinical experience with intensity modulated whole-pelvis radiation therapy in women with gynecologic malignancies. Gynecol Oncol 2001;82:456–63.
8. Mundt AJ, Lujan AE, Rotmensch J, et al. Intensity-modulated whole pelvic radiotherapy in women with gynecologic malignancies. Int J Radiat Oncol Biol Phys 2002;52:1330–37.
9. Mundt AJ, Mell LK, Roeske JC. Preliminary analysis of chronic gastrointestinal toxicity in gynecology patients treated with intensity-modulated whole pelvic radiation therapy. Int J Radiat Oncol Biol Phys 2003;56:1354–60.
10. Roeske JC, Bonta D, Lujan AE, et al. A dosimetric analysis of acute gastrointestinal toxicity in women receiving intensity-modulated whole-pelvic radiation therapy. Radiother Oncol 2003;69:201–7.
11. Ellis RE. The distribution of active bone marrow in the adult. Phys Med Biol 1961;5:255–63.
12. Keys HM, Bundy BN, Stehman FB, et al. Cisplatin, radiation, and adjuvant hysterectomy compared with radiation and adjuvant hysterectomy for bulky stage IB cervical carcinoma. N Engl J Med 1999;340:1154–61.
13. Kavanagh BD, Fischer BA, Segreti EM, et al. Cost analysis of erythropoietin versus blood transfusions for cervical cancer patients receiving chemoradiotherapy. Int J Radiat Oncol Biol Phys 2001;51:435–41.
14. Mauch P, Constine L, Greenberger J, et al. Hematopoietic stem cell compartment: acute and late effects of radiation therapy and chemotherapy. Int J Radiat Oncol Biol Phys 1995;12:1861–5.
15. Lhomme C, Fumoleau P, Fargeot P, et al. Results of a European Organization for Research and Treatment of Cancer/early clinical studies group phase II trial of first-line irinotecan in patients with advanced or recurrent squamous cell carcinoma of the cervix. J Clin Oncol 1999;17:3136–42.
16. Piver MS, Ghamande SA, Eltabbakh GH, et al. First-line chemotherapy with paclitaxel and platinum for advanced and recurrent cancer of the cervix—a phase II study. Gynecol Oncol 1999;75:334–7.
17. Brixey C, Roeske JC, Lujan AE, et al. Impact of intensity modulated whole pelvic radiation therapy on acute hematologic toxicity in women with gynecologic malignancies. Int J Radiat Oncol Biol Phys 2002;54:1388–96.
18. Salama JK, Roeske JC, Mehta N, et al. Intensity modulated radiotherapy therapy in gynecologic malignancies. Curr Treat Options Oncol 2004;5:97–108.
19. Lujan AE, Mundt AJ, Yamada SD, et al. Intensity-modulated radiotherapy as a means of reducing dose to bone marrow in gynecologic patients receiving whole pelvic radiotherapy. Int J Radiat Oncol Biol Phys 2003;57:516–21.
20. Mundt AJ, Rotmensch J, Waggoner SE, et al. Phase I trial of concomitant vinorelbine, cisplatin, and pelvic irradiation in cervical carcinoma and other advanced pelvic malignancies. Gynecol Oncl 2004;92:801–5.
21. Piney A. The anatomy of the bone marrow with special reference to the distribution of the red marrow. BMJ 1922;28:792–5.
22. Datz FL, Taylor A. The clinical use of radiocolloid bone marrow imaging. Semin Nucl Med 1985;15:239–59.
23. Desai AG, Thakur ML. Radiopharmaceuticals for spleen and bone marrow studies. Semin Nucl Med 1985;15:229–38.
24. Roeske JC, Lujan AE, Reba RC, et al. Incorporation of SPECT bone marrow imaging into intensity modulated whole-pelvic radiation therapy treatment planning for gynecologic malignancies. Radiother Oncol 2004. [In press]
25. Vandeberg B, Lecouvet F, Moysan P, et al. MR assessment of red marrow distribution and composition in the proximal femur: correlation with clinical and laboratory parameters. Skeletal Radiol 1997;26:589–96.
26. Ishijima H, Ishizaka H, Horikoshi H, et al. Water fraction of lumbar vertebral bone marrow estimated from chemical

shift misregistration on MR imaging: normal variations with age and sex. AJR Am J Roentgenol 1996;39:369–90.

27. Roeske JC, Mundt AJ. Incorporation of MR imaging into intensity modulated whole-pelvic radiation therapy treatment planning to reduce the volume of pelvic bone marrow irradiated. In: Proceedings of the 18th International Congress on Computer Assisted Radiology and Surgery. 2004;307-312.

APPLICATOR-GUIDED IMRT

EMERGING TECHNOLOGY

DANIEL A. LOW, PHD

Intracavitary brachytherapy (ICB) is frequently used to treat locally advanced cervical cancer. The direct placement of radioactive sources within the tumor-bearing tissues provides precise radiation localization and reproducibility, yielding excellent clinical results.[1–3] However, owing to the close proximity of the surrounding normal tissues (the bladder and rectum), ICB is associated with both early and late complications. Additionally, the rapid dose falloff limits the dose to the distal portions of the tumor, causing local failures to remain a clinical challenge, particularly tumors along the uterosacral ligament.[4,5] Dose optimization is desirable for these patients; however, once the treatment device is in place, optimization is limited to modifying the radioactive source strengths.

It has been suggested that intensity-modulated radiation therapy (IMRT) could improve the dose distributions in patients receiving ICB.[6] However, one of the most important considerations in evaluating IMRT for this disease site is not eliminating the localization advantage of the intracavitary applicator. We thus proposed the use of an applicator substitute in a technique known as applicator-guided intensity-modulated radiation therapy (AG-IMRT). The hypothesis is that through the use of AG-IMRT, highly conformal dose distributions could be accurately localized to the applicator substitute and address the limitations of ICB.

Treatment Planning Studies

In evaluating AG-IMRT, we initially compared ICB and IMRT dose distributions. Patients were scanned with custom-fabricated aluminum tandems and colpsotats with afterloadable bladder and rectal shields. Therefore, image artifacts caused by steel tandems, transfer tubes, and the bladder and rectal shields were avoided. The brachytherapy source positions were localized within the colpostats based on the internal cavity used to hold the sources. The source positions in the tandem were determined by examination of treatment planning radiographs acquired with radiopaque dummies in place.

Soft tissue contrast in this disease site is inherently poor using computed tomography (CT). Thus, accurate delineation of the tumor is difficult. Therefore, the ability of IMRT to reproduce the pear-shaped isodose distribution delivered by the intracavitary applicator was assessed. IMRT dose distributions were planned and delivered with a serial tomotherapy approach. Using this technique, a tertiary computer-controlled collimator (MIMiC, North American Scientific, NOMOS Radiation Oncology Division, Cranberry Township, PA) containing 20 pairs of opposed leaves is attached to the linear accelerator while treatment is delivered in the arc mode. As the linear accelerator rotates, the collimator leaves are opened and closed rapidly (transition time < 100 milliseconds), allowing fluence modulation each 5° or 10°, depending on user preferences. The projected size of the leaves is 1 cm wide at the isocenter, and the other dimension is user selectable to approximately 0.84 cm or 1.85 cm (termed 1 cm and 2 cm modes, respectively). Thus, the maximum target length that can be treated with the dynamic multileaf collimator is 1.68 cm or 3.7 cm, respectively. To treat targets of greater length, sequential dose deliveries are abutted, with the fluence modulation independently customized for the tumor and normal organs presented in those slices. The patient is moved between each slice delivery.

The *CORVUS* planning system (North American Scientific) was used to optimize the dose distributions for this study. First, the point A isodose surface was identified from the brachytherapy dose calculations. Next, this volume was outlined, and the contours were transferred to the treatment planning system. The bladder and rectum were delineated using conventional methods. The IMRT dose distributions were compared against a high–dose rate (HDR) regimen of 38 Gy. The bladder and rectal doses were based on the patient receiving 19.8 Gy from the whole-pelvis fields and an additional 38 Gy from the IMRT boost. We conducted the treatment planning study on three patients, two with the pear-shaped target volumes and one that had an unusually shaped uterus, which was contoured as the target. Figure

23.5-1 shows the dose-volume histograms from one of the patients with the target volume corresponding to the point A isodose surface. To show the relative flexibility of IMRT, two treatment plans were run, each with different optimization parameters. Our study demonstrated that when the brachytherapy isodose surface is used as the target volume, IMRT could provide equivalent target coverage with improved critical structure sparing.[6] However, this study was limited by the lack of a defined tumor volume; hence, the resultant treatment plan did not necessarily conform to the shape of the target volume.

Positron Emission Tomography

The lack of a well-defined target volume has hampered quantitative studies of the dose distributions delivered by ICB or IMRT. Recently, the use of ^{18}F-labeled fluorodeoxyglucose (^{18}FDG) positron emission tomography (PET) has been investigated as a method for delineating cervical cancer tumors.[7,8] ^{18}FDG-PET highlights the metabolically active regions, including active tumor growth. This technique was used by Wahab and colleagues[9] to continue the earlier study by Low and colleagues.[6] Rather than use the point A isodose surface as the target volume, ^{18}FDG-PET was used to define tumors in 10 patients with cervical cancer. An automated count threshold technique developed by Miller and Grigsby[8] was used to determine the primary tumor surface by defining as tumor any voxels with counts greater than a fixed threshold fraction (40%) of the peak tumor intensity.[8] Because the bladder and rectum also absorb ^{18}FDG, they were excluded by selecting a seed voxel within the tumor and expanding the regions based on the threshold criterion.[10]

The bladder and rectum were delineated on the PET image using standard software tools. To localize the tandem and colpostats in the PET image, catheters filled with ^{18}FDG were inserted in the locations corresponding to the source positions. The tandem and colpostat positions were distinguished by their respective anatomic positions. These image and contour data were transferred to a commercial treatment planning system (*XiO*, Computerized Medical Systems, St. Louis, MO). Note that CT scans were not used in this study, and the external patient contour was approximated by the PET-defined external contour. Although this contour was less accurately delineated using PET than conventional methods, the effect of inaccurate delineation is to modify the monitor units and fluence distribution to account for the inaccurate surface definition. In principle, the IMRT optimization should compensate for surface definition errors in the PET image.

Recently, Wahab and colleagues compared AG-IMRT and ICB treatment plans.[9] Unlike the previous study, the IMRT treatment plans were produced using a conventional multileaf collimator with five and nine equally spaced coplanar portals. Both 6 and 18 MV beams were examined. As

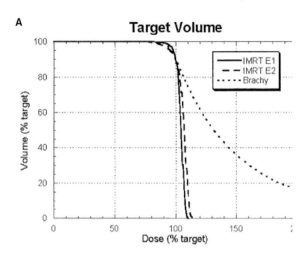

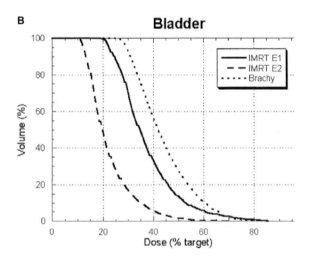

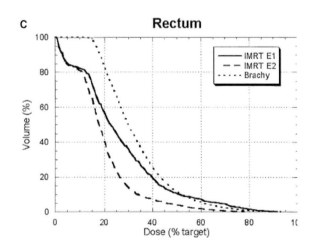

FIGURE 23.5-1. Representative dose-volume histograms (DVHs). The DVHs compare intracavitary brachytherapy against intensity-modulated radiation therapy (IMRT) with the point A isodose surface as the target volume. (*A*) Target volume DVH; (*B*) bladder DVH; (*C*) rectum DVH. Reproduced with permission from Low DA et al.[6]

in the earlier study, it was assumed that the patients received 19.8 Gy to the whole pelvis prior to the ICB or IMRT procedure. For this study, a more sophisticated method for determining the target dose prescription and critical structure tolerances was used. The IMRT prescription to the target was 6.5 Gy in six fractions based on our HDR prescription. Rectal and bladder tolerances were obtained from the three-dimensional conformal therapy literature and scaled to the HDR fractionation schedule using the linear-quadratic model (α/β = 3 for bladder and rectum late effects).[11] To aid in the interpretation of these results, the IMRT plans were scaled to a conventional fractionation scheme, again using the linear-quadratic model (α/β = 10 for the tumor). Composite dose distributions were produced by adding the whole-pelvis and AG-IMRT distributions.

Figures 23.5-2 and 23.5-3 show examples of the conventional brachytherapy and IMRT dose distributions superimposed on three-dimensional reconstructions of the tumor, bladder, and rectum for a small tumor and a large tumor, respectively. The dose distributions in Figures 23.5-2 and 23.5-3 clearly indicate the improved flexibility that IMRT has to offer with respect to target volume coverage. The target volume dose-volume histograms are shown for all 10 patients in Figure 23.5-4. Note that for all patients, the IMRT plans provide significantly better coverage of the tumor volume compared with ICB. However, ICB plans typically irradiate a larger volume of tumor to doses greater than the prescription dose.

Future Directions

Thus far, our studies have focused on the dosimetric properties of AG-IMRT. To clinically implement such an approach, an applicator substitute must be designed and fabricated. There are several important properties that such a device should have. First, it should be radiopaque so that it can be localized using fluoroscopy or planar imaging. Second, it should be positioned through the cervix and within the uterine cavity so that the localized region will be within the tumor-bearing tissues. There are a few possible candidates for these substitutes, including the tandem and

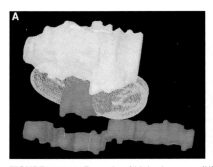 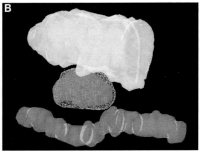

FIGURE 23.5-2. Example of high–dose rate (HDR) dose distribution for a patient with a small tumor volume (37.3 cm³). The tumor volume is shown in red, the bladder is shown in yellow, and the rectum is shown in gray. The image has been rotated to match the supine treatment position. (*A*) HDR brachytherapy; (*B*) applicator-guided intensity-modulated radiation therapy. (To view a color version of this image, please refer to the CD-ROM). Reproduced with permission from Wahab SH et al.[9]

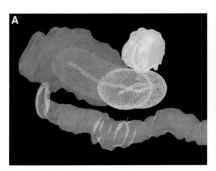 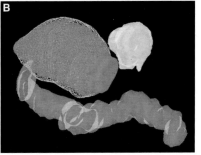

FIGURE 23.5-3. Example of high–dose rate (HDR) dose distribution for a large tumor volume (217.9 cm³). The tumor volume is shown in red, the bladder is shown in yellow, and the rectum is shown in gray. The image has been rotated to match the supine treatment position. (*A*) HDR brachytherapy; (*B*) applicator-guided intensity-modulated radiation therapy. (To view a color version of this image, please refer to the CD-ROM). Reproduced with permission from Wahab SH et al.[9]

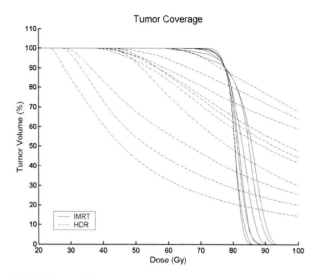

FIGURE 23.5-4. Target volume coverage (dose-volume histograms) for the 10 patients studied by Wahab and colleagues.[9] HDR = high dose rate; IMRT = intensity-modulated radiation therapy. Reproduced with permission from Wahab SH et al.[9]

colpostats themselves. However, the process of inserting the tandem and colpostats manipulates the vagina and uterus such that reproducibility of internal organ placement is compromised. Plastic stents are currently used to aid in repeated tandem placement for HDR remote afterloading of tandems, and these stents could be modified to be radiopaque and used as applicator substitutes. Unfortunately, there have been no imaging studies investigating the reproducibility of organ positioning with respect to stent placement, so this hypothesis has not yet been adequately tested.

One significant limitation with AG-IMRT, however, is the reduced high-dose region that IMRT offers with respect to ICB. It is possible that part of the relatively good local control obtained with brachytherapy is due to the very high doses near the sources, a feature that IMRT cannot provide. This high dose may be coupled with tumor regression during the beginning of therapy such that much of

even a large tumor receives high doses for the latter implants.[12] Clinical trials will be required to determine the efficacy of this approach for cervical cancer treatments.

References

1. Komaki R, Brickner T, Hanlon A, et al. Long-term results of treatment of cervical carcinoma in the United States in 1973, 1978 and 1983: a Patterns of Care Study (PCS). Int J Radiat Oncol Biol Phys 1995;31:973–82.
2. Corn B, Galvin J, Soffen E, et al. Positional stability of sources during low-dose-rate brachytherapy for cervical carcinoma. Int J Radiat Oncol Biol Phys 1993;26:513–8.
3. Perez CA. Uterine cervix. In: Perez CA, Brady LWS, editors. Uterine cervix. Philadelphia: JB Lippincott; 1992. p. 1143–202.
4. Corn B, Lanciano R, D'Agostino R, et al. The relationship of local and distant failure from endometrial cancer: defining a clinical paradigm. Gynecol Oncol 1997;66:411–6.
5. Chao KS, Williamson JF, Grigsby PW, et al. Uterosacral space involvement in locally advanced carcinoma of the uterine cervix. Int J Radiat Oncol Biol Phys 1998;40:397–403.
6. Low DA, Grigsby PW, Dempsey JF, et al. Applicator-guided intensity-modulated radiation therapy. Int J Radiat Oncol Biol Phys 2002;52:1400–6.
7. Grigsby PW, Dehdashti F, Siegel BA. FDG-PET evaluation of carcinoma of the cervix. Clin Positron Imaging 1999;2:105–9.
8. Miller TR, Grigsby PW. Measurement of tumor volume by PET to evaluate prognosis in patients with advanced cervical cancer treated by radiation therapy. Int J Radiat Oncol Biol Phys 2002;53:353–9.
9. Wahab SH, Malyapa RS, Mutic S, et al. A treatment planning study comparing HDR and AGIMRT for cervical cancer. Med Phys 2004;31:734-43.
10. Castleman K. Digital image processing. Englewood Cliffs (NJ): Prentice Hall; 1996.
11. Joiner MC, Vander Logel AJ. The linear-quadratic approach to fractionation and calculation of isoeffect relationships. In: Steel GG, editor. Basic clinical radiobiology. New York: Oxford University Press; 1997. p. 106–22.
12. Perez CA, Brady LW. Gynecologic malignancies. In: Perez CA, Brady LW, editors. Gynecologic malignancies. Philadelphia: Lippincott-Raven; 1998. p. 1733–834.

Lymphoma

Overview

Billy W. Loo Jr, MD, PhD, Richard T. Hoppe, MD, FACR

Hodgkin's disease (HD) and non-Hodgkin's lymphoma (NHL) are relatively uncommon malignancies, representing about 5% of new cancer cases in the United States annually.[1] This heterogeneous group of diseases tends to be radioresponsive compared with other malignancies and is well treated with doses within the tolerance range of many normal tissues. Not surprisingly, intensity-modulated radiation therapy (IMRT), often used for dose escalation or normal tissue dose reduction, is used infrequently in these patients. In a recent survey, fewer than 10% of the approximately one-third of radiation oncologists who employ IMRT have used it for this indication, all of them at academic centers.[2] Likewise, there is currently no published literature on the outcomes of IMRT for lymphoma.

Nevertheless, there are clinical situations in which IMRT may be useful in patients with lymphoma. Given the important, often central, role of radiation therapy (RT) in lymphoid neoplasms, the rising incidence of NHL,[1] and the increasing adoption of IMRT,[2] its use in patients with lymphoma will likely grow substantially.

In this chapter, the role and evolution of RT in the treatment of lymphoma, potential applications of IMRT in this setting, clinical and technical issues, and anticipated future directions are reviewed.

Rationale

RT for Lymphoma

The history of RT in the management of lymphoma stretches back more than a century. In 1901, A. J. Ochsner referred a young boy with HD to William Allen Pusey at the University of Illinois. Although a dermatologist, Pusey appreciated the potential beneficial effects of Roentgen rays not only in the treatment of skin diseases but also in more deeply situated tumors.

According to his mother, the boy had experienced "eight months of increasing swelling of the glands on the left side of his neck, followed by similar swelling on the right side."

Ochsner resected the glands on the right. However, when Pusey saw the child, swelling was evident on the left side "as large as a fist." Under x-ray exposures, it rapidly subsided and in 2 months was reduced to the size of an almond. At the same time, the boy changed from a "cachectic, sluggish child to a bright lively one." The results of this case (complete with a series of before and after photographs) were published by Pusey in 1902.[3]

In their 1904 textbook, Pusey and Caldwell concluded that there was no question as to the beneficial effect of x-rays in HD.[4] "There can surely be no doubt," they wrote, "that cases of Hodgkin's disease should be given the benefit of x-ray exposures as soon as possible after the disease is diagnosed. There seems to be a reasonable hope that, by the use of x-rays, years of usefulness may be added to the lives of these patients."[4]

Another series of patients was reported by Nicholas Senn in 1903.[5] One case was a 43-year-old male with extensive bilateral cervical, axillary, and inguinal involvement. He had dullness over the anterior chest, and his spleen was considerably enlarged. Within a month of the initiation of treatment, "all of the glands subjected to the x-ray treatment [had] nearly disappeared."[5] The clinical description and response in this patient suggest a diagnosis of follicular lymphoma.

Impressed by the outcome of this patient and another he reported in the same article, Senn concluded that

the eminent success attained in these two cases by the use of the x-ray can leave no further doubt of the curative effect of the Röntgen therapy... Additional experience will give us more definite information as to the best methods for using the Röntgen ray in the treatment of this disease, with a view of preventing burns and toxic symptoms without reducing its curative effect.[5]

This general philosophy is one that radiation oncologists have followed in the ensuing century!

RT continued to be the most effective treatment for the lymphomas during the first part of the twentieth century but, essentially, remained a palliative approach. More effective therapy followed advances in imaging allowing more precise identification of disease and technology permitting comprehensive treatment with good quality control. The Coolidge tube was developed in the 1920s and provided a more reliable treatment beam with improved hardness compared with gas tubes, making orthovoltage x-ray therapy in the energy range of 200 to 250 kV possible. For many years, this provided state-of-the-art therapy. Later, the cobalt-60 machine and, finally, the linear accelerator made true curative RT for lymphomas a reality.

One of the first radiologists to appreciate the curative potential for RT in HD was Rene Gilbert, a Swiss radiologist. Gilbert was among the first to note the predictable clinical behavior of HD, and he attempted to adapt his treatment techniques accordingly.[6] He wrote, "Many times I have seen recurrence developing in the immediate vicinity of a field too narrowly irradiated."[7] Gilbert advocated irradiation of suspected disease in apparently uninvolved adjacent lymph node regions and the clinically evident involved sites.

Dramatic advances in the use of RT had to await the work of two preeminent North American radiation oncologists, M. Vera Peters from the Princess Margaret Hospital and Henry S. Kaplan from Stanford University. Following up on the earlier observations of her predecessor, Gordon Richards at the University of Toronto, Peters advocated extended-field irradiation in HD, including prophylactic treatment of adjacent sites. In an analysis of patients treated between 1924 and 1942, she reported improved outcomes with extended fields and higher doses.[8]

A co-inventor of the medical linear accelerator, Henry Kaplan was chair of the Department of Radiology at Stanford University. He was a strong advocate of high-dose extended-field irradiation for HD. At the 1961 meeting of the Radiological Society of North America, Kaplan presented his seminal paper ("Radical Radiotherapy of Regionally Localized Hodgkin's Disease"), in which he reported dramatic differences in outcome for patients with HD who underwent radical versus palliative treatment.[9] More than 70% of patients treated radically remained free of disease recurrence, whereas all who received palliative therapy experienced a recurrence within 4 years.

The superiority of extended-field RT was subsequently demonstrated in prospective, randomized clinical trials at Stanford University.[10] However, the advantage of more intensive treatment was noted only in freedom from relapse because patients who relapsed were often successfully treated with chemotherapy. Nevertheless, the more aggressive initial radiation program became standard. Large single-institution reports and cooperative group studies achieved 10-year survival rates of 85 to 90% and 10-year freedom-from-relapse rates of 75 to 80% for patients with stage I–II disease.[11]

As systemic therapies became more effective and less toxic, treatment of early-stage HD began to combine brief chemotherapy with limited (involved field) RT. These programs have resulted in survival rates equal to or better than those of programs of RT alone, and the freedom-from-relapse rates have been excellent.[11,12]

In addition to its role in stage I–II disease, RT is used in some patients with stage III–IV HD. Although its benefit remains unclear in patients achieving a complete response to chemotherapy, it may "convert" partial responders to complete responders, who then have an excellent prognosis.[13] In addition, it is routinely incorporated into programs for advanced HD together with abbreviated chemotherapy regimens, such as with Stanford V.[14] Finally, limited radiation may be a useful component in patients receiving high-dose therapy and hematopoietic cell rescue after relapse.[15]

In NHL, the situation with respect to treatment was much more complicated. Not until the early 1970s were clinically useful classification systems developed. It soon became evident that effective treatments varied by histology. At first, radiation programs analogous to HD were used for the most common types of NHL, follicular lymphoma (also known as nodular lymphoma) and diffuse large B-cell lymphoma (also known as diffuse histiocytic or diffuse large cell). However, the patterns of relapse for these diseases were different from those for HD, tending to be more commonly systemic and less predictable.[16] This led to an earlier incorporation of systemic therapy, even with stage I–II disease. For patients with stage I–II diffuse large B-cell NHL, chemotherapy followed by involved-field RT has proved to be the treatment of choice.[17] However, for stage I–II follicular lymphomas (grade 1–2), involved-field RT alone remains an effective therapy.[18]

As with HD, RT serves many other roles in the NHL, beyond primary therapy. It has been employed as local treatment or total-body irradiation as a component of high-dose therapy and hematopoietic cell rescue.[19,20] It also plays a very important role in palliative treatment.

Conventional RT for Lymphoma

Although the tumoricidal dose for HD and NHL is relatively modest, especially in the context of combined-modality therapy, and organ tolerance is usually not exceeded, the wide-field treatment used in the past and long follow-up of patients have permitted identification of significant late effects related to radiation exposure.[21] Therefore, careful consideration of both short-term toxicity and long-term morbidity is essential in treatment planning. For supradiaphragmatic treatment, there is potential toxicity involving the salivary glands, thyroid, soft tissues of the neck and shoulder girdle (especially in young patients), brachial plexus, spinal cord, heart, and lungs. For subdiaphragmatic fields, dose-limiting organs include the kidneys, spinal cord, liver, bone marrow, gastrointestinal tract, and gonads.

In adults, the most radiosensitive of these organs is the lungs, where radiographic evidence of acute pulmonary reactions may be observed with doses to large lung volumes in excess of 15 Gy. However, the lungs may be treated safely to a dose of 16.5 Gy if protracted fractionation techniques are employed. Function may be ablated in areas of the lung treated to doses in excess of 25 Gy, and areas of the lung treated to 40 to 44 Gy often demonstrate fibrosis during long-term follow-up; however, the severity varies remarkably among patients.

Subclinical pericardial injury may develop at lower doses, but symptomatic pericarditis is rare unless the dose to the entire pericardium exceeds 30 Gy. Partial-field blocking (apical portion of the heart at 15 Gy, subcarinal portion of the heart at 30 Gy) reduces that risk. Although the myocardium is slightly more resistant, doses > 35 Gy may be associated with myocardial dysfunction. The coronary arteries are moderately radiation resistant; however, doses > 30 Gy increase the risk of coronary artery disease and myocardial infarction.[22]

Tolerance doses of the other organs at risk vary considerably. Doses ≥ 40 Gy may be associated with soft tissue and muscle atrophy, even in adults. Children experience adverse effects on growth or soft tissue development with doses as low as 15 Gy. Xerostomia may develop in patients treated to the Waldeyer's ring region. Thyroid gland function may be diminished, despite partial thyroid shielding with a larynx block.[23] Although spinal cord tolerance should not be an issue with standard approaches, the length of spinal cord included and use of contiguous fields overlapping the cord demand conservative dose guidelines and attention to detail. Brachial plexus injury should not be expected. However, for older techniques that employed larger daily doses, failed to take into account variations in body thickness, or ignored previous treatment when planning therapy for recurrence, doses of 44 Gy have been associated with long-term brachial plexopathy.

In the abdomen, dose-limiting organ toxicity is rarely an issue. Only a small portion of the total renal volume is within a conventional para-aortic–splenic pedicle field. If the spleen is treated, the proportion of renal volume is much greater, but with computed tomography (CT) planning, it is generally ≤ 30% of the left kidney. Although 30 to 36 Gy is sufficient to ablate renal function in that portion of the kidney, this should not impact on normal renal function. One must be alert, however, to the presence of underlying renal disease that may already compromise renal function.

A portion of the left lobe of the liver is included in the para-aortic field, which may cause transient hepatic dysfunction (accompanied by an elevation of the serum alkaline phosphatase level) but is not associated with late sequelae. In fact, the entire liver may be treated safely to a dose of 25 Gy using protracted fractionation. The gastrointestinal tract generally tolerates doses up to 44 Gy.

However, patients who have undergone abdominal surgical procedures such as staging laparotomy and have formed intra-abdominal adhesions may develop evidence of bowel injury with doses of ≥ 36 Gy. In the pelvis, the gonads are the most sensitive organ. The ovaries are exquisitely sensitive, especially in older (> 30 years) women. Fractionated doses of 4 Gy or more should be avoided.

In addition, a significant risk for patients is the development of treatment-related malignancies.[24] Long-term follow-up is essential to define this risk. Leukemia may develop in about 5% of patients, with a latent period of 3 to 7 years after chemotherapy that includes an alkylating agent such as MOPP, which consists of nitrogen mustard, vincristine, prednisone, and procarbazine. The occurrence of leukemia after treatment with RT alone is exceedingly rare, and it remains controversial as to whether the risk is greater after combined-modality therapy. Secondary solid tumors may be related to either chemotherapy or radiation and generally have a longer latent period (at least 7–10 years). Smokers are at high risk of developing lung cancer after radiation exposure. The relative risk that a female patient with HD will develop breast cancer after treatment is 4.1, primarily in women who are younger than 30 years at diagnosis.[25] Other solid tumors that may be increased include thyroid, salivary gland, pancreas, stomach, bone and soft tissue, and melanoma.

Potential Roles for IMRT

Given the long follow-up that many patients with lymphoma are likely to have, they are at risk of developing injuries that may be associated with even modest radiation doses. IMRT is thus appealing because it may limit the dose selectively to sensitive organs, reducing the risk of treatment-related toxicities.

Depending on the lymphoma type, stage, and clinical situation, RT may be used alone or in combination with chemotherapy. When used alone for curative treatment of HD, extended fields generally must be treated even in patients with early-stage disease because of the high incidence of clinically unapparent disease outside the gross tumor volume (GTV). Systemic therapy can serve as a substitute for extended fields to treat microscopic disease, allowing restriction of RT fields to involved regions and dose reduction. Salvage treatment of recurrent disease within previously irradiated sites requires further restriction of the dose and volume of tissues treated. In each of these situations, IMRT has potential advantages.

Extended-Field Treatment

Classically, treatment fields for lymphoma are based on lymph node regions defined by the Ann Arbor staging system (Figure 24-1)[26] and typically employ shaped opposed beams. Examples include the mantle field, encompassing the bilateral neck; supraclavicular, infraclavicular, and axillary regions;

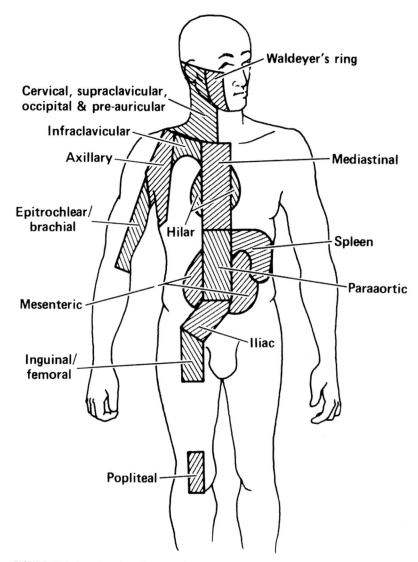

FIGURE 24-1. Lymph node regions used in the Ann Arbor staging system for Hodgkin's disease. Reproduced with permission from Hoppe RT.[68]

mediastinum and bilateral hila; the spade field encompassing the spleen, para-aortic, and common iliac regions; and subtotal lymphoid irradiation, the sum of all of these.

Treatment of such comprehensive fields to high dose, once standard for managing HD, is now used uncommonly given the availability and success of combined-modality treatment. It remains, however, an acceptable treatment for selected patients who are unable to receive or refuse chemotherapy. Also, lower-dose treatment to large or comprehensive fields is used as part of the preparative regimen for certain hematopoietic cell and organ transplant regimens and continues to be a core component of current protocols for advanced-stage pediatric HD. Dosimetric studies have shown that IMRT reduces the dose to normal tissues at risk of late complications while maintaining or improving coverage of the target in patients treated with extended fields.[27,28]

Combined-Modality Programs

The current standard management of both HD and NHL, particularly in early stages, involves combining systemic therapy with RT limited to sites of gross involvement or, in some cases, only to sites of bulky disease. When the disease is adjacent to particularly sensitive normal tissues or when it is bulky, dose-volume constraints for uninvolved critical structures may be exceeded using conventional field arrangements, even given the relatively modest doses prescribed to the targets. IMRT may make it possible to meet prescription goals and dose constraints in such cases.

In-Field Recurrences

RT is commonly employed as a component of salvage therapy for HD and NHL, either alone or more often combined with chemotherapy or high-dose chemotherapy with hematopoietic cell rescue. Particularly when disease relapse is in a previously irradiated area, dose-volume constraints for sensitive structures become more difficult to satisfy because even otherwise relatively tolerant tissues have already received a significant fraction of their tolerance dose. The spinal cord, for example, is frequently a dose-limiting organ in this setting. In addition, the effects of chemotherapy and other biologic factors may reduce tolerance doses to unexpectedly low levels, resulting in untoward sequelae.[29,30] Although these are rare occurrences, conservatism with respect to protecting critical structures is warranted for patients who may have a long survival, and IMRT may be a useful tool for achieving it.

Issues and Challenges
Patient Selection

Patients with lymphoma who might benefit from IMRT are those for whom RT is indicated and whose disease is anatomically located such that adjacent uninvolved tissues are at significant risk of acute or late injury at the doses required for treatment. Depending on the specific clinical situation, including tumor burden and response to chemotherapy, standard doses for HD range from 20 to 36 Gy and for aggressive NHL from 30 to 40 Gy or higher in daily fractions of 1.5 to 2 Gy. A number of normal tissues have tolerances within these dose ranges and must be considered when treating disease sites in the corresponding anatomic regions. Some selected scenarios are discussed below that are encountered relatively frequently.

Lymphoma may involve a number of head and neck sites, including Waldeyer's ring, the paranasal sinuses, and cervical nodes. Conventional fields may resemble those for carcinomas of the head and neck, such as nasopharyngeal carcinoma. Sensitive structures include the salivary glands, with xerostomia as a common late toxicity. A whole-organ dose to the parotid gland of only 28 Gy can be expected to result in a 50% incidence of permanent reduction of salivary production. In the case of partial organ or nonuniform irradiation, a mean dose of 24 to 26 Gy appears to be the threshold.[31] With IMRT, it is generally possible to restrict the mean dose to at least one parotid gland to less than this limit; several studies of parotid-sparing IMRT for head and neck carcinoma demonstrating preservation of salivary function are reviewed in Chapter 18, "Head and Neck Cancer: Overview." These results should apply to head and neck lymphomas as well.

The mediastinum is a common site of bulky lymphadenopathy. Although chemotherapy usually results in substantially decreased tumor volumes, bulky residual masses may remain, resulting in large volumes of lung irradiated when using conventional ports. A greater than 20% risk of pneumonitis is associated with a mean lung dose of > 20 Gy or if > 18% of the lung volume receives > 30 Gy.[32] These limits frequently are exceeded in this situation and require either accepting a greater risk of pulmonary toxicity or compromising on the tumor coverage. IMRT may be valuable in this setting, but, as discussed below, some means of addressing intrathoracic organ motion would be critical for its success. Figure 24-2 illustrates the dose distribution for a hypothetical IMRT mantle treatment with emphasis on lung and breast sparing.

Bulky para-aortic lymphadenopathy is a frequent presentation of abdominal disease. In addition, the spleen is often either involved or must be treated for potential microscopic involvement. In this region, the kidneys frequently limit the dose and/or volume treated. A whole-organ dose of 20 Gy is associated with a ~ 10% incidence of late symptomatic radiation nephropathy, rising to 50% at about 27 Gy.[33] These effects may become manifest only after a latency period of many years. Functional changes detectable by scintigraphy

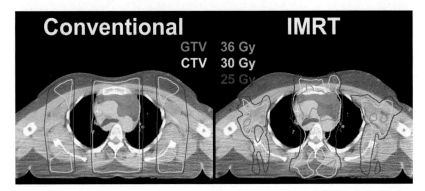

FIGURE 24-2. Conventional versus intensity-modulated radiation therapy (IMRT) dose distributions for a hypothetical mantle treatment. The patient is a young woman with a bulky mediastinal mass from nodular sclerosing Hodgkin's disease. The conventional treatment was planned using full three-dimensional compensation, with a prescription dose of 30 Gy to the midplane. The IMRT plan, designed to emphasize lung and breast sparing, demonstrates improved target coverage, sparing of at-risk normal tissues, and an integrated boost to 36 Gy to the gross tumor volume (GTV). CTV = clinical target volume. (To view a color version of this image, please refer to the CD-ROM.)

appear at lower doses, appearing in 50% of kidneys receiving 27 Gy to 10% of the volume, or 7.6 Gy to the entire organ.[34] The discrepancy between these measures probably reflects the reserve capacity of residual functional kidney tissue. A dosimetric study has demonstrated the ability of IMRT to spare the kidneys when treating a spade field for bulky para-aortic involvement of HD (see the accompanying case study in Chapter 24.1, "Hodgkin's Disease: Case Study").[27]

Other organs at risk after modest radiation doses include the lens,[35] thyroid gland,[36,37] coronary arteries,[22] ovary,[38] and bone marrow.[39] In selected cases, attempting to exclude these structures from the high-dose region may be warranted. Also, it is important to note that the doses discussed above pertain to adults receiving conventionally fractionated (1.8–2 Gy daily fractions) RT. In children or patients receiving chemotherapy or altered fractionation schedules, tolerance doses are lower, sometimes considerably so, and may depend strongly on the patient's age. Other considerations in children include, for example, that the threshold dose for significant growth abnormalities is about 20 to 25 Gy,[40] so skeletal growth regions may be reasonable avoidance structures in selected cases.

Target Delineation

Classically, lymphomas were treated with radical RT, in which the clinical target volume (CTV) consisted of all of the major lymph node–bearing regions (total or subtotal lymphoid irradiation) even when gross disease was limited in extent. Although distant sites are at risk of microscopic involvement, current chemotherapy regimens are, in general, effective for managing subclinical disease. RT is directed at the highest-risk regions using involved fields. The definition of involved fields varies somewhat between institutions. At Stanford University, the (high risk) CTV for nodal disease consists of the entire lymph node region or regions containing gross

disease, with some modifications. For example, when treating disease in the mediastinum, the CTV also includes the bilateral supraclavicular and hilar areas; when the axilla is irradiated, the ipsilateral supraclavicular and infraclavicular areas are included. Although somewhat arbitrary, these definitions of CTV are straightforward and easy to apply consistently. The CTV for extralymphatic disease is necessarily less well defined and consists of a rationally designed margin around the GTV (the original extent of disease prior to chemotherapy). In most situations, the prescription dose to the CTV is the same as that to the GTV.

Conventional fields defined in this manner are relatively straightforward to design and can be shaped using classic skeletal landmarks on planar radiographs. For IMRT, the target volumes and nearby normal structures must be defined in three dimensions using a planning CT scan, which involves contouring all of the lymph node–bearing volumes within the anatomic regions of interest (see the accompanying case study in Chapter 24.1). This is complicated by the fact that normal-sized lymphatic structures may not be visible on routine imaging. Thus, the associated vascular structures are used as a guide for target definition. Published cross-sectional imaging atlases of lymph node regions are also helpful,[41–43] as are lymphangiograms, when available.

Imaging modalities other than CT are often helpful for target and normal tissue delineation in selected cases. For disease near the base of the skull, such as in the nasopharynx or parapharyngeal areas, or in the paranasal sinuses, the superior soft tissue contrast of magnetic resonance imaging (MRI) can improve visualization of the relevant structures. In such cases, we have used the image fusion capability of the treatment planning system to register diagnostic MRIs to the treatment planning CT scan. Segmentation of normal and target structures is then performed using the combination of the scans (Figure 24-3).

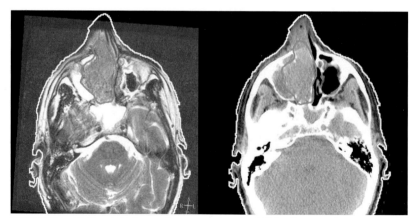

FIGURE 24-3. Multimodality (magnetic resonance imaging [MRI] and computed tomography [CT]) image fusion for treatment planning. In this case of plasmablastic lymphoma of the right maxillary sinus and nasal cavity, three-dimensional fusion of the diagnostic T2-weighted MRI (*left*) to the treatment planning CT scan (*right*) permits more accurate delineation of the gross tumor volume (highlighted in *red*). The external contour is highlighted in yellow. (To view a color version of this image, please refer to the CD-ROM.)

Because of the relatively rigid anatomy in the head, reproducing the treatment position within the magnetic resonance scanner is not essential for satisfactory image registration when questions about disease extent are confined to this region.

Positron emission tomography (PET) using the tracer ^{18}F-labeled fluorodeoxyglucose ([18]FDG) characterizes tissues based on their degree of glucose metabolism, which is markedly increased in many tumors. It has proven to be more accurate than conventional imaging methods, including CT and gallium scanning for staging HD and many NHL subtypes,[44,45] and is now considered part of the standard initial staging evaluation for most lymphomas. Because [18]FDG-PET is often capable of detecting disease in otherwise unenlarged lymph nodes, it can also be a useful adjunct to the planning CT scan for delineating the initial (prechemotherapy) extent of disease and the target volumes. To use it most effectively, the patient should be immobilized in the treatment position during both the diagnostic PET and the planning CT scans. Fiducial markers on the patient and/or immobilization device that are visible in both modalities help make the image fusion more accurate. Without their use, the lower resolution of the PET scan may compromise the quality of registration. This is less of an issue if a combined PET-CT scanner is used because in such an instrument, there is a fixed relationship between the coordinate systems of the two modalities (Figure 24-4).[46] On a practical note, given the degree of coordination required, the radiation oncologist should be involved early in the evaluation and management of the patient.

Treatment Reproducibility

The high conformity of IMRT planning depends on both the ability to localize accurately structures of interest in three dimensions and the reproducibility of the positions of those structures when treatment is delivered. Use of immobilization aids, which should be as rigid as possible, helps to reduce variability in patient positioning between treatments (interfraction variability). For treatment of the head, neck, and supraclavicular areas, a combination of a customized thermoplastic mask and molded neck and shoulder supports is useful. Custom supports such as binary foam or vacuum-lock molds may be helpful for immobilizing other body regions. Reference marks on the patient (tattoos) and the immobilization aids should be made in adequate number to verify visually the correct position of the isocenter and appropriately align mobile body parts at each treatment. Imaging verification of at least the isocenter should be performed frequently. The setup margins used to define the planning target volume and planning organ at risk volumes should be appropriate to the immobilization system used.

Particularly in the thorax and upper abdomen, internal organ motion from respiration produces intrafraction position variability up to 2 cm with regular breathing and substantially more with deep breathing.[47] Even when it can be done safely, simply expanding the treatment margin may not adequately compensate for this motion with respect to target coverage when using IMRT. Because IMRT is often delivered dynamically, with small portions of any field exposed sequentially, motion of the target during the delivery may result in a significantly different dose from that

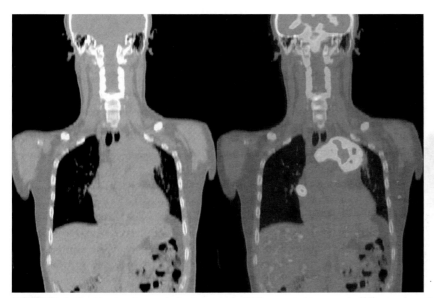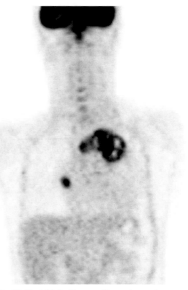

FIGURE 24-4. Combined positron emission tomography (PET)-computed tomography (CT) scan of a patient with Hodgkin's disease. Fluorodeoxyglucose-PET reveals a large centrally necrotic anterior mediastinal mass and a smaller lesion at the right cardiac border. The combined scanner permits nearly exact registration of these metabolic imaging data with the high-resolution anatomic and physical (electron density) data from the CT portion of the scan. (To view a color version of this image, please refer to the CD-ROM.)

predicted based on the static treatment plan. Gating the planning scan and treatment delivery to the respiratory cycle may localize structures during treatment in nearly their same positions as those on which the treatment was planned and may be necessary for successful application of IMRT treatment.

Differential Dose Fractionation

An inherent feature of IMRT is a large degree of dose heterogeneity within the irradiated volume. Ideally, the high-dose region conforms to areas of disease, excluding sensitive structures. Consequently, different subvolumes of tissue receive different doses per fraction, resulting in even greater differentials in biologically equivalent dose. The implications of this have been discussed in detail with respect to IMRT for head and neck cancer.[48]

The prescribed dose per fraction in conventional treatment of lymphoma tends to be relatively low, often 1.5 to 1.8 Gy in daily fractions, mainly to reduce the risk of late complications in exposed normal tissues. Using IMRT creates many options for prescription specification. These include keeping the dose per fraction to critical structures in this range while substantially increasing the dose per fraction to target structures. This would result in the acceleration of the treatment course, a reduction in total normal tissues doses, and possibly also a reduction in the total dose to the targets for the same probability of tumor control. Alternatively, the daily dose to the targets and the overall treatment time could be in the conventional range, permitting lower dose fractions and thus even lower total biologically equivalent doses to nontarget structures. Furthermore, IMRT permits multiple prescription doses within a single treatment plan so that targets felt to confer lower or higher risk to the patient can be treated simultaneously to different doses. For example, the GTV could receive a higher dose than the CTV. Again, this could be structured either as an integrated boost to escalate the dose to subregions at higher risk of treatment failure or as a means to reduce the dose to lower-risk portions of the targets and minimize toxicity to adjacent structures.

Integral Dose to Nontarget Tissues

A serious late complication of RT for lymphoma is radiation-induced secondary malignancies. These are of greater concern in this patient population, particularly those with HD, because of their relatively high probability of long-term survival. In general, when compared with dose distributions of conventional RT, the conformal IMRT dose distributions are characterized by a smaller volume of tissue receiving high doses and a larger volume receiving low doses. The latter is due to two factors. The first is not inherent to IMRT but due to the fact that IMRT often uses a greater number of beams from different angles, spreading the dose over a larger volume of tissue. The second is that in most currently available systems, modulating the beam

intensity involves sequentially exposing only a small fraction of the field aperture at any time. Because most of the beam energy is deposited in the head of the accelerator, a larger number of monitor units (MUs) is required for a given dose. Both the in-field background dose from transmission through the multileaf collimator leaves and the total-body dose owing to leakage from the head of the accelerator are roughly proportional to the total number of MUs delivered. When high-energy beams (> 6–8 MV) are used, there may be additional total-body effective dose from leakage photoneutrons.[49] It is unclear a priori whether this trade-off in dose distribution would result in a greater or lesser risk of secondary malignancy induction.

Recently, Hall and Wuu estimated that IMRT may nearly double the small risk of secondary malignancies compared with three-dimensional conformal radiation therapy (3DCRT), although they felt that 3DCRT might also have a less certain advantage over conventional RT.[50] Their analysis was based on theoretical models in which the risk of solid tumor induction is linear with a dose up to a few grays (based on atomic bomb survivor data),[51,52] beyond which it either declines or reaches a plateau with increasing dose, presumably because of cell killing (extrapolated from animal and some human data).

In such a model, any increase in the volume of tissue receiving more than a few grays is detrimental, whereas a reduction in the volume receiving high doses is not beneficial. Moreover, the dose from leakage radiation would likely have a dominant adverse effect. However, recent analyses of secondary breast and lung cancers in an international cohort of treated patients with HD, in whom secondary cancer risk was correlated with the doses received at specific sites, suggested that the cancer induction risk continues to increase with the dose, probably in a linear fashion, up to at least 40 Gy for breast cancer and 30 Gy for lung cancer.[53-55] If true, the ability of IMRT to exclude most of the normal tissues from high-dose regions would be an advantage and could have the dominant effect. In addition, to the extent that reducing the dose per fraction to normal tissues may decrease the risk of cancer induction, IMRT should have an advantage as well. Comparisons of the effects of atomic bomb exposure with those of repeated fluoroscopy have substantiated this effect of fractionation on secondary lung cancer but not breast cancer induction.[56,57] The uncertainty about the potential risks or advantages of IMRT with respect to secondary malignancies highlights the need for clinical studies with long-term follow-up.

Published Data

Two reports evaluating IMRT in the treatment of patients with lymphoma have been presented. Both are dosimetric comparisons of different forms of IMRT versus conventional treatment: IMRT for mantle-type and spade-type fields[27] and helical tomotherapy for a mantle field.[28] (See

Chapter 24.2, "Helical Tomotherapy—A New Mantle: Emerging Technology"). Compared with a standard mantle, both conventional IMRT and helical tomotherapy resulted in substantial sparing of normal tissues, including the larynx, thyroid, heart, lungs, breasts, and spinal cord, while maintaining or improving coverage of the target nodal regions. Similarly, IMRT for para-aortic–splenic treatment resulted in both improved target coverage and sparing of the kidneys, stomach, bowel, and vertebral column. In principle, these results suggest that IMRT would be expected to result in equal or improved disease control and decreased short- and long-term toxicity, although, as discussed above, the potential impact on the incidence of late second malignancies is unclear. The treatment approaches used in these two studies are highlighted in the two accompanying case studies. To date, there have been no published reports evaluating the clinical outcome of patients with lymphoma treated with IMRT.

Future Directions

Metabolic Imaging

As discussed above, IMRT makes it possible to prescribe different doses to different targets in an integrated manner based on an assessment of their risk to the patient. To make effective use of this feature requires tools that permit this assessment. Recent advances in various forms of imaging that characterize different aspects of tumor metabolism suggest that they may be useful for this purpose.

When [18]FDG-PET is used to define target volumes, as described above, the effect is to redefine the GTV as parts of what might otherwise have been included in the CTV or to exclude from the GTV areas that lack evidence of disease. This should allow a greater likelihood that the resulting CTV contains only truly microscopic disease, making it a target volume that may be adequately treated with chemotherapy. Consequently, it may be reasonable to treat only the [18]FDG-PET–defined GTV to the conventional dose while treating the CTV to a lower dose and possibly decreasing its volume.

Conversely, [18]FDG-PET may define targets at higher risk of treatment failure, allowing them to be treated to a higher dose. Persistent [18]FDG uptake following chemotherapy is predictive of treatment failure in both patients with HD and patients with NHL (mostly aggressive subtypes), with relapses occurring in the sites of abnormal metabolism.[58-61] In one study, eight patients with HD with abnormal [18]FDG-PET scans after the chemotherapy portion of combined modality therapy subsequently received their initially prescribed RT. Six had reversal of the imaging abnormalities and remained disease free, whereas two had persistent abnormalities and relapsed in those sites.[60] Of note, a normal scan following chemotherapy is not sufficient to exclude treatment failure. [18]FDG-PET scans earlier in the course of

chemotherapy are more sensitive for predicting the outcome of both HD and NHL[62,63] and may have the highest negative predictive value as early as after a single cycle of chemotherapy.[64] Thus, residual areas of abnormal [18]FDG uptake early in the course of chemotherapy may represent sites that are at higher risk of treatment failure and that might be treated more effectively with a higher radiation dose.

[18]FDG has been the most validated metabolic imaging agent for staging, response assessment, and outcome prediction of a wide range of malignancies. However, many other imaging agents currently under development may be useful for assessing specific aspects of tumor metabolism and hold promise for the applications discussed above. Fluorodeoxythymidine (FLT) is a synthetic nucleoside analog that is metabolized preferentially by proliferating cells. Its uptake, as measured by FLT-PET, correlated strongly on a per lesion basis with cellular proliferation measured by the degree of labeling of the Ki-67 antigen in biopsy samples in patients with NHL.[65] As measured by single-photon emission computed tomography (SPECT), the degree of uptake of ^{99m}Tc-labeled recombinant human annexin V, a marker of apoptosis, after one cycle of chemotherapy correlated strongly with treatment response and survival in a small group of patients that included three patients with lymphomas (two with NHL, one with HD).[66] Another study using this agent in 11 patients with low-grade follicular lymphoma treated with 2 x 2 Gy involved field RT demonstrated correlation between imaging, cytologic measures of apoptosis, and clinical response.[67] These and other novel imaging agents may ultimately prove useful for differentiating lymphomas by biologic behavior and stratifying lesions by risk.

Clinical Trials

Clinical trials of IMRT in the treatment of other malignancies have demonstrated both improved efficacy from its ability to safely escalate tumor dose and reduced short- and long-term toxicity from improved sparing of nontarget tissues. Similar data are lacking for the treatment of lymphomas, partly because IMRT has been used infrequently in these patients so far. However, the long-term toxicities following RT for lymphomas are perhaps better described than for any other malignancies, largely because of the higher long-term survival of this patient population overall. Acknowledging this risk, the strategy in many clinical trials for lymphoma has been to emphasize the use of systemic therapy, often to the exclusion of RT. However, this strategy may backfire, and the risk for local recurrence may become greater if RT is omitted. This was observed in the European Organization for the Research and Treatment of Cancer (EORTC) H9 trial, in which the chemotherapy-alone arm for patients with favorable prognosis, early-stage HD who had an apparent complete remission following chemotherapy was discontinued because of an excessive number of relapses (E. M. Noordijk, personal communication, October 2003). The appropriate use of IMRT has the potential to further decrease the risk of normal tissue injury without necessarily reducing the dose to disease sites and may expand the range over which the competing toxicities of RT and chemotherapy can be balanced. Well-designed clinical trials with adequate long-term follow-up are needed to assess whether the use of IMRT in lymphoma achieves a reduction in acute and subacute toxicity without increasing the risk of secondary cancer. Given its highly conformal nature, assessment of its efficacy requires meticulous attention to the documentation of patterns of failure in three dimensions, and follow-up imaging performed in the original treatment position should be considered.

Acknowledgments

We would like to thank our colleagues, Dr. Daniel S. Kapp, Dr. Todd A. Pawlicki, Dr. Steven M. Crooks, Dr. Thomas M. Guerrero, Dr. Lei Xing, Dr. Cristian Cotrutz, Raymond Wu, Linda Yuen, Sherri Thornton, Maria Vega, and Wendy Chang, for their valuable discussions, input, and assistance in the preparation of this chapter and accompanying case study.

References

1. Jemal A, Murray T, Samuels A, et al. Cancer statistics, 2003. CA Cancer J Clin 2003;53:1:5–26.

2. Mell LK, Roeske JC, Mundt AJ. A survey of intensity-modulated radiation therapy use in the United States. Cancer 2003;98:1:204–11.

3. Pusey WA. Cases of sarcoma and of Hodgkin's disease treated by exposures to x-rays—a preliminary report. JAMA 1902;38:3:166–9.

4. Pusey WA, Caldwell EW. The practical application of the röntgen rays in therapeutics and diagnosis. 2nd ed. Philadelphia: Saunders; 1904.

5. Senn N. The therapeutical value of the röntgen ray in the treatment of pseudoleucæmia. N Y Med J 1903;77:16:665–8.

6. Gilbert R, Babaiantz L. Notre méthode de roentgenthérapie de la lymphogranulomatose (Hodgkin): résultats éloignés. Acta Radiol 1931;12:523–9.

7. Gilbert R, Radiotherapy in Hodgkin's Disease (malignant granulomatosis): anatomic and clinical foundations, governing principles, results. AJR Am J Roentgenol 1939; 41:198-241.

8. Peters MV. A study of survivals in Hodgkin's disease treated radiologically. AJR Am J Roentgenol 1950;63:3:299–311.

9. Kaplan HS. The radical radiotherapy of regionally localized Hodgkin's disease. Radiology 1962;78:553–61.

10. Rosenberg SA, Kaplan HS. The evolution and summary results of the Stanford randomized clinical trials of the management of Hodgkin's disease: 1962-1984. Int J Radiat Oncol Biol Phys 1985;11:1:5–22.

11. Mauch PM, Connors JM, Pavlovsky S, et al. Treatment of favorable prognosis stage I-II Hodgkin's disease. In: Mauch PM, Armitage JO, Diehl V, et al, editors. Hodgkin's disease. Philadelphia: Lippincott Williams & Wilkins; 1999. p. 435–58.

12. Horning SJ, Hoppe RT, Breslin S, et al. Very brief (8 weeks) chemotherapy and low dose (30 Gy) radiotherapy for limited stage Hodgkin's disease: preliminary results of the Stanford-Kaiser G4 study of Stanford V plus radiotherapy [abstract]. Blood 1999;94:10 Suppl.

13. Aleman BM, Raemaekers JM, Tirelli U, et al. Involved-field radiotherapy for advanced Hodgkin's lymphoma. N Engl J Med 2003;348:2396–406.

14. Horning SJ, Hoppe RT, Breslin S, et al. Stanford V and radiotherapy for locally extensive and advanced Hodgkin's disease: mature results of a prospective clinical trial. J Clin Oncol 2002;20:630–7.

15. Poen JC, Hoppe RT, Horning SJ. High-dose therapy and autologous bone marrow transplantation for relapsed/refractory Hodgkin's disease: the impact of involved field radiotherapy on patterns of failure and survival. Int J Radiat Oncol Biol Phys 1996;36:1:3–12.

16. Hoppe RT. Patterns of failure after treatment for the non-Hodgkin's lymphomas. Cancer Treat Symp 1983;2:133–6.

17. Miller TP, Dahlberg S, Cassady JR, et al. Chemotherapy alone compared with chemotherapy plus radiotherapy for localized intermediate- and high-grade non-Hodgkin's lymphoma. N Engl J Med 1998;339:21–6.

18. MacManus MP, Hoppe RT. Is radiotherapy curative for stage I and II low-grade follicular lymphoma? Results of a long-term follow-up study of patients treated at Stanford University. J Clin Oncol 1996;14:4:1282–90.

19. Mundt AJ, Williams SF, Hallahan D. High dose chemotherapy and stem cell rescue for aggressive non-Hodgkin's lymphoma: pattern of failure and implications for involved-field radiotherapy. Int J Radiat Oncol Biol Phys 1997;39:617–25.

20. Horning SJ, Negrin RS, Chao JC, et al. Fractionated total-body irradiation, etoposide, and cyclophosphamide plus autografting in Hodgkin's disease and non-Hodgkin's lymphoma. J Clin Oncol 1994;12:2552–8.

21. Hoppe RT. Hodgkin's disease. In: Perez CA, Brady LW, Halperin E, et al, editors. Principles and practice of radiation oncology. 4th ed. Philadelphia: Lippincott Williams & Wilkins; 2003. p. 2043–63.

22. Hancock SL, Tucker MA, Hoppe RT. Factors affecting late mortality from heart disease after treatment of Hodgkin's disease. JAMA 1993;270:16:1949–55.

23. Hancock SL, Cox RS, McDougall IR. Thyroid diseases after treatment of Hodgkin's disease. N Engl J Med 1991;325:599–605.

24. van Leeuwen FE, Klokman WJ, Veer MB, et al. Long-term risk of second malignancy in survivors of Hodgkin's disease treated during adolescence or young adulthood. J Clin Oncol 2000;18:487–97.

25. Hancock SL, Tucker MA, Hoppe RT. Breast cancer after treatment of Hodgkin's disease. J Natl Cancer Inst 1993;85:25–31.

26. Carbone PP, Kaplan HS, Musshoff K, et al. Report of the Committee on Hodgkin's Disease Staging Classification. Cancer Res 1971;31:1860–1.

27. Loo BW Jr, Crooks SM, Xing L, et al. A dosimetric comparison of conventional and intensity modulated radiation therapies

for the treatment of Hodgkin's disease. Int J Radiat Oncol Biol Phys 2002;54(2 Suppl):323.

28. Welsh JS, Tannehill S, Olivera G, et al. Conformal avoidance radiotherapy for Hodgkin's disease and non-Hodgkin's lymphoma: a new mantle [abstract]. In: Proceedings of the 39th Annual Meeting of the American Society of Clinical Oncology; 2003 May 31–June 3; Chicago.

29. Chao MW, Wirth A, Ryan G, et al. Radiation myelopathy following transplantation and radiotherapy for non-Hodgkin's lymphoma. Int J Radiat Oncol Biol Phys 1998;41:1057–61.

30. Schwartz DL, Schechter GP, Seltzer S, et al. Radiation myelitis following allogeneic stem cell transplantation and consolidation radiotherapy for non-Hodgkin's lymphoma. Bone Marrow Transplant 2000;26:1355–9.

31. Eisbruch A, Ten Haken RK, Kim HM, et al. Dose, volume, and function relationships in parotid salivary glands following conformal and intensity-modulated irradiation of head and neck cancer. Int J Radiat Oncol Biol Phys 1999;45:577–87.

32. Hernando ML, Marks LB, Bentel GC, et al. Radiation-induced pulmonary toxicity: a dose-volume histogram analysis in 201 patients with lung cancer. Int J Radiat Oncol Biol Phys 2001;51:650–9.

33. Cassady JR. Clinical radiation nephropathy. Int J Radiat Oncol Biol Phys 1995;31:1249–56.

34. Kost S, Dorr W, Keinert K, et al. Effect of dose and dose-distribution in damage to the kidney following abdominal radiotherapy. Int J Radiat Biol Phys 2002;78:695–702.

35. Gordon KB, Char DH, Sagerman RH. Late effects of radiation on the eye and ocular adnexa. Int J Radiat Oncol Biol Phys 1995;31:1123–39.

36. Sklar C, Whitton J, Mertens A, et al. Abnormalities of the thyroid in survivors of Hodgkin's disease: data from the Childhood Cancer Survivor Study. J Clin Endocrinol Metab 2000;85:3227–32.

37. Hancock SL, McDougall IR, Constine LS. Thyroid abnormalities after therapeutic external radiation. Int J Radiat Oncol Biol Phys 1995;31:1165–70.

38. Grigsby PW, Russell A, Bruner D, et al. Late injury of cancer therapy on the female reproductive tract. Int J Radiat Oncol Biol Phys 1995;31:5:1281–99.

39. Mauch P, Constine L, Greenberger J, et al. Hematopoietic stem cell compartment: acute and late effects of radiation therapy and chemotherapy. Int J Radiat Oncol Biol Phys 1995;31:1319–39.

40. Eifel PJ, Donaldson SS, Thomas PR. Response of growing bone to irradiation: a proposed late effects scoring system. Int J Radiat Oncol Biol Phys 1995;31:1301–7.

41. Martinez-Monge R, Fernandes PS, Gupta N, et al. Cross-sectional nodal atlas: a tool for the definition of clinical target volumes in three-dimensional radiation therapy planning. Radiology 1999;211:815–28.

42. Som PM, Curtin HD, Mancuso AA. Imaging-based nodal classification for evaluation of neck metastatic adenopathy. AJR Am J Roentgenol 2000;174:837–44.

43. Cymbalista M, Waysberg A, Zacharias C, et al. CT demonstration of the 1996 AJCC-UICC regional lymph node classification for lung cancer staging. Radiographics 1999;19:899–900.

44. Schiepers C, Filmont JE, Czernin J. PET for staging of Hodgkin's disease and non-Hodgkin's lymphoma. Eur J Nucl Med Mol Imaging 2003;30 Suppl 1:S82–8.

45. Elstrom R, Guan L, Baker G, et al. Utility of FDG-PET scanning in lymphoma by WHO classification. Blood 2003;101:3875–6.

46. Ciernik IF, Dizendorf E, Baumert BG, et al. Radiation treatment planning with an integrated positron emission and computer tomography (PET/CT): a feasibility study. Int J Radiat Oncol Biol Phys 2003;57:853–63.

47. Langen KM, Jones DT. Organ motion and its management. Int J Radiat Oncol Biol Phys 2001;50:265–78.

48. Mohan R, Wu Q, Manning M, et al. Radiobiological considerations in the design of fractionation strategies for intensity-modulated radiation therapy of head and neck cancers. Int J Radiat Oncol Biol Phys 2000;46:619–30.

49. Followill D, Geis P, Boyer A. Estimates of whole-body dose equivalent produced by beam intensity modulated conformal therapy. Int J Radiat Oncol Biol Phys 1997;38:667–72.

50. Hall EJ, Wuu CS. Radiation-induced second cancers: the impact of 3D-CRT and IMRT. Int J Radiat Oncol Biol Phys 2003;56:83–8.

51. Preston DL, Shimizu Y, Pierce DA, et al. Studies of mortality of atomic bomb survivors. Report 13: solid cancer and noncancer disease mortality: 1950-1997. Radiat Res 2003;160:381–407.

52. Land CE, Tokunaga M, Koyama K, et al. Incidence of female breast cancer among atomic bomb survivors, Hiroshima and Nagasaki, 1950-1990. Radiat Res 2003;160:707–17.

53. Travis LB, Hill DA, Dores GM, et al. Breast cancer following radiotherapy and chemotherapy among young women with Hodgkin disease. JAMA 2003;290:465–75.

54. van Leeuwen FE, Klokman WJ, Stovall M, et al. Roles of radiation dose, chemotherapy, and hormonal factors in breast cancer following Hodgkin's disease. J Natl Cancer Inst 2003;95:971–80.

55. Gilbert ES, Stovall M, Gospodarowicz M, et al. Lung cancer after treatment for Hodgkin's disease: focus on radiation effects. Radiat Res 2003;159:161–73.

56. Howe GR. Lung cancer mortality between 1950 and 1987 after exposure to fractionated moderate-dose-rate ionizing radiation in the Canadian Fluoroscopy Cohort Study and a comparison with lung cancer mortality in the Atomic Bomb Survivors Study. Radiat Res 1995;142:295–304.

57. Howe GR, McLaughlin J. Breast cancer mortality between 1950 and 1987 after exposure to fractionated moderate-dose-rate ionizing radiation in the Canadian Fluoroscopy Cohort Study and a comparison with breast cancer mortality in the Atomic Bomb Survivors Study. Radiat Res 1996; 145:694–707.

58. de Wit M, Bohuslavizki KH, Buchert R, et al. [18]FDG-PET following treatment as valid predictor for disease-free survival in Hodgkin's lymphoma. Ann Oncol 2001;12:29–37.

59. Jerusalem G, Beguin Y, Fassotte MF, et al. Whole-body positron emission tomography using ^{18}F-fluorodeoxyglucose for posttreatment evaluation in Hodgkin's disease and non-Hodgkin's lymphoma has higher diagnostic and prognostic value than classical computed tomography scan imaging. Blood 1999;94:429–33.

60. Spaepen K, Stroobants S, Dupont P, et al. Can positron emission tomography with [18F]-fluorodeoxyglucose after first-line treatment distinguish Hodgkin's disease patients who need additional therapy from others in whom additional therapy would mean avoidable toxicity? Br J Haematol 2001;115:272–8.

61. Spaepen K, Stroobants S, Dupont P, et al. Prognostic value of positron emission tomography (PET) with fluorine-18 fluorodeoxyglucose ([18F]FDG) after first-line chemotherapy in non-Hodgkin's lymphoma: is [18F]FDG-PET a valid alternative to conventional diagnostic methods? J Clin Oncol 2001;19:414–9.

62. Jerusalem G, Beguin Y, Fassotte MF, et al. Persistent tumor 18F-FDG uptake after a few cycles of polychemotherapy is predictive of treatment failure in non-Hodgkin's lymphoma. Haematologica 2000;85:613–8.

63. Spaepen K, Stroobants S, Dupont P, et al. Early restaging positron emission tomography with 18F-fluorodeoxyglucose predicts outcome in patients with aggressive non-Hodgkin's lymphoma. Ann Oncol 2002;13:9:1356–63.

64. Kostakoglu L, Coleman M, Leonard JP, et al. PET predicts prognosis after 1 cycle of chemotherapy in aggressive lymphoma and Hodgkin's disease. J Nucl Med 2002;43:8:1018–27.

65. Wagner M, Seitz U, Buck A, et al. 3′-[18F]fluoro-3′-deoxythymidine ([18F]-FLT) as positron emission tomography tracer for imaging proliferation in a murine B-cell lymphoma model and in the human disease. Cancer Res 2003;63:10:2681–7.

66. Belhocine T, Steinmetz N, Hustinx R, et al. Increased uptake of the apoptosis-imaging agent (99m)Tc recombinant human annexin V in human tumors after one course of chemotherapy as a predictor of tumor response and patient prognosis. Clin Cancer Res 2002;8:9:2766–74.

67. Haas RL, De Jong D, Valdés Olmos R, et al. In vivo imaging of radiation-induced apoptosis in follicular lymphoma patients. Int J Radiat Oncol Biol Phys 2004; 59:3:782-7.

68. Hoppe RT. The non-Hodgkin's lymphomas: pathology, staging, treatment. Curr Probl Cancer 1987;11:6:363–447.

HODGKIN'S DISEASE

CASE STUDY

BILLY W. LOO JR, MD, PHD, RICHARD T. HOPPE, MD, FACR

Patient History

An 8-year-old boy with no significant past medical history presented with fevers to 39°C, fatigue, and abdominal pain with a palpable abdominal mass. Abdominal ultrasonography revealed multiple large para-aortic masses. A computed tomography (CT) scan of the neck, chest, abdomen, and pelvis revealed a left supraclavicular mass, massive retroperitoneal lymphadenopathy extending from the diaphragmatic hiatus to the pelvis, and mesenteric lymphadenopathy. The thorax was unremarkable. An excisional biopsy of the left supraclavicular lymph nodes revealed nodular sclerosing Hodgkin's disease (CD15 and CD30 positive, CD20 equivocal). The pathologic diagnosis was confirmed by expert review. Bone marrow biopsy and cytogenetics were normal. Lymphangiography revealed abnormally enlarged lymph nodes in the iliac and para-aortic areas. ^{18}F-labeled fluorodeoxyglucose (^{18}FDG) positron emission tomography (^{18}FDG-PET) revealed glucose hypermetabolism in the left supraclavicular, para-aortic, and left iliac areas. Laboratory studies at the time of diagnosis included white blood cell count of 7,800 per microliter, lymphocyte count of 1,500 per microliter, hemoglobin of 8.1 grams/deciliter, albumin of 3.7 grams/deciliter, and an erythrocyte sedimentation rate of 73 millimeters/hour.

The patient was assigned an Ann Arbor stage of IIIB and was enrolled in the unfavorable-risk arm of the St. Jude Children's Research Hospital risk-adapted therapy protocol for pediatric Hodgkin's disease (HOD99), with treatment consisting of three cycles of alternating VAMP/COP (VAMP = vinblastine, doxorubicin, methotrexate, prednisone; COP = cyclophosphamide, vincristine, procarbazine) chemotherapy followed by involved field radiation therapy (RT). Restaging studies were obtained per protocol following one cycle of VAMP/COP. CT revealed a complete response in the left supraclavicular area and a marked but partial response in the para-aortic and pelvic

areas with significant residual bulk. ^{18}FDG-PET demonstrated no residual areas of hypermetabolism. According to protocol, he was to receive 15 Gy to the left supraclavicular area and 25.5 Gy to the spleen, para-aortic, and iliac areas in 1.5 Gy daily fractions following the completion of chemotherapy.

He was treated with conventional CT-planned RT. An attempt was made to use a shrinking field technique to achieve maximal sparing of the kidneys given their close proximity to the bulk of the disease. He received 15 Gy to the supraclavicular field and 16.5 Gy to the infradiaphragmatic field delivered using opposed anterior-posterior ports. A repeat treatment planning CT scan revealed no significant reduction in tumor volume, and an additional 9 Gy was delivered to the inferior field via slightly oblique opposed portals. Significant underdosing of portions of the tumor mass was accepted to restrict the dose to the kidneys. His treatment course was complicated by nausea and vomiting, which were adequately managed with conservative measures. We present here the conventional plan compared with a hypothetical intensity-modulated radiation therapy (IMRT) plan that demonstrates some dosimetric advantages.

Simulation

The patient was positioned in the supine position, with arms in a slight akimbo position. A custom binary foam anatomic mold (Alpha Cradle, Smithers Medical Products, Inc., Hudson, OH), extending from above the head to the level of the buttocks, was used for immobilization. Custom handholds for reproducing the position of the upper extremities were integrated into the mold. CT simulation was performed using an AcQSim PQ5000 scanner (Philips Medical Systems, Andover, MA). CT slices from the base of the skull to the upper thighs were acquired with 4 mm spacing. Intravenous contrast was not used. The same procedure was repeated for planning the cone-down treatment.

Target and Tissue Delineation

All target and normal tissue segmentation was performed manually using an AcQSim VoxelQ workstation (Philips Medical Systems). In the abdomen, the grossly involved nodal mass was contoured as the gross tumor volume (GTV). To define the clinical target volume (CTV), a uniform 1 cm expansion was created around the GTV. This volume was modified to prevent expansion into adjacent normal structures; expansion into surrounding fat and muscle was allowed. Consequently, in the vicinity of the kidneys, where the GTV abutted the critical structures, there was little to no expansion. The spleen and remainder of the para-aortic and common iliac nodal chains were included as contiguous sites of potential microscopic disease. Because unenlarged lymphatic structures cannot be visualized reliably by CT, we used the corresponding vascular structures (ie, aorta, inferior vena cava, and iliac vessels) as surrogate anatomic landmarks. In this case, the presence of residual contrast from the previous lymphangiogram also aided target definition. The following normal tissues were delineated and included in the IMRT optimization process: left and right lungs, left and right kidneys, liver, stomach, bowel, spinal cord (contoured from the T8 to L3 levels), and vertebrae (T8 to S3). Representative slices from the treatment planning CT scan are shown in Figure 24.1-1.

Treatment Planning

For the conventional treatment plan, an internal margin for organ motion (eg, from breathing) was not considered for most structures of interest. However, for quality assurance, we perform an additional fluoroscopic simulation with blocks in place prior to treatment. At that time, we also verify that there is an adequate margin on the left hemidiaphragm at natural end-expiration to ensure coverage of the spleen superiorly throughout the respiratory cycle. In this case, there was essentially no planning target volume (PTV) expansion in the vicinity of the kidneys, and the block edges projected very close to the edges of the segmented GTV. This can be seen in Figure 24.1-2, the anterior port of the conventional treatment field.

Given the presumably greater sensitivity of IMRT treatments to organ motion, basing the PTV expansion on a measurement of organ motion would be desirable. This could be accomplished by acquiring CT scans at natural end-inspiration and end-expiration. In the case presented

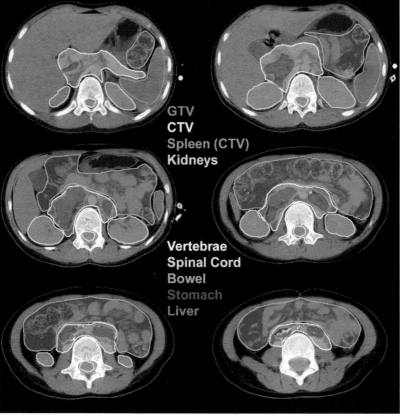

FIGURE 24.1-1. Sections from the treatment planning computed tomography scan, with targets and anatomic structures segmented. CTV = clinical target volume; GTV = gross tumor volume. (To view a color version of this image, please refer to the CD-ROM.)

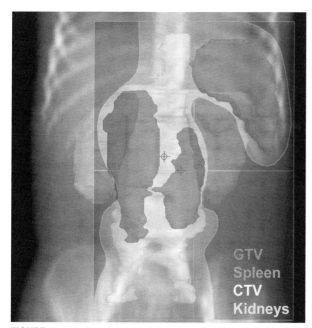

FIGURE 24.1-2. Anterior port of the conventional spade field. CTV = clinical target volume; GTV = gross tumor volume. (To view a color version of this image, please refer to the CD-ROM.)

here, the initial and subsequent cone-down planning scans were performed without controlling for breathing. However, the initial scan was acquired in relative expiration, whereas the cone-down scan was acquired in relative inspiration, providing a retrospective estimate of organ motion. The two scans were fused using bony anatomy, and the corresponding structures were contoured on both scans. This revealed that with respect to the targets, the spleen was the most mobile and on inspiration moved inferiorly and posteromedially, with a maximum displacement of approximately 2 cm superior-inferior, 2.3 cm left-right, and 1.2 cm anterior-posterior; the superior part of the GTV had approximately 0.4 cm superior-inferior and minimal anterior-posterior and left-right excursions; the remainder of the CTV and GTV was relatively stationary. Among nontarget tissues, the liver had approximately 2 cm superior-inferior and 1.5 cm left-right excursions; the kidneys had approximately 0.6 cm superior-inferior and minimal anterior-posterior and left-right excursions. These measurements are consistent with published data on organ motion and were used for defining the internal margin parameters.[1] It is important to note, however, that unlike for static conventional fields, accounting for organ motion simply by PTV expansion may be inadequate for IMRT, which is a dynamic delivery modality. We are currently implementing respiratory cycle gating of planning scans and treatment delivery and investigating other methods of breathing adapted treatment as well.

We used *CORVUS*, version 4.0 (North American Scientific, NOMOS Radiation Oncology Division, Cranberry Township, PA), IMRT treatment planning software. The input parameters described here are specific to this software package, and are shown in Table 24.1-1. Tissue heterogeneity correction was used for both optimization and dose calculation. To demonstrate the general applicability of IMRT, an attempt to fine-tune the choices of input parameters (other than to emphasize kidney sparing in the dose specification) was not made.

For the IMRT plan, we chose five coplanar beams with uniformly spaced beam angles at 36, 108, 180, 252, and 324 degrees (where 180 degrees corresponds to an anterior-posterior beam). At three of the above beam angles, the treatment field was divided in two by the *CORVUS* planning system because the field width is limited by the maximum travel of the Varian multileaf collimator (Varian Medical Systems, Palo Alto, CA) leaves in dynamic delivery mode. Thus, there were 8 fields and 808 field segments. We chose a beam energy of 6 MV (same as in the conventional plan) to enable a more direct comparison. A significant improvement in dose conformity can be achieved by using a larger number of beam angles (eg, seven to nine; not shown) or by optimizing the choice of beam angles.[2] A smaller improvement can be achieved by using higher beam energy (eg, 15 MV; not shown) at the potential cost of a higher total-body effective dose from photoneutrons produced in the head of the linear accelerator. Of note, we often deliver IMRT treatments employing up to 15 or more fields in our clinic with total treatment times (including patient positioning and treatment delivery) of approximately 30 to 40 minutes.

TABLE 24.1-1. Input Parameters

Target	Goal, Gy	Volume below Goal, %	Minimum, Gy	Maximum, Gy	Target Type
GTV	25.5	5	20	27	Homogeneous
CTV	25.5	5	20	27	Homogeneous
Spleen	25.5	5	20	27	Homogeneous

Structure	Limit, Gy	Volume above Limit, %	Minimum, Gy	Maximum, Gy	Structure Type
R kidney	8.0	10	3	20	Critical
L kidney	8.0	10	3	20	Critical
Spinal cord	15.0	10	5	20	Basic
Vertebrae	15.0	10	5	20	Basic
Bowel	15.0	20	5	20	Basic
Stomach	15.0	20	5	25	Basic
Liver	15.0	20	5	25	Basic
R lung	15.0	20	5	25	Basic
L lung	15.0	20	5	25	Basic

CTV = clinical target volume; GTV = gross tumor volume; R = right; L = left.
These parameters and their definitions are specific to the *CORVUS* 4.0 treatment planning system.

Dose-volume histograms of target structures and normal tissues comparing the conventional plan with the IMRT plan are shown in Figures 24.1-3 to 24.1-6. The corresponding isodose curves for selected slices are shown in Figure 24.1-7. These demonstrate that compared with the conventional treatment plan, IMRT results in improved target coverage and kidney sparing simultaneously. In principle, this should result in improved probability of disease control and decreased risk of late kidney dysfunction. In addition, there is better exclusion of the spinal cord, vertebrae, stomach, bowel, and liver from the high-dose regions. The reduction in normal tissue irradiated may decrease short-term toxicities such as nausea, diarrhea, and marrow suppression; intermediate-term symptoms such as L'hermitte's sign; and late complications such as bowel obstruction. Whether such improved clinical end points are realized remains to be borne out by clinical studies.

Treatment Delivery and Quality Assurance

The conventional treatment consisted of five fields (anterior, posterior open, posterior with wedge, right anterior oblique, left posterior oblique), requiring 2,989 monitor

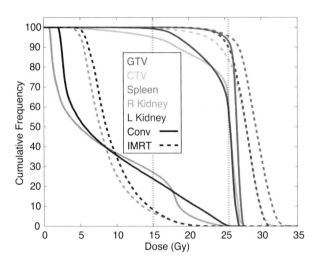

FIGURE 24.1-3. Dose-volume histograms of conventional versus intensity-modulated radiation therapy (IMRT) treatment plans. IMRT results in both improved target coverage and kidney sparing. (To view a color version of this image, please refer to the CD-ROM.)

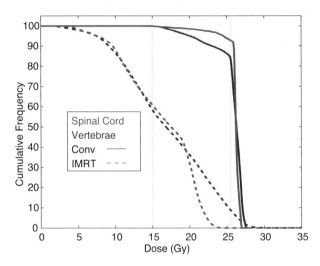

FIGURE 24.1-4. Intensity-modulated radiation therapy (IMRT) results in substantially lower doses to the spinal cord and vertebrae. (To view a color version of this image, please refer to the CD-ROM.)

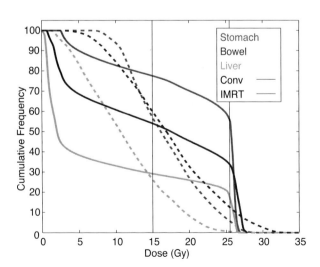

FIGURE 24.1-5. With intensity-modulated radiation therapy (IMRT), a smaller volume of abdominal organs receives higher doses (above 10–17 Gy), whereas a larger volume receives lower doses. (To view a color version of this image, please refer to the CD-ROM.)

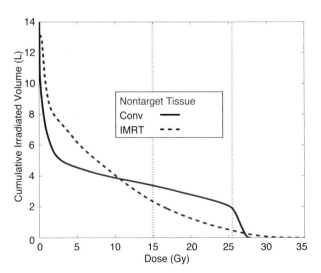

FIGURE 24.1-6. Intensity-modulated radiation therapy (IMRT) results in a reduction in the volume of all nontarget tissues receiving higher doses (> 10 Gy) at the cost of an increase in the volume receiving lower doses. (To view a color version of this image, please refer to the CD-ROM.)

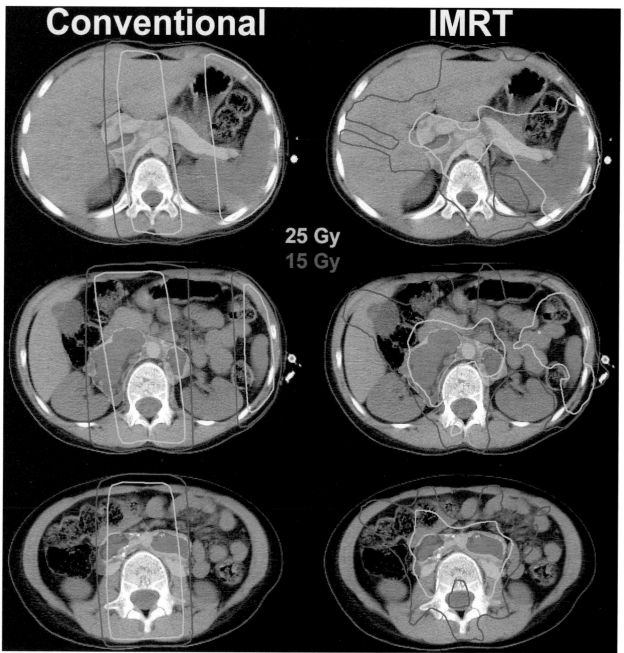

FIGURE 24.1-7. Isodose curves of conventional versus intensity-modulated radiation therapy (IMRT) treatment plans demonstrate improved dose conformity with IMRT. (To view a color version of this image, please refer to the CD-ROM.)

units over the entire treatment course to deliver 25.5 Gy to the reference point in the target. The IMRT treatment plan above would comprise eight fields (five beam angles, with three fields split in two, as described above), with 808 segments requiring 17,425 monitor units over the treatment course to deliver 25.5 Gy to the 69.5% isodose line, which encompasses 90% of the GTV. The 5.8 times greater number of monitor units required by IMRT in this case would result in similarly increased leakage radiation from the head of the linear accelerator, contributing to a higher total-body

dose. On the other hand, the total-body dose from internal scatter from the irradiated tissues is slightly lower with IMRT owing to the smaller volume of tissue receiving the highest doses. Within the irradiated field, IMRT results in a smaller volume of nontarget tissues receiving higher doses (above 10 Gy) at the cost of a larger volume receiving lower doses (see Figure 24.1-6). However, there are insufficient data to predict whether these dosimetric results would result in a greater or lesser risk of radiation-induced secondary malignancies with IMRT compared with conventional RT, and well-designed clinical trials are needed to evaluate this important question in this highly curable patient population.

Of note, improvements in IMRT planning and delivery have the potential to greatly improve its efficiency and decrease the excess radiation to nontarget tissues. Optimizing the choice of beam angles may result in improved dose conformity. Additionally, fewer beam angles may achieve the same degree of conformity, which could result in a smaller volume of tissue irradiated even to lower doses.[2] Direct optimization of the beam apertures as opposed to the beamlet intensities can reduce the treatment complexity and thereby the required number of monitor units substantially (potentially by over 70%) without compromising dose conformity.[3,4] Both of these improvements could significantly reduce the total-body doses from IMRT without diminishing its dosimetric advantages over conventional treatment.

Clinical Outcome

At nearly 2 years follow-up after completing treatment with conventional RT, the patient had no clinical or radiographic evidence of disease recurrence and no symptoms referable to late treatment-related toxicity.

Our dosimetric planning study of IMRT in Hodgkin's disease was presented earlier.[5] In that review, conventional and IMRT planning was compared in three patients (two adults with bulky mediastinal disease and a child with bulky para-aortic disease). Compared to conventional planning, treating the periphery of the GTV using IMRT resulted in an effective dose escalation to most of the GTV due to the inherent heterogeneity of GTV coverage with IMRT. Coverage of the CTV was improved, particularly in the supraclavicular region. As shown above in the case of bulky para-aortic disease, IMRT planning resulted in better GTV coverage as well as sparing of the kidneys.

References

1. Langen KM, Jones DT. Organ motion and its management. Int J Radiat Oncol Biol Phys 2001;50:265–78.
2. Pugachev A, Xing L. Pseudo beam's-eye-view as applied to beam orientation selection in intensity-modulated radiation therapy. Int J Radiat Oncol Biol Phys 2001;51:1361–70.
3. Shepard DM, Earl MA, Li XA, et al. Direct aperture optimization: a turnkey solution for step-and-shoot IMRT. Med Phys 2002;29:1007–18.
4. Cotrutz C, Xing L. Segment-based dose optimization using a genetic algorithm. Phys Med Biol 2003;48:2987–98.
5. Loo BW Jr, Crooks SM, Xing L, et al. A dosimetric comparison of conventional and intensity modulated radiation therapies for the treatment of Hodgkin's disease. Int J Radiat Oncol Biol Phys 2002;54(suppl 2):323.

Chapter 24.2

HELICAL TOMOTHERAPY— A NEW MANTLE

EMERGING TECHNOLOGY

JAMES S. WELSH, MS, MD, CHRISTOPHER PETERSON, MD, BRAD KAHL, MD, GUSTAVO OLIVERA, PHD

The mantle represents a cornerstone of the radiotherapeutic treatment of patients with lymphoma, particularly those with Hodgkin's disease. For decades, the mantle has been delivered with opposed anterior-posterior–posterior-anterior fields irradiating nodal regions in the neck, mediastinum, and supraclavicular, infraclavicular, and axillary regions. Blocks are used to shape the fields minimizing the dose to the humeral heads, mouth, and lungs.

Despite judicious blocking, considerable volumes of normal tissues are irradiated. For example, much of the spinal cord, a serial organ, receives the full dose, whereas the dose to 20% of the total lung volume (D_{20}) often exceeds 20 Gy. Unsurprisingly, irradiated patients are exposed to a wide variety of acute and chronic sequelae, notably radiation pneumonitis, hypothyroidism, cardiac disease, and second malignancies.[1–8] Although doses are typically well below the tolerance for severe late effects such as transverse myelitis, patients may develop the L'hermitte's sign, presumably secondary to transient demyelination. Although doses administered today are lower than in the past, the potential remains for significant radiation therapy (RT)-related adverse effects in these patients.

In an effort to improve on the classic mantle approach, we have been evaluating the role of intensity-modulated radiation therapy (IMRT) delivered with helical tomotherapy at our institution.[9] Unlike conventional RT approaches, IMRT offers the ability to conform the dose to the target tissues, sparing the surrounding normal structures and thus potentially reducing the risk of RT-related sequelae. Unlike other IMRT delivery methods, helical tomotherapy offers distinct advantages in these patients, given its ability to deliver IMRT rapidly to large, complex fields and to perform image-guided therapy. The purpose of this chapter is to present an overview of the new mantle approach delivered with helical tomotherapy.

Helical Tomotherapy

Helical tomotherapy (TomoTherapy, Inc., Middleton, WI) is a form of IMRT in which treatment is delivered in a continuous helix similar in technique to that of spiral computed tomography (CT). The tomotherapy unit consists of a 6 MV linear accelerator mounted on a rotating ring gantry. The treatment beam is modulated by a multileaf collimator consisting of 64 leaves. This multileaf collimator can project a field size up to 40 cm wide and 5 cm long at the isocenter. Each leaf opens and closes independently at 50-millisecond intervals as the gantry rotates and the patient is translocated through the gantry bore. These modulated rotating pencil beams create highly conformal dose distributions. Further descriptions of IMRT planning and delivery using helical tomotherapy are provided in Chapter 10, "Treatment Planning," and Chapter 12, "Delivery Systems."

The unique features of the helical tomotherapy unit make it ideal for the delivery of the new mantle. As noted above, the classic mantle entails irradiation of a large volume composed of multiple targets (axilla, mediastinum, neck, and supraclavicular regions). The continuous helical delivery approach of tomotherapy allows the delivery of treatment to such a complex, large volume in a reasonable timeframe. Rapid treatment delivery translates into better efficiency and also reduces the risk of "geographic misses" owing to patient motion. Moreover, recent data have suggested that prolonged delivery times may compromise tumor control in patients undergoing IMRT.[10]

An additional feature of helical tomotherapy in this setting is its ability to deliver image-guided IMRT.[11] The tomotherapy unit consists of a megavoltage CT detector array mounted 180° from the beam source. This detector array uses the megavoltage treatment beam to create a CT image of the patient. Using very few monitor units, a megavoltage

CT scan can be obtained immediately before treatment to verify patient setup. The patient position can be adjusted or the software used to adapt the treatment plan to the new patient position. Such an approach not only helps to minimize geographic misses but also ensures sparing of surrounding normal tissues. This unique feature of helical tomotherapy distinguishes it from other forms of IMRT and sets the stage for adaptive RT, the reconstruction of the actually delivered daily dose (as opposed to planned dose) accompanied by prescription and delivery modifications when appropriate.

Creation of a Helical Tomotherapy Mantle

Creation of the new mantle begins with a CT-based simulation. The patient is positioned supine with the arms placed overhead rather than akimbo. This is important not only because larger patients may not easily fit within the bore of the CT simulator and tomotherapy unit but, more importantly, because the continuous helical delivery of treatment might result in radiation going directly through the patient's arms if the akimbo position is used. In principle, the planning could be done with the arms entered as avoidance structures in the optimization process if the arms cannot be raised overhead, but the resultant plan might be less conformal.

Following the CT simulation, the various anatomic structures and regions of interest are contoured. In the new mantle, this involves the spinal cord, larynx, thyroid gland, lungs, and heart. In selected cases, other normal tissues can be contoured, including the breasts in young women and the vertebrae in children.

Once the normal tissues are delineated, the regions known or suspected to harbor gross or microscopic disease are then contoured. Specifically, this involves contouring the regions containing nodal chains in the axillae, supraclavicular and infraclavicular areas, mediastinum, and neck. Rather than contouring the vessels in these regions, we advocate contouring the general regions in which these nodal chains exist. Thus, instead of attempting to specifically locate the axillary or supraclavicular nodal chains, for example, we contour the axillary and supraclavicular nodal regions with generous margins (Figure 24.2-1). This is a reasonable strategy because adequate coverage of the nodal chains is of paramount importance, and the creation of generous nodal regions of interest ensures that the nodes of concern are covered whether or not they are visible. For example, we have been contouring the entire axilla as defined anatomically. We have also used the dosimetrically defined axilla (as covered by the standard mantle technique) to serve as a guide for ensuring proper coverage.

The next step in the treatment planning process is the prescription of dose to the regions of interest (eg, 30 Gy in 2 Gy daily fractions) and requesting appropriate dose-volume restrictions on the normal tissues (eg, $D_{20} < 20$ Gy). The normal tissue restrictions can be adjusted for each individual case depending on the clinical situation. For example, in a patient with poor pulmonary function, greater priority can be given to minimize the lung rather than the spinal cord doses, or, in a young female, greater priority might be given to breast avoidance than larynx dose reductions. The final plan will thus provide full dosimetric coverage of all of the disease-harboring regions, just as the mantle does, but with greatly reduced doses to normal tissues. A note of caution is that the final plan must provide full coverage of the involved sites, and this should take priority over avoidance of normal tissues.

Dose-volume histograms show that the new mantle using helical tomotherapy significantly reduces radiation dose to the spinal cord, lungs, thyroid gland, larynx, and heart (> 50% dose reduction) compared with the conventional mantle (Figure 24.2-2). Depending on the desired results, customization in planning and delivery is easily obtained. However, as mentioned earlier, given the success of the mantle and its derivatives, it is imperative that the first priority be providing an adequate dose to the lymphatic regions at risk. In our preliminary virtual planning investigations, dose-volume histogram analysis confirmed that coverage of the nodal regions at risk of gross or occult disease was equal to or better than that of the mantle approach.[12]

Once the plan is optimized, the patient will begin routine treatment on the helical tomotherapy unit. As noted above, megavoltage CT images can be obtained as often as desired to provide image guidance. Megavoltage CT imaging replaces the port films used in linear accelerator–based RT and can (in principle) also be used for dose reconstruction. Preliminary work has shown that megavoltage CT is generally adequate for the purposes of patient setup and visualization of gross tumor volumes.[13]

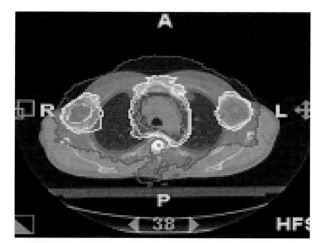

FIGURE 24.2-1. Dose distribution in the axillae and upper mediastinum using helical tomotherapy treatment planning. The general axillary and mediastinal regions are targeted rather than any specific nodes or vessels. (To view a color version of this image, please refer to the CD-ROM.)

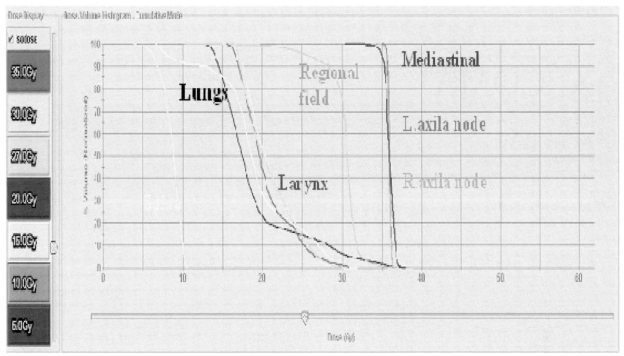

FIGURE 24.2-2. Dose-volume histogram of helical tomotherapy treatment planning for the mantle. Greater priority could be given to avoid, in particular, the spinal cord, thyroid, lungs, and breasts, depending on the specific clinical situation.

Conclusion

A mantle planned and delivered with helical tomotherapy appears to be a feasible and effective means of reducing radiation dose to critical normal tissues in patients with lymphoma compared with conventional techniques. Currently, a drawback of this approach is that it is quite labor intensive. Contouring all of the key normal structures and defining and generously contouring the general nodal regions of concern can take several hours per case with existing software technology. Despite this, we believe that it is worthy of further exploration because of the prospect of reducing complications while preserving high control rates. Clinical implementation of this new mantle should begin in the near future.

References

1. Ng AK, Bernardo MP, Weller E, et al. Long-term survival and competing causes of death in patients with early-stage Hodgkin's disease treated at age 50 or younger. J Clin Oncol 2002;20:2101–8.
2. Hudson MM, Poquette CA, Lee J, et al. Increased mortality after successful treatment for Hodgkin's disease. J Clin Oncol 1998;16:3592–600.
3. Berthe MP, van den Belt-Dusebout AW, Klockman WJ, et al. Long-term cause specific mortality of patients treated for Hodgkin's disease. J Clin Oncol 2003;21:3431–9.
4. Hoppe RT, Coleman CN, Cox RS, et al. The management of stage I-II Hodgkin's disease with irradiation alone or combined modality therapy: the Stanford experience. Blood 1982;59:455–65.
5. Mauch PM, Kalish LA, Marcus KC. Second malignancies after treatment for laparotomy staged IA-IIB Hodgkin's disease: long term analysis of risk factors and outcome. Blood 1996;16:536–44.
6. van Leeuwen FE, Klokman WJ, van't Veer MB, et al. Long-term risk of second malignancy in survivors of Hodgkin's disease treated during adolescence or young adulthood. J Clin Oncol 2000;18:487–97.
7. Hancock SL, Tucker MA, Hoppe RT. Breast cancer after treatment of Hodgkin's disease. J Natl Cancer Inst 1993;85:25–31.
8. Hancock SL, Tucker MA, Hoppe RT. Factors affecting late mortality from heart disease after treatment of Hodgkin's disease. JAMA 1993;270:1949–55.
9. Welsh JS, Tannehill S, Olivera G, et al. Conformal avoidance radiotherapy with helical tomotherapy for lymphoid malignancies: a new mantle. Proc Am Soc Clin Oncol 2003;22:593.
10. Fowler JF, Welsh JS, Howard SP. Loss of biological effect in prolonged fraction delivery. Int J Radiat Oncol Biol Phys 2004;59:242–9.
11. Welsh JS, Patel RR, Ritter MA, et al. Helical tomotherapy: an innovative technology and approach to radiation therapy. Techn Cancer Res Treat 2002;1:55–63.
12. Welsh J, Olivera G, Hui S, et al. Helical tomotherapy with conformal avoidance appears superior to 3-D CRT and IMRT for treatment of complex tumor volumes. Radiother Oncol 2002;64 Suppl 1:S124.
13. Welsh JS, Bradley K, Manon R, et al. Megavoltage CT imaging for adaptic helical tomotherapy of lung cancer. Clin Lung Cancer 2004;5:303–6.

Sarcoma

Overview

Kaled M. Alektiar, MD, Linda Hong, PhD

Radiation therapy (RT) occupies an important role in the management of patients with soft tissue sarcomas.[1] In particular, RT is used in conjunction with conservative surgery as a means of limb preservation in patients with extremity soft tissue sarcomas.[2–4] RT is also often combined with surgery in patients with retroperitoneal sarcomas.[5,6]

A concern, however, with the use of RT in these patients is the risk of untoward treatment sequelae, given that high doses are typically administered even in completely resected patients. Fortunately, the risk of edema and contracture can be minimized in patients with extremity sarcoma by paying strict attention to proper RT techniques, for example, sparing a portion of the circumference of the extremity and avoiding high radiation doses over joint spaces, respectively.[7] Given the proximity of many tumors to long bones, however, it is inevitable that considerable portions of these bones receive high doses. Although the overall risk of bone fracture is low, the rate may be as high as 24% in patients who undergo periosteal stripping and receive chemotherapy. Unfortunately, the management of RT-induced bone fracture is rather complicated and not always satisfactory.[8,9] Close proximity of retroperitoneal sarcomas to multiple normal tissues, including the small bowel, kidneys, and liver, exposes patients with retroperitoneal tumors to multiple potential acute and chronic toxicities.[10] Moreover, concerns regarding normal tissue injury limit the total dose delivered.[11]

A potential means of improving the delivery of RT in patients with soft tissue sarcoma is the use of intensity-modulated radiation therapy (IMRT). Unlike conventional approaches, IMRT conforms the dose to the shape of the target in three dimensions, thereby sparing surrounding normal tissues. The ability to produce concave dose distributions is particularly appealing in patients with extremity sarcoma in whom the target volume is juxtaposed to long bones.[12–14] Highly conformal IMRT plans may also provide a means of reducing the volume of normal tissues irradiated in patients with retroperitoneal sarcomas, allowing the safe delivery of higher doses.[15–17]

The purpose of this chapter is to examine the application of IMRT in soft tissue sarcomas. The primary focus is on patients with extremity sarcomas; in particular, the issues and challenges surrounding the use of IMRT in these patients, including target delineation, immobilization, and treatment planning. Interested readers should also refer to Chapter 26.3, "Rhabdomyosarcoma: Case Study," for a presentation of a pediatric patient with an extremity rhabdomyosarcoma. Accompanying case studies in this section include a paraspinal sarcoma (see Chapter 25.1, "Paraspinal Soft Tissue Sarcoma: Case Study") and a retroperitoneal soft tissue sarcoma (see Chapter 25.2, "Retroperitoneal Sarcoma: Case Study").

IMRT Studies
Dosimetric (Planning) Studies

Treatment planning and delivery with IMRT have been used successfully for sites such as the prostate, head and neck, breast, and gynecologic malignancies.[18–22] The feasibility of IMRT for large-field irradiation, an important aspect in the treatment of sarcoma of the extremity, has not been well established.

At Memorial Sloan-Kettering Cancer Center (MSKCC), we conducted a dosimetric study to determine whether IMRT could achieve the goal of sparing as much of the femur as possible while maintaining adequate coverage of the target volume. Additional goals included minimizing the dose to the surrounding normal soft tissue and skin located outside the target volume and avoiding other normal structures, such as the contralateral thigh.[12]

Treatment planning was performed using both three-dimensional conformal radiation therapy (3DCRT) and IMRT techniques in 10 patients with soft tissue sarcoma of the thigh with tumors approaching the femur. None of the patients had bony involvement. For all, the gross total volume (GTV) and the femur were contoured. The clinical target volume (CTV) consisted of the GTV with a 1.5 cm margin axially, except at the bone interface, where this interface was used as CTV if the 1.5 cm axial margin extended beyond the bone interface. In the superior-inferior direction, the CTV margin placed around the GTV varied from 5 to 10 cm. The planning target volume (PTV) was defined as the CTV with a uniform 5 mm margin. The 3DCRT technique consisted primarily of two to three beams with wedges or partial transmission blocks as compensators. For the IMRT technique, five coplanar beams were used, chosen to maximally spare the surrounding soft tissue and to clear the other extremity and/or groin areas. IMRT plans were designed to adequately treat the PTV and spare the femur as much as possible.

Dose distributions (Figure 25-1) and dose-volume histograms were analyzed. PTV coverage was comparable with both IMRT and 3DCRT. However, IMRT dose distributions were more conformal, especially for patients with large variations of contours. The volume of the femur receiving at least the full prescription of 63 Gy (the volume covered by 100% of the isodose [V_{100}]) decreased, on average, by 57%, from 44.7 ± 16.8% with 3DCRT to 18.6 ± 9.2% with IMRT ($p < .01$). For three patients with a GTV surrounding less than half of the circumference of the femur, the reduction in the V_{100} to the femur ranged from 61 to 79%. The hot spots in the femur, as measured by the dose encompassing 5% of the volume (D_5), were reduced, on average, from 67.2 ± 1.8 Gy with 3DCRT to 65.0 ± 1.2 Gy with IMRT ($p < .01$). The mean dose to the femur was, on average, 38.5 ± 11.5 Gy with IMRT compared with 40.9 ± 12.7 Gy with 3DCRT.

Benefits were also seen in other normal tissues. The volume of the surrounding soft tissues, defined as the ipsilateral limb excluding the PTV and the femur, receiving at least the prescription dose was reduced, on average, by 78%, from 997 ± 660 cc with 3DCRT to 201 ± 144 cc with IMRT ($p < .01$). The D_5 to the surrounding soft tissues was reduced by 13%. The volume of the skin (from the surface to a depth of 5 mm) receiving the prescription dose declined by 45%, with IMRT providing full-skin dose coverage to scars. The hot spots in the skin were also decreased with IMRT.

The conclusion from this study was that IMRT can reduce the dose to the femur without compromising target coverage by achieving concave dose distributions around the interface of the PTV and the femur. At the same time, IMRT can reduce the hot spots significantly in the surrounding soft tissues and skin.

Other studies have been published focusing on patients with extremity sarcoma. In an earlier report from MSKCC, IMRT and 3DCRT planning were compared in a patient with an extremity extraskeletal chrondrosarcoma.[13] As in patients in the above study,[12] the target volume in this

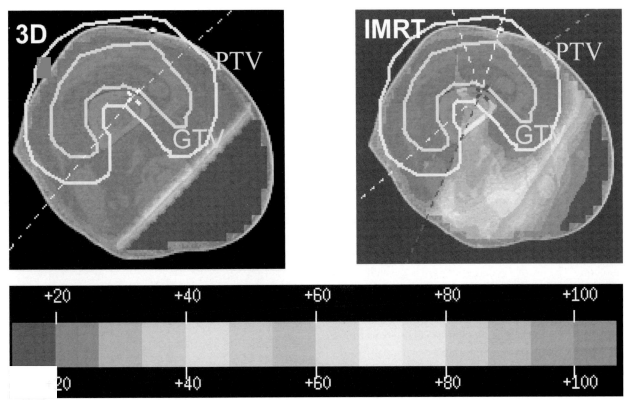

FIGURE 25-1. Comparison of conventional and intensity-modulated radiation therapy (IMRT) dose distributions for a patient with an extremity soft tissue sarcoma (dose wash level in %). Gross tumor volume (GTV) contours in yellow; planning target volume (PTV) contours in cyan. (To view a color version of this image, please refer to the CD-ROM.)

patient was large and in close proximity to the bone. IMRT was associated with improved conformity and less heterogeneity than 3DCRT. Moreover, the maximum bone dose was lower in the IMRT plan.

Millar and colleagues compared IMRT and 3DCRT planning in nine patients with soft tissue sarcoma, four of whom had extremity tumors.[14] In the extremity patients, IMRT was associated with an improved conformity index. Moreover, in patients with considerable volumes of normal tissues within the treatment volume, IMRT reduced the dose to bone and subcutaneous tissues by up to 20%.

Clinical (Outcome) Studies

We recently presented the outcome of the first 10 extremity soft tissue sarcoma patients treated with IMRT at our institution.[23] Median tumor size was 17 cm (the range being 3–21 cm). Seven patients had high-grade tumors and three had low-grade tumors. Preoperative IMRT (50 Gy) was administered to four patients to avoid treatment of the entire limb circumference, and postoperative IMRT (63 Gy) was administered to six to avoid treatment of the entire bone circumference. At a median follow-up of 13 months (the range being 6 to 22 months), all patients remained locally controlled. Two patients failed distantly. Significant wound complications were noted in two patients. Of note, none have developed a fracture. Overall, morbidity was limited. Moderate joint stiffness was noted in three patients (two were resolved with physical therapy). Two patients developed edema (one grade 1 and one grade 2). Of note, the patient with grade 2 edema had the femoral vein resected at surgery. These preliminary results suggest that IMRT is feasible in extremity soft tissue sarcoma patients. However, longer follow-up and more patients are needed to truly evaluate the role of IMRT in this setting.

Challenges of Implementing IMRT in Extremity Sarcoma

Definition of Target Volumes and Critical Structures

The definition of the target volume using IMRT is similar, for the most part, with that using 3DCRT. The only exception is the axial margin around the interface of the GTV and bone. The use of a generous margin is the hallmark of adjuvant RT in soft tissue sarcoma of the extremity. However, when considering the size of the margin in these patients, it is important to realize that bone, interosseous membranes, and the fascial plane are barriers to tumor spread and the margins employed are principally in the long axis of the extremity.[24] As Suit and Spiro pointed out, "The margins need to be viewed with respect to the direction of most likely spread, viz. the margin can be a centimeter or so where there is bone…"[1]

In our dosimetric study, the margin was 5 to 10 cm along the long axis of the thigh.[12] The circumferential margin, however, was varied. The CTV had a 1.5 cm axial margin around the GTV, except at the bone interface. Because none of the patients had bony involvement, the bone provided a natural barrier to tumor spread. The bone interface was considered CTV if the 1.5 cm axial margin around GTV extended beyond the bone interface. The PTV had an additional 5 mm axial margin around the CTV (Figure 25-2).

Immobilization

Immobilization is an integral part of optimal delivery of RT in all extremity sarcomas whether RT is delivered with 3DCRT or IMRT. To ensure the reproducibility and adequate immobilization of the treated region, custom molds should be used to immobilize the patient from the pelvic area to below the knee. In addition, longitudinal and axial alignment tattoos should be placed at the central axis, pelvic area, and knee. Horizontal alignment marks should be traced on the mold. Pretreatment and weekly portal images are also needed for treatment verifications with IMRT.

Despite all of these precautions, the question remains whether a 5 mm CTV-to-PTV margin, in the axial direction, is adequate to account for the setup uncertainties in this disease site. When considering this question, it is important to keep in mind the following realities with conventional RT. First, with a large field, the dose coverage is often

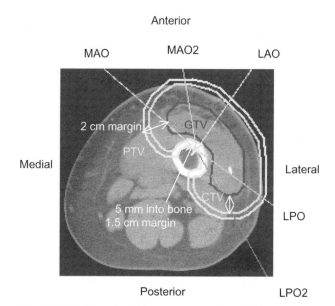

FIGURE 25-2. Illustration of the gross tumor volume (GTV), clinical target volume (CTV), planning target volume (PTV), and beam arrangement for a representative patient with an extremity soft tissue sarcoma. LAO = left anterior oblique; LPO = left posterior oblique; MAO = medial anterior oblique. (To view a color version of this image, please refer to the CD-ROM.)

poor owing to the significant variation in the tissue thickness between the proximal thigh on one end and the distal thigh on the other. Second, with conventional RT, tighter margins around the bone are routinely used where it is often recommended to bisect the femur at the expense of PTV coverage.[25]

IMRT Beam Arrangements

It could be argued that if one were to use multiple beam arrangements with conventional 3DCRT planning, a better dose distribution could be achieved without the need for IMRT. For example, beam angles could be selected using beam's eye view planning to avoid the opposite limb and genitalia. The high-dose regions in the surrounding soft tissues and the skin could also be reduced by introducing more beams. But what cannot be achieved with conventional RT, even with multiple beams, is a concave dose distribution. Furthermore, multiple beam arrangements are possible only if the target volume could be treated at a 100 cm SAD. For those patients requiring either an extended field setup or fields matching to cover the target volume, the use of extended distance setup, by default, limits the beam arrangement mainly to anterior or posterior. The employment of more than two oblique fields at an extended distance is clinically impractical. With conventional field matching, there is also the difficulty of the dosimetric match in the gap region, thus creating either cold or hot spots. With IMRT, however, use of multiple isocenters and incorporating intensity optimization in the field junction eliminate the need to treat at an extended distance. Thus, the resulting dosimetric match in the junction is superior to any conventional gapping method. This was demonstrated in this study and for whole-abdomen RT.[18]

Normal Tissue Dose

The goal of femur sparing using IMRT in our dosimetric study was achieved without exceeding the tolerance to the other surrounding normal structures.[12] In fact, other dosimetric aspects of the treatment plan were also improved with IMRT. With 3DCRT, an average of 115 cc (range 37–167 cc) of skin tissue received at least the prescription dose of 63 Gy (V_{100}), and the hot spots (D_5) were 68.0 ± 1.7 Gy. Significant reduction of skin tissues receiving high doses was achieved with IMRT; the V_{100} was, on average, 61 cc (range 18–85 cc), and the D_5 was 65.2 ± 1.2 Gy. Such a reduction in skin dose could help decrease the likelihood of skin breakdown during RT, which often requires a treatment break. Furthermore, reducing the hot spot may have an effect on subsequent fibrosis, with its impact on functional outcome. The reduction in skin dose might be an appealing aspect of IMRT, especially for preoperative RT, when the risk of wound complication is high.[4]

Sparing a segment of the circumference of the extremity from the full radiation dose is imperative if lymphedema is to be avoided.[7] Again, in the cases planned with 3DCRT, the V_{100} of surrounding soft tissues was, on average, 997 cc (range 424–2,433 cc), and the D_5, on average, was 67.8 ± 1.3 Gy. With IMRT, the V_{100} of the surrounding soft tissue was, on average, 201 cc (range 54–434 cc), 78% less than that of the 3DCRT. The D_5 was, on average, 58.7 ± 4.7 Gy with IMRT, a reduction of 13% compared with 3DCRT. The mean doses to the surrounding soft tissue, however, were not significantly different. Because of the multiple beam arrangement, IMRT irradiated a larger volume of soft tissue at lower doses compared with 3DCRT (see Figure 25-2). There is no information available in the literature on the specific dose constraints for preventing lymphedema. It would be useful to collect these data based on dosimetric calculations from modern treatment planning systems. The potential risk of secondary malignancies from the increased low-dose regions with IMRT needs to be investigated.[19]

Nonextremity Sarcomas

Several investigators have evaluated IMRT in patients with nonextremity sarcomas.[15–17,25,26] Most attention has focused on retroperitoneal soft tissue sarcomas.[15–17] Fiveash and colleagues at the University of Alabama-Birmingham (UAB) treated 14 patients with retroperitoneal sarcoma with preoperative IMRT.[15] In all patients, the GTV was expanded by 1 to 1.5 cm to generate a PTV. A separate boost volume was identified, which included the volume judged to be at risk of positive margins at the time of surgical resection. IMRT plans were generated using a simultaneous integrated boost (SIB) approach: 45 Gy in 1.8 Gy fractions to the PTV and 57.5 Gy in 2.3 Gy fractions to the boost volume. At the time of the review, all 14 patients completed preoperative IMRT and 12 had undergone laparotomy and attempted resection. IMRT was well tolerated, with only 1 patient developing grade ≥ 3 sequelae (nausea and emesis, requiring hospitalization). Of the 12 patients who underwent surgery, 11 had a complete resection with negative margins. Surgery was aborted in one secondary to peritoneal disease. At a median follow-up of 48 weeks, 8 of 11 patients who underwent curative surgery remain without disease recurrence. Only 1 patient developed a local recurrence. No chronic toxicities secondary to IMRT were noted.

As a separate part of this study, three patients were replanned to evaluate the feasibility of further dose escalation using the SIB-IMRT approach.[15] It was found that the doses could be escalated to the boost volume to a median of 75.2 to 82.8 Gy in 25 fractions without exceeding tolerance of nearby normal structures.

In two separate reports, investigators at Emory University reported outcomes of patients with retroperitoneal sarcoma treated with IMRT.[16,17] In their most recent analysis, eight patients (seven with retroperitoneal sarcomas, one with inguinal sarcoma) were included.[16] Compared with 3DCRT planning, IMRT planning was associated with a lower small bowel dose and improved tumor coverage. The mean small bowel dose in the 3DCRT and IMRT plans was 40.18 and 34.7 Gy, respectively. The tumor volume receiving 95% of the prescription dose in the 3DCRT and IMRT plans was 95.3% and 97.5%, respectively. IMRT planning increased the maximum and minimum PTV doses by 7% ($p = .01$) and 130% ($p = .006$). Of the eight patients analyzed, six received IMRT and two received 3DCRT. Grade 2 nausea and emesis, diarrhea, and cutaneous and liver toxicities were noted in four, two, one, and one patient, respectively. At a median follow-up of 58 weeks, no patient experienced a local recurrence. One patient developed recurrent disease in the liver.

Both of these reports clearly demonstrate that IMRT planning improves both target coverage and normal tissue sparing compared with 3DCRT techniques in patients with retroperitoneal soft tissue sarcomas. However, given the limited follow-up and small number of patients treated, no conclusions can be drawn regarding tumor control and late toxicity in these patients. Additional patients with longer follow-up are needed to assess the full benefits and risks of IMRT in these patients, particularly the use of dose escalation. The UAB approach using IMRT in patients with retroperitoneal sarcoma is described in detail in Chapter 25.2.

In a recent report, Weber and colleagues at the Paul Scherrer Institute evaluated different IMRT approaches in five patients with paraspinal sarcomas.[26] IMRT plans consisted of either seven-field photon (IM-photon) or three-field proton (IM-proton) beams. IM-proton plans were generated using the *KonRad* inverse treatment planning system (developed at the German Cancer Research Center). The prescribed dose was 77.4 Gy or cobalt Gray equivalent (CGE) for protons to the GTV. GTV coverage was equally homogeneous with both techniques. However, IM-proton planning significantly reduced the integral dose in the low- to mid-dose range to all organs at risk. The improved normal tissue sparing achieved with IM-proton planning allowed significant dose escalation (to 92.9 CGE to the GTV) without exceeding the normal tissue dose limits. Interested readers should refer to Chapter 28, "Intensity Modulated Proton Therapy," for further discussion of IM-proton therapy and clinical experience at the Paul Scherrer Institute.

References

1. Suit HD, Spiro I. Role of radiation in the management of adult patients with sarcoma of soft tissue. Semin Surg Oncol 1994;10:347–56.
2. Rosenberg S, Tepper J, Glatstein E, et al. The treatment of soft-tissue sarcoma of the extremities: prospective randomized evaluations of (1) limb-sparing surgery plus radiation therapy compared with amputation and (2) the role of adjuvant chemotherapy. Ann Surg 1982;196:305–5.
3. Yang JC, Chang AE, Baker AR, et al. Randomized prospective study of the benefit of adjuvant radiation therapy in the treatment of soft tissue sarcomas of the extremity. J Clin Oncol 1998;16:197–203.
4. O'Sullivan B, Davis AM, Turcotte R, et al. Preoperative versus postoperative radiotherapy in soft-tissue sarcoma of the limbs: a randomised trial. Lancet 2002;359:2235–41.
5. Kinsella TJ, Sindelar WF, Lack E, et al. Preliminary results of a randomized study of adjuvant radiation therapy in resectable adult retroperitoneal soft tissue sarcomas. J Clin Oncol 1988;6:18–25.
6. Tepper JE, Suit HD, Wood WC, et al. Radiation therapy of retroperitoneal soft tissue sarcomas. Int J Radiat Oncol Biol Phys 1984;10:825–30.
7. Stinson SF, DeLaney TF, Greenberg J, et al. Acute and long-term effects on limb function of combined modality limb sparing therapy for extremity soft tissue sarcoma. Int J Radiat Oncol Biol Phys 1991;21:1493–9.
8. Lin PP, Schupak KD, Boland PJ, et al. Pathologic femoral fracture after periosteal excision and radiation for the treatment of soft tissue sarcoma. Cancer 1998;82:2356–65.
9. Lin PP, Boland PJ, Healey JH. Treatment of femoral fractures after irradiation. Clin Orthop 1998;352:168–78.
10. Clark JA, Tepper JE. Role of radiation therapy in retroperitoneal sarcomas. Oncology (Huntingt) 1996;10:1867–72.
11. Fein DA, Corn BW, Lanciano RM, et al. Management of retroperitoneal sarcomas: does dose escalation impact on locoregional control? Int J Radiat Oncol Biol Phys 1995;31:129–34.
12. Hong L, Alektiar KM, Hunt M, et al. Intensity modulated radiotherapy for soft tissue sarcoma of the thigh. Int J Radiat Oncol Biol Phys 2004;59:752–9.
13. Chan MF, Chui CS, Schupak K, et al. The treatment of large extraskeletal chondrosarcoma of the leg: comparison of IMRT and conformal radiotherapy techniques. J Appl Clin Med Phys 2001;2:3–8.
14. Millar BM, Bragg CM, Conway J, et al. Investigation of the use of intensity modulated radiotherapy (IMRT) in comparison with conformal radiotherapy in the management of soft tissue sarcoma [abstract]. Int J Radiat Oncol Biol Phys 2001;51:412.
15. Fiveash JB, Hyatt MD, Caranto J, et al. Preoperative IMRT with dose escalation to tumor subvolumes for retroperitoneal sarcomas: initial clinical results and potential for future dose escalation [abstract]. Int J Radiat Oncol Biol Phys 2002;54:140.
16. Landry JC, Koshy M, Lawson JD, et al. Intensity modulated radiation therapy (IMRT) for retroperitoneal sarcoma: a case for dose escalation and organ at risk (OAR) toxicity [abstract]. Proc Am Soc Clin Oncol 2003;22:297.
17. Koshy M, Landry JC, Lawson JD, et al. Potential for toxicity reduction using intensity modulated radiation therapy (IMRT) for retroperitoneal sarcoma [abstract]. Int J Radiat Oncol Biol Phys 2003;57:S448.
18. Hunt MA, Zelefsky MJ, Wolden S, et al. Treatment planning and delivery of intensity-modulated radiation therapy for primary nasopharynx cancer. Int J Radiat Oncol Biol Phys 2001;49:623–32.
19. Ling CC, Burman C, Chui CS, et al. Conformal radiation treatment of prostate cancer using inversely-planned intensity-modulated photon beams produced with dynamic multileaf collimation. Int J Radiat Oncol Biol Phys 1996;35:721–30.
20. Sultanem K, Shu HK, Xia P, et al. Three-dimensional intensity-modulated radiotherapy in the treatment of nasopharyngeal

carcinoma: the University of California-San Francisco experience. Int J Radiat Oncol Biol Phys 2000;48:711–22.

21. Hong L, Hunt M, Chui C, et al. Intensity-modulated tangential beam irradiation of the intact breast. Int J Radiat Oncol Biol Phys 1999;44:1155–64.

22. Mundt AJ, Lujan AE, Rotmensch J, et al. Intensity-modulated whole pelvic radiotherapy in women with gynecologic malignancies. Int J Radiat Oncol Biol Phys 2002;52:1330–37.

23. Alektiar K, Hong L, Brennan MF, et al. Intensity Modualted Radiation Therapy (IMRT) for primary soft tissue sarcoma of the extremity: preliminary results [abstract]. Presented at the 10th Annual Meeting of the Connective Tissue Oncology Society, 11-14 November 2004, Montreal, Quebec, Canada.

24. Wylie JP, O'Sullivan B, Catton C, et al. Contemporary radiotherapy for soft tissue sarcoma. Semin Surg Oncol 1999;17:33–46.

25. Ballo MT. Radiation therapy for soft tissue sarcomas. In: Markman M, editor. Atlas of cancer. Philadelphia: Lippincott Williams & Wilkins; 2003. p. 360–3.

26. Weber DC, Trofimov AV, Delaney TF, et al. A treatment planning comparison of intensity modulated photon and proton therapy for paraspinal sarcomas. Int J Radiat Oncol Biol Phys 2004;58:1596–606.

Chapter 25.1

PARASPINAL SOFT TISSUE SARCOMA CASE STUDY

BRIAN O'SULLIVAN, MD, FRCPC, RAMANI RAMASESHAN, PHD, MOHAMMAD ISLAM, PHD, ROBERT HEATON, PHD

Patient History

A 53-year-old male presented with a 4-year history of left posterior shoulder discomfort. No formal evaluation was undertaken until his wife noticed a mass and the patient became unable to lie flat. A resection was attempted at an outside hospital but was aborted owing to the extensive nature of the lesion, and only an incisional biopsy was performed. Although the initial diagnosis suggested dermatofibrosarcoma protruberans, the pathology review at our center confirmed the diagnosis of a low-grade fibrosarcoma.

A physical examination demonstrated a large upper posterior left chest mass extending from the midline to the medial scapular margin. The scapula appeared to move adjacent to the mass, which itself was fixed to the chest wall. No neurologic deficits, adenopathy, organomegaly, or other significant findings were noted.

Magnetic resonance imaging (MRI) revealed involvement of all of the paraspinal muscles in the vicinity of the mass with extension through multiple left thoracic interspaces into the chest cavity (Figure 25.1-1). The intrathoracic component abutted the aortic arch and extended into the epidural space, displacing the thoracic spinal cord from T2 to T5. The extrapulmonic mass measured 7 × 2.5 × 7.5 cm. The main component of the

paraspinal mass measured 16 cm in the largest dimension, although evidence of the mass was seen measuring 25 cm in length from the upper cervical to the midthoracic spine.

Surgical resection was considered problematic but potentially possible following preoperative radiation therapy (RT). Conventional RT would involve treatment of a large volume of the lungs and heart, resulting in a high risk of toxicity. Moreover, the dose delivered would be compromised by the proximity of the spinal cord. It was therefore elected to treat this patient with preoperative intensity-modulated radiation therapy (IMRT).

Simulation

The patient was positioned prone on a medulla board and was immobilized with a Vac-Lok evacuation bag (MEDTEC, Orange City, IA) on the chest and abdominal area while a thermoplastic mask was applied to the head and neck region (Figure 25.1-2). Because the tumor was protruding visibly, the patient could not tolerate the supine position. The immobilization used normal tissue surfaces to ensure positioning reproducibility and eliminate sensitivity to anticipated changes in the mass. The isocenter was placed on the vertebral body, which is a stable point and is unaffected by tumor shrinkage.

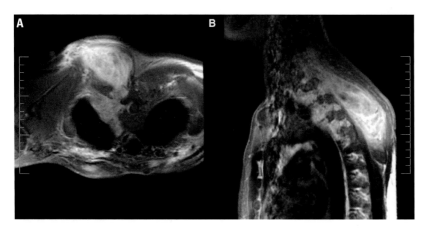

FIGURE 25.1-1. Magnetic resonance images (T1 fat-saturated postgadolinium) of the case described. (*A*) The paraspinal mass can be seen extending inside the chest cavity, where it abuts the posterosuperior aspect of the aortic arch. Note the partial encasement of the dural sac and displacement of the thoracic cord. (*B*) The sagittal view of the enormous mass reveals extension through multiple left thoracic interspaces.

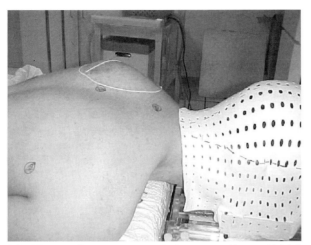

FIGURE 25.1-2. Setup of the patient in the prone position on a Vak-Lok bag with thermoplastic immobilization of the head and neck. Radiopaque skin markings have been placed surrounding the mass for simulation, and reference tattoos were also used. (To view a color version of this image, please refer to the CD-ROM.)

To determine the planning target volume (PTV) margin accounting for breathing motion (see below), a wire was placed on the top of the tumor and motion was observed under fluoroscopy. Breathing motion was measured to be less than 0.5 cm.

The patient then underwent planning computed tomography (CT) in the treatment position on an AcQSim CT simulator (Philips Medical Systems, Andover, MA). The scan extended the level of the tentorium in the posterior fossa of the skull to the L2 vertebral body. No contrast was administered at simulation.

Target and Tissue Delineation

After correlation with diagnostic images, the gross tumor volume (GTV), clinical target volume (CTV), and normal structures were contoured on an AcQSim VoxelQ workstation. The GTV consisted of all gross tumor seen on imaging studies. The CTV margin superiorly and inferiorly was approximately 5 cm, with additional margin added to account for edematous changes noted on the MRI in the longitudinal phase (see Figure 25.1-1). In the axial plane, the CTV margin on the GTV was based on a margin of 1 cm where possible, provided that this incorporated intact musculature. For areas not protected by muscle, the margin was expanded to 2 cm. Also, areas protected by an intact and durable barrier to tumor extension (eg, bone) generally had narrower margins and did not require additional clearance other than that provided by the PTV. Based on the measurement of respiratory motion, a 0.5 cm margin was added to the CTV to generate the PTV.

The normal structures contoured included the lungs, heart, spinal cord, and larynx. The planning organ at risk volumes (PRVs) for the spinal cord were defined using the 0.5 cm margin based on fluoroscopic measurements. Two PRVs were generated from the spinal cord: a high-risk PRV_{cord} (composed of the five levels at which the tumor abutted the thoracic cord) and a PRV_{cord} that contained the entire spinal cord, including the high-risk region. Three-dimensional renderings of the PTV and spinal cord PRVs are shown in Figure 25.1-3.

Treatment Planning

A two-phase IMRT plan was generated using *CadPlan*, version 6.15, inverse planning software (Varian Medical Systems, Palo Alto, CA). Phase I and II used similar geometric beam

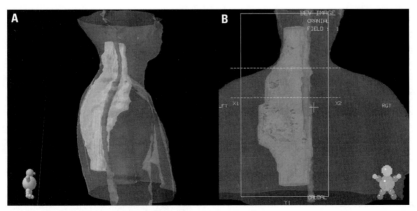

FIGURE 25.1-3. Three-dimensional rendering of the planning target volume (PTV) (*green*), planning organ at risk volume for the spinal cord (PRV_{cord}) (*pink*), and high-risk PRV_{cord} (*orange/red*). (*A*) Sagittal view from the patient's right side showing fingerlike extensions of the PTV encompassing the high-risk PRV_{cord} to include the disease shown in the magnetic resonance images. (*B*) Anterior view of the PTV and PRV spinal cord structures. The dashed lines show the locations of the axial slices depicted in Figure 25.1-5A (*upper line*) and 25.1-5B (*lower line*). The projection shows portions of the PTV (*blue*) overlying the PRV_{cord}. However, these do not encroach on the structure other than at the high-risk PRV_{cord}. (To view a color version of this image, please refer to the CD-ROM.)

configurations composed of six coplanar mixed photon energy beams of 4 MV and 10 MV. The dose-volume constraint parameters (minimum and maximum limits to the PTV and normal structures) specified in this case are summarized in Table 25.1-1.

In phase I, the PTV received 45 Gy in 25 daily fractions. In phase II, the area of the involved cord and intrathoracic extension received an additional 5.4 Gy in three fractions (because these areas were felt to be at highest risk of close or involved surgical margins).

The six-field IMRT plan (Figure 25.1-4) was generated using five posteriorly directed 4 MV beams and a 10 MV anterior beam. The 10 MV beam was angled to improve the PTV coverage in the region of maximal anterior extent while avoiding the majority of the lung. The field size was approximately 10×10 cm^2 and passed through the uniform thickness of the medulla board. The remaining field sizes were approximately 38 cm wide and 40 cm long in phase I and 28 cm long in phase II.

All beams used a neutral couch position and comprised the following gantry angles: posterior (0°), right posterior oblique (50°), left posterior oblique (330°), right posterior oblique (80°), left posterior oblique (285°), and the 10 MV right anterior oblique (170°). The plan incorporated heterogeneity corrections using the modified Batho method during plan optimization and the final calculation with the deliverable fluences.

The high-risk PRV$_{cord}$, comprising a 12 cm length in which the tumor displaced the spinal cord, was constrained to receive a dose between 49.5 and 50 Gy, with a high-priority assignment. The PRV$_{cord}$, which included the high-risk region, was constrained to receive 45 Gy to a volume level that excluded the high-risk PRV$_{cord}$.

The cumulative doses from both phases are presented in Table 25.1-2, and the high-dose region overlaid on axial CT images is shown in Figure 25.1-5. The plan delivered mean doses of 49.3 Gy and 48.2 Gy to the GTV and PTV and maximum doses (to at least 5% of the volume of interest) of 52 Gy and 52.5 Gy, respectively. The high-risk PRV$_{cord}$ received a mean dose of 47.3 Gy (maximum 50.2 Gy to a 1 cc volume), and the PRV$_{cord}$ received a mean dose of 31 Gy. Dose-volume histograms for the targets and normal tissues are shown in Figure 25.1-6. The IMRT fluence map for one of the beams coregistered with the PTV and showing avoidance of the spinal cord is shown in Figure 25.1-7.

Treatment Delivery and Quality Assurance

The treatment parameters were transferred from the planning system to the record and verify system (Multi-Access Integrated Oncology Management System, IMPAC Medical Systems Inc., Mountain View, CA). Treatment fields were delivered using a dynamic sliding window technique on a Varian Clinac 2100C linear accelerator (Varian Medical Systems) equipped with a Millennium 120 multileaf collimator (MLC).

Orthogonal portal films were taken during the trial setup on the first 2 days of treatment and then subsequently twice weekly to verify the isocenter and patient positioning. The patient position was adjusted to correct discrepancies of ≥ 4 mm when compared with digitally reconstructed radiographs.

TABLE 25.1-1. Intensity-Modulated Radiation Therapy Planning Constraints

Target/ Critical Structure Priority	Dose, Gy	Priority	Dose Limit, Gy	Percent Volume	
Right lung					
Minimum	0	0	12	50	80
Maximum	20	80			
Left lung					
Minimum	0	0	15	50	50
Maximum	50.4	80	30	30	50
Heart					
Minimum	0	0	45	66	90
Maximum	50.4	90			
Larynx					
Minimum	0	0			
Maximum	50.4	50			
PRV$_{cord}$					
Minimum	0	0	45	30	80
Maximum	48	95	39.9	51.4	50
High-risk PRV$_{cord}$					
Minimum	49	100			
Maximum	49.5	100			
PTV					
Minimum	50	100			
Maximum	50.5	100			

IMRT = intensity-modulated radiation therapy; PRV$_{cord}$ = planning organ at risk volume for the spinal cord; PTV = planning target volume.

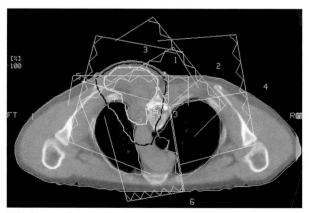

FIGURE 25.1-4. Axial view of the geometric beam arrangement for the six-field intensity-modulated radiation therapy plan. The contoured areas are the gross tumor volume in pale blue and the planning target volume in black (with a stippled white line through the dark lung region). (To view a color version of this image, please refer to the CD-ROM.)

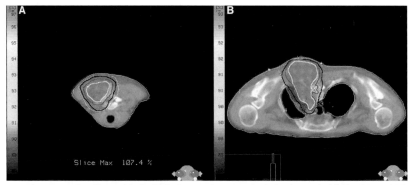

FIGURE 25.1-5. Axial computed tomography slices with the high-dose region as a shaded colorwash. (*A*) The 88 to 100% dose range (*orange/red*) in the cervical region shows the sharp dose gradient. This axial image corresponds to the level indicated in Figure 25.1-3B (*upper dashed line*). (*B*) Axial image of the 88 to 100% dose range in the middle of the target corresponding to the lower dashed line of Figure 25.1-3B taken through the area of the high-risk planning organ at risk volume for the spinal cord (PRV$_{cord}$). The gross tumor volume (*pale blue*), clinical target volume (*royal blue*), and planning target volume (*black*) are displayed in both. Note the target partially enveloping the high-risk PRV$_{cord}$. (To view a color version of this image, please refer to the CD-ROM.)

TABLE 25.1-2. Cumulative Doses: Phases I and II

Structure	Mean Dose, Gy	Maximum Dose,* Gy
GTV	49.3	52.0
PTV	48.2	52.5
Right lung	9.7	19.0
Left lung	24.7	48.4
High-risk PRV$_{cord}$	47.3	50.2
PRV$_{cord}$	31.0	50.2
True spinal cord	38.1	48.6
Heart	11.1	18.6
Larynx	25.85	42.3

GTV = gross tumor volume; PRV$_{cord}$ = planning organ at risk volume for the spinal cord; PTV = planning target volume.
*Maximum dose is defined as the dose to at least 5% of the volume of interest, except for spinal cord volumes, for which a 1 cc volume was used to define the maximum dose.

Daily treatment delivered approximately 1,000 monitor units (MU) and required a beam-on time of ~ 6 minutes at a dose rate of 250 MU/min. The IMRT plan required approximately four times the MU that would be required using conventional RT. The first treatment day occupied a 1-hour time slot, including a mock beam delivery prior to patient setup to verify the overall delivery process. Subsequent sessions, including patient setup, position verification, and treatment delivery, were performed within a 30-minute time slot.

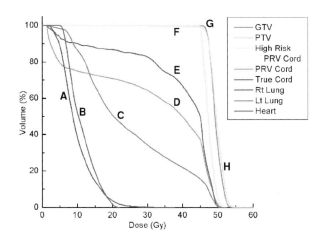

FIGURE 25.1-6. Dose-volume histograms of the critical structures and targets. A = right lung; B = heart; C = left lung; D = PRV cord; E = true cord; F = high risk PRV cord; G = GTV; H = PTV. GTV = gross tumor volume; PRV = planning organ at risk volume; PTV = planning target volume. (To view a color version of this image, please refer to the CD-ROM.)

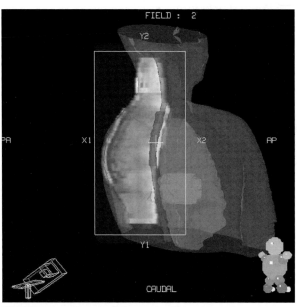

FIGURE 25.1-7. Intensity-modulated radiation therapy fluence map for the right posterior oblique (beam 2) coregistered and rendered over the planning target volume. Avoidance of the remainder of the planning organ at risk volume for the spinal cord (PRV$_{cord}$) exists while maintaining the high-risk PRV$_{cord}$ within prescribed tolerances. (To view a color version of this image, please refer to the CD-ROM.)

Patient-specific dosimetric quality assurance (QA) included three sets of related dose measurements for each field. The assessments consisted of an in-phantom absolute dose measurement in the high-dose region of each field, a relative dose measurement across the two-dimensional fluence map of each field, and an assessment of dosimetric uncertainties owing to patient heterogeneities.

QA measurements were performed using the prescribed fields within the record and verify system. Measurements of absolute dose were performed in a flat, water-equivalent phantom with a standard Farmer-type chamber at a 5 cm depth. The phantom was shifted to position the chamber within a high-dose, low-dose gradient region. Measurements were compared with the calculated doses for the same geometry using the patient fields and MU settings. Volume averaging effects were taken into account by using the average calculated dose delivered to the chamber volume modeled within the planning system.

Relative dose measurements with film were performed for each field at a depth of 5 cm within a water-equivalent phantom. The MU settings were scaled to deliver a maximum dose of 50 cGy to maintain optical densities within the approximately linear dose-response region for Kodak XV-Omat film (Eastman Kodak, Rochester, NY). Comparisons between film measurements and calculated distributions were performed using the *RIT* software package (Radiological Imaging Technology, Colorado Springs, CO). Absolute dose measurements for each field were found to agree with calculations within a 3% tolerance, whereas relative dose measurements in high gradient regions agreed to within 2 mm of their calculated position.

In addition to these standard QA measurements, a measurement was performed to verify the accuracy of the dose calculation near lung heterogeneities. The pencil beam algorithm within *CadPlan* is subject to known limitations in modeling small-field radiation transport through low-density regions such as the lung. Previous studies[1–3] recommended using low-energy (4–6 MV) beams to minimize calculation discrepancies. Because the high-dose gradients contained within IMRT fields generate similar issues to those encountered in small fields, an independent assessment of the treatment field within the lung material was performed.

Phantom measurements were performed using metal oxide semiconductor field effect transistor (MOSFET, Thomson and Neilson, Ottawa, Canada) sensors in a composite water- and lung-equivalent rectangular phantom. The phantom was assembled to simulate the heterogeneous patient geometry along the beam path, traversing the largest thickness of the lung. The phantom consisted of a 10 cm thickness of lung-equivalent material overlaid with 8 cm of water-equivalent material and followed by another 4 cm of water-equivalent material. MOSFET sensors were placed at the depth of maximum dose (D_{max}), at both lung interfaces, at 5 cm within the lung material,

and 0.5 cm beyond the lung interface within the second water-equivalent layer. Measurements within the high-dose regions of both the 4 MV and 10 MV beams at the first interface and within the lung material agreed with the calculated dose to within 5%. A larger difference of 15% between calculation and measurements was observed at the second lung interface, whereas agreement returned to within 5% at 0.5 cm beyond the second lung interface. It was concluded that acceptable dose accuracy over the treatment volume had been achieved based on these measurements.

The accuracy of leaf motion during the actual treatment delivery was verified through an examination of the MLC controller log file. In addition, system-wide QA procedures were performed at regular intervals to ensure the accuracy and consistency of treatment delivery. These now routine measurements were developed using an in-house designed and manufactured two-dimensional chamber array referred to as the matrix dosimeter.

The matrix dosimeter is a 7 × 7 ion chamber array designed to allow quick and accurate checks of beam flatness and calibration. Covering a field size of approximately 30 × 30 cm^2, the chamber assembly can be positioned reproducibly at any gantry and collimator angle using a rigid jig attached to the accelerator tray mount. The matrix is used as a constancy monitor in the delivery of a custom-designed leaf motion sequence and is capable of detecting impending failures of the dynamic MLC system before problems develop enough to interfere with treatment delivery. Factors monitored by the matrix include MLC transmission, dose constancy, partial treatment dose delivery, leaf positioning, and leaf bank positioning. Leaf position accuracy was routinely tested (monthly) using a standard picket fence test pattern at 1 cm intervals capable of detecting leaf position errors of 0.5 mm.

Clinical Outcome

During treatment, dexamethasone was administered to minimize edema that might compromise the spinal cord. Overall, treatment was well tolerated, apart from mild esophagitis. After 2 weeks of treatment, an objective reduction in the size of the mass was noted and the patient noted an increased ability to lie flat without discomfort.

Following completion of IMRT, the patient developed radiation pneumonitis with visible changes in the left lung, which delayed surgery. At surgery, the tumor was found throughout the thoracic epidural space. Dissection was required around the left brachial plexus, carotid, and subclavian vessels. The esophagus, T1 nerve root, and part of the scapula were resected. In addition, paraspinal and intrathoracic tumor resections were performed with extensive rib removal, left anterior and posterior vertebrectomies from T1 through T7, and laminectomies with thoracic epidural decompression at the same levels. Anterior and posterior spinal fusion with instrumentation was accomplished from C7 through T9, and the chest wall was repaired with a polypropylene mesh and a latissimus dorsi rotation flap. The entire operating time was 18 hours.

The patient's postoperative course was complicated, requiring an extensive intrahospital recovery and rehabilitation. He suffered from numbness related to the T1 nerve root sacrifice and needed a cervical brace for a prolonged period. These problems continue to compromise his performance and quality of life to this day. However, he was without evidence of recurrence more that 36 months since completion of combined-modality treatment. No evidence of ongoing RT-induced sequelae has been noted.

References

1. Ekstrand KE, Barnes WH. Pitfalls in the use of high energy X rays to treat tumors in the lung. Int J Radiat Oncol Biol Phys 1990;18:249-252.

2. Kornelsen RO, Young ME. Changes in the dose-profile of a 10 MV x-ray beam within and beyond low density material. Med Phys 1982;9:114-116.

3. Wang L, Yorke E, Desobry G, Chui CS. Dosimetric advantage of using 6 MV over 15 MV photons in conformal therapy of lung cancer: Monte Carlo studies in patient geometries. J Appl Clin Med Phys 2002;3:51-59.

RETROPERITONEAL SARCOMA

CASE STUDY

JOHN B. FIVEASH, MD, RICHARD A. POPPLE, PhD, MARTIN J. HESLIN, MD

Patient History

A 60-year-old female presented with a 2-month history of abdominal pain and a 25 lb weight loss. On physical examination, an abdominal mass was palpated. A computed tomography (CT) scan of the abdomen and pelvis revealed an 8 cm retroperitoneal mass and right-sided hydronephrosis. A core needle biopsy was consistent with a high-grade leiomyosarcoma. The remainder of the metastatic workup was negative.

At our institution, radiation therapy (RT) is used in such cases prior to surgical resection. A large tumor mass displaces the small bowel and other critical structures partially out of the treatment volume. The margin at greatest risk is typically away from the small bowel on the posterior or posteriomedial aspect of the tumor, whereas the anterior margin adjacent to the bowel is generally not at risk of positive margins after resection. Intensity-modulated radiation therapy (IMRT) planning and treatment were used in this patient to simultaneously boost the volume at greatest risk of positive margins while sparing surrounding organs at risk.

Simulation

At the University of Alabama-Birmingham, patients with retroperitoneal sarcoma undergoing IMRT are typically simulated in the supine position and immobilized in a custom alpha cradle device. Although prone positioning may help displace small bowel out of the treatment volume, it is used only in selected cases.

After fabrication of the immobilization device, a planning CT scan (PQ 5000, Philips Medical Systems, Andover, MA) was performed of the entire peritoneal cavity using 3 mm slices. If the tumor is very superior or inferior in the abdomen, a larger volume is imaged, allowing for the potential use of noncoplanar beam arrangements. Intravenous and oral contrast is used in all patients.

Target and Tissue Delineation

A gross tumor volume (GTV) was contoured on the planning CT scan consisting of all gross disease. Magnetic resonance imaging was also performed to aid in the delineation of the GTV. In general, a separate clinical target volume (CTV) is not defined in patients with retroperitoneal sarcoma undergoing preoperative RT. Exceptions include patients who have undergone subtotal resection or whose tumors have hemorrhaged. In such cases, the GTV is expanded by 3 cm, generating the CTV. However, this CTV should respect and follow the possible patterns of dissemination and does not need to extend through solid organs, such as bone. In patients diagnosed by core needle biopsy (such as this case), the CTV is equivalent to the GTV.

The organs at risk (OAR) delineated in this patient included the small bowel, kidneys, liver, and spinal cord. In most cases, the large bowel is generally not considered dose limiting and is not included in the optimization process as an avoidance structure. In selected cases, other OAR are included. In one case, we contoured the contralateral ovary in a premenopausal patient. If the resection of the ipsilateral kidney is planned, it is not included as an OAR. The GTV and OAR for this patient are shown in Figure 25.2-1.

Treatment Planning

As mentioned above, a simultaneous integrated boost approach was used in this case. Two planning target volumes (PTVs) were thus generated. PTV$_1$ was created by adding a 1 to 1.5 cm margin to the CTV, accounting for organ motion and setup uncertainty. PTV$_2$ included areas judged to be at highest risk of microscopic tumor involvement targeted for dose escalation and included a small margin for setup uncertainty. PTV$_2$ was delineated in consultation with the operating surgeon.

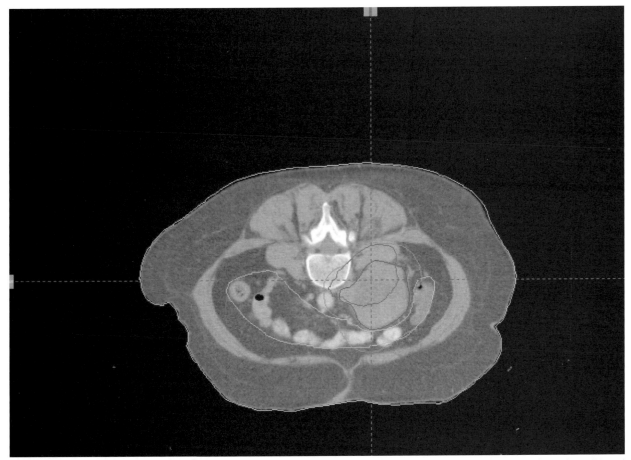

FIGURE 25.2-1. Target volumes and organs at risk: gross tumor volume (*blue*), planning target volume (PTV)₁ (*magenta*), PTV₂ (*brown*), small bowel (*red*), and spinal cord and cauda equina (*green*). (To view a color version of this image, please refer to the CD-ROM.)

The CTV-to-PTV margins may be reduced in some aspects to avoid neighboring OAR. Note that although these margins may result in smaller treatment volumes (than conventional treatment fields), marginal recurrences have not been seen in our patients who have not undergone prior incisional biopsy or subtotal resection. For tumors very near the spinal cord, a planning organ at risk volume should be considered based on the specifications of Report 62 of the International Commission on Radiation Units and Measurements (ICRU).

Our experience is that five to seven coplanar beams result in an acceptable IMRT plan in such patients. Treatment beams may be equally spaced, or their orientation may be intelligently selected by omitting gantry angles that pass through large volumes of sensitive normal tissues. The addition of an anterior-inferior oblique beam often improves sparing of the anterior bowel and may produce modest dosimetric benefits over coplanar beam arrangements in selected patients. In this patient, six coplanar 15 MV beams were used (gantry angles of 40, 80, 140, 200, 250, and 340 degrees).

Total doses of 45 Gy (in 1.8 Gy daily fractions) and 57.5 Gy (in 2.3 Gy daily fractions) were prescribed to the PTV₁ and PTV₂, respectively. Treatment planning was performed using the *Helios* inverse planning system, version 6.27 (Varian Medical Systems, Palo Alto, CA). Input parameters for the optimization process in this patient are shown in Table 25.2-1.

TABLE 25.2-1. Input Parameters and Suggested Dose Limits

Volume	Dose Limit, Gy	Volume	Priority, %	Comment
PTV₁	> 45 < 70	100%	50	95% coverage is accepted
PTV₂	> 57.5 < 70	100%	90	
Small bowel	< 45	Maximum	50	54 Gy to 20 cc is absolute dose limit
Kidney	< 23	One-third	90	Depends on need for resection and contralateral function
Liver	< 33	Whole	50	NTCP model available
Spinal cord	45	Maximum	80	

NTCP = normal tissue complication probability; PTV = planning target volume.

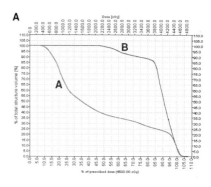
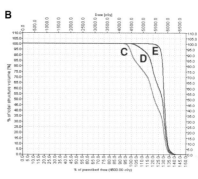

FIGURE 25.2-2. Cumulative dose-volume histograms (DVHs) for (*A*) organs at risk and (*B*) targets. The color of the DVH line corresponds to the organ or target color in Figure 25.2-1. (To view a color version of this image, please refer to the CD-ROM.)

The dose-volume histograms for the targets and normal tissues are shown in Figure 25.2-2. In this case, a significant portion of the GTV within PTV$_2$ could be dose escalated. Such hot spots are acceptable within the GTV. When using the simultaneous integrated boost technique, one should not attempt to force dose homogeneity within PTV$_1$.

Isodose curves superimposed on representative axial CT slices are shown in Figure 25.2-3. All plans should be carefully reviewed for high-dose gradients near critical structures. The partial volume tolerance of the small bowel at low volumes is unknown. We have limited 20 cc of small bowel to 54 Gy and have not had any significant untoward late toxicity. In patients who have had previous abdominal surgery and whose bowel is thought to be fixed or nonmobile, a dose limit of 50 Gy is used.

Treatment Delivery and Quality Assurance

IMRT treatment was delivered on a Varian 2100 EX linear accelerator (Varian Medical Systems) equipped with a 120 multileaf collimator. Treatment was delivered using the dynamic (sliding window) technique. All fields were filmed on the first treatment day. On subsequent weeks, orthogonal pairs of port films were obtained to confirm isocenter placement.

The treatment plan was verified by applying the beams to a near water equivalent polystyrene phantom. These beams were applied in the same geometry as the patient to a CT scan of the phantom in the treatment planning system. Dose was calculated and the expected mean dose to the ionization chamber was noted. Four transverse planes were selected for placement of film. The ionization chamber measurement agreed with the calculated value to within 3%. In the high-dose region, film dosimetry agreed to within 3% or 2 mm and to within 5% or 5 mm in the low-dose region.

On average, the total treatment time was 15 to 20 minutes (including patient setup). In many patients with retroperitoneal sarcoma, however, two carriage groups may be needed owing to the large treatment volume. In such cases, intelligent selection of beams may help minimize the number of fields, reducing overall treatment time.

Patient Outcome

The patient tolerated IMRT treatment well, with only grade 2 nausea, which responded to oral antiemetics. Approximately 6 weeks following the completion of IMRT, she underwent resection of the residual tumor mass. No viable tumor was present in the surgical specimen. At 12 months post-IMRT, the patient developed distant progression in the lungs. She underwent bilateral thoracotomies and is responding to systemic chemotherapy. The patient was alive 30 months after completion of IMRT. She is without evidence of local or regional progression and has not experienced any significant late toxicity.

Our experience to date using this technique was recently presented.[1] Between June 1999 and January 2002, 14 consecutive patients were treated. The first seven patients were treated with forward planned multiple static segmented fields. Inverse planning with dynamic multileaf collimator delivery was used in the remainder. All patients completed preoperative IMRT as planned, and 12 patients underwent laparotomy with planned resection. Only one patient experienced grade 3 or higher toxicity. This patient had the largest tumor in the series (> 35 cm in greatest diameter) and developed nausea and vomiting, leading to dehydration, and required admission for intravenous fluids.

Of the 12 patients who underwent laparotomy and attempted resection, 11 had a complete resection with negative margins. In the remaining case, surgery was aborted when peritoneal spread was found. At a median follow-up of 71 weeks, 4 of the 12 patients who underwent a curative resection developed disease recurrence (1 locally, 3 distantly). No patients developed chronic RT-related toxicity, although one patient had severe edema after resection of the inferior cava. Others have similarly reported favorable experiences using preoperative IMRT in patients with retroperitoneal sarcomas.[2]

FIGURE 25.2-3. ***Opposite*** Axial isodose curves demonstrating dose escalation to planning target volume 2 to 57.5 Gy in 25 fractions. The 100% isodose line corresponds to 45 Gy. (To view a color version of this image, please refer to the CD-ROM.)

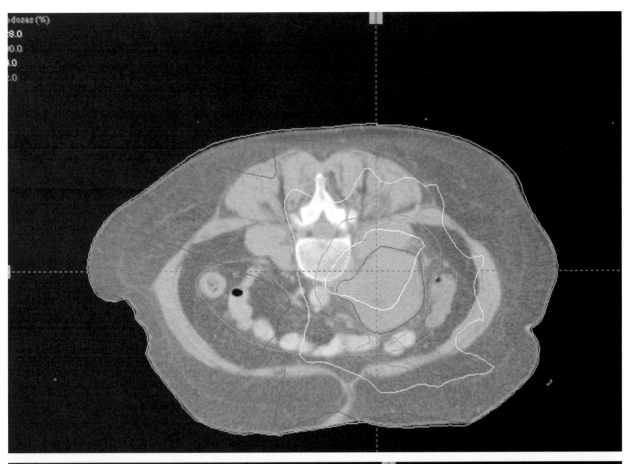

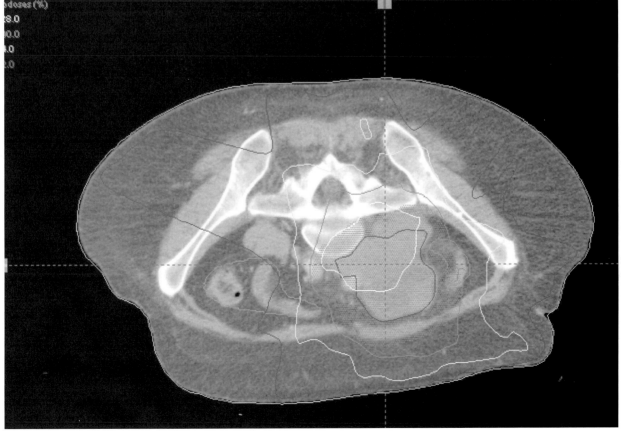

As part of our initial report, three patients were replanned to evaluate the potential of further dose escalation beyond 57.5 Gy in 25 fractions while maintaining acceptable normal tissue dosimetry.[1] Our results suggest that the PTV_2 dose could be escalated to a total dose of 75.2 to 82.8 in 25 fractions without exceeding tolerance of nearby sensitive structures. Clearly, prospective clinical trials are needed to evaluate the benefits and risks of further dose escalation in these patients.

References

1. Fiveash JB, Hyatt MD, Caranto J, et al. Preoperative IMRT with dose escalation to tumor subvolumes for retroperitoneal sarcomas: initial clinical results and potential for future dose escalation [abstract]. Int J Radiat Oncol Biol Phys 2002;54:140.

2. Koshy M, Landry JC, Lawson JD, et al. Potential for toxicity reduction using intensity modulated radiation therapy (IMRT) for retroperitoneal sarcoma [abstract]. Int J Radiat Oncol Biol Phys 2003;57:S448–9.

Pediatric Tumors

Overview

Shiao Y. Woo, MD, FRCP, FACR

The role of radiation therapy (RT) in the treatment of childhood malignancies continues to evolve. RT is undoubtedly an effective locoregional treatment for many pediatric tumors, but there is a great concern about the late effects of radiation in a growing child, especially in infants. The most worrisome late effects include growth defects, organ dysfunction, and second malignancies. On the other hand, the avoidance of RT in the treatment of certain cancers has led to an increase in both recurrence and death rates.

Conformal RT approaches, including intensity-modulated radiation therapy (IMRT), are an attempt to limit the volume of normal tissues from receiving high radiation doses. The hypothesis is that the normal tissues exposed to high doses are more likely to manifest late effects than those exposed to low doses, and a reduction of the volume of normal tissues receiving high doses would decrease the incidence or severity of the late effects.

IMRT is a versatile tool for conformal RT. Conceptually, it creates around the target (tumor) an elastic dose envelope that can be manipulated depending on the location of and the dose constraint to the adjacent normal structures. Since 1993, IMRT has been used to treat children with a variety of tumors. This technology is now widely available and is being used in many institutions. At our institution, from 1993 to 2002, approximately 150 children have been treated with IMRT. The purpose of this chapter is to review the published literature and issues and challenges surrounding the use of IMRT in children. Interested readers should also refer to the accompanying case studies illustrating the use of IMRT in a variety of tumor sites (Chapter 26.1, "Retinoblastoma;" Chapter 26.2, "Neuroblastoma;" and Chapter 26.3, "Rhabodomyosarcoma").

Rationale

Medulloblastoma

Craniospinal irradiation (CSI) is the cornerstone of treatment for children with medulloblastoma. The posterior fossa, where the tumor usually originates, is given additional doses of radiation to decrease the risk of recurrence. In recent years, cisplatinum-containing chemotherapy regimens, when added to RT, have significantly improved cure rates.[1]

Cisplatinum, however, is an ototoxic agent. When used in conjunction with RT to the posterior fossa, the combination may produce significant hearing loss in children with medulloblastoma.[2] The conventional technique of posterior fossa irradiation involves the use of parallel opposed lateral fields, which, when added to CSI, results in a total dose of 54 to 55.8 Gy to the posterior fossa and the cochlea. Ototoxicity from either radiation or cisplatinum is a dose-dependent phenomenon. Hence, it is reasonable to assume that a reduction of the dose of either agent to the cochleas could reduce ototoxicity.

There is currently no reliable method for differential delivery of cisplatinum in the treatment of medulloblastoma. The ability of amifostine (Ethyol, MedImmune Inc., Gaithersburg, MD) to ameliorate otoxicity is also uncertain. It is therefore logical to investigate the use of IMRT to reduce the radiation dose to the cochleas. In a published study, it has been demonstrated that IMRT could reduce the dose to the cochlea in children with medulloblastoma while irradiating the tumor bed to 55.8 Gy.[3] When compared with the conventional parallel opposed technique, the mean dose to the cochleas was reduced by approximately one-third. The clinical outcome using this approach is discussed in a later section.

Head and Neck Tumors

In children, malignant tumors of the head and neck region generally consist of rhabdomyosarcoma, Ewing's sarcoma, lymphomas, and metastatic tumors, such as neuroblastoma. A relatively uncommon tumor, juvenile angiofibroma, occurs in the nasopharynx or upper nose. RT plays an integral role in the treatment of rhabdomyosarcoma. Most non-Hodgkin's lymphomas do not need RT. Juvenile angiofibroma, although difficult to remove surgically because of the high vascularity, is readily controlled by RT.

Conventional RT to the head and neck region may produce a range of long-term morbidities, especially in children. IMRT may allow the delivery of full therapeutic doses to the target while reducing the dose to the organs at risk (OAR). Figure 26-1 shows an example of an IMRT plan in a patient with a nasopharyngeal tumor that minimizes the dose to the parotid glands. Figure 26-2 demonstrates a conformal dose distribution treatment of an orbital rhabdomyosarcoma.

Issues and Challenges
Immobilization and Anesthesia

The planning target volume (PTV) accounts for setup inconsistencies and target motion. It is used in addition to the gross tumor volume (GTV) and the clinical target volume (CTV). Patient immobilization reduces setup uncertainties and therefore requires a smaller PTV expansion.

Young children may not tolerate immobilization devices awake; thus, conscious sedation or short general anesthesia is needed. The introduction of short intubation tubes that do not extend past the vocal cords and short-acting anesthetic agents render daily anesthesia not only safe but relatively nonmorbid. If treated more than once a day, special attention should be paid to the child's fluid and nutritional intake.

In the treatment of head and neck tumors, the head needs to be well immobilized. Fortunately, there is very little target motion. Several immobilization devices (invasive and noninvasive) have been developed (Figure 26-3). It is important for each institution to evaluate its immobilization devices. At our institution, the invasive screws and talon used in older children and adults have produced a reproducible daily variation of within 1 mm. Two types of masks have been evaluated, and the results are summarized in Table 26-1.

Target Delineation

Accurate target delineation in medulloblastoma requires knowledge of the anatomy of the posterior cranial fossa. The posterior fossa is well defined on computed tomography (CT) by the posterior clinoid, tentorium, and occipital skull bone. The inferior border is at the level of the foramen magnum unless the tumor extends past the foramen; then the border will extend more inferiorly.

An issue that has been debated for some time and is now being actively studied is whether the entire posterior foramen needs to be irradiated to the full doses of 54 to 56 Gy. An analysis of the recurrence pattern in the posterior fossa demonstrated that the vast majority of local failures occurred at or adjacent to the original tumor.[4] A multi-institutional phase I–II trial used conformal RT techniques to deliver (in addition to CSI) 36 Gy to the posterior fossa and 55.8 Gy to the tumor bed plus a 2 cm margin (Figure 26-4).[5] The 2-year progression-free survival rates were 93.6% and 84.2% for children with average-risk and high-risk disease, respectively. At Baylor College of Medicine (one of the participat-

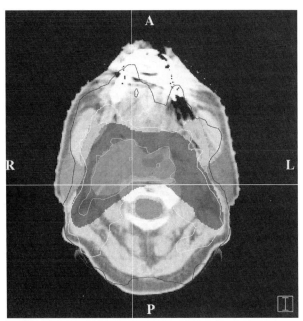

FIGURE 26-1. Intensity-modulated radiation therapy plan for a nasopharyngeal tumor. Planning target volume (*red*), clinical target volume (*dark purple*), right parotid gland (*blue*), and left parotid gland (*light purple*). (To view a color version of this image, please refer to the CD-ROM.)

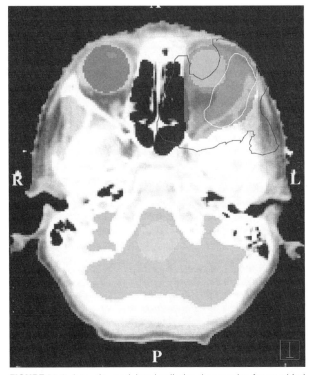

FIGURE 26-2. Intensity-modulated radiation therapy plan for an orbital rhabdomyosarcoma.

TABLE 26-1. Result of Variability Tests of Two Different Thermoplastic Masks

Action	Maximum Motion, mm	
	Type A	Type B
At rest	0.00	0.00
Chin up	0.97	0.30
Chin down	0.64	0.43
Return to at rest	0.08	0.20
At rest	0.00	0.00
Rotate right	0.76	0.33
Rotate left	1.14	0.64
Return to at rest	0.25	0.15

Adapted from Woo SY, et al. Int J Radiat Oncol Biol Phys 2003;56(1):274–86.

ing institutions), the isolated posterior fossa failure rate was 0% at a median follow-up of 35 months. It appears that irradiating only a portion of the posterior fossa to 54 to 56 Gy has not increased local recurrence. A randomized trial is currently being conducted by the Children's Oncology Group (COG) comparing irradiation of the entire posterior fossa versus irradiation of the tumor bed (plus margin) only. A defined subset of children with average-risk medulloblastoma is included in this trial. A similar trial is being proposed by the International Society of Pediatric Oncology.

In contrast, juvenile pilocytic astrocytomas, well-differentiated ependymomas, and craniopharyngiomas generally do not have a deep infiltrating border. In single-institution trials, conformal RT of these tumors using a 1 cm GTV-to-CTV margin has produced excellent results.[6] It has been suggested that the CTV expansion could be further reduced to 0.5 cm. A trial is being prepared by the COG evaluating conformal RT in low-grade gliomas using a 1 cm margin around the GTV. It is, however, important to bear in mind that when delineating the CTV on imaging slices, the same margin should be added superiorly and inferiorly. When the GTV is not well visualized on CT, magnetic resonance (MR)-CT fusion is helpful in the definition of the target and normal structures. One should, however, also remember the slight geometric inaccuracy of MR and that current fusion software is not precise. The emerging "flexible" fusion algorithms are likely to improve the technology significantly.

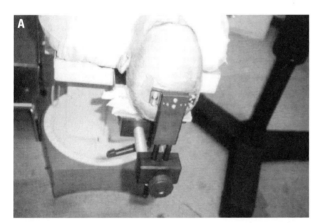 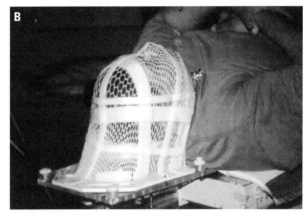

FIGURE 26-3. (*A*) Invasive immobilization device (screws and talons). (*B*) Noninvasive immobilization device (thermoplastic mask). (To view a color version of this image, please refer to the CD-ROM.)

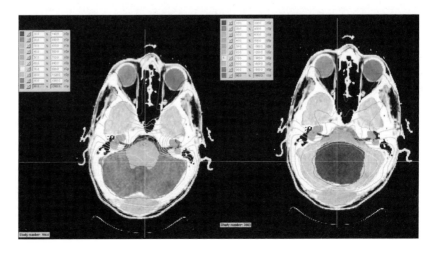

FIGURE 26-4. Intensity-modulated radiation therapy plan for a posterior fossa boost and tumor bed boost in a patient with medulloblastoma. Note the curving of the high isodose lines around the cochleas and anterior brainstem. (To view a color version of this image, please refer to the CD-ROM.)

A peculiar feature of central nervous system germinomas is that they can present with more than one discrete tumor. It is not agreed on whether these tumors represent an embryologic "field change" or discrete microscopic extensions. However, it is impossible to recognize the region at risk, which extends anteriorly from the pineal gland to the floor of the third ventricle and the suprasellar area and to the frontal horn of the lateral ventricles.

If one considers using RT as the primary modality in a patient with a central nervous system germinoma, one has to first exclude overt leptomeningeal spread because routine CSI is generally considered unnecessary in the absence of demonstrable leptomeningeal involvement. The primary target is the region at risk defined above. A secondary boost target is the tumor(s) visualized on images. Some IMRT planning systems allow irradiation of both targets simultaneously, with each receiving a different dose. An example is given in Figure 26-5.

Target delineation for pediatric head and neck tumors depends on the individual tumor type. Lymphomas in children, with the exception of Hodgkin's disease, seldom need RT. Hodgkin's disease is generally treated with conventional RT techniques using large fields. Sarcomas are, however, suitable for IMRT. In these patients, the GTV is generally well defined on imaging studies, and a 1.5 to 2 cm GTV-to-CTV expansion is used. For parameningeal rhabdomyosarcoma, it is important to recognize that the tumor could infiltrate the skull base. Therefore, a margin of at least 2 cm around the GTV at the skull base is recommended.

Benign tumors such as neuromas, neurofibromas, and juvenile angiofibromas are rare and do not always require RT. Nasopharyngeal juvenile angiofibroma, which causes epistaxis, may not be easily excised. A moderate radiation dose (45 Gy) is very effective in controlling bleeding and halting tumor progress. IMRT is a suitable technology for this lesion. A 0.5 to 1 cm margin around the GTV is sufficient.

Plan Evaluation

To determine if an IMRT plan satisfies the prescribed dose delivery and maintains the constraints of doses to the normal structures, one needs to carefully evaluate the isodose dose distribution, statistical panel, and dose-volume histograms of the target and the OAR. In addition, if the tumor control probability and normal tissue complication probability data are available, they have to be considered.

It is generally recommended that the prescribed isodose covers at least 95% of the PTV. However, this is entirely arbitrary. A plan that delivers 100% of the prescribed dose to 95% of the PTV but almost 0% to the remainder of the target is obviously bad because clonogens in the 5% volume will almost certainly cause regrowth of the tumor. Fortunately, for all practical purposes, this situation does not occur. As mentioned earlier, IMRT produces an elastic dose envelope that allows the planner at different directions to "indent" the boundary depending on the dose constraint on the adjacent OAR. If a target touches an OAR that has lower tolerance than the prescribed dose to the target, one can "push" the dose envelope into the target. In such a situation, the volume of the target receiving less than the prescribed dose could be more than 5%, but the minimal dose to the PTV would be the dose received by the OAR. One has to apply clinical judgment as to whether to accept such a plan or take the risk of exceeding the presumed "tolerance" of one or more of the OAR.

When evaluating the dose to the normal structures, several factors need to be considered, namely, the presumed tolerance of the entire organ or part of the organ (partial volume tolerance), the accepted notions on the arrangements of the functional subunits, the presence of radiation-enhancing drugs, other medical conditions of the patient, and, to a certain extent, the patient's age (infant or older child). Unfortunately, the available data on some of

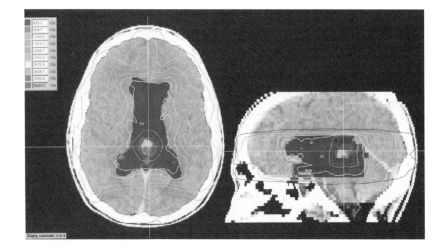

FIGURE 26-5. Intensity-modulated radiation therapy plan to treat a pineal germinoma simultaneously with the region at risk at two dose levels. (To view a color version of this image, please refer to the CD-ROM.)

these factors, for instance, partial volume tolerance and the radiation repair mechanisms, are incomplete, but the data are accumulating.[7,8]

Published Data

Medulloblastoma

Since 1997, IMRT has been used in children with medulloblastoma as part of a multi-institutional phase I–II study. In this study, average-risk patients received 23.4 Gy CSI followed by a 12.6 Gy conformal boost to the posterior fossa and then a tumor bed boost of 19.8 Gy. All patients received high-dose chemotherapy with stem cell rescue. The 2-year progression-free survival rate was 93.6%.[5] A recent updated analysis of 73 children with average-risk medulloblastoma in this trial showed an isolated posterior fossa failure rate of < 3% at a median follow-up of 32.4 months.[9] A patterns of failure analysis after a conformal tumor bed boost at the Memorial Sloan-Kettering Cancer Center also demonstrated one posterior fossa recurrence in 32 children.[10]

In addition, as mentioned earlier, those patients treated with IMRT received a significantly lower mean dose to the cochlea compared with children treated with conventional techniques (36.7 vs 54.2 Gy). These children also experienced significantly less ototoxicity, despite having received a higher cumulative dose of cisplatinum than conventionally treated children.[3] This report highlights the important contribution of IMRT in reducing treatment-related morbidity in children. A similar experience was recently reported by investigators at the Los Angeles Children's Hospital.[11]

Juvenile Angiofibroma

One report described three cases of recurrent or unresectable juvenile angiofibroma treated with IMRT (34–45 Gy).[12] The tumor responded radiographically in all three cases, and there was no endoscopic evidence of disease in two cases at 15 and 40 months, respectively. Minimal morbidity was encountered. Even though the experience is limited, IMRT appears to be an excellent radiotherapeutic modality for this condition.

Future Directions

IMRT plans generally produce some degree of inhomogeneity in the high-dose region. The hot spots can potentially be a problem if a normal structure traverses within the PTV, for example, a cranial nerve or the prostatic urethra. Therefore, it is important to identify such normal structures and place a dose constraint on them or to create as homogeneous a dose distribution within the PTV as possible. In the treatment of medulloblastoma, part of the normal cerebellum (included within the CTV) is in the high-dose region. MR changes have been observed in about 10% of children 4 to 6 months after IMRT. Such abnormalities, although usually asymptomatic, raise the concerns of tumor recurrence. Our experience, however, has shown that these abnormalities gradually subside within 9 to 12 months with little or no intervention. It remains conjectural as to whether the underlying pathology is transient breakdown of the blood-brain barrier, subacute demyelination, or another mechanism.

One could also take advantage of hot spots in the IMRT plans, placing them at sites of high clonogen density or in regions of hypoxia if identifiable. This technique has been investigated in the treatment of prostate cancer using magnetic resonance spectroscopy to identify regions of higher tumor burden within the prostate.[13] Regions of hypoxia can also be imaged.[14] With the advent of molecular imaging technologies, such an approach could be applied and studied in many tumors.

A feature common to practically all IMRT plans is that a relatively large volume will receive a low dose of radiation. This low-dose volume may not cause acute or subacute clinical morbidity but could potentially be carcinogenic, especially in children.[15] Theoretically, the use of helical tomotherapy to treat large tumors could exaggerate this problem. This potential for increasing the rate of second malignancy has thus far not been observed owing to the relatively short duration of clinical application of IMRT, but it remains a concern. Long-term follow-up of children treated with IMRT needs to be performed on a continual basis to determine the extent of this potential morbidity.

As mentioned earlier, IMRT generates an elastic dose envelope that can be indented at the location of the identified OAR. The laws of physics, however, dictate that the dose envelope will then protrude somewhere else by the displaced radiation dose. This displaced dose could be another factor for late morbidity, the so-called trade-off. In the treatment of brain tumors in children, such displaced doses to certain regions of the brain could cause a decline in neurocognitive function. An example is the treatment of the posterior fossa in children with medulloblastoma. To reduce the dose to the cochleas, some of the dose could be "squeezed" anteriorly to the supratentorial cerebrum. An argument has been raised that reduced ototoxicity may be replaced by neurocognitive impairments.[16]

However, the direction of the radiation dose displacement can be manipulated by an experienced planner. One tactic is to place a severe dose constraint for structures situated anterior to the target so that the radiation is displaced posteriorly. In a recent analysis of children in the previously cited ototoxicity report, it was noted that children treated with the above IMRT technique had better nonverbal intelligence and visual motor integration scores than children treated with the conventional approach (N. Jain, personal communication, December 2003).

Therefore, it appears that the benefit of decreased ototoxicity associated with IMRT may not come at the cost of increased neurocognitive deficits. Nevertheless, it is vitally important that we continue to investigate potential trade-offs in morbidity in children undergoing IMRT.

References

1. Packer RJ, Sutton LN, Elterman R, et al. Outcome for children with medulloblastoma treated with radiation and cisplatin, CCNU, and vincristine chemotherapy. J Neurosurg 1994;81:690–8.

2. Miettinen S, Laurikainen E, Johansson R, et al. Radiotherapy enhanced ototoxicity of cisplatin in children. Acta Otolaryngol Suppl (Stockh) 1997;529:90–4.

3. Huang E, Teh BS, Strother DR, et al. Intensity-modulated radiation therapy for pediatric medulloblastoma: early report on the reduction of ototoxicity. Int J Radiat Oncol Biol Phys 2003;52:599–605.

4. Fukunaga-Johnson N, Lee JH, Sandler HM, et al. Patterns of failure following treatment for medulloblastoma: is it necessary to treat the entire posterior fossa? Int J Radiat Oncol Biol Phys 1998;42:143–6.

5. Strother D, Ashley D, Kellie SJ, et al. Feasibility of four consecutive high-dose chemotherapy cycles with stem-cell rescue for patients with newly diagnosed medulloblastoma or supratentorial primitive neuroectodermal tumor after craniospinal radiotherapy: results of a collaborative study. J Clin Oncol 2001;19:2696–704.

6. Merchant TE, Zhu Y, Thompson SJ, et al. Preliminary results from a phase II trial of conformal radiation therapy for pediatric patients with localized low-grade astrocytoma and ependymoma. Int J Radiat Oncol Biol Phys 2002;52:325–32.

7. Bijl HP, van Luijk P, Coppes RP, et al. Unexpected changes of rat cervical spinal cord tolerance caused by inhomogeneous dose distributions. Int J Radiat Oncol Biol Phys 2003;57:274–81.

8. Withers R. Migration and myelination. Int J Radiat Oncol Biol Phys 2003;57:9–10.

9. Merchant TE, Kun LE, Krasin MJ, et al. A multi-institution prospective trial of reduced-dose craniospinal irradiation (23.4 Gy) followed by conformal posterior fossa (36 Gy) and primary site irradiation (55.8 Gy) and dose-intensity chemotherapy for average-risk medulloblastoma. Int J Radiat Oncol Biol Phys 2003;57:S194–5.

10. Wolden SL, Dunkel IJ, Souweidane MM, et al. Patterns of failure using a conformal radiation therapy tumor bed boost for medulloblastoma. J Clin Oncol 2003;21:3079–83.

11. Kim SH, Olch J, Villablanca E, et al. Posterior fossa boost by intensity-modulated radiation therapy (IMRT) vs lateral beams (LB): impact on cisplatin dosing and ototoxicity. Int J Radiat Oncol Biol Phys 2002;54 Suppl:202–3.

12. Kuppersmith RB, Teh BS, Donovan DT, et al. The use of intensity modulated radiotherapy for the treatment of extensive and recurrent juvenile angiofibroma. Int J Pediatr Otorhinolaryngol 2000;52:261–8.

13. Pickett B, Kurhanewicz J, Fein B, et al. Use of magnetic resonance imaging and spectroscopy in the evaluation of external beam radiation therapy in prostate cancer. Int J Radiat Oncol Biol Phys 2003;57:S163–4.

14. Perez CA Bradley J Chao CK, et al. Functional imaging in treatment planning in radiation therapy: a review. Rays 2002;27:157–73.

15. Hall EJ, Wim CS. Radiation-induced second cancers: the impact of 3D-CRT and IMRT. Int J Radiat Oncol Biol Phys 2003;56:83–8.

16. Soomal R, Mosleh-Shirazi MA, Saran F, et al. What is the cost of cochlear avoidance in pediatric medulloblastoma? Evaluation of 3-D conformal planning techniques for the posterior fossa boost. Int J Radiat Oncol Biol Phys 2002;54 Suppl:204.

RETINOBLASTOMA

CASE STUDY

ROBERT S. LAVEY, MD, MPH, ARTHUR J. OLCH, PhD

Case 1: Treatment of Both Eyes

Patient History

A 13-month-old boy presented with a 1-month history of right eye strabismus. Examination under anesthesia revealed complete retinal detachment with subretinal tumor and vitreous seeding with clumps of tumor (group E retinoblastoma) in the right eye and several large retinal tumors without vitreous seeding (group C retinoblastoma) in the left eye. There was no evidence of disease outside the globes on the head computed tomography (CT) scan, in the cerebrospinal fluid, or in the bone marrow.

The patient was treated with laser photoablation and six cycles of intravenous carboplatin, etoposide, and vincristine chemotherapy, with carboplatin administered subconjunctivally during the first three cycles. Multiple recurrences of retinal tumors in the left eye after the fourth and fifth chemotherapy cycles were treated with additional laser photoablation and cryotherapy. Owing to an inability to control the left retinal recurrences, the patient was subsequently referred for radiation therapy (RT). Although active disease was present in the left retina only, it was elected to also irradiate the entire right globe owing to prior vitreous seeding in the right eye. Intensity-modulated radiation therapy (IMRT) was used to maximize sparing of the surrounding normal tissues.

Simulation

The patient was sedated during simulation (and treatment) using intravenous continuous-infusion propofol because of his young age. His head was positioned in a custom-molded, bead-filled, evacuated headrest and the HeadFix immobilization system (Medical Intelligence, Schwabmünchen, Germany). This system secures the head using a mouthpiece containing a custom impression of the maxillary teeth and palate. Proper fit is ensured by attainment of a vacuum seal between the mouthpiece and the palate (Figure 26.1-1).

A planning CT scan (Lightspeed QX/I, GE Medical Systems, Waukasha, WI) of the orbits with 3 cm margins inferiorly and superiorly was obtained, with the patient in his head positioning apparatus. A slice thickness of 1.25 mm was used throughout the scan. A 10 mm thick tissue-equivalent bolus was placed over each orbit during the planning CT scan (and every treatment). It should be noted that we currently make a custom bolus for our retinoblastoma cases to better match the patient's periorbital skin contour (see Case 2).

Target and Tissue Delineation

Two gross tumor volumes (GTVs) were delineated. GTV_1 consisted of the entire right globe, whereas GTV_2 consisted of the left retina. The left lens was not included in the target volume because there had never been evidence of vitreous

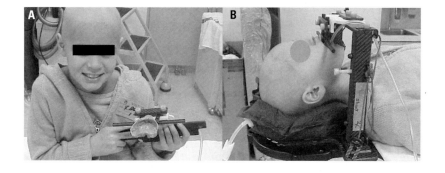

FIGURE 26.1-1. (*A*) A patient with retinoblastoma holding his custom mouthpiece. (*B*) The patient in the HeadFix immobilization system with the mouthpiece inserted and in the custom headrest. (To view a color version of this image, please refer to the CD-ROM.)

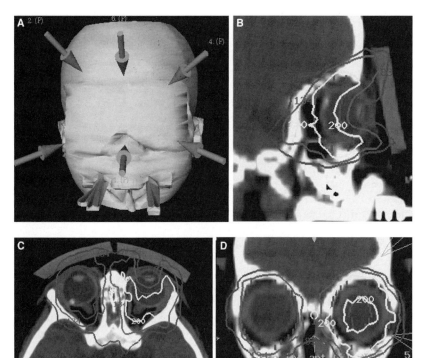

FIGURE 26.1-2. Case 1. (*A*) Three-dimensional reconstruction of the child's head, showing the custom mouthpiece, bolus over the orbits, and entry directions of the six treatment beams. (*B*) Sagittal computed tomography (CT) slice showing isodose distribution through the left orbit with sparing of the left lens. (*C*) Axial CT slice with bolus overlying the orbits, showing isodose distribution through both orbits. (*D*) Coronal CT slice showing isodose distribution through both orbits. The planning target volumes are outlined in blue, the 200 cGy isodose line (corresponding to a cumulative dose of 3,600 cGy) is yellow, the 134 cGy isodose line (corresponding to a cumulative dose of 2,400 cGy) is green, and the 83 cGy isodose line (corresponding to a cumulative dose of 1,500 cGy) is purple. (To view a color version of this image, please refer to the CD-ROM.)

involvement in the left eye. The left lens with a 3 mm margin was the sole organ at risk (OAR). GTV_1, GTV_2, and the left lens were contoured manually on each axial CT slice on which they were present. No clinical target volume (CTV) was specified in this case separately. Two planning target volumes (PTVs) were generated, each consisting of one GTV plus a 2 mm margin, as shown in Figure 26.1-2.

Treatment Planning

IMRT planning was performed using the *Plato* Inverse Treatment Planning software, version 1.0, and *Plato* Radiation Treatment Planning System software, version 2.4, modules (Nucletron BV, Veenendaal, the Netherlands).

The two PTVs were planned to receive different daily doses. PTV_2, which contained progressive disease, received 36 Gy in 2 Gy daily fractions. The dose to the left lens was to be minimized, with the provision that the dose to the left retina plus a 2 mm margin would not be compromised. The entire right globe was included in PTV_1 because disease seeded its corpus vitreum at presentation. The planned dose to the right globe, 24 Gy given in 133.3 cGy daily fractions, was less than that to the left retina because there was no active disease in the right eye. The input parameters used in this patient are listed in Table 26.1-1.

Six noncoplanar beam angles, all from anterior to the patient, were selected to deliver the IMRT plan. The six anteriorly oriented beam angles were inferior sagittal (couch angle 90°, gantry angle 169°), superior sagittal (couch 90°, gantry 220°), right inferior oblique (couch 193°, gantry 232°),

right superior oblique (couch 130°, gantry 235°), left inferior oblique (couch 166°, gantry 135°), and left superior oblique (couch 220°, gantry 130°). The beams were 3.0 to 3.5 cm long at 100 cm source-axis distance (SAD). We currently treat our retinoblastoma cases with eight noncoplanar beams to achieve a better dose distribution (see case 2).

One hundred fifty beam segments were used. The beamlets were 5.0 × 2.5 mm. The photon energy of each beam was 6 MV. The resultant isodose distributions overlaid on axial and coronal CT slices through the middle of both orbits and a sagittal CT slice through the middle of each orbit are shown in Figure 26.1-2. The final plan gave a minimum of 100% of the prescribed dose to 99% of the right orbit PTV and a minimum of 95% of the prescribed dose to 96% of the left retina PTV. The dose-volume histograms of the PTVs and left lens are shown in Figure 26.1-3.

TABLE 26.1-1. Input Parameters, Case 1: Treatment of Both Eyes

Organ	Maximum Dose, Gy	Weight, %	Minimum Dose, Gy	Weight, %
PTV right orbit	35	80	24	80
PTV left retina	37	100	36	100
Left lens	16	60	—	—
Body	28	40	—	—

PTV = planning target volume. Body refers to all tissues inside the skin surface that were not contoured as gross tumor volume, planning target volume, or an organ at risk.

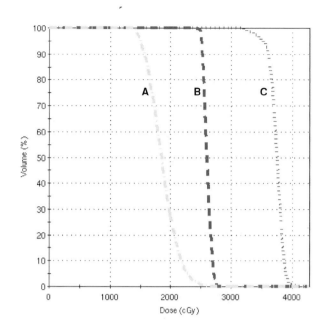

FIGURE 26.1-3. Case 1. Cumulative dose-volume histogram of the planning target volumes (PTV) and the left lens (organ at risk). Lens (*A*), PTV right orbit (*B*), PTV left retinal (*C*). (To view a color version of this image, please refer to the CD-ROM.)

Treatment Delivery and Quality Assurance

The dose calculations from the *Plato* treatment planning software were verified by both ionization chamber and film measurements prior to delivery of the first treatment. The IMRT plan was applied to a 30 × 30 × 10 cm phantom with the isocenter in the center of the phantom. The ionization chamber air volume (0.6 cc chamber) was contoured into the center of the phantom, permitting calculation of the mean dose in the air volume. The three-dimensional dose grid was calculated by the *Plato* treatment planning software and stored as a single file. The file was transferred to *RIT* (Radiological Imaging Technology, Colorado Springs, CO) film dosimetry software to permit extraction of isodoses in a coronal plane 1 cm anterior to the isocenter.

The plan was transferred to a Varian linear accelerator (Varian Medical Systems, Palo Alto, CA), and a 30 × 30 × 10 cm solid water phantom was positioned on the treatment couch such that the center of the phantom was at the gantry isocenter. A 0.6 cc ionization chamber was placed in the center of the phantom, and a film (EDR2, Eastman Kodak, Rochester, NY) was placed in the same coronal plane as was calculated by the treatment planning software. The phantom (with chamber and film) was given a mock IMRT treatment, delivering the exact beams and monitor of units of the patient's plan. The charge recorded by the electrometer was converted into dose and compared with that calculated by the planning system. The allowed difference was 3%. A calibration film was processed along with the EDR2

film. Both films were scanned by a Vidar 16-bit Dosimetry Pro scanner (Vidar Systems Corporation, Herndon, VA), and scanner units were converted to dose using the calibration film. The EDR2 film and the *Plato* coronal plane dose patterns were then registered and digitally overlaid using the *RIT* software. Visual and analytic comparisons were made for doses above 20% of the isocenter dose. The tolerance for agreement in the high dose gradient areas was 3 mm and in the high dose/low gradient areas was 3%.

In addition to dual verification of the dose calculations, multiple system-wide quality assurance tests were conducted. The performance of the multileaf collimator was checked daily by measuring the dose delivered to the central channel of a Keithley Tracker (Keithley Instruments, Inc, Cleveland, OH) irradiated by a standard dynamic plan. A film consisting of a composite of two complex patterns, the first of which is the negative of the second, was taken once weekly. The appropriate result is a series of uniformly dark bars separated by unexposed bars. If any result was found to be outside tolerance limits, the error would be located and corrected.

Treatment was delivered on a Varian 2100C linear accelerator equipped with the integrated Millennium 120-leaf collimator (Varian Medical Systems) in the "step-and-shoot" mode. Orthogonal anterior-posterior and left lateral digital images of the treated region were taken on the first day of treatment and at least once weekly throughout the treatment course. These images were compared with digitally reconstructed radiographs of the same projections made from the treatment planning CT scan. The field position was adjusted if there was a 2 mm or greater disparity in the anterior-posterior, superior-inferior, or medial-lateral direction between the digital Portal Vision (Varian Medical Systems) images and the digitally reconstructed radiographs.

Clinical Outcome

The patient was last examined at age 3.8 years, 2.2 years following IMRT. He had age-appropriate behavior, neurocognitive function, and facial development without orbital hypoplasia. No additional chemotherapy or local control measure (radioactive plaque, laser, or cryotherapy) has been administered. There had been no evidence of active disease in either globe, as determined by periodic examinations under anesthesia. Visual acuity has been difficult to measure because of the patient's young age. However, he fixes and follows objects with his left eye better than his right eye and does not require corrective lenses. No retinopathy, keratitis, or other complications have been detected.

Case 2: Treatment of One Eye
Patient History

A 12-month-old boy was noted to have a white pupillary reflex in both eyes by his pediatrician. Examination under anesthesia revealed subretinal seeds with retinal detachment and small vitreous seeds (group D retinoblastoma) in the right eye and several large retinal tumors without vitreous seeding (group C retinoblastoma) in the left eye. There was no evidence of disease outside the globes on head CT scan, in the cerebrospinal fluid, or in the bone marrow.

The patient was treated with laser photoablation, cryotherapy, and six cycles of intravenous carboplatin, etoposide, and vincristine chemotherapy, with carboplatin administered subconjunctivally during the first three cycles.

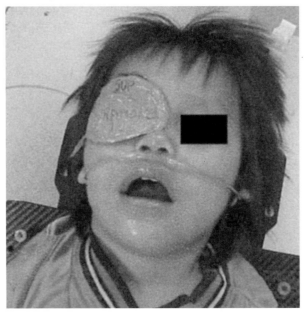

FIGURE 26.1-4. Case 2. Custom bolus material covering the treated orbit. (To view a color version of this image, please refer to the CD-ROM.)

Multiple recurrences of retinal tumors in the right eye were treated with laser photoablation. The left eye remained continuously free of active disease following regression of its retinal tumors during chemotherapy. When recurrence of vitreous seeding was found in the right eye, the patient was referred for irradiation of the entire right globe. As in the previous case, IMRT was used to maximize sparing of the surrounding normal tissues.

Simulation

The simulation parameters were the same as described in the case above, except that a custom 5 to 7 mm–thick bolus (effective thickness 8–11 mm) was created to match the contour of the patient's right periorbital skin surface (Figure 26.1-4). The bolus was made using Correct VPS (Jeneric/Pentron, Inc., Wallingford, CT), the heavy-viscosity vinyl polysiloxane impression material used to form the dental impression in the patient's HeadFix immobilization system. A custom bolus is currently used for all of our IMRT retinoblastoma cases, rather than standard bolus material, because it results in less of an air gap between the bolus and the patient's periorbital skin surface.

Target and Tissue Delineation

The GTV consisted of the entire right globe because there was active disease in both the corpus vitreum and the retina. The right globe was contoured manually on each axial CT slice on which it was present. No other organs were contoured. As in the above case, a CTV was not delineated separately. The PTV in this case consisted of the GTV plus a 3 mm margin (Figure 26.1-5).

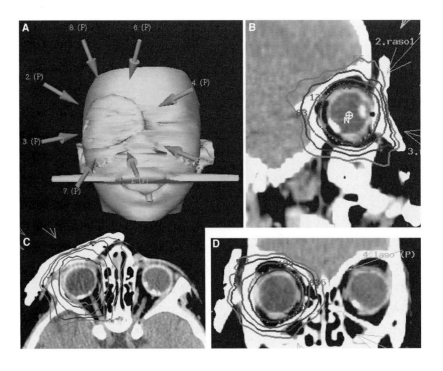

FIGURE 26.1-5. Case 2. (*A*) Three-dimensional reconstruction of the child's head, showing the custom mouthpiece, custom bolus over the right orbit, and entry directions of the eight treatment beams. (*B*) Sagittal computed tomography (CT) slice showing isodose distribution surrounding the right orbit. (*C*) Axial CT slice with bolus overlying the right orbit, showing isodose distribution surrounding the orbit. (*D*) Coronal CT slice showing isodose distribution surrounding the right orbit. The planning target volume is outlined in red, the 200 cGy isodose line (corresponding to a cumulative dose of 3,600 cGy) is purple, the 134 cGy isodose line (corresponding to a cumulative dose of 2,400 cGy) is green, the 83 cGy isodose line (corresponding to a cumulative dose of 1,500 cGy) is blue, and the 55 cGy isodose line (corresponding to a cumulative dose of 1,000 cGy) is brown. (To view a color version of this image, please refer to the CD-ROM.)

TABLE 26.1-2. Input Parameters, Case 2: Treatment of One Eye

Organ	Maximum Dose, Gy	Weight, %	Minimum Dose, Gy	Weight, %
Planning target volume	37	50	36	100
Body	18	20	—	—

Body refers to all tissues inside the skin surface that were not contoured as gross tumor volume or planning target volume.

Treatment Planning

The IMRT plan was generated using the *Plato* Inverse Treatment Planning software, version 1.0, and *Plato* Radiation Treatment Planning System software, version 2.5.1, modules.

The PTV was planned to receive a dose of 36 Gy given in 2 Gy daily fractions. The input parameters used in this case are listed in Table 26.1-2. Eight noncoplanar beam angles, all anterior to the patient, were selected to deliver IMRT. There were two right superior oblique beams (couch angle 150°, gantry angle 245°, and couch angle 110°, gantry angle 240°), two right inferior oblique beams (couch 193°, gantry 232° and couch 240°, gantry 220°), two left superior oblique beams (couch 200°, gantry 130° and couch 250°, gantry 130°), and two left inferior oblique beams (couch 115°, gantry 148° and couch 155°, gantry 135°). The beams were 3.0 to 3.5 cm long at 100 cm SAD. Ninety-seven beam segments were used. The beamlets were 5.0 × 2.5 mm. The photon energy of each beam was 6 MV. The resultant isodose distributions overlaid on axial, sagittal, and coronal CT slices through the middle of the orbit are shown in Figure 26.1-5. The final plan gave a minimum of 95% of the prescribed dose to 95% of the PTV. The dose-volume histogram of the PTV is shown in Figure 26.1-6.

Treatment Delivery and Quality Assurance

The treatment delivery parameters were the same as described above for case 1. Treatment was also delivered on a Varian 2100C linear accelerator equipped with the integrated Millennium 120-leaf collimator in the step-and-

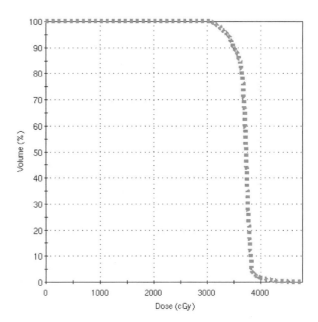

FIGURE 26.1-6. Case 2. Cumulative dose-volume histogram of the right globe planning target volume.

shoot mode. Quality assurance procedures performed at our institution in our patients with retinoblastoma were described in the previous case.

Clinical Outcome

The patient was last examined at age 2.8 years, 8 months following IMRT. At that time, he had age-appropriate behavior, neurocognitive function, and facial development without orbital hypoplasia. No chemotherapy or local control measure (radioactive plaque, laser, or cryotherapy) has been administered. There has been no evidence of active retinoblastoma in either globe since the completion of IMRT, as determined by periodic examinations under anesthesia. Visual acuity has been difficult to measure because of the patient's young age. The patient fixes and follows objects with both eyes well. No retinopathy, keratitis, or other complications have been detected.

Chapter 26.2

NEUROBLASTOMA

CASE STUDY

ROBERT S. LAVEY, MD, MPH, ARTHUR J. OLCH, PhD

Patient History

A 4-year-old boy presented with a 1-month history of progressive fatigue, anorexia, weight loss, pallor, and intermittent abdominal pain. A computed tomography (CT) scan demonstrated a 10 × 9 × 9 cm heterogeneous, moderately enhancing, lobulated retroperitoneal mass encasing the aorta and inferior vena cava and extending from the level of the T9 to the L5 vertebral body. A 1 × 1 × 3 cm left paraspinous mass was also noted at the level of the T4 and T5 vertebral bodies, consistent with neuroblastoma. Laboratory tests revealed significant anemia and elevated serum homovanillic acid and vanillylmandelic acid levels. Metastatic workup included a bone scan and ^{123}I-metaiodobenzylguanidine (MIBG) scan, both of which showed widely disseminated bone metastases. Bone marrow biopsy confirmed the diagnosis of neuroblastoma.

The patient was enrolled in the Children's Oncology Group (COG) protocol A3973 for high-risk neuroblastoma and received six cycles of induction chemotherapy, including cyclophosphamide, doxorubicin, and vincristine in cycles 1, 2, 4, and 6 and cisplatin and etoposide in cycles 3 and 5. A repeat CT scan following the fourth cycle of chemotherapy showed resolution of the left paraspinous mass and a decrease in size of the retroperitoneal mass to 4 × 4 × 6 cm with calcific areas.

The abdominal tumor was subtotally resected following the fifth cycle of chemotherapy, with residual unresectable disease in the porta hepatis. A postoperative CT scan showed a residual tumor mass 3.5 × 3 × 2 cm in the porta hepatis region. Repeat ^{123}I-MIBG scanning demonstrated resolution of all metastatic sites but persistence of increased uptake in the right upper quadrant. Following consolidation myeloablative chemotherapy (melphalan, etoposide, and carboplatin) with autologous stem cell rescue, the patient was referred for radiation therapy (RT) of the preoperative retroperitoneal tumor volume per the guidelines of the COG high-risk neuroblastoma protocol. In an effort to spare the surrounding normal tissues, intensity-modulated radiation therapy (IMRT) was used in this patient.

Simulation

The patient was sedated during simulation (and daily RT) using intravenous continuous-infusion propofol because of his young age. His trunk and lower extremities were positioned in the BodyFix cushion, a custom-molded, bead-filled, evacuated vinyl bag (Medical Intelligence, Schwabmünchen, Germany) shown in Figure 26.2-1. Marks were drawn on the patient and the bag for reproducibility of positioning. A planning CT scan (Lightspeed QX/I, GE Medical Systems, Waukasha, WI) of the abdomen was obtained with the patient in the BodyFix using a slice separation and thickness of 2.5 mm.

Target and Tissue Delineation

The gross tumor volume (GTV) consisted of the primary tumor volume (visualized on the CT scan done between the fourth cycle of chemotherapy and partial resection). The planning target volume (PTV) consisted of the GTV plus a 5 mm margin. Organs at risk (OAR) delineated in this patient included the kidneys, liver, and vertebral bodies. The GTV and OAR were contoured manually on each axial CT slice. The PTV was generated from the GTV by the treatment planning software and was altered manually to give a 2 mm rather than a 5 mm margin on the kidneys and vertebral bodies. A three-dimensional reconstruction of the GTV and PTV is shown in Figure 26.2-2A and outlines of the PTV in the sagittal, axial, and coronal planes are given in Figure 26.2-2B–D.

Treatment Planning

The IMRT plan was generated using the *Plato* Inverse Treatment Planning software, version 1.1, and *Plato* Radiation Treatment Planning System software, version 2.6, modules (Nucletron BV, Veenendaal, the Netherlands). The input parameters for the PTV were weighted maximum and minimum doses. The liver and nonspecified tissues (body) had input parameters that were weighted maximum doses (Tables 26.2-1 and 26.2-2). For the kidneys and vertebrae, desired

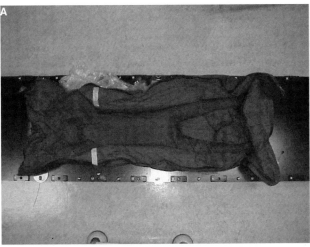 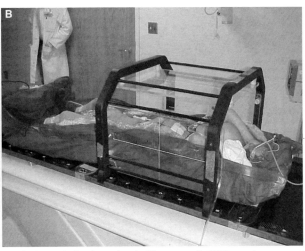

FIGURE 26.2-1. (*A*) The custom-molded BodyFix positioning and immobilization device made for the patient in this case study. (*B*) The patient secured in his BodyFix on the computed tomography scan platform with the target localizer box mounted for positioning the couch. The target localizer box was removed prior to treatment daily. (To view a color version of this image, please refer to the CD-ROM.)

dose-volume histograms were constructed by inputting six dose-volume points into the planning software. The PTV was planned to receive a cumulative dose of 2,160 cGy given in 12 equal daily fractions of 180 cGy.

Eight coplanar beams, all with a couch angle of 180°, were selected to deliver the IMRT plan. The beam angles were chosen to avoid the passage of any entry beam through the couch rails. The gantry angles for beam delivery were 35, 85, 125, 165, 200, 240, 275, and 325 degrees. The beams were 16.5 to 17.0 cm long at 100 cm source-axis distance. One hundred seventeen beam segments were used. The beamlets were 5 × 5 mm. The photon energy of each beam was 6 MV. The resultant isodose distributions overlaid on sagittal, axial, and coronal CT slices are shown in Figure 26.2-2. The final plan gave a minimum of 100% of the prescribed dose to 95% of the PTV. The dose-volume histograms of the PTV and OAR are shown in Figure 26.2-3.

Treatment Delivery and Quality Assurance

The dose calculations from the *Plato* treatment planning software were verified by both ionization chamber and film measurements prior to delivery of the first treatment. The IMRT plan was applied to a 30 × 30 × 10 cm phantom with the isocenter in the center of the phantom. The ionization chamber air volume (0.6 cc chamber) was contoured into the center of the phantom, permitting calculation of the mean dose in the air volume. The three-dimensional dose grid was calculated by the *Plato* treatment planning software and stored as a single file. The file was transferred to *RIT* (Radiological Imaging Technology, Colorado Springs, CO) film dosimetry software to permit extraction of isodoses in a coronal plane 1 cm anterior to the isocenter.

The plan was transferred to a Varian linear accelerator (Varian Medical Systems, Palo Alto, CA), and a 30 × 30 × 10 cm solid water phantom was positioned on the treatment couch such that the center of the phantom was at the gantry isocenter. A 0.6 cc ionization chamber was placed in the center of the phantom, and a film (EDR2, Eastman Kodak, Rochester, NY) was placed in the same coronal plane as was calculated by the treatment planning software. The phantom (with chamber and film) was given a mock IMRT treatment, delivering the exact beams and monitor of units of the patient's plan. The charge recorded by the electrometer was converted into dose and compared with that calculated by the planning system. The allowed difference was 3%. A calibration film was processed along with the EDR2 film. Both films were scanned by a Vidar 16-bit Dosimetry Pro scanner (Vidar Systems Corporation, Herndon, VA), and scanner units were converted to dose using the calibration film. The EDR2 film and the *Plato* coronal plane dose patterns were then registered and digitally overlaid using the *RIT* software. Visual and analytic comparisons were made for doses above 20% of the isocenter dose. The tolerance for agreement in the high dose gradient areas was 3 mm and in the high dose/low gradient areas was 3%.

In addition to dual verification of the dose calculations, multiple system-wide quality assurance tests were conducted. The performance of the multileaf collimator was checked daily by measuring the dose delivered to the central channel of a Keithley Tracker (Keithley Instruments, Inc, Cleveland, OH) irradiated by a standard dynamic plan. A film consisting of a composite of two complex patterns, the first of which is the negative of the second, was taken once weekly. The appropriate result is a series of uniformly dark bars separated by unexposed bars. If any result was

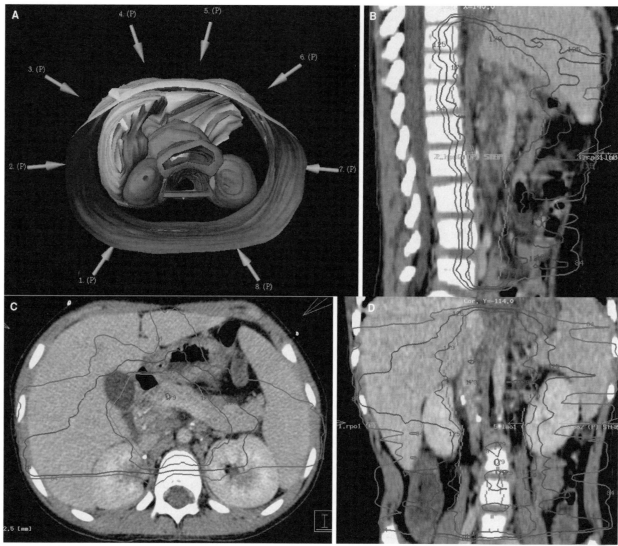

FIGURE 26.2-2. (*A*) Three-dimensional reconstruction of the child's abdomen, showing the gross tumor volume in blue, planning target volume (PTV) in red, vertebral bodies in purple, kidneys in green, liver in yellow, and entry directions of the eight treatment beams. (*B*) to (*D*) Computed tomography (CT) slices (*B*) sagittal; (*C*) axial; (*D*) coronal) showing isodose distribution in the abdomen. The PTV is outlined in red, the 180 cGy isodose line (corresponding to a cumulative dose of 2,160 cGy) is green, the 125 cGy isodose line (corresponding to a cumulative dose of 1,500 cGy) is green, and the 84 cGy isodose line (corresponding to a cumulative dose of 1,000 cGy) is blue. (To view a color version of this image, please refer to the CD-ROM.)

TABLE 26.2-1. Input Parameters: Specified Doses and Weighting for the Planning Target Volume, Body, and Liver*

Organ	Maximum Dose, Gy	Weight, %	Minimum Dose, Gy	Weight, %
Planning target volume	22	50	21.6	100
Body	15	25	—	—
Liver	15	50	—	—

*All tissues inside the skin surface that were not contoured as gross tumor volume, planning target volume, or an organ at risk.

TABLE 26.2-2. Input Parameters: Weighting and Dose-Volume Points for the Kidneys and Vertebral Bodies

Organ	Weight, %	Gy/%V	Gy/%V	Gy/%V	Gy/%V	Gy/%V	Gy/%V
Kidneys	80	4/100	5/75	11/27	15/14	19/3	20/0
Vertebrae	20	3/100	8/34	10/14	17/10	20/7	23/0

%V indicates the maximum percent volume of the organ at risk that is permitted to receive the specified dose.

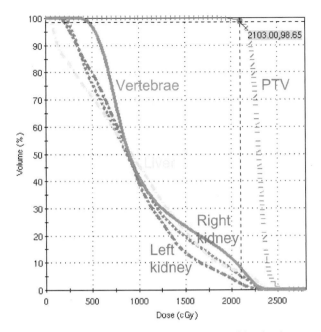

FIGURE 26.2-3. Cumulative dose-volume histogram of the planning target volume (PTV) and the specified organ at risk (liver, kidneys, and vertebral bodies).

found to be outside tolerance limits, the error would be located and corrected.

Treatment was delivered on a Varian 2100C linear accelerator equipped with the integrated Millennium 120-leaf collimator (Varian Medical Systems) in the "step-and-shoot" mode. Orthogonal anterior-posterior and left lateral digital images of the treated region were taken on the first day of treatment and at least once weekly throughout the treatment course. These images were compared with digitally reconstructed radiographs of the same projections made from the treatment planning CT scan. The field position was adjusted if there was a 2 mm or greater disparity in the anterior-posterior, superior-inferior, or medial-lateral direction between the digital Portal Vision (Varian Medical Systems) images and the digitally reconstructed radiographs.

Clinical Outcome

The patient tolerated IMRT well, without experiencing nausea or fatigue. He has been taking 13-*cis*–retinoic acid orally as maintenance therapy per protocol guidelines since the completion of IMRT. Body CT and ^{123}I-MIBG scans obtained at 4 months following IMRT showed no evidence of residual or recurrent disease. He was last examined at age 5.5 years, 6 months following completion of IMRT. At that time, he remained asymptomatic with normal diet, behavior, and physical activity.

Chapter 26.3

RHABDOMYOSARCOMA

CASE STUDY

JOSEPH K. SALAMA, MD, PHILIP P. CONNELL, MD

Patient History

A newborn boy's mother palpated a 3 mm nodule on his right leg after an uneventful pregnancy and a normal spontaneous vaginal delivery. By 1 month of age, the lesion had grown to 2 × 4 cm in size. When brought to the attention of the family's primary care physician, it was described as a well-circumscribed, raised, mobile lesion on the lateral aspect of the right leg, midway between the knee and the ankle. Presumed to be a benign cyst, the mass was excised at 2 months of age.

Surprisingly, pathology revealed a small round blue cell tumor. Immunohistochemistry staining was strongly positive for myogenin, muscle-specific actin, and desmin, supporting the diagnosis of rhabdomyosarcoma. CD45, CD43, CD99, and FLI-1 were negative, making the diagnoses of lymphoid malignancy and Ewing's sarcoma unlikely. Cytogenetic studies were negative for t(2;13), but positive for t(1;13), consistent with alveolar rhabdomyosarcoma. Microscopic malignant foci invaded the lateral and deep margins.

Because subcutaneous rhabdomyosarcoma is a rare diagnosis, the patient was evaluated for an alternative primary disease site. However, infused computed tomography (CT) of the chest, abdomen, and pelvis; bone scan; and magnetic resonance imaging (MRI) of the brain revealed no evidence of disease. A bone marrow biopsy and aspirate were negative. A T_2-weighted MRI of the right lower extremity demonstrated increased signal within the subcutaneous fat adjacent to the extensor halucis longus tendon, consistent with residual tumor.

The patient was classified as having a group II, stage II rhabdomyosarcoma. He was treated with induction vincristine, actinomycin D, and cyclophosphamide (VAC) chemotherapy. At the completion of induction chemotherapy, the patient was deemed a candidate for

a radical re-resection. The remaining skin and subcutaneous tissues surrounding the prior surgical cavity were removed, and a skin graft was placed. Pathologic evaluation revealed microscopic foci of residual alveolar rhabdomyosarcoma with negative surgical margins.

For this clinical situation, Intergroup Rhabdomyosarcoma Study V (IRS-V) mandates local radiation therapy (RT) of the tumor bed (36 Gy) with concurrent vincristine and cyclophosphamide, followed by 24 weeks of VAC. RT was particularly challenging in this patient because the target volume wrapped around approximately one-third of the limb's circumference. This made an electron-based plan difficult, and a photon-based approach with opposed oblique fields would expose the underlying bones to high doses. Therefore, an intensity-modulated radiation therapy (IMRT) approach was developed to cover this challenging target while minimizing the dose to the underlying bones and epiphyseal growth plates.

Simulation

Given the patient's young age, the patient was simulated under general endotracheal anesthesia. He was positioned supine with his legs spread apart. A custom body immobilization device (Alpha Cradle, Smithers Medical Products, Inc., Hudson, OH) was fabricated to ensure reproducible daily setup. The proximal and distal ends of the surgical scar were demarcated with metallic makers to aid in target volume definition. Axial CT slices from the mid-femur to past the foot were acquired with 3 mm spacing using a Marconi AcQSim scanner (Philips Medical Systems, Andover, MA). Intravenous contrast infusion was deemed unnecessary because there was no gross tumor and there was no plan to treat the draining lymph nodes.

Target and Tissue Delineation

IRS-V guidelines define the presurgical extent of disease as the gross tumor volume (GTV). The clinical target volume

---

Editor's Note: This is not an actual case but is based on a patient with a similar clinical situation. This chapter demonstrates how one might approach the challenge of treating an infant with an extremity soft tissue sarcoma.

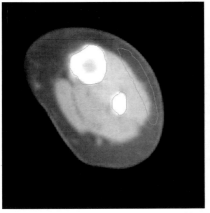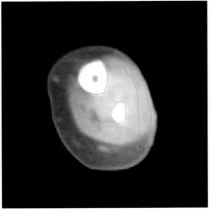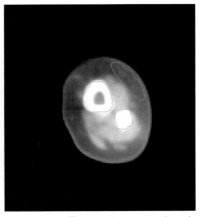

FIGURE 26.3-1. Contoured target and avoidance structures overlaid on the planning computed tomography scan. The planning target volume is shown in orange, and the tibia and fibula are blue. (To view a color version of this image, please refer to the CD-ROM.)

(CTV) for extremity tumors requires a 2 cm volumetric expansion of the GTV. Subsequently, the CTV is expanded by an "institution-specific" margin, accounting for patient motion and daily setup error. The protocol emphasizes the discretion of the radiation oncologist to avoid treatment across a joint, circumferential limb irradiation, and treatment of a volume outside the patient.

The target and normal tissues were delineated on a VoxelQ workstation (Philips Medical Systems). For this case, the postsurgical T2-weighted MRI was referenced while contouring the surgical bed. CT-MRI fusion is routinely used at our institution to assist in accurate contouring of treatment volumes. In this case, it was not because positional differences between the MRI and CT simulation left too few anatomic landmarks to serve as surrogate fiducial markers. Furthermore, no radiologic studies had been performed prior to the initial surgery. Definition of the tumor bed was also complicated by age-appropriate growth between the initial MRI (obtained at 3 months of age) and the imaging obtained 3 months later (after chemotherapy and second surgery). Given these limitations, the CTV was defined as the resection cavity (now covered with a skin graft) and a rim of the underlying muscular compartment. This volume was expanded by 0.5 cm to generate the planning target volume (PTV). Figure 26.3-1 illustrates volumes contoured on representative slices of the planning CT in this patient.

The deleterious effects of RT on growing bones are well known. Radiation doses as low as 2 to 20 Gy can inhibit proliferation of cartilage cells, disrupting normal growth at the epiphyseal plate and arresting chondrogenesis. Within a given bone, known growth rates can be used to predict the magnitude of RT-induced growth disturbances. The tibia, for example, grows 60% from the proximal epiphysis and 40% from the distal epiphysis. Therefore, generous avoidance structures were contoured in this patient for each epiphyseal plate of the tibia and fibula. Irradiation is also known to inhibit the absorption of bone and cartilage in

the metaphysis, alter periosteal physiology, and hinder normal bone remodeling in the diaphysis.[1] To reduce the probability of these events occurring in this child, the entire tibia and fibula were entered as avoidance structures. A three-dimensional representation of the PTV and all avoidance structures are shown in Figure 26.3-2.

Treatment Planning

The *CORVUS* software package, version 5.0 (North American Scientific, NOMOS Radiation Oncology Division,

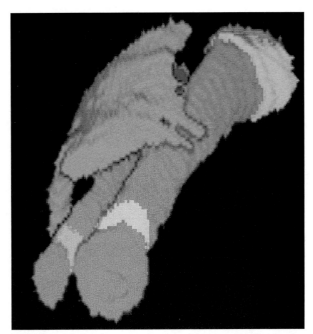

FIGURE 26.3-2. Inferior to superior view of the lower leg. The planning target volume is orange, and the tibia and fibula are blue. Generous avoidance structures representing the epiphyseal plates of the tibia and fibula are displayed as green, yellow, brown, and purple structures at either end of the bones. (To view a color version of this image, please refer to the CD-ROM.)

Cranberry Township, PA), was used for inverse treatment planning. The input parameters for this case are summarized in Table 26.3-1. An additional sparing structure was generated to further promote conformity of treatment. Given that several of the epiphyseal plates were located outside the treatment fields, they were included in the prescription only as reference structures (not shown in Table 26.3-1), whereby the planning system does not attempt to optimize the dose to these structures.

It should be noted that *CORVUS* generally places the isocenter at the geometric center of the treatment volume. In this case, owing to the curvature of the PTV, the isocenter was placed at its edge. We selected seven coplanar beams with uniformly spaced gantry angles (0, 51, 103, 154, 206, 257, and 308 degrees). The seven beams required 188 segments and 722 monitor units to deliver each 1.8 Gy fraction. Six-megavolt photons were used for this plan.

The 95% isodose surface (34.2 Gy) covered 99% of the PTV. The majority of the PTV (95%) received the 36 Gy prescription dose. Although this plan was highly conformal, the small size of the infant's anatomy resulted in considerable dose inhomogeneity. However, these hot spots were located within the target volume, and only 0.74 cc of the PTV volume received > 20% (43.2 Gy) of

the prescription dose. Dose-volume histograms of the target and critical structures are displayed in Figure 26.3-3. Isodose curves in representative axial planes are shown in Figure 26.3-4. These illustrate dose sparing around the tibia and the fibula while conforming to the semi-lunar-shaped target.

TABLE 26.3-1. Input Parameters

	CORVUS 5.0 Prescription				
Target	Goal, Gy	Volume below Goal, %	Minimum, Gy	Maximum, Gy	Target Type
Planning target volume	34.2	1	32.5	36.5	Basic

Structure	Limit, Gy	Volume above Limit, %	Minimum, Gy	Maximum, Gy	Structure Type
Tissue	13.9	35	1.0	32.5	Basic
Tibia and fibula	6.7	10	2.9	32.5	Basic
Fibula distal epiphyseal	1.7	3	0.7	32.5	Basic
Sparing structure	30.0	0	4.8	32.5	Critical

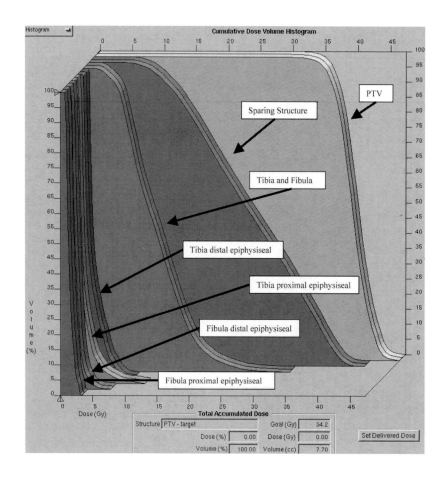

FIGURE 26.3-3. Dose-volume histograms of the planning target volume (PTV) and surrounding normal structures for this patient. (To view a color version of this image, please refer to the CD-ROM.)

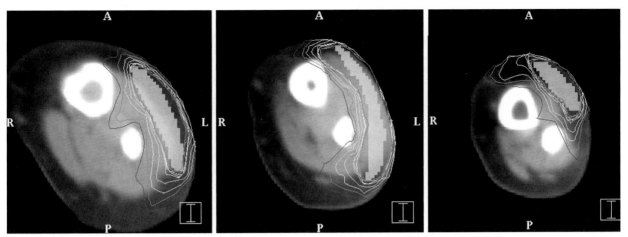

FIGURE 26.3-4. Isodose curves overlaid on axial computed tomography slices of the planned patient. The planning target volume (PTV) is shaded in green. Note the conformity of the high-dose lines to the shape of the PTV and the subsequent sparing of the tibia and fibula. (To view a color version of this image, please refer to the CD-ROM.)

Treatment Delivery and Quality Assurance

Daily treatments were performed under general anesthesia. Treatments were conducted in the early morning when the clinic schedule was relatively light to ensure adequate time to induce anesthesia, properly position the patient, and reverse anesthesia. The patient was set up with his feet toward the gantry. A Millennium 120-leaf multileaf collimator on a CL 2100 C/D (Varian Medical Systems, Palo Alto, CA) was used to deliver the treatments. The fields were treated sequentially in a clockwise direction starting at 206°.

Careful quality assurance was performed prior to the first treatment. A monitor unit verification calculation (*RadCalc*, Version 4.3, Lifeline Software, Inc., Tyler, TX) was used to verify the dose delivered to the isocenter. Previous investigations from our institution have demonstrated that the average discrepancy between *RadCalc* and *CORVUS* is +1.4% with a 1.2% SD.[2] Based on this work, our departmental standard requires a +4%, −2% agreement between *RadCalc* and *CORVUS*. Disparities outside this range are checked and resolved prior to treatment. On this particular plan, a −4.7% dose discrepancy between *RadCalc* and *CORVUS* was noted at the isocenter. Given that this type of error can occur in regions with a steep dose gradient, a point 9 mm off-axis (within a low dose gradient) was chosen, and the calculation was repeated. The subsequent disparity between the two systems was +1.9%.

In addition, a phantom plan was generated using the fluence maps for this patient. A cylindrical acrylic phantom (diameter 9 cm, mass density 1.18 g/cm³, effective density to water 1.15) was used to represent the shape of the limb treated. The phantom was scanned and irradiated with a 0.1 cm³ ion chamber (PTW, Nuclear Associates, Hicksville, NY) in

place. A dose of 196 cGy, in acrylic, was measured with the ion chamber. The dose to water was 202 cGy, based on the appropriate correction factors. The calculated dose to the ion chamber (based on water equivalence) was 195 cGy (SD = 16 cGy), agreeing within 3.7% of the measurement. The axial dose distributions of the phantom quality assurance plan are shown in Figure 26.3-5. Because of the relatively large standard deviation in the ion chamber dose, this discrepancy was considered acceptable to proceed with treatment.

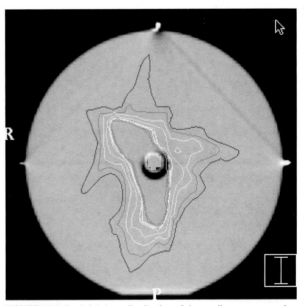

FIGURE 26.3-5. Axial dose distribution of the quality assurance plan overlaid on a CT slice of the acrylic phantom. The green shaded area is the ion chamber. The phantom was accurately positioned on the treatment table using metallic markers on the surface. (To view a color version of this image, please refer to the CD-ROM.)

Outcome

This case demonstrates how IMRT can be effectively used to treat a limb while sparing nearby critical structures. Every attempt should be made to avoid the devastating consequences that asymmetric limb growth can have on a child. The plan presented here exhibits the capability of IMRT to conformally irradiate targets with challenging shapes and locations. Although not specifically demonstrated in this plan, sparing dose to the long bones results in a reduced volume of irradiated bone marrow. Theoretically, this may decrease the severity of hematologic toxicity and may reduce the incidence of leukemic second malignancies attributable to concurrent chemotherapy and radiotherapy.

For this particular patient, brachytherapy could have been an alternative method to deliver conformal therapy while sparing nearby structures. However, implantation of radioactive sources in a child has its own set of challenges. Patient cooperation is key to the success of brachytherapy. This infant could not have been left alone with radioactive sources in place, so exposure of caretakers would be an important concern. Furthermore, the inhomogeneity of brachytherapy would almost certainly be greater than the IMRT plan described here.

References

1. Halperin E, Constine L, Tarbell N, et al. Pediatric radiation oncology. 3rd ed. Philadelphia: Lippincott Williams & Wilkins; 1999.
2. Haslam JJ, Bonta DV, Lujan AE, et al. Comparison of dose calculated by an intensity modulated radiotherapy treatment planning system and an independent monitor unit verification program. J Appl Clin Med Phys 2003;4:224–30.

Chapter 27

METASTATIC AND RECURRENT TUMORS OVERVIEW

JOHNNY KAO, MD, ARNO J. MUNDT, MD

Radiation therapy (RT) occupies an important role in the treatment of cancer patients with metastastic and recurrent disease.[1] Palliative RT is commonly used in patients with metastatic disease to the bone, brain, and visceral sites.[2–4] Palliative RT is also administered to the primary tumor when cure is no longer possible.[4] Moreover, radiation oncologists are often called on to reirradiate primary and metastatic sites if progression occurs.[5]

Although the role of intensity-modulated radiation therapy (IMRT) is rapidly growing in the definitive treatment of a large number of tumor sites in both adults and children, little attention has been focused on its role in metastatic and recurrent disease. Given its increased time requirements and added costs, it is not surprising that many feel that such patients should not receive IMRT. Ironically, these may be the very patients most likely to benefit. The highly conformal isodose distributions achieved with IMRT offer distinct advantages in patients with recurrent or metastatic disease, providing a means of safely delivering higher than conventional doses and allowing reirradiation of selected sites.

The purpose of this chapter is to explore potential roles for IMRT in patients with metastatic and recurrent disease. Particular attention is given to its use in patients with recurrent tumors within a prior radiation field. In addition, outcome studies and future directions of IMRT planning in the treatment of patients with metastatic and recurrent disease are discussed.

Metastatic Disease
Bone Metastasis

RT is commonly used in the treatment of bone metastases from a wide variety of primary sites, notably breast, lung, and prostate cancer.[2] Treatment typically involves short-course external beam approaches delivered with large daily fractions, for example, 30 Gy in 10 fractions. Patients with multiple bone metastases may also be treated with radioactive colloids, such as strontium 89.[6]

Palliative RT is associated with high response rates in the majority of patients with bone metastases. Overall, 66 to 83% experience subjective improvement, with 17 to 54% obtaining complete relief.[2,7–9] As long as normal tissue tolerances are respected, toxicity is rare. Strontium 89 therapy is similarly associated with high response rates. Apart from transient hematologic toxicity, it is generally well tolerated.[6]

Given the efficacy and tolerance of such approaches, IMRT is unlikely to occupy a major role in the primary treatment of patients with bone metastases. Moreover, conventional approaches are easily administered and do not require complex treatment planning, allowing treatment to be initiated almost immediately.

Nonetheless, IMRT may prove useful in a subset of patients with bone metastases. One role may be in the delivery of higher than conventional doses. With current approaches, approximately 60% of patients experience sustained pain relief for over 1 year or until death.[2] Some data, however, suggest that higher doses may result in more durable control rates. In an analysis of the Radiation Therapy Oncology Group (RTOG) trial 74-02, complete pain relief was noted in 55% of patients treated with 40.5 Gy in 15 fractions compared with 37% using 20 Gy in 5 fractions, suggesting a benefit to higher doses.[10] Although feasible in most sites using conventional techniques, IMRT provides the ability to escalate the dose in sites that are in close proximity to radiosensitive normal tissues, for example, the lumbar spine and base of the skull.

It is imperative that any patient with bone metastases undergoing such an approach be carefully selected. In one series, the survival of patients with bone metastasis undergoing palliative RT was only 25% at 1 year and 8% at 2 years, suggesting that most patients with metastatic disease do not survive long enough to experience a benefit from dose escalation.[11] However, some patients with metastatic disease may live long enough to benefit. Singh and colleagues reported that 36% of patients with prostate cancer with fewer than five bony metastatic sites are alive at 10 years.[12] Similarly, 45% of women with metastatic breast cancer limited to bone are alive at 5 years.[13] Additional studies suggest that histology, sensitivity to systemic therapy, extent of disease, performance status, and serum markers may be used to select favorable cohorts who would likely have prolonged survival rates.[4] Efforts to maximize long-term tumor control in patients with a favorable prognosis are clearly warranted.

Limited experience exists using dose-escalated IMRT in patients with bone metastases. Ryu and Yin and their colleagues recently described an intensity-modulated radiosurgical approach in 10 patients with spinal metastases.[14,15] All received conventional external beam RT (25 Gy in 10 fractions) followed by a 6 to 8 Gy intensity-modulated radiosurgical boost. Complete pain relief was achieved in five patients, whereas partial pain relief was noted in four patients. Of two paraplegic patients, one had a complete neurologic recovery and one had a partial recovery of strength. At a mean follow-up of 6 months, no acute toxicity was noted. A full discussion of this approach is provided in an accompanying case study (see Chapter 27.3, "Intensity-Modulated Radiosurgery for Spinal Metastasis: Emerging Technology").

Brain Metastases

Brain metastases are commonly treated with palliative RT. Patients typically receive whole-brain irradiation alone or following surgical resection.[16] Those with a limited number of brain metastases may undergo stereotactic radiosurgery (SRS) alone or in combination with whole-brain RT.[17]

RT is associated with high response rates in most patients with brain metastases. Headache, seizure, nausea, and neurologic symptoms are palliated in 50 to 85% of patients undergoing whole-brain irradiation, with a doubling of their median survival compared with using corticosteroids alone.[18] SRS is associated with control rates exceeding 85% in most series.[19,20] As in patients with bone metastases, significant toxicity using whole-brain RT or SRS is infrequent when attention is given to proper treatment techniques.[18,20]

Despite the efficacy and tolerance of such approaches, several potential roles for IMRT exist in patients with brain metastases. One role is in SRS treatment planning. Several investigators have performed detailed dosimetric studies comparing IMRT and conventional planning in patients undergoing linear accelerator–based SRS. Singh and colleagues noted that IMRT planning resulted in superior homogeneity and conformity, although the mean target dose was lower and the nontarget tissue dose was marginally greater.[21] Investigators at the Medical College of Virginia compared multiple-isocenter SRS with six-field, noncoplanar, three-dimensional conformal RT and six-field, noncoplanar IMRT.[22] IMRT planning resulted in superior conformity and reduced high and low isodoses to normal brain for irregularly shaped and hemispheric tumors. A full discussion of IMRT planning in patients

undergoing SRS is provided in Chapter 17.4, "Intensity-Modulated Radiosurgery: Emerging Technology."

IMRT may represent an alternative to SRS in selected patients.[23] Using the simultaneous integrated boost technique, the entire brain could be treated with conventional fractions to a modest total dose, whereas the gross lesions could receive higher total doses with large fraction sizes. This approach has been widely studied in a number of disease sites, notably head and neck and prostate cancers.[24,25] However, no reports have been published applying this technique to the treatment of brain metastases.

A provocative role for IMRT may also be in the delivery of prophylactic whole-brain RT. Although the entire brain is currently irradiated, most metastases occur in the watershed areas in the gray-white junction.[26] IMRT could be used to focus treatment on this region while reducing the dose to the outer cortex. Such an approach may help reduce the risk of cognitive dysfunction. A possible avoidance region could be the hippocampus because injury to stem cells may contribute to radiation-induced cognitive dysfunction.[27] Prospective clinical trials are needed to test the efficacy of such an approach.

Visceral Metastases

Metastatic disease may occur in a number of visceral sites, notably the lung and liver. Metastatic disease in these sites is not commonly treated with RT. These sites can be treated with surgical resection, particularly in cases of solitary metastases. Other treatment modalities include radiofrequency ablation and cryotherapy.

Interest exists in the treatment of liver metastases with focal RT. Investigators at the University of Michigan have studied the use of high-dose RT (median dose 59.5 Gy).[28] Such a treatment is well tolerated if the mean liver dose is kept below 31 Gy. Lung metastases are rarely treated with palliative RT.

IMRT is not an appealing approach in the treatment of liver and lung metastases. Although IMRT conforms the dose to the shape of the target tissues, reducing the volume of normal tissues irradiated to high doses, it increases the volume of normal tissues receiving low doses. Given the exquisite radiosensitivity of the liver and lung tissues, unless this "dose-dumping" effect can be reduced, concerns exist regarding the potential increase in the risk of toxicity using an IMRT approach.[29] Moreover, the impact of organ motion in these sites needs to be studied.

Nonetheless, promising results have been reported using IMRT in the treatment of liver and lung metastases. Fuss presented a series of lung and liver metastases patients treated with an intensity-modulated hypofractionated tomotherapy approach.[30] Radiation doses were 3 × 12 Gy for small tumors and 3 × 16 Gy for stage I lung cancer lesions. Two patients with large liver lesions received 6 × 6 Gy. Patients were immobilized using a vacuum-assisted whole-body immobilization system (Bodyfix, Medical Intelligence,

Schwabmünchen, Germany). Of 22 lesions treated, 16 showed a complete response and 6 a partial response or stable disease. Toxicity was minimal, with only localized pneumonitic reactions and fibrotic changes.

IMRT may also prove beneficial in the treatment of other visceral sites, particularly metastases in close proximity to critical normal tissues. Examples include the orbit, adrenal glands, and bulky lymph nodes in the abdomen or pelvis (Figure 27-1).

Locally Advanced Disease

Unlike metastatic disease sites, less attention has been focused on the use of palliative RT for patients with locally advanced disease, when cure is no longer possible. Published data, however, provide strong evidence supporting the efficacy of palliative RT in a wide number of locally advanced patients, including lung cancer, head and neck cancer, and pelvic malignancies.

A potential role for IMRT in such patients is to reduce the volume of normal tissues irradiated. Most patients receive short-course, hypofractionated RT delivered with large daily fractions. Unsurprisingly, significant normal tissue toxicity may result, particularly in patients with longer life expectancies. Onsrud and colleagues irradiated 64 locally advanced gynecology patients with one to three fractions of 10 Gy to the entire pelvis over a 4-week period. A benefit was seen in the majority of patients, with decreased bleeding noted in 90%. However, severe gastrointestinal toxicity was seen in patients surviving 9 months or more.[31] Reducing the volume of the small bowel and rectum treated in these patients using IMRT may help reduce this risk (Figure 27-2).

Normal tissue sparing using IMRT may also provide a safe means of escalating the dose in patients with locally advanced disease. Multiple investigators have noted improved responses in such patients using higher total doses. Lankford and colleagues at the M. D. Anderson Cancer Center treated regionally localized hormone-refractory prostate cancer with palliative RT. With a median follow-up of 43 months, symptom-free local control was 90% for patients receiving ≥ 60 Gy versus 29% for those receiving lower doses.[32] Crane and colleagues reported that palliative RT (plus sensitizing chemotherapy) in locally advanced or metastatic rectal cancer relieved pelvic symptoms in 81 to 91% of patients. Of note, a biologically equivalent dose of > 35 Gy in 2 Gy fractions was associated with improved pelvic control.[33] These results support the development of clinical trials examining the efficacy and toxicity of dose escalation using IMRT in these patients.

Recurrent Disease

RT is commonly used at the time of disease recurrence, particularly when it was not used initially. In addition, radiation oncologists are commonly confronted with recurrent

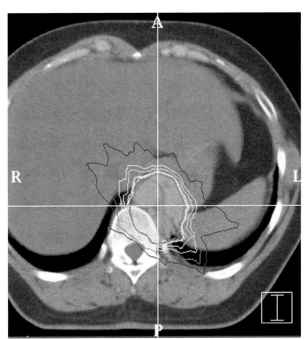

FIGURE 27-1. Example intensity-modulated radiation therapy (IMRT) plan in a patient with stage IIIc ovarian cancer with an isolated abdominal (paraspinal) recurrence (15 years after her diagnosis). Initial treatment consisted of primary surgery and adjuvant chemotherapy. Following partial resection of the paraspinal mass, a total dose of 59.4 Gy was delivered using this IMRT plan. Note the considerable sparing of the spinal cord, liver, and kidneys. (To view a color version of this image, please refer to the CD-ROM.)

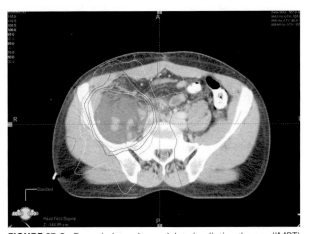

FIGURE 27-2. Example intensity-modulated radiation therapy (IMRT) plan in a patient with locally advanced (T3N1) bladder cancer with an isolated right pelvic recurrence. Initial treatment consisted of cysto-prostatectomy, lymph node dissection, and adjuvant chemotherapy. A recurrent pelvic mass was noted 1 year later invading the surrounding muscles and bone, resulting in intractable pelvic pain. Palliative IMRT (50 Gy) was delivered, combined with gemcitabine. IMRT was elected to minimize the risk of gastrointestinal toxicity owing to the use of concomitant gemcitabine. (To view a color version of this image, please refer to the CD-ROM.)

tumors within a prior RT field. Unsurprisingly, many elect not to reirradiate such patients owing to concerns over untoward normal tissue toxicity.

Despite such concerns, reirradiation is gaining interest for both palliation and cure.[5] The largest experience is in head and neck cancer, often combined with chemotherapy. Although promising results have been reported in terms of tumor control, toxicity is considerable.[34] IMRT represents an appealing approach in these patients owing to the highly conformal dose distributions sparing the surrounding normal tissues. An example of an IMRT plan used in a patient with recurrent head and neck cancer is shown in Figure 27-3.

Limited published data exist on using IMRT in recurrent head and neck cancer. Chen and colleagues at the University of California at Irvine treated 12 previously irradiated patients with head and neck cancer (median dose 63 Gy) with IMRT using doses of 30 to 70 Gy (median 60 Gy).[35] At 4 to 16 months of follow-up, 5 of 12 patients were free of disease, with none experiencing ≥ grade 3 acute toxicity. One death occurred secondary to aspiration pneumonia.

Another possible use of IMRT in patients with recurrent disease is in the irradiation of spinal metastases. Few radiation oncologists elect to reirradiate such patients owing to the high potential of gastrointestinal and neurologic toxicity. However, IMRT may overcome these concerns by minimizing the dose to the neighboring small bowel and spinal cord (Figure 27-4).

Increasing data have been published using IMRT in this setting. Milker-Zabel and colleagues treated 18 previously irradiated patients with 19 sites of recurrent spinal metastases.[36] The median dose of prior spinal irradiation was 38 Gy. The median reirradiation dose was 39.6 Gy. With a median follow-up of 12.3 months, 95% were locally controlled, with 81% experiencing pain relief and 42% obtaining neurologic improvement. No grade 3 acute or late toxicities were noted. The treatment of recurrent spinal metastases using this technique is outlined in detail in the accompanying case study (see Chapter 27.1, "Recurrent Spinal Metastasis: Case Study").

Kuo and colleagues reported their experience using IMRT to irradiate 8 patients with 10 recurrent spinal metastases.[37] Five patients were treated with palliative intent, and five patients were reirradiated. Treatment efficacy was difficult to assess because of 10 sites irradiated, irradiation was discontinued in 3 before completion owing to deterioration in the patients' medical condition, and 1 patient was lost to follow-up. Three of four lesions treated with primary irradiation were locally controlled at a mean follow-up of 9 months. IMRT allowed doses as high as 75 Gy to be delivered to the primary tumor while limiting the maximum spinal cord dose to 48 Gy. For reirradiation cases, despite a mean previous spinal dose of 41.5 Gy, the median prescribed PTV dose was 36.7 Gy. No neurologic complications occurred.

Increasing interest has been focused on IMRT in the retreatment of gynecologic and other pelvic tumors within a prior irradiation field.[38] In the past, few radiation oncol-

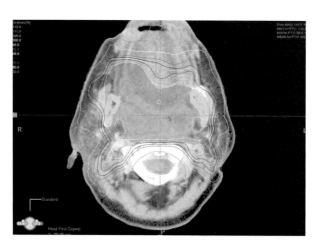

FIGURE 27-3. Example intensity-modulated radiation therapy (IMRT) plan in a patient with recurrent head and neck (T3N3 pharyngeal) cancer. Initial treatment consisted of total laryngectomy, radical neck dissection, and postoperative radiotherapy (total dose 66 Gy). A localized recurrence was noted 4 years later in the tumor bed and regional lymph nodes. Reirradiation was performed using this IMRT plan (45 Gy) combined with concomitant chemotherapy. Note considerable sparing of the spinal cord. (To view a color version of this image, please refer to the CD-ROM.)

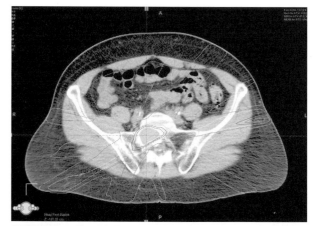

FIGURE 27-4. Example intensity-modulated radiation therapy (IMRT) plan in a patient with locally advanced prostate cancer (T3b, Gleason grade 5 + 4, prostate-specific antigen level 234) with an isolated bony recurrence. In addition to hormonal ablation, initial treatment consisted of whole-pelvis irradiation (45 Gy), followed by a boost to the prostate and seminal vesicles (total dose 70.2 Gy). An isolated S1 vertebral body recurrence was noted 2 years later within the prior radiotherapy field. IMRT was used to reirradiate this patient (total dose 30 Gy). Note significant sparing of the small bowel and cauda equina. (To view a color version of this image, please refer to the CD-ROM.)

ogists would consider irradiating such tumors, except perhaps with brachytherapy.[39] However, the highly conformal isodose distributions achieved with IMRT planning provide a potential means of delivering meaningful total doses to these sites (Figure 27-5).

Future Directions

Numerous issues and challenges need to be addressed if IMRT is ever to occupy a meaningful role in the treatment of patients with metastatic or recurrent disease. First, the available data using IMRT in these patients remain limited. Additionally, published reports include small patient numbers, with limited follow-up, treated at only a few institutions. More data are needed involving well-controlled, large, multicenter cohorts to fully investigate the potential role for IMRT in this setting. It is imperative that such trials include objective toxicity and detailed quality-of-life measures as outcomes to allow the full assessment of the benefits and risks of treatment.

A unique challenge in applying IMRT in patients with metastatic and/or recurrent disease is that many are in considerable pain. Given the high dose gradients inherent in IMRT treatment plans, accurate patient setup is imperative. Unfortunately, patients in pain may not tolerate prolonged planning and treatment sessions. Considerable attention should thus be given to obtaining optimal pain control prior to irradiation.[40] Moreover, careful positioning and immobilization are important to maximize patient tolerance.

A final important issue is cost. Although third-party payers may be willing to accept the added cost of IMRT in definitive patients, they may not accept it in palliative patients.

Data demonstrating decreased toxicity and improved quality of life in the palliative setting with IMRT are clearly needed to justify the added expense. However, as IMRT becomes widely accepted, the cost of IMRT may decrease because capital expenditures for technology acquisition have already been made.[41] Further innovations in automating many of the labor-intensive components of IMRT planning and treatment delivery also may decrease the cost of treatment.

References

1. Janjan NA. Palliative therapy. Semin Radiat Oncol 2000; 10:169–74.
2. Gilbert HA, Kagan AR, Nussbaum H, et al. Evaluation of radiation therapy for bone metastases: pain relief and quality of life. AJR Am J Roentgenol 1977;129:1095–6.
3. Gaspar L, Scott C, Rotman M, et al. Recursive partitioning analysis (RPA) of prognostic factors in three Radiation Therapy Oncology Group (RTOG) brain metastases trials. Int J Radiat Oncol Biol Phys 1997;37:745–51.
4. Janjan NA. Palliative care. In: Cox JD, Ang KK editors. Radiation oncology: rationale, technique, result. 8th ed. Philadelphia: Mosby; 2003. p. 954–86.
5. Morris DE. Clinical experience with retreatment for palliation. Semin Radiat Oncol 2000;10:210–21.
6. Hamdy NA, Papapoulos SE. The palliative management of skeletal metastases of prostate cancer: use of bone-seeking radionuclides and biphosphonates. Semin Nucl Med 2001;31:62–8.
7. Wu JS, Wong R, Johnston M, et al. Meta-analysis of dose-fractionation radiotherapy trials for the palliation of painful bone metastases. Int J Radiat Oncol Biol Phys 2003;55:594–605.
8. Hartsell WF, Scott C, Bruner DW, et al. Phase III randomized trial of 8 Gy in 1 fraction vs. 30 Gy in 10 fractions for palliation of painful bone metastases: preliminary results of RTOG 97-14. Int J Radiat Oncol Biol Phys 2003;57(2 Suppl):S124.
9. Steenland E, Leer JW, van Houwelingen H, et al. The effect of a single fraction compared to multiple fractions on painful bone metastases: a global analysis of the Dutch Bone Metastasis Study. Radiother Oncol 1999;52:101–9.
10. Blitzer PH. Reanalysis of the RTOG study of the palliation of symptomatic osseous metastasis. Cancer 1985;55:1468–72.
11. Bates T. A review of local radiotherapy in the treatment of bone metastases and cord compression. Int J Radiat Oncol Biol Phys 1992;23:217–21.
12. Singh D, Yi WS, Brasacchio FA, et al. Is there a favorable subset of patients with metastatic prostate cancer who have oligometastases? Int J Radiat Oncol Biol Phys 2003;54 Suppl 1:193.
13. Sherry MM, Greco FA, Johnson DH, et al. Breast cancer with skeletal metastases at initial diagnosis. Distinctive clinical characteristics and favorable prognosis. Cancer 1986;58:178–82.
14. Ryu S, Fang Yin F, Rock J, et al. Image-guided and intensity-modulated radiosurgery for patients with spinal metastasis. Cancer 2003;97:2013–8.
15. Yin FF, Ryu S, Ajlouni M, et al. A technique of intensity-modulated radiosurgery (IMRS) for spinal tumors. Med Phys 2002;29:2815–22.

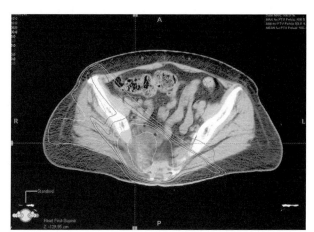

FIGURE 27-5. Example intensity-modulated radiation therapy (IMRT) plan in a patient with recurrent rectal cancer. Initial treatment consisted of surgery alone. The patient subsequently developed an unresectable pelvic recurrence and received palliative irradiation (total dose 36 Gy). Symptoms returned the following year, and this IMRT plan was used to reirradiate the pelvic mass (30 Gy in 2.5 Gy daily fractions). (To view a color version of this image, please refer to the CD-ROM.)

16. Patchell RA, Tibbs PA, Walsh JW, et al. A randomized trial of surgery in the treatment of single metastases to the brain. N Engl J Med 1990;322:494–500.

17. Sneed PK, Suh JH, Goetsch SJ, et al. A multi-institutional review of radiosurgery alone vs. radiosurgery with whole brain radiotherapy as the initial management of brain metastases. Int J Radiat Oncol Biol Phys 2002;53:519–26.

18. Wen PY, Black PM, Loeffler JJ. Metastatic brain cancer. In: Devita VT, Hellman S, Rosenberg SA, editors. Cancer, principles and practice of oncology. 6th ed. Philadelphia: Lippincott Raven; 2001. p. 2655–70.

19. Sperduto PW, Scott C, Andrews D, et al. Stereotactic radiosurgery with whole brain radiation therapy improves survival in patients with brain metastases: report of Radiation Therapy Oncology Group phase III study 95-08. Int J Radiat Oncol Biol Phys 2002;54 Suppl 1:3.

20. Varlotto JM, Flickinger JC, Niranjan A, et al. Analysis of tumor control and toxicity in patients who have survived at least one year after radiosurgery for brain metastases. Int J Radiat Oncol Biol Phys 2003;57:452–64.

21. Singh RR, Ayyangar KM, Shen B, et al. Comparative study between IMRT with NOMOS BEAK and linac-based radiosurgery in the treatment of intracranial lesions. Med Dosim 2001;26:47–53.

22. Cardinale RM, Benedict SH, Wu Q, et al. A comparison of three stereotactic radiotherapy techniques: ARCS vs. non-coplanar fixed fields vs. intensity modulation. Int J Radiat Oncol Biol Phys 1998;42:431–6.

23. Teh BS, Woo SY, Butler EB. Intensity modulated radiation therapy (IMRT): a new promising technology in radiation oncology. Oncologist 1999;4:433–42.

24. Wu Q, Mohan R, Morris M, et al. Simultaneous integrated boost intensity-modulated radiotherapy for locally advanced head-and-neck squamous cell carcinomas. I: dosimetric results. Int J Radiat Oncol Biol Phys 2003;56:573–85.

25. Dogan N, King S, Emami B, et al. Assessment of different IMRT boost delivery methods on target coverage and normal-tissue sparing. Int J Radiat Oncol Biol Phys 2003;57:1480–91.

26. Delattre JY, Krol G, Thaler HT, et al. Distribution of brain metastases. Arch Neurol 1988;45:741–4.

27. Monje ML, Mizumatsu S, Fike JR, et al. Irradiation induces neural precursor-cell dysfunction. Nat Med 2002;8:955–62.

28. Dawson LA, McGinn CJ, Normolle D, et al. Escalated focal liver radiation and concurrent hepatic artery fluoro-deoxyuridine for unresectable intrahepatic malignancies. J Clin Oncol 2000;18:2210–8.

29. Cheng JC, Wu JK, Huang CM, et al. Dosimetric analysis and comparison of three-dimensional conformal radiotherapy and intensity-modulated radiation therapy for patients with hepatocellular carcinoma and radiation-induced liver disease. Int J Radiat Oncol Biol Phys 2003;56:229–34.

30. Fuss M. Intensity-modulated hypofractionated extracranial radioablation techniques for lung and liver lesions: adding a new treatment option [abstract]. Cancer J 2003;9:498.

31. Onsrud M, Hagen B, Strickert T. 10-Gy single-fraction pelvic irradiation for palliation and life prolongation in patients with cancer of the cervix and corpus uteri. Gynecol Oncol 2001;82:167–71.

32. Lankford SP, Pollack A, Zagars GK. Radiotherapy for regionally localized hormone refractory prostate cancer. Int J Radiat Oncol Biol Phys 1995;33:907–12.

33. Crane CH, Janjan NA, Abbruzzese JL, et al. Effective pelvic symptom control using initial chemoradiation without colostomy in metastatic rectal cancer. Int J Radiat Oncol Biol Phys 2001;49:107–16.

34. Kao J, Garofalo MC, Milano MT, et al. Reirradiation of recurrent and second primary head and neck malignancies: a comprehensive review. Cancer Treat Rev 2003;29:21–30.

35. Chen YJ, Kuo JV, Ramsinghani NS, et al. Intensity-modulated radiotherapy for previously irradiated, recurrent head-and-neck cancer. Med Dosim 2002;27:171–6.

36. Milker-Zabel S, Zabel A, Thilmann C, et al. Clinical results of retreatment of vertebral bone metastases by stereotactic conformal radiotherapy and intensity-modulated radiotherapy. Int J Radiat Oncol Biol Phys 2003;55:162–7.

37. Kuo JV, Cabebe E, Al-Ghazi M, et al. Intensity-modulated radiation therapy for the spine at the University of California, Irvine. Med Dosim 2002;27:137–45.

38. Implementation of intensity modulated radiation therapy for patients with carcinoma of the cervix. Panel 6. Presented at the 45th Annual Meeting of the American Society for Therapeutic Radiology and Oncology (ASTRO); 2003 Oct 20; Salt Lake City, UT.

39. Monk BJ, Tewari KS, Pethawala AA, et al. Treatment of recurrent gynecologic malignancies with iodine-125 permanent interstitial irradiation. Int J Radiat Oncol Biol Phys 2002;52:806.

40. Jacox A, Carr DB, Payne R. New clinical-practice guidelines for the management of pain in patients with cancer. N Engl J Med 1994;330:651–5.

41. Mell LK, Roeske JC, Mundt AJ. A survey of intensity-modulated radiation therapy use in the United States. Cancer 2003; 98:204–11.

RECURRENT SPINAL METASTASIS CASE STUDY

STEFANIE MILKER-ZABEL, MD

Patient History

A 38-year-old female with a history of breast cancer presented in August 1992 with a painful osteolytic metastasis at the level of the tenth thoracic (T10) vertebral body. She was treated with conventional palliative radiation therapy (RT) on a cobalt 60 unit using an arc technique. A dose of 36 Gy was prescribed in 2 Gy daily fractions.

Nine years later, the patient returned with recurrent midback pain. No other neurologic symptoms were noted.

A computed tomography (CT) scan demonstrated a recurrent osteolytic metastasis in the T10 vertebral body (Figure 27.1-1). Magnetic resonance imaging (MRI) revealed a hyperintense mass (on the T$_2$-weighted images) involving the left lateral transverse process without evidence of spinal cord compression (Figure 27.1-2). In light of her previous RT, we chose to reirradiate this site using intensity-modulated radiation therapy (IMRT) to minimize the dose to the previously treated spinal cord.

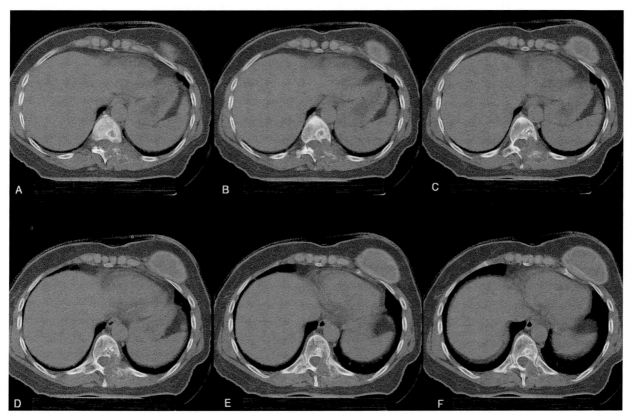

FIGURE 27.1-1. Computed tomography (CT) scans (bone window) of the recurrent vertebral bone metastasis located at the level of T10.

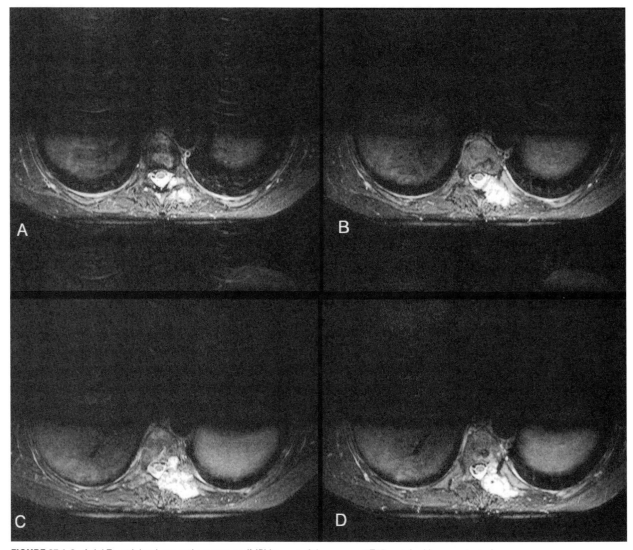

FIGURE 27.1-2. Axial T₂-weighted magnetic resonance (MR) images of the recurrent T10 vertebral bone metastasis.

Simulation

For immobilization, a noninvasive immobilization device was fabricated consisting of a carbon fiber compound base plate and a custom-made wraparound body cast extending from the abdomen to the thighs with a separate head mask (Scotch-Cast, 3M, St. Paul-Minneapolis, MN) (Figure 27.1-3). The patient was placed on a 20 cm–wide board with a custom lumbar support, and the body cast was formed by wrapping the patient together with the board. The body cast and narrow board were then placed on the adaptor plate and secured with nylon screws. The adaptor plate was secured with precisely fitting bolts on the carbon fiber base plate supporting the extracranial stereotactic frame.[1,2]

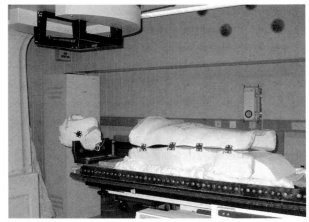

FIGURE 27.1-3. Custom-made wraparound body cast with a separate head mask fixation for patient immobilization.

After becoming rigid, the cast was opened with an oscillating saw, and closing devices were mounted. The cast was filled with a thin layer of polyurethane foam, and a metal arch was attached to the base plate. A V-shaped indicator was mounted on the base plate, and three other V-shaped indicators were attached to the lateral and anterior aspects of the metal arch. The metal wires on the indicators can be seen on the planning CT scan and are used for stereotactic target point definition. These indicators can be moved along the longitudinal axis of the base plate to define a stereotactic system around the region of interest. Metric scales, which are mounted on the stereotactic frame, are used for setup of stereotactic coordinates. The mean setup accuracy of this approach is < 3.6 mm.[3]

In this patient, T_1- and T_2-weighted axial and sagittal MRIs were obtained in the treatment position. MRIs were then fused to the planning CT scan using an anatomic matching algorithm. Both the CT scan and MRI were obtained with 3 mm slices and extended from the diaphragm to the bladder. Note that the stereotactic body frame cannot be used in the MRI environment. However, given that the body cast or adaptor plate is MRI compatible, MRIs of the patient can be obtained in the same position as that of the planning CT scan.

Target and Tissue Delineation

The gross tumor volume (GTV) in this case consisted of the macroscopic tumor visualized on MRI. The planning target volume (PTV) included the GTV plus the entire vertebral body. A separate clinical target volume (CTV) was not defined in this patient.

Organs at risk (OAR) included the spinal cord, right and left lungs, right and left kidneys, and right and left ureters. The PTV and OAR were contoured manually on all axial CT slices (Figure 27.1-4). The spinal cord was segmented with a safety margin of 2 to 3 mm.

Treatment Planning

IMRT plans were generated using the *KonRad* inverse planning system (MRC System GmbH, Heidelberg, Germany), developed at the German Cancer Research Center.[4,5] Eight coplanar treatment beams (gantry angles of 218, 250, 280, 310, 85, 105, 135, and 163 degrees) were selected owing to the complex geometry of the target. Each beam group consists of 6 to 13 subfields. The input parameters used in this case are shown in Table 27.1-1.

The goal of treatment planning was to cover the PTV with a minimum of 90% of the prescribed dose. The resultant dose-volume histograms of the PTV and critical structures are shown in Figure 27.1-5. Isodose distributions overlaid on axial CT slices are shown in Figure 27.1-6. The total prescribed dose was 39.6 Gy in 1.8 Gy daily fractions.

Treatment Delivery and Quality Assurance

Treatment was delivered using 15 MV photon beams on a Siemens linear accelerator (Siemens AG, Erlangen, Germany) equipped with an integrated multileaf collimator. This accelerator and treatment couch have a combined geometric error at the isocenter of less than 1 mm. Treatment was delivered in the "step-and-shoot" mode.[6]

Before the initial treatment, the IMRT plan was verified extensively. A phantom plan was created by casting the intensity maps onto a CT-scanned, water-equivalent phantom, and the doses were recalculated according to the phantom dimensions. The absolute dose was measured, and the relative dose distribution was filmed and verified.

On the first treatment day, the isocenter was verified with a double-exposure portal image. The intensity maps of each delivered treatment portal were acquired with the *BeamView Plus* (Siemens Oncology Systems, Concord, CA), enabling one to compare treated and calculated intensity maps.

As part of the quality assurance process, the patient underwent weekly CT with the body cast fixation and stereotactic localization system. These scans were performed with 3 mm slices, extending 1 cm above to 1 cm below the isocenter. Prior to scanning, fiducial markers were placed on the patient corresponding to the isocenter location. Deviations between the planned and treated isocenters were measured and recorded.

Clinical Outcome

At 25.8 months following completion of treatment, the patient is alive and well. The reirradiated bone metastasis remains controlled and asymptomatic. Unfortunately, the patient subsequently presented with a new bone metastasis at the level of T7 (outside the irradiated volume). A course of conventional palliative irradiation is planned.

Our clinical experience treating recurrent spinal metastases with IMRT was published earlier.[7] The outcome of 18 previously irradiated patients with 19 sites of recurrent disease was reviewed. The median dose of prior spinal irradiation was 38 Gy. The median reirradiation dose was 39.6 Gy. With a median follow-up of 12.3 months, 95% were locally controlled, with 81% experiencing pain relief and 42% obtaining neurologic improvement. No grade 3 acute or late toxicities were noted.

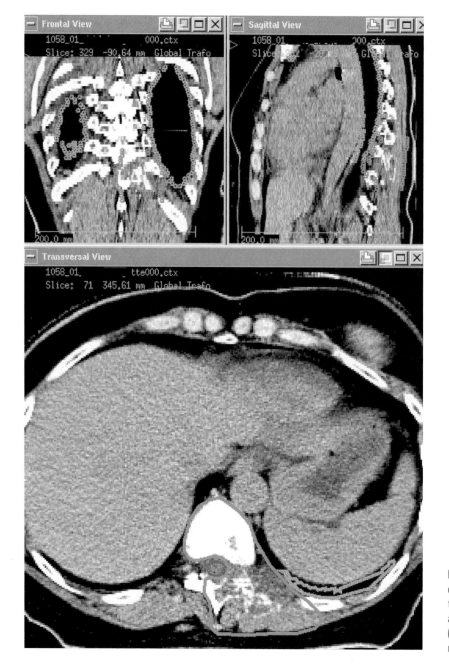

FIGURE 27.1-4. Axial, sagittal, and coronal computed tomography slices with contours of the planning target volume (*pink*) and organs at risk (lung left/right [*lilac*]; spinal cord [*blue*]). (To view a color version of this image, please refer to the CD-ROM.)

TABLE 27.1-1. Input Parameters

Organ	Overlap Priority	Maximum Dose, Gy	Maximum Penalty	Minimum Penalty
PTV	1	40	1000	1500
Right lung	6	15	600	
Left lung	5	15	600	
Spinal cord	2	15	3000	
Right kidney	3	20	400	
Left kidney	4	20	400	-
Left ureter	7	15	100	
Right ureter	8	15	100	

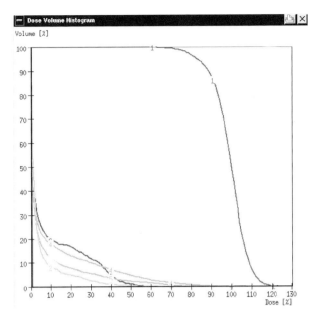

FIGURE 27.1-5. Dose-volume histograms of the treated patient. 1 = planning target volume; 2 = left kidney; 3 = right kidney; 4 = left lung; 5 = right lung; 6 = spinal cord; 7 = left ureter; 8 = right ureter.

References

1. Schlegel W, Pastyr O, Bortfeld T, et al. Stereotactically guided fractionated radiotherapy: technical aspects. Radiother Oncol 1993;31:467–76.
2. Debus J, Engenhart-Cabilic R, Knopp MV, et al. Image-oriented planning of minimally invasive conformal radiotherapy in the head and neck. Radiologe 1996;36:732–6.
3. Lohr F, Debus J, Frank C, et al. Noninvasive patient fixation for extracranial stereotactic radiotherapy. Int J Radiat Oncol Biol Phys 1999;45:521–7.
4. Preiser K, Bortfeld T, Hartwig K, et al. Inverse treatment planning for intensity modulated photon beams. Radiologe 1998;38:228–34.
5. Bortfeld T. Optimized planning using physical objectives and constraints. Semin Radiat Oncol 1999;9:20–39.
6. Keller-Reichenbecher MA, Bortfeld T, Levegrün S, et al. Intensity modulation with the "step and shoot" technique using a commercial MLC: a planning study. Int J Radiat Oncol Biol Phys 1999;45:315–24.
7. Milker-Zabel S, Zabel A, Thilmann C, et al. Clinical results of retreatment of vertebral bone metastases by stereotactic conformal radiotherapy and intensity-modulated radiotherapy. Int J Radiat Oncol Biol Phys 2003; 55:315–24.

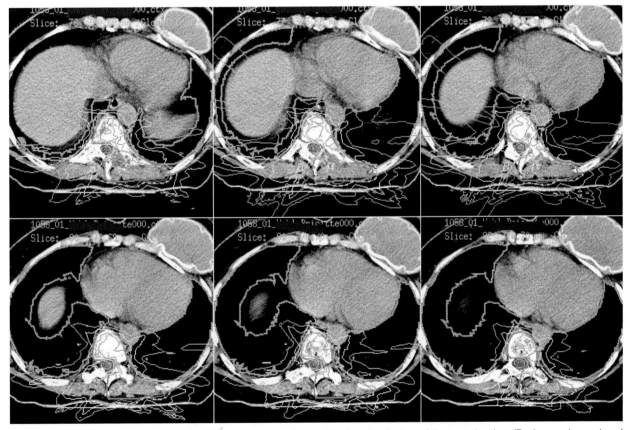

FIGURE 27.1-6. Axial computed tomography (CT) slices with superimposed isodose distributions of the treated patient. (To view a color version of this image, please refer to the CD-ROM.)

RECURRENT NASOPHARYNGEAL CANCER CASE STUDY

WEI-YUAN MAI, MD, TAI-XIANG LU, MD, XIAO-WU DENG, PhD

Patient History

A 34-year-old male presented in February 1998 with a 1-month history of right-sided tinnitus. Clinical examination revealed bilateral palpable enlarged lymph nodes in the upper neck (right 1.8 × 1.8 cm, left 1.5 × 1.5 cm). Endoscopic examination demonstrated a nasopharyngeal lesion, and a biopsy was performed. The pathology was consistent with a World Health Organization type III undifferentiated carcinoma. A computed tomography (CT) scan revealed extension of the nasopharyngeal mass into the right parapharygneal space. The remainder of the workup was negative for metastases. The tumor was thus staged as T2bN2M0.

The patient was treated with conventional radiation therapy (RT). Total doses to the nasopharynx and the neck lymph node were 70 and 60 Gy, respectively, delivered in 2 Gy daily fractions. Chemotherapy was not administered. The patient achieved a complete response based on clinical and follow-up CT examinations.

In December 2000, the patient presented with recurrent right-sided tinnitus and progressive diplopia. Clinical examination demonstrated a nasopharyngeal mass and a right cranial nerve VI deficit. A biopsy was performed, and the pathology confirmed a local recurrence. Restaging CT and magnetic resonance imaging (MRI) scans demonstrated a nasopharyngeal mass involving the oropharynx and right cavernous sinus with erosion of the skull base (foramen lacerum, apex of the petrous temporal bone, clivus). A metastatic workup, including chest radiography, liver ultrasonography, and liver function tests, was negative. His Karnofsky Performance Score at the time of recurrence was 80. Salvage RT was performed using intensity-modulated radiation therapy (IMRT).

Simulation

The patient was immobilized in the supine position using a thermoplastic face mask (Figure 27.2-1). A customized "pillow" made of molded polyurethane foam was used to support his head and neck. A planning CT scan was performed in the treatment position on a Somatom Plus 4 CT simulator (Siemens Medical Systems, Munich, Germany) with 3 mm slices. The anatomic extent of the scan was from the vertex of the head to below the clavicles. Intravenous contrast was administered.

Target and Tissue Delineation

Target volumes were delineated on each axial slice of the planning CT scan. The gross tumor volume (GTV) in this patient was defined as the gross extent of the tumor visualized on imaging (CT and MRI) studies. The clinical target volume (CTV) was defined as the GTV plus a 1 cm margin for potential microscopic spread, except in regions adjacent to the brainstem and/or spinal cord, where the margin was reduced to 0.5 cm. A planning target volume (PTV) was generated by expanding the CTV by 0.5 to 1.5 cm. Adjacent to the brainstem and spinal cord, a 0.5 cm expansion was used. Figure 27.2-2 illustrates the GTV, margin 1, and margin 2 delineated in this patient.

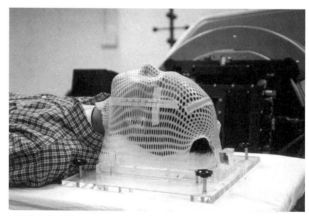

FIGURE 27.2-1. A thermoplastic face mask was used for immobilization with a customized "pillow" to support the patient's head and neck. (To view a color version of this image, please refer to the CD-ROM.)

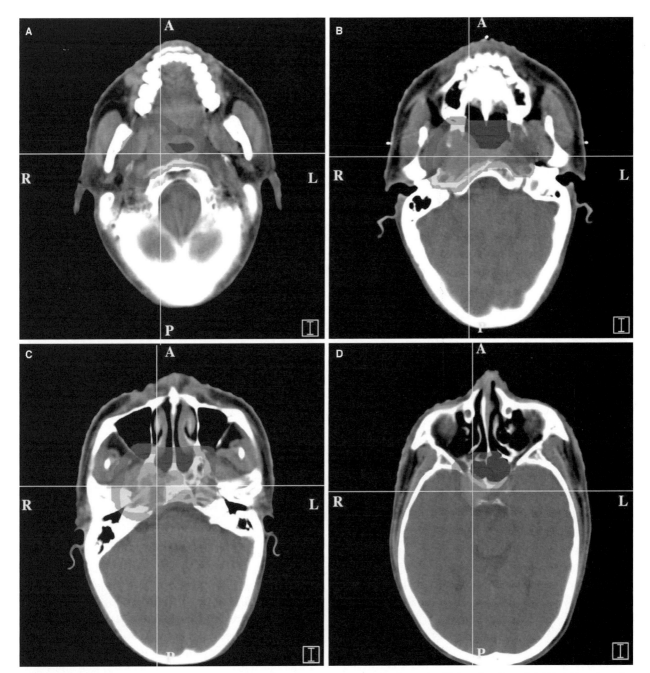

FIGURE 27.2-2. Axial computed tomography slices illustrating the gross tumor volume (*red*), margin 1 (*light red*), and margin 2 (*blue*). Note that adjacent to the brainstem, a smaller expansion margin (0.5 cm) was used for both the CTV and the PTV. (*A*) Oropharynx; (*B*) nasopharynx; (*C*) skull base; (*D*) cavernous sinus. (To view a color version of this image, please refer to the CD-ROM.)

Organs at risk (OAR) in this patient included the brainstem, spinal cord, optic nerves, optic chiasm, eyes, temporal lobes, parotid glands, temporomandibular joints, and mandible.

Treatment Planning

Inverse treatment planning was performed using the *CORVUS* planning system, version 3.0 (North American

Scientific, NOMOS Radiation Oncology Division, Cranberry Township, PA). The input parameters for IMRT planning for the GTV, margin 1, and margin 2 in this patient are summarized in Table 27.2-1. The total prescribed doses for GTV, margin 1, and margin 2 were 70, 60, and 50 Gy, respectively. Corresponding daily fractions were 2.3, 2.0, and 1.7 Gy, respectively. Threshold doses to the OAR were based on the publication of Emami and colleagues.[1] In general, we used more restricted dose limits because the

TABLE 27.2-1. Input Parameters

Targets and Critical Structures	Goal and Limit, Gy	Minimum Dose, Gy	Maximum Dose, Gy
GTV	70	68	74
Margin 1	60	56	64
Margin 2	50	48	54
Brainstem	30	10	46
Spinal cord	30	10	40
Optic chiasm	40	30	50
Optic nerves	40	30	50
Eye	15	10	20
Lens	3	1	5
Temporal lobe	30	10	40
Parotid gland	26	20	30
Temporomandibular joint	30	10	40
Mandible	30	20	40

GTV = gross tumor volume.

patient had undergone RT. The targets were given priority over normal structures in the planning process.

A treatment plan was generated, reviewed, and accepted. Each axial image was evaluated for dosimetric coverage of the target volumes and avoidance of normal structures. An optimized treatment plan is shown in Figure 27.2-3. Dose-volume histograms for the GTV, margin 1, margin 2, and OAR are summarized in Table 27.2-2 and Figure 27.2-4. The CTV is denoted as GTV plus margin 1, and the PTV is denoted as CTV plus margin 2.

Treatment Delivery and Quality Assurance

The treatment was delivered with a dynamic multileaf intensity-modulating collimator using a segmental tomotherapy technique (North American Scientific). The gantry rotation arc was 105° to 255°, and beamlet patterns changed every 5°. The patient was treated on a Varian Clinic 600C (Varian Medical Systems, Palo Alto, CA) using 6 MV photons.

The treatment plan was verified using a film phantom. Commercial prepackaged film (XV-2, Eastman Kodak Co., Rochester, NY) in a transverse orientation was used to confirm that the dose pattern was correct relative to the isocenter of the linear accelerator. These films were qualitatively compared for the shape and intensity with images generated by the computer.

Port films were taken for the first two fractions and weekly thereafter to verify isocenter placement. Six 1 cm treatment arcs were used in this patient. Daily treatment delivery time for the patient was approximately 20 minutes.

Clinical Outcome

The patient tolerated treatment well, without interruptions. A follow-up clinical examination revealed the complete response of the recurrent tumor. However, the cranial nerve VI deficit did not resolve. At 3 months following completion of IMRT, MRI demonstrated resolution of the nasopharyngeal lesion. However, persistent skull base destruction was noted. MRI performed at 9 months revealed identical results.

When last seen (32 months post-treatment), the patient remained clinically without evidence of disease recurrence. His mucous membrane was slightly atrophic and dry. He needed to sip liquids to swallow dry food and carry a water bottle. However, there were no obvious RT-related side effects to his eyes, spinal cord, or brain.

Our initial experience using IMRT in 49 patients with recurrent nasopharyngeal carcinoma was recently presented.[2] The median dose to the nasopharynx in the initial conventional RT treatment was 70 Gy (range 60.9–78 Gy). Using our IMRT approach, a mean dose of 71.4 Gy was delivered to the GTV. Three patients with positive nodes received adjuvant chemotherapy (cisplatin, 5-fluorouracil) following IMRT; the remainder were treated with IMRT alone.

At a median follow-up of 9 months (range 3–13 months), the locoregional control rate was 100%. Three patients developed metastases at a distant site (two in bone, one in the liver and lung). Overall, treatment was well tolerated. The percentages of patients with acute grade 2 skin and mucosal toxicities were 2% and 43%, respectively. Grade 3 mucosal toxicity was seen in 4% of patients. Twenty-three patients (47%) experienced grade 2 xerostomia (18 moderate, 5 severe). All patients are being followed closely to assess late toxicity and treatment outcome.

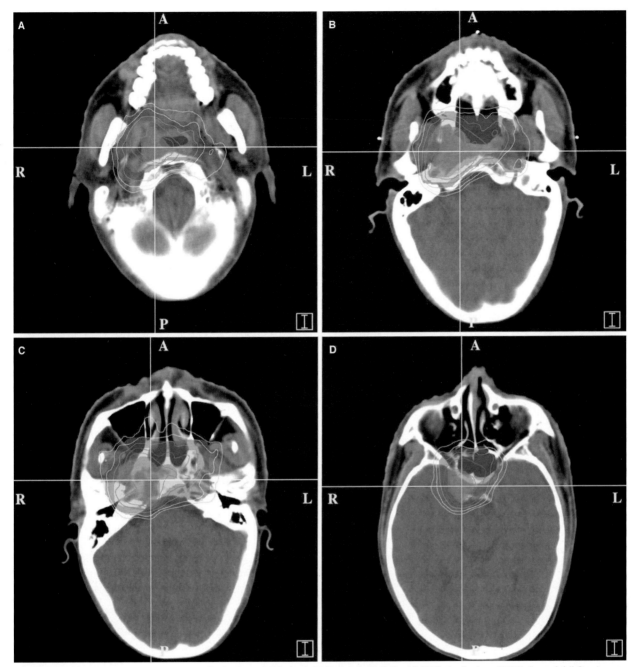

FIGURE 27.2-3. Treatment plan and isodose distributions: 70 Gy (*red*), 65 Gy (*pink*), 60 Gy (*gold*), 55 Gy (*yellow*), and 50 Gy (*green*). (*A*) Oropharynx; (*B*) nasopharynx; (*C*) skull base; (*D*) cavernous sinus. (To view a color version of this image, please refer to the CD-ROM.)

TABLE 27.2-2. Target and Normal Tissue Doses

Critical Structures	Volume, cm³	Mean Dose, Gy	Minimum Dose, Gy	Maximum Dose, Gy
GTV	38.1	70.1	63.5	74.3
Margin 1	55.6	65.4	50.9	73.1
Margin 2	89.5	57.5	36.8	72.4
Brainstem	31.3	32.1	11.1	63.5
Spinal cord	3.0	24.9	9.7	36.4
Optic chiasm	0.5	41.4	29.3	49.0
Optic nerve				
L	0.8	31.2	14.9	47.9
R	0.6	32.7	14.5	56.4
Eye				
L	9.8	9.3	1.5	24.1
R	9.9	10.8	1.9	28.2
Lens				
L	0.2	3.0	1.9	5.2
R	0.2	3.2	2.2	5.6
Temporal lobe				
L	34.5	24.5	3.3	59.7
R	27.3	28.4	3.7	67.9
Parotid gland				
L	8.5	20.0	6.3	37.1
R	9.2	25.0	9.3	50.1
Temporomandibular joint				
L	3.1	25.7	17.1	41.2
R	3.7	29.9	20.8	52.3
Mandible				
L	37.0	19.1	0.7	42.7
R	37.0	23.6	0.7	58.3

GTV = gross tumor volume, R = right, L = left.

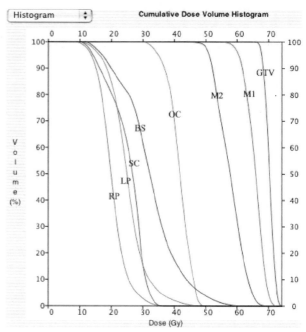

FIGURE 27.2-4. Dose-volume histograms of the target and normal tissues. M1 = margin 1; M2 = margin 2; OC = optic chiasm; BS = brainstem; LP = left parotid gland; RP = right parotid gland; SC = spinal cord; GTV = gross tumor volume.

Acknowledgments

We thank Bin S. Teh, MD, and E. Brian Butler, MD (Baylor College of Medicine, Houston, TX), for their assistance and recommendations regarding the planning and treatment of this patient.

References

1. Emami B, Lyman J, Brown A, et al. Tolerance of normal tissue to therapeutic irradiation. Int J Radiat Oncol Biol Phys 1991;21:109–22.
2. Lu TX, Mai WY, Teh BS, et al. Initial experience using intensity-modulated radiotherapy for recurrent nasopharyngeal carcinoma. Int J Radiat Oncol Biol Phys 2004;58:682–7.

INTENSITY-MODULATED RADIOSURGERY FOR SPINAL METASTASIS EMERGING TECHNOLOGY

FANG-FANG YIN, PHD, SAMUEL RYU, MD, JAE HO KIM, MD, PHD

Patient History

A 54-year-old male with a history of stage IIIa squamous cell carcinoma of the lung presented with a lumbar spine metastasis. Three years previously, the patient was treated with concomitant external beam radiation therapy (RT) to the right lung and mediastinum (total dose 65.8 Gy) combined with chemotherapy (docetaxel, carboplatin, and gemcitabine).

He did well until recently, when he developed pain in his low back (9 on a 10-point scale), radiating to his left flank and iliac region. On physical examination, focal tenderness was noted along the lumbar spine. A computed tomography (CT) scan demonstrated a destructive lesion in the L1 vertebral body consistent with a metastasis. The remainder of his workup revealed no evidence of disease, including the primary site. In light of his isolated spinal metastasis, it was elected to treat the patient with image-guided intensity-modulated radiosurgery.

Simulation

The patient was immobilized in the supine position using a BodyFix immobilization device (Medical Intelligence, Schwabmünchen, Germany) to minimize setup uncertainty and target motion (Figure 27.3-1). The BodyFix device combines a vacuum cushion and a piece of special plastic foil.[1] The vacuum cushion is used to stabilize the patient in a comfortable position while the plastic foil is used to constrain the patient by evacuating the region between the patient and the plastic foil. The supine setup helps to minimize the vertebral body motion owing to breathing. After the immobilization device was fabricated, motion of the involved vertebral body was examined under fluoroscopy and was noted to be less than 1 mm.

A planning CT simulation (AcQSim, Philips Medical Systems, Andover, MA) was then performed with the patient in the treatment position using 3 mm slices.

Infrared sensitive markers (used for patient setup and localization) were placed on the patient's skin prior to the CT scan. Intravenous contrast was administered to enhance imaging of the tumor on the CT images. The patient was scanned from T9 to S5 to accurately identify vertebral bodies and to provide sufficient anatomy for the use of noncoplanar beams.

Target and Tissue Delineation

The gross tumor volume (GTV) in this case was the entire L1 vertebral body. To aid in the delineation of the GTV, contrast-enhanced magnetic resonance imaging (MRI) was used. Image fusion between the CT scan and MRI was performed manually to ensure accurate anatomic matching. Figure 27.3-2 shows both the CT scan and MRI and their fusion result for this specific case. The GTV is indicated by an arrow. In this case, the clinical target volume (CTV) was the GTV.

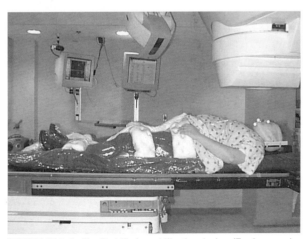

FIGURE 27.3-1. The BodyFix immobilization device. (To view a color version of this image, please refer to the CD-ROM.)

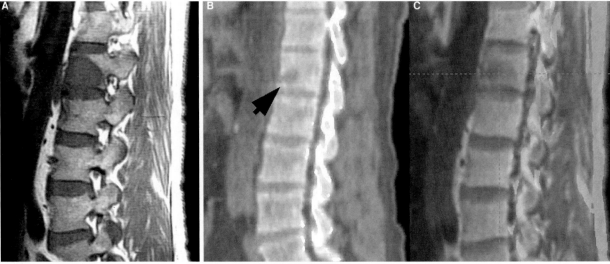

FIGURE 27.3-2. (*A*) Magnetic resonance image (MRI); (*B*) computed tomography (CT) scan; and (*C*) image fusion of MRIs and CT scans. The arrow indicates the gross tumor volume.

Because the BodyFix device was used for immobilization, the planning target volume (PTV) in this patient was generated by adding a 3 mm margin to the GTV to accommodate patient positioning and target localization variations. This expansion did not extend into the spinal cord. Critical normal tissues, including the spinal cord and kidneys, were contoured on the planning CT scan as avoidance structures (Figure 27.3-3).

Treatment Planning

Six treatment beams were selected for this patient, primarily from the posterior direction, to minimize doses to the crit-

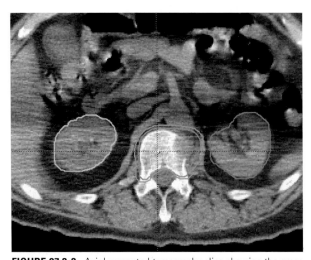

FIGURE 27.3-3. Axial computed tomography slice showing the gross tumor volume (*purple*), planning target volume (*magenta*), spinal cord (*green*), right kidney (*yellow*), and left kidney (*orange*). (To view a color version of this image, please refer to the CD-ROM.)

ical normal organs. All six beams were coplanar (295, 220, 195, 170, 145, and 120 degrees), and the collimator was set to 90°. The total prescribed dose was 18 Gy in a single fraction delivered using 6 MV photons. Treatment planning was performed using *BrainSCAN* software, version 5.21 (BrainLAB AG, Heimstetten, Germany).

Each beam was optimized using an inverse treatment planning algorithm based on the dynamically penalized likelihood method and a pencil beam dose calculation algorithm.[2,3] Dose-volume histograms (DVHs) were used to specify the dose constraints for both the target volume and critical organs (Figure 27.3-4). In this case, both the target volume and the critical organs were given the same priority weights. An additional parameter, the conformity index $[C = 1 + (V_n/V_t)]$, was also calculated to evaluate the treatment plan. Here V_n is the volume of the normal tissue and V_t is the volume of the target receiving the indicated dose.[1] The conformity index provides a relative measure of the amount of normal tissue within the prescription isodose. Typically, we require this value to be < 2.0. For this particular case, the conformity index was 1.45.

Figure 27.3-5A shows the 90%, 80%, 50%, and 30% isodose lines. The isodose was normalized to the isocenter, and the dose was prescribed to the volume included by the 90% isodose line. Inhomogeneity corrections were included in the dose calculation for this plan. The corresponding DVHs actually achieved after optimization are shown in Figure 27.3-5B.

After the radiation oncologist selected a suitable inverse treatment plan, all treatment data were electronically transferred to the treatment unit through the Varis record and verify system (Varian Medical Systems, Palo Alto, CA) and to the image guidance system (Novalis Body System, BrainLAB AG).

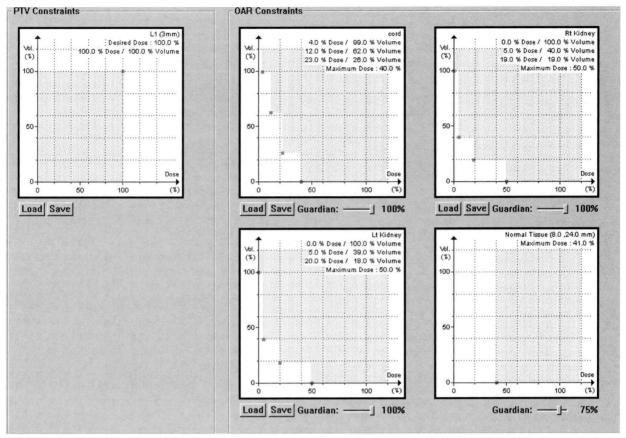

FIGURE 27.3-4. Input dose-volume histograms used for intensity-modulated radiation therapy planning in this patient. OAR = organ at risk; PTV = planning target volume.

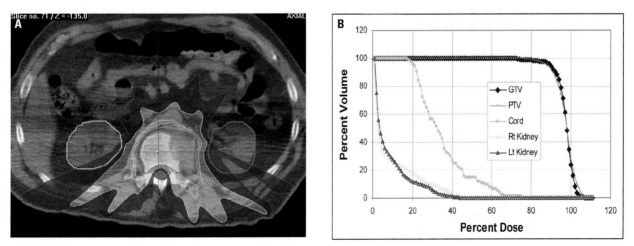

FIGURE 27.3-5. (*A*) An inverse plan using six predominantly posterior beams and (*B*) corresponding dose-volume histograms for target and critical organs. GTV = gross tumor volume; PTV = planning target volume. (To view a color version of this image, please refer to the CD-ROM.)

Treatment Delivery and Quality Assurance

On completion of treatment planning, the patient was repositioned on the linear accelerator couch in the treatment position to align the planned isocenter to the accelerator isocenter. Image-guided techniques, including infrared camera imaging and KV x-ray imaging techniques, were used for patient setup and target (or isocenter) localization.[1,4] This procedure was achieved using the Novalis Body System, which consists of dual infrared and single video cameras and two KV x-ray imaging systems (Figure 27.3-6).

After the patient was immobilized on the treatment couch, the infrared camera system guided the patient setup to the planned treatment position based on the localization of infrared sensitive markers on the patient's skin. Given that the infrared markers reflect only the patient's surface information, two KV radiographs were acquired. Digitally reconstructed radiographs (DRRs) were then generated from the planning CT images at the same orientations as the KV radiographs. Internal structures such as the vertebral bodies were subsequently compared to indicate the relative isocenter deviations from the planned isocenter position. Patient shift and rotational information were identified using a rigid-body three-dimensional to two-dimensional image fusion technique in which DRRs were iteratively generated with different angulations to simulate potential patient deviations in all directions.[5] Note that the accuracy of image fusion depends on the reliability of those structures used for matching both sets of images. Image fusion based on the implanted markers is often more accurate and reliable.[5,6]

After reviewing the comparison result, the radiation oncologist decides whether an adjustment of the isocenter position is necessary. If so, the infrared camera system will guide the patient to the adjusted position. With this image-guided patient localization technique, an accuracy of 1 mm is achievable in a rigid-body phantom, as shown in a previous study.[6] However, depending on the immobilization technique used for the actual patient treatment, a 2 mm isocenter deviation can be realistically achieved. This accuracy is considered to be acceptable for spine radiosurgery if a proper margin can be added.

The intensity-modulated beams were delivered using a dedicated radiosurgical unit (Novalis) equipped with a micromultileaf collimator (MLC).[1,7] The maximal leaf width is 5.5 mm, and the minimal leaf width is 3 mm. For inverse plans delivered using different MLCs, the leaf width may potentially affect the dose distribution. However, the dosimetric difference of IMRT beams delivered using the MLC leaf width of 5 mm or less is negligible.[8] A single isocenter can be used for any target shape unless the target size exceeds the maximal field size (10 × 10 cm) of the Novalis unit. A sliding window (or dynamic MLC) technique was used to deliver the IMRT beams through the micro-MLC, and a dose rate of 480 monitor units (MU)/min was used for efficient and accurate delivery. Because the entire process, from simulation to delivery, can be completed within a few hours, the procedure is noninvasive, frameless, accurate, and efficient.

Quality assurance (QA) in intensity-modulated radiosurgery is both machine specific and patient specific. Machine-specific QA involves examination of leaf travel accuracy, isocenter accuracy, and dose output consistency. As part of the commissioning process, dose distributions and delivery accuracy have been carefully verified.[1]

Our patient-specific QA protocol uses an independent dose calculation algorithm based on a modified Clarkson method used to calculate the isocenter dose contributed by each micro-MLC segment and its corresponding MUs.[9] Next, each intensity map was checked by delivering a given amount of radiation to a film (XV and EDR2 ready packs, Eastman Kodak, Rochester, NY) and was compared with the planned intensity map. To verify the absolute point dose, the planned intensity maps were exported to a verification phantom and the isocenter point dose in the phantom was calculated. The phantom was then irradiated with all planned beams. The point dose in the phantom was measured using a micro–ion chamber (CC01, Scanditronix-Wellhofer, Bartlett, TN) and was compared with the planned point dose. Under normal conditions, the deviation between these is less than 3%.

The imaging devices used for patient setup and target localization were calibrated prior to each application based on the requirements specified by the manufacturers.[6] Independent patient positioning verification was achieved by taking orthogonal images and comparing them with simulation images. Alternatively, this verification could also be accomplished by comparing the two verification KV radiographs to the corresponding DRRs.

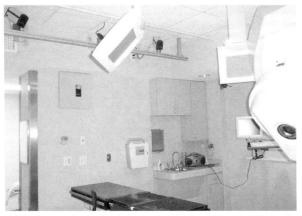

FIGURE 27.3-6. Image-guided target localization systems on the Novalis treatment unit. (To view a color version of this image, please refer to the CD-ROM.)

Clinical Outcome

The patient tolerated treatment well. One month following the intensity-modulated radiosurgery, the patient walked into the clinic without a wheelchair. He was fully ambulatory. On physical examination, there was no tenderness over the L1 region. The pain decreased significantly to the level of 5 of 10, with reduced pain medication requirements. However, a follow-up CT scan demonstrated evidence of disease progression within the chest.

The clinical efficacy of the spinal radiosurgery was recently analyzed in 49 patients with 61 lesions of spinal metastasis treated at Henry Ford Hospital from May 2001 to May 2003. Most patients had back pain as the primary presenting symptom. Doses of 10 to 16 Gy were delivered in a single fraction. Complete and partial pain relief was achieved in 37.7% and 47.6% of the lesions treated, respectively.[10] The median time to pain relief was 14 days, and the earliest time of pain relief was obtained within 24 hours. The median duration of pain relief was 13.3 months. Progressive metastasis in the adjacent spine was observed in only 4.9%. There was no acute or subacute radiation toxicity detected clinically during the maximum follow-up of 24 months.[11]

Single spinal metastasis may be optimally treated with intensity-modulated radiosurgery alone. Pain relief was rapid and durable, and there was satisfactory neurologic improvement in patients with cord compression.[10] Radiosurgery can also be used for patients with multiple isolated spinal metastases, for example, metastasis to C5, T7, and L3 spinal segments. These patients would otherwise have been treated to almost the entire spine. Patient tolerance has been excellent, and this treatment was convenient to the patient because it was given in a single outpatient hospital visit. Moreover, the volume of bone marrow could also be preserved by reducing the volume of RT, thus possibly making chemotherapy more feasible in this group of patients when the need arises. In addition, radiosurgery can also be used for selected cases of primary spine tumors[12] and other organ sites, such as head and neck cancers, with excellent tumor control.[13]

References

1. Yin FF, Ryu S, Ajlouni M, et al. A technique of intensity-modulated radiosurgery (IMRS) for spinal tumors. Med Phys 2002;29:2815–22.
2. Llacer J. Inverse radiation treatment planning using the dynamically penalized likelihood method. Med Phys 1997;24:1751–64.
3. Llacer J, Solberg TD, Promberger C. Comparative behavior of the dynamically penalized likelihood algorithm in inverse radiation therapy planning. Phys Med Biol 2001;46:2637–63.
4. Ryu S, Yin FF, Rock J, et al. Image-guided and intensity-modulated radiosurgery for patients with spinal metastases. Cancer 2003;97:2013–8.
5. Kim JK, Yin FF, Kim JH. Characteristics of a CT/dual x-ray image registration method using 2D texture map based DRR, gradient ascent, and mutual information. ICCR 2004 (Seoul, Korea).
6. Yan H, Yin FF, Kim JH. A phantom study on the positioning accuracy of the Novalis Body system. Med Phys 2003;30:3052–60.
7. Yin FF, Zhu JH, Yan H, et al. Dosimetric characteristics of Novalis shaped beam surgery unit. Med Phys 2002;29:1729–38.
8. Fiveash JB, Murshed H, Duan J, et al. Effect of multileaf collimator leaf width on physical dose distributions in the treatment of CNS and head and neck neoplasms with intensity modulated radiation therapy. Med Phys 2002;29:1116–9.
9. Zhu J, Yin FF, Kim JH. Point dose verification for intensity-modulated radiosurgery using Clarkson's method. Med Phys 2003;30:2218–21.
10. Ryu S, Yin FF, Rock J, et al. Image-guided radiosurgery for single spinal metastasis [abstract]. Proc Am Soc Clin Oncol 2004. [In press].
11. Ryu S, Sharif A, Yin FF, et al. Tolerance of human spinal cord to single dose radiosurgery. Proc Int Congress Radiat Res 2003.
12. Rock J, Kole M, Yin FF, et al. Radiosurgical treatment for Ewing's sarcoma of the lumbar spine. Spine 2002;27:471–5.
13. Ryu S, Khan M, Yin FF, et al. Image-guided radiosurgery of head and neck cancers. Otolaryngol Head Neck Surg 2004;130:690–7.

IV. Invited Commentaries

Chapter 28

INTENSITY-MODULATED PROTON THERAPY

TONY LOMAX, PhD, EROS PEDRONI, PhD, DOELF CORAY, PhD, GUDRUN GOITEIN, MD, MARTIN JERMANN

Robert Wilson first suggested the use of protons for radiation therapy (RT) in 1946.[1] The physical characteristics of protons dictate that, for any delivered field, substantially less dose will be delivered to normal tissues positioned proximally to the target than with photons, and immediately beyond the distal end of the target, the delivered dose rapidly drops to zero. After the first patients were treated with protons at Lawrence Berkeley Laboratories in 1954, these characteristics have been exploited for more than 40 years to deliver highly conformal dose distributions in a number of research facilities. By 2004, more than 35,000 patients had been treated with protons worldwide.[2]

Although there is an inherent dynamic component to any form of proton therapy, the most predominant form, passive scattering, depends only on a fast modulation of the proton beam in depth, achieved through a rapidly rotating, varying thickness wheel.[3,4] However, the potential for the dynamic delivery of proton therapy has also been proposed.[5] Such methods have been pioneered at the Paul Scherrer Institute (PSI), where the world's first spot scanning gantry was developed in the early 1990s and the first patient was treated in 1996.[6] More recently, this spot scanning technology was further refined to allow for the delivery of intensity-modulated proton therapy (IMPT), which was first used clinically in 1999.[7,8]

IMPT can be considered to be the direct equivalent of intensity-modulated radiation therapy (IMRT) with photons in that each field delivers an optimized and highly irregular fluence pattern. The desired dose distribution in the patient is then achieved when all such fields are combined. For both IMRT and IMPT, the ability to deliver arbitrarily complex fluence patterns allows for considerably greater flexibility in tailoring the dose distribution to the target and in selectively avoiding critical structures than conventionally delivered photon or proton treatments, respectively. Comparative computer-based studies between photon IMRT

and both spot scanning[9–13] and IMPT[14–16] have shown the potential of such advanced proton delivery methods and suggest that protons have the potential to further increase the efficacy of RT beyond that which is presently achievable with state-of-the-art photon therapies.

Spot Scanning Proton Therapy

Non-IMRT conformal RT relies on two main methods to concentrate the high dose onto the tumor region: the selection of angularly spaced beams converging onto the target volume and the shaping of these beams to conform to the target. Conventionally, whether using photons, electrons, or protons, beam shaping has been achieved through the use of field-specific collimators, which take the same form as the projected shape of the target volume along the beam direction. In addition, for protons and, to a lesser extent, for electrons, the dose falloff at the distal end of the volume can be formed to match the distal surface through the use of a field-specific compensator.[17,18] With spot scanning, the use of such hardware is not normally necessary, and conformation of single-field dose distributions to the lateral and distal aspects of the target volume is achieved through the automatic selection and optimization of individual and discretely deposited Bragg peaks.[6,19] This process is demonstrated in Figure 28-1.

For any given field direction (incident from the right side of Figure 28-1), the treatment planning software uses the patient's CT data to calculate all possible positions of Bragg peaks within the patient for the nominal energy selected for the field. These are shown as the set of red crosses in Figure 28-1A. The uneven border at the left of the image indicates the maximum range of 138 MeV protons (the beam energy selected for this example). To confine the dose to the target volume, however, only a subset of these Bragg peaks is required, and the treatment plan-

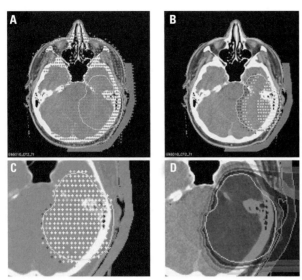

FIGURE 28-1. A step-by-step guide to the calculation of a spot-scanned proton field. (*A*) The calculation of the positions of all deliverable Bragg peaks (represented by the crosses) for a 138 MeV field (maximum range 13.15 cm in water), accounting for the relative stopping power of the patient anatomy and the scanning limits of the delivery system. (*B*) Computer-based selection of Bragg peaks within the target volume or a defined distance outside (eg, 5 mm). This step emulates a "virtual" collimator but operates in three dimensions. Cross colors represent the first-guess relative weights of the selected Bragg peaks. (*C*) The relative weights after the optimization process and (*D*) the optimized dose distribution. (To view a color version of this image, please refer to the CD-ROM.)

ning system automatically selects all Bragg peaks that lie within the target volume or a certain distance outside. This step is critical to the planning process because it emulates the effect of a collimator in conventional RT. That is, it "blocks Bragg" peaks outside the target volume. Thus, this process can be considered to be akin to a "virtual" three-dimensional collimation of the beam.

The result of this Bragg peak selection is shown in Figure 28-1B, where the colors of the crosses now indicate the "first-guess" relative weights of the individual Bragg peaks. These are calculated using conventional methods required to produce a flat spread-out Bragg peak in passive scattering proton therapy.[3] For all but the simplest target volumes, however, this initial set of weights does not result in a homogeneous dose throughout the target volume. Thus, an iterative optimization method is required to calculate the set of beam weights necessary to deliver a homogeneous dose within the entire target volume. In the PSI system, this is a gradient-based method initially developed for Pion therapy[20] and subsequently modified for proton treatment planning.[19,21] The result of this optimization is shown in Figure 28-1C, together with the resultant dose distribution in Figure 28-1D. For conventional spot scanning, a plan consists of the weighted linear combination of one or more individually homogeneous single-field dose distributions similar to that shown in Figure 28-1D. Through a combination of magnetic scanning, table motion, and fast energy variation, spot scanned proton therapy has been implemented clinically at our center using a custom-designed gantry system,[6] providing a flexibility in the choice of incident beam angles similar to what is available with a conventional linear accelerator.

Clinical Implementation of Spot Scanning

Presently, dynamic particle therapy is being used clinically in only two institutes worldwide: at PSI, with protons using the spot scanning method,[6] and at the German Heavy Ion Research Institute (GSI), with carbon ions using raster scanning.[22] By the end of 2003, 166 patients of varying indications had been treated at our center with spot-scanned protons[23] and nearly 200 at GSI with carbon ions. In addition, there is some interest from commercial companies in developing dynamic systems for protons.[24]

To illustrate the potential of spot scanning proton therapy, two cases treated at PSI are presented here. The first case is a patient with an adenoid carcinoma of the skull base treated in 2001. The gross tumor volume (GTV) was close to the brainstem and lateral to the parotid glands. However, such tumors may involve regional lymph nodes in the neck; thus, it was decided that the neck nodes should be irradiated for at least the initial part of the treatment. The delivered spot-scanned proton plan is shown in Figure 28-2. Three fields (one lateral and two superior lateral oblique) were used to irradiate the primary tumor bed while avoiding the brainstem and parotid gland. An additional, nonoverlapping, single lateral field was used to treat the neck nodes. Thus, with no more than four fields, a highly conformal dose distribution could be delivered to this complex case, with total sparing of the contralateral normal tissues and excellent sparing of the ipsilateral parotid gland and brainstem.

Figure 28-3 illustrates a comparison between a single-field spot-scanned plan and a nine-field IMRT plan calculated for a sarcoma in a 12-year-old boy treated with the plan shown in Figure 28-3A at the end of 2002. Owing to the sharp falloff of the distal Bragg peaks, this plan has an almost perfect dose distribution, conforming to the target volume in all dimensions; dropping off sharply before the spinal column, spinal cord, and kidney; and delivering minimal integral dose to the nontarget tissues. This can be compared with the nine-field IMRT plan shown in Figure 28-3B. Although, as may be expected, IMRT can deliver a highly conformal dose at the 90% dose level, there is a significantly higher dose delivered to the spinal cord and, perhaps more importantly, to the entire kidney. In addition, calculation of the total integral dose delivered to the

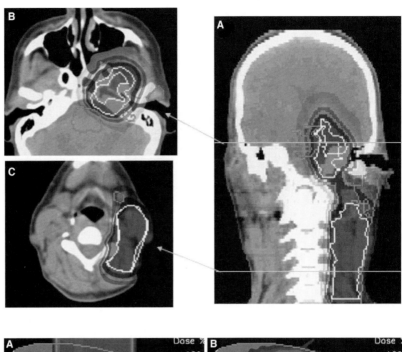

FIGURE 28-2. A four-field spot scanning technique applied to a patient with an adenoid cystic carcinoma. (*A*) A frontal view through the dose distribution showing the primary tumor bed in the area of the skull base and the irradiated nodal chain along the neck. (*B*) A transaxial view through the distribution at the level of the skull base showing the dose conformity to the primary tumor bed and sparing of the brainstem and parotid gland. (*C*) A similar slice through the cervical nodal region. (To view a color version of this image, please refer to the CD-ROM.)

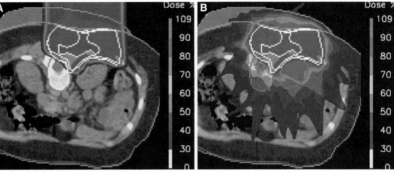

FIGURE 28-3. A single-field spot-scanned proton plan (*A*) and nine-field intensity-modulated radiation therapy (IMRT) photon plan (*B*) in a 12-year-old boy with a soft tissue sarcoma. Note the high degree of dose conformation in the proton plan, with excellent sparing of the spinal cord and kidney compared with the nine-field IMRT plan. In addition, the total dose to the nontarget tissues is reduced by more than a factor of 6 in the proton plan compared with the IMRT plan. (To view a color version of this image, please refer to the CD-ROM.)

nontarget tissues demonstrated that the IMRT plan delivers six times more dose to the child than the proton treatment shown in Figure 28-3A.

Intensity-Modulated Proton Therapy

As discussed above, the optimization process in spot scanning is a necessary step for achieving a variable spread-out Bragg peak and, as such, is used only to emulate the type of field that can be applied across the target volume by passive scattering techniques. IMPT, on the other hand, is analogous to IMRT in that arbitrarily complex fluences—or, more strictly, doses—are applied from different field directions with the aim of applying a homogeneous and highly conformal dose across the target volume only when all fields are combined. In contrast to IMRT with photons, however, given that the depth of the individually weighted Bragg peaks can also be varied, the form of the dose along any given beamlet can, in effect, also be modulated in depth. Put another way, with IMPT, it is not solely the

in-plane particle fluence that can be varied but also the effective shape of the depth dose curve.

This characteristic is demonstrated in Figure 28-4 using a four-field IMPT plan calculated for a patient with a cervical chordoma. The combined dose is shown in the middle dose distribution and the individual fields and their incidences by the surrounding distributions. Notice, in particular, fields 1 and 3, each of which delivers small high-dose areas toward the proximal or central portions of the planning target volume (PTV) near the spinal cord. The dose distribution along these beamlets is selectively increased at one particular depth, compensating for the missing dose in these areas from the other fields, which have been reduced in this area to avoid overdosing the spinal cord. Thus, IMPT provides, in its most general form, the ability to vary the delivered dose in three dimensions for any given field direction and is consequently often referred to as 3DIMPT.[7] From a treatment planning perspective, IMPT differs in one subtle but critical aspect from the simple spot scanning approach: instead of optimizing the Bragg peak weights

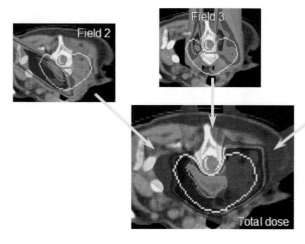

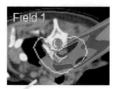

FIGURE 28-4. A three-field three-dimensional intensity-modulated proton therapy (3DIMPT) plan calculated for a cervical chordoma. The individual field dose distributions are highly inhomogeneous but, when combined, form a homogeneous and highly conformal dose distribution to the target, with almost complete sparing of the spinal cord. Note the variation in the dose along the field directions of the incident fields, indicating the capability of 3DIMPT to vary the effective depth dose curves for the individually applied beamlets. (To view a color version of this image, please refer to the CD-ROM.)

of each field independently, in IMPT, all Bragg peaks from all selected fields are optimized simultaneously. Similar to photon IMRT planning, the dose-volume constraints of all critical structures can be defined in the optimization process.

At first glance, the distinction between spot scanning and IMPT may seem rather arbitrary; after all, both involve the application of individually positioned and optimized Bragg peaks within the patient. There are, however, two significant differences between the two approaches. First, IMPT provides greater flexibility in where the dose is applied (ie, to better avoid deep-seated critical structures). Second, the resulting plans can be more sensitive to delivery uncertainties.

Given the three-dimensional nature of the modulation, IMPT has a large number of degrees of freedom available to it—indeed, considerably many more than photon IMRT. For example, for a typical 10 × 10 cm photon IMRT field, approximately 400 individual beamlets can be modulated (assuming a beamlet size of 5 × 5 mm). For a 10 × 10 × 10 cm field with protons, however, approximately 8,000 beamlets are available to the optimization procedure per beam given that Bragg peaks will also be distributed in depth (with a separation of 5 mm). Thus, a 20-fold increase in the degrees of freedom is available for IMPT treatments per field. For simple cases, such a large number of degrees of freedom may well be many more than required. Consider, for example, the case shown in Figure 28-5. A and B illustrate two five-field dose distributions calculated for a skull base angiosarcoma treated with identical incident beam directions. Qualitatively, the dose distributions appear to be quite similar. C and D, however, show the distributions and relative weights of the individual Bragg peaks calculated for the left anterior lateral oblique field in the two plans. The differences in the number and weightings of the two fields are considerable but, nevertheless, result (when combined with the doses applied from the other four fields) in similar resultant dose distributions. Thus, the large number of Bragg peaks that can be delivered from each field results in a large degeneracy of solutions for delivering a specific dose to the tumor.

The example of Figure 28-5, B and D, indicates one way in which the degeneracy of solutions inherent in IMPT can be used. Indeed, this solution has been proposed as a potential method of delivering proton therapy. The concept of distal edge tracking for proton therapy was first suggested by Deasy and colleagues and has subsequently been investigated in detail by Lomax, Oelfke and Bortfeld, and Nill and colleagues.[7,25–27] These latter authors argued that the optimization of IMPT can be simplified and the results improved when just considering a two-dimensionally distributed set of single Bragg peaks, each of which is delivered with an energy that is just sufficient to place the Bragg peak at the distal end of the target volume. Although the distal edge tracking approach can never provide a homogeneous dose to the entire target from a single field direction, it can provide clinically acceptable solutions, applying four to five angularly spaced and individually modulated fields (Figure 28-5D). Proponents of this approach claim that (at least for centrally situated tumors) this method minimizes the total integral dose delivered to the patient, sharpens the lateral falloff of the resulting three-dimensional dose distribution, and can be more rapidly calculated and delivered.[26] On the other hand, this large degeneracy can be exploited in other ways, for instance, by providing greater flexibility for sculpting dose around the target volume and critical structures, particularly in complex cases. Examples of such cases are presented in the following section.

Clinical Potential

Of the 166 patients treated with dynamic proton therapy at PSI, 15 have been treated using IMPT as part of their treatment. Figure 28-6 illustrates the three-field IMPT plan used to treat a 10-year-old girl with a lumbar chordoma. Although the clinical target volume (CTV) was relatively small, we elected to treat the entire vertebrae to at least 20 Gy to reduce the risk of asymmetric bone growth. However, to keep the dose to the spinal cord below tolerance, 3DIMPT was used to "sculpt" the dose away from the spinal cord, despite the

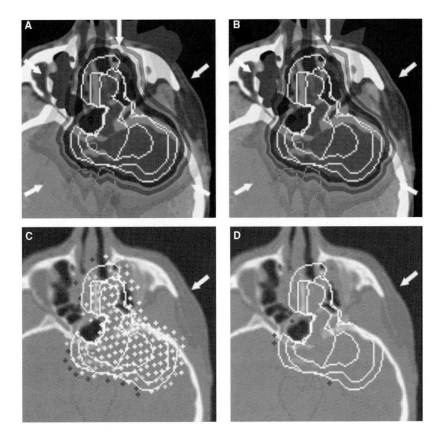

FIGURE 28-5. Two intensity-modulated proton therapy (IMPT) plans in a patient with an angiosarcoma (*A*) and (*B*). The corresponding Bragg peak distributions are shown in (*C*) and (*D*). Although the two dose distributions are very similar, they have been calculated using very different Bragg peak distributions and weights, indicating the considerable amount of degeneracy available to IMPT optimization schemes. Arrows indicate the the field directions used for the plan. (To view a color version of this image, please refer to the CD-ROM.)

fact that this structure was within the PTV. An interesting aspect of this plan is that the three fields used were all applied from the posterior aspect of the patient (as indicated in the figure), reducing both the dose to the intestine and the normal tissues as a whole. The ability to produce "doughnut"-like dose distributions with a small number of incident beams, with each beam incident from a single aspect of the patient, is a unique characteristic of 3DIMPT.

Figure 28-7 illustrates a three-field 3DIMPT plan in a patient with a chondrosarcoma of the skull base. The PTV is particularly large in this case and completely overlaps with the optic chiasm and partially with both optic nerves. The PTV is also in close proximity to the brainstem. Note that planning volumes to the organs at risk have been added, accounting for setup uncertainties. Despite the complexity of the case and the demands made on the plan as a result of the overlapping critical structures, the delivered IMPT plan was able to reduce the doses to the brainstem and chiasm to below 30% and 70% of the prescription dose, respectively, while maximally irradiating the remaining portions of the PTV. This case clearly demonstrates the ability of 3DIMPT for delivering highly conformal and, indeed, conformally avoided distributions in difficult clinical situations.

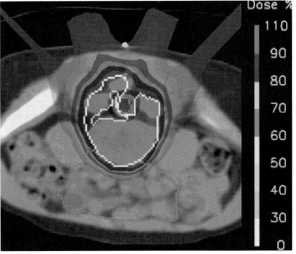

FIGURE 28-6. A three-field three-dimensional intensity-modulated proton therapy plan applied to a 10-year-old girl with a lumbar chordoma. All three fields are incident from the posterior aspect (thus minimizing the dose to the intestines that lie anteriorly to the target volume). Through three-dimensional modulation of the individual Bragg peaks, it is possible to "sculpt" the dose out of the spinal cord, which is embedded within the planning target volume. (To view a color version of this image, please refer to the CD-ROM.)

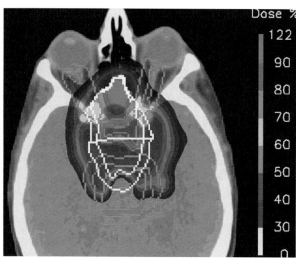

FIGURE 28-7. A three-field three-dimensional intensity-modulated proton therapy plan calculated and applied to a patient with a skull base chordoma. Note the excellent sparing of the brainstem (dose below the 30% level) and the sparing of the chiasm and optic nerves (between 60 and 70%). The concentric contours around the different organs at risk are planning organ at risk volumes, defined to apply a safety margin around these structures. (To view a color version of this image, please refer to the CD-ROM.)

Summary

Dynamic approaches to delivering proton therapy can be considered to be the current state of the art. Although, currently, spot scanning and IMPT can be delivered at only one institute, the potential of both methods is attracting great interest in both the academic and the commercial proton communities. Based on this experience, all new proton therapy facilities, either currently under construction or planned in the near future, will have a scanning capability. Both methods have considerable potential to conform the dose to complex target geometries while simultaneously reducing the overall dose delivered to the patient.

However, a number of challenges remain. In particular, the application of a large number of narrow and individually modulated proton pencil beams is particularly sensitive to organ motions.[28] Before such methods can be applied in areas of mobile tumors, methods have to be developed for reducing the sensitivity of this delivery technique to motion artifacts. Rescanning is one option,[29] and this is currently being investigated at PSI as part of the development of a second-generation scanning gantry.[30] Nevertheless, proton therapy is increasingly being seen as the next logical step in the development of external beam RT. Over the next several years, many new facilities, mostly hospital based, are expected.

References

1. Wilson RR. Radiological use of fast protons. Radiology 1946;47:487–91.
2. Sisterson J. World wide charged particle patient totals 2003. Particles Newsletter 2003;32.
3. Koehler AM, Schneider RJ, Sisterson JM. Range modulators for protons and heavy ions. Med Phys 1975;131:437–40.
4. Koehler AM, Schneider RJ, Sisterson JM. Flattening of proton dose distributions for large fields. Nucl Instrum Meth 1977;4:297–301.
5. Kanai T, Kanai K, Kumamoto Y, et al. Spot scanning system for radiotherapy. Med Phys 1980;7:365–9.
6. Pedroni E, Bacher E, Blattmann H, et al. The 200 MeV proton therapy project at PSI: conceptual design and practical realization. Med Phys 1995;22:37–53.
7. Lomax AJ. Intensity modulated methods for proton therapy. Phys Med Biol 1999;44:185–205.
8. Lomax AJ, Boehringer T, Coray A, et al. Intensity modulated proton therapy: a clinical example. Med Phys 2001;28:317–24.
9. Miralbell R, Lomax AJ, Russo M. Potential role of proton therapy in the treatment of paediatric medulloblastoma/primitive neuroectodermal tumors: spinal theca irradiation. Int J Radiat Oncol Biol Phys 1997;38:805–11.
10. Zurlo, A, Lomax AJ, Hoess A, et al. The role of proton therapy in the treatment of large irradiation volumes: a comparative planning study of pancreatic and biliary tumours. Int J Radiat Oncol Biol Phys 2000;48:277–88.
11. Cozzi L, Fogliata A, Lomax AJ, et al. A treatment planning comparison of 3D conformal therapy, intensity modulated photon therapy and proton therapy for treatment of advanced head and neck tumours. Radiother Oncol 2001;61:287–97.
12. Fogliata, A, Bolsi A, Cozzi L. Critical appraisal of treatment techniques based on quasi-conventional, intensity modulated photon beams and proton beams for therapy of intact breast. Radiother Oncol 2002;62:137–45.
13. Lomax AJ, Cella L, Weber D, et al. Potential role of IMRT and protons in the treatment of the breast and regional nodes. Int J Radiat Oncol Biol Phys 2003;55:785–92.
14. Miralbell R, Cella L, Weber D, et al. Optimizing radiotherapy of orbital and paraorbital tumors: intensity modulated x-ray beams versus intensity modulated proton beams. Int J Radiat Oncol Biol Phys 2000;47:1111–9.
15. Cella L, Lomax AJ, Miralbell R. Potential role of intensity modulated proton beams in prostate cancer radiotherapy. Int J Radiat Oncol Biol Phys 2001;49:217–23.
16. Lomax AJ, Goitein M, Adams J. Intensity modulation in radiotherapy: photons versus protons. Radiother Oncol 2003;66:11–8.
17. Petti PL, Lyman JT, Renner TR, et al. Design of beam-modulating devices for charged-particle therapy. Med Phys 1991;18:513–8.
18. Petti PL. New compensator design options for charged-particle radiotherapy. Phys Med Biol 1997;42:1289–300.
19. Lomax AJ, Pedroni E, Schaffner B, et al. 3D treatment planning for conformal proton therapy by spot scanning. In: Proceedings of the 19th L. H. Gray Conference. London: BIR Publishing; 1996. p. 67–71.

20. Pedroni E. Therapy planning system for the SIN-pion therapy facility. Strahlenther Onkol 1981;77:60–9.

21. Scheib S. Spot-scanning mit Protonen: experimentelle Resultate und Therapieplanung [dissertation]. Zurich: Technical High School (ETH); 1993.

22. Harberer T. Magnetic scanning system for heavy ion therapy. Nucl Instr Meth 1993;330:296–305.

23. Lomax AJ, Boehringer T, Bolsi A, et al. Treatment planning and verification of proton therapy using spot scanning: initial experiences. Med Phys 2004.

24. Marchand B, Prieels D, Bauvir B, et al. IBA proton pencil beam scanning: an innovative solution for cancer treatment. In: Proceedings of the 7th European Particle Accelerator Conference (EPAC2000); Vienna, Austria. Madison, WI: Medical Physics Publishing; 2000.

25. Deasy JO, Shephard DM, Mackie TR. Distal edge tracking: a proposed delivery method for conformal proton therapy using intensity modulation. In: Leavitt DD, Starkschall GS, editors. Proceedings of the XIIth ICCR, Salt Lake City. Madison (WI): Medical Physics Publishing; 1997. pp. 406–9.

26. Oelfke U, Bortfeld T. Intensity modulated radiotherapy with charged particle beams: studies of inverse treatment planning for rotation therapy. Med Phys 2000;27:1246–57.

27. Nill S, Bortfeld T, Oelfke U. Inverse planning of intensity modulated proton therapy. Z Med Phys 2004;24:35–40.

28. Philips MH, Pedroni E, Blattmann H, et al. Effects of respiratory motion on dose uniformity with a charged particle scanning system. Phys Med Biol 1992;37:223–34.

29. Bortfeld T, Jokivarsi K, Goitein M, et al. Effects of intra-fraction motion on IMRT dose delivery: statistical analysis and simulation. Phys Med Biol 2002;47:2203–20.

30. Pedroni E, Bearpark R, Boehringer T, et al. The PSI gantry 2: a second generation proton scanning gantry. Z Med Phys 2004;14:25–34.

Chapter 29

BIOLOGIC MODIFIERS AND IMRT

KENNETH DORNFELD, MD, PhD, JOHN BUATTI, MD

Biologic modifiers of radiation response comprise a large number of agents and compounds, including traditional (known) radiation sensitizers, radiation sensitizing agents under development, gene therapy approaches, and radiation protecting agents. The purpose of this chapter is to review issues regarding the combination of these biologic modifiers with intensity-modulated radiation therapy (IMRT). Particular attention is focused on the problems and opportunities arising from the unique features of IMRT. In addition, the available clinical data on combining IMRT and radiation response modifiers are reviewed.

There are two fundamental differences between IMRT and conventional RT in regard to biologic modifiers. First, an increased volume of normal tissue receives low-dose radiation with IMRT. The significance of this phenomenon through both the use of multiple fields and increased collimator leakage during IMRT has been described and quantified elsewhere.[1] Second, IMRT offers the potential to generate more heterogeneous dose distributions across treatment and target tissues. The possibility of delivering different doses to different regions within a field creates issues of gradient matching within treatment fields, and this has been described by Butler and colleagues.[2] These authors combined treatment to high risk and subclinical risk for head and neck cancer treatment. The gross disease received 2.4 Gy per fraction concurrently with 2.0 Gy to the subclinical disease. These two properties of IMRT have significant implications for how radiation and its modifiers interact in tissue.

Radiation Sensitizers

Biologic modifications of radiation response are meant to increase the therapeutic ratio of radiation therapy (RT), that is, the ratio of toxicity to tumor versus normal tissues. Increasing this ratio can be accomplished by either increasing toxicity selectively for tumor tissues or decreasing toxicity selectively for normal tissues. Many agents with diverse modes of action have been used to modify radiation toxicity for tumor tissues. A brief list of radiation sensitizers includes halogenated pyrimidines, hydroxyurea, cisplatin, mitomycin C, misonidazole, paclitaxel, carmustine, epidermal growth factor receptor (EGFR) inhibitors, and several others. By far, most information regarding radiation sensitizing agents is derived from in vitro experiments, usually clonogenic survival studies, assessing the effect of radiation over a range of doses. A modifier's effect is expressed as the dose enhancement ratio (DER) and is calculated by dividing the dose of radiation necessary to achieve a defined effect, such as 10% survival, by the dose of radiation used with the modifier (Figure 29-1).

Although in vitro data are essential when initially characterizing radiation modifiers, more relevant data regarding the effect of sensitizers on tissue and organ tolerance are necessary. Animal models bearing xenograft tumors now serve as the primary source of preclinical data on radiation sensitizers. Although animal models provide important information for in vivo interactions for tumor tissue, they are rarely able to provide information regarding normal orthotopic tissue effects. Reports on clinical human data using radiation sensitizers with conventional RT typically include treatment effects on tumor tissues, but the effects on normal tissues are usually less well characterized. The current challenge in integrating biologic modifiers with IMRT is using existing information regarding the impact of modifiers on increased volumes of normal tissue receiving low-dose radiation and the effects of potentially higher doses per fraction within the target tissues. Some examples of clinical data are offered as an illustration.

Fluorodeoxyuridine (FUdR) has been used as a radiation sensitizer for decades. FUDR delivered via hepatic artery infusion has been combined with partial liver irradiation.[3] This approach has enabled safe dose escalation to a portion of the liver, although not resulting in undue liver toxicity from lower yet still significant doses of radiation delivered by beam entrance and exit to the normal (FUdR perfused) liver.[3] In addition, the radiation tolerance for whole-organ

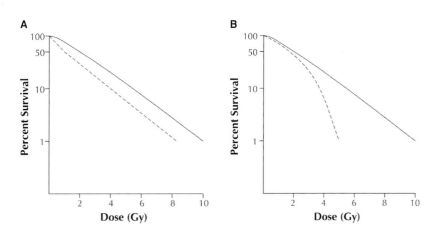

FIGURE 29-1. Examples of dose-response curves for a fictitious cell line exposed to radiation in the presence and absence of a radiosensitizing drug. In the absence of a drug, these cells show a 50% survival rate at 2 Gy and a 1% survival rate at 10 Gy. In (*A*) the dose enhancement ratio (DER) is greater at low doses, such that combined treatment leads to 50% survival at 1 Gy (DER 2.0) and 1% survival at 8.3 Gy (DER 1.2). In (*B*) the DER is greater at higher doses such that combined treatment leads to 50% survival at 1.7 Gy (DER 1.2) and 1% survival at 5 Gy (DER 2.0).

treatment of the liver was not altered by concurrent use of FUdR. Without FUdR, 33 Gy to the whole liver in 1.5 Gy twice-daily fractions results in a 10% risk of radiation-induced liver disease.[4] This is comparable to the dose found by investigators at the University of Michigan using 1.5 Gy twice daily delivered with concurrent FUdR.[5] Therefore, FUdR appears to be a reasonable agent to combine with IMRT for hepatic irradiation because adjacent normal tissues can tolerate the sensitizer and radiation.

Iododeoxyuridine (IUdR) is a radiosensitizer that acts via a mechanism distinct from FUdR. Whereas FUdR acts primarily through thymidylate synthase inhibition, IUdR appears to engender radiosensitization through incorporation into deoxyribonucleic acid (DNA). Miller and colleagues reported that the radiation sensitizing effects of IUdR occur predominantly by affecting the lower-dose portion of the survival curve.[6] Normal tissues surrounding tumor will be sensitized to radiation if they are proliferating and incorporating IUdR into their DNA. Therefore, the increased volume of normal (but sensitized) tissue receiving a low dose with IMRT may lead to increased toxicity for adjacent normal proliferating tissues when using IUdR. Indeed, the toxicity of adjacent proliferating normal tissue was observed when using IUdR in patients with head and neck cancer treated with conventional RT[7] and would be a concern for combining IMRT with IUdR.

IMRT with concurrent chemotherapy for pancreatic cancer provides another example of how properties of the sensitizing agent are important in combining IMRT with modifiers. Ben-Josef and colleagues used capecitabine with IMRT for pancreatic cancer and found concurrent treatment tolerable.[8] Bai and colleagues used IMRT concurrently with 5-fluorouracil for pancreatic cancer and likewise found concurrent treatment tolerable.[9] In contrast, gemcitabine delivered concurrently with IMRT was not tolerable, as reported by Crane and colleagues. A pilot study reported by Crane and colleagues showed the maximum tolerated dose of gemcitabine to be 350 mg/m[2] in combination with 30 Gy in 3 Gy fractions delivered with

conventional four-field conformal RT.[10] In a subsequent dose escalation trial using IMRT, these same authors used the identical radiation schedule and found that gemcitabine at 250 mg/m[2] was not tolerated.[11] The two trials were reported separately and were not intended to address the effects of conventional RT versus IMRT by direct comparison. However, their data may suggest that the gemcitabine and RT combination was less tolerable when the radiation was delivered via IMRT. For sensitizing agents that have effects on adjacent normal tissues at low doses, combined use with IMRT may result in increased toxicity. The pancreatic experience may serve to highlight the complexity of combining IMRT with different sensitizers.

Newer Radiation Modifiers and IMRT

Increased understanding of the molecular changes involved in carcinogenesis should lead to therapies exploiting the molecular differences between normal and cancerous tissues.[12] Antiangiogenic factors, cyclooxygenase inhibitors, polyribose polymerase inhibitors, cell-cycle modulators, and farnesyl transferase inhibitors are among the many agents developed to exploit specific differences in tumor cell biology. Many of these agents have been investigated as radiation response modifiers.[12,13] The list of agents is too extensive to review each class of agents here. One example of agents designed to exploit molecular changes present in cancer cells is the EGFR inhibitors.[14,15] The specificity of these approaches should increase the therapeutic ratio of radiation treatments and minimize normal tissue toxicity. These agents have been combined with radiation.

The combination of EGFR inhibition and RT has been studied in vitro, in vivo, and in several clinical trials.[16] The appeal of manipulating EGFR for radiosensitization is that many tumors, particularly high-grade glioma and head and neck cancers, have a high rate of EGFR overexpression. EGFR signaling enhances radioresistance.[17] Several agents have been described that can inhibit EGFR signaling.[16] These include the low-molecular-weight compound that inhibits EGFR tyrosine kinase activity, gefitinib (ZD1839, Iressa), and the monoclonal antibody recognizing and inhibiting EGFR, C225 (cetuximab). The activity of gefitinib against non–small cell lung cancers has been modest.[18] However, in a recent report analyzing patients' genotype for EGFR, a marked response was found in patients with certain genetic alterations in EGFR.[19] The observed significant difference in responses highlights the need to use targeted therapies against appropriately selected patients. Combined irradiation and EGFR blockade will also most likely benefit from selecting patients with alterations in EGFR signaling.

The EGFR signal inhibitor ZD1839 has been studied extensively. Strikingly greater than additive effects were observed with combined fractionated RT and ZD1839 in tumor growth delay studies using the A431 vulvar squamous cell cancer line in the mouse xenograft system.[20] This cell line overexpresses EGFR. Interestingly, the DER for tumor growth delay was dose dependent. For a single 10 Gy dose, the DER was 1.5, whereas a schedule of 4 × 2.5 Gy produced a DER of 4.[20] Although these dosing schemes have slightly different biologically effective doses, the pronounced effect of fractionation and dose per fraction are still worth noting. If substantiated in relevant preclinical and clinical situations in vivo, the effect of fraction size on DER could be significant, particularly for IMRT applications. One method of delivering IMRT for head and neck cancer uses a so-called "SMART" (simultaneous modulated accelerated radiation therapy) boost technique that delivers a differential dose rate across target tissues.[2] In this approach, high-risk areas (gross disease) receive 2.4 Gy per fraction, whereas subclinical disease sites receive 2.0 Gy per fraction. If the DER for ZD1839 is dose dependent and decreases with increased dose per fraction, the SMART boost IMRT scheme may actually diminish the radiosensitizing effects of ZD1839 in the gross tumor.

Altering the signals produced by aberrant EGFR signaling in selected tumors would potentially widen the therapeutic ratio because normal tissues do not have an abnormality in this pathway. This appears to be the case for head and neck cancers. A phase III trial conducted with C225 and radiation for patients with head and neck cancer was recently reported by Bonner and colleagues at the 2004 meeting of the American Society for Clinical Oncology.[21] Their results demonstrated a significant survival advantage with the addition of C225. Interestingly, the combined therapy did not result in increased skin or other toxicity, an important finding because anti-EGFR agents by themselves have produced a mild skin reaction. Low-molecular-weight inhibitors such as ZD1839 and CI1033, as well as C225, are in various stages of clinical investigation. As anti-EGFR agents are combined with IMRT, the effects on normal tissues exposed to the agent and lower doses of radiation should be monitored and reported with dose-volume metrics.

Few clinical data exist that directly address the relative toxicity of conventional RT versus IMRT when delivered concurrently with a radiation sensitizing agent. The points raised above argue that as IMRT and radiosensitizers are brought together in the clinic, special attention should be paid to the mechanism of action of the sensitizer, the effects of the sensitizer at low doses of radiation, the effect of fraction size on the DER, and the volume and type of normal tissue exposed to low-dose radiation.

The effects of radiation sensitizers on normal tissues have been difficult to study.[22] Subjective end points, variable amounts of treated tissues, comorbid illnesses, and a focus on tumor control rather than toxicity are all reasons why a thorough understanding of the effect of radiosensitizers on normal tissue is lacking. As IMRT is combined with the plethora of available modifying agents, special attention should be paid to normal tissue toxicity and then reported in clinical trials as a function of dose and volume. The variation in volume of normal tissue irradiation between patients afforded by IMRT should provide a rich source of data to further our understanding of the effect of radiosensitizers on normal tissues. These analyses will need to be performed for each agent but should also make use of dose-volume analysis tools readily available during IMRT planning.

Besides the increase in the volume of normal tissues receiving low-dose radiation, IMRT also varies from conventional delivery by the ability to deliver high doses within a portion of the treatment volume. Again, the potential gains in combining this feature of IMRT with sensitizing agents are dependent on the therapeutic ratio of the sensitizing agent. The DER, as defined previously, is typically reported for a single effect, such as a certain colony survival fraction, and is usually based on in vitro data. The DER typically varies for different doses in an agent-specific manner such that for many agents, higher doses yield proportionately more killing. In contrast, for some agents, the DER decreases as the dose per fraction increases, so that although radiation plus a sensitizer kills more cells than radiation alone at high doses, the combination may kill proportionately fewer tumor cells than with lower doses of radiation. Few data address how the effects of sensitizing agents on tumor versus normal tissues vary with fraction size, but given the potential of IMRT to exploit this variable, sensitizers should be analyzed for the variation of the DER at high and low doses.

Conformal Chemotherapy

As the delivery of RT becomes more precise in an effort to reduce normal tissue toxicity, efforts to deliver chemotherapy in a more anatomically precise manner are also under way. Among the approaches being used to deliver targeted chemotherapy are intra-arterial infusion, liposomal or carrier-complexed chemotherapy, and gene therapy.

The utility of intra-arterial delivery of chemotherapy for intrahepatic[23] and head and neck cancers[24] has been clearly established. Worthy of a full review on their own, these treatment approaches are mentioned here to highlight the potential use of combining anatomically limited combined-modality therapy. Robbins and colleagues described the use of selective arterial catheterization to infuse cisplatin into vessels supplying the tumor with radiation therapy (termed RADPLAT).[25] Intravenous delivery of sodium thiosulfate is used to counter systemic distribution of the cisplatin. The appeal of this method is that the chemotherapy delivered to normal systemic structures, such as bone marrow, can be minimized. Quality-of-life assessments in patients undergoing RADPLAT therapy appear to support its use and indicate reasonable toxicity.[26] Given the significant short- and long-term toxicity of combined-modality therapy for head and neck cancer treatment, it is appealing to consider the possibilities of limiting radiation dose and chemotherapy dose to sensitive, uninvolved sites during head and neck cancer treatment. Anatomically confined chemotherapy would also limit radiosensitization produced in the increased volume of normal tissue irradiated via IMRT.

Other methods to deliver radiation sensitizing agents to a limited amount of treated tissue are currently being developed. Two examples include chemotherapeutic agents in matrix, such as carmustine[27] or cisplatin embedded in polymers for slow release.[28] Several other chemotherapy agents have been complexed into a solid form for slow, localized release.[29] Complexed radiosensitizing agents would provide an additional means to limit the toxic effects of chemotherapy to tumor tissues. Localized delivery of chemotherapy may decrease the amount of normal tissue being sensitized to low-dose irradiation in IMRT delivery.

Gene therapy also holds promise as a method to deliver radiation sensitizing drugs to target tissues. Gene therapy typically involves transfer of a gene into target tissues by injection of a modified adenovirus into tissues to be modified. Although many other methods have been investigated, adenoviral delivery appears to offer the most efficient approach. Even with adenovirus, the efficiency of gene transfer is very limited.[30] Therefore, successful gene therapy methods must currently alter a target cell not only to affect itself but also surrounding cells. This so-called bystander effect is meant to amplify the effects of gene therapy; thus, the rare cells that do become altered and express the exogenous gene are able to affect several adjacent cells.

One such example is the use of gene therapy to impart cytosine deaminase or thymidine kinase activity to tumor tissue. This approach, termed enzyme-dependent prodrug therapy, allows an innocuous prodrug such as fluorocytosine or a thymidine analog (typically ganciclovir) to be delivered to the patient. Only the tissues expressing the gene would convert the prodrug to the cytotoxic or radiation sensitizing agent, fluorouracil in the case of cytosine deaminase or phosphorylated ganciclovir in the case of thymidine kinase. This approach has been used in the treatment of prostate cancer.[31,32] As for infusional or complexed chemotherapeutics, this application of gene therapy is a means to limit the effects of chemotherapy to the anatomic site being treated.

Another attractive potential use of gene therapy is to modify tumor cells in such a way that they become uniquely able to concentrate a radioactive isotope. This could be achieved by delivering the gene for the sodium iodide symporter that concentrates iodide in thyroid tissue. This method seeks to modify tumor tissues to have the ability to concentrate ^{131}I. In essence, this approach could convert tumor tissue to be avid for ^{131}I and amenable to iodide ablation, as is currently used for thyroid cancer. Termed cellular brachytherapy,[33] the sodium-iodide symporter may provide a means to deliver a boost of radiation over a very limited anatomic region. The anatomic precision of IMRT may allow a unique combination and dose escalation with these two techniques.

IMRT and Radiation Protectors

If IMRT increases the volume of normal tissues irradiated to lower doses, the potential for increased acute and late side effects is increased, as discussed above. Possible radiation protective agents would therefore be particularly useful for IMRT delivered alone or with concurrent chemotherapy. Supporting its use with IMRT, amifostine (Ethyol, MedImmune Inc., Gaithersberg, MD) appears to be most effective as a radiation protective agent for lower doses of radiation.[34] The utility of amifostine with IMRT is currently under investigation in head and neck cancer treatment.[35] In their study, Thorstad and colleagues delivered amifostine subcutaneously. Unfortunately, nausea appeared to be a persistent problem, with 5 of 15 patients discontinuing amifostine because of nausea.[35] The final results of this study are currently pending.

Conformal RT and amifostine are also being combined in the treatment of prostate cancer. An ongoing study is evaluating the utility of endorectal delivery of amifostine and RT.[36] Amifostine appears to accumulate preferentially in rectal mucosa, whereas prostate and systemic levels appear to be quite limited. Early results in the first 10 patients suggest that the acute side effects of radiation are not significantly reduced compared with historical controls not treated with amifostine. It remains to be seen if a difference will be found as more patients are enrolled. The late tissue effects of radiation are more typically dose-limiting events, and these toxicities are still being determined.

The question of late-term toxicities, including second malignancies, following IMRT alone or with chemotherapy remains open. In vivo animal study data suggest that amifostine is able to reduce mutation rates following radiation exposure[37] and therefore may play an important role in reducing both the long-term and short-term toxicity of IMRT. If the finding of lower mutation rates is confirmed using additional in vivo modeling systems, amifostine may be able to reduce second cancers after IMRT. The increased amount of normal tissue receiving low-dose radiation has prompted some concern over the possibility of increased second malignancy rates using IMRT compared with conventional RT.[38]

Amifostine also appears to be able to limit the toxicity of chemoradiation, at least within in vitro systems.[39] The use of amifostine in this setting is particularly important, again given the concerns mentioned above regarding IMRT and chemotherapy and the increased amount of normal tissue receiving lower doses of RT.

Other radiation protective agents, such as manganese superoxide dismutase (MnSOD), may also show benefit in combination with IMRT. Gene therapy using either liposomal or adenoviral delivery of the MnSOD gene to various normal tissues in rodent models has shown increased radiation tolerance.[40] Given that many of the effects of ionizing radiation are mediated through generation of oxidative species, superoxide dismutase, by detoxifying superoxide, should lead to decreased radiation effects in tissues expressing increased amounts of MnSOD. The encouraging preclinical data have led to currently ongoing clinical trials using plasmid or liposomal delivery of MnSOD to reduce mucositis in head and neck treatment and esophagitis in non–small cell lung cancer treatment.[40] As described above, this protection could be particularly useful for IMRT treatments.

Summary

Biologic modifiers of radiation response are being developed and used more commonly in both laboratory research and clinical practice. The combination of biologic modifiers and IMRT poses unique opportunities and challenges. To best realize opportunities and meet these challenges, the tools developed to understand the combined effects of modifying agents with radiation should be applied. Not only must the unique properties of the biologic agent be understood but also the properties of the cancer and normal tissues being treated and the unique properties of IMRT. In particular, the features of IMRT that merit close attention are the increased volume of normal tissue receiving low-dose radiation and the potential to deliver increased fraction sizes within a treatment volume. Whether these features of IMRT will be important in combination with a biologic agent will depend on the individual properties of the agent. The tools necessary to study these questions include dose-volume histograms, careful determinations of DER, and other standard techniques used to study radiation effects but now applied with attention to the characteristic features of IMRT.

References

1. Meeks SL, Paulino AC, Pennington EC, et al. In vivo determination of extra-target doses received from serial tomotherapy. Radiother Oncol 2002;63:217–22.

2. Butler EB, Teh BS, Grant WH III, et al. SMART (simultaneous modulated accelerated radiation therapy) boost: a new accelerated fractionation schedule for the treatment of head and neck cancer with intensity modulated radiotherapy. Int J Radiat Oncol Biol Phys 1999;45:21–32.

3. Dawson LA, McGinn CJ, Normolle D, et al. Escalated focal liver radiation and concurrent hepatic artery fluorodeoxyuridine for unresectable intrahepatic malignancies. J Clin Oncol 2000;18:2210–8.

4. Russell AH, Clyde C, Wasserman TH, et al. Accelerated hyperfractionated hepatic irradiation in the management of patients with liver metastases: results of the RTOG dose escalating protocol. Int J Radiat Oncol Biol Phys 1993;27:117–23.

5. Lawrence TS, Ten Haken RK, Kessler ML, et al. The use of 3-D dose volume analysis to predict radiation hepatitis. Int J Radiat Oncol Biol Phys 1992;23:781–8.

6. Miller EM, Fowler JF, Kinsella TJ. Linear-quadratic analysis of radiosensitization by halogenated pyrimidines. I. Radiosensitization of human colon cancer cells by iododeoxyuridine. Radiat Res 1992;131:81–9.

7. Epstein AH, Lebovics RS, Van Waes C, et al. Intravenous delivery of 5′-iododeoxyuridine during hyperfractionated radiotherapy for locally advanced head and neck cancers: results of a pilot study. Laryngoscope 1998;108:1090–4.

8. Ben-Josef E, Shields AF, Vaishampayan U, et al. Intensity-modulated radiotherapy (IMRT) and concurrent capecitabine for pancreatic cancer. Int J Radiat Oncol Biol Phys 2004;59:454–9.

9. Bai YR, Wu GH, Guo WJ, et al. Intensity modulated radiation therapy and chemotherapy for locally advanced pancreatic cancer: results of feasibility study. World J Gastroenterol 2003;9:2561–4.

10. Crane CH, Abbruzzese JL, Evans DB, et al. Is the therapeutic index better with gemcitabine-based chemoradiation than with 5-fluorouracil-based chemoradiation in locally advanced pancreatic cancer? Int J Radiat Oncol Biol Phys 2002;52:1293–302.

11. Crane CH, Antolak JA, Rosen II, et al. Phase I study of concomitant gemcitabine and IMRT for patients with unresectable adenocarcinoma of the pancreatic head. Int J Gastrointest Cancer 2001;30:123–32.

12. Ma BB, Bristow RG, Kim J, et al. Combined-modality treatment of solid tumors using radiotherapy and molecular targeted agents. J Clin Oncol 2003;21:2760–76.

13. Brown JM. Therapeutic targets in radiotherapy. Int J Radiat Oncol Biol Phys 2001;49:319–26.

14. Harari PM, Huang SM. Combining EGFR inhibitors with radiation or chemotherapy: will preclinical studies predict clinical results? Int J Radiat Oncol Biol Phys 2004;58:976–83.

15. Milas L, Fan Z, Andratschke NH, et al. Epidermal growth factor receptor and tumor response to radiation: in vivo preclinical studies. Int J Radiat Oncol Biol Phys 2004;58:966–71.

16. Sartor CI. Epidermal growth factor family receptors and inhibitors: radiation response modulators. Semin Radiat Oncol 2003;13:22–30.

17. Ang KK, Andratschke NH, Milas L. Epidermal growth factor receptor and response of head-and-neck carcinoma to therapy. Int J Radiat Oncol Biol Phys 2004;58:959–65.

18. Fukuoka M, Yano S, Giaccone G, et al. Multi-institutional randomized phase II trial of gefitinib for previously treated patients with advanced non-small-cell lung cancer. J Clin Oncol 2003;21:2237–46.

19. Lynch TJ, Bell DW, Sordella R, et al. Activating mutations in the epidermal growth factor receptor underlying responsiveness of non-small-cell lung cancer to gefitinib. N Engl J Med 2004;350:2129–39.

20. Solomon B, Hagekyriakou J, Trivett MK, et al. EGFR blockade with ZD1839 ("Iressa") potentiates the antitumor effects of single and multiple fractions of ionizing radiation in human A431 squamous cell carcinoma. Epidermal growth factor receptor. Int J Radiat Oncol Biol Phys 2003;55:713–23.

21. Bonner JA, Giralt J, Harari PM, et al. Cetuximab prolongs survival in patients with locoregionally advanced squamous cell carcinoma of head and neck: a phase III study of high dose radiation therapy with or without cetuximab. J Clin Oncol 2004;22(14S):489.

22. Poggi MM, Coleman CN, Mitchell JB. Sensitizers and protectors of radiation and chemotherapy. Curr Probl Cancer 2001;25:334–411.

23. Lawrence TS, Dworzanin LM, Walker-Andrews SC, et al. Treatment of cancers involving the liver and porta hepatis with external beam irradiation and intraarterial hepatic fluorodeoxyuridine. Int J Radiat Oncol Biol Phys 1991;20:555–61.

24. Wilson WR, Siegel RS, Harisiadis LA, et al. High-dose intra-arterial cisplatin therapy followed by radiation therapy for advanced squamous cell carcinoma of the head and neck. Arch Otolaryngol Head Neck Surg 2001;127:809–12.

25. Robbins KT, Doweck I, Samant S, et al. Factors predictive of local disease control after intra-arterial concomitant chemoradiation (RADPLAT). Laryngoscope 2004;114:411–7.

26. Ackerstaff AH, Tan IB, Rasch CR, et al. Quality-of-life assessment after supradose selective intra-arterial cisplatin and concomitant radiation (RADPLAT) for inoperable stage IV head and neck squamous cell carcinoma. Arch Otolaryngol Head Neck Surg 2002;128:1185–90.

27. Brem H, Ewend MG, Piantadosi S, et al. The safety of interstitial chemotherapy with BCNU-loaded polymer followed by radiation therapy in the treatment of newly diagnosed malignant gliomas: phase I trial. J Neurooncol 1995;26:111–23.

28. Yapp DT, Lloyd DK, Zhu J, et al. The potentiation of the effect of radiation treatment by intratumoral delivery of cisplatin. Int J Radiat Oncol Biol Phys 1998;42:413–20.

29. Shikani AH, Domb AJ. Polymer chemotherapy for head and neck cancer. Laryngoscope 2000;110:907–17.

30. Lang FF, Bruner JM, Fuller GN, et al. Phase I trial of adenovirus-mediated p53 gene therapy for recurrent glioma: biological and clinical results. J Clin Oncol 2003;21:2508–18.

31. Freytag SO, Stricker H, Pegg J, et al. Phase I study of replication-competent adenovirus-mediated double-suicide gene therapy in combination with conventional-dose three-dimensional conformal radiation therapy for the treatment of newly diagnosed, intermediate- to high-risk prostate cancer. Cancer Res 2003;63:7497–506.

32. Teh BS, Ayala G, Aguilar L, et al. Phase I-II trial evaluating combined intensity-modulated radiotherapy and in situ gene therapy with or without hormonal therapy in treatment of prostate cancer-interim report on PSA response and biopsy data. Int J Radiat Oncol Biol Phys 2004;58:1520–9.

33. Gaut AW, Niu G, Krager KJ, et al. Genetically targeted radiotherapy of head and neck squamous cell carcinoma using the sodium-iodide symporter (NIS). Head Neck 2004;26:265–71.

34. Rojas A, Denekamp J. The influence of x ray dose levels on normal tissue radioprotection by WR-2721. Int J Radiat Oncol Biol Phys 1984;10:2351–6.

35. Thorstad WL, Haughey B, Chao KS. Pilot study of subcutaneous amifostine in patients undergoing postoperative intensity modulated radiation therapy for head and neck cancer: preliminary data. Semin Oncol 2003;30(6 Suppl 18):96–100.

36. Menard C, Camphausen K, Muanza T, et al. Clinical trial of endorectal amifostine for radioprotection in patients with prostate cancer: rationale and early results. Semin Oncol 2003;30(6 Suppl 18):63–7.

37. Grdina DJ, Kataoka Y, Basic I, et al. The radioprotector WR-2721 reduces neutron-induced mutations at the hypoxanthine-guanine phosphoribosyl transferase locus in mouse splenocytes when administered prior to or following irradiation. Carcinogenesis 1992;13:811–4.

38. Hall EJ, Wuu CS. Radiation-induced second cancers: the impact of 3D-CRT and IMRT. Int J Radiat Oncol Biol Phys 2003;56:83–8.

39. Komaki R, Lee JS, Milas L, et al. Effects of amifostine on acute toxicity from concurrent chemotherapy and radiotherapy for inoperable non-small-cell lung cancer: report of a randomized comparative trial. Int J Radiat Oncol Biol Phys 2004;58:1369–77.

40. Greenberger JS, Epperly MW, Gretton J, et al. Radioprotective gene therapy. Curr Gene Ther 2003;3:183–95.

Chapter 30

Pros and Cons of IMRT

What's Been Swept Under the Rug?

Roberto J. Santiago, MD, Eli Glatstein, MD

Perspective

Before embarking on a discussion of the merits and disadvantages of intensity-modulated radiation therapy (IMRT), it is worthwhile to reflect on the role of radiation in the treatment of cancer. The main goal in all cancer therapy is improvement of survival, in terms of both duration and quality of life. Ultimately, cancer survival is a reflection of five factors: aggressiveness of the tumor, intrinsic efficacy of the therapies, applicability of the therapies, toxicities secondary to treatment, and, finally, the clinical judgment and experience of the physician(s) who carries out the treatment.

It is clear that cancers are very heterogeneous in their biologic behavior. This is true not only when comparing different types of cancer but also when comparing the same type of cancer in different patients. In fact, it is well known that there are biologic differences among cells within the same tumor. These differences are well illustrated by the development of metastatic capability in some cells.

The ability of a particular therapy to control a specific tumor is also affected by cell heterogeneity. Routinely, diagrams plotted on linear scales have been used to illustrate the probabilities of tumor control and normal tissue injury as very steep functions of radiation dose. Moreover, the corresponding sigmoid dose-response curves are assumed to parallel each other, with the tumor shown as being more radiosensitive than normal tissues (ie, the tumor curve to the left of the normal tissue curve). These theoretical curves are depicted in most textbooks (Figure 30-1A); unfortunately, there are virtually no clinical data that confirm these theoretical dose-response curves. However, the radiosensitivity for most tumors cannot be uniformly expected to parallel normal tissue owing to the inherent genetic heterogeneity of cancer cells. Considering this heterogeneity, one would predict tumor radiosensitivity to be correspondingly diverse. This would be depicted as a less

steep dose-response curve for tumor, crossing that of normal tissues (Figure 30-1B). The latter case is more consistent with clinical reality; not all tumors of a particular type respond equally to a specific therapy. The same can be expected from the cells within a particular tumor.

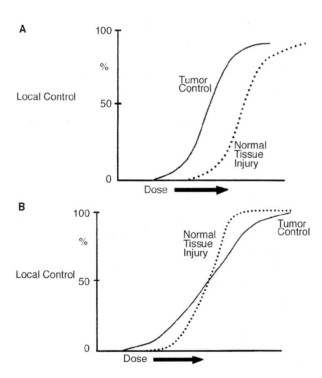

FIGURE 30-1. (*A*) A theoretical diagram of normal tissue injury and local control as functions of increasing dose in linear scale. The curves are conveniently drawn as steep and parallel. (*B*) A more realistic portrayal of normal tissue injury and local control as functions of dose in the clinical setting. The curves are not parallel with less steep tumor control. Reproduced with permission from Glatstein E.[72].

The scope of radiation therapy (RT) has, for the most part, been limited to the treatment of local and regional disease. In other words, RT is used for areas involved with gross tumor or those that, based on the natural history of the disease, are deemed to be at high risk of harboring subclinical disease. Appropriately, its efficacy is best assessed by its impact on locoregional control. However, it is important to emphasize that the majority of cancer patients develop hematogenous metastases and that, typically, these imply widespread, incurable disease. Unfortunately, radiation has proven too toxic to be exploited as a systemic therapy. On the other hand, radiation oncologists should not react by focusing exclusively on local control. It is more appropriate to emphasize RT as an important component of the modern multidisciplinary approach to cancer treatment. This is a conceptually sound approach that addresses both local and systemic disease and in which patient outcome is truly dependent on many disciplines.

Treatment-related toxicities can negate the full benefits of a therapy. In fact, that seems to be the case for patients with early-stage breast carcinoma treated with adjuvant RT after lumpectomy. An overview of randomized trials in patients treated with this strategy revealed that RT significantly reduced cancer-related deaths but not overall mortality.[1] The benefit in cancer-specific survival was offset by an excess in vascular deaths, presumably because of treatment. However, treatment-related toxicity is a difficult topic to dissect. On the one hand, meticulous long-term follow-up is essential to ascertain the incidence of toxicity and the impact of these morbidities on patients' lives. On the other hand, the relevance of long-term toxicity data in regard to current treatment techniques is controversial because RT has improved over time technically. Undeniably, the major contribution of recent technical advances in radiation oncology has been a reduction in toxicity far more than improved tumor control.

IMRT

IMRT entails the manipulation of the radiation fluence as a selected function over time. This is accomplished by dividing a radiation field into a series of segments that are irradiated for different time spans. Integration of these segments achieves modulation of the radiation intensity. In addition, IMRT typically employs multiple, nonopposed radiation beams intersecting within the target volume. This approach essentially spreads modest doses of radiation over normal tissues that integrate to a higher dose throughout the tumor. Often an odd number of coplanar beams (typically between five and nine) is employed; sometimes additional noncoplanar beams are used.

IMRT encompasses a variety of RT planning and delivery techniques. In general, treatment planning for IMRT can be approached in two ways: a forward method or an inverse method. In both methods, the planner, not the computer, determines the appropriate beam directions with which to treat the target. However, in forward planning, the beams are manually conformed to the target and divided into different segments to be irradiated. Subsequently, the weights of the segments are optimized to achieve an appealing dose distribution. In contrast, inverse planning involves optimization of the beam profiles by a computer. This is achieved by providing the computer with a list of constraints describing the desired dose distribution. The process also includes translation of each optimized beam profile into an appropriate sequence of segments delivered by a multileaf collimator (MLC).

Just as IMRT planning can be done in one of two ways, so it can be delivered through one of two methods: a static mode or a dynamic mode. In the static mode, the MLC moves to a preset position and stops, and the beam is turned on for a set period of time. On completion of a segment, the beam is turned off, and the process is repeated. In the dynamic mode, the MLC moves on a continual basis while the beam is on. The point to emphasize here is that there are a range of options under the heading of IMRT, and, as a result, some of the issues discussed in this chapter do not apply equally to all of its variants. However, most of them do.

There are clearly some technical benefits to be obtained from this new tool. Numerous reports show that IMRT can result in improved dose distributions compared with those obtained using other forms of conformal RT. Obviously, the appeal of this capability is in its application to currently problematic clinical situations. However, we encourage radiation oncologists to recognize that every new development has negative and positive aspects. It is very important that both sides of the issue be discussed openly because, thus far, the potential pitfalls have received little attention.

In addition, it is important to acknowledge that because these new technologies represent a major investment of time and resources by vendors, they are here to stay. Conversely, one has to recognize that IMRT has been heavily marketed by both vendors and investigators directly to patients, who, in most cases, cannot truly comprehend the issues and the potential gains (or lack thereof). The media presents it as a major "breakthrough" in treatment. Yet these technologies are refinements of linear accelerator–based RT, not breakthroughs. Treatment still depends on exactly the same interactions between photons and biologic tissues. Furthermore, the planning of this breakthrough is based on stacks of two-dimensional computed tomography (CT) snapshots, which have been in use for over 20 years. Most importantly, prospective data demonstrating unequivocal and clear superiority in clinical outcomes over conformal therapy are presently lacking.

There is no doubt that some patients will benefit from IMRT. However, the answers to the following relevant questions are less clear: How many will truly benefit beyond the accomplishments of conformal RT? Are the substantial health care costs associated with IMRT implementation and use justified? Last but not least, what proportion of patients might actually be harmed by it? Before proclaiming IMRT as the "new standard" in RT, the responsibility of the radiation oncology community is to scour thoroughly (and objectively) for the potential pitfalls of IMRT. Surely, they are to be found somewhere beneath the putative virtues, swept under a proverbial rug.

This chapter reviews the positive and the negative aspects of the development of IMRT. Theoretical, practical, and cost considerations are also discussed.

Theoretical Considerations
Positive

The dose heterogeneity inherent in IMRT can be theoretically exploited by forcing all hot spots within the tumor volume. When this manipulation is combined with the use of multiple nonopposed fields intersecting at the target, the tumor receives radiation at a higher daily dose rate than the normal tissues surrounding it.[2–5] This inherent dose heterogeneity can be used to deliver a simultaneous integrated boost to selected regions of the tumor volume. This approach is theoretically advantageous, not only by shortening the overall treatment time but also by preferentially delivering a presumably more cytotoxic dose per fraction. The result is analogous to accelerated fractionation, which, in some cases, may overcome the problem of accelerated repopulation.[6] Although the survival benefits of such treatment may not be huge, hyperfractionation studies in head and neck cancer already suggest that there will be some modest benefit in outcome by such exploitation.[7]

Another positive theoretical consideration is the potential for safer tumor dose escalation. The capacity to decrease the dose received by normal tissues with IMRT has encouraged escalation of tumor doses. The underlying assumption is that increasing the dose delivered to the tumor will improve local control and, potentially, survival. Tumor dose escalation efforts are not new; IMRT simply facilitates them with its promise of decreasing side effects. As a result, radiation oncologists previously content with prescribing low tumor doses, which, in some cases, may be inappropriate, may be persuaded to increase their doses to more adequate levels. In reality, this is a logical strategy whenever a radiation regimen results in suboptimal local control but not severe toxicity. However, there have been randomized studies in breast, lung, and rectal cancer in which, following a complete surgical resection, RT markedly improved local control without any noticeable impact on survival.[8–10] To a certain extent, this inconsistency is explained by the presence of undetectable micrometastatic disease, which is usually the ultimate determinant of clinical outcome. Consequently, it is simply erroneous to assume that dose escalation will uniformly translate into progressively better survival. Such a presumption is a non sequitur.

Negative

Spreading lower doses over a larger volume may safeguard the function of normal tissues, but it compromises their genetic integrity. It is well known that genetic mutations play a central role in carcinogenesis. Therefore, it is conceivable that IMRT will increase the incidence of secondary malignancies. However, it is prudent to point out some relevant issues regarding radiation-induced carcinogenesis before discussing the impact of IMRT on this problem.

Radiation-induced mutagenesis and, thus, carcinogenesis are stochastic processes. In other words, the induction of these processes appears to be random, and the frequency increases partly as a function of dose.[11] Radiation-induced carcinogenesis is best fit by a time-related model of relative risk.[12,13] This model maintains that the risk of radiation-induced cancer is directly correlated with age at exposure and time from exposure. However, in vitro and in vivo studies suggest that radiation is not a particularly efficient carcinogen compared with other agents.[14] Considering the huge numbers of cells routinely included in a radiation portal, the astonishing thing is how infrequently such treatment-induced cancers are seen.

Human data on the incidence of radiation-induced cancers are available over a limited dose range and are of questionable quality.[15] This is especially true for nontherapeutic exposure. In the case of therapeutic exposures, the issue is subject to controversy mainly because cancer patients appear to be predisposed to the development of additional cancers.[16] Possible explanations for this include genetic or immunologic predisposition, environmental or lifestyle factors, and exposure to other carcinogenic treatments. In addition, most of the data from RT are retrospective and often incomplete.

The relationship between radiation dose and secondary leukemia is surprisingly best fitted by a linear-quadratic function of dose in which intermediate doses are actually more carcinogenic than higher doses. This paradox stems from two simultaneous and competing processes as a function of dose: exponentially increasing mutagenesis versus exponentially decreasing cell survival. The net result is a bell-shaped curve in which peak carcinogenesis is expressed at an intermediate-dose level. A dose-response relationship with this general shape describes the incidence of leukemia in atomic bomb survivors, as well as leukemogenesis in irradiated mice.[17,18] In contrast, the data for solid tumors may be fitted to a linear function of dose up to approximately 2.5 Sv.[17,19] However, it is speculated that the actual relationship for solid tumors also follows a linear-quadratic function of dose in which the peak and subsequent decline in carcinogenesis occur at higher doses than those associated with leukemia.[20] The precise dose levels corresponding to these peaks are unclear.[21] Finally, data suggest that fewer malignancies are induced if a given dose is spread out over a period of time at a low-dose rate than if it is delivered in an acute exposure.[22] The quantitative magnitude of this dose-rate effect in humans is unclear and further confounded by articles that quote the treated tumor dose and do not try to recreate dose where the induced tumor was thought to originate. A few meticulous studies suggest that secondary carcinomas appear most often at the margins of treated areas, where doses are intermediate.[23,24] In contrast, secondary sarcomas are usually found in the heavily irradiated areas.

The fact remains that IMRT exposes larger volumes of tissue to lower but still mutagenic doses of radiation compared with other forms of conformal RT. This is a consequence of the numerous fields used and an increase in total-body doses from greater radiation leakage from the linear accelerator (see below). Logically, this is almost certainly likely to increase mutagenesis and the incidence of radiation-induced cancers.[24,25] Compared with conventional RT, IMRT is predicted to more than double the 10-year incidence of second malignancies.[26–28] The most noticeable rises are predicted to occur in secondary leukemias and secondary solid tumors in survivors of pediatric cancer, and favorable cancers of adulthood, such as patients with breast or prostate cancer. It is critical that patients treated with IMRT are followed closely regarding this issue.

Another theoretical problem with IMRT is uncertainty and the heterogeneity of the dose at the tumor level, especially for small targets. Logically, there must be some imperfection in matching adjacent, small segmental exposures. Presumably, these imperfections will be smeared out over time by fractionating these exposures. However, the smaller the segment being exposed, the greater the issue of penumbra within the treated segments at depth becomes and hence the uncertainty of the dose.[29,30] By adding any degree of movement within the patient, dose calculations truly become variable and quite uncertain, especially at the periphery of the target, where the dose gradient is the steepest.[31–33] Leakage through the MLC is another consideration and has been described to be as high as 4%.[34] When multiple fields are involved, the leakage problem will integrate to greater numbers and further confound dose reliability. Perhaps the homogeneity of the dose, as traditionally thought of in radiation oncology, is less important than we have all been taught, but that remains to be seen.[35] A possible explanation is that injury in irradiated cells induces them to release noxious signals damaging to neighboring unirradiated cells. This "bystander effect" may be important in RT, as has been demonstrated by Sawant and colleagues in elegant tissue culture experiments.[36,37]

Practical Considerations
Positive

Successful RT depends on the auspicious balance of two competing goals: irradiating the target to tumoricidal doses and respecting the radiation tolerance of normal tissues. By spreading the path of radiation delivery over larger volumes,

IMRT can substantially reduce the dose to normal tissues compared with the dose to the tumor volume. Further reduction can be accomplished by lowering the dose through segments in close proximity to sensitive normal tissues. The potential to decrease RT side effects is among the most appealing aspects of IMRT.[2,3,38,39] However, it cannot be assumed that IMRT will always decrease the dose and, thus, injury to normal tissues. Actually, IMRT may simply exchange a particular toxicity for another in certain situations. This results from practical limitations in the planning of IMRT and the typical intention of escalating the tumor dose. These limitations include the number and angles of beams used, the number and location of critical normal tissues or organs, and the degree of constraint imposed on the normal tissue or organ doses in comparison with the tumor dose. The physician and physicist, not the computer, choose the number and angle of the beams to be used based on anatomic knowledge and experience. Furthermore, the number of tissues that the physician lists on the planning system and the dose constraints imposed on them are finite, subjective, and often estimates rather than known facts.[40–42] Yet every tissue other than the tumor is presumably "normal." In addition, photon beams must enter the patient, traverse normal tissues on their path across the tumor, and exit, even in IMRT. Consequently, most of the radiation will enter through tissues or organs lower in priority or not listed during IMRT planning. Depending on the ultimate dose (often escalated in IMRT), normal tissues previously neglected can manifest unexpected, clinically significant toxicity.

Unfortunately, this phenomenon has already been encountered in the clinic. Efforts to limit the dose to the parotid glands, central nervous system, larynx, and mandible during treatment of pharyngeal tumors with IMRT have resulted in severe mucositis and skin toxicity.[39] Chao and colleagues reported that almost 25% of patients treated with IMRT for oropharyngeal carcinoma required gastrostomy tube placement; 41% had severe mucosal toxicities.[43] Likewise, Lee and colleagues reported comparable results in patients being treated for nasopharyngeal carcinoma with IMRT.[44] Lee and colleagues also described how the tangential beams used in IMRT, as well as the bolus effect of the immobilization mask, the imprecise delineation of neck nodes, and the omission of the skin as a sensitive structure in the planning process, can result in a marked increase in cutaneous toxicity.[45] Similar results have been observed at the Washington University Medical Center, where higher rates of severe skin toxicity were reported in patients treated for oropharyngeal tumors with IMRT compared with conventional therapy.[46] These data are partly explained by the fact that the mucosa, skin, and other normal tissues are often overlooked in the planning process; consequently, the software presumes that delivering substantial doses through these structures will not cause clinical problems.

However, focusing on complications overlooks the fact that RT-induced morbidities have markedly declined from those of 30 years ago. The primary reasons for this decline include better fractionation (ie, treating all fields each day), better localization of the target volume (ie, performing formal simulation, especially CT simulation), and the availability of multiple energies (both photon and electron), permitting the tailoring of RT to individual patient and tumor characteristics.

Although IMRT will undoubtedly contribute to the reduction of radiation injury, its benefits are likely to parallel, not supersede, the magnitude of the advances discussed above. Actually, there is concern that an increase in secondary malignancies and atypical normal tissue toxicities could negate the presumed benefits to be obtained in terms of local control.

Another attractive feature of IMRT is its ability to enhance dose distributions compared with those obtained with conformal RT. Radiation can be easily conformed to complex shapes, even concave and circular distributions.[2] Until recently, the treatment of tumors in difficult locations (eg, tumors involving the cavernous sinus, suprasellar region, and vertebral bodies) would require treatment with multiple fields, complicated weightings, and sophisticated blocking. Even then, recommended doses were frequently limited by the tolerances of abutting normal tissues. Now one can devise an IMRT plan whereby a tight dose distribution can be conformed to virtually any irregular shape, allowing for adequate treatment of these difficult problems.

Negative

The advent of IMRT presents new challenges in the way in which tumor and dose-limiting organs are delineated. IMRT planning requires precise delineation of numerous target and normal tissue volumes. Depending on the case, this can be a difficult and time-consuming task. In addition, predefined volumes are frequently expanded or contracted in an attempt to manipulate the computerized optimization of dose distributions. Artificial dose-limiting volumes (ie, dummy organs) are sometimes created in an effort to steer radiation in a particular direction. However, the delineation of treatment volumes is neither taught nor practiced in a standardized manner. Guidelines applicable to certain anatomic sites have been published.[47] Nonetheless, more research and education on this matter are necessary.

Although IMRT has been demonstrated in many publications to achieve steep dose gradients conforming tightly to virtually any irregular shape, it is unclear whether such improvements will translate into clinically significant benefits. This uncertainty is largely due to the fact that IMRT treatment planning is based on images with significant limitations.

Obviously, a fundamental principle of radiation oncology is to know exactly where the radiation needs to be deposited. However, CT and magnetic resonance imaging (MRI) still have significant limitations in their ability to image the true extent of a cancer. It is well known that tumors have microscopic extensions projecting outward from the main mass. Modern imaging does not reveal these "offshoots"; they are beyond the resolution of CT and MRI. In fact, the accuracy of CT and MRI for most cancers is only about 65 to 75% when compared with true surgical findings.[48,49] Although this is better than the technologies available 30 years ago, the results are still far from ideal. This is well illustrated by the fact that imaging modalities cannot reliably discriminate a tumor volume measuring 1 mm^3, yet a tumor deposit of the same volume is composed of approximately 1 million cells. Unfortunately, treatment failure can theoretically result from a single surviving cell, either because it was not treated or because of an inherent radioresistance.

Furthermore, successful RT often involves irradiation of either abnormal lymph nodes or lymphatic basins at high risk of harboring tumors. Yet the main radiologic criterion for classifying a lymph node as "abnormal" is an arbitrary level of gross nodal enlargement. The logic of this definition is debatable because tumor deposits do not appear overnight but rather grow over time. Positron emission tomography (PET) may offer some improvement based on metabolic information,[50] but the resolution is still suboptimal for subcentimeter lesions.

In patients with unresectable lung cancer, some have begun to use PET and CT to restrict the target volume to only those areas that appear to be positively involved.[51,52] Their goal is to escalate doses safely by decreasing the "standard" volume of treatment. Of note, there are no data supporting the assumption that the dose can be escalated only by reducing the target volume. Although only approximately two-thirds of patients received the escalated doses intended for their mediastinal lymphadenopathy, early reports with this strategy suggested little in the way of nodal recurrence or persistence.[51,52] However, this has to be interpreted with caution because the results lack pathologic confirmation. These days, the development of metastases frequently overshadows assessment of locoregional control. In addition, autopsies in patients with documented metastases are rarely performed. Yet metastases are coming from somewhere; it is possible that some originate from subclinically involved lymph nodes. Given that lung cancer has the greatest predilection for dissemination of all of the common solid tumors, the wisdom of this approach for lung cancer at this time remains to be seen. Presently, convincing data of improved long-term survival or even long-term local control (ie, minimum 5-year figures) resulting from such a strategy are lacking.

Finally, the old trial of breast cancer from King's College in Great Britain calls into question exactly what defines malignant nodal disease, both clinically and radiologically, when the only discriminator is an arbitrary size cutoff.[53] As implied earlier, survival is the critical end point; surrogate end points are of far lesser importance.

Another shortcoming of CT and MRI is that they represent a static snapshot of what is, in fact, a moving target. Therefore, blind trust in CT scans belies another major challenge in our field: accounting for tumor motion. Some of the movement is voluntary and some is involuntary; but, whatever its cause, movement will definitely confound dose calculations, tumor definition, and interpretation of real-time dose-volume histograms. Considering the highly conformal and steep dose gradients frequently employed, one can infer that movement is a worse problem for IMRT than for conventional RT. In fact, movement may be IMRT's worst problem.[31–33] We wonder what a dose-volume histogram based on such plans truly means when the target or organ in question moves a couple of centimeters or more. Moreover, movement in the setting of tight dose distributions may increase the risk of marginal misses, especially for thoracic and abdominal cancers.

The value of IMRT without accurate localization and immobilization of the tumor volume is dubious at best. Much more attention needs to be focused on immobilization and patient positioning techniques. Perhaps stepping back and thinking outside the box will yield some answers. For example, let us pose the following question: Is every patient best treated in the recumbent position? Investigators at the National Cancer Institute in Bethesda, MD, described a design for a chair allowing isocentric simulation and treatment.[54] The design was partly inspired by physiologic considerations suggesting that pulmonary exposure during mediastinal irradiation could be minimized by treating patients in the upright position. This approach allows gravity to work to our advantage. When a patient lies down, the diaphragms move upward and the thoracic cavity volume is decreased. The lungs are compressed in this position, not the tumor. As a consequence, when a patient is recumbent, the ratio of pulmonary parenchymal cells being irradiated compared with the tumor volume will always be greater than would be the case if the patient was upright. Furthermore, some mediastinal tumors significantly expand in volume when the patient lies down owing to changes in vascular pressures related to this position.[54]

Of course, this approach would require patients to be CT-simulated in the upright position. This conceptual obstacle was ingeniously circumvented at Fermilab (Batavia, IL), where vertical CT scanning was developed. This resulted from the necessity to perform sophisticated treatment planning well suited for the fixed, horizontal neutron beam at that facility (Arlene Lennox, PhD, personal communication, 2001). Thus, there is more than one possible way to decrease the risk of pulmonary injury as a result of RT for lung cancer.

One of the concerns is that significant respiratory motion, classically seen at fluoroscopic simulation, may not be taken into account in IMRT. Physicians planning treatment based on these snapshots are often fooled into thinking that they know exactly where the tumor is, even though fluoroscopy might show that it moves 2 cm or more.

We encourage readers to recognize this delusion and keep their "eyes on the doughnut, not on the hole"—in other words, understand that "virtual reality" is not reality.

Efforts are presently ongoing to gate treatment to respiratory movement with the goal of decreasing the amount of pulmonary volume irradiated and, hence, the risk of pneumonitis. Of course, other things besides dose and volume have an impact on the probability of developing radiation pneumonitis. These include medications, coexistent medical diseases, smoking history, baseline pulmonary function, life expectancy, performance status, and transforming growth factor $\beta 1$.[40,55,56] Furthermore, it is unclear how much can be gained by gating to respiration. It has already been suggested that systematic setup errors are more important.[57]

Another serious downside to IMRT is a significant increase in total-body dose to patients and, possibly, radiation therapists.[58–62] IMRT requires radiation fluence (ie, beam-on time) for much longer periods of time than conventional RT. As a consequence of that increased beam-on time, there will be significantly greater radiation leakage from the machine head, yielding greater total-body exposure.[58–62] This is especially true when IMRT involves a high number of segments per field, typical of inverse planning. For some machines, there may be additional radiation resulting from a "pause" state of the machine. This is due to so-called "dark current." This dark current radiation is nearly seven times greater than traditional leakage radiation.[63] Moreover, if one were to plan IMRT with energies of 15 MV or greater, there would be significant neutron contamination within that total-body dose.[64] Because neutrons have higher linear energy transfer and relative biologic effectiveness than x-rays, the mutagenic potential of this contamination is very worrisome. Greater shielding could conceivably reduce (but not eliminate) this problem. However, this would require a considerable increase in machine weight and expense. Of course, there is really no advantage to using high energies (> 6 MV) for IMRT because, when using multiple fields, the greater exit doses from the higher photon energies effectively negate some of the potential depth dose advantages.

As discussed previously, the potential consequence of this greater whole-body dose is an increase in radiation-induced neoplasms, especially leukemia. Traditionally, radiation-induced cancers from therapeutic exposures have been defined as those occurring within radiation fields. However, if the total-body dose is increased by a factor of 3 (or more), this may no longer be a fair or realistic definition. The increase in total-body dose with IMRT is real; its predictable serious consequences await careful, long-term follow-up and documentation among surviving patients.

Despite the potential disadvantages of using very tight margins, they have often been advocated arbitrarily to allow for safer dose escalation throughout the tumor in an attempt to improve local control. Supporting this approach, a subset analysis of 301 patients with prostate cancer (median pretreatment prostate-specific antigen [PSA] of 7.8 ng/mL) treated with conformal RT has suggested that increasing the dose from 70 to 78 Gy significantly reduces the rates of PSA failure and distant metastases in those with intermediate-risk disease (pretreatment PSA > 10 ng/mL). Patients with low-risk disease (pretreatment PSA ≤ 10 ng/mL) did not benefit from this approach.[65] The study did not contain enough patients with high-risk disease to draw conclusions in that subgroup (only 5% had pretreatment PSA > 20 ng/mL, 80% had T1–T2 tumors, and < 18% had Gleason grades ≥ 8).

The reader is strongly cautioned not to extrapolate to other sites on the basis of these data. First, the large proportion of patients with prostate cancer diagnosed today because of abnormal PSA levels in the absence of palpable disease results in a major shift in lead-time from diagnosis. In addition, the relatively thick prostatic capsule is not representative of most primary sites. Both of these features are highly atypical of other carcinomas. Furthermore, if the intention is simply to maximize the dose to the prostate, surely, a combination of external RT plus brachytherapy will achieve doses well beyond what can be delivered by any plan with external beam alone, as has been standard for decades in the management of cervical cancer.

Still another drawback to IMRT is a major difficulty in validating or verifying fields and ports in vivo. Phantom measurements are useful but not necessarily accurate in their representation of dose distribution within living, breathing, coughing, sneezing, scratching, wiggling, litigious patients. This is well illustrated by the occasional weekly port film demonstrating a significant yet inexplicable deviation (1 cm or more) in the treatment of a patient. It remains to be seen if newly designed rapid portal imaging systems can keep up with the fluence of the IMRT in real time.[66–68] Nonetheless, at the moment, this is still an important area in which IMRT lags behind other conformal approaches. The potential medical and legal implications are obvious.

Despite its heavy reliance on automation, IMRT has not simplified the RT workplace. Several years ago, there was some concern among dosimetrists regarding an adverse impact of IMRT on their field. Today, it is clear that IMRT did not decrease the demand or workload of dosimetrists and physicists across the nation. In fact, there is concern about a shortage of dosimetrists and other RT staff. In addition, IMRT has required the prompt addition of new responsibilities for radiation therapists (eg, performing sonograms for target localization on a daily basis) and other personnel. The proficient fulfillment of these roles requires proper training and is associated with a learning curve. Logically, the risk of committing errors increases as the degree of complexity increases. Unfortunately, this is easily overlooked because the computerized nature of these technologies can seem deceptively infallible.

Cost Considerations
Positive

There can be little question that IMRT is presently being driven largely by marketing forces and reimbursement issues. However, it is doubtful that the presently generous reimbursement scale will continue unless clearly convincing and unequivocal data on improved outcomes can be shown, especially gains in survival.

Negative

It should be obvious that the initial costs of IMRT are expensive in terms of the space, hardware, and software that are required. Less obvious and perhaps more exorbitant are the requirements in terms of human resources and time involved in its planning and delivery. Multiple different plans are routinely generated to "optimize" the treatment. One can only question if such efforts are going on at centers that claim to do IMRT but where planning responsibilities may fall to the physicist, who may be at that hospital 1 or 2 days a week. Furthermore, IMRT implies additional expenditure in sophisticated equipment for patient or target immobilization, target tracking, quality assurance, and radiation shielding.

MLCs, because of their motorized nature, will probably lead to increases in downtime and repairs. It is reasonable to assume that a similar problem will have an impact on the performance of the equipment simply because the beam is on for longer periods of time in IMRT than in conformal RT.

Finally, there is the major concern that as radiation oncologists become more involved with the technical components of clinical care, they will be perceived less as physicians and more as mere technicians by both patients and other physicians. That particular outcome would be most unfortunate because it could ultimately erode the independence of radiation oncologists. Considering the high costs of IMRT and the paucity of clinical data supporting it, one can wonder if its use would be as popular and indiscriminate if it were not for the presently generous reimbursement.

Conclusions

IMRT techniques can yield very intricate dose distributions deemed "superior" to those obtained with conformal RT. Clearly, this capability will prove beneficial for certain clinical problems. However, just like every new development, IMRT is not without several major potential disadvantages. Unfortunately, our field has thus far embraced its virtues and ignored its pitfalls. Perhaps this stems from the heavy marketing by vendors, the allure of its technologic sophistication, the generous level of reimbursement, and the frustration with the rate of progress in oncology. Whatever the case may be, there is a true need to evaluate prospectively both the advantages and disadvantages of IMRT compared with those of other forms of conformal therapy.

Although undoubtedly a valuable tool, it remains to be seen whether these arbitrarily "improved" dose distributions on paper translate into meaningful improvements in the outcome of patients. We encourage the prudent use of IMRT because the highly conformal and steep dose distributions resulting from CT-based IMRT planning belie two major difficulties in our field: accounting accurately for both the extent and the motion of tumors. The snug margins advocated to allow for safer dose escalation of the tumor volume introduce considerable uncertainty into the dose calculations. This is especially true at the periphery of the tumor volume and in areas subject to movement. In addition, such tight margins predispose IMRT to marginal misses. The true worth of IMRT without accurate localization and immobilization of the tumor volume is, at best, dubious.

Patterns of care data suggest that only a modest fraction of the overall patient load undergoing RT may benefit from IMRT over the offerings of "conventional" therapy. It has been estimated that approximately 50% of all RT is given with palliative intent.[69–71] Undeniably, the potential advantage of IMRT in this group is dubious because there is no real case for dose escalation on a routine basis. Furthermore, it is reasonable to assume that a substantial proportion of the remaining 50% is very unlikely to benefit. This includes patients with unresectable and/or highly aggressive tumors frequently associated with poor performance status and dismal systemic control in which treatment expectations are very low.

Another group of patients unlikely to benefit are those treated in the adjuvant setting for tumors with good prognosis and who currently achieve excellent disease control with moderate doses of radiation (45–54 Gy). Given the fact that there is no gross tumor volume and the good results currently achieved in this group, the likelihood of major survival benefit from IMRT is limited. Of course, such a discussion overlooks the value of a potential benefit in toxicity. However, RT-related toxicity has been markedly decreased over the last 30 years. Therefore, the potential benefits in terms of major side effects, both early and late, also need prospective quantification.

The most sinister aspect of IMRT is the fact that, over the long run, it may actually harm some patients. This possibility could offset all of the potential benefits to be gained. Larger volumes of tissue exposed to lower but still mutagenic doses of radiation, together with higher total-body doses from machine leakage, may result in a significant increase in RT-induced carcinogenesis (especially leukemia) compared with that observed with conformal RT. Such events are most likely to occur in young patients and in those with relatively favorable cancers. It is reasonable to assume that any noteworthy increase in the incidence of secondary malignancies will adversely impact referral patterns for RT and the overall image of the specialty.

The concreteness of IMRT technology unfortunately overshadows the greater gains to be obtained at this time from biologic and combined-modality treatments. The greatest future gains in survival will be obtained through better systemic management simply because that is where success is poorest today. Paradoxically, any long-term systemic benefit afforded by these newer biologic therapies will only magnify the importance of local control. Epidemiologic data suggest that if we had a truly effective radiation sensitizer in the clinic, it would provide a greater benefit to patient outcome than all of the dosimetric fine-tuning presently under way. The reason for this is that RT, a physical modality, is nonspecific to the pathophysiology of cancer; thus, it will never be the entire answer to the problem of cancer therapy. Yet, without question, it remains an important component of the answers. Radiation oncologists need to maintain a strong biologic and cellular orientation. Failure to do so will almost certainly herald a decline of our field within an oncologic world that is rapidly moving toward more biologic and molecular orientations.

We consider IMRT a new, sophisticated, valuable tool whose exact value remains to be quantitatively established. Its advent presents new therapeutic options and new challenges. We need to assess, thoroughly and without bias, both its advantages and disadvantages against those of the technology that it intends to substitute. Until then, IMRT should not be considered the new standard in RT but only a new, potentially valuable tool needing confirmation. Perhaps it would be better scrutinized and used less liberally if it were not for the existing economic enticement. We trust that the field of radiation oncology, in keeping with its tradition, will recognize the issues at hand and rise to the challenge.

References

1. Early Breast Cancer Trialists' Collaborative Group. Favourable and unfavourable effects on long-term survival of radiotherapy for early breast cancer: an overview of the randomized trials. Lancet 2000;355:1757–70.

2. Teh BS, Woo S, Butler EB. Intensity modulated radiation therapy (IMRT): a new promising technology in radiation oncology. Oncologist 1999;4:433–43.

3. Butler EB, Teh BS, Grant WH, et al. SMART boost: a new accelerated fractionation schedule for the treatment of head and neck cancer with intensity modulated radiotherapy. Int J Radiat Oncol Biol Phys 1999;45:21–32.

4. Wu Q, Manning M, Schmidt-Ullrich R, et al. The potential for sparing of parotids and escalation of biologically effective dose with intensity-modulated radiation treatments of head and neck cancers: a treatment design study. Int J Radiat Oncol Biol Phys 2000;46:195–205.

5. Mohan R, Wu Q, Manning M, Schmidt-Ullrich R. Radiobiological considerations in the design of fractionation strategies for intensity-modulated radiation therapy of head and neck cancers. Int J Radiat Oncol Biol Phys 2000;46:619–30.

6. Rosenthal DI, Pistenmaa DA, Glatstein E. A review of neoadjuvant chemotherapy for head and neck cancer: partially shrunken tumors may be both meaner and leaner. Int J Radiat Oncol Biol Phys 1994;28:315–20.

7. Fu KK, Pajak TF, Trotti A, et al. A Radiation Therapy Oncology Group (RTOG) phase II randomized study to compare hyperfractionation and two variants of accelerated fractionation to standard fractionation radiotherapy for head and neck squamous cell carcinomas: first report of RTOG 9003. Int J Radiat Oncol Biol Phys 2000;48:7–16.

8. Fisher B, Redmond C, Fisher E, et al. Ten-year results of a randomized clinical trial comparing radical mastectomy and total mastectomy with or without irradiation. N Engl J Med 1985;312:674–9.

9. Lung Cancer Study Group. Effects of post-operative mediastinal radiation on completely resected stage II and stage III epidermoid cancer of the lung. N Engl J Med 1986;315:1377–81.

10. Gastrointestinal Tumor Study Group. Prolongation of the disease free interval in surgically treated rectal carcinoma. N Engl J Med 1985;312:1465–71.

11. Little MP. Risks associated with ionizing radiation. Br Med Bull 2003;68:259–75.

12. Boice JD Jr. Carcinogenesis—a synopsis of human experience with external exposure in medicine. Health Phys 1988;55:621–30.

13. Little MP, Muirhead CR, Charles MW. Describing time and age variations in the risk of radiation-induced solid tumour incidence in the Japanese atomic bomb survivors using generalized relative and absolute risk models. Stat Med 1999;18:17–33.

14. Hall EJ, Hei TK. Oncogenic transformation with radiation and chemicals. Int J Radiat Biol Relat Stud Phys Chem Med 1985;48:1–18.

15. Samet JM. Epidemiologic studies of ionizing radiation and cancer: past successes and future challenges. Environ Health Perspect 1997;105 Suppl 4:883–9.

16. Little MP. Cancer after exposure to radiation in the course of treatment for benign and malignant disease. Lancet Oncol 2001;ii:212–20.

17. Little MP, Muirhead CR. Curvature in the cancer mortality dose response in Japanese atomic bomb survivors: absence of evidence of threshold. Int J Radiat Biol 1998;74:471–80.

18. Upton AC. The dose response relation in radiation induced cancer. Cancer Res 1961;21:717–29.

19. Preston DL, Shimizu Y, Pierce DA, et al. Studies of mortality of atomic bomb survivors. Report 13: solid cancer and non-cancer disease mortality: 1950-1997. Radiat Res 2003;160:381–407.

20. Hall EJ. Radiation, the two-edged sword: cancer risks at high and low doses. Cancer J 2000;6:343–50.

21. Lindsay KA, Wheldon EG, Deehan C, et al. Radiation carcinogenesis modeling for risk of treatment-related second tumours following radiotherapy. Br J Radiol 2001;74:529–36.

22. Relative biological effectiveness (RBE), quality factor (Q), and radiation weighting factor (w(R)). A report of the International Commission on Radiological Protection. Ann ICRP 2003;33:1–117.

23. Hall EJ. Do no harm—normal tissue effects. Acta Oncol 2001;40:913–6.

24. Dorr W, Herrmann T. Cancer induction by radiotherapy: dose dependence and spatial relationship to irradiated volume. J Radiol Prot 2002;22:A117–21.

25. Meeks SL, Paulino AC, Pennington EC, et al. In vivo determination of extra-target doses received from serial tomotherapy. Radiother Oncol 2002;63:217–22.

26. Hall EJ, Wuu CS. Radiation-induced second cancers: the impact of 3D-CRT and IMRT. Int J Radiat Oncol Biol Phys 2003;56:83–8.

27. Followill D, Geis P, Boyer A. Estimates of whole-body dose equivalent produced by beam intensity modulated conformal therapy. Int J Radiat Oncol Biol Phys 1997;38:667–72.

28. Verellen D, Vanhavere F. Risk assessment of radiation-induced malignancies based on whole-body equivalent dose estimates for IMRT treatment in the head and neck region. Radiother Oncol 1999;53:199–203.

29. Sohn JW, Dempsey JF, Suh TS, et al. Analysis of various beamlet sizes for IMRT with 6 MV photons. Med Phys 2003;30:2432–9.

30. Cheng CW, Das IJ, Huq MS. Lateral loss and dose discrepancies of multileaf collimator segments in intensity modulated radiation therapy. Med Phys 2003;30:2959–68.

31. Langen KM, Jones DT. Organ motion and its management. Int J Radiat Oncol Biol Phys 2001;50:265–78.

32. Chui CS, Yorke E, Hong L. The effects of intra-fraction organ motion on the delivery of intensity-modulated field with a multileaf collimator. Med Phys 2003;30:1736–46.

33. Bortfeld T, Jiang SB, Rietzel E. Effects of motion on the total dose distribution. Semin Radiat Oncol 2004;14:41–51.

34. Klein EE, Low DA. Interleaf leakage for 5 and 10 mm dynamic multileaf collimation systems incorporating patient motion. Med Phys 2001;28:1703–10.

35. Langer M, Kijewski P, Brown R, et al. The effect on minimum tumor dose of restricting target-dose on homogeneity in optimized three-dimensional treatment of lung cancer. Radiother Oncol 1991;21:245–56.

36. Sawant SG, Randers-Pehrson G, Geard CR, et al. The bystander effect in radiation oncogenesis: I. Transformation in C3H 10T1/2 cells in vitro can be initiated in the unirradiated neighbors of irradiated cells. Radiat Res 2001;155:397–401.

37. Sawant SG, Randers-Pehrson G, Metting NF, et al. Adaptive response and the bystander effect induced by radiation in C3H 10T(1/2) cells in culture. Radiat Res 2001;156:177–80.

38. Shu HKG, Lee TT, Vigneault E, et al. Toxicity following high dose three-dimensional conformal and intensity-modulated radiation therapy for clinically localized prostate cancer. Urology 2001;57:102–7.

39. Chao KS, Ozyigit G, Thorsdad WL. Toxicity profile of intensity-modulated radiation therapy for head and neck carcinoma and potential role of amifostine. Semin Oncol 2003;30 Suppl 18:101–8.

40. Glatstein E. Personal thoughts on normal tissue tolerance or what the textbooks don't tell you. Int J Radiat Oncol Biol Phys 2001;57:1185–9.

41. Johansson S, Svensson H, Denekamp J. Timescale evolution of late radiation injury after postoperative radiotherapy of breast cancer patients. Int J Radiat Oncol Biol Phys 2000;48:745–50.

42. Johansson S, Per-Olov L, Denekamp J. Left-sided vocal cord paralysis: a newly recognized late complication of mediastinal irradiation. Radiother Oncol 2001;58:287–94.

43. Chao KS, Ozyigit G, Blanco AI, et al. Intensity-modulated radiation therapy for oropharyngeal carcinoma: impact of tumor volume. Int J Radiat Oncol Biol Phys 2004;59:43–50.

44. Lee N, Xia P, Quivey JM, et al. Intensity-modulated radiotherapy in the treatment of nasopharyngeal carcinoma: an update of the UCSF experience. Int J Radiat Oncol Biol Phys 2002;53:12–22.

45. Lee N, Chuang C, Quivey JM, et al. Skin toxicity due to intensity-modulated radiotherapy for head-and-neck carcinoma. Int J Radiat Oncol Biol Phys 2002;53:630–7.

46. Chao KS, Majhail N, Huang CJ, et al. Intensity-modulated radiation therapy reduces late salivary toxicity without compromising tumor control in patients with oropharyngeal carcinoma: a comparison with conventional techniques. Radiother Oncol 2001;61:275–80.

47. Gregoire V, Levendag P, Ang KK, et al. CT-based delineation of lymph node levels and related CTVs in the node-negative neck: DAHANCA, EORTC, GORTEC, NCIC, RTOG consensus guidelines. Radiother Oncol 2003;69:227–36.

48. Rifkin MD, Zerhouni EA, Gatsonis CA, et al. Comparison of magnetic resonance imaging and ultrasonography in staging early prostate cancer. N Engl J Med 1990;323:621–6.

49. Webb WR, Gatsonis C, Berhouni EA, et al. CT and MRT imaging in staging non-small cell bronchogenic carcinoma: report of the Radiologic Diagnostic Oncology Group. Radiology 1991;178:705–13.

50. Pieterman RM, van Patten JWG, Meuzelaar JJ, et al. Preoperative staging of non-small cell lung cancer with positron emission tomography. N Engl J Med 2000;343:254–61.

51. Rosenzweig KE, Mychalczak B, Fuks Z, et al. Final report of the 70.2 Gy and 75.6 Gy dose levels of a phase I dose escalation study using three-dimensional conformal radiotherapy in the treatment of inoperable non-small cell lung cancer. Cancer J 2000;6:82–7.

52. Rosenzweig KE, Sim SE, Mychalczak B, et al. Elective nodal irradiation in the treatment of non-small cell lung cancer with three-dimensional conformal radiation therapy. Int J Radiat Oncol Biol Phys 2001;50:681–5.

53. Brinkley D, Haybittle JL, Houghton J. The Cancer Research Campaign (King's/Cambridge) trial for early breast cancer: an analysis of the radiotherapy data. Br J Radiol 1980;57:309–21.

54. Miller RW, Raubitschek AA, Harrington FS, et al. An isocentric chair for the simulation and treatment of radiation therapy patients. Int J Radiat Oncol Biol Phys 1991;21:469–73.

55. Robnett TJ, Machtay M, Vines E, et al. Factors predicting severe radiation pneumonitis receiving definitive chemoradiation for lung cancer. Int J Radiat Oncol Biol Phys 2000;48:89–94.

56. Anscher MS, Marks LB, Schafman TD, et al. Using plasma transforming growth factor beta-l during radiotherapy to select patients for dose escalation. J Clin Oncol 2001;19:3758–65.

57. Engelsman M, Damen EMF, DeJaeger K, et al. The effect of breathing and set-up errors on the cumulative dose to a lung tumor. Radiother Oncol 2000;60:95–105.

58. Lillicrap SC, Morgan HM, Shakeshaft JT. X-ray leakage during radiotherapy. Br J Radiol 2000;73:793–4.

59. Williams PO, Hounsell AR. X-ray leakage considerations for IMRT. Br J Radiol 2001;74:98–100.

60. Mutic S, Low DA, Klein EE, et al. Room shielding for intensity-modulated radiation therapy treatment facilities. Int J Radiat Oncol Biol Phys 2001;50:239–46.

61. Rodgers JE. Radiation therapy vault shielding calculational methods when IMRT and TBI procedures contribute. J Appl Clin Med Phys 2001;2:157–64.

62. Rawlinson JA, Islam MK, Galbraith DM. Dose to radiation therapists from activation at high-energy accelerators used for conventional and intensity-modulated radiation therapy. Med Phys 2002;29:598–608.

63. Cheng CW, Das IJ. Comparison of beam characteristics in intensity modulated radiation therapy (IMRT) and those under normal treatment condition. Med Phys 2002;29:226–30.

64. Dong L, McGary J, Bellezza D, et al. Whole body dose from Peacock-based IMRT treatment [2158]. Proceedings of the ASTRO 42nd annual meeting. Int J Radiat Oncol Biol Phys 2000;48:342.

65. Pollack A, Zagars GK, Starkschall G, et al. Prostate cancer radiation dose response: results of the M. D. Anderson phase III randomized trial. Int J Radiat Oncol Biol Phys 2002;53:1097–105.

66. Antonuk LE, Yorkston J, Huang W, et al. Megavoltage imaging with a large area, flat-panel, amorphous silicon imager. Int J Radiat Oncol Biol Phys 1996;36:661–72.

67. Van Esch A, Vanstraelen B, Verstraete J, et al. Pretreatment dosimetric verification by means of a liquid filled electronic portal imaging device during dynamic delivery of intensity modulated treatment fields. Radiother Oncol 2001;60:181–90.

68. Greer PB, Popescu CC. Dosimetric properties of an amorphous silicon electronic portal imaging device for verification of dynamic intensity modulated radiation therapy. Med Phys 2003;30:1618–27.

69. Hoegler D. Radiotherapy for palliation of symptoms in incurable cancer. Curr Probl Cancer 1997;21:129–83.

70. Anderson PR, Coia LR. Fractionation and outcomes with palliative radiation therapy. Semin Radiat Oncol 2000;10:191–9.

71. Nielsen OS. Present status of palliative radiotherapy. Eur J Cancer 2001;37 Suppl 7:S279–88.

72. Glatstein E. Intensity-modulated radiation therapy: the inverse, the converse, and the perverse. Semin Radiat Oncol 2002;12Suppl3:272–81.

INDEX